Basic Pharmacology for Nurses

eleventh edition

Basic Pharmacology for Nurses

eleventh edition

Bruce D. Clayton
Pharm D, RPh

**Professor of Pharmacy Practice,
College of Pharmacy & Health Sciences,
Butler University,
Indianapolis, Indiana**

Yvonne N. Stock
RN, MS

**Professor of Nursing,
Health Occupations Department,
Iowa Western Community College,
Council Bluffs, Iowa**

with 216 illustrations

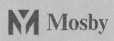

St. Louis Baltimore Boston
Carlsbad Chicago Naples New York Philadelphia Portland
London Madrid Mexico City Singapore Sydney Tokyo Toronto Wiesbaden

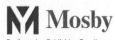

Mosby
Dedicated to Publishing Excellence

A Times Mirror
Company

Vice President and Publisher: Nancy Coon
Editor: Robin Carter
Developmental Editor: Jeanne Allison
Project Manager: Dana Peick
Production Editor: Dottie Martin
Manuscript Editors: Chris DeVito, Clare Genovese
Designer: Amy Buxton
Manufacturing Manager: Betty Mueller

A NOTE TO THE READER

The authors and publisher have made every attempt to check dosages and nursing content for accuracy. Because the science of pharmacology is continually advancing, our knowledge base continues to expand. Therefore we recommend that the reader always check product information for changes in dosage or administration before administering any medication. This is particularly important with new or rarely used drugs.

Printed in the United States of America

Composition by Carlisle Communications, Ltd.
Illustrations by Jack Reuter
Printing/binding by Rand McNally

Mosby–Year Book, Inc.
11830 Westline Industrial Drive
St. Louis, Missouri 63146

Library of Congress Cataloging-in-Publication Data

ISBN 0–8151–1512–1 (pbk.)

96 97 98 99 00 / 9 8 7 6 5 4 3 2 1

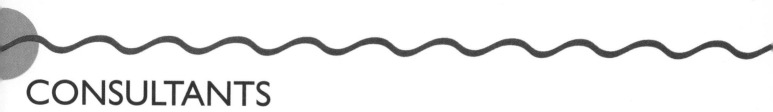

CONSULTANTS

Laura H. Clayton, RN, MSN, FNP
Instructor of Nursing Education,
Shepherd College,
Shepherdstown, West Virginia;
Staff Nurse, Intensive Care Unit,
City Hospital, Inc.,
Martinsburg, West Virginia

Mondella Woods, RN, MS
Coordinator, Practical Nursing Program,
Regional Medical Center at Memphis,
Memphis, Tennessee

PREFACE

The eleventh edition of Clayton and Stock's **Basic Pharmacology for Nurses** upholds the standards first established by the book in 1957—the administration of medication with concern for safety and precision and attention to important physiologic factors. However, as the practice of nursing continues to evolve through the 1990s, the demands have been expanding to include much more than the preparation and administration of drugs with an understanding of drug action at the physiologic level. In today's practice setting the nurse also must understand the disease process, along with the assessment needed to establish a solid data base from which to analyze and develop nursing diagnoses relevant to the individual's care needs. The nurse also must plan and implement patient care in a manner that involves the patient as an active participant in decisions affecting each individual's care needs. Therefore a primary concern throughout is the integration of patient teaching of pharmacology so the patient can choose an optimal level of health to attain and be provided with the information needed to maximize the potential of reaching the therapeutic goal. The nurse must provide patient education and verify the degree of mastery attained to ensure that the individual has the ability to provide safe self-care and monitoring of the prescribed regimen, including the pharmacologic aspects of care.

ORGANIZATION

The text consists of two parts. **Part One: *Principles of Basic Pharmacology*** has two units. Unit I: *Foundations of Pharmacology* comprises five chapters. Chapter 1, *Definitions, Names, Standards, and Sources,* provides an introductory discussion of pharmacology, drug nomenclature, drug and patient information sources, legal standards for both the United States and Canada, and the use of an electronic database. Chapter 2, *Principles of Drug Action and Drug Interaction,* is a foundational chapter on understanding drug actions and variables that influence drug actions and drug interactions. Chapter 3, *Drug Action Across the Life Span,* is a *new chapter* that allows the learner to explore the basic physiology underlying drug action that occurs as a result of variables in drug absorption, drug distribution, drug metabolism, and drug excretion occurring in individuals of different ages across the life span. Chapter 4, *The Nursing Process and Pharmacology,* provides an overview of the nursing process and contains a section that focuses on the application of the nursing process to the study of pharmacology. Chapter 5, *Patient Education and Health Promotion,* another new chapter, presents the three domains of learning: cognitive domain, affective domain, and psychomotor domain. Principles of learning such as focusing learning, learning styles,

motivation of the learner, organization of the content, spacing of learning sessions, repetition to enhance learning, the patient's education level, and the importance of incorporating cultural and ethnic diversity into the delivery of health teaching is addressed in this chapter. The information contained in this chapter is foundational to planning and implementing patient education and health promotion. As stated earlier, *patient education* and *health promotion* remain strong features of this book.

Unit II: *Illustrated Atlas of Medication Administration and Math Review,* comprising Chapters 6 through 10, features photographs and illustrations to assist the learner in mastering proper techniques of medication administration. Chapter 6, *A Review of Arithmetic,* provides an extensive review of mathematics including examples of fractions, decimals, and conversions between the metric and avoirdupois systems of weights and measures to assist the learner in mastering dosage calculations. Chapter 7, *Principles of Medication Administration,* describes drug distribution systems, use of medication administration records and medication profiles used in the acute care and long-term care settings, the content of the patient chart, the types of drug orders, and associated nursing responsibilities. The text emphasizes the need for inclusion of a sixth Right of Medication Administration—*documentation*—by identifying the appropriate nursing actions needed to chart the details of drug administration, the therapeutic effectiveness of each medication administered, the patient teaching performed, and the degree of understanding of the medication regimen attained. Chapters 8 through 10, which discuss enteral administration, parenteral administration, and percutaneous administration, have comprehensive, illustrated sections on dosage forms, administration sites, and techniques of administration. A new addition in Chapter 8 is the inclusion of the method of administration of *enteral feedings.*

Part Two: *Application of the Nursing Process to Pharmacology,* comprising Units III through IX, has been completely revised to use a *more user-friendly* format that clearly labels each category relating to the drug therapy, providing the learner with easy access to content. All of these units have been updated with new drugs and have been reviewed to eliminate drugs no longer available or in use. The format used in Part Two has undergone major revision so that students can find information more easily. All chapters in both parts start with *chapter content, objectives,* and *key words.* In Part Two, these are followed by a discussion of the *anatomy* and *physiology* of the body system or disease process to provide a better understanding of the treatment modalities used. Next is a discussion of the *drug therapy* used to treat a particular disease and the effects of that drug therapy on the appropriate body system. *Nursing process* relating to the disease, disorder, or body system is then presented as a synopsis of relevant information the nurse needs to assess, plan, develop nursing diagnoses, implement care, teach patient education and health promotion, and evaluate the therapeutic effectiveness of the drug therapy. A new addition to this edition is the inclusion of *premedication assessment* to assist the novice to focus on important assessment relating to the particular drug to be administered. Finally, the importance of *fostering health maintenance* through the inclusion of all aspects of care to treat the disease, not just the pharmacologic aspects, is addressed. By educating the patient regarding the desired therapeutic response of the drug therapy and explaining the need to contact the physician when this response is not occurring, it allows the patient to achieve some degree of control over the treatment of the disease process for which the drugs are prescribed. Furthermore, as the nurse examines the drug monographs, it becomes apparent what side effects to drug therapy are to be anticipated. By giving the patient concrete suggestions to alleviate the bothersome side effects, the possibility of increased adherence to the prescribed regimen is enhanced. Information on adverse drug effects needs to be taught to the patient in a manner that does not unduly upset the patient but emphasizes the need for prompt reporting of the adverse effects to the physician should they occur so the needed modifications in the regimen can be made. When individuals do not master their self care, it must be validated in the chart and reported to a physician so necessary referrals can be made.

FEATURES

Color The addition of color is used throughout the book for both functionality and visual enhancement. Color has been used in headings to make content easier to locate, in tables and boxes to draw attention to special topics, in figures to add clarity, and in pedagogy to add emphasis. The use of color is an important addition because it will more fully engage students in the content.

New Life Span Chapter (Chapter 3) This new chapter alerts the nurse to differences in pharmacology between different age groups, such as pediatrics and geriatrics.

New Patient Education Chapter (Chapter 5) With the advent of shorter hospital stays, education of the patient and significant others is even more important than in the past. This new chapter emphasizes this important nursing role.

Pedagogy Learning objectives, key word lists, and math review questions for each chapter reinforce key content.

Critical Thinking Questions Critical thinking questions are included for each drug chapter to promote the development of clinical decision-making skills.

Life Span Issues Boxes These boxes are interspersed throughout the book, providing important information about drug administration to various age groups, specifically the pediatric and geriatric patient populations.

Patient Education and Monitoring Forms These forms are included throughout Part Two as examples for the student to adapt to the individual needs of the patient when providing patient education, and they may be copied from the book for student use. These written records may assist the individual in understanding the monitoring parameters needed to per-

form and should include information on the signs and symptoms that need to be reported to the physician.

ANCILLARIES

Instructor's Resource Manual The Instructor's Resource Manual has been completely updated to include information on the newly added drugs and the new chapters added to this edition. It consists of four parts: drug classification review, syllabi, test bank, and answer section. The drug classification section contains a quick review of the drug classification in easy-to-understand language. This is a tool instructors can use to help students grasp important information on drug classes. The syllabi include chapter objectives and outlines, key words, math review questions and critical thinking questions from the book, and new collaborative activities and projects. The test bank has added math review questions. The answers to the math review questions and the test bank questions are included in the answer section. Also included are reproducible forms of patient education and monitoring forms, illustrated shaded syringes, and a blank medication administration record.

Student Learning Guide The Student Learning Guide is new to the instructional package and is available separately or packaged with the book. The study guide includes drug classification review, chapter assignments from the syllabi in the instructor's manual, content review questions, math review worksheets, collaborative activities and projects, critical thinking questions, and practice quizzes for each chapter. Also included are an answer section and reproducible patient education and monitoring forms.

Transparency Acetate Package This package contains 36 completely updated color illustrations, including approximately 10 medication administration illustrations in full color.

Pharmacology Newsletter: *Mosby's Pharmacology Update* This is a biannual publication of new drugs, drug news, and feature articles.

This revised eleventh edition reflects the nurse's responsibilities during the preparation, administration, and monitoring of medication therapy in the health care settings of the 1990s. Each chapter in this edition has been thoroughly reviewed and updated. We have tried to clarify content and reinforce learning throughout the text. We also have placed emphasis on assisting the patient to improve his or her health by educating nursing students on the importance of their role in providing appropriate physical care, emotional and social support, and information necessary for self-care. It is our hope that this revision will motivate the learner to administer medication with concern for safety, precision, and attention to important physiologic factors and will teach and assist nurses in providing the best possible nursing care to their patients.

Bruce D Clayton

Yvonne N. Stock

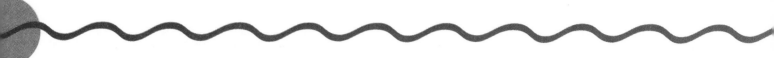

CONTENTS

PART TWO

APPLICATION OF
THE NURSING PROCESS
TO **PHARMACOLOGY 150**

PART **ONE**

PRINCIPLES OF
BASIC
PHARMACOLOGY

Unit One
FOUNDATIONS OF PHARMACOLOGY

CHAPTER 1

Definitions, Names, Standards, and Information Sources

CHAPTER CONTENT

DEFINITIONS

Objectives

1. State the origin and definition of pharmacology.
2. Explain the meaning of therapeutic methods.

Key Words

pharmacology   medicine
therapeutic methods   drug

Pharmacology

Pharmacology (Greek *pharmakon,* "drugs," and *logos,* "science") deals with the study of drugs and their actions on living organisms.

Therapeutic Methods

Diseases may be treated in several different ways. The approaches to therapy are called **therapeutic methods.** Most illnesses require a combination of therapeutic methods for successful treatment. Examples of therapeutic methods include the following:
* Drug therapy—treatment with drugs
* Diet therapy—treatment by diet, such as a low-salt diet for patients with cardiovascular disease
* Physiotherapy—treatment with natural physical forces such as water, light, and heat
* Psychologic therapy—identification of stressors and methods to reduce or eliminate stress or the use of drugs

Drugs

Drugs (Dutch *droog,* "dry") are chemical substances that have an effect on living organisms. Therapeutic drugs, often called **medicines,** are those drugs used in the prevention or treatment of diseases. Until a few decades ago, dried plants were the greatest source of medicines; thus the word **drug** was applied to them.

DRUG NAMES (UNITED STATES)

Objectives

1. Describe the process used to name drugs.

2. Differentiate among the *chemical, generic, official,* and *brand* names of medicines.

chemical name

generic name

trademark

brand name

proprietary name

drug classifications

over-the-counter (OTC) drugs

illegal drugs

official name

Many drugs have a variety of names. This may cause confusion to the patient, physician, and nurse; therefore care must be taken in obtaining the exact name and spelling for a particular drug. When administering the prescribed drug, the *exact* spelling on the drug package must correspond exactly to the spelling of the drug ordered.

Chemical Name

The **chemical name** is most meaningful to the chemist. By means of the chemical name, the chemist understands exactly the chemical constitution of the drug and the exact placing of its atoms or molecular groupings.

Generic Name (Nonproprietary Name)

Before a drug becomes official, it is given a **generic name,** or common name. A generic name is simpler than the chemical name. It may be used in all countries and by any manufacturer. It is not capitalized.

Generic names are provided by the United States Adopted Names (USAN) Council, an organization sponsored by the United States Pharmacopeial Convention, the American Medical Association, and the American Pharmaceutical Association.

Official Name

The **official name** is the name under which the drug is listed by the United States Food and Drug Administration (FDA). The FDA is empowered by federal law to name drugs for human use in the United States.

Trademark (Brand Name)

A **trademark,** or **brand name,** is followed by the symbol ®. This indicates that the name is registered and that its use is restricted to the owner of the drug, who is usually the manufacturer of the product. Some drug companies place their official drugs on the market under trade names, or **proprietary names,** instead of official names. The trade names are deliberately made easier to pronounce, spell, and remember. The first letter of the trade name is capitalized.

EXAMPLE:

Chemical name: 4-dimethylamino-1,4,4a,5,5a,6,11,12a-octahydro-3, 6,10,12,12a-pentahydroxy-6-methyl-1,11,dioxo-2-naphthacenecarboxamide
Generic name: tetracycline
Official name: Tetracycline, USP
Brand names: Achromycin, Panmycin, Tetracyn

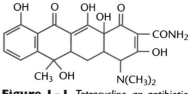

Figure 1 - 1 *Tetracycline, an antibiotic.*

Drug Classifications

Drugs may be classified according to the body system they affect, for example, drugs affecting the central nervous system, drugs affecting the cardiovascular system, drugs affecting the gastrointestinal system.

Drugs may also be classified by *therapeutic use* or *clinical indications,* for example, antacids, antibiotics, antihypertensives, diuretics, laxatives.

Drugs may be classified using the *physiologic* or *chemical action,* for example, anticholinergics, beta adrenergic blockers, calcium channel blockers, and cholinergics.

Drugs may be further classified as prescription or nonprescription, also known as **over-the-counter** (OTC) drugs. Prescription drugs require an order by a health care professional licensed to prescribe, such as a physician or dentist. Nonprescription, or OTC, drugs are sold without a prescription in a pharmacy or the drug section of department stores and grocery stores.

Illegal drugs are drugs or chemical substances used for nontherapeutic purposes. These substances are obtained illegally or have not received approval for use by the FDA.

DRUG NAMES (CANADA)

Objective

1. Differentiate between the *official* and *proper* names of medicines.

Official Drug

The term *official drug* pertains to any drug for which a standard is described either specifically in the *Food and Drug Regulations* or in any publication named in the Food and Drugs Act as satisfactory for officially describing the standards for drugs in Canada. Most commonly used are the generic and brand names of drugs. Although many of the drug names are the same in both Canada and the United States, there are some dissimilarities, especially in brand names.

Proper Name

The *proper name* is the nonproprietary (generic) name used to describe an official drug in Canada.

SOURCES OF DRUG STANDARDS (UNITED STATES)

Objective

1. List official sources of drug standards.

Key Word

The United States Pharmacopeia/National Formulary (USP/NF)

Standardization is needed to ensure that drug products made by different manufacturers, or in different batches by the same manufacturer, are uniformly pure and potent. Before 1820 many drugs were manufactured with varying degrees of purity in different parts of the United States. This problem was solved by the establishment of an authoritative book that set forth required standards of purity for drugs and methods to determine purity. It is called the *Pharmacopeia—National Formulary of the United States of America.*

The United States Pharmacopeia (USP), 23rd Revision, and the National Formulary (NF), 18th Revision

The *USP* and *NF* are now published as a single volume by the United States Pharmacopeial Convention, a nonprofit, nongovernmental corporation. The latest edition, published in 1995, is the fourth edition in which these two established reference books have been combined into one volume. This book is revised every 5 years. Supplements are published more frequently to keep it up to date. The latest edition contains 3410 monographs and 147 general chapters. The most notable of the new contents is the section on nutritional supplements.

The primary purpose of this volume is to provide standards for identity, quality, strength, and purity of substances used in the practice of health care. The standards set forth in the *USP/NF* have been adopted by the FDA as official standards for the manufacture and quality control of medicines and nutritional supplements produced in the United States.

USP Dictionary of USAN and International Drug Names

The *USP* dictionary is a compilation of more than 8274 drug names. Each drug monograph contains the United States Adopted Name (USAN), a pronunciation guide, the

molecular and graphic formula, chemical and brand name, manufacturer, and therapeutic category. It also contains the Chemical Abstracts Service registry numbers for drugs.

Manufacturers submit a proposal for a name to the USAN Council, in which they announce that a certain chemical compound has therapeutic potential and that they plan to investigate its use in human beings. The Council studies the chemical name, applies a series of nomenclature guidelines, and then selects the USAN (generic name). It is now customary for the FDA to accept the adopted generic name as the FDA official name for a chemical compound.

SOURCES OF DRUG STANDARDS (CANADA)

Objective

1. List official sources of drug standards.

Key Words

British Pharmacopoeia   *Pharmacopee Francaise*

The Food and Drugs Act recognizes the standards described by seven international authoritative books to be acceptable for official drugs in Canada. The acceptable publications are the **British Pharmacopoeia,** the *Pharmacopoeia of the United States of America,* the *Pharmacopoeia Internationalis,* the **Pharmacopee Francaise,** the *British Pharmaceutical Codex,* the *National Formulary* (United States), and the *Canadian Formulary.*

SOURCES OF DRUG INFORMATION (UNITED STATES)

Objectives

1. List and describe examples of literature resources for researching prescription and nonprescription medications.

2. List and describe examples of literature resources for researching drug interactions and drug incompatibilities.

Key Words

American Drug Index
American Hospital Formulary Service
Drug Interaction Facts
Facts and Comparisons
Handbook on Injectable Drugs

Handbook of Nonprescription Drugs
Martindale—The Extra Pharmacopoeia
Medical Letter
Physicians' Desk Reference (PDR)

American Drug Index

The *American Drug Index* is edited annually by Norman F. Billups, Ph.D., and is published by Facts and Comparisons. It is an index of all drugs available in the United States.

Drugs in the *Index* are listed alphabetically by generic name and brand name. The generic name monographs indicate that the drug is recognized in the *United States Pharmacopeia—National Formulary* or *United States Adopted Names* and give the chemical name, use, and cross-references to brand names. Each brand name monograph lists the manufacturer, composition and strength, pharmaceutical forms available, package size, dosage, and use. Other features of this reference book include a list of common medical abbreviations; tables of weights, measures, and conversion factors; normal laboratory values; a glossary to aid in interpretation of the monographs; a labeler code index to identify drug products; and a list of manufacturers' addresses. The book is useful for a quick comparison of brand names and generic names and also a check of the availability of strengths and dosage forms.

American Hospital Formulary Service

The *American Hospital Formulary Service, Drug Information,* is a comprehensive reference book published annually by the American Society of Health System Pharmacists in Bethesda, Maryland. Four updated supplements are published yearly. This volume contains monographs on virtually every single-drug entity available in the United States. The monographs emphasize rational therapeutic use of drugs. Each monograph is subdivided into sections on chemistry and stability, pharmacology, pharmacokinetics, uses, cautions, toxicity, drug interactions, laboratory test interferences, dosage and administration, and available products. The index is cross-referenced by both generic and brand names.

The *American Hospital Formulary Service, Drug Information* has been adopted as an official reference by the U.S. Public Health Service and the Veterans Administration. It has also been approved for use by the American Health Care Association, the American Hospital Association, the Catholic Health Care Association of the United States, the National Association of Boards of Pharmacy, and the American Pharmaceutical Association. It is recognized by the U.S. Congress, Health Care Financing Administration, and various third-party health care insurance providers and is included as a required or recommended standard reference in pharmacies in many states.

Drug Interaction Facts

Drug Interaction Facts is published by Facts and Comparisons. This three-ring, loose-leaf, approximately 800-page book, first published in 1983, is currently the most comprehensive book available on the subject of drug interactions. The format is somewhat different from that of most other books: the index is in the front, and the book is not divided into chapters but divided every 100 pages by a plastic tab sheet. Each page is a single monograph describing a drug interaction. Each monograph is subdivided into a table that lists the onset and severity of the drug interaction, expected outcomes, a statement on the

expected effects, the proposed mechanism, and management of the interaction. A short discussion (with references) on the relevance of the interaction follows.

One of the most meaningful, although not obvious, benefits is the source of information used to develop *Drug Interaction Facts*. All the information reviewed is from the MEDIPHOR Group of the Stanford University School of Medicine. This internationally renowned group of physicians and pharmacists has the personnel, clinical experience, scientific background, library, and computer resources to collect, collate, review, and evaluate the scientific accuracy of descriptions of drug interactions from the world literature. Thus the book is an extremely reliable source of information. Subscribers receive an updated supplement four times yearly.

Facts and Comparisons

Facts and Comparisons is a large, loose-leaf compendium of over 3000 pages published by Facts and Comparisons. The book is divided by organ system into 12 chapters. At the beginning of each chapter is a detailed table of contents. All drugs within each chapter are subdivided by therapeutic classes. For each therapeutic class of drug, a monograph provides a brief description of drug action, pharmacokinetics, metabolism, uses, contraindications, warnings, precautions, adverse effects reported, treatment of overdosage, patient information in brief, and administration. The database for the monographs is the most current FDA-approved package insert and publications from official groups such as the Centers for Disease Control and the National Academy of Sciences. The editors have reformatted the information and added additional information from the medical literature on investigational uses of the drugs.

At the end of each monograph are tables of all drugs in that therapeutic class. The tables are particularly valuable because they are designed to allow comparison of similar products, brand names, manufacturers, cost index, and available dosage forms.

The index is comprehensive and is updated both monthly and quarterly. Within each chapter, there is an excellent cross-referencing system as well, which makes it easy to gain information on drugs that may be categorized by more than one therapeutic class. Updated supplements for the entire book are provided monthly.

Handbook on Injectable Drugs

The *Handbook on Injectable Drugs,* the most comprehensive reference available on the topic of compatibility of injectable drugs, is written by Lawrence A. Trissel and published by the American Society of Health System Pharmacists of Bethesda, Maryland. It is a collection of monographs on almost 300 injectable drugs. Each monograph is subdivided into sections on availability of concentrations, stability, pH, dosage and rate of administration, compatibility information, and other useful information about the drug.

Handbook of Nonprescription Drugs

The *Handbook of Nonprescription Drugs* is prepared and published by the American Pharmaceutical Association,

Washington, D.C. It is the most comprehensive text available on medications that can be purchased over the counter in the United States.

Chapters are divided by therapeutic activity, such as antacid products, cold and allergy products, nutritional supplements, mineral and vitamin products, and feminine hygiene products. Each chapter provides a brief review of anatomy and physiology, evaluation of the symptoms being treated, suggested treatments with appropriate dosages, and a list of medications and their ingredients.

This book has three particular advantages for the health care professional: (1) a list of questions to ask the patient to determine whether treatment should be recommended; (2) product selection guidelines for determining the most appropriate products; and (3) counseling to be conveyed to the patient on proper use of the recommended product.

Martindale—The Extra Pharmacopoeia

Martindale—The Extra Pharmacopoeia is a 2400-page volume edited by James E. F. Reynolds and published by The Pharmaceutical Press in London. It is one of the most comprehensive texts available for information on drugs in current use throughout the world. Part 1 contains extensive referenced monographs on the pharmacologic activity and side effects of about 5100 medicinal agents. Part 2 contains short monographs on another 832 agents that are considered either obsolete or too new for inclusion in Part 1. Part 3 gives the composition and manufacturers of more than 46,000 preparations or groups of preparations from 14 countries, including the United Kingdom, North America, Australia, South Africa, and Japan.

The index contains more than 153,500 entries. Medicinal agents are indexed by official names, chemical names, synonyms, and proprietary names.

Medical Letter

The *Medical Letter,* published by Medical Letter, Inc., New Rochelle, New York, is a biweekly periodical newsletter. It contains brief comments on newly released drug products and related topics by an independent board of competent authorities. The board relies on the knowledge of specialists in various fields for their experience with certain drugs. The primary purpose of the newsletter is to report new data on drug action and comparative clinical efficacy. The *Medical Letter* presents timely and critical summaries of data on new drugs during their early period of promotion. Such appraisals must necessarily be tentative.

Package Inserts

Before a new drug is marketed, the manufacturer develops a comprehensive, concise description of the drug, indications and precautions in clinical use, recommendations for dosage, known adverse reactions, contraindications, and other pharmacologic information relating to the drug. Federal law requires that this material be approved by the FDA before the product is released for marketing and that it be presented on an insert that accompanies each package of the product.

Physicians' Desk Reference

The *Physicians' Desk Reference (PDR)* is published annually by Medical Economics, Inc., of Oradell, New Jersey. It is made up of seven sections and lists approximately 2500 therapeutic agents. Each section uses a different page color for easy access.

Section 1 (White), Manufacturers' Index
This section is an alphabetic listing of each manufacturer, its addresses, emergency phone numbers, and a partial list of available products.

Section 2 (Pink), Product Name Index
This section contains a comprehensive alphabetic listing of the generic and brand name products that are discussed in the Product Information section of the book.

Section 3 (Blue), Product Category Index
Products are subdivided by therapeutic classes, such as analgesics, laxatives, oxytocics, and antibiotics.

Section 4 (Gray), Product Identification Guide
Each manufacturer has provided actual-size color pictures of tablets and capsules. These are invaluable aids in product identification.

Section 5 (White), Product Information Section
This contains reprints of the package inserts for the major products of manufacturers, with information on action, uses, administration, dosages, contraindications, composition, and how each drug is supplied.

Section 6 (Green), Diagnostic Product Information
Many diagnostic tests used in hospital and office practice are listed alphabetically by manufacturer.

Section 7, Miscellaneous
The last section of the book contains a listing of certified poison control centers, discontinued products, the FDA telephone directory, definitions of controlled substances categories, definitions of FDA Use-in-Pregnancy ratings, and adverse event report forms.

Nursing Journals

Many specialty journals have articles on drug therapy relating to a specific field (for example, *Geriatric Nursing, Heart and Lung.*) Nursing journals such as *RN, AJN,* and others present articles on drugs, drug update information, and articles that stress nursing considerations relating to the drug therapy.

The nurse must keep in mind the purpose of using resources and be mindful of the accuracy of the information contained. Nurses should check the dates on articles to validate the currency of the information. Reliable sources to validate drug information are listed earlier in this section.

SOURCES OF DRUG INFORMATION (CANADA)

Objectives

1. Describe the organization of *Compendium of Pharmaceuticals and Specialties* and the information contained in each colored section.
2. Describe the organization of *Canadian Self-Medication*.

Key Words

Compendium of Pharmaceuticals and Specialties

Self-Medication
electronic databases

Compendium of Pharmaceuticals and Specialties

The *Compendium of Pharmaceuticals and Specialties (CPS)* is published annually by the Canadian Pharmaceutical Association. It provides an extensive list of the pharmaceutical products distributed in Canada and other information of practical value to health care professionals. Manufacturers voluntarily submit information concerning their products for this text. The entire *CPS* is available in print in both English and French. The book is divided into six color-coded sections.

Pink Pages—Therapeutic Guide

The Therapeutic Guide is a clinical guide for the use of single-entity drugs listed in the *CPS*. Most products listed are single entity, but there are some combination products (e.g., oral contraceptives, antacids). The guide uses the Canadian version of the World Health Organization's Anatomic Therapeutic Chemical Classification. Drugs are classified under 16 anatomic groups (for example, gastrointestinal tract) and then subdivided into therapeutic categories (for example, antacids, antiemetics, digestive enzymes, laxatives). Drugs are then further subclassified under specific therapeutic, pharmacologic, or chemical subheadings within the therapeutic category (for example, antacids—aluminum containing, calcium containing). Medicines may be classified under more than one section if used for more than one indication. Once a generic name has been identified, the corresponding brand name can be found in the Brand/Nonproprietary Name Index (Green Section).

Green Pages—Drug Listing of Brand and Nonproprietary Names

This section is an alphabetic cross-reference that lists drugs by both nonproprietary and brand names and also indicates whether the product was available in Canada at the time of publication. Brand names that are in boldface type have a product monograph in the *CPS* White Section.

Photograph Pages—Product Recognition Section

This section contains color photographs of drug products arranged according to the size and color shadings of indi-
vidual dosage forms (tablets, capsules, liquids). Products are cross-referenced in the white pages monograph section. This section is also printed in French.

Yellow Pages—Manufacturers' Index

This section contains names, addresses, and telephone numbers of the manufacturers and distributors of pharmaceutical products in Canada; it also contains product listings for many of the manufacturers.

Lilac Pages—Clin-Info

This section contains tables, charts, and text describing a wide range of information of interest to health care professionals that otherwise would seldom be easily accessible, particularly in a single reference book. Topics include the nonmedicinal ingredients of selected pharmaceuticals (for example, sulfite, gluten, alcohol, tartrazine content), SI unit conversion factors, drugs and sports competition, clinical monitoring (for example, anticoagulant drug monitoring, body surface area nomograms, serum drug concentration monitoring), clinical information on cardiac arrest, travel (drinking water purification, immunization schedules, malaria prevention and treatment), drug interactions, dietary recommendations, poison control centers in Canada and a summary of Canadian regulations for narcotics and controlled drugs, and the procedure to obtain on an emergency basis a drug not cleared for use in Canada.

Blue Pages—Patient Information

This section lists the information to be conveyed to patients on almost 200 individual products. The information is arranged alphabetically by brand name. Margins are wider in this section to allow photocopying of the patient information.

White Pages—Monographs of Pharmaceuticals and Specialties

This unit is an alphabetic arrangement of manufacturer's brand information. It also contains numerous general monographs for common multisource drugs; a few medical devices are described.

Self-Medication

Self-Medication is a two-volume text published by the Canadian Pharmaceutical Association. Volume 1, *Self-Medication: Reference for Health Professionals,* is published approximately every 4 years. Volume 2, *Self-Medication: Compendium of Nonprescription Drugs,* is published annually. The text provides comprehensive information about the nonprescription drug products that are available in Canada. As in the *CPS,* manufacturers voluntarily submit monographs for publication.

In volume 1, the chapters are organized by therapeutic category, such as ophthalmic products, constipation and laxatives, diabetes care, ostomy care and incontinence, herbal medicines, and poisoning and overdose. Each provides a review of anatomy and physiology and the conditions suitable for self-medication. Treatment measures include both general and pharmacologic management suggestions and a review of the nonprescription drug alternatives available. Appendixes include a table of chemicals with assorted pharmaceutical uses (e.g., alum, compound benzoin tincture) and key counseling tools to encourage communication between health care professionals and patients.

Volume 2 focuses on product information in the form of drug monographs (alphabetically listed) and extensive product comparison tables. There is also a manufacturers' and distributors' index with names, addresses, phone and fax numbers, and products listed.

Electronic Databases

There is an ever-growing increase in the use of **electronic databases** as a resource for drug information. On-line services can now be accessed for a nominal fee through the National Library of Medicine. Most of the drug information sources listed previously are available through electronic retrieval at libraries. Many college libraries subscribe via CD-ROM disks to CINAHL, a cumulative index of nursing and allied health literature. By using these sources, nurses have access to a wealth of information from sources published in the United States and other countries.

SOURCES OF PATIENT INFORMATION

Objective

1. Cite a literature resource for reviewing information to be given to the patient concerning prescribed medication.

Key Word

United States Pharmacopeia Dispensing Information (USPDI)

Over the past two decades, it has become evident that health care providers must do a better job of informing patients of what they must do to assume responsibility for their own health care. The following material is an excellent source of information for teaching patients how to use their medications properly.

United States Pharmacopeia Dispensing Information

United States Pharmacopeia Dispensing Information (USPDI) is an annual publication written by the United States Pharmacopeial Convention, Inc.

The *USPDI* is a two-volume set supplemented with bimonthly updates. The first volume includes information for health care providers arranged in alphabetically ordered monographs. Each monograph is subdivided into sections on the drug's use, mechanism of action, precautions, side effects, patient consultation information, general dosing information, and dosage forms available.

The second volume, *Advice for the Patient,* provides the layman's language for the patient consultation guidelines found in the first volume. The second volume is designed to be used at the discretion of the health care provider as an aid to counseling the patient if written information is to be given to the patient. The publisher permits all health care practitioners to reproduce the pages of advice for their patients receiving the prescribed drug. Generic and brand names are cross-referenced in the index of *Advice for the Patient.*

DRUG LEGISLATION (UNITED STATES)

Objectives

1. List legislative acts controlling drug use and abuse.
2. Differentiate among Schedule I, II, III, IV, and V medications and describe nursing responsibilities associated with the administration of each type.

Key Words

Federal Food, Drug, and Cosmetic Act

Controlled Substances Act

scheduled drugs

Drug legislation protects the consumer and patient. The need for such protection is great because manufacturers and advertising agents may make unfounded claims about the benefits of their products.

Federal Food, Drug, and Cosmetic Act, June 25, 1938 (Amended 1952, 1962)

The 1938 **Food, Drug, and Cosmetic Act** authorizes the federal Food and Drug Administration of the Department of Health and Human Services to determine the safety of drugs before marketing and to ensure that certain labeling specifications and standards in advertising are met in the marketing of products. Manufacturers are required to submit new drug applications to the FDA for review of safety studies before products can be released for sale.

The Durham-Humphrey Amendment in 1952 tightened control by restricting the refilling of prescriptions.

The Kefauver-Harris Drug Amendment in 1962 was passed as a result of the thalidomide tragedy. Thalidomide was an incompletely tested drug approved for use as a sedative-hypnotic during pregnancy. Infants exposed to thalidomide were born with serious birth defects. This amendment provides greater control and surveillance of the distribution and clinical testing of investigational drugs and requires that a product be proved both safe and effective before release for sale.

Harrison Narcotic Act, 1914

The Harrison Narcotic Act regulated the importation, manufacture, sale, and use of opium, cocaine, and all their compounds and derivatives. Its purpose was to limit the indiscriminate use of such drugs and to prevent the spread of the drug habit. The act was amended many times. However, it has been repealed and replaced by the Controlled Substances Act of 1970.

Controlled Substances Act, 1970

The Comprehensive Drug Abuse Prevention and Control Act was passed by Congress in 1970. This new statute, commonly referred to as the **Controlled Substances Act,** repealed almost 50 other laws written since 1914 that relate to the control of drugs. The new composite law is designed to improve the administration and regulation of manufacturing, distributing, and dispensing of drugs found necessary to be controlled.

The Drug Enforcement Administration (DEA) was organized to enforce the Controlled Substances Act, to gather intelligence, and to train and conduct research in the area of dangerous drugs and drug abuse. The DEA is a bureau of the Department of Justice. The director of the DEA reports to the Attorney General of the United States.

The basic structure of the Controlled Substances Act consists of five classifications, or **schedules,** of controlled substances. The degree of control, the conditions of record keeping, the particular order forms required, and other regulations depend on these classifications. The five schedules, their criteria, and examples of drugs in each schedule are listed in the following.

Schedule I ℂ Drugs

1. A high potential for abuse
2. No currently accepted medical use in the United States
3. A lack of accepted safety for use under medical supervision

EXAMPLES: lysergic acid diethylamide (LSD), marijuana, peyote, heroin, hashish

Schedule II ℂ Drugs

1. A high potential for abuse
2. A currently accepted medical use in the United States
3. An abuse potential that may lead to severe psychologic or physical dependence

EXAMPLES: secobarbital, pentobarbital, amphetamines, morphine, meperidine, methadone, Percodan

Schedule III ℂ Drugs

1. A high potential for abuse, but less so than drugs in schedules I and II
2. A currently accepted medical use in the United States
3. An abuse potential that may lead to moderate or low physical dependence or high psychologic dependence

EXAMPLES: Empirin with codeine, Doriden, Fiorinal, paregoric, Noludar, Tylenol with codeine

Schedule IV ℂ Drugs

1. A low potential for abuse, compared with those in schedule III
2. A currently accepted medical use in the United States
3. An abuse potential that may lead to limited physical or psychologic dependence, compared with drugs in schedule III

EXAMPLES: phenobarbital, Equanil, chloral hydrate, paraldehyde, Librium, Valium, Dalmane, Tranxene

Schedule V ℂ Drugs

1. A low potential for abuse, compared with those in schedule IV
2. A currently accepted medical use in the United States
3. An abuse potential of limited physical or psychologic dependence liability, compared with drugs in schedule IV

EXAMPLES: Lomotil, Robitussin A-C

The Attorney General, after public hearings, has authority to reschedule a drug, bring an unscheduled drug under control, or remove controls on scheduled drugs.

Every manufacturer, physician, dentist, pharmacy, and hospital that manufactures, prescribes, or dispenses any of the drugs listed in the five schedules must register biannually with the Drug Enforcement Administration.

A physician's prescription for substances named in this law must contain the physician's name, address, DEA registration number and signature, the patient's name and address, and the date of issue. The pharmacist cannot refill such prescriptions without the approval of the physician.

All controlled substances for ward stock must be ordered on special hospital forms that are used to help maintain inventory and dispersion control records of the schedule drugs. When a nurse administers a Schedule II drug, under a physician's order, the following information must be entered on the controlled substances record: name of the patient, date of administration, drug administered, and drug dosage.

Possession of Controlled Substances

Federal and state laws make the possession of controlled substances a crime, except in specifically exempted cases. The law makes no distinction between professional and practical nurses in regard to possession of controlled drugs. Nurses may give controlled substances only under the direction of a physician or dentist who has been licensed to prescribe or dispense these agents. Nurses may not have controlled substances in their possession unless they are giving them to a patient under a doctor's order, the nurse is a patient for whom a doctor has prescribed schedule drugs, or the nurse is the official custodian of a limited supply of controlled substances on a ward or department of the hospital. Controlled substances ordered but not used for patients must be returned to the source from which they were obtained (the doctor or the pharmacy). Violation or failure to comply with the Controlled Substances Act is punishable by fine, imprisonment, or both.

DRUG LEGISLATION (CANADA)

Objectives

1. List legislative acts controlling drug use and abuse.
2. Differentiate between Schedule F and G, and describe nursing responsibilities with each.

Food and Drugs Act 1927   nonprescription drugs

Food and Drug
  Regulations 1953, 1954,
  1979

Food and Drugs Act 1927; the Food and Drug Regulations 1953 and 1954, Revised 1979 and Periodic Amendments

The **Food and Drugs Act** and the **Food and Drug Regulations** empower the Department of National Health and Welfare of Canada to protect the public from foreseeable risks relating to the manufacture and sale of drugs. The administration of this legislation is carried out by the Health Protection Branch. It provides for a review of the safety and efficacy of drugs before their clearance for marketing in Canada as either prescription or nonprescription products. Also included in this legislation are requirements for good manufacturing practices, adequate labeling, and fair advertising.

Drugs requiring a prescription, except for narcotics, are listed on Schedule F or Schedule G of the Food and Drug Regulations.

Schedule F Prescription Drugs

Schedule F drugs may be prescribed only by qualified practitioners (physicians, dentists, or veterinarians) because they would normally be used most safely under supervision.

> EXAMPLES: most antibiotics, antineoplastics, corticosteroids, cardiovascular drugs, antipsychotics

Schedule G Controlled Drugs

Schedule G drugs may be prescribed only by qualified practitioners. Because of a recognized abuse potential, these drugs are subject to additional requirements of record keeping for purchase, sale, or administration to a patient in a hospital.

> EXAMPLES: amphetamines, barbiturates, diethylproprion, methaqualone, methylphenidate

The legitimate use of amphetamines in Canada is restricted to specific disorders such as narcolepsy or hyperkinetic disorders in children. It does not include obesity control.

Narcotic Control Act (1960–1961) and Narcotic Control Regulations (Amended 1978)

The Narcotic Control Act and the Narcotic Control Regulations establish the requirements for the control and sale of narcotic substances in Canada.

Generally, because of their abuse potential, narcotics are subject to more stringent requirements for inventory control than other prescription drugs.

> EXAMPLES: meperidine (Demerol), morphine, propoxyphene (Darvon), codeine, oxycodone, hydrocodone

Recently, despite considerable controversy, special provision was made for the limited medical use of heroin in Canada for intractable pain.

The Narcotic Control Regulations also provide for the nonprescription sale of certain codeine preparations. The content must not exceed the equivalent of 8 mg of codeine phosphate per solid dosage unit or 20 mg per 30 ml of a liquid, and the preparation must also contain two additional nonnarcotic medicinal ingredients. These preparations may not be advertised or displayed and may be sold only by pharmacists. In hospitals, the pharmacy usually requires strict inventory control of these products, as well as other narcotics.

> EXAMPLES: Tylenol No. 1, Frosst "222," Benylin with codeine

Requirements for the legitimate administration of drugs to patients by nurses are generally similar in Canada and the United States. Individual hospital policy determines specific record-keeping requirements based on federal and provincial laws. Violations of these laws would be expected to result in fines or imprisonment in addition to the loss of professional license.

Drug Legislation

In 1972 the FDA initiated the use of criteria to evaluate nonprescription, or over-the-counter, drugs. This legislation has resulted in the removal of some drugs from the market and the reformulation of other drugs. In addition, some drugs that formerly required a prescription can now be purchased as nonprescription drugs.

Nonprescription Drugs

In Canada, the Health Protection Branch acknowledges two classes of **nonprescription drugs.** Provision is made in Division 10 of the Food and Drug Regulations for "proprietary medicines" that can be adequately labeled by manufacturers for direct use by consumers. Laws in each of the 10 provinces determine the actual conditions of distribution of nonprescription drugs. Proprietary medicines can generally be sold through any retail outlet, whereas other nonprescription drugs in some provinces may be sold only in pharmacies. In fact, a few provinces require the direct involvement of a pharmacist in the sale of certain nonprescription drugs. Most hospitals do not differentiate between prescription and nonprescription drugs, requiring physician's orders for both.

EFFECTIVENESS OF DRUG LEGISLATION

The effectiveness of drug legislation depends on the interest and determination used to enforce these laws, the appropriation by government of adequate funds for enforcement, the vigor used by proper authorities in enforcement, the interest and cooperation of professional people and the public, and the education of the public concerning the dangers of unwise and indiscriminate use of drugs in general. Many organizations help in this education, including the National Coordinating Council on Patient Information and Education, the American Medical Association, the American Dental Association, the American Pharmaceutical Association, the American Society of Health System Pharmacists, and local, state, and county health departments.

NEW DRUG DEVELOPMENT

1. Describe the procedure outlined by the FDA to develop and market new medicines.

preclinical research

clinical research

new drug application
  review

postmarketing surveillance

Health care professionals and consumers alike often ask why it takes so long from the time a drug is discovered to the time it is brought to the market. It now takes an average of 100 months and over $200 million in research and development costs to bring a single new drug to market. The Pharmaceutical Manufacturers Association estimates that only 1 of 10,000 chemicals investigated will actually be found to be "safe and effective" and brought to the pharmacist's shelf.

The Food, Drug, and Cosmetic Act of 1938 charged the FDA with the responsibility of regulating new drugs. Rules and regulations evolved by the FDA divide new drug development into four stages: (1) preclinical research and development; (2) clinical research and development; (3) new drug application review; and (4) postmarketing surveillance (Figure 1-2).

Preclinical Research and Development Stage

The **preclinical phase** of new drug development begins with discovery, synthesis, and purification of the drug. The goal at this stage is to use laboratory studies to determine whether the experimental drug has therapeutic value and whether the drug appears to be safe in animals. Enough data must be available to justify testing the experimental drug in humans. The preclinical phase of data collection may require 1 to 3 years, although the average length of time is 18 months. Near the end of this phase, the investigator (often a pharmaceutical manufacturer) submits an Investigational New Drug Application (IND) to the FDA, which describes

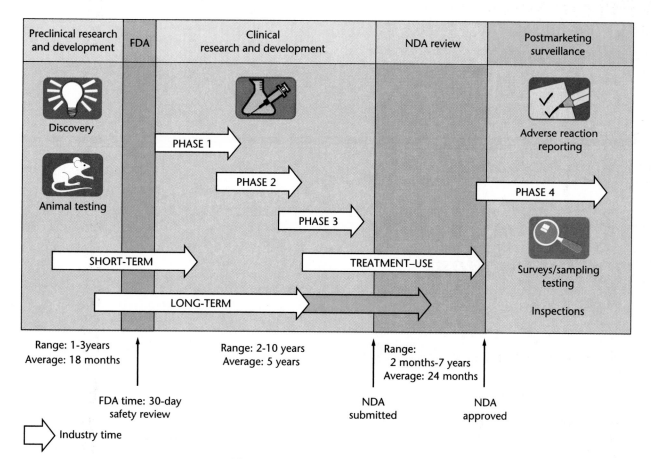

Figure 1-2 *New drug review process.*

all studies completed to date and the safety and testing planned for human subjects. The FDA must make a decision based on safety considerations within 30 days on whether to allow the study to proceed. Only about 20% of the chemicals tested in the preclinical phase advance to the clinical testing phase.

Clinical Research and Development Stage

The "testing in humans" stage, the **clinical stage,** or IND stage, is usually subdivided into three phases, generally described as phases 1, 2, and 3. Phase 1 studies determine an experimental drug's pharmacologic properties, such as its pharmacokinetics, metabolism, and potential for toxicity at a certain dosage. The study population is either normal volunteers or the intended treatment population, such as patients with certain cancers or arrhythmias. Phase 1 studies usually require 20 to 100 subjects who are treated for 4 to 6 weeks. If phase 1 trials are successful, the drug is moved to phase 2, in which a larger population of several hundred patients is used. Studies are conducted to determine the success rate of a drug for its intended use. If successful, the drug is advanced to phase 3 trials, in which larger patient populations are used to ensure statistical significance of the results. Phase 3 studies also provide additional information on proper dosing and safety. The clinical research phase may require 2 to 10 years, with the average experimental drug requiring 5 years. Each study completed is reviewed by the FDA to help ensure patient safety. Only one of five drugs that enter the clinical trials will eventually be approved for sale. The others are eliminated because of efficacy or safety problems or lack of commercial interest.

New Drug Application Review

When sufficient data have been collected to demonstrate that the experimental drug is both safe and effective, the investigator submits a **New Drug Application** (NDA) to the FDA, formally requesting approval to market a new drug for human use. Thousands of pages of NDA data are reviewed by a team of pharmacologists, toxicologists, chemists, physicians, and others, as appropriate, who then recommend to the FDA whether the drug should be approved for use. The average NDA review takes 24 months. Once a drug is approved by the FDA, it is the manufacturer's decision as to when to bring a product to the marketplace.

Postmarketing Surveillance

If the manufacturer decides to market the medicine, the **postmarketing surveillance** phase, or fourth phase of drug product development, begins. It consists of an ongoing review of adverse effects of the new drug and periodic inspections of the manufacturing facilities and products. Other studies completed during the fourth phase include identification of other patient populations in whom the drug may be useful, refinement of dosing recommendations, and exploration of potential drug interactions. Health care practitioners make a significant contribution to the knowledge of drug safety by reporting adverse effects of drugs to the FDA by using the MEDWATCH program for voluntary reporting of adverse event and product problems (see Appendix F).

CHAPTER 2

Principles of Drug Action and Drug Interactions

CHAPTER CONTENT

BASIC PRINCIPLES

Objectives

1. Identify five basic principles of drug action.

2. Explain nursing assessments necessary to evaluate potential problems associated with the absorption of medications.

3. Describe nursing interventions that can enhance drug absorption.
4. List three categories of drug administration, and state the routes of administration for each category.
5. Differentiate between general and selective types of drug distribution mechanisms.
6. Name the process that inactivates drugs.
7. Identify the meaning and significance to the nurse of the term *half-life* when used in relation to drug therapy.

Key Words

receptors	percutaneous
agonists	distribution
antagonists	drug blood level
partial agonists	metabolism
ADME	biotransformation
absorption	excretion
enteral	half-life
parenteral	

How do drugs act in the body? The following are a few key facts to remember:

1. Drugs do not create new responses but alter existing physiologic activity. Thus drug response must be stated in relation to what the physiologic activity was before the response to drug therapy (that is, an antihypertensive agent is successful if the blood pressure is lower during therapy than before therapy). Therefore it is important to perform a thorough nursing assessment to identify the baseline data. Thereafter, regular assessments are performed by the nurse and compared with the baseline data by the physician, the nurse, and the pharmacist in order to evaluate the effectiveness of the drug therapy.
2. Drugs interact with the body in several different ways. The most common way in which drugs act is formation of chemical bonds with specific sites called **receptors** within the body. Bonding occurs only if the drug and its receptor have similar shapes. The relationship between a drug and a receptor is like that between a key and a lock (Figure 2-1, *A*).
3. Most drugs have several different atoms within the molecule that interlock into several locations on the receptor. The better the "fit" between the receptor and the drug, the better the response. The intensity of a drug response is related not only to how well the drug molecule fits in the receptor but also to the number of receptor sites occupied.
4. Drugs that interact with a receptor to stimulate a response are called **agonists** (Figure 2-1, *B*). Drugs that attach to a receptor but do not stimulate a response are called **antagonists** (Figure 2-1, *C*). Drugs that interact with a receptor to stimulate a response but

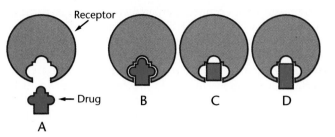

Figure 2-1 **A**, *Drugs act by forming a chemical bond with specific receptory sites, similar to a key and lock.* **B**, *The better the "fit," the better the response. Those with complete attachment and response are called agonists.* **C**, *Drugs that attach but do not elicit a response are called antagonists.* **D**, *Drugs that attach, elicit a small response, and also block other responses are called partial agonists.*

inhibit other responses are called **partial agonists** (Figure 2-1, *D*).
5. Once administered, all drugs go through four stages: absorption, distribution, metabolism, and excretion (**ADME**). Each drug has its own unique ADME characteristics.

Absorption

Absorption is the process by which a drug is made available to the body fluids for distribution. Absorption is the way in which a drug is transferred from its site of entry into the body to the circulating fluids of the body, the blood, and the lymphatic system. The rate at which this occurs depends on the route of administration, the blood flow through the tissue at the point of drug administration, and the solubility of the drug. It is therefore important to (1) administer oral drugs with an adequate amount of fluid, (2) give parenteral forms properly so they are deposited in the correct tissue for enhanced absorption, and (3) reconstitute and dilute drugs only with the diluent recommended by the manufacturer in the package literature so that drug solubility is not impaired. Equally important are nursing assessments that imply poor absorption (for example, if insulin is administered subcutaneously and a "lump" remains at the site of injection 2 to 3 hours later, absorption from that site may be impaired).

There are three categories of drug administration: the enteral, the parenteral, and the percutaneous routes. The **enteral** route is administration directly into the gastrointestinal (GI) tract by oral, rectal, or nasogastric routes. **Parenteral** routes of administration bypass the GI tract by subcutaneous (SC), intramuscular (IM), or intravenous (IV) injection. Methods of **percutaneous** administration are inhalation or sublingual or topical administration. Absorption of topical drugs applied to the skin can be influenced by the drug concentration, length of contact time, size of affected area, thickness of skin surface, hydration of tissue, and degree of skin disruption. Percutaneous absorption is greatly increased in newborns and young infants who have thin, well-hydrated skin. Inhalation of drugs and their absorption can be influenced by depth of respirations and fineness of the droplet particles, available surface area of mucous membrane, contact time, hydration state, blood supply to the area, and concentration of the drug itself.

The rate of absorption by parenteral routes is partially dependent upon the rate of blood flow through the tissues. Circulatory insufficiency and respiratory distress may lead to hypoxia and further complicate this situation by resulting in vasoconstriction. (The nurse should therefore not give an injection in situations in which circulation is known to be impaired. Another site on the rotation schedule should be used.) SC injections have the slowest absorption rate, especially if peripheral circulation is impaired. IM injections are absorbed more rapidly because of greater blood flow per unit weight of muscle. (Depositing the medication into the muscle belly is important. Nurses must carefully assess the individual patient for the correct length of needle to ensure that this occurs.) Cooling an area of injection will slow the rate of absorption while heat or massage will hasten the rate of absorption. When administered by IV injection, the drug is dispersed throughout the body most rapidly. (Nurses must be thoroughly educated regarding the responsibilities and techniques associated with administering IV medications. Once the drug enters the bloodstream, it cannot be retrieved.)

Regardless of the route of administration, a drug must be dissolved in body fluids before it can be absorbed into body tissues. For example, before a solid drug taken orally can be absorbed into the bloodstream for transport to the site of action, it must disintegrate and dissolve in the GI fluids and be transported across the stomach or intestinal lining into the blood. The process of converting the drug into a soluble form can be partially controlled by the pharmaceutical dosage form used (that is, solution, suspension, capsule, and tablets with various coatings) or can be influenced by the time of administration in relation to the presence or absence of food in the stomach.

Distribution

The term **distribution** refers to the ways in which drugs are transported by the circulating body fluids to the sites of action (receptors), metabolism, and excretion. Drug distribution is both transport throughout the entire body by the blood and lymphatic systems and transport from the circulating fluids into and out of the fluids that bathe the receptor sites. Organs having the most extensive blood supply, such as the heart, liver, kidneys, and brain, receive the distributing drug most rapidly. Areas with less extensive blood supply, such as the muscle, skin, and fat, receive the drug more slowly.

Once a drug has been dissolved and absorbed into the circulating blood, its distribution is determined by the chemical properties of the drug and how it is affected by the blood and tissues it contacts. Two of the factors that influence drug distribution are protein binding and lipid (fat) solubility. Most drugs are transported in combination with plasma proteins, especially albumin, which act as carriers for relatively insoluble drugs. Drugs bound to plasma proteins are pharmacologically inactive because the large size of the complex keeps them in the bloodstream and prevents them from reaching the sites of action, metabolism, and excretion. Only the free or unbound portion of a drug is able to diffuse into tissues, interact with receptors, and produce biologic effects (or be metabolized and excreted). The same proportion of bound and free drug is maintained in the blood at all times. Thus as the free drug acts on receptor sites, the decrease in serum drug levels causes some of the bound drug to be released from protein to maintain the ratio between bound and free drug.

When a drug is circulating in the blood, a blood sample may be drawn and assayed to determine the amount of drug present. This is known as a **drug blood level.** It is important for certain drugs (for example, anticonvulsants, aminoglycoside antibiotics) to be measured to ensure that the drug is in the therapeutic range. If the blood level is low, the dosage must either be increased or the medicine must be administered more frequently. If the drug blood level is too high, the patient may develop toxicities; either the dosage must be reduced or the medicine must be administered less frequently. See Appendix D for therapeutic blood levels for selected medicines.

Once a drug leaves the bloodstream, it may become bound to tissues other than those with active receptor sites. The more lipid-soluble drugs have a high affinity for adipose tissue, which serves as a repository site for these agents. Because there is relatively low blood circulation to fat tissues, the more lipid-soluble drugs tend to stay in the body for much longer. An equilibrium is established between the repository site (lipid tissue) and circulation, so that as the amount of drug in the blood drops as a result of binding at the sites of biologic activity, metabolism, or excretion, more drug is released from the lipid tissue. By contrast, if more drug is given, a new equilibrium will be established between the blood, activity sites, lipid tissue repository sites, and metabolic and excretory sites.

Distribution may be general or selective. Some drugs cannot pass certain types of cell membranes, such as the central nervous system (blood-brain barrier) or the placenta (placental barrier), while other types of drugs will readily pass into these tissues. The distribution process is important, because the amount of drug that actually reaches the receptor sites determines the extent of pharmacologic activity. If little of the drug actually reaches and binds to the receptor sites, the response will be only minimal.

Metabolism

Metabolism, also called **biotransformation,** is the process by which the body inactivates drugs. The enzyme systems of the liver are the primary sites of metabolism of drugs, but other tissues and organs metabolize certain drugs to a minor extent.

Excretion

Elimination of metabolites of drugs and, in some cases, the active drug itself from the body is called **excretion.** The primary routes are through the GI tract to the feces and through the renal tubules into the urine. Other routes of excretion include evaporation through the skin, exhalation from the lungs, and secretion into the saliva and mother's milk.

Because the kidneys are a major organ of drug excretion, it is appropriate for the nurse to review the chart for the results of the urinalysis and renal function tests. The patient with renal failure will often experience an increase

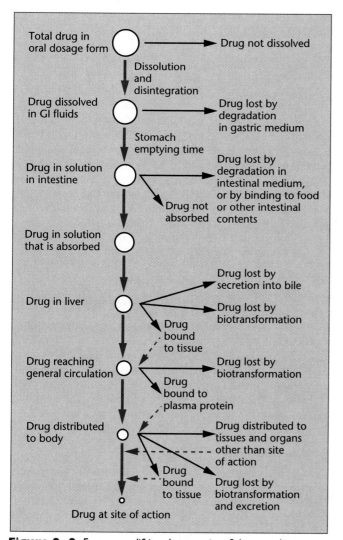

Figure 2-2 *Factors modifying the quantity of drug reaching a site of action after a single oral dose.* (Modified from Levine RR: *Pharmacology, drug actions, and reactions,* Boston, 1973, Little, Brown).

Time (Hours)	Half-life	Drug Remaining in Body
0	—	100 mg (100%)
12	1	50 mg (50%)
24	2	25 mg (25%)
36	3	12.5 mg (12.5%)
48	4	6.25 mg (6.25%)
60	5	3.12 mg (3.12%)

Note that as each 12 hours (one half-life) passes, the amount remaining is 50% of the amount present 12 hours earlier. After six half-lives, more than 98% of the drug is eliminated from the body.

The half-life is determined by an individual's ability to metabolize and excrete a particular drug. Because most patients metabolize and excrete the same drug at approximately the same rate, the approximate half-lives of most drugs are now known. When the half-life of a drug is known, dosages and frequency of administration can be calculated. Drugs with a long half-life, such as digoxin at 36 hours, need to be administered only once daily; while drugs with a short half-life, such as aspirin at 5 hours, need to be administered every 4 to 6 hours to maintain therapeutic activity. In patients who have impaired hepatic or renal function, the half-life may become considerably longer because of the inability to metabolize or excrete the drug. An example is digoxin, which has a half-life of approximately 36 hours in a patient with normal renal function but as long as 105 hours in a patient in complete renal failure. Monitoring diagnostic tests that measure renal or hepatic function is important. Whenever laboratory data reflect impairment of either function, the nurse should notify the physician.

DRUG ACTION

Objective

1. Compare and contrast the following terms used in relationship to medications: desired action, side effects, adverse effects, allergic reactions, and idiosyncratic reactions.

Key Words

desired action	urticaria
side effects	hives
adverse effects	carcinogenicity
idiosyncratic reaction	teratogen
allergic reactions	

in the action and duration of a drug if the dosage and frequency of administration are not adjusted to the patient's renal function.

Figure 2-2 is a schematic review of the absorption, distribution, metabolism, and excretion process of an oral medication. It is important to note how little of the active ingredient actually reaches the receptor sites for action.

Half-life

Elimination of drugs occurs by metabolism and excretion. A measure of the time required for elimination is the half-life. The **half-life** is defined as the amount of time required for 50% of the drug to be eliminated from the body. For example, if a patient were given 100 mg of a drug that had a half-life of 12 hours, the following would be observed:

No drug has a single action. When a drug enters a patient and is absorbed and distributed, the **desired action,** (that is, the expected response) usually occurs. All drugs, however, have the potential to affect more than one body system simultaneously, producing reactions known as **side effects** or **adverse effects.** Most of these side effects are predictable, and patients should be monitored so that dosages can be adjusted to allow the maximum therapeutic benefits with a minimum of side effects. As described in Part Two of this text, each drug has a series of *parameters* (such as therapeutic actions to expect, side effects to expect, adverse effects to report, and probable drug interactions) that should be monitored by the nurse, physician, pharmacist, and patient in order to optimize therapy while reducing the possibility of serious adverse effects.

Two other types of drug action are much more unpredictable. These are idiosyncratic reactions and allergic reactions. An **idiosyncratic reaction** occurs when something unusual or abnormal happens when a drug is first administered. The patient usually shows an *overresponse* to the action of the drug. This type of reaction is usually caused by a patient's inability to metabolize a drug as a result of a genetic deficiency of certain enzymes. Fortunately, this type of reaction is rare.

Allergic reactions, also known as hypersensitivity reactions, occur in approximately 6% to 10% of patients taking medications. Allergic reactions occur in patients who have previously been exposed to a drug and have developed antibodies to it in the immune system. Upon reexposure, the antibodies cause a reaction, most commonly seen as raised, irregular-shaped patches on the skin with severe itching, known as **urticaria** or **hives.** Occasionally, a patient will have a severe, life-threatening reaction that causes respiratory distress and cardiovascular collapse, known as an *anaphylactic reaction.* This condition is a medical emergency and must be treated immediately. Fortunately, anaphylactic reactions occur much less frequently than the more mild urticarial reactions. If a patient has a mild reaction, it should be taken as a warning that the medication should not be administered again. The patient is much more likely to have an anaphylactic reaction at the next exposure to the drug. Patients should receive information regarding the drug name and be told to tell health care professionals (such as nurses, physicians, pharmacists, and dentists) that they have had a reaction and must not receive the drug again. In addition, patients should wear an identification bracelet or necklace explaining the allergy.

Carcinogenicity is the ability of a drug to induce living cells to mutate and become cancerous. Many drugs have this potential, so all drugs are tested in several animal species before human investigation to help eliminate this potential.

A drug that induces birth defects is known as a **teratogen.** Organs of the body are particularly susceptible to malformation if exposed to a drug while they are being formed in the fetus. Because most organ systems are formed during the first trimester of pregnancy, the greatest potential for birth defects caused by drugs occurs during this period.

VARIABLE FACTORS INFLUENCING DRUG ACTION

Objective

1. List factors that cause variations in absorption, metabolism, distribution, and excretion of drugs.

Key Words

placebo	drug dependence
tolerance	drug accumulation

Many times we have heard patients say "That drug really knocked me out!" or "That drug didn't touch the pain!" The effects of drugs are unexpectedly potent in some patients, while other patients show little response to the same dose. In addition, some patients will react differently to the same dose of a drug administered at different times. Because of individual patient variation, exact responses to drug therapy are difficult to predict. The following factors have been identified as contributors to a variable response to drugs.

Age

Infants and the very elderly tend to be the most sensitive to the response of drugs. There are important differences in the absorption, distribution, metabolism, and excretion of drugs in premature neonates, full-term newborns, and older children. The aging process brings about changes in body composition and organ function that can affect the elderly patient's response to drug therapy. See Chapter 3 for a more complete discussion of age-related variables influencing drug action.

Body Weight

Considerably overweight patients will usually require an increase in dosage to attain the same therapeutic response. Conversely, patients who are underweight (compared with the general population) tend to require lower doses for the same therapeutic response. Most pediatric doses are calculated by milligrams of drug per kilogram of body weight to adjust for growth rate.

Metabolic Rate

Patients with a higher metabolic rate tend to metabolize drugs more rapidly, thus requiring either larger doses or more frequent administration. The converse is true for those with lower metabolic rates. Chronic smoking enhances the metabolism of some drugs (e.g., theophylline), thus requiring higher doses to be administered more often for a therapeutic effect.

Illness

Pathologic conditions may alter the rate of absorption, distribution, metabolism, and excretion. For example, patients in shock will have reduced peripheral vascular circulation and will absorb IM or SC injected drugs slowly; patients who are vomiting may not be able to retain a medication in the stomach long enough for dissolution and absorption; patients with diseases such as nephrotic syndrome or malnutrition may have reduced amounts of serum proteins in the blood necessary for adequate distribution of drugs; patients with kidney failure must have significant reductions in the dosages of those medications that are excreted by the kidneys.

Psychologic Aspects

Attitudes and expectations play a major role in a patient's response to therapy and the willingness to take medication as prescribed. Patients with diseases that have relatively rapid consequences if therapy is ignored, such as insulin-dependent diabetes, usually have a good rate of compliance. Patients with "silent" illnesses, such as hypertension, tend to be much less compliant with the treatment regimen.

Another psychologic consideration is the "placebo effect." A **placebo** is a drug dosage form, such as a tablet or capsule, that has no pharmacologic activity because it contains no active ingredients. When taken, the patient may report a therapeutic response. This response can be beneficial in patients being treated for illnesses such as anxiety, because the patient tends to take fewer potentially habit-forming drugs.

Tolerance

Tolerance occurs when a person begins to require higher doses to produce the same effects that lower doses once provided. An example is the person addicted to heroin. After a few weeks of use, larger doses will be required to provide the same "high." Tolerance can be caused by psychologic dependence, or the body may metabolize a particular drug more rapidly than before, causing the effects of the drug to diminish more rapidly.

Dependence

Drug dependence, also known as "addiction" or "habituation," occurs when a person is unable to control the ingestion of drugs. The dependence may be physical (in which the person develops withdrawal symptoms if the drug is withdrawn for a certain period of time) or psychologic (in which the patient is emotionally attached to the drug). Drug dependence occurs most commonly with the use of the schedule, or controlled, medications listed in Chapter 1, such as opiates and barbiturates.

Cumulative Effect

A drug may accumulate in the body if the next doses are administered before previously administered doses have been metabolized or excreted. Excessive **drug accumulation** may result in drug toxicity. An example of drug accumulation is the excessive ingestion of alcoholic beverages. A person becomes "drunk" or "inebriated" when the rate of consumption exceeds the rate of metabolism and excretion of the alcohol.

DRUG INTERACTIONS

Objectives

1. State the mechanism by which drug interactions may occur.

2. Differentiate among the following terms used in relationship to medications: additive effect, synergistic effect, antagonistic effect, displacement, interference, and incompatibility.

Key Words

drug interaction	antagonistic effect
unbound drug	displacement
additive effect	interference
synergistic effect	incompatibility

A **drug interaction** is said to occur when the action of one drug is altered by the action of another drug. Drug interactions are cited in two ways: (1) those agents that when combined *increase* the actions of one or both drugs; and (2) those agents that when combined *decrease* the effectiveness of one or both of the drugs. Some drug interactions are beneficial, such as the use of caffeine, a central nervous system (CNS) stimulant, with an antihistamine, a CNS depressant. The stimulatory effects of the caffeine counteract the drowsiness caused by the antihistamine without eliminating the antihistaminic effects.

The mechanisms of drug interactions can be categorized as altering the absorption, distribution, metabolism, and excretion of a drug or enhancing the pharmacology of a drug. Most drug interactions that alter absorption occur in the GI tract, usually the stomach. Examples of this type of interaction include the following:
- Antacids inhibit the dissolution of ketoconazole tablets by increasing the gastric pH. The interaction is managed by administration of antacids at least 2 hours after ketoconazole administration.
- Aluminum-containing antacids inhibit the absorption of tetracycline. Aluminum salts form an insoluble chemical complex with tetracycline. The interaction is managed by separating the administration of tetracycline and antacids by 3 to 4 hours.

Drug interactions that cause an alteration in distribution usually affect the binding of a drug to an inactive site, such as circulating plasma albumin or muscle protein. Once a drug is absorbed into the blood, it is usually transported throughout the body bound to plasma proteins. It will often bind to other proteins such as those of muscle. A drug that is highly bound (that is, >90% bound) to a protein-binding site may be displaced by another drug that has a higher affinity for the binding site. Very significant interactions can occur this way because very little displacement is required to produce a significant impact. Remember that only **unbound drug** is pharmacologically active. If a drug is 90% bound to a protein, 10% of the drug is providing the pharmacologic effect. If another drug with a stronger affinity for the protein-binding site displaces just 5% of the bound drug, there is now 15% unbound for pharmacologic activity. This is the equivalent of a 50% increase in dose, from 10% to 15% active drug. For example, the anticoagulant action of warfarin is increased by administration with furosemide and ethacrynic acid. These loop diuretics displace warfarin from albumin-binding sites, increasing the free fraction of anticoagulant. This interaction is managed by lowering the warfarin dose.

The most common ways in which drug interactions result from an alteration in metabolism are either inhibition or induction (stimulation) of enzymes responsible for metabolism of a drug. Medicines known to bind to enzymes and slow the metabolism of other drugs are verapamil, chloramphenicol, ketoconazole, amiodarone, cimetidine, and erythromycin. Serum levels usually increase as a result of inhibited metabolism, and dosages usually must be reduced to prevent toxicity. An example is that of erythromycin inhibiting the metabolism of theophylline. The dose of theophylline must be reduced based upon theophylline serum levels and signs of toxicity. Because erythomycin (an antibiotic) is usually administered only in short courses, the theophylline dose will probably have to be increased again after erythromycin is discontinued.

Common enzyme inducers are phenobarbital, carbamazepine, rifampin, and phenytoin. Examples of drugs whose metabolism is stimulated are disopyramide, doxycycline, griseofulvin, warfarin, metronidazole, mexiletine, quinidine, theophylline, and verapamil. When administered with enzyme inducers, the dosage of the more rapidly metabolized drug must usually be increased to provide therapeutic activity. It is crucial that the patient be monitored closely for adverse effects, especially if the enzyme inducer is discontinued. The metabolism of the induced drug will decelerate, leading to accumulation and toxicity if the dosage is not reduced. An example of this type of interaction is that of a woman receiving oral contraceptives (e.g., Ortho-Novum, Lo/Ovral) who requires a course of rifampin antimicrobial therapy. Rifampin induces enzymes that metabolize both the progestational and estrogenic components of the contraceptives, causing an increased incidence of menstrual abnormalities and reduced effectiveness of conception control. This interaction is managed by advising the patient to use an additional form of contraception while receiving rifampin therapy.

Drugs that interact by altering excretion usually act in the kidney tubules by altering the pH to enhance or inhibit excretion. The classic example of altered urine pH is with acetazolamide, a drug that elevates urine pH, and quinidine. The alkaline urine produced by acetazolamide causes quinidine to be reabsorbed in the renal tubules, potentially increasing the pharmacologic and toxic effects of quinidine. Frequent monitoring of quinidine serum levels and toxicity is used as a guide for reducing quinidine dosages.

The last major mechanisms of drug interactions enhance the pharmacologic effect of a drug. Examples of enhanced pharmacologic effect are those that cause CNS potentiation of neuromuscular blockage between an aminoglycoside antibiotic and a neuromuscular blocking agent such as tubocurarine.

The following terminology is used in describing drug interactions:

Additive effect: Two drugs, with similar actions, are taken for a doubled effect.

EXAMPLE: Propoxyphene + aspirin = added analgesic effect

Synergistic effect: The combined effect of two drugs is greater than the sum of the effect of each drug given alone.

EXAMPLE: Aspirin + codeine = much greater analgesic effect

Antagonistic effect: One drug interferes with the action of another.

EXAMPLE: Tetracycline + antacid = decreased absorption of the tetracycline

Displacement: The displacement of a drug by a second drug increases the activity of the first drug.

EXAMPLE: Warfarin + aspirin = increased anticoagulant effect

Interference: One drug inhibits the metabolism or excretion of a second drug, causing increased activity of the second drug.

EXAMPLE: Probenecid + spectinomycin = prolonged antibacterial activity from spectinomycin caused by blocking renal excretion by probenecid

Incompatibility: One drug is chemically incompatible with another drug (causing deterioration) when the two drugs are mixed in the same syringe or solution; incompatible drugs should not be mixed together or administered together at the same site. Signs of incompatibility are haziness, a precipitate, or a change in color of the solution when drugs are mixed.

EXAMPLE: Ampicillin + gentamicin = ampicillin inactivates gentamicin

The side effects of medicines are perhaps better tolerated by younger persons than elderly persons. Dizziness in the elderly may cause a decrease in activity because of fear of falling; a dry mouth can initiate poor tolerance of dentures, along with alterations in taste and chewing, thus reducing nutritional intake. Even a minor, subtle alteration in mental or behavioral functioning deserves to be investigated for the possibility of a drug-induced change before any additional medicines are prescribed for the symptomatology. Drug-induced side effects are frequently mistaken for disease symptoms. Many medicines (for example, reserpine, beta blockers, antiparkinsonian drugs, and corticosteroids) cause depression. Confusion may be the first and only symptom of a drug accumulation. Because confusion and delirium are frequently observed in the elderly population (for example, in the nursing home), what actually may be a drug-induced symptom is often treated with another agent.

Because it is impossible to memorize all of the possible drug interactions, it is the nurse's responsibility to check for drug interactions when suspected. It requires taking the time to consult drug resource books and pharmacists to ensure that patients receiving multiple medications do not suffer from unplanned drug interactions.

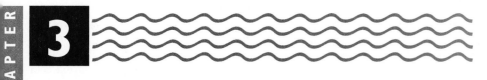

CHAPTER 3

Drug Action Across the Life Span

CHAPTER CONTENT

Objectives

1. Discuss the effects of age on drug action.
2. Cite major factors associated with drug absorption, distribution, metabolism, and excretion in the young and the older aged populations.

Key Words

passive diffusion	metabolism
hydrolysis	metabolites
intestinal transit	polypharmacy
protein binding	

CHANGING DRUG ACTION ACROSS THE LIFE SPAN

Age of the patient and impact on drug therapy can be significant. When discussing the effect of age and drug therapy, it is helpful to divide the population into the following categories:

Age		Title
<38	weeks	Premature
0-1	month	Newborn, neonate
1-24	months	Infant, baby
1-5	years	Young child
6-12	years	Older child
13-18	years	Adolescent
19-54	years	Adult
55-64	years	Older adult

Age		Title	
65-74	years	Elderly	Geriatric population
75-84	years	Aged	
85+	years	Very old	

As described in Chapter 2, drug action depends on four factors: absorption, distribution, metabolism, and excretion (ADME). Each of these factors varies depending on age.

Drug Absorption

Before a medicine can be absorbed, it must first be administered. Both pediatric and geriatric patients require special considerations for medication administration. Medicines administered by the intramuscular route are usually erratically absorbed in both neonatal and geriatric populations. Differences in muscle mass, blood flow to muscles, and muscular inactivity in bedridden patients make absorption unpredictable.

Topical administration with percutaneous absorption is usually effective in infants because the outer layer of skin (stratum corneum) is not fully developed and the skin is more fully hydrated at this age, causing water-soluble drugs to be absorbed more readily. Infants wearing plastic-coated diapers are also more susceptible to skin absorption because the plastic forms the equivalent of an occlusive dressing that increases hydration of the skin. Inflammation (for example, diaper rash) also increases the amount of drug absorbed. Transdermal administration in geriatric patients is difficult to predict. Although there is a decrease in dermal thickness with aging that may enhance absorption, conversely, there is drying, wrinkling, and a decrease in hair follicles that may diminish absorption. With aging, there is decreased cardiac output and diminishing tissue perfusion that may also affect transdermal drug absorption.

In most cases, medicines are administered orally. However, tablet and capsule dosage forms are often too large for either pediatric or geriatric populations to swallow. It is frequently necessary to crush a tablet for administration with food or use a liquid formulation for easier administration. Taste also becomes a factor when administering oral liquids, because the liquid comes in contact with the taste buds. Sustained-release tablets (p. 82), enteric-coated tablets (p. 82), and sublingual tablets (p. 142) should not be crushed because of changes in the absorption rate and the potential for toxicity. Infants and older adults often do not have a sufficient amount of teeth for chewable medicines. Geriatric patients frequently have a reduced salivary flow, making chewing and swallowing more difficult.

Two major factors affecting drug absorption from the gastrointestinal (GI) tract are **passive diffusion** and gastric emptying time. Both are dependent upon the pH of the environment. Newborn infants and geriatric patients have altered gastric acidity and transit time compared with adults. Premature infants have a high gastric pH (6 to 8) because of immature acid-secreting cells in the stomach. In a full-term newborn, the gastric pH is also 6 to 8, but within 24 hours it decreases to 2 to 4 because of gastric acid secretion. Infants are approximately 1 year of age before the stomach pH approximates that of adults (1 to 3). Geriatric patients frequently have a higher gastric pH because of loss of acid-secreting cells. Drugs that are destroyed by gastric acid (for example, ampicillin, penicillin) are more readily absorbed and have higher serum concentrations because of the lack of acid destruction. In contrast, drugs that depend on an acidic environment for absorption (for example, phenobarbital, aspirin) are more poorly absorbed and have lower serum concentrations than those in patients with normal gastric acidity. Premature infants and geriatric patients also have a slower gastric emptying time, partly because of the lack of acid secretion. A slower gastric emptying time may allow the drug to stay in contact with the absorptive tissue longer, allowing more absorption with a higher serum concentration. There is also the potential for toxicity caused by more contact time in the stomach for potentially ulcerogenic drugs (for example, nonsteroidal antiinflammatory drugs).

Another factor affecting drug absorption in the newborn is the absence of enzymes needed for **hydrolysis.** Infants do not have the ability to hydrolyze palmitic acid from chloramphenicol palmitate, thus preventing absorption of the chloramphenicol. Oral phenytoin doses are also greater than one would expect for infants less than 6 months of age, caused by poor absorption (neonates— 15 to 20 mg/kg/24 hr versus infants; children—4 to 7 mg/kg/24 hr).

The **intestinal transit** rate also varies with age. As the neonate matures into infancy, the GI transit rate increases, causing some medicines to be poorly absorbed. Sustained-release capsules (for example, TheoDur Sprinkles) move through the intestines so rapidly that only approximately 50% of a dose is absorbed in infants compared with children more than 5 years of age. The elderly develop decreased GI motility and intestinal blood flow. This has the potential for altered absorption of medicines and either constipation or diarrhea, depending on the medicine.

Drug Distribution

Distribution refers to the ways in which drugs are transported by the circulating body fluids to the sites of action (receptors), metabolism, and excretion. Distribution is dependent upon pH, body water concentrations (intracellular, extracellular, and total body water), presence and quantity of fat tissue, protein binding, cardiac output, and regional blood flow.

Most medicines are transported either dissolved in the circulating water (in blood) of the body or bound to plasma proteins within the blood. Body water composition as a percentage of weight changes substantially with age (Table 3-1). Note that the total body water content of a preterm infant is 83%, whereas that of an adult man is 60%. The significance of this is that infants have a larger volume of distribution for water-soluble drugs and will require a higher dose on a milligram per kilogram basis than an older child or adult.

As we age, lean body mass and total body water decrease, while total fat content increases. Preterm infants may have body weight composed of only 1% to 2% fat, while a full-term newborn may have 15% fat. Adults increase from 18% up to 36% fat content for men and 33% to 48% for women between ages 18 and 35. Drugs that are highly fat soluble (for example, antidepressants, phenothiazines, benzodiazepines, calcium channel blockers) require a longer onset of action and accumulate in fat tissues, prolonging their action and potential toxicity. Highly fat-soluble medicines (for example, diazepam) must be given in smaller milligram per kilogram doses for infants with low birth weight because there is less fat tissue to bind the drug, leaving more drug to be active at receptor sites.

Drugs that are relatively insoluble are transported in the circulation by binding to plasma proteins, especially albumin. **Protein binding** is reduced in preterm infants because of decreased plasma protein concentrations, lower binding capacity of protein, and decreased affinity of proteins for drug binding. Drugs known to have lower protein binding in neonates compared with an adult are phenobarbital, phenytoin, theophylline, propranolol, lidocaine, penicillin, and chloramphenicol. Because serum protein binding is diminished, the drugs are distributed over a wider area of the body and a larger loading dose is required than that in older children to achieve therapeutic serum concentrations. There may also be competition for binding sites from several drugs

Table 3-1

Percentages of Body Water*			
AGE (WEIGHT)	**EXTRACELLULAR WATER (%)**	**INTRACELLULAR WATER (%)**	**TOTAL BODY WATER (%)**
Premature infant (1.5 kg)	60	40	83
Full-term infant (3.5 kg)	56	44	74
5-month-old (7 kg)	50	50	60
1-year-old (10 kg)	40	60	59
Male adult	40	60	60

*Developmental changes from birth to adulthood. The extracellular and intracellular water are expressed as a percentage of total body weight. (Data from Friis-Hansen B: Body composition during growth, *Pediatrics* 47:264, 1971.)

used to treat neonatal conditions. Sulfisoxazole is well known for displacing bilirubin from protein-binding sites, which allows the bilirubin to accumulate and pass into the brain, causing kernicterus.

In adults more than 40 years of age, the composition of body proteins begins to change. Whereas the total body protein concentration is unaffected, albumin concentrations gradually decrease and other proteins (for example, the globulins) increase. As albumin levels diminish, there is an increase in unbound, active drug. Increased levels of naproxen, diflunisal, salicylate, and valproate have been found in the elderly, presumably as a result of decreased albumin levels. Disease states such as cirrhosis, renal failure, and malnutrition can lower albumin levels. Initial dosages of highly protein-bound drugs (for example, warfarin, phenytoin, tolbutamide, propranolol, digitoxin, diazepam) should be reduced and increased slowly if there is evidence of decreased serum albumin.

Drug Metabolism

Metabolism is the process by which the body inactivates medicines. Enzyme systems, primarily in the liver, are the major pathway of drug metabolism. All enzyme systems are present at birth but mature at different rates, taking several weeks to a year to fully develop. Monitoring of serum concentrations to ensure therapeutic levels is more common (for example, aminoglycosides, phenytoin, theophylline) in the first few weeks after birth because medicines are more rapidly metabolized as the enzyme systems mature. Dosages and frequency of administration or both must often be increased to help maintain therapeutic serum concentrations.

Liver weight, the number of functioning hepatic cells, and hepatic blood flow decrease with increasing age. This results in a slower metabolism of drugs in the elderly. This can be seriously aggravated by the presence of liver disease or heart failure. Drugs that are extensively metabolized by the liver (for example, morphine, lidocaine, propranolol) can have substantially prolonged duration of action if hepatic blood flow is reduced. Dosages usually must be reduced or the time interval between doses extended to prevent accumulation of active medicine and potential toxicity. Drug metabolism can also be affected at all ages by genetics, smoking, diet, gender, other medicines, and disease. Unfortunately, there are no specific laboratory tests, like renal function tests, to directly measure liver function to adjust dosages of medicines.

Drug Excretion

Metabolites of drugs and, in some cases, the active drug itself are eventually excreted from the body. The primary routes are through the renal tubules into the urine and the GI tract to the feces. Other generally minor routes of excretion include evaporation through the skin, exhalation from the lungs, and secretion into the saliva and mother's milk.

At birth, a preterm infant has up to 15% of the renal capacity of an adult, while a full-term newborn has approximately 35%. The filtration capacity of an infant increases to approximately 50% at 4 weeks of age and is equivalent to adult function at 9 to 12 months. As previously discussed

with maturation of enzyme systems, drugs that are excreted primarily by the kidneys (penicillin, gentamicin, tobramycin) must be administered in larger dosages or more frequently to maintain adequate therapeutic serum concentrations as renal function matures. As already stated, serum drug concentrations must be monitored regularly.

With the passage of time, important physiologic changes that take place in the kidneys include decreased renal blood flow caused by atherosclerosis and reduced cardiac output, loss of glomeruli, and decreased tubular function and concentrating ability. There is, however, a great degree of individual variation in changes in renal function, and no prediction of renal function can be made only on the basis of a person's age. Renal function of elderly patients should be, at a minimum, estimated using mathematic equations that factor in the patient's age. More optimally, it should be measured by collecting urine creatinine specimens over time. Serum creatinine can give a general estimate of renal function, but in elderly patients these methods tend to overestimate actual functional capability. This happens because the production of creatinine is dependent upon muscle mass that is diminished in the elderly. Significant elevations occur only when there has been major deterioration of renal function. Blood urea nitrogen (BUN) concentration is also a poor predictor of renal function because it is significantly altered by diet, status of hydration, and blood loss either externally or into the GI tract.

MONITORING DRUG THERAPY

Whereas many of the same monitoring parameters (for example, vital signs, urine output, renal function tests) are used to plan dosages and monitor the effects of drug therapy in all ages of patients, it is absolutely crucial that the normal values for these monitoring parameters and laboratory tests be used for the age of the patient being monitored. For example, neonates have a greater respiratory and heart rate and lower normal blood pressure than adults. It is also important that measuring devices be appropriate for the individual patient (for example, appropriately sized blood pressure cuff).

Infants are not smaller versions of adults, and we cannot extrapolate the principles of drug therapy to infants only on the basis of size. Dosages must be adjusted to age, weight, and liver and kidney function. Measuring serum concentrations of medicines is particularly important in those drugs with potentially serious adverse effects. Usually, if a pediatric dosage is not readily available in reference texts, it may not be appropriate for pediatric use.

Geriatric patients represent an ever-increasing portion of the population. It is important that health care professionals understand the physiologic and pathologic changes that develop with advancing age and adjust drug therapy for the individual patient. Factors that place the elderly patient at greater risk for drug interactions or drug toxicity are reduced renal and hepatic function, chronic illnesses that require multiple drug therapy (**polypharmacy**), and a greater likelihood of malnourishment. All of these factors lead to accumulation of active drugs with the potential for serious adverse effects in these patients.

The Nursing Process and Pharmacology

THE NURSING PROCESS

Objectives

1. Identify the purpose for using the nursing process methodology.
2. State the five steps in the nursing process and describe these steps in terms of a problem-solving method used in nursing practice.

Key Word

nursing process

The practice of nursing is an art and science that uses a systematic approach to identify and solve the potential problems individuals may experience as they strive to maintain basic human function along the wellness-illness continuum. The focus of all nursing care is to help individuals maximize their potential for maintaining the highest possible level of independence in meeting self-care needs. Conceptual frameworks of the basis of nursing practice such as Henderson's Complementary-Supplement Model (1980), Roger's Life Process Theory (1979, 1980), Roy's Adaptation Model (1976), and the Canadian Nurses' Association Testing Service (1980) are examples of models used today.

The **nursing process** is the foundation for the clinical practice of nursing. It provides the framework for consistent nursing actions, using a problem-solving approach rather than an intuitional approach. It provides a systematic method of working with patients to identify actual and potential patient problems, particularly those related to drug therapy, and helps determine what actions must be taken to correct the problems. When implemented properly, it also provides a method to evaluate the outcomes of the therapy delivered. In addition to quality of care, the nursing process provides a scientific, transferable method for health care planners to assign nursing staff to patients and to determine and justify the cost of providing nursing care in this age of soaring health care expense. As computerization of patient care records increases, the ability to retrieve data based on nursing diagnosis statements and to analyze the nursing care delivered will become easier. Accountability for nursing care and for developing new methodologies will also be enhanced by the use of this technology.

Many nursing education programs and health care facilities use a five-step model that includes assessment, nursing diagnosis, planning, implementation, and evaluation. Other programs prefer a four-step model, in which analysis of data (nursing diagnosis in the five-step model) is the final part of the assessment phase, followed by the planning, intervention, and evaluation phases (Table 4-1). The five-step model is used here for purposes of discussion. Regardless of the model used, it is not the number of steps but the quality of nursing care provided and documented by the process that counts.

Nurses should examine the nurses' practice act in the state in which they practice to identify the educational and experiential qualifications necessary to perform physical assessment and develop nursing diagnoses. Formulation of nursing diagnoses requires a broad knowledge base from which to make discriminating judgments needed to identify the individual patient's care needs. All members of the health care team must contribute data regarding the patient's care needs and response to the prescribed treatment regimen.

Just as bodily functions are constantly undergoing adjustments to maintain homeostasis in the internal and external environment, the nursing process is an ongoing, cyclic process that must respond to the changing requirements of the patient. The nurse must continually interact with people in a variety of settings to creatively and cooperatively establish and execute nursing functions to meet the holistic care needs of patients (Figure 4-1).

Assessment

Objectives

1. Describe the components of the assessment process.
2. Compare current methods used to collect, organize, and analyze information about the health care needs of patients and their significant others.

Key Word

assessment

Table 4-1

Principles of the Nursing Process

ASSESSMENT	PLANNING	INTERVENTION	EVALUATION
Collect all relevant data associated with the individual patient's diagnosis to detect actual, high-risk or possible problems needing intervention. Primary data sources Secondary data sources Tertiary data sources Based on the data collected, formulate a statement of the behaviors or problems of concern and the cause. This is referred to as an "actual" nursing diagnosis when the defining characteristics are present; as a "high-risk" nursing diagnosis when there is a likelihood of the diagnosis developing or being prevented; or a "possible" nursing diagnosis when more data are required to substantiate or refute the problem. A wellness nursing diagnosis is a one-part diagnosis statement used for persons desiring and capable of attaining a higher level of wellness who currently have an effective status. (Check hospital policy for the level of nursing required to perform this function.)	Prioritize the problems identified from the assessment data, with the most severe or life-threatening first. Other problems are arranged in descending order of importance. (Maslow's hierarchy is frequently used as a basis for prioritizing; other approaches may be equally valid.) Develop short- and long-term patient goals in measurable statements to describe the behavior to be observed. Identify the monitoring parameters to be used to detect possible complications of the disease process or treatments being used. Plan nursing approaches to correlate with each identified long-term goal. More than one short-term goal may be required to actually lead to the broader, more encompassing long-term goals.	Perform the nursing intervention planned to achieve the individualized short- and/or long-term goals. Monitor the patient's response to treatments, and monitor for complications related to existing pathophysiology. Provide for patient safety. Perform ongoing assessments on a continuum. Document care given and additional findings on the chart.	Evaluation is an ongoing process that occurs at every phase of the nursing process. Establish target data to review and analyze data. Review and analyze the data regarding the patient and modify the care plan so that goals of care (usually, returning the patient to the highest level of functioning) are attained. Unrealistic goals may require revision or discontinuation. Follow a systematic approach to recording progress, depending on the setting and charting methods used. Document goal attainment, partial attainment, or failure to achieve goals. Continue the nursing process, initiate referral to a community-based health agency, or execute discharge procedures as ordered by the physician

*Nursing Diagnosis: Because not all patient problems are amenable to resolution by nursing actions, those complications associated with medical diagnosis or from treatment-related complication are placed in a category known as *collaborative problems* that the nurse monitors. A wellness diagnosis is a one part diagnosis statement used for persons desiring and capable of attaining a high level of wellness who currently have an effective status. Check hospital policies for the level of nursing required to perform this function.

Assessment is an ongoing process that starts with the admission of the patient and is completed at the time of dismissal. It is the problem-identifying phase of the nursing process. The initial assessment must be performed by registered nurses who have the necessary assessment skills to perform the physical examination and the knowledge base to analyze the data assembled and identify patient problems based on defining characteristics (signs, symptoms, clinical evidence). In addition, the nurse should identify risk factors that cause an individual or group of persons to be more vulnerable to the development of certain problems in response to a disease process or to the prescribed therapeutic interventions when used (for example, side effects to drugs that may require modification of the regimen).

During the assessment phase, the nurse collects a comprehensive information base about the patient from the physical exam, the nursing history, the medication history, and professional observation. Formats commonly used for data collection, organization, and analysis are the "head-to-toe" assessment, "body systems" assessment, or Gordon's Functional Health Patterns Model. Both the "head-to-toe" and "body systems" approaches focus on physiology and thereby limit the nurse's knowledge of sociocultural, psychologic, spiritual, and developmental factors affecting the individual's needs. The box on p. 24 shows Gordon's Functional Health Patterns Model.

Nursing Diagnosis

Objectives

1. Define "nursing diagnosis" and discuss the wording used in formulating nursing diagnosis statements.
2. Define a "collaborative problem."

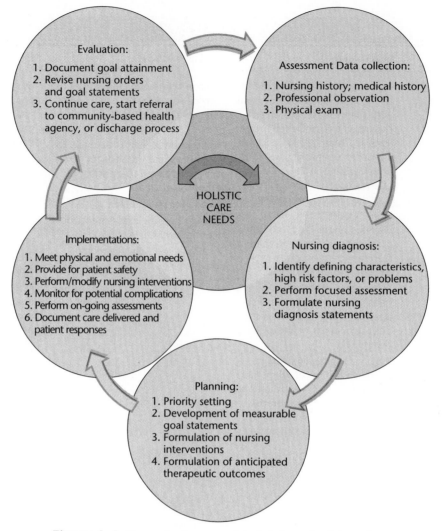

Figure 4-1 *The nursing process and the holistic needs of the patient.*

Gordon's Functional Health Patterns Model

1. Health Perception–Health Management Pattern
2. Nutrition-Metabolic Pattern
3. Elimination Pattern
4. Activity-Exercise Pattern
5. Sleep-Rest Pattern
6. Cognitive-Perceptual Pattern
7. Self-Perception–Self Concept Pattern
8. Role-Relationship Pattern
9. Sexuality-Reproductive Pattern
10. Coping–Stress Tolerance Pattern
11. Value-Belief Pattern

3. Differentiate between a "nursing diagnosis" and a "medical diagnosis."

4. Differentiate between problems that require formulation of a nursing diagnosis and those categorized as collaborative problems, which may not require nursing diagnosis statements.

Key Words

nursing diagnosis

actual nursing diagnosis

risk nursing diagnosis

wellness nursing diagnosis

defining characteristics

medical diagnosis

collaborative problem

focused assessment

Nursing diagnosis is the second phase of the five-step nursing process. The North American Nursing Diagnosis Association (NANDA) approved the following official definitions relating to nursing diagnosis.

Nursing diagnosis: A clinical judgment about individual, family, or community response to actual or potential health problems and life processes. Nursing diagnosis provides the basis for selection of nursing intervention to achieve outcomes for which the nurse is accountable (approved at the 9th NANDA conference, 1990).

Actual nursing diagnosis: Describe human responses to health conditions and life processes that exist in an individual, family, or community. It is supported by defining characteristics (manifestations or signs and symptoms) that cluster in patterns of related cues or inferences.

Risk nursing diagnosis: Describe human responses to health conditions and life processes that may develop in a vulnerable individual, family, or community. It is supported by risk factors that contribute to increased vulnerability.

Wellness nursing diagnosis: Describe human responses to levels of wellness in an individual, family, or community that have a potential for enhancement to a higher state.

Using the knowledge and skill (in anatomy, physiology, nutrition, psychology, pharmacology, microbiology, nursing practice skills, and communication techniques), the nurse analyzes the data collected to identify whether certain major and minor **defining characteristics** (signs, symptoms, and clinical evidence) that may be present relate to a particular patient problem. If so, the nurse may conclude that certain actual problems are present. These patient-related problems are referred to as "nursing diagnosis."

It should be noted that not all patient problems identified during an assessment are treated by the nurse alone. Many of the identified problems require a multidisciplinary approach. When the nurse cannot legally order the definitive interventions required under the circumstances, a collaborative problem exists (Figure 4-2).

As nursing care has gained recognition as a cognitive process in planning patient care, several national conferences have been held to identify the diagnostic terms that describe areas of potential health problems that nurses should anticipate and may treat. As of 1994, the NANDA has recognized the approved listing of nursing diagnoses that appears in the box on p. 26.

There is a difference between a medical diagnosis and a nursing diagnosis. A **medical diagnosis** is a statement of the patient's alterations in structure and function and results in a diagnosis of a disease or disorder that impairs normal physiologic function. A nursing diagnosis usually refers to the patient's ability to function in activities of daily living in relation to the impairment induced by the medical diagnosis; it identifies the individual's or group's response to the illness. A medical diagnosis also tends to remain unchanged throughout the illness, whereas nursing diagnoses may vary depending upon the patient's state of recovery. Concepts that help distinguish a nursing diagnosis from a medical diagnosis include the following:

- Conditions described by nursing diagnoses can be accurately identified by nursing assessment methods.
- Nursing treatments or methods of risk factor reduction can resolve the condition described by a nursing diagnosis.
- Because the necessary treatment to resolve nursing diagnoses are within the scope of nursing practice, nurses assume accountability for outcomes.
- Nursing assumes responsibility for the research required to clearly identify the defining characteristics and etiologic factors and to improve methods of treatment and treatment outcomes for conditions described by nursing diagnoses (Gordon, 1987, p. 15).

The wording of an "actual" nursing diagnosis takes the form of a three-part statement. These statements consist of the following: (1) a diagnostic label (from the NANDA-approved list), (2) the contributing factors (cause if known or stated as etiology unknown), and (3) the defining characteristics (signs and symptoms). As of January 1992, problems previously referred to as "potential" problems are referred to as "risk" nursing diagnoses.

The risk nursing diagnosis statement consists of the diagnostic label (from the NANDA-approved list) and the risk factors that make the individual or group more susceptible to the development of the problem. Validation of a risk diagnosis is the presence of the risk factors that would contribute to the individual or group developing the stated problem. "Possible" nursing diagnosis identifies a problem that may occur, but the assembled data are insufficient to confirm it.

A "wellness" nursing diagnosis statement has only a one-part label. It is initiated by "Potential for Enhanced" followed by the nursing diagnosis being applied to the situation or group. The individual or group must understand that the higher level of functioning is feasible. This can be applied only to individuals or groups when the capability for attainment of a higher level of wellness is realistic.

Further discussion of the philosophy and clinical use of nursing diagnoses; the specifics regarding the wording of "actual," "risk," and "possible" nursing diagnoses; and the new categories of "wellness" nursing diagnoses and "syndrome" nursing diagnoses can be found in other primary texts and reference works, especially those developed solely for the purpose of explaining nursing diagnosis.

Collaborative Problems

Not all patient problems identified by the nurse can be resolved by nursing actions. The nurse is, however, responsible

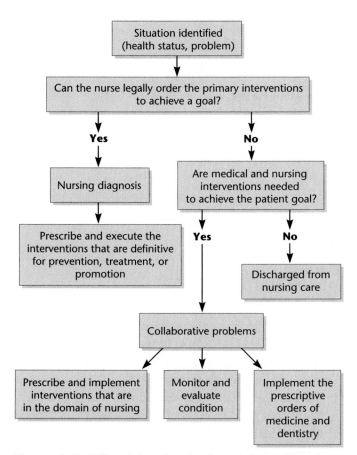

Figure 4-2 *Differentiation of nursing diagnosis from collaborative problems.* (From Carpenito LJ: *Nursing diagnosis application to clinical practice,* ed 6, Philadelphia, 1995, Lippincott.)

North American Nursing Diagnosis Association (NANDA) Accepted Nursing Diagnoses	
Activity Intolerance	Family Coping: Disabling, Ineffective
Activity Intolerance, Risk for	Family Coping: Potential for Growth
Adjustment, Impaired	Family Processes, Altered
Airway Clearance, Ineffective	Family Processes, Altered: Alcoholism
Anxiety	Fatigue
Aspiration, Risk for	Fear
Body Image Disturbance	Fluid Volume Deficit
Body Temperature, Risk for Altered	Fluid Volume Deficit, Risk for
Breastfeeding, Effective	Fluid Volume Excess
Breastfeeding, Ineffective	Gas Exchange, Impaired
Breastfeeding, Interrupted	Grieving, Anticipatory
Breathing Pattern, Ineffective	Grieving, Dysfunctional
Cardiac Output, Decreased	Growth and Development, Altered
Caregiver Role Strain	Health Maintenance, Altered
Caregiver Role Strain, Risk for	Health-Seeking Behaviors (Specify)
Communication, Impaired Verbal	Home Maintenance Management, Impaired
Confusion, Acute	Hopelessness
Confusion, Chronic	Hyperthermia
Constipation	Hypothermia
Constipation, Colonic	Incontinence, Bowel
Constipation, Perceived	Incontinence, Functional
Coping, Defensive	Incontinence, Reflex
Coping, Ineffective Community	Incontinence, Stress
Coping, Ineffective Individual	Incontinence, Total
Decisional Conflict (Specify)	Incontinence, Urge
Decreased Adaptive Capacity: Intracranial	Infant Behavior, Disorganized
Denial, Ineffective	Infant Behavior, Risk for Disorganized
Diarrhea	Infant Behavior, Potential for Enhanced
Disuse Syndrome, Risk for	Organized
Diversional Activity Deficit	Infant Feeding Pattern, Ineffective
Dysreflexia	Infection, Risk for
Energy Field Disturbance	Infection Transmission, Risk for
Enhanced Community Coping, Potential for	Injury, Risk for
Environmental Interpretation Syndrome,	Injury, Risk for Perioperative Positioning
Impaired	Knowledge Deficit (Specify)
Family Coping: Compromised, Ineffective	Loneliness, Risk for

continued

for *monitoring* the patient on a continuum for potential complications that are associated with the medical diagnosis, diagnostic procedures, or treatments prescribed. To differentiate between a problem requiring a nursing diagnosis and a **collaborative problem,** the nurse must judge whether the definitive interventions can be ordered to prevent or treat the problem to maintain the health status of the patient (Carpenito, 1985, 1987, 1990, 1995). See Figure 4-2 for an illustration of this decision-making process.

Focused Assessment

A **focused assessment** is the process of collecting additional data specific to a patient or family that would validate a suggested problem or nursing diagnosis. The questions asked or data collected would be used to confirm or rule out the defining characteristics associated with a specific nursing diagnosis statement.

Planning

Objectives

1. Identify the steps included in the planning of nursing care.

2. Explain the process of prioritizing individual patient needs using Maslow's hierarchy of needs.

3. Formulate measurable goal statements for a patient for whom you are actively caring in the clinical practice setting.

4. State the behavioral responses around which goal statements revolve when the discharge of a patient is planned.

5. Identify the purposes and uses of a "patient care plan."

6. Differentiate between nursing interventions and therapeutic outcomes.

North American Nursing Diagnosis Association Accepted Nursing Diagnoses—cont'd

Memory, Impaired
Noncompliance (Specify)
Nutrition, Altered: Less Than Body Requirements
Nutrition, Altered: More Than Body
　Requirements
Nutrition, Altered: Potential for More Than Body
　Requirements
Oral Mucous Membrane, Altered
Pain, Acute
Pain, Chronic
Parent-Infant Attachment, Risk for Altered
Parental Role Conflict
Parenting, Altered
Parenting, Risk for Altered
Peripheral Neurovascular Dysfunction, Risk for
Personal Identity Disturbance
Physical Mobility, Impaired
Poisoning, Risk for
Post-Trauma Response
Powerlessness
Protection, Altered
Rape Trauma Syndrome
Rape Trauma Syndrome: Compound Reaction
Rape Trauma Syndrome: Silent Reaction
Relocation Stress Syndrome
Role Performance, Altered
Self-Care Deficit
　Bathing/Hygiene
　Feeding
　Dressing/Grooming
　Toileting
Self-Esteem, Chronic Low
Self-Esteem, Situational Low
Self-Esteem Disturbance
Self-Mutilation, Risk for

Sensory/Perceptual Alterations (Specify) (visual,
　auditory, kinesthetic, gustatory, tactile, olfactory)
Sexual Dysfunction
Sexuality Patterns, Altered
Skin Integrity, Risk for Impaired
Skin Integrity, Impaired
Sleep Pattern Disturbance
Social Interactions, Impaired
Social Isolation
Spiritual Distress
Spiritual Well-Being, Potential for Enhanced
Suffocation, Risk for
Swallowing, Impaired
Therapeutic Regimen, Effective Management of:
　Individual
Therapeutic Regimen, Ineffective Management of
Therapeutic Regimen, Ineffective Management
　of: Community
Therapeutic Regimen, Ineffective Management
　of: Family
Thermoregulation, Ineffective
Thought Processes, Altered
Tissue Integrity, Impaired
Tissue Perfusion, Altered (Specify Type) (renal,
　cerebral, cardiopulmonary, gastrointestinal, pe-
　ripheral)
Trauma, Risk for
Unilateral Neglect
Urinary Elimination, Altered
Urinary Retention
Ventilation, Inability to Sustain Spontaneous
Ventilatory Weaning Response, Dysfunctional
Violence, Risk for: Self-Directed or Directed at
　Others

Key Words

priority setting
measurable goal
　statements
nursing actions
nursing interventions
nursing orders
anticipated therapeutic
　outcomes

Once the patient has been assessed and problems have been diagnosed, plans should be formulated to meet the patient's needs. Planning usually encompasses four phases: (1) priority setting, (2) development of measurable goal statements, (3) formulation of nursing interventions, and (4) formulation of anticipated therapeutic outcomes that can be used to evaluate the patient's status. The written document that evolves from this planning process is called the *nursing care plan*. When completed, it is placed in the patient's Kardex or chart, where it serves as a communication system for all health care providers. Because care needs are constantly changing, the care plan and priorities also must be evaluated and modified on a continuing basis to meet the patient's needs.

Priority Setting

After the nursing diagnoses and collaborative problems have been identified, they must be prioritized. The box below shows Maslow's hierarchy of needs, which is a model frequently used to establish priorities. Using Maslow's hierarchy to perform **priority setting** of an individual's needs focuses on organizing the needs in relation to their direct effect on the maintenance of homeostasis. Usually, physiologic needs such as oxygenation, temperature maintenance, or nutritional and fluid requirements would take precedence over psychologic needs. The box on p. 28 lists the priority ranking of Maslow's subcategories of human needs.

Maslow's Hierarchy of Needs

High	Self-Actualization Needs
	Esteem Needs
	Social Needs
	Safety Needs
Low	Physiologic Needs

Priority Ranking of Maslow's Subcategories of Human Needs

Physiologic needs
Oxygen, circulation
Water-salt balance
Food balance
Acid-base balance
Waste elimination
Normal temperature
Sleep, rest, relaxation
Activity, exercise
Energy
Comfort
Stimulation
Cleanliness
Sexuality

Safety needs
Protection from physical harm
Protection from psychologic threat
Freedom from pain
Stability
Dependence
Predictable, orderly world

Belonging needs
Love and affection
Acceptance
Warm, communicating relationship
Approval from others
Unity with loved ones
Group companionship

Self-esteem needs
Recognition
Dignity
Appreciation from others
Importance, influence
Reputation of good character
Attention
Status
Dominance over others

Self-actualization needs
Personal growth and maturity
Awareness of potential
Increased learning
Full development of potential
Improved values
Religious, philosophic satisfaction
Increased creativity
Increased reality perception and problem-solving abilities
Less rigid conventionality
Less of the familiar, more of the novel
Greater satisfaction in beauty
Increased pleasantness
Less of the simple, more of the complex

From Campbell C: *Nursing diagnosis and intervention in nursing practice*, New York, 1978, John Wiley & Sons.

Measurable Goal Statements

After priorities of needs have been set, goals must be established and statements written. Goals are usually divided into short-term and long-term plans. The **measurable goal statements** start with an action word (verb), followed by the behavior(s) to be performed by the patient or family with a specific time allocated for attainment.

All goal statements must be individualized and based on the patient's abilities. Statements must also take into consideration the degree of rehabilitation that is realistic for the person. It is sometimes difficult to accept that not everyone can return to their preillness health status; therefore the nurse must be realistic in setting a measurable goal and strive to assist the individual to an optimal degree of functioning consistent with personal capabilities.

When goals are being established, it is important to include the patient and appropriate significant others in decision making because the patient and the support persons will be responsible for the accomplishment of the goals. Involvement of the patient is essential to promote cooperation and compliance with the therapeutic regimen and a sense of control over the disease process and course of treatment. The goals established should be *patient goals,* not nursing goals for the patient.

With the advent of shorter hospital stays, most of the goal statements will be short-term goals. The nurse must keep in mind the usual length of hospitalization and be realistic about the number and types of goals being established. Short-term goals should serve as a bridge to meet the long-term goals established in a care plan. Long-term goals can be established with assistance from referral agencies as appropriate to the individual's needs and circumstances. The long-term goals are then implemented in long-term care settings, rehabilitation centers, mental health facilities, and community-based and home health care delivery settings.

The planning process may be scheduled with all significant persons present at one or more meetings. It is important to establish an openness that conveys a willingness to consider each person's input into the final plan. The strengths and weaknesses of each participant in the final care plan must be analyzed, and the goal statements must be realistically achievable for the group. Most goal statements are based on the patient's need to do the following:

• Reduce or resolve the symptoms (usually the chief complaint) of the disease that caused the person to seek medical attention
• Understand the disease process and its effect on lifestyle and activities of daily living
• Gain knowledge and skills associated with the treatment procedures in order to attain the highest level of function possible (nutrition, comfort measures, medication regimen, physical therapy)
• Understand reasonable expectations of the therapy, including signs and symptoms of improvement versus complications requiring physician consultation
• Identify monitoring parameters that should be maintained on a written record that reflects the response to the prescribed therapy
• Establish a schedule for follow-up evaluation

The beginning practitioner should consult a text on nursing diagnosis for further information on the correct wording of measurable goal statements associated with nursing diagnosis and collaborative problems.

Nursing Actions or Nursing Interventions

Nursing action or **intervention** statements list in a concise form exactly what the nurse will do to achieve each goal developed for each nursing diagnosis. A nursing action is a statement that describes nursing interventions applicable to any patient (for example, "promote adequate respiratory ventilation"). **Nursing orders** describe how specific actions will be implemented for an individual patient.

EXAMPLE:

(date): Cough, turn, deep breath: 0800, 1000, 1200, 1600, 1800, 2000, 2200.

(date): Educate patient re: abdominal breathing, splinting the abdomen and pursed-lip breathing, assuming correct position to facilitate breathing.

(date): Auscultate breath sounds: 0800, 1200, 1600, 2000.

(date): Increase fluid intake to at least 2000 ml/24 hr:
           0700-1500: 1000 ml.
           1500-2300: 800 ml.
           2300-0700: 200 ml.

(date): Assess respiratory depth and rate at 0800, 1200, 1600, 2000, 2400.

Anticipated Therapeutic and Expected Outcome Statements

Measurable **anticipated therapeutic** and expected **outcome statements** are also developed to document the effectiveness of the care delivered. In the previous example, the patient will do the following:
- Improve in the ability to perform coughing technique.
- Maintain adequate fluid intake as evidenced by achieving a mutually set goal of 2000 ml within 24 hours.
- Attain a respiratory rate between 18 and 24 per minute.
- Perform activities of daily living without feeling fatigued.

Therapeutic and expected outcomes have been developed throughout this book for each drug classification. These can be used by the student to identify the outcomes anticipated from the use of the drugs listed in a particular classification.

EXAMPLE: The primary therapeutic outcome expected from the benzodiazepine antianxiety agents is a decrease in the level of anxiety to a manageable level (for example, coping is improved, physical signs of anxiety such as look of anxiety, tremor, and pacing are reduced).

Nursing Intervention or Implementation

Objective

1. Compare the types of nursing functions classified as dependent, interdependent, and independent, and give examples of each.

Key Words

nursing interventions and implementation
dependent actions

interdependent actions
independent actions

Nursing intervention or **implementation** is the actual process of carrying out the established plan of care. Nursing care is directed at meeting the physical and emotional needs of the patient, providing patient safety, monitoring for potential complications, and performing ongoing assessments as a part of the continual process of data collection and evaluation to identify changes in the patient's care needs. Nursing actions are suggested by the etiologies of the problems identified in the nursing diagnoses and are used to implement plans. They may include activities such as counseling, teaching, providing comfort measures, coordinating, referring, using communication skills, and performing a physician's orders. Documentation of all care given, including patient education and the patient's apparent response, should be done regularly both to assist in evaluation and reassessment and to make other health care professionals aware of the patient's changing needs.

Nursing Actions

Within the nursing process, there are three types of nursing actions: (1) dependent, (2) interdependent, and (3) independent. **Dependent actions** are those performed by the nurse based on the physician's orders (such as the administration of prescribed medications and treatments). It is important to note that, although this is a dependent function, the nurse is still responsible for exercising professional judgment in performing the orders. **Interdependent actions** are nursing actions that the nurse implements cooperatively with other members of the health care team for restoration or promotion of health maintenance. This allows nurses to coordinate the interventions with those of other health care professionals to maximize knowledge and skills from various disciplines for the well-being of the patient. **Independent actions** are nursing actions not prescribed by a physician that a nurse can provide by virtue of the education and licensure attained. These actions are usually written in the nursing care plan and originate from the nursing diagnosis.

Evaluating and Recording Therapeutic and Expected Outcomes

Objective

1. Describe the evaluatory process used to establish whether patient behaviors are consistent with the identified short-term or long-term goals.

The final step of the nursing process is evaluation of the expected outcomes of the patient's behavior. All care is evaluated against the established nursing diagnoses (goal statements), planned nursing actions, and anticipated therapeutic outcomes. In order for the evaluation process to be successful, the participants (patient, family, nurse) must be willing to receive the feedback. Therefore plans for evaluation must involve the patient and family from the beginning.

Although the evaluation phase is the last step in the nursing process, it is not an end in itself. Evaluation recognizes successful completion of previously established goals, but it also provides a means for input of new, significant data indicating the development of additional problems or a lack of therapeutic responsiveness that may require additional nursing diagnoses or collaboration with the physician or other professionals on the health care team as plans for therapy are revised.

RELATING THE NURSING PROCESS TO PHARMACOLOGY

Assessment

Objectives

1. State the information that should be obtained as a part of a medication history.
2. Identify primary, secondary, and tertiary sources of information used to build a patient information base.

Key Words

drug history   secondary sources
primary sources   tertiary sources
subjective data

Assessment is an ongoing process that starts with the admission of the patient and is completed at the time of discharge. In relating the nursing process to the nursing functions associated with medications, assessment includes taking a **drug history** for three reasons: (1) to evaluate the patient's need for medication; (2) to obtain the patient's current and past use of over-the-counter medication, prescription medication, and street drugs; and (3) to identify problems related to drug therapy. Nurses will also want to identify risk factors such as allergy to certain medications (for example, penicillins) or the presence of other diseases (such as hypertension) that may limit the use of certain types of drugs (as with sympathomimetic agents).

The nurse draws upon three sources to build the medication-related information base. Whenever the patient is able to provide reliable information, the patient should be used as the **primary source** of information. Subjective and objective data serve as the baseline for the formulation of drug-related nursing diagnoses. **Subjective data** come from information provided by the patient (e.g., "Whenever I take this medicine I feel sick to my stomach"). Objective data are gained from observations that the nurse makes using physiologic parameters (such as "skin pale, cold, and moist"; "temperature 99.2° F orally"). Other objective information needed will be the patient's height and weight, which may be needed to select dosages of medications and later as a monitoring parameter for drug therapy.

In some cases it is necessary to obtain information from **secondary sources** (for example, relatives, significant others, medical records, laboratory reports, nursing notes, or other health care professionals). Secondary sources of information are subject to interpretation by someone other than the patient. Data collected from secondary sources should be analyzed using other portions of the data base to validate the conclusions reached.

Tertiary sources of information, such as a literature search, provide a "textbook picture" of the characteristics of

a disease, nursing interventions, diagnostic tests used, pharmacologic treatment prescribed, diets, physical therapy, and other factors pertinent to the patient's care requirements. (When using these sources, the student should be aware that the patient has individual needs and that the plan of care must be adapted to the patient's identified needs.)

Assessment related to drug therapy continues on an ongoing basis throughout the hospitalization period. Examples of ongoing assessment activities include visiting with the patient, the need for "as needed" (prn) medication, monitoring vital signs, and observation for therapeutic effects, side effects to expect, side effects to report, and potential drug interactions.

In preparation for the patient's eventual discharge and need for education about new health-related responsibilities, the assessment process should include collection of data related to the patient's health beliefs, existing health problems, prior compliance with prescribed regimens, readiness for learning both emotionally and experientially, and ability to learn and execute the skills required for self-care.

Nursing Diagnoses

Objectives

1. Define "problem."
2. Describe the process that is used to identify factors that could result in patient problems when medications are prescribed.
3. Review the content of several drug monographs to identify information that may result in patient problems from the medication therapy.

Key Words

drug monographs   pathophysiology
side effects   (indications)

To deal effectively with identified problems (diagnoses), the nurse must recognize the etiology and contributing factors.

The etiological and contributing factors are those clinical and personal situations that can cause the problem or influence its development.... Situations can be pathophysiological, treatment related, situational, or maturational (Carpenito, 1987).

When identifying problems related to medication therapy, the nurse should review the **drug monographs** given later in this text for each prescribed drug. Several nursing diagnoses can be formulated based on the patient's drug therapy. Although the most commonly observed are those associated with drug *treatment* of a disease or the **side effects** from drug therapy, nursing diagnoses can also originate from **pathophysiology** caused by drug interactions.

EXAMPLE: Drugs prescribed for Parkinson's disease are administered to provide relief of symptoms (muscle tremors, slowness of movement, muscle weakness with rigidity, and alterations in posture and equilibrium). An actual nursing diagnosis of "Mobility, impaired physical: related to neuromuscular impairment (Parkinson's disease)" would be formulated based on the defining characteristics established for this nursing diagnosis. These nursing diagnoses are labeled (as indications) in the nursing diagnosis subsection of the nursing process related to drug therapy sections throughout this book, meaning that the diagnosis is associated with the medical diagnosis or signs and symptoms of the disease process for which the medications are being prescribed. Evaluation of the therapeutic and expected outcomes from the prescribed medications are based on the degree of improvement noted in the symptoms present.

A second nursing diagnosis would be "Injury, risk for: related to amantadine side effects (confusion, disorientation, dizziness, light-headedness)." Nursing diagnoses of this type are labeled as *side effects* in the nursing diagnosis subsection of the nursing process related to drug therapy sections throughout the book.

In this example, the drug amantadine, prescribed to *treat* the symptoms of the disease, is also the basis of the first nursing diagnosis. The second nursing diagnosis is a collaborative problem that requires the nurse to *monitor* the development of these side effects. In other words, a patient with Parkinson's disease is at risk of developing the defining characteristics that can cause this to occur. When the defining characteristics are observed, notification of the physician is required, and the nurse would need to intervene to provide for the patient's safety.

Two nursing diagnoses that apply to all types of medications prescribed are as follows:
- Knowledge deficit (actual, risk, or possible), related to: the medication regimen (patient education).
- Noncompliance (actual, risk, or possible) related to: the patient's value system, cognitive ability, cultural factors, or economic resources.

Planning

Objectives

1. Identify steps used to plan nursing care in relation to a medication regimen prescribed for a patient.

2. Describe an acceptable method of organizing, implementing, and evaluating the patient education delivered.

3. Practice developing short-term and long-term patient education objectives, and have them critiqued by the instructor.

Key Words

therapeutic intent   side effects to report
side effects to expect

Planning, with reference to the prescribed medications, must include the following steps:
1. Identification of the **therapeutic intent** for each prescribed medication. (Why was the drug prescribed? What symptoms should be relieved?)
2. Review of the drug monograph in this text to identify the **side effects to expect** (symptoms that can be alleviated or prevented by actions of the nurse or patient will require immediate planning for patient education).
3. Review of the drug monograph in this text to identify the **side effects to report** (a collaborative problem in which the nurse has a responsibility to *monitor* the patient for adverse effects of drug therapy and report suspected adverse effects to the physician).
4. Identification of the recommended dosage and route of administration (compare the recommended dosage with the dosage ordered; confirm that the route of administration is correct and that the dosage form ordered can be tolerated by the patient).
5. Scheduling of the administration of the medication based on the physician's orders and the policies of the health care facility (medications prescribed must be reviewed for drug-drug interactions and drug-food interactions; laboratory tests may also need to be scheduled if serum levels of the drug have been ordered).
6. Teaching the patient to keep written records of responses to the prescribed medications (see Appendix I).
7. Additional education as needed on techniques of self-administration (such as injection, topical patches, instillation of drops).
8. Information as needed on proper storage, how to refill a medication, or how to fill out an insurance claim for reimbursement.

Priority ranking in preparation for health education may encompass several factors: (1) the patient's concerns and priorities; (2) the urgency or time available for the learning to take place; (3) a sequence that allows the patient to move from the simple to the more complex concepts; and (4) a review of the overall needs of the individual. The content taught to the patient should be well planned in advance and delivered in increments that the patient is capable of mastering. The complete teaching plan should be in the Kardex or on the patient's chart.

EXAMPLE: Mr. Jones will be able to state the following:
1. Drug name
2. Dosage
3. Route and administration times
4. Anticipated therapeutic response
5. Side effects to expect
6. Side effects to report
7. What to do if a dosage is missed
8. When, how, or if to refill the medication for each prescribed medication (by *date*) and show retention of this information by repeating it on *date*.

To attain this goal, the patient's ability to name all these factors would need to be checked at the initial time of exposure and on subsequent meetings to validate retention. Once the goals have been formulated, they should not be considered final but should be reevaluated as needed throughout the course of treatment.

Nursing Intervention or Implementation

Objective

1. Differentiate among dependent, interdependent, and independent nursing actions, and give an example of each.

Nursing actions applied to pharmacology may be categorized as dependent, interdependent, or independent.

Dependent Nursing Actions

The physician admits the patient, states the admitting diagnosis, and orders diagnostic procedures and medications for the immediate well-being of the patient. The physician reviews data on a continuing basis to determine the risks and benefits of maintaining or modifying the medication orders. Maintenance or modification of the medication orders is the physician's responsibility; however, the data collected and recorded by the nurse on the patient's chart are essential for evaluation of the effectiveness of the medications prescribed.

Interdependent Nursing Actions

The nurse will perform baseline and subsequent assessments that will be valuable in establishing therapeutic goals, duration of therapy, detection of drug toxicity, and frequency of reevaluation.

The nurse should approach any problems related to the medication prescribed collaboratively with appropriate members of the health care team. Whenever the nurse is in doubt about medication calculations, monitoring for therapeutic efficacy and side effects, or the establishment of nursing interventions or patient education, another qualified professional should be consulted.

The pharmacist reviews all aspects of the drug order, then prepares the medications and sends them to the unit for storage in a medication room or a unit dose medication cart. If any portion of the drug order or the rationale for therapy is unclear, the nurse and pharmacist may consult with each other or the physician for clarification.

The frequency of medication administration is defined by the physician in the original order. The nurse and pharmacist establish the schedule of the medication based on the standardized administration times used at the practice setting. The nurse and occasionally the pharmacist also coordinate the schedule of the medication administration and the collection of blood samples with the laboratory phlebotomist to monitor drug serum levels.

The nurse completes laboratory test requisitions based on the physician's orders to monitor drug therapy, establish dosages, and identify the most effective medication for pathogenic microorganisms.

As soon as laboratory and diagnostic test results are available, the nurse and pharmacist review them to identify values that could have an influence on drug therapy. The results of the tests are conveyed to the physician. The nurse should also have current assessment data available for collaborative discussion of signs and symptoms that may relate to the medications prescribed, dosage, therapeutic efficacy, or adverse effects.

Patient education (including discharge medications) requires that an established plan be developed, written in the patient's medical record, implemented, documented, and reinforced by all persons delivering care to the patient (see the sample teaching plan on p. 44).

Independent Nursing Actions

The nurse visits with the patient and obtains the nursing history, which includes a medication history. The history of current and past medications—including prescription, over-the-counter, and street drugs—is reviewed to identify treatment-related problems.

The nurse verifies the drug order and assumes responsibility for correct transcription of the drug order to the nurse's Kardex, medication administration record (MAR), or com-

puter. As part of this process, the nurse makes professional judgments concerning the class of drug, therapeutic intent, usual dosage, and the patient's ability to tolerate the drug dosage form ordered. If all aspects of the verification and transcription procedure are considered to be correct, the carbon copy of the original order is sent to the pharmacy.

The nurse formulates appropriate nursing diagnoses and actions to monitor for therapeutic effects and side effects of medications. (The nurse may need to review drug monographs to formulate the diagnoses and goal statements.) Criteria for therapeutic responses should describe the improvement expected in symptoms of the disease for which the medication was prescribed.

The nurse prepares the prescribed medications using procedures to ensure patient safety. As part of this process, nursing professional judgments required include the following:

1. Selection of the correct supplies (needle gauge, length, type of syringe) for administration of the medications.
2. Verification of all aspects of the medication order before preparing the medication; the order should be verified again immediately following preparation and again before actual patient administration. Patients should always be identified immediately before administration of the medication each time a medication is to be administered.
3. Collection of appropriate data to serve as a baseline for later assessments of therapeutic effectiveness and to detect adverse effects of drugs.
4. Administration of the medication by the correct route at the correct site (selection and rotation of sites for medication should be based on established practices for rotation of sites and on principles of drug absorption, which in turn may be affected by the presence of pathophysiology, such as poor tissue perfusion).
5. Documentation in the chart of all aspects of medication administration; subsequent assessments should be documented to identify the drug efficacy, the development of expected side effects, or any adverse effects.
6. Implementation of nursing actions to minimize expected side effects and to identify side effects to be reported promptly.
7. Education of patients as appropriate for the medications prescribed, in addition to other facets of the therapeutic regimen; when noncompliance is identified, the nurse should attempt to ascertain the patient's reasons for not following the regimen and collaboratively discuss approaches to the problems viewed by the patient as hindrances to following the prescribed regimen.

Evaluating Therapeutic and Expected Outcomes

Objective

1. Describe the procedure for evaluating the therapeutic outcomes obtained from prescribed therapy.

Evaluation associated with drug therapy is an ongoing process that assesses response to the medications prescribed, observation for signs and symptoms of recurring illness or the development of adverse effects of the medication, determination of the patient's ability to receive patient education and self-administer medications, and the potential for compliance. Table 4-2 illustrates an overview of the application of the nursing process to the nursing responsibilities associated with drug therapy.

Table 4-2

The Nursing Process Applied to the Patient's Pharmacologic Needs

ASSESSMENT	PLANNING	INTERVENTION	EVALUATION
Data collection Collect data on patient symptoms; disease process is based on the history and physical, patient, and/or family information; nursing assessments and interview	Identify and prioritize: ■ Patient problems ■ Baseline assessment data to be monitored to evaluate the patient's symptoms ■ Anticipated drug side effects and those to report ■ Examine drug monograph and data to determine the therapeutic outcomes.	Perform the identified baseline patient assessments on a regularly scheduled basis (such as blood pressure, pulse, respirations, pain level [frequency, duration, activity associated with onset], leg pain).	Analyze data collected on a continuum; chart and report *changes* of significance in the baseline data and/or patient's status; report escalating of symptoms or ineffective response to drug therapy.
Drug history: ask questions in a simple, direct manner to elicit information regarding drugs currently being taken, or those taken during the preceding year; ask about over-the-counter drugs used on a regular or casual basis	Plan to monitor patient's total drug needs; develop goals to deal with any drug interactions, incompatibilities, or diagnostic tests potentially affected by drugs being administered. Examine drug monograph to identify premedication data needed.	Perform drug preparation, scheduling, and administration to coincide with specific patient needs or problems.	Analyze data collected on a continuum.
Ask about any prior drug "allergies" and specifics of the "reaction" and treatment used	Plan to monitor patient at risk for the development of an allergic reaction.	Perform premedication assessment, and implement monitoring parameters.	Analyze observed symptoms for potential drug reaction or interactions. Report alterations to the prescribing physician.
Age and disease process present	Plan modifications in dosage, administration technique, and observations based on the individual's age and physiologic status that may indicate a problem with drug absorption, distribution, metabolism, or excretion; confirm drug dosages BEFORE administering any drug in question.	Implement the proper administration of confirmed drug dosages.	As therapy continues, analyze the patient's weight, mental status, and disease processes that may be indicative of a problem with drug absorption, distribution, metabolism, or excretion; report abnormal laboratory values or *changes* from the patient's baseline assessment data.
Body weight	Plan to weigh the patient daily or as needed.	Perform the procedure of weighing the patient at the same time, in the same weight clothing, on the same scale at the intervals ordered.	Report weight gains or losses (this is of particular importance with some types of drugs such as digitalis glycosides, corticosteroids, thyroid medications, and chemotherapy)
Metabolic rate	Plan nursing intervention to correlate with diseases that alter metabolic rate (such as hyperthyroidism, hypothyroidism, heart failure).	Institute nursing measures directed at nutritional status, activity/exercise needs, environmental alterations needed.	Analyze effectiveness of approaches utilized; observe closely for an increase or decrease in therapeutic effect.

continued

Table 4-2

The Nursing Process Applied to the Patient's Pharmacologic Needs—cont'd

ASSESSMENT	PLANNING	INTERVENTION	EVALUATION
Monitoring parameters Laboratory data (see Appendix D for normal values): review data to determine potential problems in the absorption, distribution, metabolism, and elimination of the prescribed drug	Follow hospital policies for order and assisting with laboratory/diagnostic test; always check for drugs that may interact with scheduled laboratory tests.		
Hepatic function	AST, ALT, Alkaline phosphatase, LDH, GGT	Complete appropriate forms to order the tests; assist in drawing of blood samples and in providing patient support during procedure.	As soon as results are received on the unit, report any diagnostic value outside the normal to the physician.
Renal function	Serum creatinine, creatinine clearance, blood urea nitrogen (BUN), urinalysis	Same as above. Collect urine sample by clean catch or, if ordered, by catheterization. Check for drugs being given and record on urinalysis slip. Send urine samples to laboratory promptly after collection. Be certain it is refrigerated/iced as appropriate. Always record the exact start date/time and end date/time on laboratory slip for 12 hr/24 hr urine collection (e.g., urine creatinine).	Elevated serum creatinine levels generally indicate renal disease. Elevated BUN levels occur in renal disease, dehydration, a high protein diet, or a catabolic state. Depressed BUN levels are found in severe hepatic damage, overhydration, and malnutrition. Urinalysis: Always report RBCs, casts, crystals, proteinuria, glycosuria, high or low pH, or specific gravity outside the normal range (1.001–1.017).
In addition to the above tests, the following tests may be used to monitor disease and drug therapy:			
Infectious disease Assessment for site/source of the infection	Culture and sensitivity (C&S)	Collect specimen properly to maintain sterility of the culture tip so that the source examined is the only surface touched. Label appropriately; take to lab immediately.	Report results of a C & S promptly; particularly important are results that indicate that the drug being administered is not effective against the organism cultured.
Complete blood count (CBC)	Plan intervention based on the organism, the site of the infection, fever, hematuria, and drainage.	Implement nursing measures to deal effectively with the patient's needs—fever, pain, drainage, and degree of precautions appropriate to the organism.	Elevated WBCs, bands, segs, lymphocytes need to be reported to the physician. Analyze subsequent CBC reports for significant changes; continue performing baseline assessments to detect degree of responsiveness to therapy.

continued

Table 4-2

The Nursing Process Applied to the Patient's Pharmacologic Needs—cont'd

ASSESSMENT	PLANNING	INTERVENTION	EVALUATION
Monitoring of drug levels Routinely monitored: digitalis glycosides, theophylline, aminoglycosides, lithium, lidocaine, phenytoin, procainamide, quinidine, vancomycin (see Appendix D)	Plan to requisition the laboratory tests ordered by the physician to monitor serum blood levels at the scheduled times; ensure that the patient will be available at the required times.	Record drug name, dosage, and times and route of administration on requisition.	Therapeutic doses of certain drugs can be established through a combination of monitoring of serum levels and patient assessments of essential data. Example: aminophylline—The patient's age and disease factors modify the dosage needs; therefore patients with cardiac, pulmonary, or renal dysfunction may require serum concentration as a guide to dosage. *The current clinical status of the patient is always important; therefore regular assessments specifically planned to detect therapeutic and toxic activity are imperative to effective patient management.* Check specific drug monographs for other drugs that may alter laboratory results; report results promptly for the physician's evaluation.
Other laboratory tests	Prothrombin time (PT) (for warfarin) Partial thromboplastin time (PTT) (for heparin)	Requisition the prescribed laboratory test so that the drug dosage can be ordered by the physician; perform nursing assessments associated with anticoagulant therapy and the disease process specifically being treated.	Be certain the correct date and patient data are relayed to the physician when seeking or confirming the anticoagulant drug order; always double check the data, time, and specific dosage of the anticoagulant drug order; anticoagulants should be checked with a second qualified nurse at the time of preparation and administration.
	Blood glucose	Withhold daily insulin until blood sugar sample is drawn; test blood for glucose as ordered or ac and hs.	Correlate the results of the laboratory reports to the patient's status and degree of response to drug therapy; carefully evaluate patient symptoms for hyper- and hypoglycemia. Report laboratory data and patient status changes to the physician.
	Glycosylated hemoglobin	Measures average blood glucose control for past 120 days. No food or fluid restriction.	
	Fructosamine	Measures average blood glucose control for previous 1 to 3 wk.	

continued

Table 4-2

The Nursing Process Applied to the Patient's Pharmacologic Needs—cont'd

ASSESSMENT	PLANNING	INTERVENTION	EVALUATION
Nurse's research of prescribed drugs			
Drug action. Review introductory nursing assessments in specific drug monographs to correlate drug action and monitoring parameters to the patient's presenting symptoms and disease process.	Develop goal statements for monitoring presence or absence of response. Plan the administration schedule to correlate with known information about time of administration in relation to food, tests, and planned sleep. Plan interventions to minimize or alleviate drug-related complications (side effects).	Assess the patient for baseline data before administering the drug; perform subsequent assessments at regular intervals to collect data to evaluate therapeutic response to the drug. Administer the prescribed drug: RIGHT patient RIGHT drug RIGHT dose RIGHT route RIGHT time RIGHT documentation	Document all assessments by carefully recording all pertinent observations in the patient's chart. Analyze the collected data and compare to the baseline data gathered before initiation of drug therapy; report significant changes in the patient's status.
Side effects to expect	Consult specific drug monographs for side effects to expect; plan assessments to detect and intervention to manage these as they occur.	Monitor the patient for development of expected side effects; implement measures designed to effectively manage or minimize effects; assist patient to understand and cope with specific symptoms as developed.	Once expected side effects develop, it is important to evaluate the nursing measures designed to minimize or reduce the effects; report lack of responsiveness; modify intervention appropriately; analyze the patient's level of tolerance of the side effects.
	Plan specific teaching that incorporates side effects to expect.	Teach which side effects to expect and how to alleviate discomfort. Encourage the patient to discuss relevant symptoms with the physician and to adhere to the medication prescribed; suggest discussion of symptoms and encourage cooperative planning for modifications in the medications taken; discourage discontinuance or self-adjusted dosages.	Document specific teaching performed and the degree of understanding observed through direct questioning; and return demonstrations. Analyze verbal and nonverbal behaviors observed to detect patient response to suggestion of cooperative goal-setting between the physician and patient.
Side effects to report	Plan nursing assessments and intervention for side effects that are serious and require reporting. Develop a specific teaching plan that incorporates teaching of side effects to report. Plan teaching of necessary monitoring parameters (blood pressure, pulse, respirations, daily weights, etc).	Perform regularly scheduled nursing assessments to detect any side effects from drug therapy that should be reported. Perform health teaching of the observations the patient should make and the findings that require reporting. Teach and repeat at appropriate intervals to achieve patient/family mastery.	Analyze data collected on a continuum; report deviations appropriately. Carefully evaluate the patient's attitude toward compliance with drug therapy and intent to report problems for discussion and needed modifications. Evaluate the degree of accuracy attained by the patient or family members; refer to social services or community agencies if assistance is needed at time of discharge.

continued

Table 4-2

The Nursing Process Applied to the Patient's Pharmacologic Needs—cont'd

ASSESSMENT	PLANNING	INTERVENTION	EVALUATION
Nurse's research of prescribed drugs—cont'd			
Patient understanding of drug therapy	Plan teaching of drug name, dosages, route of administration, and exact time schedule; record overall teaching plan on the Kardex or chart. Plan teaching of medications taken on a prn basis (such as nitroglycerin) and establish goals to evaluate understanding of frequency of dose, repeating of dose, lack of response. Plan teaching of any self-administration techniques (oral, inhalation, injection, rectal, etc.).	Throughout the hospitalization, discuss medication information and how it will benefit the course of treatment; seek cooperation and understanding of the following points so that medication compliance may be enhanced: 1. Name 2. Dosage 3. Route and administration times 4. Anticipated therapeutic response 5. Side effects to expect 6. Side effects to report 7. What to do if a dosage is missed 8. When, how, or if to refill the medication prescription Teach name of drug being taken, symptoms that can be relieved by the prn drug, when to take it, amount to take, what to do if not effective. Teach administration techniques to be used at home; give simple written instructions to follow at home.	Document teaching and understanding achieved; try role-playing a situation or, when appropriate during hospitalization, have the patient describe what needs to be done. Document the individual's understanding of the directions given; try role-playing a situation or, when appropriate during hospitalization, have the patient describe what needs to be done. Validate the patient/significant other's understanding by return demonstration; document teaching of administration techniques and degree of understanding in nurse's notes.
Patient understanding of entire treatment plan	Develop goal statements for teaching the individual's care that will assist the patient in gaining knowledge of all aspects of self-care for the disease process present (nutritional status, activity or exercise modifications, psychologic, medication, physical therapy, etc.). Incorporate assessments to determine the individual's readiness and capability to learn, degree of understanding, and tolerance for needed alterations.	Implement planned nursing measures appropriate to the specific disease process affecting the individual. Incorporate teaching techniques (visual aids, demonstrations and return demonstrations, role playing, etc.).	Analyze the patient's response to *each* component of the entire treatment plan. Throughout the course of teaching establish target dates to evaluate the degree of understanding exhibited by having the patient perform appropriate activities (for example, choose the therapeutic diet from the hospital menu). Evaluate the tolerance exhibited to restrictions and modifications implemented, or to drug side effects expected and present; document all facets of health teaching performed, degree of understanding attained, or intolerances observed or experienced.

ac, Before meals, *ALT*; alanine aminotransferase; *AST*, aspartate aminotransferase; *GGT*, gamma-glutamyltransferase; *hs*, at bedtime, *LDH*, lactic dehydrogenase; *RBCs*, red blood cells; *WBCs*, white blood cells.

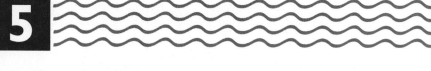

Patient Education and Health Promotion

Objectives

1. Differentiate between the meanings of cognitive, affective, and psychomotor learning.

2. Identify the main principles of learning that must be applied during the teaching of patient, family, or group.

3. Apply the principles of learning to the content learned in pharmacology.

Key Words

cognitive domain

affective domain

psychomotor domain

objectives

ethnocentrism

scientific-biomedical
 paradigm

magicoreligious paradigm

holistic paradigm

THE THREE DOMAINS OF LEARNING

Cognitive Domain

The **cognitive domain** is the level at which basic knowledge is learned and stored. It is the thinking portion of the process and incorporates a person's previous experiences and perceptions.

One's previous experiences with health and wellness can influence the learning of new materials. Prior knowledge and experience forms the foundation for adding new concepts. The learning process is thus started by identifying what prior experiences the person has had with the subject.

Thinking involves much more than just the delivery of new information or concepts. During the thinking process a person must build relationships between prior experiences and the new concepts to formulate new meanings. At a higher level in the thinking process, the new information must be used to question when uncertain, to recognize when to seek additional information, and to make decisions during real-life situations.

Affective Domain

Affective behavior is conduct that reflects attitudes, values, beliefs, needs, and emotional responses (Davis, 1981). The **affective domain** is the most intangible portion of the learning process. It is well known that individuals view events from different perspectives. Persons frequently do not express feelings, choosing instead to internalize them. The nurse must be willing to approach patients nonjudgementally, listen to their needs, be cognizant of the nonverbal messages being given, and assess their needs with an open mind.

Developing a sense of trust and confidence among the professionals providing health care can have a powerful impact on the attitude of the patient and family members. This will influence the learner's response to the new information being taught. Be positive, be accepting, and involve the learner in a discussion to draw out his or her views toward the solution to problems.

Psychomotor Domain

The **psychomotor domain** involves the learning of a new procedure or skill. It is often referred to as the *doing* domain. Learning is usually done by demonstration of the procedure or task using a step-by-step approach, with return demonstrations by the patient to validate the degree of mastery obtained.

PRINCIPLES OF LEARNING

Focus the Learning

The patient must be allowed to focus on the material or task to be learned. The environment must be conducive to learning; it must be quiet, well lighted, and have the essential equipment needed to complete the lesson.

The person will need repetition of new information to master it. Many times nurses feel a responsibility to teach the patient or family everything they know about a disease or procedure, overwhelming them with information. It is a good idea to ask yourself what information is essential. Second, consider what the patient wants to know. It is best to start with the questions the individual has and proceed from there. Otherwise you may be explaining things the individual is not interested in knowing, and the individual may not be focused on the presentation. By starting with the learner's needs you give the person some control over the learning, and thereby increase the learner's participation in the process. Active participation in the learning process increases learning.

Learning Styles

People's learning styles vary. Some can read and readily comprehend directions, whereas others need to see, feel, hear, touch, and think to master a task. To be effective the nurse must fit the teaching techniques used to the learner's style. Therefore, a variety of materials must be available to perform health education. The nurse can select the instructional approach to be used from written materials such as pamphlets, video recordings, motion pictures, models, slides, filmstrips, audiocassettes, photographs, charts, transparencies, and computer-aided instruction. These materials supply the audio and visual component that may be essential to the learning style.

Organization Fosters Learning

In most clinical settings today, patient education materials are developed by staff and then reviewed by a committee for adoption. Specific objectives should be formulated for the patient education sessions. The **objectives** should state the purpose of the activities and the expected outcomes. Objectives may be developed in conjunction with a nursing diagnosis statement (for example, Nutrition, Altered: Less than Body Requirements). Or they can be developed for common conditions requiring care delivery (for example, Care of the Patient Receiving Chemotherapy). Regardless of the format used, these instructional programs have established content given in outline form and are arranged such that one nurse can initiate the teaching and document the degree of understanding, and another nurse can continue the teaching on a different shift or day. By checking off what has been accomplished, the next nurse knows where to begin the next lesson. At the start of a subsequent teaching session it is important to review what has been covered previously and to affirm the retention of the information from the previous lessons. Organizing materials this way (1) standardizes the content, (2) allows for more than one nurse to be able to teach the same patient, (3) allows for the material to be covered in increments the patient can handle, and (4) makes documentation easier. This information is then readily available for review before discharge and can support the need for additional home care when a patient has not mastered self-care needs.

When psychomotor skills are being taught, return demonstrations are particularly useful for ensuring mastery. It helps to allow the individual to practice a task several times. Giving the person immediate feedback on skills mastered and then giving time to practice skills that are more difficult allows for growth in manual dexterity and mastery of the sequencing of the procedure. If appropriate, the equipment

may be left with the person for practice before the next session. Sometimes it is particularly useful to set up a videotape player for the patient to view alone at a convenient time. At the next meeting, the videotape can be reviewed together with discussion of important points for clarification when the patient expresses confusion or uncertainty. This technique reinforces what has been said, reviews what has been learned, and provides the individual with repetition, which may be necessary for learning.

Motivating the Individual to Learn

All teaching is not done in a formal setting. Some of the most effective teaching can be done while care is being delivered. The patient can be exposed to a skill, a treatment, or facts that must be comprehended in small increments. The nurse who explains a procedure and informs the patient why certain procedures are being done reinforces the need for it and motivates the individual to learn. If patients understand the personal benefits of performing a task, their willingness to do it is strengthened. As the patient practices using the new skill or procedure, the nurse can reinforce the benefits and the technique for mastery.

Readiness to Learn

A patient's perception of health and his or her health status may not be the same as that of the nurse; therefore the values of health to each individual may differ greatly. The patient may not be aware of his or her health needs and may not realize that a healthy lifestyle provides significant benefits. Persons who commonly indulge in alcohol, smoking, and high-fat diets, and have a sedentary lifestyle may not consider the consequences of these practices in relation to health. Not everyone is interested in the concept of healthy living. The nurse must respect the individuality of the patient, family, or group and should accept that not everyone is motivated by the possibility of a higher level of wellness.

The nurse can positively influence the learning process by being enthusiastic about the content to be taught. A patient's response to the new information will be variable and depends on several influences, for example, the need to know, life experiences, self-concept, the impact of the illness on lifestyle, prior experience with learning new materials, and readiness to learn. In research by Kaluger and Kaluger (1984) it was discovered that readiness or the ability to engage in learning depends on motive, relevant preparatory training, and physiologic maturation. In other words, is the individual motivated to learn? Is the individual willing to make behavioral changes? Is the individual at a point in the state of illness or wellness at which learning is beneficial and appropriate?

In teaching activities undertaken with children, psychosocial, cognitive, and language abilities must be considered. Cognitive and motor development and the individual's language usage and understanding must be assessed. Age definitely influences the types and amount of self-care activities the child is capable of learning and executing independently. Consult a text in developmental theory for further information.

Adult education is usually oriented toward learning what is necessary to maintain a personal lifestyle. In general, adults must understand why there is a need to learn something before they expend the effort to learn it. When planning the educational needs of the patient, the nurse must assess what the patient already knows and what additional information is desired. It is imperative that the teacher make the content relevant to the individual and that the patient's health beliefs be incorporated into the overall plan.

The older adult needs additional assessments before implementation of health teaching. Assess vision, hearing, and short- and long-term memory. If a task is to be taught, fine and gross motor abilities must be evaluated as well. An older patient may also have major concerns over the cost of the proposed treatments in relation to available resources. Individuals frequently evaluate the benefits of planned medical interventions and the overall impact of these on the quality of their lives. Any of these situations can affect the ability to focus on the new information to be taught and influence responses and the overall outcome of the teaching. Older adults have frequently experienced losses and may also be facing social isolation, physical (functional) losses, and financial constraints. Because the elderly frequently suffer more chronic health problems, a new diagnosis, exacerbation of a disease, or a new crisis may be physically or emotionally overwhelming. The timing of the teaching is therefore of great significance.

When teaching an elderly patient it is prudent to slow the pace of the presentation and limit the length of each session to prevent overtiring. The elderly can learn the material, but they often process things more slowly than younger persons because short-term memory may be limited. The nurse must work with the individual to develop ways to remember what is being taught. The more the older person is involved in forming the associations that will help him or her remember new ideas and connect these ideas with past experiences, the better the outcome. Many individuals are embarrassed by the inability to master a task. Asking them if they understand is useless because they will not reveal embarrassment. Provide information in small increments, allow for practice, review, practice, review, practice until success is achieved. Stop at appropriate intervals and reschedule sessions to meet the learning needs.

When the learner becomes anxious, slow the presentation of new information, repeat, or stop and reschedule the session for later. Be sure to extend a compliment on positive aspects of the session before ending it. Fear and anxiety often impair the ability to focus on the task or content being presented; creating an environment that is conducive to learning is important. Consider the lighting so that glare is not on materials to be read, face the individual for better eye contact, and speak directly in a clear voice without shouting. Be calm; use tact and diplomacy if frustrations develop, and try to instill confidence in the patient's ability to surmount any problems.

Spacing the Content

Spacing the amount of material given in one session should be considered when teaching patients of all ages. People tend to remember what is learned first best. Based on this principle, multiple short sessions are usually better than longer sessions that overwhelm the person. Beginning teachers tend to focus on giving all the materials to the individual and checking off on checklists that the materials were taught. The giving of information is not synonymous with the learning of the information.

Assess the individual's learning style to determine if he or she likes to read materials and then discuss them or prefers other methods of study such as audiovisuals. After this is done, the spacing of the content can be tailored to the types of learning materials available to teach the content.

Repetition Enhances Learning

Repetition is known to enhance learning. Making a plan that incorporates multiple practice sessions reinforces this principle. Because of limited duration of hospitalization, the feasibility of multiple practice sessions may be limited; therefore it is important to validate in the charting those aspects of the patient's educational needs that have been mastered and those that still require assistance from home health care agencies.

Education Level

Vocabulary and reading level used during the teaching sessions must be tailored to the patient's ability to comprehend what is being presented. It is imperative that the information be presented at an appropriate educational level. Medical terms may not be understood, and written instructions left at the bedside to be read independently may be misinterpreted, if read at all. Some persons are illiterate; others may read at grade one, grade seven, or collegiate level. Therefore, if written materials are used, it is important to consider these wide variations in literacy.

Cultural and Ethnic Diversity

Many health care professionals have limited understanding of what persons of other cultures believe and of the importance of these beliefs to the learning process. **Ethnocentrism** is the assumption that one's culture provides the right way, the best way, the only way to live. In short, people who believe in the theory of ethnocentrism assume that one's way of viewing the world is superior to that of others (Leininger, 1978). As understanding of cultural diversity increases, health care professionals must expand their knowledge of the basic tenants of the belief systems of the consumers with whom they work.

Albers Herberg (1989) described scientific, magicoreligious, and holistic paradigms as three ways people explain life events. Table 5-1 is a summary of belief systems about health and illness. The **scientific-biomedical paradigm** is the one most familiar to health care workers educated in the United States. The basic tenant of this health care system is that all disease has a cause. When the etiology is unknown, scientific research is directed toward finding a cure because one exists even though yet undiscovered.

The **magicoreligious paradigm** views the world and its inhabitants as being under the control of supernatural, mystical forces. People who attribute their illnesses to this model

Table 5-1

Summary of Belief Systems about Health and Illness

	MAGICORELIGIOUS	SCIENTIFIC-BIOMEDICAL	HOLISTIC
World view	Fate of world is under control of supernatural forces. God(s) or other supernatural forces for good or evil are in control; humans are at the mercy of natural forces.	Life is controlled by physical and biochemical processes that can be studied and manipulated by humans.	Harmony, natural balance. Human life is only one aspect of nature and part of the general order of the cosmos. Everything in universe has a place and role according to laws that maintain order.
Illness/disease	Initiated by supernatural agent with or without justification, via sorcery. Cause of health or illness is not organic, it is mystical. Causes: possession by evil spirits, breaching a taboo, supernatural forces (sorcery, witchcraft).	Wear and tear, accident, injury, pathogens, and fluid and chemical imbalance. Cause-effect relationship exists for natural events. Life related to structure and functions like machines. Life can be reduced or divided into smaller parts. Mind and body two distinct entities. Cause exists, if only it were known.	Disease, imbalance, and chaos result when these laws are disturbed.
Health	Gift or reward given as a sign of God's blessing and good will.	Illness prevention activities; restoration through exercise, medication, treatments, and other means.	Environment, behavior, and sociocultural factors are influential in maintenance of health and prevention of disease. Maintaining and restoring balance are important to health.
Ethnic group	Hispanic Americans, African Americans; components found in other groups	White Americans	Native Americans, Asian Americans; components found in other groups
Other concepts			Yin/yang Hot/cold Harmony/disharmony

Modified from Albers cited in Herberg P: Theoretical foundations of transcultural nursing. In Boyle JS, Andrews MM: *Transcultural concepts in nursing care,* Boston, 1989, Scott, Foresman. Data from Babcock DE, Miller MH: *Client education: theory and practice,* St Louis, 1995, Mosby.

believe in evil spirits and gods, witchcraft, spells, and other forces that impart illness on a person. Health can be a gift or a blessing from God, and an illness may be punishment from God or, conversely, a way of God showing the individual that he or she has been chosen to carry out God's will. Illnesses are natural, intended by God, or unnatural, or not a part of God's plan.

The **holistic paradigm** recognizes harmony among the body, mind, and spirit. This model identifies disease as a direct result of an imbalance between these natural components. Health is restored by bringing these three components—body, mind, and spirit—into balance.

Because there are differing beliefs, it is important that the nurse explore the meaning of an illness with the patient. Members of other cultures do not always express themselves when their views are in conflict with those of another. Unless a careful assessment of psychosocial needs is done, the true meaning of an illness or of the proposed intervention may never be uncovered. Even the assessment process has obstacles attached. People in some cultures do not believe that family information should be shared outside the family, and still others, such as those of the Indian culture, believe that only the individual may reveal personal information.

Communication is vitally important within any cultural group, yet verbal and nonverbal communication mean different things to different cultures. For example, white Americans tend to value eye contact, but in other cultures direct eye contact is a sign of disrespect or rudeness (Native Americans, Asian Americans).

Apparent aggressiveness, paranoia, and other behaviors experienced when interrelating with some ethnic groups may be a result of defensiveness arising from conditioning during life's experiences and from perceptions of racial prejudice. When these behaviors are exhibited, the nurse must remain calm and nonjudgemental and intervene to clarify what is causing the miscommunication.

If working with an interpreter when a language barrier exists, remember that this presents several additional variables for interpretation. Does the interpreter understand what you are asking or saying and have experience with medical terminology? Are there comparable words in the patient's language that can be used to interpret what you are saying? Is the interpreter telling you what the individual is saying? Any time a third person enters into the communication cycle, there are more chances for lack of clarity and misinterpretation. Keep questions brief, and ask questions one at a time to give the interpreter an opportunity to rephrase the question and obtain a response. Sometimes supplementing your questioning with pictures and pantomime may be helpful. When using an interpreter look directly at the patient while conversing, not the interpreter.

As part of the cultural assessment, determine who makes the decisions within the family. Include the decision maker in the teaching session, otherwise all of the teaching may be for naught.

Today, as cultural mixes become more common, educational materials are being adapted to meet a variety of cultural needs. Unfortunately, this does not solve all problems; interpreting what is written still leaves the chance for misunderstanding because many persons cannot read or do not read at the level at which the materials are written.

Compliance

Health care professionals and educators tend to think an individual should change behaviors and adhere to a new therapeutic regimen simply because the educator said it. However, we must recognize that patients have the right to make their own life choices and frequently do. Unfortunately, there is no way to ensure compliance unless the patient sees the value of it.

Success with a health regimen is enhanced when the educator conveys an enthusiastic attitude, appears positive about the subject matter, and shows confidence in the abilities of the participants to understand the lesson. Reinforcing positive accomplishments is imperative to fostering successful achievement.

The response to the therapeutic regimen and degree of compliance is influenced by several variables, including the following:

- Beliefs about the seriousness of the illness
- Perception of the benefits to be derived from the proposed treatment plans
- Personal beliefs, values, and attitudes toward health and the health care system, including prior experience within the system
- Impact of the proposed changes on personal life
- Acceptance (or denial) of the illness and its associated problems
- Comprehension and understanding of the health regimen
- Cost of treatment in relation to resources
- Support of significant others
- Amount of control the individual experiences over the disease or condition and, ultimately, over life as a result of the changes

- Side effects from the treatment and degree of inconvenience, annoyance, or impairment in functioning they produce
- Degree of positive response achieved

The ability of an individual to comply with a proposed health regimen is a complex process requiring the evaluator to reach conclusions based on established criteria. The ultimate goal is to assist patients in achieving the greatest degree of control possible within the context of their beliefs, values, and needs. Health care professionals can offer support and encouragement, be complimentary in response to positive achievements, and encourage examination of the available options and benefits of a healthy lifestyle. It is vital to assist patients in exploring options when a problem or complication is experienced rather than giving up the treatment because they are uninformed about the alternatives. Financial costs may be a deciding factor in the decisions made.

Needs are constantly changing; it is necessary to modify the learning objectives on a continuum and adapt the plan of care to the individual's needs. The plan of care should evolve as a result of the nurse and patient discussing the available options and then establishing objectives with which the patient is willing and able to live.

PATIENT EDUCATION ASSOCIATED WITH MEDICATION THERAPY

Objectives

1. Describe essential elements of patient education in relation to the prescribed medications.

2. Describe the nurse's role in fostering patient responsibility for the maintenance of well-being and for compliance with the therapeutic regimen.

3. Identify the types of information that should be discussed with the patient or significant others in order to establish reasonable expectations for the prescribed therapy.

4. Discuss specific techniques used in the practice setting to document the patient education performed and degree of achievement attained.

During the past two decades, health teaching has evolved from an abstract form of intervention that occurred only if a specific need existed at discharge (and if the physician approved of providing the information to the patient) to the current state of formalized development of learning objectives to direct the individual toward attainment of goals based on the needs of the patient. Today, health teaching is an important nursing responsibility that carries with it legal implications for failure to provide and document education.

The content taught to the patient should be thoroughly planned in advance (see the sample teaching plan on p. 44), and delivered in increments that the patient is capable of mastering. The complete teaching plan should be in the Kardex or on the patient's chart. Each segment should be expressed in measurable behavioral terms. Once the goals have been formulated, they should not be considered final but should be reevaluated on established target dates throughout the course of treatment and modified if necessary. All teaching should be documented in the nurse's notes or on the health teaching record, along with observations that verify the patient's degree of understanding or proficiency of skill mastered. As mastery of an item is attained, it should be checked off on the Kardex or health teaching form in the patient's chart.

Assessing the patient's readiness for learning is crucial to success. When anxiety is high, the ability to focus on details is reduced. The nurse should anticipate periods during the hospitalization when teaching can be more effectively implemented. Some teaching is most successful when done spontaneously, such as when the patient asks direct questions regarding progress toward discharge. The nurse also must learn to anticipate inopportune times to initiate teaching, such as during times of withdrawal after learning of a diagnosis with a poor prognosis. With reduced hospital stays, the ability to time patient education ideally and to perform actual teaching is a challenge. It is imperative that the nurse document those aspects of the health teaching that have been mastered and, of equal importance, document what has not been accomplished and request referral to an appropriate agency for follow-up teaching and assistance.

During the process of patient education, the nurse should address the areas of communication and responsibility, expectations of therapy, changes in expectation, and changes in therapy through cooperative goal setting.

Communication and Responsibility

Nurses tend to think that patients will do what is suggested simply because they have been told it is beneficial. In the hospital, the nurse and other health team members reinforce the basic therapeutic regimen. At dismissal, however, the patient leaves the controlled environment and is free to choose to follow the prescribed treatment or to alter it as is deemed appropriate based on personal values and beliefs. For learning to take place, the patient must perceive the information as relevant. Whenever possible, start with simple, attainable teaching goals to build the patient's confidence. It is important to correlate the teaching with the patient's perspective on the illness and ability to control the signs and symptoms or course of the disease process.

Expectations of Therapy

Before dismissal, discuss reasonable responses to the planned therapy. The patient should know what signs and symptoms can be expected to be altered by the prescribed medications. The precautions necessary when taking a medication must be explained by the nurse and understood by the patient (for example, caution in operating power equipment or a motor vehicle, avoidance of direct sunlight, or the need for follow-up laboratory studies).

Changes in Expectations

Assess changes in expectations as therapy progresses and the patient gains understanding and skill in the management of the diagnosis. The expectations about therapy of patients with acute illnesses may vary widely from those of patients with chronic illnesses.

Changes in Therapy through Cooperative Goal Setting

An attitude of shared input into the goals can encourage the patient into therapeutic alliance. Therefore the patient should be taught to help monitor the parameters used to evaluate therapy. It is imperative that the nurse nurture a cooperative environment that encourages the patient to (1) keep records of the essential data needed to evaluate the prescribed therapy and (2) contact the physician for advice rather than altering the medication dosages or schedule or discontinuing the medication entirely. For each major class of drugs in this book, written records are provided to help the nurse identify essential data that the patient must understand and record on a regular basis to assist the physician in monitoring therapy. (See Appendix I and the box on p. 44 for a sample teaching plan for a patient with diabetes mellitus receiving one type of insulin.) In the event that the patient, family, or significant others do not understand all aspects of the continuing therapy prescribed, they may be referred to a community-based agency for the achievement of long-term health care requirements.

At Dismissal

A summary statement of the patient's unmet needs must be written and placed in the medical chart. The physician should be consulted concerning the possibility of a referral to a community-based agency for continued monitoring or treatment. The nurse's dismissal notes must identify the nursing diagnoses that are unmet and potential collaborative problems that require continued monitoring and intervention. All counseling information should be carefully written out in a manner that the patient can read and understand.

Understanding of health condition
- Assess the patient's and family's understanding of diabetes mellitus.
- Clarify the meaning of the disease in terms the patient is able to understand.
- Establish learning goals through mutual discussion. Arrange to teach most important data first. Set dates for teaching of content after discussion with patient.

Food and fluids
- Arrange for the patient, family members, and significant others to attend nutrition lectures and demonstrations on food preparation.
- Reinforce knowledge of exchange lists (or other dietary method) by tactful questioning and by giving the patient a chance to practice food selections for daily meals from menus provided.
- Explain management of the diabetic diet during illness (that is, nausea and vomiting, need for increase in fluid) and when to contact the physician.
- Stress interrelationship of food and onset, peak, and duration of the prescribed insulin.

Monitoring tests
- Demonstrate the collection and testing of blood glucose samples and, as appropriate, urine testing.
- Validate understanding by having the patient collect, test, and record results of the testing for the remainder of the hospitalization.
- Stress performing serum glucose testing and urine tests (for example, ketones) before meals and at bedtime.
- Explain the importance of regular follow-up laboratory studies (that is, fasting plasma glucose testing or postprandial, glycosylated hemoglobin) to monitor the patient's degree of control.

Medications and treatments
- Teach the name, dose, route of administration, desired action, storage, and refilling of the type of insulin prescribed.
- Explain the principles of insulin action, onset, peak, and duration (see Chapter 33)
- Demonstrate preparation and administration of the prescribed dose of insulin.
- Teach site location and self-administration of insulin.
- Give specific instructions on reading the syringe to be used at home.
- Teach how to obtain disposable syringes.
- Cite usual times for "reactions," signs and symptoms of hypoglycemia or hyperglycemia, and management of each complication.
- Validate the patient's understanding of the side effects to expect and those that require reporting.
- Teach and validate family members' and significant others' understanding of the signs and symptoms of hypoglycemia and hyperglycemia and management of each complication.

- Teach general approach to management of illnesses (for example, if nausea and vomiting or fever occur—actions required; stress glucose monitoring before meals and at hour of sleep; and need to call physician).

Personal hygiene
Discuss the management of personal hygiene measures of great importance to the patient with diabetes mellitus:
- Regular foot care.
- Meticulous oral hygiene and dental care.
- Care of cuts, scratches, minor and major injuries.
- Stress the management and needed alterations in insulin dosage during an illness; emphasize the need to consult the physician for guidance and discussion.

Activities
- Help the patient develop a detailed time schedule for usual activities of daily living. Incorporate diabetic care needs into the schedule.
- Encourage maintenance of all usual activities of daily living; discuss anticipated problems and possible interventions.
- Correlate personal care needs not only in the home environment, but also in the work setting as appropriate. (Consider involvement of the industrial nurse if available in the work setting.)
- Discuss effects of an increase or decrease in activity level on the management of the diabetes mellitus.

Home or follow-up care
- Arrange for outpatient or physician follow-up appointments and for scheduling ordered laboratory tests.
- Tell the individual to seek assistance from the physician or from the nearest emergency room service for problems that may develop.
- Arrange appropriate referral to community health agencies if needed.
- Complete a Diabetic Alert card or other means of alerting people to the individual's needs (such as an identification necklace or bracelet).

Special equipment and instructional material
- Develop a list of equipment and supplies to be purchased; have a family member purchase and bring to the hospital for use during teaching sessions (ketone testing and blood glucose monitoring supplies, syringes, needles and sterilizing equipment, alcohol, cotton balls, and so on).
- Show audiovisual materials available on insulin preparation, storage, administration on serum glucose and urine testing, and so on.
- Develop a written record (see Chapter 33) and assist the patient to maintain data during hospitalization.

Other
- Teach measures to make travel easier.
- Tell the patient of the American Diabetes Association and material available through this resource.

---

*Each item listed must be assessed for the individual's current knowledge base and level of understanding throughout the course of teaching. The process is reassessed and the teaching continued until the patient masters all facets of self-care needs. With the advent of shorter hospitalizations, inpatient and outpatient teaching may be necessary with referral to community-based health care agencies as necessary. Discharge charting and referral should carefully document those facets of the teaching plan mastered and those to be taught. The physician should be notified of deficits in learning ability or mastery of needed elements in the teaching plan.

Unit Two
ILLUSTRATED ATLAS OF MEDICATION ADMINISTRATION AND MATH REVIEW

A Review of Arithmetic

Although many hospitals are using the "unit dosage" system in dispensing drugs, it continues to be the nurse's responsibility to ascertain that the medication administered is exactly as prescribed by the physician. To give an accurate dosage, the nurse must have a working knowledge of basic mathematics. This review is offered so that individuals may determine areas in which improvement is needed.

ROMAN NUMERALS

Objective

1. Read and write selected numerical values using Roman numerals.

Toward the end of the sixteenth century two systems of numbers emerged—Roman and Arabic. They are the basis for our communications in mathematics today, are used interchangeably, and are occasionally used by the physician in prescribing drugs. Roman numerals 1 through 100 are used frequently in medicine. Key symbols are

$$I = 1, V = 5, X = 10, L = 50,$$
$$C = 100, D = 500, M = 1000$$

Whenever a Roman numeral is repeated, or when a smaller numeral follows, the numerals are added.

EXAMPLES:

I = 1,	II = 2,	III = 3,	VI = 6,
(1 + 0 = 1)	(1 + 1 = 2)	(1 + 1 + 1 = 3)	(5 + 1 = 6)
VII = 7,		XI = 11,	XII = 12
(5 + 1 + 1 = 7)		(10 + 1 = 11)	(10 + 1 + 1 = 12)

Whenever a smaller Roman numeral appears before a larger Roman numeral, subtract the smaller numeral.

EXAMPLES:

IV = 4,	IX = 9,	XC = 90
(5 − 1 = 4)	(10 − 1 = 9)	(100 − 10 = 90)

Whenever a smaller Roman numeral appears between two larger Roman numerals, subtract the smaller number from the numeral following it.

EXAMPLES:

XIX = 19	XIV = 14
(10 + 10 − 1 = 19)	(10 + 5 − 1 = 14)
XCIX = 99	
(100 − 10 + 10 − 1 = 99)	

The most common Roman numerals associated with medication administration are śś = ½, i = 1, ii = 2, iii = 3, iv = 4, v = 5, vi = 6, vii = 7, viiśś = 7½, viii = 8, ix = 9, x = 10 and xv = 15.

Express the following in Roman numerals:

3 ________	20 ________	101 ________
9 ________	18 ________	499 ________
10 ________	49 ________	1979 ________

Express the following in Arabic numerals:

iv ________	xxxix ________	xix ________
vi ________	ix ________	xv ________

FRACTIONS

Objective

1. Demonstrate proficiency in calculating mathematic problems using the addition, subtraction, multiplication, and division of fractions.

Key Words

numerator   denominator

Fractions are one or more of the separate parts of a substance, or less than a whole number or amount.

EXAMPLE: $1 - \frac{1}{2} = \frac{1}{2}$

Common Fractions

A common fraction is part of a whole number. The **numerator** (dividend) is the number above the line. The **denominator** (divisor) is the number below the line. The line separating the numerator and denominator tells us to divide.

$$\frac{\text{Numerator (Names how many parts are used)}}{\text{Denominator (Tabulates the pieces, or tells how many pieces the whole is divided into)}}$$

EXAMPLES:

The denominator represents the number of parts or pieces the whole is divided into.

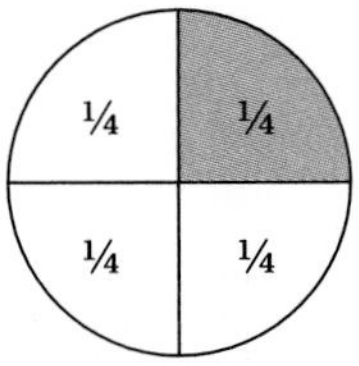

$1/4$ means graphically that the whole circle is divided into four (4) parts; one (1) of the parts is being used.

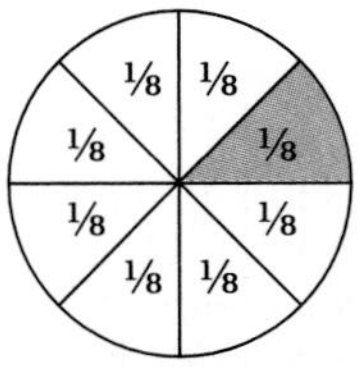

$1/8$ means graphically that the whole circle is divided into eight (8) parts; one (1) of the parts is being used.

From these two examples, $1/4$ and $1/8$, you can see that the *larger* the *denominator* number, the *smaller* the *portion* is. (Each section in the $1/8$ circle is smaller than each section in the $1/4$ circle.) This is an important concept to understand for persons who will calculate drug dosages. The drug ordered may be $1/4$ gr and the drug source available on the shelf $1/2$ gr. Before proceeding to do any formal calculations you should first decide if the dose you need to give is smaller or larger than the drug source available on the shelf.

EXAMPLES:

Visualize:

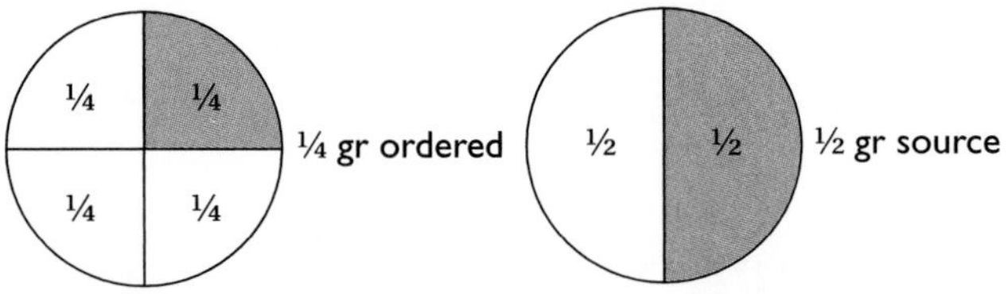

Decide: "Is what I need to administer to the patient a larger or smaller portion than the drug available on the shelf?"
Answer: $1/4$ is smaller; thus it would be less than one tablet.

Try a second example: $1/8$ gr is ordered; the drug source on the shelf is $1/2$ gr.
Visualize:

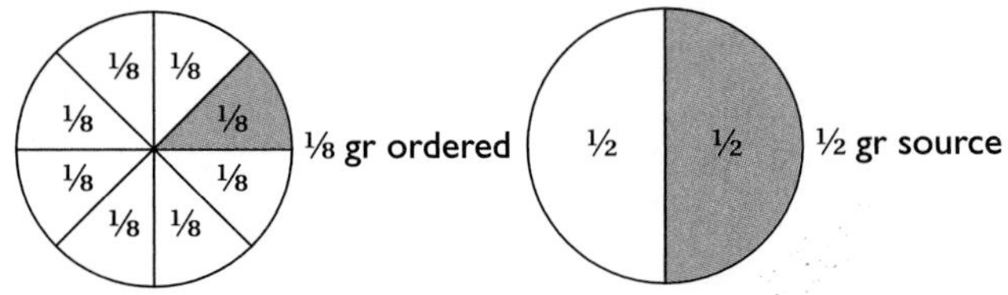

Decide: "Is what I need to administer to the patient a larger or smaller portion than the drug available on the shelf?"
Answer: $1/8$ is smaller than the drug source; thus it would be less than one tablet.

Types of Common Fractions

1. *Simple:* contains *one* numerator and *one* denominator: $1/4$, $1/20$, $1/60$, $1/100$
2. *Complex:* may have a simple fraction in the numerator or denominator:
3. *Proper:* numerator is smaller than denominator: $1/8$, $2/5$, $1/100$

$$1/2 \text{ over } 4 = \frac{1/2}{4}$$

or

$$1/2 \div 4 =$$
$$1/2 \div 4/1 =$$
$$1/2 \times 1/4 = 1/8$$

4. *Improper:* numerator is larger than denominator: $4/3$, $6/4$, $100/10$
5. *Mixed number:* a whole number and a fraction: $4\,5/8$, $6\,2/3$, $1\,5/100$
6. *Decimal:* fractions written on the basis of a multiple of ten: $0.5 = 5/10$, $0.05 = 5/100$, $0.005 = 5/1000$
7. *Equivalent:* fractions that have the same value: $1/3$ and $2/6$

Working with Fractions

Reducing to Lowest Terms

Divide both the numerator and the denominator by a number that will divide into both evenly (a common denominator).

EXAMPLE: $\dfrac{25}{125} \div \dfrac{25}{25} = \dfrac{1}{5}$

Reduce the following:

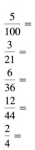

$$\dfrac{5}{100} =$$

$$\dfrac{3}{21} =$$

$$\dfrac{6}{36} =$$

$$\dfrac{12}{44} =$$

$$\dfrac{2}{4} =$$

Finding the lowest common denominator of a series of fractions is not always easy. Here are some points to remember:

If the numerator and denominator are both even numbers, 2 will work as a common denominator but may not be the smallest one.

If the numerator and denominator end with 0 or 5, 5 will work as a common denominator but may not be the smallest one.

Check to see if the numerator divides evenly into the denominator; this will be the smallest term. When all else fails, use the prime number method to find the lowest common denominator. A prime number is a whole number, greater than 1, that can be divided only by itself and 1 (2, 3, 5, 7, 11, 19, 23, etc.).

Steps: (1) Write down all the denominators in a row, then proceed to divide each denominator by the lowest prime number until you can no longer use that number. Proceed to the next higher prime number and divide using it until it can no longer be used. Continue this procedure until all 1s are obtained. (2) Multiply all the prime numbers used to divide and you will have the lowest common denominator.

EXAMPLE:

Fractions: $\dfrac{7}{16}$ $\dfrac{5}{9}$ $\dfrac{13}{30}$ $\dfrac{7}{22}$

Write down all denominators:

Prime numbers:		16	9	30	22
	2	8	9	15	11
	2	4	9	15	11
	2	2	9	15	11
	2	1	9	15	11
	3	1	3	5	11
	3	1	1	5	11
	5	1	1	1	11
	11	1	1	1	1

2 is the smallest prime number. Keep dividing by this number until it no longer will divide into the denominators evenly. Proceed to the next higher prime and reuse if possible. Go to the next higher prime that will divide in evenly; continue until all 1s are obtained.

The lowest common denominator is

$$2 \times 2 \times 2 \times 2 \times 3 \times 3 \times 5 \times 11 = 7920$$

Addition

Adding Common Fractions

When denominators are the same figure, add the numerators.

EXAMPLE: $\dfrac{1}{4} + \dfrac{2}{4} + \dfrac{3}{4} = \dfrac{6}{4} = 1\dfrac{1}{2}$

Add the following:

$$\dfrac{2}{6} + \dfrac{3}{6} + \dfrac{4}{6} = \dfrac{9}{6} = 1\dfrac{1}{2}$$

$$\dfrac{1}{100} + \dfrac{3}{100} + \dfrac{5}{100} = \dfrac{9}{100}$$

When the denominators are unlike, change the fractions to equivalent fractions by finding the lowest common denominator.

EXAMPLE: $\dfrac{2}{5} + \dfrac{3}{10} + \dfrac{1}{2} = ?$

1. Determine the lowest common denominator. (Use 10 as the common denominator.)
2. Divide the denominator of the fraction being changed into the common denominator and multiply the product (answer) by the numerator.

$\dfrac{2}{5} = \dfrac{4}{10}$ [Divide 5 into 10 and multiply the answer (2) by 2]

$\dfrac{3}{10} = \dfrac{3}{10}$ [Divide 10 into 10 and multiply the answer (1) by 3]

$\dfrac{1}{2} = \dfrac{5}{10}$ [Divide 2 into 10 and multiply the answer (5) by 1]

$\dfrac{12}{10} = 1\dfrac{1}{5}$ [Add the numerators and place the total over the denominator (10); then convert the improper fraction to a mixed number and reduce to lowest terms.]

Add the following:

a.
$$\dfrac{2}{8} = \dfrac{}{64}$$
$$+ \dfrac{4}{64} = \dfrac{}{64}$$
$$+ \dfrac{5}{16} = \dfrac{}{64}$$
$$\dfrac{}{64} \qquad \text{Answer: } \dfrac{5}{8}$$

b.
$$\dfrac{3}{7} = \dfrac{}{28}$$
$$\dfrac{9}{14} = \dfrac{}{28}$$
$$+ \dfrac{1}{28} = \dfrac{}{28}$$
$$\dfrac{}{28} \qquad \text{Answer: } 1\dfrac{3}{28}$$

Adding Mixed Numbers

Add the fractions first; then add the whole numbers.

EXAMPLE: $2\frac{3}{4} + 2\frac{1}{2} + 3\frac{3}{8} = ?$

1. Determine the lowest common denominator. (Use 8 as the common denominator.)
2. Divide the denominator of the fraction being changed into the common denominator and multiply the product (answer) by the numerator.

$2\frac{3}{4} = \frac{6}{8}$ [Divide 4 into 8 and multiply the answer (2) by 3]

$2\frac{1}{2} = \frac{4}{8}$ [Divide 2 into 8 and multiply the answer (4) by 1]

$+\ 3\frac{3}{8} = \frac{3}{8}$ [Divide 8 into 8 and multiply the answer (1) by 3]

$\frac{13}{8}$ [Add the numerators and place the total over the denominator (8)]

$7 + 1\frac{5}{8} = 8\frac{5}{8}$ $\left(\frac{13}{8}\right)$ [Convert the improper fraction to a mixed number $\left(1\frac{5}{8}\right)$ and add it to the whole numbers]

Add the following:

a.
$+\frac{1}{4}$
$+\frac{3}{4}$
$\frac{\ }{4}$ Answer: $\frac{4}{4} = 1$

b.
$\frac{1}{2} = \frac{\ }{6}$
$+\frac{1}{3} = \frac{\ }{6}$
$+\frac{1}{6} = \frac{\ }{6}$
$= \frac{\ }{6}$ Answer: $\frac{6}{6} = 1$

c.
$\frac{3}{5} = \frac{\ }{50}$
$+\frac{4}{50} = \frac{\ }{50}$ Answer: $\frac{34}{50} = \frac{17}{25}$
$= \frac{\ }{50}$ (Reduced to lowest term.)

Subtraction

Subtracting Fractions

When the denominators are unlike, change the fractions to an equivalent fraction by finding the lowest common denominator.

EXAMPLE: $\frac{1}{4} - \frac{3}{16} =$

1. Determine the lowest common denominator. (Use 16 as the common denominator.)
2. Divide the denominator of the fraction being changed into the common denominator and multiply the product (answer) by the numerator.

$\frac{1}{4} = \frac{4}{16}$ [Divide 4 into 16 and multiply the answer (4) by 1]

$-\frac{3}{16} = \frac{3}{16}$ [Divide 16 into 16 and multiply the answer (1) by 3]

$\frac{1}{16}$ [Subtract the numerators and place the total over the denominator (16)]

Subtract the following:

a.
$\frac{3}{8}$
$-\frac{2}{8}$
$\frac{\ }{8}$ Answer: $\frac{1}{8}$

b.
$\frac{1}{100} = \frac{\ }{300}$
$-\frac{1}{150} = \frac{\ }{300}$
$\frac{\ }{300}$ Answer: $\frac{1}{300}$

Subtracting Mixed Numbers

Subtract the fractions first; then subtract the whole numbers.

EXAMPLE: $4\frac{1}{4} - 1\frac{3}{4} = ?$

$4\frac{1}{4} = 3\frac{5}{4}$ [NOTE: You cannot subtract $\frac{3}{4}$ from $\frac{1}{4}$;

$-\ 1\frac{3}{4} = 1\frac{3}{4}$ therefore borrow 1 (which equals $\frac{4}{4}$) from

the whole numbers and add $\frac{4}{4} + \frac{1}{4} = \frac{5}{4}$.]

$2\frac{2}{4} = 2\frac{1}{2}$ [Subtract the numerators, place answer over the denominator (4); reduce to lowest terms; subtract the whole numbers]

When the denominators are unlike, change the fractions to equivalent fractions by finding the lowest common denominator.

EXAMPLE: $2\frac{5}{8} - 1\frac{1}{4} = ?$

1. Determine the lowest common denominator. (Use 8 as the common denominator.)
2. Divide the denominator of the fraction being changed into the common denominator and multiply the product (answer) by the numerator.

$2\frac{5}{8} = 2\frac{5}{8}$ [Divide 8 into 8 and multiply the answer (1) by 5]

$-\ 1\frac{1}{4} = 1\frac{2}{8}$ [Divide 4 into 8 and multiply the answer (2) by 1]

$1\frac{3}{8}$ [Subtract the numerators and place the total over the denominator (8); reduce to lowest terms; subtract the whole numbers.

Subtract the following:

a.
$\frac{7}{8} = \frac{\ }{24}$
$-\frac{3}{6} = \frac{\ }{24}$
$\frac{\ }{24}$ Answer: $\frac{9}{24} = \frac{3}{8}$

b.
$6\frac{7}{8} = \frac{\ }{16}$
$-\ 3\frac{1}{16} = \frac{\ }{16}$
$\frac{\ }{16}$ Answer: $3\frac{13}{16}$

Multiplication
Multiplying a Whole Number by a Fraction

EXAMPLE: $3 \times \dfrac{5}{8} = ?$

1. Place the whole number over 1. $\left(\dfrac{3}{1}\right)$
2. Multiply the numerators (top numbers) and multiply the denominators (bottom numbers).

$$\frac{3}{1} \times \frac{5}{8} = \frac{15}{8}$$

3. Change the improper fraction to a mixed number.

$$\frac{15}{8} = 1\frac{7}{8}$$

Multiply the following:

a. $2 \times \dfrac{3}{4} = ?$ Answer: $\dfrac{3}{2} = 1\dfrac{1}{2}$

b. $15 \times \dfrac{3}{5} = ?$ Answer: $\dfrac{9}{1} = 9$

Multiplying Two Fractions

EXAMPLE: $\dfrac{1}{4} \times \dfrac{2}{3} = ?$

1. Use cancellation to speed the process.

$$\frac{1}{\underset{2}{\cancel{4}}} \times \frac{\overset{1}{\cancel{2}}}{3} =$$

2. Multiply the numerators (top numbers); multiply the denominators.

$$\frac{1}{2} \times \frac{1}{3} = \frac{1}{6}$$

Multiplying Mixed Numbers

EXAMPLE: $3\dfrac{1}{2} \times 2\dfrac{1}{5} = ?$

1. Change the mixed numbers (a whole number and a fraction) to an improper fraction (numerator is larger than denominator).

$3\dfrac{1}{2} \times 2\dfrac{1}{5} = ?$ (Multiply the denominator times the whole number and add the numerator.)

$\dfrac{7}{2} \times \dfrac{11}{5} = ?$

2. Multiply the numerators; multiply the denominators.

$$\frac{7}{2} \times \frac{11}{5} = \frac{77}{10}$$

3. Change the product (answer), an improper fraction, to a mixed number by dividing the denominator into the numerator; reduce to lowest terms.

$$\frac{7}{2} \times \frac{11}{5} = \frac{77}{10} = 7\frac{7}{10}$$

Multiply the following:

a. $1\dfrac{2}{3} \times \dfrac{3}{6} = ?$ Answer: $\dfrac{5}{6}$

b. $1\dfrac{7}{8} \times 1\dfrac{1}{4} = ?$ Answer: $\dfrac{75}{32} = 2\dfrac{11}{32}$

Division
Dividing Fractions

EXAMPLE: $4 \div \dfrac{1}{2} = ?$

1. Change the division sign to a multiplication sign.
2. Invert the divisor, the number after the division sign.
3. Reduce the fractions using cancellation.
4. Multiply the numerators and the denominators.

$$4 \div \frac{1}{2} = \frac{4}{1} \times \frac{2}{1} = \frac{8}{1} = 8$$

Dividing with a Mixed Number

1. Change the mixed number to an improper fraction.
2. Change the division sign to a multiplication sign.
3. Invert the divisor.
4. Reduce whenever possible.

EXAMPLES:

$$4\frac{1}{2} \div \frac{3}{4} = \frac{9}{2} \div \frac{3}{4} = \frac{\overset{3}{\cancel{9}}}{\underset{1}{\cancel{2}}} \times \frac{\overset{2}{\cancel{4}}}{\underset{1}{\cancel{3}}} = \frac{6}{1} \text{ or } 6$$

$$6\frac{1}{4} \div 1\frac{1}{4} = \frac{25}{4} \div \frac{5}{4} = \frac{\overset{5}{\cancel{25}}}{\underset{1}{\cancel{4}}} \times \frac{\overset{1}{\cancel{4}}}{\underset{1}{\cancel{5}}} = \frac{5}{1} \text{ or } 5$$

Fractions as Decimals

Fractions can be changed to a decimal form by dividing the numerator by the denominator.

EXAMPLE: $\dfrac{1}{2} = 2\overline{)1.0}\,^{0.5}$

Change the following fractions to decimals:

a. $\dfrac{1}{100} = ?$ Answer: 0.01

b. $\dfrac{5}{8} = ?$ Answer: 0.625

c. $\dfrac{1}{2} = ?$ Answer: 0.5

Using Cancellation to Speed Your Work

1. Determine a number that will divide evenly into both a numerator and a denominator.
2. Continue the process of dividing both a numerator and denominator by the same number until all numbers are reduced to the lowest terms.
3. Complete the multiplication of the problem.

EXAMPLES: $\dfrac{\overset{1}{\cancel{5}}}{\underset{2}{\cancel{6}}} \times \dfrac{\overset{3}{\cancel{9}}}{\underset{2}{\cancel{10}}} = ?$

$$\frac{1}{2} \times \frac{3}{2} = \frac{3}{4}$$

4. Complete the division of the problem.

EXAMPLE: $\dfrac{6}{9} \div \dfrac{5}{8} = ?$ (Change the division sign to a multiplication sign; invert the number after the division sign; reduce and complete the multiplication of the problem.)

$$\frac{2}{3} \times \frac{8}{5} = \frac{16}{15} = 1\frac{1}{15}$$

DECIMAL FRACTIONS

Objectives

1. Demonstrate proficiency in calculating mathematic problems using the addition, subtraction, multiplication, and division of decimals.
2. Convert decimals to fractions and fractions to decimals.

When fractions are written to decimal form, the denominators are not written. The word *decimal* means "10."

When reading decimals, the numbers to the left of the decimal point are whole numbers. It helps to think of them as whole dollars.

EXAMPLES:

1. =	one
11. =	eleven
111. =	one hundred eleven
1111. =	one thousand one hundred eleven

Numbers to the right of the decimal point are read as follows:

EXAMPLES:

Decimal(s):		Fraction(s):
0.1 = one tenth		1/10
0.01 = one hundredth		1/100
0.465 = four hundred sixty-five thousandths		465/1000
0.0007 = seven ten thousandths		7/10,000

Here is another way to view reading decimals:

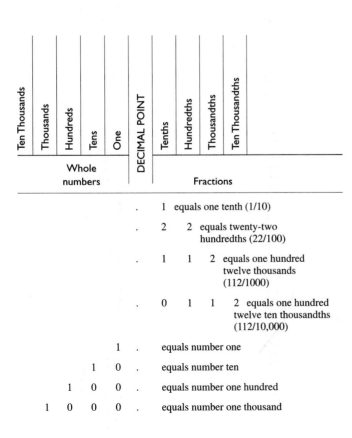

On prescriptions another way of expressing the decimal is by using a slanted line.

EXAMPLES:

1	mg	=	0.001	g	=	0/001	g
0.1	mg	=	0.0001	g	=	0/0001	g
30	mg	=	0.030	g	=	0/030	g
100	mg	=	0.100	g	=	0/100	g
1000	mg	=	1.000	g	=	1/0	g
250	mg	=	0.250	g	=	0/250	g

Multiplying Decimals

Multiplying Whole Numbers and Decimals

1. Count as many places in the answer, starting from the right, as there are places in the decimal involved in the multiplication.
2. The multiplier is the bottom number with the × or multiplication sign before it.
3. The multiplicand is the top number.

EXAMPLES:

500	1000	1000
× .02	× .04	× .009
10.00 (10)	40.00 (40)	9.000 (9)

7.25	500
× 4	× .009
29.00 (29)	4.500 (or 5)

Rounding the Answer

Note in the last example that the first number after the decimal point in the answer is 5. Instead of the answer remaining 4.5 it becomes the next whole number, 5. This would be true if the answer were 4.5, 4.6, 4.7, 4.8, or 4.9. In each case the answer would become 5. If the answer were 4.1, 4.2, 4.3, or 4.4 the answer would remain 4.

When the first number after the decimal point is 5 or above, the answer becomes the next whole number. When the first number after the decimal point is less than 5, the answer becomes the whole number in the answer.

Multiply the following:

1200	575	515	510
× 0.009	× 0.02	× 0.02	× 0.04

Multiplying a Decimal by a Decimal

1. Multiply the problem as if the numbers were both whole numbers.
2. Count decimal places in the answer, starting from the right, as many decimal places as there are in both of the numbers that were to be multiplied.

EXAMPLE:

3.75
× 0.5
1.875 = 2

There are two decimal places in 3.75 and one decimal place in 0.5, making three decimal places. Count three decimal places from the right. Round off the answer to 2.

Multiplying Numbers with Zero

EXAMPLES:

1. Multiply 223 by 40.
   a. Multiply 223 by 0. Write the answer, 0, in the unit column of the answer.
   b. Then multiply 223 by 4. Write this answer in front of the 0 in the product.

$$\begin{array}{r} 223 \\ \times\ 40 \\ \hline 8920 \end{array}$$

2. Multiply 124 by 304.
   a. First multiply 124 by 4. The answer is 496.
   b. Now multiply 124 by 0. Write the answer, 0, under the 9 in 496.
   c. Multiply 124 by 3. Write this answer in front of the 0 in the product.

$$\begin{array}{r} 124 \\ \times\ \ \ 304 \\ \hline 496 \\ 37\ 20 \\ \hline 37,696 \end{array}$$

Dividing Decimals

1. If the divisor (number by which you divide) is a decimal, make it a whole number by moving the decimal point to the right of the last figure.
2. Move the decimal point in the dividend (the number inside the bracket) as many places to the right as you move the decimal point in the divisor.
3. Place the decimal point for the quotient (answer) directly above the new decimal point of the dividend.

EXAMPLES:

$$0.25)\overline{10} = 25)\overline{1000.}^{\ 40.} \qquad 0.3)\overline{99.3} = 3)\overline{993.}^{\ 331.}$$

$$0.4)\overline{1.68} = 4)\overline{16.8}^{\ 4.2}$$

Changing Decimals to Common Fractions

1. Remove the decimal point.
2. Place the appropriate denominator under the number.
3. Reduce to lowest terms.

EXAMPLES:

$$0.2 = \frac{2}{10} = \frac{1}{5} \qquad 0.20 = \frac{20}{100} = \frac{1}{5}$$

Change the following:

$$0.3 = \underline{\hspace{1cm}} \qquad 0.25 = \underline{\hspace{1cm}}$$
$$0.4 = \underline{\hspace{1cm}} \qquad 0.50 = \underline{\hspace{1cm}}$$
$$0.5 = \underline{\hspace{1cm}} \qquad 0.75 = \underline{\hspace{1cm}}$$
$$0.05 = \underline{\hspace{1cm}} \qquad 0.002 = \underline{\hspace{1cm}}$$

Changing Common Fractions to Decimal Fractions

Divide the numerator of the fraction by the denominator.

EXAMPLE: $\frac{1}{4}$ means $1 \div 4$ or $4)\overline{1.00}^{\ 0.25}$

Change the following:

$$\frac{1}{2} \text{ means } \underline{\hspace{1cm}} \qquad \frac{3}{4} \text{ means } \underline{\hspace{1cm}}$$
$$\frac{1}{6} \text{ means } \underline{\hspace{1cm}} \qquad \frac{1}{50} \text{ means } \underline{\hspace{1cm}}$$
$$\frac{2}{3} \text{ means } \underline{\hspace{1cm}}$$

PERCENTS

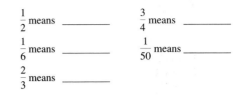

Objectives

1. Demonstrate proficiency in calculating mathematic problems using percentages.
2. Convert percents to fractions, percents to decimals, decimal fractions to percents, and common fractions to percents.

Determining Percent One Number Is of Another

1. Divide the smaller number by the larger number.
2. Multiply the quotient by 100 and add the percent sign.

EXAMPLE: A certain 1000 parts solution is 10 parts drug. What percent of the solution is drug?

$$1000)\overline{10.00}^{\ 0.01}$$
$$0.01 \times 100 = 1.\ \text{or}\ 1\%$$

Changing Percents to Fractions

1. Omit the percent sign to form the numerator.
2. Use 100 for the denominator.
3. Reduce the fraction.

EXAMPLES: $5\% = \frac{5}{100} = \frac{1}{20} \qquad 75\% = \frac{75}{100} = \frac{3}{4}$

Change the following:

$$25\% = \frac{25}{100} = \qquad 2\% = \frac{2}{100} =$$
$$15\% = \frac{15}{100} = \qquad 12\tfrac{1}{2}\% = \frac{12.5}{100} =$$
$$10\% = \frac{10}{100} = \qquad \tfrac{1}{4}\% = \frac{\tfrac{1}{4}}{100} =$$
$$20\% = \frac{20}{100} = \qquad 150\% = \frac{150}{100} =$$
$$50\% = \frac{50}{100} = \qquad 4\% = \frac{4}{100} =$$

Changing Percents to Decimal Fractions

1. Omit the percent signs.
2. Insert a decimal point *two places to the left* of the last number, or express as hundredths, decimally.

EXAMPLES: $5\% = .05 \qquad 15\% = .15$

Change the following:

$$4\% = \qquad 25\% =$$
$$1\% = \qquad 50\% =$$
$$2\% = \qquad 10\% =$$

Note in these examples that those numbers that were already hundredths, such as 10%, 15%, 25%, 50%, merely need to have the decimal point placed in front of the first number, because they are already expressed in hundredths; whereas 1%, 2%, 4%, 5% needed to have a zero placed in front of the number to express them as hundredths.

Change these percents to decimal fractions:

$$12\tfrac{1}{2}\% = \qquad \tfrac{1}{4}\% =$$

If the percent is a mixed number, it should have the fraction expressed as a decimal. Then change the percent to a decimal by moving the decimal point two places to the left.

EXAMPLES:

$$12\tfrac{1}{2}\% = 12.5\% \text{ or } 0.125$$

$$\tfrac{1}{4}\% = 0.25\% \text{ or } 0.0025$$

Changing Common Fractions to Percents

1. Divide the numerator by the denominator.
2. Multiply the quotient by 100 and add the percent sign.

EXAMPLE: $\dfrac{1}{50} = 50\overline{)1.00}^{\,0.02} = 0.02 \times 100 = 2\%$

Change the following:

$$\frac{1}{400} =$$

$$\frac{1}{8} =$$

Changing Decimal Fractions to Percents

1. Move the decimal point two places to the right.
2. Omit the decimal point if a whole number results.
3. Add the percent signs. (This is the same as multiplying the decimal fraction by 100 and adding the percent sign.)

EXAMPLE: $0.01 = 1.00 = 1\% \left(\text{or } \dfrac{1}{100}\right)$

Change the following:

$$0.05 \quad =$$
$$0.25 \quad =$$
$$0.15 \quad =$$
$$0.125 \quad =$$
$$0.0025 \quad =$$

Points to Remember in Reading Decimals

1. 1. is the whole number 1. When it is written 1.0, it is still one or 1.
2. The whole number is usually written like this: 1 or 2 or 3 or 4, and so on.

3. The whole number also can be written with the decimal point after the number: 1.0, 2.0, 3.0, 4.0.
4. Can you read this one? 0.1. This is one tenth. There is one number after the decimal point.
5. Can you read this one? .1. This is also one tenth. The zero in front of the decimal point does not change its value. One tenth can be written, then, in two ways: 0.1 and .1.
6. Remember that in writing the number 1. or 1.0, the decimal point is after the number. This makes the number a whole number. It is read the whole number 1.

RATIOS

Objective

1. Demonstrate proficiency in converting ratios to percentages and percentages to ratios, in simplifying ratios, and in use of the proportion method for solving problems.

A ratio expresses the relationship that one quantity bears to another.

EXAMPLES:

1:5 means 1 part of a drug to 5 parts of a solution.
1:100 means 1 part of a drug to 100 parts of a solution.
1:500 means 1 part of a drug to 500 parts of a solution.

A common fraction can be expressed as a ratio.

EXAMPLE: $\tfrac{1}{5}$ is the same as 1:5

The ratio of one amount to an amount expressed in terms of the same unit is the number of units in the first divided by the number of units in the second. The ratio of 2 ounces of a disinfectant to 10 ounces of water is 2 to 10 or 1 to 5 or ⅕. This ratio may be written ⅕ or 1:5.

The two numbers compared are referred to by using the term *ratio*. The first term of a true ratio is always one, or 1. This is the simplest form of a ratio.

Changing Ratio to Percent

1. Make the first term of the ratio the numerator of the fraction whose denominator is the second term of the ratio.
2. Divide the numerator by the denominator.

EXAMPLE: $5{:}1 = \dfrac{5}{1} \times 100 = 500\%$

3. Multiply by 100 and add the percent sign.
Change the following:

$$1{:}5 =$$

Changing Percent to Ratio

1. Change the percent to a fraction and reduce the fraction to lowest terms.
2. The numerator of the fraction is the first term of the ratio, and the denominator is the second term of the ratio.

EXAMPLE: $\tfrac{1}{2}\% = \dfrac{\tfrac{1}{2}}{100} = \dfrac{1}{2} \div \dfrac{100}{1}$

$$= \dfrac{1}{2} \times \dfrac{1}{100} = \dfrac{1}{200} = 1{:}200$$

Change the following:

$$2\% =$$
$$50\% =$$
$$75\% =$$

Simplifying Ratios

Ratios can be simplified as ratios or as fractions.

EXAMPLE: $25:100 = 1:4$ or $\dfrac{25}{100} = \dfrac{1}{4}$

Simplify the following:

$$4:12 =$$
$$5:10 =$$
$$10:5 =$$
$$75:100 =$$
$$\tfrac{1}{4}:100 =$$
$$15:20 =$$
$$3:9 =$$

Proportions

A proportion shows how two *equal* ratios are related. This method is good because it is possible to prove that your answer is correct, and it is especially useful in solutions.
1. Three factors are known. The fourth *unknown* (what you are looking for) is represented by x.
2. The first and fourth terms of a proportion are called extremes. The second and third are the means. The product of the means equals the product of the extremes, or multiplying the first and fourth equals the second and third.

EXAMPLE:

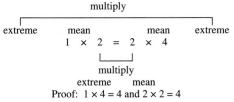

Proof: $1 \times 4 = 4$ and $2 \times 2 = 4$

If you did not know one number, you could solve for it as follows:

EXAMPLE:

$$1:2 = 2:x$$
$$1x = 4$$
$$x = 4 \div 1 = 4$$
$$x = 4$$
Proof: $1 \times 4 = 4$ and $2 \times 2 = 4$

Solve the following:

a. $9 : x : : 5 : 300$ _____
b. $x : 60 : : 4 : 120$ _____
c. $5 : 3000 : : 15 : x$ _____
d. $0.7 : 70 : : : x : 1000$ _____
e. $\tfrac{1}{400} : : x: : 2 : 1600$ _____
f. $0.2 : 8 : : x : 20$ _____
g. $100{,}000 : 3 : : 1{,}000{,}000 : x$ _____
h. $\tfrac{1}{4} : x : : 20 : 400$ _____

NOTE: x is the unknown factor. It may be a mean or an extreme in any of the four positions in any problem.

SYSTEMS OF WEIGHTS AND MEASURES

Objectives

1. Memorize the basic equivalents of the household, apothecary, and metric systems.
2. Demonstrate proficiency in performing conversion of medication problems using the household, apothecary, and metric systems.

Key Words

household	apothecary
measurements	measurements
grains	minim
metric system	milliliter
centimeter	liter
milligram	gram
kilogram	

Three systems of measurement are used during the calculation, preparation, and administration of drugs: household, apothecary, and metric.

Household Measurements

Household measurements are the least accurate. However, they are often the way pharmacologic agents are administered at home. The patient has grown up using this system of measurement and therefore understands it best. Household measurements include drops, teaspoons, tablespoons, teacups, cups, glasses, pints, quarts, and gallons. The first three measurements—drops, teaspoons, and tablespoons—would be used for medications, depending on the amount prescribed.

Common Household Equivalents

1 quart	=	4 cups
1 pint	=	2 cups
1 cup	=	8 ounces
1 teacup	=	6 ounces
1 tablespoon	=	3 teaspoons
1 teaspoon	=	approximately 60 drops

Apothecary Measurements

The **apothecary system** of measurement is an ancient system; the word *apothecary* means "pharmacist" or "druggist." Physicians rarely order medicine using the apothecary system. The metric system is the preferred system of measurement because it is more accurate.

Apothecary Weight

For weighing solids, the units of apothecary weight are, in increasing order of magnitude (smallest to largest), as follows:

```
              20 grains (gr) = 1 scruple
3 scruples or 60 grains = 1 dram (ℨ)
                              (1 dram = 4 ml or 4 cc)
   8 drams or 480 grains = 1 ounce (℥)
              12 ounces = 1 pound (lb)
```

The **grain** was originally derived from the average weight of a grain of wheat. The symbol for grain is gr. The dram (originally, drachma or drachm) was a Greek silver coin. The symbol for dram is ℨ. The ounce, whose symbol is ℥, is ¹⁄₁₂ of a troy pound. The pound is of Roman origin and signifies a balance. The symbol lb is the abbreviation for the Latin word *libra*, which means pound.

In apothecary weight, 12 ounces equals 1 pound (same weight as those of troy weight). In avoirdupois weight, 16 ounces equal 1 pound. Avoirdupois weight is used in weighing all articles *except* drugs, gold, silver, and precious stones.

Apothecary Volume

For measuring fluids the units of apothecary volume are, from smallest to largest, as follows:

```
      60 minims (♏) = 1 fluidram (f ℨ)
8 fluidrams or 480 minims = 1 fluidounce (f ℥)
         16 fluidounces = 1 pint (pt or O)
               2 pints = 1 quart (qt)
              4 quarts = 1 gallon (C)
```

The unit of fluid measure is a minim (Figure 6-1). This is approximately the quantity of water that would weigh a grain. The symbol of minim is ♏. The symbol O is the abbreviation for the Latin word *octarius*. It means an eighth of a gallon and is the same as a pint. The symbol C is taken from the Latin word *congius*. It means a vessel or container that holds a gallon.

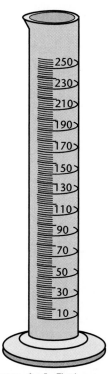

Figure 6-1 *Fluid measures.*

It might be of aid to visualize a dram as approximately equal to one teaspoonful in household measure.

The **minim** (♏) is the approximate equivalent of the drop, but it is not identical to the drop. Minims are not an accurate method of measuring medicines and, wherever possible, **milliliters** or cubic **centimeters** should be used.

Imperial System of Volume

In Canada, the imperial system of volume measurement is used. The names of the units (that is, minims, fluidounces, pints, quarts, gallons) are the same as those used in the apothecary system, but the volumes are somewhat different.

```
                60 minims = 1 fluidram
8 fluidrams or 480 minims = 1 fluidounce
           20 fluidounces = 1 pint
                  2 pints = 1 quart
                 4 quarts = 1 gallon
```

NOTE: In the imperial system, 20 fluidounces equals 1 pint; in the apothecary system, 16 fluidounces equals 1 pint.

Metric System

The **metric system** was invented by the French in the late eighteenth century. A committee of the Academy of Sciences, working under government authority, recommended a standard unit of linear measure. For a basis of measurement they chose a quarter of the earth's circumference measured across the poles. One ten-millionth of this distance was accepted as the standard unit of linear measure.

The committee calculated the distance from the equator to the North Pole from surveys that had been made along the meridian that passes through Paris. The distance divided by 10,000,000 was chosen as the unit of length, or the meter.

Metric standards were adopted in France in 1799. The International Metric Convention met in Paris in 1875, and as a result of this meeting the International Bureau of Weights and Measures was formed. The first task of the International Bureau of Weights and Measures was the preparation of an international standard meter bar and an international standard kilogram weight. Duplicates of these were made for all countries participating in the convention.

A measurement line was selected on the international standard meter bar. The distance between the two lines of measurement on the bar is the official unit of the metric system. The standards given to the United States are preserved at the National Institute of Standards and Technology, Gaithersburg, Maryland. There are 25.4 millimeters in 1 inch (2.5 centimeters).

The metric system uses the meter as the unit of length, the **liter** as the unit of volume, and the **gram** as the measurement of weight.

Units of Length (Meter)		
1 millimeter = 0.001	meaning 1/1000
1 centimeter = 0.01	meaning 1/100
1 decimeter = 0.1	meaning 1/10
1 meter = 1	meter

Units of Volume (Liter)

1 milliliter = 0.001	meaning 1/1000
1 centiliter = 0.01	meaning 1/100
1 deciliter = 0.1	meaning 1/10
1 liter = 1	liter

Units of Weight (Gram)

1 microgram = 0.000001	meaning 1/1,000,000
1 milligram = 0.001	meaning 1/1000
1 centigram = 0.01	meaning 1/100
1 decigram = 0.1	meaning 1/10
1 gram = 1	gram

Other Prefixes

Deca means ten or 10 times as much. *Hecto* means one hundred or 100 times as much. *Kilo* means one thousand or 1000 times as much. These three prefixes can be combined with the words meter, gram, or liter.

EXAMPLES:

> 1 decaliter = 10 liters
> 1 hectometer = 100 meters
> 1 kilogram = 1000 grams

Arabic numbers are used to write metric doses.

EXAMPLES: 500 milligrams, 5 grams, 15 milliliters

Prefixes added to the units (meter, liter, or gram) indicate smaller or larger units. All units are derived by dividing or multiplying by 10, 100, or 1000.

Common Metric Equivalents

> 1 milliliter (ml) = 1 cubic centimeter (cc)
> 1000 milliliters (ml) = 1 liter (L) = 1000 cubic centimeters (cc)
> 1000 milligrams (mg) = 1 gram (g)
> 1000 micrograms (μg) = 1 milligram (mg)
> 1,000,000 micrograms (μg) = 1 gram (g)
> 1000 grams (g) = 1 kilogram (kg)

Differentiate between metric and apothecary weights. Mark each of the following M for metric or A for apothecary.

1. grain = _____
2. microgram = _____
3. milligram = _____
4. dram = _____
5. gram = _____

Differentiate between metric and apothecary volume. Mark each of the following M for metric or A for apothecary.

1. minim = _____
2. milliliter = _____
3. fluidram = _____
4. fluidounce = _____
5. liter = _____

Differentiate among metric weight, metric volume, apothecary weight, and apothecary volume. Mark each of the following MW for metric weight, MV for metric volume, AW for apothecary weight, or AV for apothecary volume.

1. minim = _____
2. microgram = _____
3. milliliter = _____
4. liter = _____
5. gram = _____

Conversion of Metric and Apothecary Units

The first step in calculating the drug dosage is to make sure that the drug ordered and the drug source on hand are *both* in the same *system of measurement* (preferably in the metric system) and in the *same unit of weight* for example, both **milligrams** or both grams). See Table 6-1.

Converting Grams (Metric) to Grains (Apothecary) or Milliliters (Metric) to Minims (Apothecary)

(1 g = 15 gr; 1 ml = 15 ℳ.)
Multiply the number of grams (or milliliters) by 15.

EXAMPLES:

1. Change 30 grams to grains
   30 × 15 = 450 gr
2. Change 1 gram to grains

$$\frac{1\text{ g} \times 15\text{ gr}}{g} = 15\text{ gr}$$

Use ratio and proportion.

$$\frac{g}{1} : \frac{gr}{1} :: \frac{g}{15} : \frac{gr}{x}$$
$$x = 15$$
$$1\text{ g} = \text{gr }15$$

Change the following grams (metric) to grains (apothecary).

> a. 15 g = _____ gr
> b. 30 g = _____ gr
> c. 1 g = _____ gr

Converting Grains (Apothecary) to Grams (Metric)

(1 gr = 0.060 g)
Divide the number of grains by 15 (or multiply by 0.060).

EXAMPLES:

1. Change 30 grains to grams.
   30 ÷ 15 = 2 g
2. Change 5 grains to grams.

$$\frac{0.060\text{ g}}{gr} \times 5\text{ gr} = 0.3\text{ g}$$

Change grains (apothecary) to grams (metric).

> a. 1 grain = _____ g
> b. 5 grains = _____ g
> c. 10 grains = _____ g
> d. 15 grains = _____ g

In the following example, both the physician's order and the medication available are in the metric system. They are

Table 6-1

Metric Doses and Apothecary Equivalents

LIQUID MEASURE		WEIGHT	
METRIC	**APPROXIMATE APOTHECARY EQUIVALENTS**	**METRIC**	**APPROXIMATE APOTHECARY EQUIVALENTS**
1000 ml	**1 quart**	**30 g**	**1 ounce**
750 ml	1 ½ pints	15 g	4 drams
500 ml	**1 pint**	100g	2 ½ drams
250 ml	8 fluidounces	7.5 g	2 drams
200 ml	7 fluidounces	6 g	90 grains
100 ml	3 ½ fluidounces	5 g	75 grains
50 ml	1 ⅔ fluidounces	3 g	45 grains
30 ml	**1 fluidounce**	2 g	30 grains (½ dram)
15 ml	4 fluidrams	1.5 g	22 grains
10 ml	2 ½ fluidrams	**1 g**	**15 grains**
8 ml	2 fluidrams	0.75 g	12 grains
5 ml	1 ¼ fluidrams	0.6 g	10 grains
4 ml	1 fluidrams	**0.5 g**	**7 ½ grains**
3 ml	45 minims	0.4 g	6 grains
2 ml	30 minims	0.3 g	5 grains
1 ml*	**15 or 16 minims**	0.25 g	4 grains
0.75 ml	12 minims	0.2 g	3 grains
0.6 ml	10 minims	0.15 g	2 ½ grains
0.5 ml	8 minims	0.12 g	2 grains
0.3 ml	5 minims	0.1 g	1 ½ grains
0.25 ml	4 minims	75 mg	1 ¼ grains
0.2 ml	3 minims	**60 mg**	**1 grain**
0.1 ml	1 ½ minims	50 mg	¾ grain
0.06 ml	**1 minim**	40 mg	⅔ grain
0.05 ml	¾ minim	**30 mg**	**½ grain**
0.03 ml	½ minim	25 mg	⅜ grain
		20 mg	⅓ grain
Metric	**✤Imperial Eqivalent**	**15 mg**	**¼ grain**
28.4 ml	1 fluidounce	12 mg	⅕ grain
568 ml	1 pint (20 fl oz)	10 mg	⅙ grain
1136 ml	1 quart	8 mg	⅛ grain
(1.136 L)	(40 fl oz)	6 mg	⅒ grain
4546 ml	1 gallon	5 mg	1/12 grain
(4.546 L)	(160 fl oz)	4 mg	1/15 grain
		3 mg	1/20 grain
		2 mg	1/30 grain
		1.5 mg	1/40 grain
		1.2 mg	1/50 grain
		1 mg	**1/60 grain**
		0.8 mg	1/80 grain
		0.6 mg	**1/100 grain**
		0.5 mg	1/120 grain
		0.4 mg	**1/150 grain**
		0.3 mg	**1/200 grain**
		0.25 mg	1/250 grain
		0.2 mg	1/300 grain
		0.15 mg	1/400 grain
		0.12 mg	1/500 grain
		0.1 mg	1/600 grain

Modified from *United States Pharmacopeia XX.* Equivalents in bold type should be memorized.

*A milliliter (ml) is approximately equivalent to a cubic centimeter (cc).

not both in the *same unit of weight* within the metric system.

> **EXAMPLE:** The physician orders the patient to have 0.250 g of a drug. The label on the bottle of medicine says 250 mg, meaning that each capsule contains 250 mg of the drug.
> To change the gram dose into milligrams multiply 0.250 by 1000 and move the decimal point three places to the right (a milligram is one thousandth of a gram); 0.250 g = 250 mg, so you would give one tablet of this drug.
> **TRY THIS ONE:** The physician orders the patient to have 0.1 g of a drug. The label on the bottle states that the strength of the drug is 100 mg/capsule.
> To change the gram dose into milligrams, move the decimal point three places to the right: 0.1 g = 100 mg, exactly what the bottle label strength states.

Convert the following grams (g) to milligrams (mg):

0.2 g = _____ mg
0.250 g = _____ mg
0.125 g = _____ mg
0.0006 g = _____ mg
0.004 g = _____ mg

Converting Milligrams (Metric) to Grams (Metric)

(1000 mg = 1 g)
Divide by 1000 or move the decimal point of the milligrams three places to the left.

> **EXAMPLES:** 200 mg = 0.2 g
> 0.6 mg = 0.0006 g

Convert the following milligrams to grams:

0.4 mg = _____ g
0.12 mg = _____ g
0.2 mg = _____ g
0.1 mg = _____ g
500 mg = _____ g
125 mg = _____ g
100 mg = _____ g
200 mg = _____ g
50 mg = _____ g
400 mg = _____ g

Can you take the gram dosages in these answers and convert them to milligrams?

Converting Grains (Apothecary) to Milligrams (Metric)

(1 gr = 60 mg)
Multiply the number of grains by 60.

> **EXAMPLE:** Change gr to mg.
> 5 grains × 60 mg/gr = 300 mg

Solid Dosage for Oral Administration

If the dosage on hand and dosage ordered are both in the same system (metric or apothecary) and in the same unit of weight, proceed to calculate the dosage using one of these methods.

> **EXAMPLE:** Physician orders patient to have 1.0 g of ampicillin. The ampicillin bottle states that each tablet in the bottle contains 0.5 g.
> **PROBLEM:** You do not have the 1.0 g as ordered. How many tablets will you give? (Both the amount ordered and the amount available are in the same system of measurement [metric] and the same unit of weight [grams]).

SOLUTION: You may use two methods.
Method 1:

1. $\dfrac{\text{Dosage desired}}{\text{Dosage on hand}} = \dfrac{1.0\text{ g}}{0.5\text{ g}} = 2$ You will give two 0.5 g capsules to give the 1.0 g ordered.

Method 2: (Proportional)
Metric dosage ordered: Drug form
Metric dosage available: Drug form

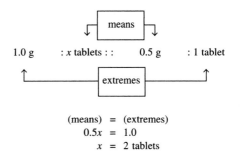

1.0 g   : x tablets : : 0.5 g : 1 tablet

(means) = (extremes)
0.5x = 1.0
x = 2 tablets

Proof: Product of means: 2 (value of x) × 0.5 = 1.0
Product of extremes: 1.0 × 1 = 1.0

If the dosage on hand and dosage ordered are both in the same system of measurement (metric or apothecary) but they are *not* in the same unit of weight within the system, the units of weight must first be converted.

> **EXAMPLE:** Physician orders 1000 milligrams (metric) of ampicillin. On hand: 0.25 grams (metric) per tablet.
>
> Rule: Converting grams (metric) to milligrams (metric) (1 g = 1000 mg) Multiply the number of grams by 1000; move the decimal point of the grams three places to the right. 0.25 g = 250 mg
>
> **SOLUTION:**

1. $\dfrac{\text{Dosage desired}}{\text{Dosage on hand}} = \dfrac{1000}{250\text{ mg}} = 4$ Give four 0.25 g tablets

2. $\dfrac{\text{mg}}{250} : \dfrac{\text{tablet}}{1} : : \dfrac{\text{mg}}{1000} : \dfrac{\text{tablet}}{x}$
   250x = 1000
   $x = \dfrac{1000}{250} = 4$ tablets

Proof: Product of means: 1 × 1000 = 1000
Product of extremes: 250 × 4 = (value of x) = 1000

Do the following conversions. (Make sure the amount ordered and source available are converted to the same system of measurement and unit of weight.)
1. Physician orders aspirin 600 mg. You have aspirin gr v per tablet. (metric and apothecary units)
2. Physician orders Gantrisin 0.25 g. You have Gantrisin 500 mg per tablet. (metric units, but different weight units)
3. Physician orders pentobarbital 200 mg. You have pentobarbital 1½ gr capsules. (metric and apothecary units)

Conversion Problems

Some students understand problems in tablet dosage for oral administration if presented with their fractional equivalents as follows:
1. Physician orders patient to receive 2 g of a drug in oral tablet forms. The medicine bottle label states that the

strength on hand is 0.5 g. This means each tablet in the bottle is the strength 0.5 g.

How many tablets would be given to the patient? 1, 2, 3, 4, or 5? Answer: 4

What strength is ordered? 2 g

What strength is on the bottle label? 0.5 g

What is the fractional equivalent of 0.5 g? ½ g

How many ½ g (0.5 g) tablets would equal 2 g? 4

$$2 \div \frac{1}{2} = \frac{2}{1} \times \frac{2}{1} = 4 \text{ tablets}$$

2. Physician orders patient to receive 0.2 mg of a drug in oral tablet form. The medicine bottle label states that the strength on hand is 0.1 mg. This means each tablet in the bottle is the strength 0.1 mg.

How many tablets would be given to the patient? 1, 2, 3, or 4? Answer: 2 tablets

What strength is ordered? 0.2 mg

What is the fractional equivalent of 0.2 mg? ²/₁₀

What strength is on the bottle label (on hand)? 0.1 mg

What is the fractional equivalent of 0.1 mg? ¹/₁₀

How many ¹/₁₀ mg (0.1 mg) tablets would equal ²/₁₀ mg (0.2 mg)? 2

```
 0.1 mg = ¹/₁₀ mg or 1 tablet
+0.1 mg = ¹/₁₀ mg or 1 tablet
 0.2 mg = ²/₁₀ mg or 2 tablets
```

Dosage desired ÷ Dosage on hand =

$$or \quad \frac{2}{10} \div \frac{1}{10} = \frac{2}{\cancel{10}} \times \frac{\cancel{10}}{1} = 2 \text{ tablets}$$

3. Physician orders patient to receive 0.5 mg of a drug in oral tablet form. The medicine bottle label states that the strength on hand is 0.25 mg. This means each tablet in the bottle is the strength 0.25 mg.

How many tablets would be given to the patient? 1, 2, 3, 4, or 5? Answer: 2 tablets

What strength is ordered? 0.5 mg

What fractional equivalent equals 0.5 mg? ½ mg

What strength is on the bottle label? 0.25 mg

What fractional equivalent equals the strength on hand? ¼ mg

How many ¼ mg (0.25 mg) tablets would equal ½ mg (0.5 mg)? 2

```
 0.25 mg = ¼ mg or 1 tablet
+0.25 mg = ¼ mg or 1 tablet
 0.50 mg = ½ mg or 2 tablets
```

Dosage desired ÷ Dosage on hand =

$$or \quad \frac{1}{2} \div \frac{1}{4} = \frac{1}{2} \times \frac{4}{1} = 2 \text{ tablets}$$

4. Physician orders patient to receive 0.25 mg of a drug in oral tablet form. The medicine bottle label states that the strength on hand is 0.5 mg. This means that every tablet in the bottle is the strength 0.5 mg.

How many tablets would be given? ½, 1, 1½, 2, 2½, 3, 4, or 5? Answer: ½ tablet

What strength did the physician order? 0.25 mg

What is the fractional equivalent of the strength the physician ordered? ¼ mg

What strength is on the bottle label? 0.5 mg

What is the fractional equivalent of the strength on the bottle label (on hand)? ½ mg

Which is less: 0.5 mg (½ mg) or 0.25 mg (¼ mg)? Answer: 0.25 mg (¼ mg)

Was the amount ordered less than the strength on hand or more? Answer: Less

$$0.5 \text{ mg} = \tfrac{1}{2} \text{ mg or 1 tablet}$$
$$0.25 \text{ mg} = \tfrac{1}{4} \text{ mg or half as much or } \tfrac{1}{2} \text{ tablet}$$
$$or \quad \frac{1}{4} \div \frac{1}{2} = \frac{1}{4} \times \frac{2}{1} = \frac{1}{2} \text{ tablet}$$

If the medication is also available in 0.25 mg tablets, request that size from the pharmacy. A tablet should be divided only when scored; even then the practice should be avoided.

Liquid Dosage for Oral Administration

1. Physician orders 60 ml of a liquid medication. How many ounces will be given?

To convert milliliters to ounces, divide milliliters by 30:

$$60 \text{ ml} \div 30 \text{ (30 ml = 1 oz)} = 2 \text{ oz}$$

2. Physician orders 45 ml. How many ounces will be given?

$$45 \div 30 = 1\tfrac{1}{2} \text{ oz}$$

3. Physician orders 6 drams. How many milliliters (cubic centimeters) will you give?

To convert drams to milliliters, multiply drams by 4:

$$4(4 \text{ ml} = 1 \text{ dram}) \times 6 = 24 \text{ ml (cc)}$$

Converting Weight to Kilograms (1 kg = 2.2 lb)

Many physicians request that the metric measure be used to record the body weight of the patient. Because the scales used in many hospitals are calibrated in pounds, conversion from pounds to **kilograms** is required.

1. To convert weight in kilograms to pounds, multiply the kilogram weight by 2.2.

EXAMPLE: 25 kg × 2.2 lb = 55 lb

Convert the following:

35 kg = _____ lb
16 kg = _____ lb
65 kg = _____ lb

2. To convert weight in pounds to kilograms, divide the weight in pounds by 2.2.

EXAMPLE: 140 lb ÷ 2.2 kg = 63.6 kg

Convert the following:

125 lb = _____ kg
9 lb = _____ kg
180 lb = _____ kg

The weight of a liter of water at 40° C is 2.2 pounds.

CALCULATION OF INTRAVENOUS FLUID AND MEDICATION ADMINISTRATION RATES

Objective

I. Use formulas to calculate intravenous fluid and medicine administration rates.

Key Words

administration set	microdrip
drip chamber	drop factor
macrodrip	rounding

Intravenous Fluid Orders, Drip Rates, Pumps, and Rounding

Intravenous (IV) solutions (fluids) consist of a liquid (solvent) containing one or more dissolved substances (solutes). The physician orders a specific type and volume of solution to be infused over a specific time span. (See Chapter 9 for a listing of common intravenous solutions and abbreviations.)

The order can be written in any of the following three ways:

1. 1000 ml 5% dextrose and water (D$_5$/W) to infuse over the next 8 hr
2. 1 L D$_5$/W IV over next 8 hr
3. Infuse 5% dextrose at 125 ml/hr

Administration sets used to deliver a specified volume of solution are different depending on the company manufacturing the set. The administration set can vary in different lengths and diameters of tubing, the presence or absence of in-line filters, and a differing number of Y-ports (sites).

The **drip chamber** of the administration set is either a **macrodrip,** a chamber that delivers large-size drips, or a **microdrip,** a chamber that delivers small-size drops.

All microdrip chambers deliver 60 drops (gtts) per ml. The microdrip administration set is used whenever a small volume of intravenous solution is ordered to be infused over a specified time (for example, neonatal, pediatric units). In some clinical settings a microdrip administration set is used whenever the volume of solution to infuse is below 100 ml per hour.

The manufacturer of the macrodrip administration set has standardized the *drops* per milliter, called the **drop factor** (DF), for the specific brand of administration set as follows:

Company name	Drop factor (gtts/ml)
Abbott	15
Baxter-Travenol	10
Cutter	20
IVAC	20
McGraw	13

The box containing the administration set always has the drop factor printed on the label.

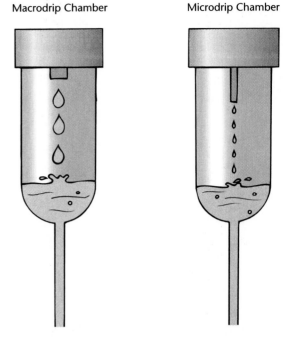

Macrodrip Chamber   Microdrip Chamber

Rounding

Not all calculations used to compute intravenous fluid administration rates divide out evenly; it is necessary to have a uniform way to **round** the answers to whole numbers. One method commonly used is to divide the numbers, carry the calculations to hundredths, and round to tenths. If the tenths is 0.5 or above, increase the answer to the next whole number. If the tenths is below 0.5, leave the whole number at the current value.

EXAMPLES:

$$
\begin{aligned}
167.57 &= 167.6 = 168\\
167.44 &= 167.4 = 167\\
32.15 &= 32.2 = 32\\
32.45 &= 32.5 = 33
\end{aligned}
$$

The nurse must be able to calculate the rate for the prescribed infusion whether it is being given as an additive in the primary intravenous fluid (using a secondary set called a piggyback or rider setup with calibrated regulators) or is being infused by means of an electronic infusion pump.

Volumetric and Nonvolumetric Pumps

When determining the flow rate for infusion pumps, the type of infusion pump must first be determined. Pumps are categorized as either volumetric or nonvolumetric. Volumetric pumps are set to measure the volume being infused in milliliters per hour, whereas nonvolumetric pumps are set in drops per minute. (Check the individual pump being used to see the type of calibration [ml/hr or gtts/min] printed on the display window of the pump.)

Calculation of Flow Rates

Milliliters per Hour (ml/hr)

The formula for the calculation of flow rates is as follows. Divide the total volume in milliliters (no. ml) of fluid ordered for infusion by the total number of *hours* (no. hr) the infusion is to run. This will equal the milliliters per hour (ml/hr) the infusion is to run.

$$\frac{\text{no. ml}}{\text{no. hr}} = \text{ml/hr}$$

EXAMPLE: Infuse 1000 ml lactated ringer's (LR) solution over 10 hr.

$$\frac{\text{no. ml} = 1000 \text{ ml}}{\text{no. hr} = 10 \text{ hr}} = 100 \text{ ml/hr}$$

Calculate the following problems:

Doctor's order:	Duration of infusion	Rate (ml/hr)
1000 ml 5% dextrose in water	12 hr	= _____ ml/hr
1000 ml lactated ringer's	6 hr	= _____ ml/hr
500 ml 0.9% sodium chloride	4 hr	= _____ ml/hr

Calculating Rates of Infusion for Other Than 1 Hour

The nurse must be able to convert infusion rates given in minutes to milliliters per hour because volumetric pumps are calibrated in millimeters. The formula is as follows: the volume of solution ordered times 60 minutes per hour divided by time (in minutes) to administer.

$$\frac{\text{no. ml to infuse} \times 60 \text{ min/hr}}{\text{time (min)}} = \text{ml/hr}$$

$$\frac{\text{no. ml to infuse} \times 60 \text{ ~~min~~/hr}}{\text{time (~~min~~)}} = \text{ml/hr}$$

Calculate the following problems:

Doctor's order	Duration of infusion	Rate (ml/hr)
50 ml 0.9% NaCl with ampicillin 1 g	20 min	= _____ ml/hr
150 ml D$_5$/W with gentamicin 80 mg	30 min	= _____ ml/hr
50 ml 0.9% NaCl with ondansetron 32 mg	15 min	= _____ ml/hr

Drops per Minute (gtts/min)

The nurse must calculate drops per minute whenever a drug infusion is given with the use of a secondary administration set, a nonvolumetric infusion pump, or a calibrated cylinder. The formula is as follows: multiply the total volume (milliliters) to infuse times the drop factor and divide by the time in minutes.

$$\frac{\text{no. ml to infuse} \times \text{DF (gtts/ml)}}{\text{time (min)}} = \text{gtts/min}$$

$$\frac{\text{no. ~~ml~~ to infuse} \times \text{DF (gtts/~~ml~~)}}{\text{time (min)}} = \text{gtts/min}$$

Remember that the answer, *drops*, cannot be given as a fraction; as previously discussed, the answer must be rounded to a whole number.

EXAMPLE: 31.4 gtts = 31 gtts; 31.5 gtts = 32 gtts.

Calculate the following problems.

Directions: Use a drop factor of 15 gtts/ml for volumes of *100 ml or greater* per hour; use a microdrip (60 gtts/hr) for volumes below 100/hr. (NOTE: Whenever a microdrip is used, milliliters per hour equals drops per minute, so no calculations are needed.)

Doctor's order	Duration of infusion	= Rate (ml/hr)
125 ml D$_5$/W	60 min	= _____ ml/hr
100 ml lactated ringer's	60 min	= _____ ml/hr
50 ml 0.9% NaCl	20 min	= _____ ml/hr

Drugs Ordered in Units per Hour or Milligrams per Hour

Physicians may order drugs in units per hour (U/hr) or in milligrams per hour (mg/hr). Drugs ordered in this way are administered by means of an electronic infusion pump. The formula is as follows. Set up a proportion:

Total volume of solution : total units or milligrams of drug added as *x* amount of solution : ordered amount of drugs in units or milligrams

EXAMPLE: U/hr

Doctor's order: mix 10,000 U heparin in 1000 ml D$_5$/W; infuse 80 units per hour.
1000 ml : 10,000 units as *x* ml : 80 U
Multiply the means: 10,000 U × *x* = 10,000 U*x*.
Multiply the extremes: 1000 ml × 80 U/hr = 80,000 ml - U/hr.
Divide both sides of equation by number with *x*.

$$\frac{10,000 \text{ U}x}{10,000 \text{ U}} = \frac{80,000 \text{ ml-U/hr}}{10,000 \text{ U}}$$

$$\frac{\cancel{10,000 \text{ U}}x}{\cancel{10,000 \text{ U}}} = \frac{\cancel{80,000} \text{ ml-}\cancel{U}\text{/hr}}{\cancel{10,000 \text{ U}}}$$

Reduce: *x* = 8 ml/hr

Set infusion pump at 8 ml per hour to deliver 80 units of heparin per hour.

EXAMPLE: ml/hr

The doctor could order the number of milliliters of heparin per hour rather than specifying the order in units per hour.
Mix 10,000 U heparin in 1000 ml D$_5$/W; infuse at 15 ml/hr. How many units of heparin is being delivered per hour?

1000 ml : 10,000 U as 15 ml : *x* U

Multiply the means: 10,000 U × 15 ml = 150,000 U–ml.
Multiply the extremes: 1000 ml × *x* = 1000 ml*x*.
Divide both sides of equation by number with *x*.

$$\frac{1000 \text{ ml}x}{1000 \text{ ml}} = \frac{150,000 \text{ U} - \text{ml}}{1000 \text{ ml}}$$

$$\frac{\cancel{1000 \text{ ml}}x}{\cancel{1000 \text{ ml}}} = \frac{\cancel{150,000} \text{ U} - \cancel{\text{ml}}}{\cancel{1000 \text{ ml}}}$$

Reduce: *x* = 150 U

EXAMPLE: milligrams/hr
Doctor's order: mix 500 mg dopamine in 500 ml of D$_5$ /0.45% NaCl to infuse at 30 mg/hr.

500 ml : 500 mg as x : 30 mg/hr

Multiply the means: 500 mg × x = 500 mg-x.
Multiply the extremes: 500 ml × 30 mg/hr = 15,000 ml–mg/hr.
Divide both sides of equation by the number with x.

$$\frac{(500 \text{ mg})(x)}{500 \text{ mg}} = \frac{(15000 \text{ ml})(\text{mg/hr})}{500 \text{ mg}}$$

$$\frac{(500 \text{ mg})(x)}{500 \text{ mg}} = \frac{(\overset{30}{\cancel{15000}} \text{ ml})(\text{mg/hr})}{\cancel{500 \text{ mg}}}$$

Reduce: x = 30 ml/hr

Set infusion pump at 30 ml/hr

Calculate the following problems:
Doctor's order:

heparin 20,000 U in 1 L lactated   =   _____ ml/hr
Ringer's
infuse at 120 U/hr

Regular insulin 100 U in 100 ml   =   _____ ml/hr
normal saline (NS)
infuse at 15 units/hour

FAHRENHEIT AND CENTIGRADE (CELSIUS) TEMPERATURES

Objective

I. Demonstrate proficiency in performing conversions between the centigrade and Fahrenheit systems of temperature measurement.

Key Words

centigrade   Celsius
Fahrenheit

It is necessary for the nurse to be familiar with both the centigrade and the Fahrenheit scales. Here are some of the main points about **centigrade** and **Fahrenheit** thermometers (Figure 6-2).
1. Centigrade **(Celsius)** and Fahrenheit thermometers look alike.
2. Both are made of the same-sized tube containing mercury.
3. The column of mercury in each thermometer rises to the same height when placed in a beaker of freezing water and to the same height in boiling water.
4. The centigrade and Fahrenheit thermometers differ from each other in the way they are graduated.
5. On the centigrade thermometer the point at which water freezes is marked "0."
6. On the Fahrenheit thermometer the point at which water freezes is marked "32."
7. The boiling point in centigrade is 100°.
8. The boiling point in Fahrenheit is 212°.
9. The space between the 0° point and the 100° point on the centigrade scale is divided into equal spaces or degrees.

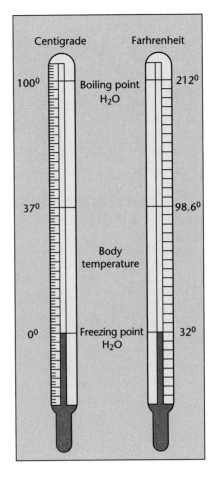

Figure 6-2 *Clinical thermometers.*

10. The value of graduations (degrees) on the centigrade thermometer differs from the value of degrees on the Fahrenheit thermometer.
11. There are 180 spaces between the freezing and boiling points on the Fahrenheit thermometer.
12. To change readings on the centigrade thermometer to the Fahrenheit scale, the centigrade reading is multiplied by 180/100 or 9/5 and then added to 32.
13. To change Fahrenheit reading to centigrade scale, subtract 32 from the Fahrenheit reading and multiply by 5/9.
   To understand why thermometer readings are interpreted in the way explained in point 12 and to understand your conversion formula better, read points 4 to 12 again several times.

Formula for Converting Fahrenheit Temperature to Centigrade Temperature

$$(\text{Fahrenheit} - 32) \times \frac{5}{9} = \text{centigrade}$$

$$(\text{F} - 32) \times \frac{5}{9} = \text{C}$$

EXAMPLE: Change 212° F to C.

$$(F - 32) \times \frac{5}{9} = C$$
$$212 - 32 = 180$$
$$180 \times \frac{5}{9} = \frac{900}{9} = 100°C$$

Convert the following Fahrenheit temperatures to centigrade:

$$98.6° \text{ F} = \underline{\hspace{2cm}} ° \text{ C}$$
$$102.4° \text{ F} = \underline{\hspace{2cm}} ° \text{ C}$$
$$95.2° \text{ F} = \underline{\hspace{2cm}} ° \text{ C}$$

Formula for Converting Centigrade Temperature to Fahrenheit Temperature

$$\left(\text{Centigrade} \times \frac{9}{5} \right) + 32 = \text{Fahrenheit}$$
$$\left(C \times \frac{9}{5} \right) + 32 = F$$

EXAMPLE: Change 100° C to F.

$$\left(C \times \frac{9}{5} \right) + 32 = F$$
$$100 \times \frac{9}{5} = \frac{900}{5} = 180$$
$$180 + 32 = 212°F$$

Convert the following centigrade temperatures to Fahrenheit:

$$37° \text{ C} = \underline{\hspace{2cm}} ° \text{ F}$$
$$35° \text{ C} = \underline{\hspace{2cm}} ° \text{ F}$$
$$41° \text{ C} = \underline{\hspace{2cm}} ° \text{ F}$$

Try these problems in converting centigrade to Fahrenheit and Fahrenheit to centigrade.

1. The nurse takes the following temperatures with Fahrenheit clinical thermometers: patient A, 104° F; patient B, 99° F; patient C, 101° F. The physician asks what the centigrade temperature is for each patient. Work your problems to convert Fahrenheit temperatures to centigrade. Check your answers. (Answers: patient A, 40° C; patient B, 37.2° C; patient C, 38.3° C.)

2. The nurse takes the following temperatures with centigrade clinical thermometers: patient D, 37° C; patient E, 37.8° C; patient F, 38° C. The physician asks what the Fahrenheit temperature is for each patient. Work your problems to convert centigrade to Fahrenheit. Check your answers. (Answers: patient D, 98.6° F; patient E, 100° F; patient F, 100.4° F.)

Many hospitals today have conversion tables available on the wards. This saves time and possibility of error in doing problems. The nurse simply refers to the particular temperature on one scale and finds the conversion listed in a column beside it. However, try to remember the formula for each conversion.

Most larger hospitals currently use electronic thermometers that give centigrade or Fahrenheit readings.

7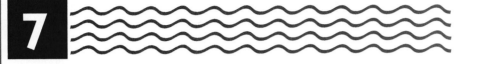

Principles of Medication Administration

CHAPTER CONTENT

Before medications are administered, it is important that the nurse understand the professional responsibilities associated with medication administration, drug orders, medication delivery systems, and the nursing process as it relates to drug therapy. Lack of knowledge of the nurse's overall responsibilities in the system will, at the least, result in delays in receiving and administering medications, but it may also result in serious administration errors. Either way, the patient loses and may suffer unnecessarily.

LEGAL AND ETHICAL CONSIDERATIONS

Objectives

1. Research the Nurse Practice Act in the state where practicing. Identify the limitations relating to medication administration placed on licensed practical nurses, registered nurses, and nurse clinicians.

2. Study the policies and procedures of the practice setting to identify specific regulations concerning medication administration by licensed practical nurses, registered nurses, and nurse clinicians.

Key Word

Nurse Practice Act

The practice of nursing under a professional license is a privilege, not a right. In accepting the privilege, the nurse must understand that this responsibility includes being held accountable for one's actions and judgments during the performance of professional duties. An understanding of the **Nurse Practice Act** and of the rules and regulations estab-

lished by the state boards of nursing for the various levels of entry (that is, practical nurse, registered nurse, and nurse practitioner) is a solid foundation for beginning practice.

In addition to state rules and regulations, nurses must be familiar with the established policies and procedures of the employing health care agency. These policies must adhere to the minimum standards of the state board of nursing, but agency policies may be more stringent than those recognized by the state. Employment within the agency implies the willingness of the professional to adhere to established standards and to work within established guidelines to make necessary changes in the standards. Examples of policy statements relating to medication administration include the following: (1) educational requirements of professionals authorized to administer medications (many health care facilities require that a written test be passed to attest to the necessary knowledge and skills of medication preparation, calculation, and administration before being granted approval to administer any medications); (2) approved lists of intravenous solutions and medications that the nurse can start or add to an existing infusion; and (3) lists of restricted medications (such as antineoplastic agents, magnesium sulfate, allergy extracts, lidocaine, RhoGAM, Imferon, and heparin) that may be administered only by certain personnel.

Before administering any medication, the nurse must have a current license to practice nursing, a clear policy statement that authorizes the act, and a medication order signed by a licensed physician or dentist. The nurse must understand the individual patient's diagnosis and the symptoms that correlate with the rationale for drug use. The nurse should also know why a medication is ordered, the expected actions, usual dosage, route of administration, minor side effects to expect, adverse effects to report, and contraindications of the use of a particular drug. If drugs are to be administered using the same syringe or at the same intravenous (IV) site, drug compatibility should be confirmed before administration. If unsure of any of these key medication points, the nurse must consult an authoritative resource or the hospital pharmacist *before* the administration of a medication. The nurse must be accurate in the calculation, preparation, and administration of medications. The nurse must assess the patient to be certain that both therapeutic and adverse effects associated with the medication regimen are reported. Nurses must be able to collect patient data at regularly scheduled intervals and to record observations in the patient's chart for evaluation of the effectiveness of the treatment. Claiming unfamiliarity with any of these nursing responsibilities when an avoidable complication arises is unacceptable; it is considered negligence of nursing responsibility.

Nurses must take an active role in the education of the patient and family in preparation for discharge from the health care environment. (A person's health will improve only to the extent that the patient understands how to take care of himself or herself.) Specific teaching goals should be developed and implemented. Nursing observations and progress toward mastery of skills should be charted to verify the degree of understanding attained.

PATIENT CHARTS

Objectives

1. Identify the basic categories of information available in a patient's chart.
2. Study the patient charts at different practice settings to identify the various formats used to chart patient data.
3. Cite the information contained in a Kardex and describe the purpose of this file.

Key Words

summary sheet	nurses' notes
physician's order form	laboratory tests record
graphic record	consultation reports
history and physical examination form	medication administration record (MAR)
progress notes	Kardex records

The patient's chart is a primary source of information that is necessary in patient assessment so that the nurse may make and implement plans for patient care. It is also the place for the nurse to provide a written record documenting nursing assessments performed, observations reported to the physician for further verification, basic nursing measures implemented (for example, daily bath and treatments), patient teaching performed, and observed responses to therapy.

This document serves as the communications link among all members of the health care team regarding the patient's status, care provided, and progress. It is a legal document that describes the patient's health, lists diagnostic and therapeutic procedures initiated, and describes the patient's response to these measures. The chart must be kept current as long as the patient is in the hospital. After the patient's discharge, it is stored in the medical records department until needed again. While in medical records, the chart may be used for research to compare responses to selected therapy in a sampling of patients with similar diagnoses.

Contents of Patient Charts

Although each health care facility uses a somewhat different format, the basic patient chart consists of the following elements.

Summary sheet. This sheet gives the patient's name, address, date of birth, attending physician, sex, marital status, allergies, nearest relative, occupation and employer, insurance carrier and other payment arrangements, religious preference, date and time of admission to the hospital, previous hospital admissions, and admitting problem or diagnosis. The date and time of discharge will be added when appropriate.

Physician's order form. The physician orders all procedures and treatments on this form (Figure 7-1). These orders include general care (activity, diet, frequency of vital signs), laboratory tests to be completed, other diagnostic procedures (such as x-rays, electrocardiogram [ECG], computed tomography [CT] scans), and all medications and treatments (such as physical therapy, occupational therapy).

Graphic record. This is a list of the vital signs, fluid intake and output, activity level, and other information used regularly for assessment of the patient's status (Figure 7-2, *A* and *B*).

History and physical examination form. On admission to the hospital, the patient is interviewed by the physician and given a physical examination. The physician records the findings here and lists the problems to be corrected (the diagnoses).

Progress notes. The physician uses this sheet to record frequent observations of the patient's health status. In some hospitals, other health professionals, such as pharmacists, dietitians, and physical therapists, may record observations and suggestions.

Nurses' notes. Although format varies between institutions, the nurses' notes is where nurses record ongoing assessments of the patient's condition: responses to nursing interventions ordered by the physician (such as treatments or medications) or those initiated by the nurse (skin care or patient education); evaluations of the effectiveness of nursing interventions; procedures completed by other health care professionals (such as wound cleaning by a physician or fitting for a prosthesis by a fitter); and other pertinent information, such as physician or family visits and the patient's responses after these visits (Figure 7-3, p. 68). Entries may be made on the nurses' notes throughout a shift, but general guidelines include the following: (1) completing records immediately after making contacts with and assessments of the patient (that is, when first admitted or returning from a diagnostic procedure or therapy); (2) recording all prn medications immediately after administration, and the effectiveness of the medication; and (3) recording immediately before leaving the patient for extended periods of times, such as lunch or coffee breaks. In addition to accurately charting the observations in a clear, concise form, the nurse should report significant changes in a patient's status or assessments to the charge nurse. The charge nurse will then make a nursing judgment regarding notification of the attending physician.

Prn medication record. Some clinical settings use a prn (from the Latin *pro re nata,* meaning "as circumstances require") medication record rather than nurses' notes to record the date, time, prn medication administered and dose, reason for administering the prn medication, and patient's response to the drug given (Figure 7-4, p. 68).

Laboratory tests record. All laboratory test results are kept together in one section of the chart. Hospitals using computerized reports may list consecutive values of the same test once that test has been repeated several times (such as the electrolytes). Other hospitals may attach small report forms to a full-sized backing sheet as each report returns

PHYSICIAN'S ORDER FORM

Addressograph here:

016-28-3978
Joseph Lorenzo
18 Bush Ave.
Hometown, U.S.A.

Martindale Hometown Hospital
Hometown, U.S.A.

Dr. M. Martin
Unit-6W, Rm. 621

Please Indicate Allergies

None	Codeine	Penicillin	Sulfa	Aspirin	Others

Date	Time	Prob. No.	Physician's Orders	Physician	Progress Record
1/6/96	3:00 p.m.	6	Erythromycin 250 mg, po		
			q6h x 8 days	M. Martin	

Figure 7-1 *Physician's order form and progress record.*

Temperature Graph
and Vital Signs Record

TEMP	0000	0400	0800	1200	1600	2000	0000	0400	0800	1200	1600	2000	0000	0400	0800	1200	1600	2000	0000	0400	0800	1200	1600	2000
°F																								
104°																								
103°																								
102°																								
101°																								
100°																								
99°																								
98°																								
97°																								
96°																								
95°																								
Date																								
Hosp./PO																								

VITAL SIGNS	Time	B/P	Pulse	Resp	Time	B/P	Pulse	Resp	Time	B/P	Pulse	Resp	Time	B/P	Pulse	Resp
11-7																
7-3																
3-11																

Figure 7-2 A *Vital signs record.*

DATE							
HT-WT							
Hygiene:							
Bedbath							
Partial							
Self							
Shower/tub							
Oral							
HS							
ACTIVITY:							
Bedrest							
BRP							
BRcBRP							
Dangle							
Chair/WC							
Amb							
Other							
Rails	7-3-11	7-3-11	7-3-11	7-3-11	7-3-11	7-3-11	7-3-11
DIET:	8-12-5	8-12-5	8-12-5	8-12-5	8-12-5	8-12-5	8-12-5
NPO							
Liquid							
Soft							
Regular							
Spec.							
HOLD							
OTHER:							

Intake	11-7	7-3	3-11	11-7	7-3	3-11	11-7	7-3	3-11	11-7	7-3	3-11	11-7	7-3	3-11	11-7	7-3	3-11	11-7	7-3	3-11
Oral																					
IV or Subq.																					
Blood																					
Other																					
Total 24 Hr (ml)																					
Output Urine																					
Total 24 Hr (ml) Urine																					
Emesis																					
Other																					
Total 24 Hr (ml)																					
Stool																					
Signature																					

Figure 7-2 B *Patient care record.*

Time	Output	MEDS/TX/VS

Figure 7-3 *Format of nurses' notes.*

Last Name: First Name: Room & Bed No.:   Patient No.:   Physician:

PRN MEDICATION RECORD

DATE	TIME	MEDICATION	REASON	RESPONSE	NAME OF NURSE

Figure 7-4 *Prn medication record.*

from the laboratory. Because some medication dosages are based on daily blood studies, it is important to understand where to locate these data within the patient's chart. Figure 7-5 shows a daily series of prothrombin time (PT) results.

Consultation reports. When other physicians (or other health care professionals) are asked to consult on a patient, the specialist's summary of findings, diagnoses, and recommendations for treatment are recorded in this section.

Other Diagnostic Reports. Reports of surgery, electroencephalograph (EEG), ECG, pulmonary function tests, radioactive scans, and x-ray reports are usually recorded in this section.

Medication administration record or **medication profile.** Today the medication administration record (MAR) or medication profile is usually computer generated. This ensures that the pharmacist and the nurse have identical medication profiles for the patient. Each clinical site arranges the MAR somewhat differently, but the following represents key components of the MAR.

The MAR lists all medications to be administered. The medications are usually grouped according to the following categories: Those *scheduled* on a regular basis (for example, every 6 hours or twice a day), *parenteral, stat* (from the Latin *statim,* "immediately"), and *preoperative*

orders. *Prn medications* are usually listed at the bottom of the MAR.

The MAR provides a space for recording the time when the medication is administered and by whom it is given. Generally the nurse records and initials the time when the medication is given. The nurse also places his or her initials, name, and title in a designated place provided within the record for documentation.

All MARs are kept in a notebook or clipboard file on the medication cart for the 24-hour period they are in use, then become a permanent part of the patient chart. In the acute-care setting, a new MAR is generated every 24 hours at the same time the unit dose cart is refilled (Figure 7-6).

In the long-term care setting the MAR uses the same principles; however, it generally provides a space for medications to be recorded for up to 1 month (Figure 7-7). The medication record also shows the name of the pharmacy dispensing the prescribed medications and the assigned prescription number. Medications prescribed for residents in the long-term care setting are required to be reviewed on a scheduled basis; therefore the MAR identifies the reviewer and date (see Figure 7-6).

Additional forms included in a patient's chart depend on the therapy prescribed. These include separate medication

Martindale Hometown Hospital
Laboratory Summary Report

PATIENT NAME: Joseph Lorenzo   Rm. 621-2   ADM: January 21
ID NO.   016-28-3978
DIAGNOSIS: Myocardial Infarction
PHYSICIAN: M. Martin, M.D.   TIME: 12:13 AM
                                                                                   DATE: 1/28

| DATE | 1/27 | 1/26 | 1/25 | 1/24 | 1/23 | Normal |
TIME	07:00	07:00	07:00	07:00	07:00	Range
ProTime	19	18	24	18	16	11.0-13.0 sec
PTT	34	33	38	34	31	0-35 sec

Figure 7-5 *Laboratory test reports. Example of the prothrombin times for a patient receiving warfarin.*

administration reports; health teaching records; operative and anesthesiology records; recovery room records; physical, occupational, or speech therapy records; inhalation therapy reports; and a diabetic's daily record of insulin dosage and urine and blood sugar test results. Each page placed in the patient's chart will be imprinted with the patient's name, registration number, and unit or room number. Nurses often use data from all of these sections to formulate a plan of nursing care.

Kardex Records

The **Kardex** (Figure 7-8) is a large index-type card usually kept in a flip-file or separate holder that contains pertinent information such as the patient's name, diagnosis, allergies, schedules of current medications with stop dates, treatments, and the nursing care plan. Because all ordered medications are listed in the Kardex, the nurse can assemble the medication cards (Figure 7-9, p. 73) for all assigned patients and verify each medication card against the Kardex. When the unit dose system is used, all medications are still listed on the Kardex or the medication profile, but individual medication cards are not necessary. Although used primarily by nurses, the Kardex makes patient data quickly accessible to all members of the health care team. The Kardex is often completed in pencil and updated by erasures. Because it is not a legal document, it is destroyed when the patient is discharged from the institution.

DRUG DISTRIBUTION SYSTEMS

Objectives

1. Cite the advantages and disadvantages of the ward stock system, the individual prescription order system, and the unit dose system of drug distribution.

2. Study the narcotic control system used at the assigned clinical practice setting, and compare it with the requirements of the Controlled Substance Act, 1970.

Key Words

ward stock system
individual prescription
  system

unit dose system
long-term care unit dose
  system

Before the administration of medications, it is important that the nurse understand the overall medication delivery system used at the employing health care agency. Although no two drug distribution systems function exactly alike, the following general types are currently being used.

Floor or **ward stock system.** In this system, all but the most dangerous or rarely used medications are stocked at the nursing station in stock containers. This system has been used most often in small hospitals and in hospitals where there are no charges directly to the patient for medications, such as in some government hospitals. Some advantages that exist with the complete floor stock system are ready availability of most drugs, fewer inpatient prescription orders, and minimal return of medications. The disadvantages of this type of system are the increased potential for medication errors because of the large array of stock medications to choose from and the lack of review by the pharmacist of each individual patient's medication order; the increased danger of unnoticed drug deterioration, jeopardizing patient safety; economic loss caused by misplaced or forgotten charges and misappropriation of medication by hospital personnel; increased amounts of expired drugs to be discarded; the need for larger stocks and frequent total drug inventories; and storage problems on the nursing units in many hospitals.

Individual prescription order system. In this system, medications are dispensed from the pharmacy upon receipt of a prescription or a drug order for an individual patient. The pharmacist usually sends a 3- to 5-day supply of medication in a bottle labeled for a specific patient. Once received at the nurses' station, medications are placed in the medication cabinet in accordance with institutional practices.

MARTINDALE HOMETOWN HOSPITAL

MEDICATION ADMINISTRATION RECORD

NAME:	Joseph Lorenzo	RM-BD: 621-2
ID NO.	016-28-3978	AGE: 62
DIAGNOSIS	Myocardial Infarction	SEX: M
PHYSICIAN	M. Martin, M.D.	Ht: 6' Wt:

Init	Signature	Title

	SCHEDULED MEDICATIONS			
DATES:	MEDICATION—STRENGTH—FORM—ROUTE	0030-0729	0730-1529	1530-0029
1/25	RANITIDINE (ZANTAC) 　　ZANTAC 　　150 MG　　TABLET ORAL 　　TWICE A DAY		0900	1800
1/25	DILTIAZEM HYDROCHLORIDE 　　CARDIZEM 　　90 MG　　TABLET ORAL 　　4 TIMES DAILY		0900 1300	1800 2100
1/25	WARFARIN SODIUM 　　COUMADIN 　　1 MG　　TABLET ORAL 　　EVERY OTHER DAY	NOT GIVEN	TODAY	
	IV AND PIGGYBACK ORDERS			
1/25	CEFTAZIDIME (FORTAZ) 1 GM IV SODIUM CHLORIDE 0.9% 50 ML EVERY 8 HOURS　　INFUSE: 20 MIN	0200	1000	1800
1/25	GENTAMICIN PREMIX　　80 MG IV ISO-OSMOTIC SOLN　　100 ML BY IV PUMP EVERY 12 HOURS　　INFUSE: 30 MIN	0200	1400	
1/25	BY IV PUMP　　1　　IV DEXT-5/0.2 NACL　　1000 ML 　　　　RATE: 100 ML/HR			
	PRN MEDICATIONS			
1/25	ACETAMINOPHEN (TYLENOL) 　　TYLENOL 　　650 MG (2×325)　　TABLET ORAL 　　Q 4H AS NEEDED　　PRN			
1/25	MAGNESIUM HYDROXIDE 　　MILK OF MAGNESIA 　　60 ML (CONC)　　ORAL CONC. ORAL 　　AS NEEDED　　PRN			
1/25	ALBUTEROL 　　PROVENTIL INHALER 　　90 MCG/INH　　AEROSOL INH 　　AS NEEDED　　PRN 　　SEE RESPIRATORY THERAPY NOTES 　　AT BEDSIDE			

Age/Sex	HT	WT	Date 1/25	ALLERGIES CODEINE
62/ M	6'0"	200 Lbs		
Room-Bd	Name			
621　2	Joseph Lorenzo			

Figure 7-6 *Example of medication administration record. Note separation of scheduled orders, IVs, and prn medications.*

MEDICATION ADMINISTRATION RECORD

| Nursing Home Name | PHARMACY PROVIDER | INIT.=GIVEN
R=REFUSED
V=VOMITED
H=HELD
O=HOME | INIT. | SIGNATURE | INIT. | SIGNATURE | INIT. | SIGNATURE | INIT. | SIGNATURE |

Mo. _____ Yr. _____

RX#—DATE ORDERED	MEDICATION—DOSE—ROUTE	TIME	1	2	3	4	5	6	7	8	9	10	11	12	13	14	15	16	17	18	19	20	21	22	23	24	25	26	27	28	29	30	31

ALLERGIES

DIAGNOSIS

| LAST NAME | FIRST | INIT. | LEVEL OF CARE | ROOM-BED | SEX | BIRTHDATE | DIET | IDENTIFICATION # | PHYSICIAN |

DATE OF MED. REVIEW

REVIEWED BY _____ (RPh)
_____ (RN)

Figure 7-7 *Example of medication administration record used in long-term care setting.*

71

JENNIE EDMUNDSON HOSPITAL
PATIENT ASSESSMENT/CARE PLAN

IN EMERGENCY CALL   Mary Doe (wife)   (Home) 323-6421
   (Name)   (Relationship)   (Phone)

John Jr. (son)   (Home) 323-0644
   (Name)   (Relationship)   (Phone)

IV THERAPY   6/1 Heparin lock   (Work) 536-1282
Rotate site 6/4 6/7 6/10 M.D.

CONSULTS/REFERRALS   Dr Krammer—cardiology

O₂ THERAPY/IPPB   6/1 O₂ 2L N.C. Continuously
6/5 O₂ PRN Chest pain 2L/N.C.

PHYSICAL THERAPY _____

SUPPORT SERVICES _____

TREATMENTS-OTHER _____

CURRENT MEDS BEING TAKEN Lanoxin 0.125 mg qid. Tenormin 50 mg qid. Procardia 20 mg qid, Transderm Nitro 1 patch 12 hr on/12 hr off, Persantine 25 mg tid, N & G 1/150 gr PRN chest pain, Tylenol gr X PRN headache, minor discomforts

OPERATIVE PROCEDURE   6/6/96 Cardiac catheterization
Outcome: 2 Grafts blocked - severe coronary artery disease

DIAGNOSIS   Angina, heart failure
Hist. 7/76 hypertension

ALLERGIES   Penicillin
REACTION   Hives on Trunk   ALLERGY BAND APPLIED   ☑

Physical Care Bath   6/1 N.O.   Daily Lab Specimens

At bedside c̄ Assistance if pain free

Diet   6/1 2 gm Na; low cholesterol diet

Fluid   As desired. Not to exceed 3000 cc/24 hr

Help Needed
N/A

Miscellaneous
B.P., basic Rhythm
6/1 sinus tachy 120-130

Activity/Limitations/Safety
6/1 Bedrest c̄ BRP c̄ pain
Up as desires when pain free. Begin 6/1/96

Elimination   N.O. Note bowel activity daily. Allow to stand to void.

Not to SMOKE IN HOSP.   D.O.
Smoker √ 1/2 pk/day   Dentures upper only
Non Smoker   Eye Glasses √ #4
Hearing Aid   Other Telemetry

I & O	BP	T.P.R.	Weight
√	q̄ 4°	q̄ 4°	D.O. Daily at breakfast

(N.O. Apical & Radial pulses q 4 hr)

PATIENT CLASSIFICATION
KEY 0-13 = I   14-18 = II   19 + = III

AMBUL	MEALS	BATH	PR/PO OP	TRTMTS	TOT
1②3	①23	1②3	2	3–1	PTS 14
BTH RM	MEDS	T&ES	UNCON'S	AGE	PT
1②34	①TO 2	1 OR③	5	21	CAT 2

PSYCHIATRIC PATIENT CLASSIFICATION
KEY 0-15=I 16-20=II 21+ = III CONSTANT CARE

AMBUL	BATHR'M	TRTMNTS	BEHAV'R	TOT PTS
123	1234	×1		
MEALS	MEDS	PR/PO-OP	5 3 1	
123	1 OR 2	2	PHYS ACT	PAT CAT
BATHE	AGE	MENT ATT		
123	+1	5 3 1	5 3 1	

CHURCH/PARISH ST. LUKES
ADM DATE 5/31/96   RELIGION CATHOLIC

NAME DOE, JOHN   HOSP.# 43641   AGE 58   PHYSICIAN FITZGERALD   ROOM NO. 425
DO, Doctor's order; *NO*, nursing order.

Figure 7-8 *Example of a nursing care plan in a Kardex.*

Generally, the medication containers are arranged alphabetically by the patient's name, but they may be arranged numerically by the patient's room or bed number. This system provides greater patient safety, due to the review of prescription orders by both the pharmacist and the nurse before administration; less danger of drug deterioration and easier inventory control; smaller total inventories; and reduced revenue loss as a result of improved charging systems and less pilferage. Although the dispensing of medication to individual patients is better than in the floor stock system, the major disadvantages of this system are the unwieldy and time-consuming procedures used to schedule, prepare, administer, control, and record the drug distribution and administration process.

Unit dose system. Unit dose drug distribution systems use single-unit packages of drugs, dispensed to fill each dosage requirement as it is ordered. Each package is labeled with generic and brand name, manufacturer, lot number, and expiration date. When dispensed by the pharmacy, the indi-

vidual packages are placed in labeled drawers assigned to individual patients. The drawers are kept in a large *unit dose cabinet* (Figure 7-10) that is kept at the nurses' station. Under most unit dose systems, the drawers are refilled by the pharmacist every 24 hours. In long-term care facilities, they are usually exchanged on 3- or 7-day schedules. The system was developed in the 1960s to overcome problems with inefficient use of nursing personnel, underutilization of pharmacists, excessively high rates of medication errors, poor drug control, waste of medications, and large inventories. The unit dose system is the safest and most economical method of drug distribution in hospitals and long-term care facilities today.

Advantages of the system include the following:
1. The time normally spent by nursing personnel in preparation of drugs for administration is drastically reduced.
2. The pharmacist has a profile of all medications of each patient and is therefore able to analyze the prescribed medications for drug interactions or contraindications.

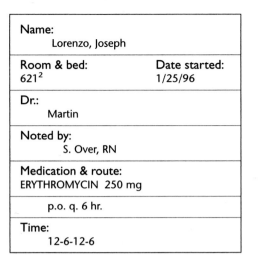

Name:	
Lorenzo, Joseph	
Room & bed: 621²	Date started: 1/25/96
Dr.: Martin	
Noted by: S. Over, RN	
Medication & route: ERYTHROMYCIN 250 mg	
p.o. q. 6 hr.	
Time: 12-6-12-6	

Figure 7-9 *Transcription of a medication order onto the Kardex or a medication card or ticket. (Modified from McKenry LM, Salerno E: Mosby's pharmacology in nursing, ed 19, St Louis, 1995, Mosby.)*

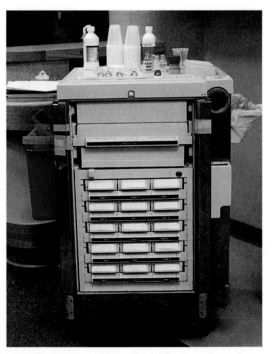

Figure 7-10 *Unit dose cabinet. (Courtesy Chuck Dresner.)*

This method increases the pharmacist's involvement and better utilizes his or her extensive drug knowledge.

3. No dosage calculations are necessary because of unit-of-use packaging, thus reducing errors.
4. The nurse may double-check drugs and dosages because each dose is individually packaged and labeled.
5. There is less waste and misappropriation because single units are dispensed.
6. Credit is given to the patient for unused medications because each dose is individually packaged. (Under the individual prescription order system, returned bottles of unused medications were destroyed because of fear of contamination.)

An argument occasionally used by nurses against the unit, or single-dose, system is that medications are prepared by someone else for the nurse to administer. Nurses have been taught: "Never administer anything you haven't prepared yourself." In principle, this is certainly true. A nurse should not administer any drug mixed and left unlabeled by another individual. However, for decades nurses have administered medications that have been prepared and labeled by the pharmacist. The unit dose medication is prepared under rigid controls and is dispensed only after quality control procedures have been completed by pharmacists. Nurses should always continue to check medications before administration. If there is a discrepancy between the Kardex and the medication in the cart, the pharmacist and the original physician's order should be consulted.

At the time of administration, the nurse should check all aspects of the medication order as stated on the medication profile against the medication container removed from the patient's drawer for administration. The number of doses remaining in the drawer for the shift should also be checked. If the number of remaining doses is incorrect, check the medication order before continuing with the drug administration. Always consider the possibility that the drug has been discontinued, that someone else has given the dose, or that someone has omitted a dose or given the wrong patient the wrong medication. In the event that an error has been made, report it in accordance with hospital policies.

Long-term care unit dose system. The unit dose medication system used in the long-term care system is an adaptation of that used in the acute care setting. The unit dose cart is designed with individual drawers to hold one resident's medication containers for 1 week. The drawer is labeled with the resident's name, room number, pharmacy name and telephone number, and the name of the facility. The pharmacist fills the medication container with the prescribed drug. Each container has enough compartments or cubicles to contain the prescribed number of doses of the drug for each day of the week. The individual compartments may be labeled with the days of the week. The medication cart has other compartments to store bottles of medication that cannot be placed in patient drawers. The cart has a storage area for medication cups, medicine crusher, drinking cups, straws, alcohol sponges, syringes, and other necessities for the preparation and administration of the medications prescribed. The entire cart has a locking system, and the cart should be kept locked when not in use and when unattended while medications are being dispensed.

The unit dose systems may use a color coding system to simplify finding the medication holder for a specific time of day; for example, purple = 6 AM (0600), pink = 8 AM (0800), yellow = noon (1200), green = 2 PM (1400) or 4 PM (1600), orange = early evening, red = p.r.n. Using this method to organize the medications allows the nurse or medication aide to remove all the pink holders to administer the prescribed 8 AM (0800) tablets or capsules. Each individual medication holder is also labeled with the resident's name, physician's name, prescription number, generic or brand name of the drug, dose, frequency of drug order (for example, four times a day), and the actual time the drug within this holder is to be administered (for example, 8 AM, or 0800). This system is easy to use unless the user is color blind. By using military time to mark the individual containers, the individual who is color blind can use the military time as the guideline.

At the time of administration, the nurse or medication aide checks all aspects of the medication order as stated on medication profile against the medication container that has been removed from one of the drawers. The number of doses remaining within the holder is checked against the days of the week that remain for the medication to be administered. If the resident refuses the medication, it must be charted on the record with the reason the medication was refused. In a long-term care setting, residents seldom wear identification bands; therefore third-party identification of the resident must be relied on until the nurse or medication aide is able to identify the residents. All medications administered should be charted as soon as given. The medication aide has specific limitations on the types of medications he or she can administer; therefore the nurse should be thoroughly familiar with the law and guidelines that exist in the state where functioning. The nurse is ultimately responsible for verifying the qualifications of the individual being supervised in the medication aide capacity and for the medications he or she is administering.

Narcotic Control Systems

As described in Chapter 1, laws regulating the use of controlled substances have been enacted and are rigidly enforced. Within hospitals, it is a standard policy that controlled substances are issued in single-unit packages and are kept in a separate, locked cabinet on each nursing unit. The key to the cabinet is controlled by the head nurse or a designated individual. When controlled substances are issued to a nursing unit, they are accompanied by an inventory sheet (Figure 7-11) that lists each type of controlled substance being supplied. This record is used to account for the disposition of each type of medication issued. At the time the controlled substance supply is dispensed to the nursing unit by the pharmacist, the nurse receiving the drug supply is responsible for counting and verifying the number and types of controlled substances received. The nurse then signs a record attesting to the accuracy and receipt of the controlled substances and locks them in the controlled substances (narcotic) cabinet.

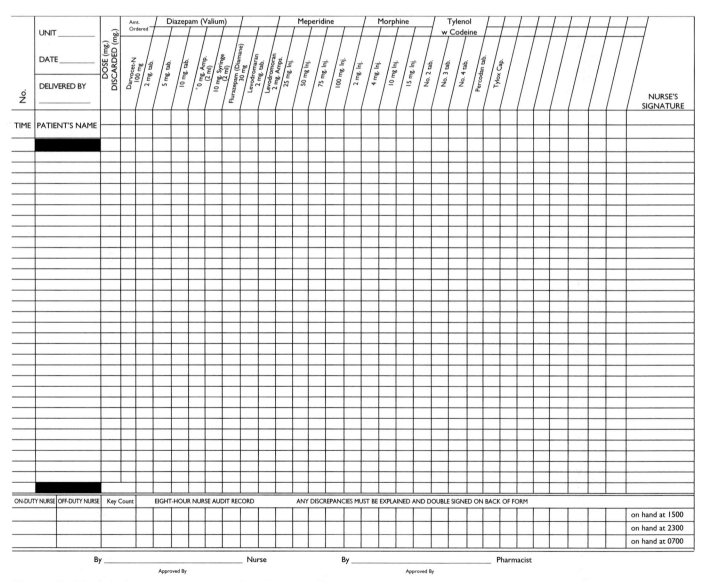

Figure 7-11 *Controlled substances inventory form. (Courtesy of University Hospital, The University of Nebraska Medical Center. Copyright, Board of Regents of the University of Nebraska, Lincoln, Nebraska.)*

When a controlled substance is ordered for a particular patient, the nurse caring for the patient requests the key to the cabinet to obtain and prepare the medication for administration. At the time of removal from the cabinet, the inventory control record (see Figure 7-11) must be completed indicating time, patient's name, drug, dose, and the signature of the nurse responsible for checking out the controlled substance. If a portion of the medication is to be discarded because of a smaller prescribed dosage, two nurses must check the dosage, preparation, and the portion discarded. Both nurses must then cosign the inventory control record to verify the transaction. The key is returned to the charge nurse after the dose is obtained and the paperwork is completed.

A newer system involves a controlled substance cart. It has a computer system for selecting and recording the patient's name, dose, drug, and the physician's name. Each time the nurse has the machine dispense a narcotic the date, time, and nurse's code (issued by the pharmacy) is entered into the computer along with data relating to patient's name, physician's name, drug name, dose, and drug form.

Before the administration of any controlled substance, the patient's chart should be checked to verify that the appropriate time interval since the last use of the drug has elapsed, as specified in the physician's orders. (See Chapter 18 for details of monitoring pain and the use of analgesics.) Immediately after the administration of a controlled substance, the chart should be completed by the nurse administering the medication. At appropriate intervals following the administration of a controlled substance, the degree and duration of effectiveness should be recorded in the nurse's notes.

At the end of each shift, the contents of the controlled substances cabinet or controlled substance cart are counted (inventoried) by two nurses, one from the shift that is about to end and the other from the oncoming shift. Each individual container is counted and the remaining number of tablets, ampules, and prefilled syringes is added to the amount used, according to the inventory control record. The amount of each drug remaining, plus the amount recorded as administered to individual patients, should equal the total number issued. During the counting procedure, packages of prefilled syringes that have not been opened are visually inspected to verify that the seal and the cellophane coverings are intact. Once the package seal is broken, closer scrutiny of the package is required. These observations should include tilting the package of prefilled syringes to observe the rate of air bubble movement inside the barrel, uniformity of color of the solutions in each of the barrels, and the similarity in fluid level in each of the barrels. The same medication in the same type of syringe should be the same color and should travel within the barrel at the same rate, and all fluid levels should be similar. Discrepancies in the number of remaining doses are checked with nursing personnel on the unit to see if all narcotics used have been charted. If this does not reveal the source of the inaccuracy, each patient's chart is checked to be certain that all controlled substances recorded on the individual patient's chart for the shift coincide with the controlled substances inventory record. If the error still is not found, the pharmacy and the nursing service office should be contacted in accordance with the policy of the institution. In the event that the count appears to be accurate but tampering with the contents of the containers is suspected, a report should be made to the pharmacy and the nursing service office. When the controlled substances inventory is complete, the two nurses doing the counting sign the inventory control shift record to verify that the records and inventory are accurate at that time. With the controlled substance cart, the computer generates an end of shift report, which is then verified in the same manner just described.

THE DRUG ORDER

Objectives

1. Define each of the four categories of medication orders used.
2. Describe the procedure used in the assigned clinical setting for taking, recording, transcribing, and verifying verbal medication orders.

Key Words

stat orders · prn order
transcription standing orders · verification
renewal order

Medications for patient use must be ordered by licensed physicians or dentists (or in some states by nurse practitioners and physician's assistants) acting within their areas of professional training. Placing an order for a medication or treatment is known as issuing a *prescription*. Initially it may be issued verbally or in written form. Prescriptions issued for nonhospitalized patients use a form similar to that shown in Figure 7-12, whereas prescriptions for hospitalized patients are written on the Physician's Order Form (see Figure 7-1). All prescriptions must contain the following elements: the patient's full name, date, drug name, route of administration, dosage, duration of the order, and signature of the prescriber. Additional information may be required for certain types of medications (for example, for intravenous administration, the

CLAYTON'S PHARMACY
213 West Third Street   Grand Island, Nebraska

NAME Joseph Lorenzo   AGE Adult
ADDRESS 18 Bush Ave., Glen Cove, NY   DATE 3/18/96
℞
ERYTHROMYCIN TABS. 250 mg ENTERIC
  #40   COATED
sig: TAB i q 6 hr.

_____ Marilyn Wells MD
DISPENSE AS WRITTEN   SUBSTITUTION PERMISSIBLE
THIS PRESCRIPTION WILL BE FILLED GENERICALLY UNLESS PHYSICIAN SIGNS ON THE LINE STATING "DISPENSE AS WRITTEN"

Figure 7-12 *A prescription showing patient name, patient address, date, drug and strength, number of tablets, directions for use, and physician's signature.*

concentration, dilution, and rate of flow should be specified in addition to the method—"IV push" or "continuous infusion").

Types of Medication Orders

Medication orders fall into four categories: the stat order, the single order, the standing order, and the prn order.

The **stat order** is generally used on an emergency basis. It means that the drug is to be administered as soon as possible, but only once. For example, if a patient is having a seizure, the physician may order "diazepam 10 mg IV stat," which is meant to be given immediately, and one time only.

The *single* order means administration at a certain time, but only one time. For example, a preoperative analgesic may order "Demerol 100 mg IM to be given at the time the patient leaves the floor for surgery." Demerol would then be administered intramuscularly (IM) at that time, but once only.

The **standing order** indicates that a medication is to be given for a specified number of doses; for example, "cefazolin 1 g q6hr × 4 doses." A standing order may also indicate that a drug is to be administered until discontinued at a later date; for example, "Ampicillin 500 mg PO q6h." In the interest of patient safety, however, all accredited health agencies have policies that automatically cancel an order after a certain number of doses are administered or a certain number of days of therapy have passed (for example, before surgery, after 72 hours for narcotics, after one dose only for anticoagulants, after 7 days for antibiotics). A **renewal order** must be written and signed by the physician before the nurse can continue to administer the medication.

A **prn order** means "administer if needed." This order allows a nurse to judge when a medication should be administered based on the patient's need and when it can be safely administered.

Verbal Orders

Health care agencies have policies regarding who may accept verbal orders and under what circumstances they should be accepted. The practice should be avoided whenever possible, but when a verbal order is accepted, the person who took the order is responsible for accurately entering it on the order sheet and signing it. The physician must cosign and date the order, usually within 24 hours.

Electronic Transmission of Patient Orders

With the advent of fax machines, many physicians' offices fax new orders to the area where the patient is admitted or transferred. These fax transmissions must have an original signature within a specified time, often 24 hours. Hospital units also find it useful to fax orders to a nursing home where the individual is being transferred. This allows the receiving agency to prepare for the patient or resident, and the original orders, signed by the physician, then accompany the individual at time of transfer.

Nurse's Responsibilities

Verification

Once a prescription has been written for a hospitalized patient, the nurse interprets it and makes a professional judgment on its acceptability. Judgments must be made regarding the type of drug, the therapeutic intent, the usual dose, and the mathematical and physical preparation of the dose. The nurse must also evaluate the method of administration in relation to the patient's physical condition, as well as any allergies and the patient's ability to tolerate the dosage form. If any part of an order is vague, the physician who wrote the order should be consulted for further clarification. Patient safety is of primary importance and the nurse assumes responsibility for **verification** and safety of the medication order. If, after gathering all possible information, it is concluded that it is inappropriate to administer the medication as ordered, the prescribing physician should be notified immediately. An explanation should be given as to why the order should not be executed. If the physician cannot be contacted or does not change the order, the nurse should notify the director of nurses, the nursing supervisor on duty, or both. The reasons for refusal to administer the drug should be recorded in accordance with the policies of the employing institution.

Transcription

Transcription of the prescriber's order is necessary to put it into action. After verification of an order, a nurse or another designated person transcribes the order from the physician's order sheet onto the Kardex or onto an MAR. These data may also be entered into a computer that produces a Kardex. When this process is delegated to a ward clerk or unit secretary, the nurse is still responsible for the verification of all aspects of the medication order. The nurse must sign the original medication order indicating that he or she received, interpreted, and verified the order. The nurse then sends a carbon copy of the original order to the pharmacy. A small supply is issued either in unit dose or in a container containing a multiday supply. The container is labeled with the date, patient's name, room number, and the drug name, strength and dose. When the supply arrives from the pharmacy it is stored in the medication room or in the patient's medication drawer of a medication cart.

In the long-term care setting, carbon copies of new medication orders are sent to the local pharmacy to be filled. If a stat. dose is needed or if the medication must be started soon, the pharmacy is notified via telephone or fax, and written verification of the medicines ordered is supplied to the pharmacy. Because the local pharmacy generates the medication administration record only on a monthly basis, new orders must be added to the current medication record by the nurse transcribing the order. Nurses also send requests to the pharmacy via fax for drug reorders (for example, prn orders).

The nurse administers a drug by following the order on the medication administration record or drug profile according to the six rights of drug administration: right drug, right time, right dose, right patient, right route, right documentation.

THE SIX RIGHTS OF DRUG ADMINISTRATION

Objectives

1. Identify specific precautions needed to ensure that the RIGHT DRUG is prepared for the patient.

2. Memorize and recite standard abbreviations associated with the scheduling of medications.

3. Identify data found in the patient's chart that must be analyzed to determine if the patient has abnormal renal or hepatic function.

4. Describe specific safety precautions the nurse should institute to ensure that correct medication calculations are performed.

5. Review the policies and procedures of the practice setting to identify drugs whose dosages must be checked by two qualified persons.

6. Describe the methods that should be used to ensure that the correct patient receives the correct medication, by the correct route, in the correct amount, at the correct time.

7. Compare each safety measure described to ensure safe preparation and administration of medications with those procedures used at the clinical practice setting.

8. Identify appropriate nursing actions to document the administration and therapeutic effectiveness of each medication administered.

Right Drug

Many drugs have similar spellings and variable concentrations. *Before* the administration of the medication, it is imperative to compare the exact spelling and concentration of the prescribed drug with the medication card or drug profile and the medication container. Regardless of the drug distribution system used, the drug label should be read at least three times:

1. Before removing the drug from the shelf or unit dose cart
2. Before preparing or measuring the actual prescribed dose
3. Before replacing the drug on the shelf or before opening a unit dose container (just before administering the drug to the patient)

Right Time

When scheduling the administration time of a medication, factors such as timing abbreviations, standardized times, consistency of blood levels, absorption, diagnostic testing, and the use of prn medications must be considered.

Standard abbreviations. The drug order specifies the frequency of drug administration. Standard abbreviations used as part of the drug order specify the times of administration (see Appendixes A and B). The nurse should also check institutional policy concerning administration of medications. Hospitals often have standardized interpretations for abbreviations (for example, *q6h* may mean 0600, 1200, 1800, and 2400; *qid* may mean 0800, 1200, 1600, or 2000). The nurse must memorize and use standard abbreviations in interpreting, transcribing, and administering medications accurately.

Standardized administration times. For patient safety, certain medications are administered at specific times. This allows laboratory work or ECGs to be completed first, so that the size of the next dose to be administered can be deter-

mined. For example, warfarin or digoxin would be administered at 1300, if ordered by the physician.

Maintenance of consistent blood levels. The schedule for the administration of a drug should be planned to maintain consistent blood levels of the drug in order to maximize the therapeutic effectiveness. If blood draws to establish the current serum blood level of a specific drug are ordered, the nurse should follow the guidelines stated in the drug monograph for the specific time when the blood sample should be drawn in relation to the drug dosage administration schedule.

Maximum drug absorption. The schedule for oral administration of drugs must be planned to prevent incompatibilities and maximize absorption. Certain drugs require administration on an empty stomach. Thus they are given 1 hour before or 2 hours after meals. Other medications should be given with foods to enhance absorption or reduce irritations. Still other drugs are not given with dairy products or antacids. It is important to maintain the recommended schedule of administration for maximum therapeutic effectiveness.

Diagnostic testing. Determine whether any diagnostic tests have been ordered for completion before initiating or continuing therapy. Before beginning antimicrobial therapy, ensure that all culture specimens (such as blood, urine, or wound) have been collected. If a physician has ordered serum levels of the drug, coordinate the administration time of the medication with the time the phlebotomist is going to draw the blood sample. When completing the requisition for a serum level of a medication, always make a notation of the date and time that the drug was last administered. Timing is important; if tests are not conducted at the same time intervals in the same patient, the data gained are of little value.

Prn medications. Before the administration of any prn medication, the patient's chart should be checked to ensure that the drug has not been administered by someone else and that the specified time interval has passed since the medication was last administered. When a prn medication is given, it should be charted immediately. Record the response to the medication.

Right Dose

Check the drug dosage ordered against the range specified in the reference books available at the nurses' station.

Abnormal hepatic or renal function. Always consider the hepatic and renal function of the specific patient who will receive the drug. Depending on the rate of drug metabolism and route of excretion from the body, certain drugs require a reduction in dosage to prevent toxicity. Conversely, patients being dialyzed may require higher than normal doses. Whenever a dosage is outside the normal range for that drug, it should be verified *before* administration. Once verification has been obtained, a brief explanation should be recorded in the nurse's notes and on the Kardex (or drug profile) so that others administering the medication will have the information and the physician will not be repeatedly contacted with the same questions. The following laboratory tests are used to monitor liver function: aspartame aminotransferase (AST), alanine aminotransferase (ALT), gamma glutamyl transferase (GGT), alkaline phosphatase, and lactic dehydrogenase (LDH). The blood urea nitrogen (BUN), serum creatinine

(Cr_s), and creatinine clearance (C_{cr}) are used to monitor renal function.

Pediatric and geriatric patients. Specific doses for some drugs are not yet firmly established for the elderly and for the pediatric patient. The nurse should question any order outside the normal range *before* administration. For pediatric patients, the most reliable method is by proportional amount of body surface area or body weight. (See Appendix C.)

Nausea and vomiting. If a patient is vomiting, oral medications should be withheld and the physician contacted for alternate medication orders, because the parenteral or rectal route may be preferred. Investigate the onset of the nausea and vomiting. If it began after the start of the medication regimen, consideration should be given to rescheduling the oral medication. Administration with food usually decreases gastric irritation. Consult a physician for changes in orders.

Accurate dose forms. Do not break a tablet unless it is scored. Consult with the pharmacy about other available dosage forms.

Accurate calculations. Safety should always be maintained when calculating a drug dose. Whenever a dosage is questionable or when fractional doses are calculated, check the dosage with another qualified individual. Most hospital policies require that certain medications (for example, insulin, heparin, IV digitalis preparations) be checked by two qualified nurses before administration.

Correct measuring devices. Accurate measurement of the volume of medication prescribed is essential. Fractional doses require the use of a tuberculin syringe, whereas insulin is always measured in an insulin syringe that corresponds to the number of units in 1 ml (U-100 insulin is measured in a U-100 syringe).

Right Patient

When using the medication card system, compare the name of the patient on the medication card with the patient's identification bracelet. With the unit dose system, compare the name on the drug profile with the individual's identification bracelet. When checking the bracelet under either system, always check for allergies. Some institutional policies require that the individual be called by name as a means of identification. This practice must take into consideration the patient's mental alertness and orientation. It is always much safer to check the identification bracelet.

Pediatric patients. Never ask children their names as a means of positive identification. Children may change beds, try to avoid the nurse, or seek attention by identifying themselves as someone else. Check identification bracelets EVERY TIME.

Geriatric patients. It is a wise policy to check identification bracelets, in addition to confirming names verbally. In a long-term care setting, residents usually do not wear identification bracelets. In these instances, only a person who is familiar with the residents should confirm their identity for administration of the medications.

Many errors may be avoided by carefully following the practices just presented. Make it a habit to check the identification bracelet EVERY TIME a medication is admin-

istered. The adverse effects of administration of the wrong medication to the wrong patient and the potential for a lawsuit can thus be avoided.

Right Route

The drug order should specify the route to be used for the administration of the medication. Never substitute one dosage form of medication for another unless the physician is specifically consulted and an order for the change is obtained. There can be great variation in the absorption rate of the medication through various routes of administration. The intravenous route delivers the drug directly into the bloodstream. This route provides the fastest onset but also the greatest danger of potential adverse effects, such as tachycardia and hypotension. The intramuscular route provides the next fastest absorption rate, based on availability of blood supply. This route can be painful, as is the case with many antibiotics. The subcutaneous route is next fastest, based on blood supply. In some instances the oral route may be as fast as the intramuscular route, depending on the medication being given, the dosage form (liquids are absorbed faster than tablets), and whether there is food in the stomach. The oral route is usually safe if the patient is conscious and able to swallow. The rectal route should be avoided, if possible, because of irritation of mucosal tissues and erratic absorption rates. In case of error, the oral and rectal routes have the advantage of recoverability for a short time after administration.

To ensure that the right drug is prepared at the right time for the right patient, using the right route, it is important to maintain the highest standards of drug preparation and administration. Focus your entire attention on the calculation, preparation, and administration of the ordered medication. A drug reconstituted by a nurse should be clearly labeled with the patient's name, the dose or strength per unit of volume, the date and time the drug was reconstituted, the amount and type of diluent used, the expiration date or time, and the initials or name of the nurse who prepared it. Once reconstituted, the drug should be stored according to the manufacturer's recommendation.

- CHECK the label of the container for the drug name, concentration, and route of appropriate administration.
- CHECK the patient's chart, Kardex, medication administration record, or identification bracelet for allergies. If no information is found, ask the patient before the administration of the medication if he or she has any allergies.
- CHECK the patient's chart, Kardex, or medication administration record for rotation schedules of injectable or topically applied medications.
- CHECK medications to be mixed in one syringe with a list approved by the hospital or the pharmacy for compatibility. Normally, all drugs mixed in a single syringe should be administered within 15 minutes after mixing. Immediately before administration, ALWAYS CHECK the contents of the syringe for clarity and the absence of any precipitate; if either is present, do not administer the contents of the syringe.
- CHECK the patient's identity EVERY TIME a medication is administered.
- DO approach the patient in a firm but kind manner that conveys the feeling that cooperation is expected.

- DO adjust the patient to the most appropriate position for the route of administration (for example, for oral medications, sit the patient upright to facilitate swallowing). Have appropriate fluids ready before administration.
- DO remain with the patient to be certain that all medications have been swallowed.
- DO use every opportunity to teach the patient and family about the drug being administered.
- DO give simple and honest answers or explanations to the patient regarding the medication and treatment plan.
- DO use a plastic container, medicine cup, medicine dropper, oral syringe, or nipple to administer oral medications to an infant or small child.
- DO reward the child who has been cooperative by giving praise; comfort and hold the uncooperative child after completing the medication administration.
- Do NOT prepare or administer a drug from a container that is not properly labeled or from a container whose label is not fully legible.
- Do NOT give any medication prepared by an individual other than the pharmacist. ALWAYS check the drug name, dosage, frequency, and route of administration against the order. Student nurses must know the practice limitations instituted by the hospital or school and which medications can be administered under what level of supervision.
- Do NOT return an unused portion or dose of medication to a stock supply bottle.
- Do NOT attempt to administer any drug orally to a comatose patient.
- Do NOT leave a medication at the patient's bedside to be taken later; remain with the individual until the drug is taken and swallowed. (There are a few exceptions to this rule. One is that nitroglycerin may be left at the bedside for the patient's use. Second, in a long-term care setting certain patients are allowed to take their own medications. In both instances, a specific physician's order is required for *self-medication,* and the nurse must still chart the medications taken and the therapeutic response achieved.)
- Do NOT dilute a liquid medication form unless there are specific written orders to do so.
- BEFORE DISCHARGE: (1) Explain the proper method of taking prescribed medications to the patient (for example, do not crush or chew enteric-coated tablets, or any capsules; sublingual medication is placed under the tongue and is not taken with water). (2) Stress the need for punctuality in the administration of medications and what to do if a dosage is missed. (3) Teach the patient to store medications separately from other containers and personal hygiene items. (4) Provide the patient with written instruc-

tions reiterating the medication names, schedules, and how to obtain refills. Write the instructions in a language understood by the patient, and use **LARGE, BOLD LETTERS** when necessary. (5) Identify anticipated therapeutic response. (6) Instruct the patient, family members, or significant others on how to collect and record data for use by the physician to monitor the patient's response to drug and other treatment modalities. (7) Give the patient, or another responsible individual, a list of signs and symptoms that should be reported to the physician. (8) Stress measures that can be initiated to minimize or prevent anticipated side effects to the prescribed medication. It is important to do this to further encourage the patient to be compliant with the prescribed regimen.

Right Documentation, the Sixth Right

Documentation of nursing actions and patient observations has always been an important ethical responsibility, but now it is becoming a major medicolegal consideration as well. Indeed, it is becoming known as the *sixth right.* Always record on the right patient's chart the following information: date and time of administration, name of medication, dosage, and route and site of administration. Documentation of drug action should be made in the regularly scheduled assessments for changes in the disease symptoms the patient is exhibiting. Promptly record and report adverse symptoms observed. Document health teaching performed and evaluate and record the degree of understanding exhibited by the patient.

- DO record when a drug is *not* administered and why.
- Do NOT record a medication until after it has been given.
- Do NOT record in the nurses' notes that an incident report has been completed when a medication error has occurred. However, data regarding clinical observations of the patient related to the occurrence should be charted to serve as a baseline for future comparisons.

Whenever a medication error does occur, an incident report is completed to describe the circumstances of the event. An incident report related to a medication error should include the following data: date, time the drug was ordered, drug name, dose, and route of administration. Information regarding the date, time, drug administered, and dose and route of administration should be given, and the therapeutic response or adverse clinical observations present should be noted. Finally, record the date, time, and physician notified of the error and any physician's orders given. Be FACTUAL; do not state opinions on the incident report.

Enteral Administration

LIFE SPAN ISSUES

ORAL MEDICATIONS

Oral medicines can be made more palatable for children and geriatric patients by mixing with foods such as fruit puree, juice, or jam. Do not mix medications with food containing essential nutrients. The patient may later refuse this food because the medication has altered its taste. Rinsing the mouth, performing oral hygiene, or offering an iced carbonated beverage after administration of a distasteful medication may enhance the acceptance of repeat doses.

The routes of drug administration can be classified into three categories: the enteral, the parenteral, and the percutaneous routes. The enteral route refers to those drugs administered directly into the gastrointestinal tract by oral, rectal, or nasogastric routes. The oral route is safe, convenient, and relatively economical, and dosage forms are readily available for most medications. In the event of a medication error or intentional drug overdose, much of the drug can be retrieved for a reasonable time after administration. Disadvantages of the oral route are that it has the slowest and least dependable rate of absorption (and thus onset of action) of the commonly used routes of administration because of the frequent changes in the gastrointestinal environment produced by food, emotion, and physical activity. Another limitation on this route is that a few drugs, such as insulin and gentamicin, are destroyed by digestive fluids and must be administered parenterally for therapeutic activity. This route should not be used if the drug may harm or discolor the teeth or if the patient is vomiting, has gastric or intestinal suction, is likely to aspirate, or is unconscious and unable to swallow.

An alternative for those patients who cannot swallow or who have had oral surgery is the nasogastric route. The primary purpose of the nasogastric route is to bypass the mouth and pharynx. Advantages and disadvantages are similar to those of the oral route. The irritation caused by the tube in the nasal passage and throat must be weighed against the relative immobility associated with continuous intravenous infusions, expense, and the pain and irritation of multiple injections.

Administration via the rectal route has the advantages of bypassing the digestive enzymes and avoiding irritation of the mouth, esophagus, and stomach. It may also be a good

alternative when nausea or vomiting is present. Absorption via this route varies depending on the drug product, the ability of the patient to retain the suppository or enema, and the presence of fecal material.

ADMINISTRATION OF ORAL MEDICATIONS

Objectives

1. Correctly define and identify oral dosage forms of medications.
2. Identify common receptacles used to administer oral medications.

Key Words

capsules	suspensions
lozenges	syrups
tablets	soufflé cup
elixirs	medicine cup
emulsions	oral syringe

Dosage Forms

Capsules

Capsules are small, cylindrical gelatin containers (Figure 8-1) that hold dry powder or liquid medicinal agents. They are available in a variety of sizes and are a convenient way of

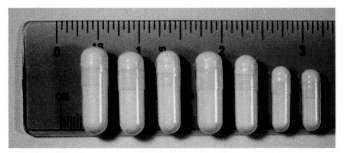

Figure 8-1 *Various sizes and numbers of gelatin capsules, actual size.* Courtesy Oscar H. Allison, Jr.

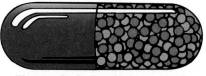

Figure 8-2 *Timed-release capsule.*

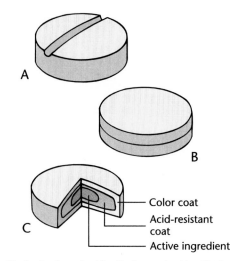

Figure 8-3 A, *Scored tablet.* **B,** *Layered tablet.* **C,** *Enteric-coated tablet.*

administering drugs with an unpleasant odor or taste. They do not require coatings or additives to improve the taste. The color and shapes of capsules, as well as the manufacturer's symbols on the capsule surface, are means of identifying the product.

Timed-Release Capsules

Timed-release or sustained-release capsules (Figure 8-2) provide a gradual but continuous release of drug because the granules within the capsule dissolve at different rates. The advantage of this delivery system is that it reduces the number of doses administered per day. Trade names indicating that the drug is a timed-release product are Spansules, Gyrocaps, and Plateau Caps. The timed-release capsules should NOT be crushed or chewed or the contents emptied into food or liquids, because this may alter the absorption rate and could result in either drug overdose or subtherapeutic activity.

Lozenges or Troches

Lozenges are flat disks containing a medicinal agent in a suitably flavored base. The base may be a hard sugar candy or the combination of sugar with sufficient mucilage to give it form. Lozenges are held in the mouth to dissolve slowly, thus releasing the therapeutic ingredients.

Pills

Pills are an obsolete dosage form that are no longer manufactured because of the development of capsules and compressed tablets. Laypersons still use the term to refer to tablets and capsules.

Tablets

Tablets are dried, powdered drugs that have been compressed into small disks. In addition to the drug, tablets also contain one or more of the following ingredients: binders (adhesive substances that allow the tablet to stick together); disintegrators (substances that encourage dissolution in body fluids); lubricants (required for efficient manufacturing); and fillers (inert ingredients to make the tablet size convenient). Tablets are sometimes scored or grooved (Figure 8-3, *A*); the

indentation may be used to divide the dosage. When possible, it is best to request the exact dosage prescribed rather than attempt to divide a tablet.

Tablets can be formed in layers (Figure 8-3, *B*). This method allows otherwise incompatible medications to be administered at the same time.

An enteric-coated tablet (Figure 8-3, *C*) has a special coating that resists dissolution in the acidic pH of the stomach but is dissolved in the alkaline pH of the intestines. Enteric-coated tablets are often used for administering medications that are destroyed in an acid pH. Enteric-coated tablets must NOT be crushed or chewed, or the active ingredients will be released prematurely and destroyed in the stomach.

Elixirs

Elixirs are clear liquids made up of drugs dissolved in alcohol and water. Elixirs are used primarily when the drug will not dissolve in water alone. After the drug is dissolved in the elixir, flavoring agents are frequently added to improve taste. The alcohol content of elixirs is highly variable, depending on the solubility of the drug.

Emulsions

Emulsions are dispersions of small droplets of water in oil or oil in water. The dispersion is maintained by emulsifying agents such as sodium lauryl sulfate, gelatin, or acacia. Emulsions are used to mask bitter tastes or provide better solubility to certain drugs.

Suspensions

Suspensions are liquid dosage forms that contain solid, insoluble drug particles dispersed in a liquid base. All suspensions should be shaken well before administration to ensure thorough mixing of the particles.

Syrups

Syrups contain medicinal agents dissolved in a concentrated solution of sugar, usually sucrose. Syrups are particularly effective for masking the bitter taste of a drug. Many

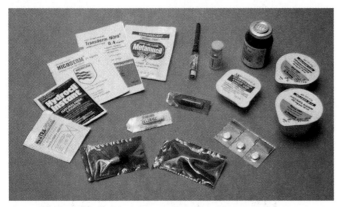

Figure 8-4 *Unit dose packages.* Courtesy Chuck Dresner.

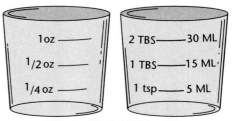

Figure 8-6 *Medicine cup.*

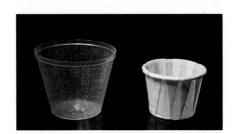

Figure 8-5 *Soufflé cup.* Courtesy Chuck Dresner.

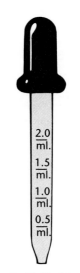

Figure 8-7 *Medicine dropper.*

preparations for pediatric patients are syrups because children tend to like the flavored base.

Equipment

Unit Dose or Single Dose

Unit dose or single dose packaging (Figure 8-4) provides a single dose of medication in one package, ready for dispensing. The package is labeled with generic and brand names, manufacturer, lot number, and date of expiration. Depending on the distribution system, the patient's name may be added to the package by the pharmacy.

Soufflé Cup

A small paper or plastic cup (Figure 8-5) may be used to transport solid medication forms, such as a capsule or tablet, to the patient to prevent contamination by handling. A tablet that must be crushed can be placed between two **soufflé cups** and then crushed with a pestle. This powdered form of the tablet can then be administered in a solution if soluble, or it may be mixed with a small amount of food, such as applesauce.

Medicine Cup

The **medicine cup** (Figure 8-6) is a glass or plastic container that has three scales (apothecary, metric, and household) for the measurement of liquid medications. The medicine cup should be carefully examined before pouring any medication to ensure that the proper scale is being used for measurement (Table 8-1). The medicine cup is inaccurate for the measure-

ment of doses smaller than 1 teaspoonful, although it is reasonably accurate for larger volumes. A syringe comparable to the volume to be measured should be used for smaller volumes. For volumes less than 1 cc, a tuberculin syringe should be used.

Medicine Dropper

The medicine dropper (Figure 8-7) may be used to administer eye drops, ear drops, and, occasionally, pediatric medications. There is great variation in the size of the drop formed, so it is important to use only the dropper supplied by the manufacturer for a specific liquid medication. Before drawing medication into a dropper, become familiar with the calibrations on the barrel. Once the medication is drawn

Table 8-1

Commonly Used Measurement Equivalent		
HOUSEHOLD MEASUREMENT	**APOTHECARY MEASUREMENT**	**METRIC MEASUREMENT**
2 Tbsp	1 oz	30 ml
1 Tbsp	½ oz	15 ml
2 tsp	⅓ oz	10 ml
1 tsp	⅙ oz	5 ml

MEASUREMENT OF ORAL MEDICATION

Liquid medications are often given to children. To obtain an accurate measurement of oral medication dosages, use a household measuring spoon or an oral syringe available from the pharmacy. Whenever a medicine dropper is to be used, only the dropper that accompanies a prescribed medication should be used to ensure accuracy of the dosage.

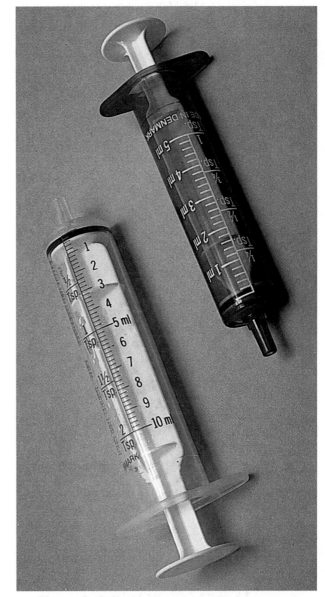

Figure 8-9 *Plastic oral syringe.* Courtesy Chuck Dresner.

into the barrel, the dropper should not be tipped upside down. The medication will run into the bulb, causing some loss of the medication. Medications should not be drawn into the dropper and then transferred to another container for administration because part of the medication will adhere to the second container, thus diminishing the dose delivered.

Teaspoons

Doses of most liquid medications are prescribed in terms using the teaspoon (Figure 8-8) as the unit of measure. However, there is great variation between the volumes measured by various teaspoons within the household. Within the hospital, 1 teaspoonful is converted to 5 ml (see Table 8-1) and is read on the metric scale of the medicine cup. For home use, an oral syringe is recommended. If not available, a teaspoon used specifically for baking may be used as an accurate measuring device.

Oral Syringes

Plastic **oral syringes** (Figure 8-9) may be used to measure liquid medications accurately. Various sizes are available to measure volumes from 0.1 ml to 15 ml. Note that a needle will not fit on the tip.

Nipples

An infant feeding nipple (Figure 8-10) with additional holes may be used for administering oral medications to infants.

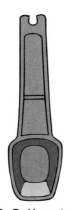

Figure 8-8 *Measuring teaspoon.*

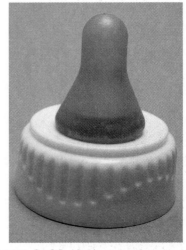

Figure 8-10 *Nipple.* Courtesy Chuck Dresner.

ADMINISTRATION OF SOLID-FORM ORAL MEDICATIONS

1. Describe general principles of administering solid forms of medications and the different techniques used with a medication card and unit dose distribution system.

Technique

Medication Card System

Equipment

Medication tray
Soufflé cup or medicine cup
Medication cards
  1. Wash hands.
  2. Gather medication cards and verify against Kardex, physician's order, or both for accuracy.
  3. Gather remainder of equipment.
  4. Read the entire medication card.
  5. Obtain the medication prescribed from the cabinet.
  6. COMPARE the label on the container against the medication card:
     RIGHT PATIENT
     RIGHT DRUG
     RIGHT ROUTE OF ADMINISTRATION
     RIGHT DOSAGE
     RIGHT TIME OF ADMINISTRATION
  7. Open lid of the bottle; pour correct number of capsules or tablets into the lid; return any extras to the container using the lid. (Do NOT touch the medication with your hands!)
  8. Transfer correct number of tablets or capsules from the lid to a soufflé cup or medicine cup.
  9. COMPARE the information on the medication card against the label on the stock bottle and the quantity of drug placed in the cup.
  10. Replace lid of container.
  11. RECHECK the FIVE RIGHTS of the medication order.
  12. Return the medication container to the shelf in the cabinet.

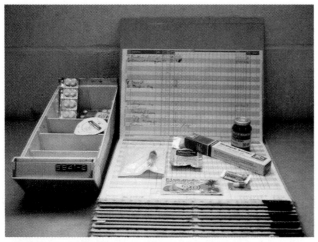

Figure 8-11 *Tray for medication card system.* Courtesy Robert Manchester, RPh.

13. Place the patient's medication cup on the medication tray with the medication card (Figure 8-11).
14. Proceed to the patient's bedside when all medications are assembled for administration.
   • Check the patient's identification bracelet and verify against the medication card.
   • Explain what you are doing.
   • Check pertinent patient monitoring parameters (apical pulse, respiratory rate, and so on).
   • Hand medication to patient for placement in the mouth.

Unit Dose System

Equipment

Medication cart
Medication profile
  1. Wash hands.
  2. Read the patient medication profile for drugs and times of administration.
  3. Obtain the medication prescribed from the drawer that is assigned to the patient in the medication cart.
  4. Check the label on the unit dose package against the patient medication profile.
     RIGHT PATIENT
     RIGHT DRUG
     RIGHT ROUTE OF ADMINISTRATION
     RIGHT DOSAGE
     RIGHT TIME OF ADMINISTRATION
  5. Check the number of doses remaining in the drawer. (If the number of doses remaining is not consistent, investigate!)
  6. Check the FIVE RIGHTS of the medication order on the patient medication profile and unit dose package as removed from drawer.
  7. Proceed to the bedside:
     • Check patient's identification bracelet and verify against the profile.
     • Explain carefully to the patient what you are doing.
     • Check pertinent patient monitoring parameters (apical pulse, respiratory rate, and so on).
  8. Hand the medication to the patient and allow him or her to read the package label.
  9. Retrieve the unit dose package and open it, placing the contents in the patient's hand for placement in the mouth.

General Principles of Solid-Form Medication Administration

1. Give the most important medication first.
2. Allow the patient to drink a small amount of water to moisten the mouth to make swallowing the medication easier.
3. Have the patient place the medication well back on the tongue. Offer appropriate assistance.
4. Give the patient liquid to swallow the medication. Encourage keeping the head forward while swallowing.
5. Drinking a full glass of fluid should be encouraged to ensure that the medication reaches the stomach and to dilute the drug to decrease the potential for irritation.
6. Always remain with the patient while the medication is taken. Do NOT leave the medication at the bedside unless an order exists to do so (medication such as nitroglycerin may be ordered for the bedside).

7. Discard the medication container (such as a soufflé cup or unit dose package).

Documentation, the Sixth Right

Provide the RIGHT DOCUMENTATION of medication administration and responses to drug therapy:

1. Chart the date, time, drug name, dosage, and route of administration.
2. Perform and record regular patient assessments for the evaluation of the therapeutic effectiveness (blood pressure, pulse, output, improvement or quality of cough and productivity, degree and duration of pain relief, and so on).
3. Chart and report any signs and symptoms of adverse drug effects.
4. Perform and validate essential patient education about the drug therapy and other essential aspects of intervention for the disease process affecting the individual.

ADMINISTRATION OF LIQUID-FORM ORAL MEDICATIONS

Objective

I. Compare techniques used to administer liquid forms of oral medication using medication card and unit dose system of distribution.

Technique

Medication Card System

Equipment
Medication tray
Plastic syringe or medicine cup
Medication cards

1. Wash hands.
2. Gather medication cards and verify against Kardex, physician's order, or both for accuracy.
3. Gather remainder of equipment.
4. Read the entire medication card.
5. Obtain the medication prescribed from the cabinet.
6. COMPARE the label on the container against the medication card:
   RIGHT PATIENT
   RIGHT DRUG
   RIGHT ROUTE OF ADMINISTRATION
   RIGHT DOSAGE
   RIGHT TIME OF ADMINISTRATION
7. Shake medication, if required.
8. Remove lid and place upside down on a flat surface to prevent contamination.
9. Proceed with one of the following measuring techniques.

Measuring with a Medicine Cup
- Hold the bottle of liquid so that the label is in the palm of the hand. This prevents the contents from smearing the label during pouring.

- Examine the medicine cup and locate the exact place to where the measured volume should be measured; place your fingernail at this level.
- While holding the medicine cup straight at eye level, pour the prescribed volume.
- Read the volume accurately at the level of the meniscus (Figure 8-12).
- COMPARE the information on the medication card against the label on the stock bottle and the quantity of drug placed in the cup.
- Replace lid on the container.
- RECHECK the FIVE RIGHTS of the medication order.
- Return the medication container to the shelf of the cabinet.
- Place the patient's medication cup on the medication tray with the medication card (see Figure 8-11).
- Proceed to the patient's bedside when all medications are assembled for administration.

Measuring with an Oral Syringe
See Chapter 9 for reading calibrations of a syringe.
- Select a syringe in a size comparable to the volume to be measured.
- *Method 1:* With a large-bore needle attached to the syringe, draw up the prescribed volume of medication. The needle is not necessary if the bottle opening is large enough to receive the syringe (Figure 8-13).
- *Method 2:* Using the cup and method 1, pour the amount of medication needed into a medicine cup, then use a syringe to measure the prescribed volume (Figure 8-14).
- COMPARE the information on the medication card against the label on the stock bottle and the quantity of drug placed in the syringe.
- Replace the lid on the container.
- RECHECK the FIVE RIGHTS of the medication order.
- Return the medication container to the shelf of the cabinet.
- Place the patient's medication syringe on the medication tray with the medication card directly under the syringe.
- Proceed to the patient's bedside when all medications are assembled for administration.

Now that the medication is ready to be administered, proceed as follows:

10. Check the patient's identification bracelet and verify against the medication card.
11. Explain what you are doing.

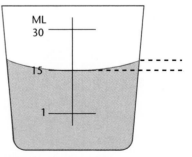

Figure 8-12 *Reading meniscus. The meniscus is caused by the surface tension of the solution against the walls of the container. The surface tension causes the formation of a concave or hollowed curvature on the surface of the solution. Read the level at the lowest point of the concaved curve.*

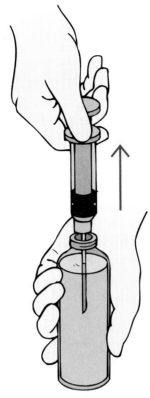

Figure 8-13 *Removing medication directly from a bottle.*

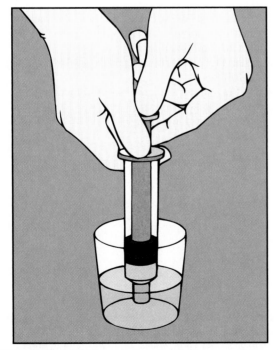

Figure 8-14 *Filling a syringe directly from a medicine cup.*

12. Check pertinent patient monitoring parameters (apical pulse, respiratory rate, and so on).
13. Hand medication cup to patient for placement of the contents in the mouth or administer via the oral syringe.

Unit Dose System

Equipment
Medication cart
Medication profile
1. Wash hands.
2. Read the patient medication profile for drugs and times of administration.
3. Obtain the medication prescribed from the drawer assigned to the patient in the medication cart.
4. Check the label on the unit dose package against the patient medication profile:
RIGHT PATIENT
RIGHT DRUG
RIGHT ROUTE OF ADMINISTRATION
RIGHT DOSAGE
RIGHT TIME OF ADMINISTRATION
5. Check the number of doses remaining in the drawer. (If the number of doses remaining is not consistent, investigate!)
6. Check the FIVE RIGHTS of the medication order on the patient medication profile and unit dose package as removed from the drawer.
7. Proceed to the bedside:
   • Check patient's identification bracelet and verify against the profile.
   • Explain what you are doing.
   • Check pertinent patient monitoring parameters (apical pulse, respiratory rate, and so on).
8. Hand the unit dose medication to the patient and allow him or her to read the package label.
9. Retrieve the unit dose package and open it, placing the container in the patient's hand for placement of the contents in the patient's mouth.

General Principles of Liquid-Form Oral Medication Administration

For an Adult or Child

1. Give the most important medication first.
2. Never dilute a liquid medication unless specifically ordered to do so.
3. Always remain with the patient while the medication is taken. Do NOT leave the medication at the bedside unless an order exists to do so.

For an Infant

1. Check the infant's identification bracelet and verify against the medication card or profile.
2. Be certain that the infant is alert.
3. Position the infant so that the head is slightly elevated (Figure 8-15).
4. Administration:
   • *Oral syringe or dropper:* Place the syringe or dropper between the cheek and gums, halfway back into the mouth. This placement will lessen the chance that the

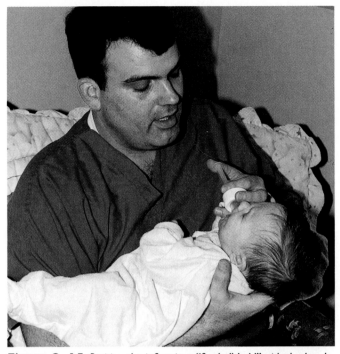

Figure 8-15 *Position the infant in a "football hold" with the head slightly elevated. Place the nipple in the infant's mouth. When the baby starts to suck, place the medication in the back of the nipple and allow the baby to suck.* Courtesy Oscar H. Allison, Jr.

infant will spit out the medication with tongue movements. Slowly inject, allowing the infant to swallow medication. (Rapid administration may cause choking and aspiration.)

* *Nipple:* When the infant is awake (and preferably hungry), place the nipple in the infant's mouth. When the baby starts to suck, place the medication in the back of the nipple with a syringe or dropper and allow the baby to suck it in (see Figure 8-15). (The size of the nipple holes may have to be enlarged for suspensions and syrups.) Follow with milk or formula, if necessary.

Documentation, the Sixth Right

Provide the RIGHT DOCUMENTATION of the medication administration and responses to drug therapy:

1. Chart the date, time, drug name, dosage, and route of administration.
2. Perform and record regular patient assessments for the evaluation of therapeutic effectiveness (blood pressure, pulse, output, improvement or quality of cough and productivity, degree and duration of pain relief, and so on).
3. Chart and report any signs and symptoms of adverse drug effects.
4. Perform and validate essential patient education about the drug therapy and other essential aspects of intervention for the disease process affecting the individual.

ADMINISTRATION OF MEDICATIONS BY THE NASOGASTRIC TUBE

Objective

1. Cite the equipment needed, techniques used, and precautions necessary when administering medications via a nasogastric tube.

Key Word

nasogastric tube

Medications are administered via a **nasogastric (NG) tube** to patients who have impaired swallowing, who are comatose, or who have a disorder of the esophagus. Whenever possible, a liquid form of a drug should be used for NG administration. If it is necessary to use a tablet or capsule, the tablet should be crushed and the capsule pulled apart and the powder sprinkled in approximately 30 ml of water. (Do NOT crush enteric-coated tablets or timed-release capsules.) When more than one medication is ordered for administration at the same time, flush between each medication with 5 to 10 ml of water.

Equipment

Glass of water
5-to 10-ml syringe (adult patient)
1-ml syringe (young child)
Stethoscope
Medication
Bulb syringe with catheter tip

Technique

Refer to the sections on the administration of solid-form or liquid-form oral medications for preparation of dosages.

1. Proceed to the patient's bedside when all medications are assembled for administration.
2. Check the patient's identification bracelet and verify against the medication card or drug profile.
3. Explain what you are going to do.
4. Sit the patient upright and check the location of the nasogastric tube before administering any liquid (Figure 8-16).
   * *Method 1:* Aspirate part of the stomach contents using the bulb syringe (Figure 8-16, *A*). Return of stomach contents confirms correct tube placement. If contents are not returned, use methods 2, 3, or both to assess the location of the tube tip.
   * *Method 2:* Place a stethoscope over the stomach area; listen as 5 to 10 ml (adult) (0.5 up to 5 ml for child) of air are inserted (Figure 8-16, *B*). A gurgling sound should be heard if the nasogastric tube is properly placed. Withdraw the amount of air inserted. (Although a bulb syringe is frequently used to insert the air, a syringe with an adapter may also be used for more accurate measurement.)

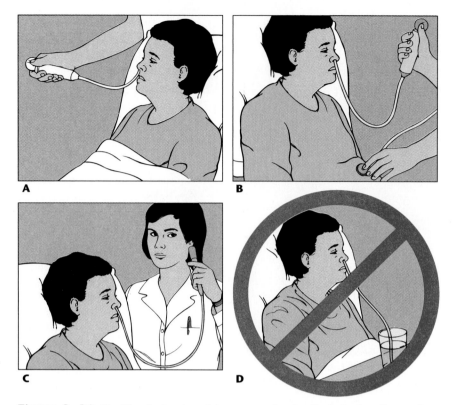

Figure 8-16 *Checking the location of the nasogastric tube.* **A,** *Aspiration of stomach contents.* **B,** *Place a stethoscope over the stomach area; listen for a gurgling sound as air is inserted.* **C,** *Listen for crackling sounds indicating placement of nasogastric tube in the lung.* **D,** *It is no longer recommended to place the end of the nasogastric tube in a glass of water. Although bubbling with respirations indicates placement of the tube in the lung, the patient may inadvertently inhale additional water from the glass into the lungs.*

- *Method 3:* Place the unclamped NG tube next to the ear and listen for any crackling noise (Figure 8-16, *C*); if the crackling sounds are heard, the tube may be in the lung. Remove and reinsert.
5. Once the placement of the NG tube in the stomach is confirmed, do the following:
   - Clamp the tubing and attach the bulb syringe; pour the medication into the syringe while the tubing is still clamped (Figure 8-17, *A*).
   - Unclamp the tubing and allow the medication to run in by gravity (Figure 8-17, *B*); add the specified amount of water (at least 50 ml) (Figure 8-17, *C*) to flush the medication through the tube and into the stomach; clamp the tubing as soon as the water has flowed through the bulb syringe (Figure 8-17, *D*).
   - Clamp the tubing at the end of the medication administration. Do NOT attach to the suction source for at least 30 minutes, or the medication will be suctioned out.
   - Give oral hygiene, if needed.

Documentation, the Sixth Right

Provide the RIGHT DOCUMENTATION of medication administration and responses to drug therapy:

1. Chart the verification of the NG tube placement.
2. Chart the date, time, drug name, dosage, and route of administration. Include all fluids administered on intake record.
3. Perform and record regular patient assessments for the evaluation of the therapeutic effectiveness (blood pressure, pulse, output, improvement or quality of cough and productivity, degree and duration of pain relief, and so on).
4. Chart and report any signs and symptoms of adverse drug effects.
5. Perform and validate essential patient education about the drug therapy and other essential aspects of intervention for the disease process affecting the individual.

ADMINISTRATION OF ENTERAL FEEDINGS

Objective

1. To meet the person's basic metabolic requirements and provide adequate nutritional intake through the use of enteral nutrition support.

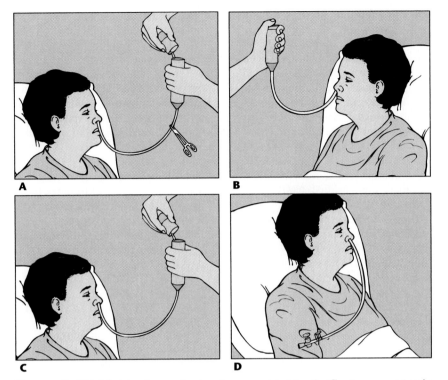

Figure 8-17 *Administering medication via nasogastric tube.* **A,** *Clamp nasogastric tube, attach a bulb syringe, and pour prescribed medication into syringe portion.* **B,** *Unclamp tubing and allow the medication to flow in by gravity.* **C,** *When medication is low in the syringe portion, pour in water to allow for thorough flushing of the medication from the tubing.* **D,** *Clamp tubing and secure end in place. Do not reattach to suction (if being used) for at least 30 minutes.*

Dosage Form

Enteral formulas are available in a variety of mixtures to meet the individual's needs. There are four general categories: (1) intact nutrient (polymeric), (2) elemental, (3) disease or condition specific, and (4) modular nutrient. The type of formula ordered will be selected by the physician to meet the patient's energy requirements to maintain body functions and growth demands and to repair tissue that is damaged or depleted by illness or injury.

Intermittent Tube Feedings

Equipment

Feeding formula
Toomey syringe
50 ml of water
Measuring container or graduate
Stethoscope
Clamp (C-clamp or ostomy plug)
Towel or small incontinent pad

Formula should be properly labeled with time, date, type of formula, and strength. Check date and time of preparation on formula mixed in hospital pharmacy: discard unused portion every 24 hours. Commercially prepared, vacuum-sealed formulas are generally stored at room temperature until used. Check the expiration date and return if outdated. If opened, refrigerate and use within 24 hours or discard.

Optional supplies to cleanse stoma area:
Sterile basin
4 × 4 gauge sponges
hydrogen peroxide
sterile saline or water
precut drain sponge
tape

Technique

Place the patient in a semi-Fowler's position, 30-degree head-of-bed (HOB) elevation for 30 minutes before starting feeding.

1. Wash hands and assemble the necessary equipment and the prescribed formula.
2. Check date, time, strength of solution, and type of formula against the physician's order:
   RIGHT PATIENT
   RIGHT DRUG (FORMULA)
   RIGHT ROUTE OF ADMINISTRATION
   RIGHT DOSAGE (AMOUNT, DILUTION, STRENGTH)
   RIGHT TIME OF ADMINISTRATION
3. Proceed to patient's bedside.
4. Check the patient's identification bracelet and verify against the medication card or drug profile.
5. Explain what you are going to do.
6. Provide for patient privacy; check patient positioning, drape to avoid unnecessary exposure. Place a towel or

small incontinent pad under feeding tube area to protect area in case of accidental spills.

7. Don disposable gloves. If stoma site needs cleansing, which should be done at least once daily or prn, proceed as follows: If crusted, place 4 × 4 gauze sponges in solution of half hydrogen peroxide and half saline or water. Place saturated sponge around stoma area, allowing solution to soften the crusted exudate. Remove sponges and wipe from tube or stoma area outward. Rinse with saline- or water-soaked 4 × 4 sponges; pat dry and apply a precut drain sponge around site. Secure with tape.

8. Attach Toomey syringe to clamped tube; release clamp. Slowly withdraw plunger to aspirate residual. Notify physician if residual is greater than 100 cc (or amount specified) since last bolus feeding 4 hours earlier. Reintroduce gastric contents aspirated. If unable to aspirate gastric contents, assess proper placement of nasogastric or gastrostomy tube by auscultation with stethoscope over midepigastric area while injecting a *small* amount of air.

9. Clamp tube; remove Toomey syringe and remove plunger. Reattach Toomey syringe to tubing while still clamped, pour formula into Toomey syringe, unclamp tubing, and allow contents to flow in by gravity. Continue filling Toomey as it drains until the prescribed amount is instilled. Do not allow air to enter the stomach and cause distention.

10. Flush tubing with 50 ml of water. This removes formula from tubing, maintains the patency of the tube, and prevents formula remaining in tube from supporting bacterial growth.

11. Clamp or plug ostomy tube; remove Toomey syringe.

12. Explain to patient that he or she must remain in a sitting position or turn on the right side for 30 minutes to 1 hour to aid in normal digestion of feeding and to prevent gastric reflux (with possible aspiration) or leakage.

13. Wash all reusable equipment, dry, and store in clean area in patient environment until the next feeding. Change equipment every 24 hours.

Documentation, the Sixth Right

Provide the RIGHT DOCUMENTATION of the formula administered, cleansing of the stoma, or therapeutic response to the enteral feedings.

1. Chart date, time, amount of residual aspirated; amount, type, and strength of formula instilled and amount of water used to rinse tubing.

2. Record formula and water instilled on intake and output sheet. Record formula type, amount, and strength on diet portion of graphic sheet.

3. Record patient's tolerance of procedure and any observations made that would indicate potential problems.

4. When stoma area is cleansed, document on chart.

Note: Day shift personnel usually reorder formula for use over next 24-hour period.

Continuous Tube Feedings

Equipment
Electronic infusion pump and compatible feeding set
Feeding formula

Stethoscope
Toomey syringe

Formula should be properly labeled with time, date, type of formula, and strength. Check date and time of preparation on formula mixed in hospital pharmacy; discard unused portion every 24 hours. Commercially prepared, vacuum-sealed formulas are generally stored at room temperature until used. Check the expiration date and return if outdated. If opened, refrigerate and use within 24 hours or discard.

Technique
Place the patient in a semi-Fowler's position, 30-degree HOB elevation for 30 minutes before starting feeding.

1. Wash hands and assemble the necessary equipment and the prescribed formula.

2. Check date, time, strength of solution, and type of formula against the physician's order:
RIGHT PATIENT
RIGHT DRUG (FORMULA)
RIGHT ROUTE OF ADMINISTRATION
RIGHT DOSAGE (AMOUNT, DILUTION, STRENGTH)
RIGHT TIME OF ADMINISTRATION

3. Proceed to patient's bedside.

4. Check the patient's identification bracelet and verify against the medication card or drug profile.

5. Explain what you are going to do.

6. Provide for patient privacy; check patient positioning, drape to avoid unnecessary exposure. Place a towel or small incontinent pad under feeding tube area to protect area in case of accidental spills.

7. Fill container with enough formula solution for 6 to 8 hours. Store remaining formula in the refrigerator. Hang container on pump pole.

8. For Flexiflow companion pump (Ross Laboratories): Fill sight chamber one third to one half full by squeezing bellows of cassette. Continue compressing bellows intermittently to move formula through tubing and expel all air; clamp tubing.

   Insert cassette into pump, being sure it is thoroughly intact. (Use shape of cassette as orientation for placement into machine.)

   Turn dial to "set rate"; select flow rate using indicators on front of pump. (Compare flow rate with doctor's order.)

   Turn dial to "hold."

   Cover tip of tubing to maintain sterility.

9. Don disposable gloves. If stoma site needs cleansing, which should be done at least once daily or prn, proceed as follows: If crusted, place 4 × 4 gauze sponges in solution of half hydrogen peroxide and half saline or water. Place saturated sponge around stoma area, allowing solution to soften the crusted exudate. Remove sponges and wipe from tube or stoma area outward. Rinse with saline- or water-soaked 4 × 4 sponges; pat dry and apply a precut drain sponge around site. Secure with tape.

10. Attach Toomey syringe to clamped tube; release clamp. Slowly withdraw plunger to aspirate residual. Notify physician if residual is greater than 100 cc (or amount specified) since last bolus feeding 4 hours earlier.

Reintroduce gastric contents aspirated. If unable to aspirate gastric contents, assess proper placement of nasogastric or gastrostomy tube by auscultation with stethoscope over midepigastric area while injecting a *small* amount of air.

11. Attach tubing to stoma site. There are adapters for jejunostomy tube size and regular gastrostomy use in set.
12. Release clamp from tubing; turn pump to "run" to start feeding.
13. Mark feeding container and tubing with date and time and initials of nurse preparing setup and feeding. Tubing and container must be changed every 24 hours. Attach label to feeding container with date, time, amount and type of formula, and nurse's initials.
14. Check patient's positioning.
15. Wash all reusable equipment, dry, and store in clean area in patient environment until next feeding. Change equipment every 24 hours.

Documentation, the Sixth Right

Provide the RIGHT DOCUMENTATION of the formula administered, cleansing of the stoma, or therapeutic response to the enteral feedings.

1. Chart date, time, and amount of residual aspirated.
2. Record type of formula, strength, and any water instilled on intake and output sheet q8h. Record formula type, amount, and strength on diet portion of graphic sheet.
3. Record patient's tolerance of procedure and any observations made that would indicate problems are or may be occurring.
4. When stoma area is cleansed, document on chart.

Note: Day shift personnel usually reorder formula for use over next 24-hour period.

ADMINISTRATION OF RECTAL SUPPOSITORIES

Objective

1. Cite the equipment needed and technique used to administer rectal suppositories.

Dosage Form

Suppositories (Figure 8-18) are a solid form of medication designed for introduction into a body orifice. At body temperature, the substance dissolves and is absorbed by the mucous membranes. Suppositories should be stored in a cool place to prevent softening. If a suppository becomes soft and the package has not yet been opened, hold the foil-wrapped

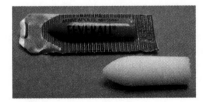

Figure 8-18 *Rectal suppositories.* Courtesy Chuck Dresner.

suppository under cold running water or place in ice water for a short time until it hardens. Rectal suppositories should generally not be used for patients who have had recent prostatic or rectal surgery or recent rectal trauma.

Equipment

Finger cot or disposable glove
Water-soluble lubricant
Prescribed suppository

Technique

1. Wash hands and assemble the necessary equipment and the prescribed rectal suppository.
2. COMPARE the label on the container against the medication card or drug profile:
   RIGHT PATIENT
   RIGHT DRUG
   RIGHT ROUTE OF ADMINISTRATION
   RIGHT DOSAGE
   RIGHT TIME OF ADMINISTRATION
3. Proceed to the patient's bedside.
4. Check the patient's identification bracelet and verify against the medication card or drug profile.
5. Explain what you are going to do.
6. Check pertinent patient monitoring parameters (time of last defecation, severity of nausea or vomiting, respiratory rate, and so on) as appropriate to the medication to be administered.
7. Whenever possible, have the patient defecate.
8. Provide for patient privacy; position and drape to avoid unnecessary exposure (Figure 8-19, *A*). Generally, the patient is placed on the left side (Sim's position).
9. Put on a disposable glove or finger cot (index finger for an adult; fourth finger for infants).
10. Ask the patient to bend the uppermost leg toward the waist.
11. Unwrap the suppository and apply a small amount of water-soluble lubricant to its tip. If lubricant is not available, use plain water to moisten; do NOT use Vaseline or mineral oil (Figure 8-19, *B* and *C*).
12. Place the tip of the suppository at the rectal entrance and ask the patient to take a deep breath and exhale through the mouth (many patients will have an involuntary rectal gripping when the suppository is pressed against the rectum). Gently insert the suppository about an inch beyond the orifice past the internal sphincter (Figure 8-19, *D*).
13. Ask the patient to remain lying on the side for 15 to 20 minutes to allow melting and absorption of the medication.
14. In children, it is necessary to gently but firmly compress the buttocks and hold in place for the same time period to prevent expulsion.
15. Discard used materials and wash hands thoroughly.

Documentation, the Sixth Right

Provide the RIGHT DOCUMENTATION of medication administration and responses to drug therapy:

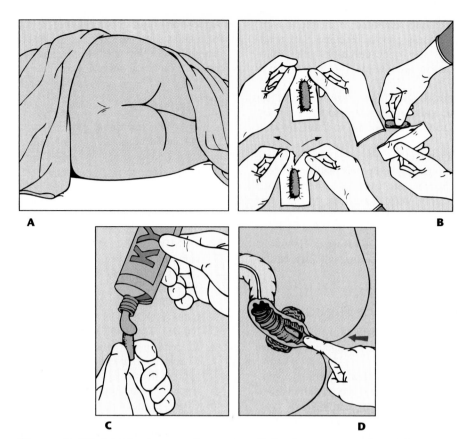

Figure 8-19 *Administering a rectal suppository.* **A,** *Position patient on side and drape.* **B,** *Unwrap suppository and remove from package.* **C,** *Apply watter-soluble lubricant to suppository.* **D,** *Gently insert suppository approximately one inch past the internal sphincter.*

1. Chart the date, time, drug name, dosage, and route of administration.
2. Perform and record regular patient assessments for the evaluation of the therapeutic effectiveness (for example, when given as a laxative, chart color, amount, and consistency of stool; if given for pain relief, chart the degree and duration of pain relief; if given as an antiemetic, the degree and duration of relief of nausea and vomiting).
3. Chart and report any signs and symptoms of adverse drug effects.
4. Perform and validate essential patient education about the drug therapy and other essential aspects of intervention for the disease process affecting the individual.

ADMINISTRATION OF DISPOSABLE ENEMA

Objective

1. Cite the equipment needed and technique used to administer a disposable enema.

Dosage Form

A prepackaged, disposable-type enema solution of the type prescribed by the physician.

Equipment

Toilet tissue
Bedpan, if patient is not ambulatory
Water-soluble lubricant
Gloves
Prescribed disposable enema kit

Technique

1. Wash hands and assemble the necessary equipment and the prescribed rectal enema.
2. COMPARE the label on the container against the medication card or drug profile:
   RIGHT PATIENT
   RIGHT DRUG
   RIGHT ROUTE OF ADMINISTRATION
   RIGHT DOSAGE
   RIGHT TIME OF ADMINISTRATION
3. Proceed to the patient's bedside.
4. Check the patient's identification bracelet and verify against the medication card or drug profile.
5. Explain what you are going to do.
6. Check pertinent patient monitoring parameters (time of last defecation).
7. Provide for patient privacy; position patient on left side; drape to avoid unnecessary exposure (Figure 8-20, *A*).
8. Don gloves, remove protective covering from the rectal tube, and lubricate (Figure 8-20, *B*).

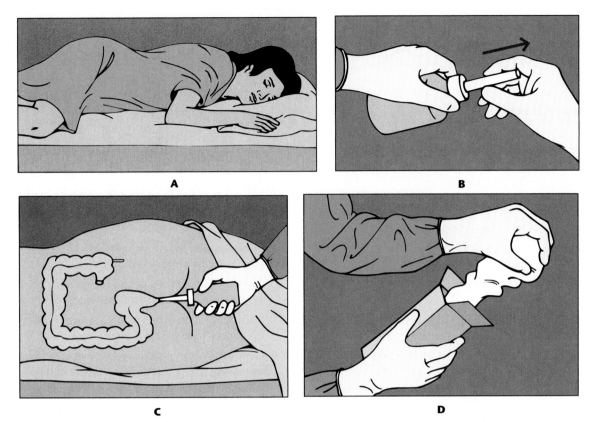

Figure 8-20 *Administering a disposable enema (Fleet enema).* **A,** *Place patient in a left lateral position, unless knee-chest position has been specified.* **B,** *Remove protective covering from rectal tube and lubricate tube.* **C,** *Insert lubricated rectal tube into rectum and dispense solution by compressing plastic container.* **D,** *Replace used container in original wrapping for disposal.*

9. Insert lubricated rectal tube into the rectum and insert solution by compressing plastic container (Figure 8-20, *C*).
10. Replace used container in its original container for disposal (Figure 8-20, *D*).
11. Encourage the patient to hold the solution for a short period of time (30 minutes) before defecating.
12. Assist the patient to a sitting position on the bedpan or to the bathroom, as orders permit.
13. Tell the patient NOT to flush the toilet until you return and can see the results of the enema. Instruct the patient regarding the location of the call light in case assistance is needed.
14. Wash hands thoroughly.

Documentation, the Sixth Right

Provide the RIGHT DOCUMENTATION of medication administration and responses to drug therapy:
1. Chart the date, time, drug name, dosage, and route of administration.
2. Perform and record regular patient assessments for the evaluation of the therapeutic effectiveness (color, amount, and consistency of stool).
3. Chart and report any signs and symptoms of adverse drug effects.
4. Perform and validate essential patient education about the drug therapy and other essential aspects of intervention for the disease process affecting the individual.

Parenteral Administration

The routes of drug administration may be classified into three categories: the enteral, the parenteral, and the percutaneous routes. The term *parenteral* means administration by any route other than the enteral, or gastrointestinal, tract. Technically, this definition could include topical or inhalation administration. However, as ordinarily used, *parenteral route* refers to intradermal, subcutaneous, intramuscular, or intravenous injections.

When drugs are given parenterally rather than orally, (1) the onset of drug action is generally more rapid but of shorter duration, (2) the dosage is often smaller because drug potency tends not to be immediately altered by the stomach or liver, and (3) the cost of drug therapy is often greater. Drugs are administered by injection when it is important that all of the drug be absorbed as rapidly and completely as possible or at a steady, controlled rate, or when a patient is unable to take a medication orally because of nausea and vomiting.

Injection of drugs requires skill and special care because of the trauma at the site of needle puncture, the possibility of infection, and the chance of allergic reaction, and because, once it is injected, the drug is irretrievable. Therefore it is important that medications are prepared and administered carefully and accurately. Precautions must be taken to ensure that aseptic technique is used to avoid infection and that accurate drug dosage, proper rate of injection, and proper site of injection are used to avoid harm such as abscesses, necrosis, skin sloughing, nerve injuries, prolonged pain, or periostitis. Thus parenteral administration of drugs requires specialized knowledge and manual skill to ensure safety and therapeutic effectiveness.

EQUIPMENT USED IN PARENTERAL ADMINISTRATION

Objectives

1. Name the three parts of a syringe.
2. Read the calibrations of the minim and cubic centimeter or milliliter scale on different types of syringes.
3. Identify the sites where the volume of medication is read on a glass syringe and a plastic syringe.
4. Give examples of volumes of medications that can be measured in a tuberculin syringe, rather than a larger volume syringe.
5. State the advantages and disadvantages of using prefilled syringes.
6. Explain the system of measurement used to define the inside diameter of a syringe.
7. Identify the parts of a needle.
8. Explain how the gauge of a needle is determined.
9. Compare the usual volume of medication that can be administered at one site when giving a medication by intradermal, subcutaneous, or intramuscular routes.
10. State the criteria used for the selection of the correct needle gauge and length.
11. Identify the parts of an intravenous administration set.
12. State where to find the number of drops per milliliter delivered by the drip chambers on intravenous administration sets purchased from different manufacturers.
13. Identify the meaning of needle protector systems.

Key Words

barrel	tuberculin syringe
plunger	prefilled syringe
minim scale	tip
milliliter scale	gauge
insulin syringe	butterfly needle

Syringes

The syringe (Figure 9-1) has three parts. The **barrel** is the outer portion on which the calibrations for the measurement

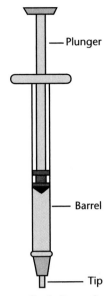

Figure 9- 1 *Parts of a syringe.*

of the drug volume are located (Figure 9-2). The **plunger** is the inner, cylindrical portion that fits snugly into the barrel. This portion is used to draw up and eject the solution from the syringe. The *tip* is the portion that holds the needle. There are two types of tips: the plain tip and the Luer-Lok.

Syringes are made of glass or a hard plastic material. Each type has advantages and disadvantages.

Glass Syringes

Advantages of the glass syringe include economy, easy-to-read calibrations, and availability in a wide range of sizes. In addition, they can be cleaned, packaged, sterilized, and reused. Disadvantages of the glass syringe are that it is easily breakable, it is time-consuming to clean and resterilize, and the plunger may become loose with extended use, which causes medication to "creep" between the plunger and the barrel. This results in an inaccurate dose being administered to the patient.

Plastic Syringes

Advantages of the plastic syringe include availability in a wide range of sizes, prepackaging with and without needles in a wide variety of gauges and needle lengths, disposability, and convenience. Disadvantages of the plastic syringe include expense, one-time use, and in some instances unclear calibrations.

Calibration

The syringe is calibrated in *minims* ($\mathfrak{m}$) and *milliliters* (ml) or *cubic centimeters* (cc) (see Figure 9-2). The most commonly used syringes are 1, 3, and 5 cc syringes, but 10, 20, and 50 cc syringes are also available. (*Note:* Technically, millimeter is a measure of volume, while cubic centimeter is a three-dimensional measure of space. Even though it is technically inappropriate, many syringes are labeled in "cc" rather than "ml.")

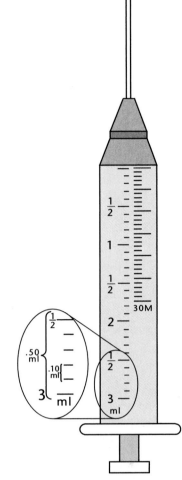

Figure 9-2 *Reading the calibrations of a 3-cc syringe.*

Reading the Calibration

Minim Scale ($\mathfrak{m}$)

Using Figure 9-2 as a guide, note that 1 minim is indicated by *each* smaller line on the calibrated scale marked ($\mathfrak{m}$). Each of the longer lines on the scale equals 5 minims. Remember that 16 minims equals 1 ml or 1 cc. The use of the **minim scale** should be discouraged. The **milliliter scale** is more accurate and represents the units by which medications are routinely ordered. For volumes of 1 ml or less, use a 1 ml, or tuberculin, syringe.

Milliliter Scale (ml)

Milliliters (or cubic centimeters) are read on the scale marked ml or cc (see Figures 9-2 and 9-4). The shorter lines represent 0.1 cc. The longer lines on this scale each represent 0.5 cc (1 ml = 1 cc).

Insulin Syringe

The **insulin syringe** has a scale specifically calibrated for the measurement of insulin. The most commonly used size is U-100, because insulin is now manufactured in this concentration.

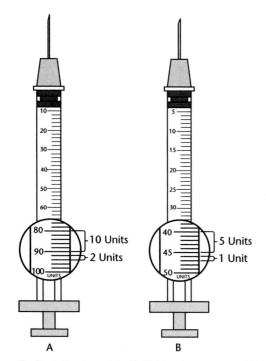

Figure 9-3 *Calibration of* **A,** *U-100 insulin syringe and* **B,** *low-dose insulin syringe.*

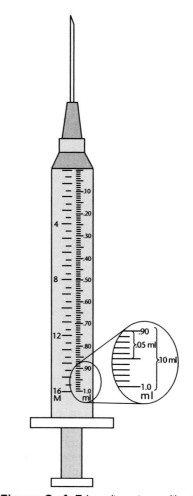

Figure 9-4 *Tuberculin syringe calibration.*

The U-100 syringe (Figure 9-3, *A*) holds 100 units of insulin per cc. On the scale, the shorter lines represent 2 units measured, and the longer lines measure 10 units of insulin. Low-dose insulin syringes (Figure 9-3, *B*) may be used for patients receiving 50 units or less of U-100 insulin. The shorter lines on the scale of the low-dose insulin syringe measure 1 unit, and the longer lines each represent 5 units.

Tuberculin Syringe

The **tuberculin syringe,** or 1 ml syringe (Figure 9-4), was originally designed to administer tuberculin. Today it is used to measure small volumes of medication accurately. The volume should be measured on the cubic centimeter scale to achieve the greatest degree of accuracy. The syringe holds a total of 1 cc or 16 minims. On the minim scale, the longer lines represent 1 minim, and the shorter lines measure 0.5 (⁵⁄₁₀ or ½) minim; however, the use of the minim scale should be discouraged. On the cubic centimeter scale, each of the longest lines represents 0.1 (¹⁄₁₀) cc, the intermediate lines equal 0.05 (⁵⁄₁₀₀) cc, and the shortest lines are 0.01 (¹⁄₁₀₀) cc.

The volumes within glass syringes are read at the point where the plunger is directly parallel with the calibration on the syringe (Figure 9-5). Volumes within disposable plastic syringes are read at the point where the rubber flange of the syringe plunger is parallel to the calibration scale of the barrel (Figure 9-6). Also note the area of the needle to keep sterile and the area on the syringe plunger to avoid touching.

Prefilled Syringes

Several manufacturers supply a premeasured amount of medication in a disposable cartridge-needle unit (**prefilled**

syringe). These units are called by brand names such as Tubex and Carpuject. The cartridge contains the amount of drug for one standard dose of medication. The drug name, concentration, and volume are clearly printed on the cartridge. Certain brands of prefilled cartridges require a holder that corresponds to the type of cartridge being used (Figure 9-7). Advantages of the prefilled syringe include the time saved in preparation of a standard amount of medication for

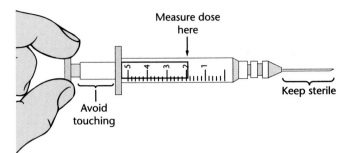

Figure 9-5 *Reading measured amount of medication in glass syringe.*

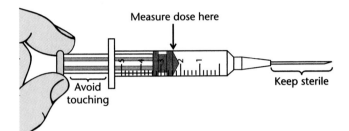

Figure 9-6 *Reading measured amount of medication in a plastic syringe.*

one injection and the diminished chance of contamination between patient and hospital personnel (the cartridge is in a sealed unit, which is used once and discarded). Disadvantages include additional expense, the need for different holders for different cartridges, and the limitation of the volume of a second medication that may be added to the cartridge.

Many hospital pharmacies "prefill" syringes for specific doses of medication for specific patients. The syringe is labeled with the drug name, dose, patient's name, room number, and date of preparation and expiration.

The Needle

Parts of the Needle

The needle parts (Figure 9-8) are the hub, shaft, and beveled **tip.** The angle of the bevel can vary; the longer the bevel, the easier the needle penetration.

Gauge

The needle **gauge** is the diameter of the hole through the needle. The larger the number (which indicates the gauge), the smaller the hole. The gauge number is marked on the hub of the needle and on the outside of the disposable package. The proper needle gauge is usually selected based on the viscosity (thickness) of the solution to be injected. A thicker solution requires a larger diameter; thus a smaller gauge number is chosen (Figure 9-9). There are finer needles (for example, 27 and 29 gauge) for specialty use.

Protector Systems

The needle protector system covers the needle to protect the user from accidental needle stick while sampling blood or administering intravenous medications. Blunt needle adapters

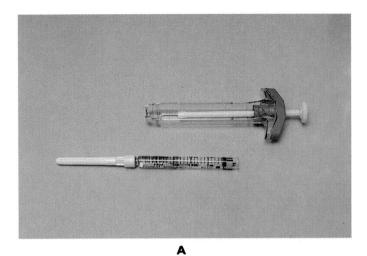

A

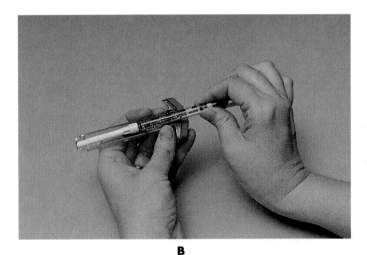

B

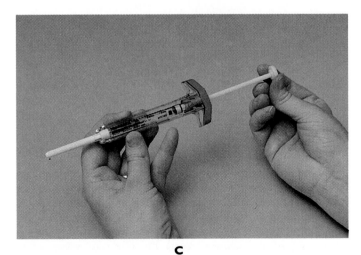

C

Figure 9-7 A, *Carpuject syringe and prefilled sterile cartridge with needle.* **B,** *Assembling the Carpuject.* **C,** *Cartridge slides into syringe barrel, turns, and locks at needle end. Plunger then screws into cartridge end.* (From Potter PA, Perry AG: *Basic nursing: theory and practice,* ed 3, 1995, St. Louis, Mosby).

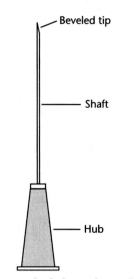

Figure 9-8 *Parts of a needle.*

Beveled tip

Shaft

Hub

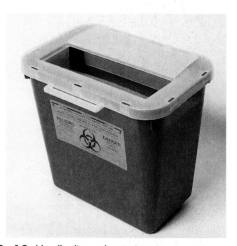

Figure 9-10 *Needle disposal container.* Courtesy Chuck Dresner.

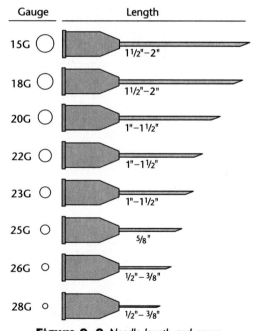

Gauge	Length
15G ◯	1½"–2"
18G ◯	1½"–2"
20G ◯	1"–1½"
22G ◯	1"–1½"
23G ◯	1"–1½"
25G ◯	⅝"
26G ○	½"–⅜"
28G ○	½"–⅜"

Figure 9-9 *Needle length and gauge.*

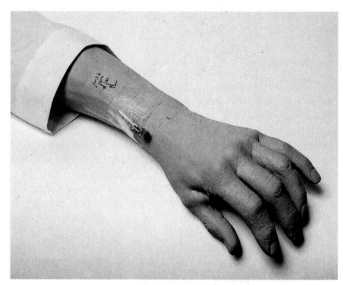

Figure 9-11 *Butterfly, scalp, or wing-tipped needle in place as a heparin lock. The tape should be labeled: date, time, and initials of person inserting the heparin lock. Some practice settings also require the date and time the lock is to be changed on the label.* Courtesy Chuck Dresner.

are available for a variety of uses, such as the male adapters on heparin locks. These accommodate the use of blunt rather than sharp needles. Other devices include a needle-free access system that has a two-way valve in place of the male adaptor cap on a heparin-lock intravenous (IV) catheter. The tapered leur end of the syringe opens the two-way valve when inserted into the valve diaphragm, thus permitting injection or aspiration of fluids. To prevent accidental needle sticks, a needle disposal container is used for all "sharps" (Figure 9-10).

Intravenous Administration

All needles, if long enough, may be used to administer medications or fluids intravenously, but special equipment has been designed for this purpose.

The **butterfly,** *scalp,* and *wing-tipped* needles (Figure 9-11) are short, sharp-tipped needles designed to minimize tissue injury during insertion. The "winged" area can be pinched together to form a handle while the needle is being inserted, then laid flat against the skin to form a base for anchoring with tape. These needles come in gauges 17 to 29. A short plastic tubing with a plastic adapter at the end is

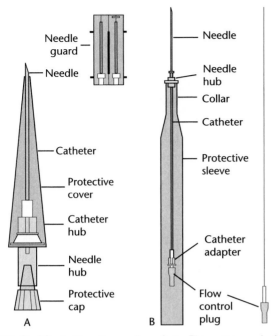

Figure 9-12 A, *Over-the-needle catheter. This unit is used when intravenous therapy is expected to continue several days.*
B, *Intracatheters use a large-bore needle for venipuncture, then a 4- to 6-inch sterile, small-gauge plastic catheter is advanced through the needle into the vein. The needle is withdrawn, and the skin forms a seal around the plastic catheter.*

attached to the needle. Butterfly needles are commonly used for venipuncture in infants and as "heparin locks" to allow patient mobility.

Plastic needles, or *over-the-catheter* needles (Figure 9-12, *A*), are actually stainless steel needles coated with a Teflon-like plastic. After penetrating the vein, the metal needle is removed, leaving the plastic catheter in place. This unit is used when IV therapy is expected to continue for several days or more. The rationale for use of the plastic catheter is that it does not have a sharp tip that may cause venous irritation and extravasation.

Intracatheters (Figure 9-12, *B*) use a large-bore needle for venipuncture. Then a 4- to 6-inch sterile, smaller-gauge plastic catheter is advanced through the needle into the vein. The needle is withdrawn and the skin forms a seal around the plastic catheter. The IV administration set is attached directly to the plastic catheter. This type of catheter is often used for hyperalimentation solutions and for IVs that will be running for a week or more.

Selection of the Syringe and Needle

The size of the syringe used is determined by the volume of medication to be administered, the degree of accuracy needed in measurement of the dose, and the type of medication to be administered.

Needle selection should be based on the correct gauge for the viscosity of the solution and the correct needle length for delivery of the medication to the correct site (subcutaneous, intramuscular, or intravenous). Table 9-1 may be used as a guideline to select the proper volume of syringe and length and gauge of needle for adult patients.

In small children and older infants, the usual maximum volume for intramuscular injection at one site is 1 ml. In small infants the muscle mass may only be able to tolerate 0.5 ($\frac{5}{10}$ or $\frac{1}{2}$) ml. For older children, the amount should be individualized; generally, the larger the muscle mass, the greater the similarity to the adult volume for one injection site. Pediatric intramuscular injections routinely use a 25- to 27-gauge needle 1 to 1½ inches long, depending on assessment of the depth of the muscle mass in the child. There are also 30-gauge, ½-inch needles available for pediatric use.

Clinical Example: Selection of Needle Length

Assess the depth of the patient's tissue for administration (muscle tissue for intramuscular administration, subcutaneous tissue for subcutaneous injection), and then choose a needle length to correspond with the findings.

> EXAMPLE: Compare the muscle depth of a 250-lb obese, sedentary female to the muscle depth of a 105-lb debilitated adult patient. The obese individual may require a 3- to 5-inch needle, the frail person a 1- to 1½-inch needle. A child may need a 1-inch needle (Figure 9-13).

Table 9-1

Selection of Syringe and Needles			
ROUTE	**VOLUME**	**GAUGE**	**LENGTH**
Intradermal	0.01-0.1 ml	26-29 g	⅜-½ inch
Subcutaneous	0.5-2 ml	25-27 g	Individualize based on depth of appropriate tissue at site of injection†
Intramuscular	0.5-2 ml*	20-22 g	
Intravenous	1-2000 ml	20-22 g (solutions)	½-1¼ inch (butterfly)
		15-19 g (blood)	½-2 inch (regular needles)

*Divided doses are generally recommended for volumes that exceed 2-3 ml, particularly for medications that are irritating to the tissues.
†When judging the needle length, allow an extra 1/4-1/2 inch length to remain above the skin surface when the injection is administered. In the rare event of a needle breaking, this allows a length of needle to protrude above the skin to grasp for removal.

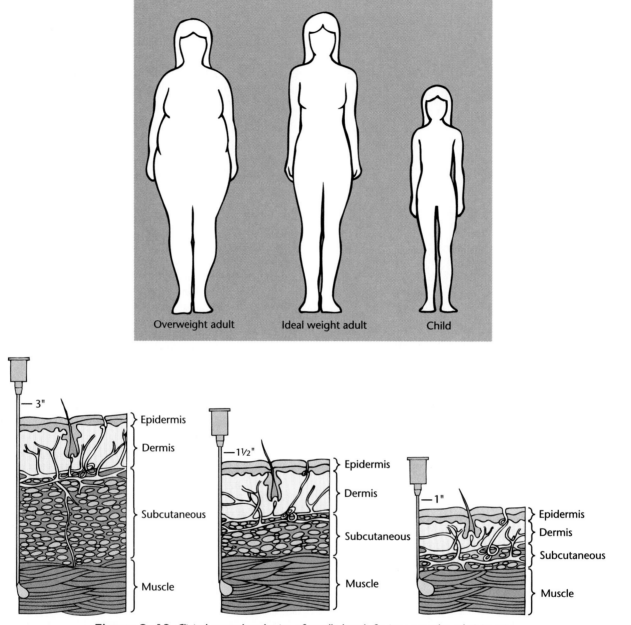

Figure 9-13 *Clinical example: selection of needle length for intramuscular administration.*

Packaging of Syringes and Needles

Always inspect and verify the sterility of the syringe and needle to be used to prepare and administer a parenteral medication. Check cloth wrappers for holes, signs of moisture penetrating the wrapper, and the date of expiration. With prepackaged disposable items, check for continuity of the wrapper, loose lids or needle guards, and for any penetration of the paper or plastic container by the needle.

Intravenous Administration Sets

Intravenous administration sets (Figure 9-14) are available with a variety of attachments (volume and size of drip chamber, "piggyback" portals, filters, drug administration chamber, clamps, or rollers), but all sets have an insertion

spike, a drip chamber, plastic tubing with a control clamp, a rubber injection portal, a needle adapter, and a protective cap over the needle adapter. The type of system used by a particular hospital is usually determined by the manufacturer of the physiologic solutions used by the institution. Each manufacturer makes adaptations to fit a specific type of glass or plastic large-volume solution container. A crucial point to remember about administration sets is that the drops delivered by drip chambers vary from different manufacturers. Macrodrip chambers (Figure 9-14, *A* and *C*) provide 10, 13, 15, or 20 drops per milliliter, and microdrip chambers (Figure 9-14, *B*) deliver 60 drops per milliliter of solution. Microdrip administration sets are used when a small volume of fluid is being administered, such as a TKO (to keep open)

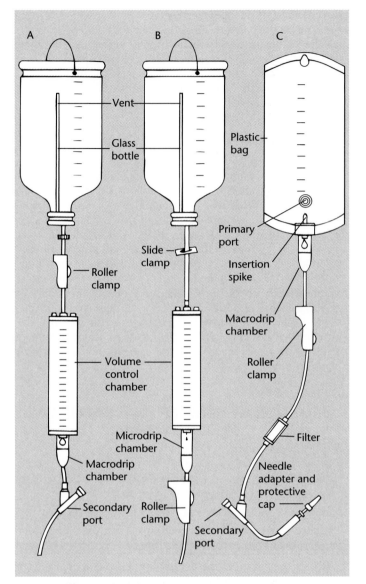

Figure 9-14 *Intravenous administration sets.*

order. In some clinical settings they are used for all volumes of IV fluid ordered that are less than 100 ml per hour. To ensure having the correct administration set it is essential to read the label box before opening it. The nurse must know the number of drops per milliliter to calculate the flow rate for the IV solution.

PARENTERAL DOSAGE FORMS

1. Differentiate among ampules, vials, and Mix-o-Vials.
2. Describe the different types of large-volume solution containers available.

ampules   piggyback
vials   IV rider
Mix-O-Vials   heparin lock
tandem setup

All parenteral drug dosage forms are packaged so that the drug is sterile and ready for reconstitution (if needed) and administration.

Ampules

Ampules are glass containers that usually contain a single dose of a medication. The container may be scored (Figure 9-15, *A*) or have a darkened ring around the neck (Figure 9-15, *B*). This marking is the location at which the ampule is broken open for withdrawing the medication.

Vials

Vials are glass containers that contain one or more doses of a sterile medication. The mouth of the vial is covered with a thick rubber diaphragm (Figure 9-16, *B*) through which a needle must be passed to remove the medication. Before use, the rubber diaphragm is sealed by a metal lid (Figure 9-16, *A*) to ensure sterility. The medication in the vial may be in solution, or it may be a sterile powder to be reconstituted just before the time of administration.

Mix-O-Vials

Mix-O-Vials are glass containers with two compartments (Figure 9-17). The lower chamber contains the drug (solute) and the upper chamber contains a sterile diluent (solvent). Between the two areas is a rubber stopper. A single dose of medication is normally contained in the Mix-o-Vial. At the time of use, pressure is applied on the top rubber diaphragm plunger. This forces the solvent and the rubber stopper to fall into the bottom chamber, dissolving the drug. A needle is then placed through the top plunger-diaphragm to withdraw the solution. (Change the needle after drug withdrawal because puncturing the plunger-diaphragm may dull the needle bevel.)

Large-Volume Solution Containers

Intravenous solutions are available in both glass and plastic containers in a variety of types and concentrations (Table 9-2) and volumes ranging from 100 to 2000 ml. Both the glass and plastic containers are vacuum sealed. The glass bottles are sealed with a hard rubber stopper, then a metal disk, followed by a metal cap. Just before use, the metal cap and disk are removed, exposing the hard rubber stopper. The insertion spike of the IV administration set is pushed into a specifically marked area on the rubber stopper. Some brands also have another opening in the rubber stopper that serves as an air vent (see Figure 9-14, *A* and *B*). As the solution runs out of the container, it is replaced with air. Other brands use a

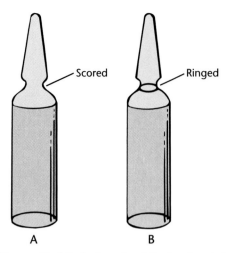

Figure 9-15 A, *Scored and* **B,** *ringed ampules.*

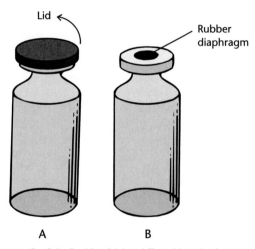

Figure 9-16 A, *Metal lid and* **B,** *rubber diaphragm vials.*

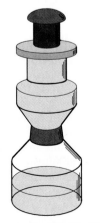

Figure 9-17 *Mix-O-Vial.*

flexible plastic container (see Figure 9-14, *C*). As the solution runs out of the bag, the flexible container collapses.

Plastic bags are somewhat different in that the entire bag and solution is sealed inside another plastic bag for removal just before administration. When the insertion spike is forced into the specifically marked portal, an internal seal is broken, allowing the solution to flow into the tubing.

Small-Volume Solution Containers

Some medicines, such as antibiotics, are administered by intermittent infusion through an apparatus known as a **tandem setup, piggyback** (IVPB), or **IV rider** (Figure 9-18). These medicines are given by a setup that is secondary to the primary IV infusion that is hung in tandem and connected to the primary setup. The secondary setup may consist of a drug infusion from a small volume of fluid in either a small bag or bottle (up to 250 ml) (see Figure 9-18) or from a volume-control set (also known as a Volutrol, Pediatrol, or Buretrol) (see Figure 9-14, *A* and *B*). A volume-control set is made up of a calibrated chamber hung under the primary IV solution container that can provide the necessary 50 to 250 ml of diluent per dose of drug. Most intermittent diluted-drug infusions are infused over 20 to 60 minutes.

PREPARATION OF PARENTERAL MEDICATION

Objectives

1. List the equipment needed for the preparation of parenteral medication.
2. Describe, practice, and perfect the preparation of medications using the various dosage forms for parenteral administration.
3. Describe, practice, and perfect the technique of preparing two different drugs in one syringe, such as insulin or a preoperative medication.

Equipment

Drug in sterile, sealed container
Syringe of the correct volume
Needles of the correct gauge and length
Antiseptic swab
Special equipment based on the route of administration (such as **heparin lock** for insertion, IV administration set for starting IV infusion)

Technique

These are standard procedures for preparing all parenteral medications:

1. Wash hands *before* preparing any medication or handling sterile supplies. During the actual preparation of a parenteral medication, the primary rule is "sterile-to-sterile and unsterile-to-unsterile" when handling the syringe and needle.

Table 9-2

Types of Intravenous Solutions*

SOLUTION	INGREDIENTS	ABBREVIATIONS
Electrolyte solutions	5% dextrose in water	D_5W
	10% dextrose in water	$D_{10}W$
	0.9% sodium chloride (normal saline)	NS or NaCl
	Ringer's lactate	RL
	5% dextrose in 0.2% sodium chloride	$D_5/.2$
	5% dextrose in 0.45% sodium chloride	$D_5/.45$
	5% dextrose in Ringer's lactate	D_5/LR
	5% dextrose in 0.2% sodium chloride + 20 mEq potassium chloride	$D_5/0.2+20$ KCl
Nutrient solutions		
Carbohydrate	Dextrose 5%-25%	D_{5-25}
Amino acids	Novamine	
	Aminosyn	
	Travasol	
	Nephramine	
	Trophamine	
	BranchAmin	
	Hepatamine	
Lipids	Intralipid	
	Liposyn	
Blood volume expanders	Hetastarch	
	Dextran	
	Albumin	
	Plasma	
Alkalinizing solutions	Sodium bicarbonate	
	Tromethamine (THAM)	
	Citrate salts	
	Sodium lactate	
Acidifying solutions	Ammonium chloride	

*A representative listing, not intended to be inclusive.

2. Use the FIVE RIGHTS of medication preparation and administration throughout the procedure:
RIGHT PATIENT
RIGHT DRUG
RIGHT ROUTE OF ADMINISTRATION
RIGHT DOSAGE (AMOUNT AND CONCENTRATION)
RIGHT TIME OF ADMINISTRATION
3. Check the drug dosage form ordered against the source you are holding to prepare.
4. Check compatibility charts or contact the pharmacist before mixing two medications or adding medication to an IV solution.
5. Check medication calculations. When in doubt about a dose, check it with another qualified nurse. (Most hospital policies require that fractional doses of medications and doses of heparin and insulin be checked by two qualified personnel before administration.)
6. Be knowledgeable of the hospital policy regarding limitations on the types of medications to be administered by nursing personnel.
7. Prepare the drug in a clean, well-lighted area, using aseptic technique throughout the entire procedure.
8. Concentrate on this procedure; ensure accuracy in preparation.

Guidelines for Preparing Medications
Preparing a Medication from an Ampule
1. Move all of the solution to the bottom of the ampule, flicking the side of the glass container with the fingers to displace the medication from the top portion of the ampule (Figure 9-19, *A*).
2. Cover the ampule neck area with a sterile gauze pledget or antiseptic swab while breaking the top off (Figure 9-19, *B*). Discard the swab and top.
3. Using an aspiration (filter) needle (Figure 9-19, *C*), withdraw the medication from the ampule (Figure 9-19, *D* and *E*). Lower needle as solution is withdrawn from ampule.
4. Remove the aspiration needle from the ampule and point the needle vertically (Figure 9-19, *F*). Pull back on the plunger (this allows air to enter the syringe) (Figure 9-19, *G*) and replace the filter needle with a new sterile needle (Figure 9-19, *H* and *I*) of the appropriate gauge and length for administration.
5. Push the plunger slowly until the medication appears at the tip of the needle (Figure 9-19, *J*), or measure the amount of air to be included to allow total clearance of the medication from the needle when injected. (Never add air to a syringe that is to be used to administer an IV medication.)

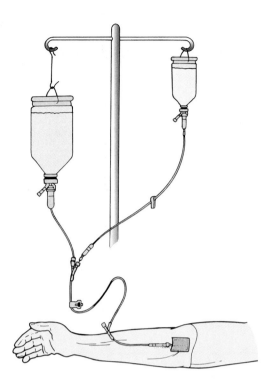

Figure 9-18 *Tandem, secondary, or piggyback intermittent administration setup. Note that the smaller bottle is hung higher than the primary bottle.*

Drugs in a *vial* may be in solution ready for administration (Figure 9-20) or may be in a powdered form for reconstitution before administration.

Preparing a Medication From a Vial
Reconstitution of a Sterile Powder
1. Read the accompanying literature from the manufacturer and follow specific instructions for reconstituting the drug ordered. Add only the diluent specified by the manufacturer.
2. Cleanse the rubber diaphragm of the vial of diluent with an antiseptic swab (Figure 9-20, *A*, p. 108).
3. Pull back on the plunger of the syringe to fill with an amount of air equal to the volume of solution to be withdrawn (Figure 9-20, *B*).
4. Insert the needle through the rubber diaphragm; inject air (Figure 9-20, *C*).
5. Withdraw the measured volume of diluent required to reconstitute the powdered drug (Figure 9-20, *D* and *E*). Remove the needle from the diaphragm of the diluent container.
6. Recheck the type and volume of diluent to be injected against the type and amount required.
7. Tap the vial containing the powdered drug to break up the caked powder (Figure 9-20, *F*). Wipe the rubber diaphragm of the vial of powdered drug with a new antiseptic swab (Figure 9-20, *G*).
8. Insert the needle in the diaphragm and inject the diluent into the powder (Figure 9-20, *H*).

9. Remove the syringe and needle from the rubber diaphragm.
10. MIX THOROUGHLY to ensure that the powder is entirely dissolved BEFORE withdrawing the dose (Figure 9-20, *I*).
11. Label the reconstituted medication, indicating date and time of reconstitution, volume and type of diluent added, name of reconstituted drug, concentration of reconstituted drug, expiration date and time, and name of person reconstituting drug. Store according to manufacturer's instructions.
12. Change the needle as described earlier (use principles illustrated in Figure 9-19, *H, I,* and *J*) . Attach a needle of the correct gauge and length to administer the medication to the patient.

Reconstitution of a Powder in a Preassembled Piggyback
Several routinely used medicines that have short expiration dates after being reconstituted (for example, ampicillin) have been preassembled by the manufacturer in a small volume parenteral solution bag that contains the sterile powder in a separate container within the bag. The primary purpose of this apparatus is to maintain sterility and minimize waste if the order for the medicine is canceled. Just before the scheduled time of administration the nurse checks all aspects of the drug order against the container, grasps the tip of the "needle" inside the IV solution container, bends it to break the tip free, and compresses the IV solution container so that the IV solution flows into the vial of medicine that is attached. This allows the IV solution to act as the diluent, and no needles are needed to reconstitute the drug. The container is shaken to dissolve the powder. The container is then inverted and compressed several times until all the drug is "pumped" from the vial into the IV solution bag ready for use. The drug is now ready for parenteral administration.

Removal of a Volume of Liquid from a Vial (Figure 9-20, A to E)
1. Calculate the volume of medication required for the prescribed dose of medication to be administered.
2. Cleanse the rubber diaphragm of the vial of diluent with an antiseptic pledget.
3. Pull back on the plunger of the syringe to fill with an amount of air equal to the volume of solution to be withdrawn.
4. Insert the needle through the rubber diaphragm; inject air.
5. Withdraw the volume of drug required to administer the prescribed dosage.
6. Recheck all aspects of the drug order.
7. Change the needle as described earlier (use principles illustrated in Figure 9-19, *H, I, J*). Attach a needle of the correct gauge and length to administer the medication to the patient.

Preparing Medication from Mix-o-Vial
1. Check the drug order against the medication you have for administration.
2. To mix:
   - Tap the container in the hand a few times to break up the caked powder.
   - Remove the plastic lid protector (Figure 9-21, *A*, p. 108).

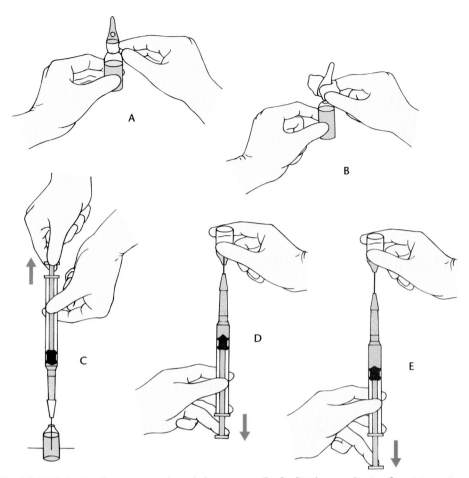

Figure 9-19 *Withdrawing from an ampule and changing needle.* **A,** *Displace medication from top portion of ampule.* **B,** *Cover ampule neck area with gauze sponge while breaking top off.* **C,** *Filter needle.* **D,** *Withdraw medication from ampule.* **E,** *Note that needle must be lowered to withdraw all solution from ampule.*

* Push firmly on the diaphragm-plunger. The downward pressure dislodges the divider between the two chambers (Figure 9-21, *B* and *C*).
* Mix thoroughly to ensure that the powder is COMPLETELY DISSOLVED before drawing up the medication for administration.
* Cleanse the rubber diaphragm and remove the drug in the same manner as described for removal of a volume of liquid from a vial (see Figure 9-20, *A-E*).

Preparing Two Medications in One Syringe

Occasionally two medications may be drawn into the same syringe for a single injection. This is most commonly done when preparing a preoperative medication or when two types of insulin are ordered to be administered at the same time. Mixing insulins is a routine procedure, so it will be used to illustrate the technique (Figure 9-22, p. 109).

1. Check the compatibility of the two drugs to be mixed before starting to prepare the medications.
2. Check the labels of the medications against the medication order.
3. Check the following:
Type: NPH, Regular, Lente, other
Concentration: U-100 (U-100 = 100 units/ml)
Expiration date: Do NOT use if outdated

Appearance: Clear, cloudy, precipitate present?
Temperature: Should be at room temperature
4. Philosophies: There are two philosophies concerning how insulins should be mixed. In one procedure, the volume of the shorter-acting insulin is drawn into the syringe first, followed by the longer-acting insulin. The rationale for this approach is that if a small amount of short-acting insulin is accidently displaced into the second (longer-acting insulin) bottle, the onset, peak, and duration of the longer-acting insulin will not be appreciably affected. If done in reverse order, the shorter-acting insulin would have its onset, peak, and duration affected because of the contamination by the longer-acting preparation.

In the second procedure, the opposite is advocated. The rationale for this approach is that because the longer-acting insulin is cloudy, a change in clarity would be immediately visible if the longer-acting insulin contaminated the normally clear second (shorter-acting) insulin during preparation.

We strongly recommend the use of the first procedure, but encourage you to check your institution's procedure manual for details.
5. Procedure:
* Roll the bottle between the palms of the hands to thoroughly mix the contents. DO NOT SHAKE.

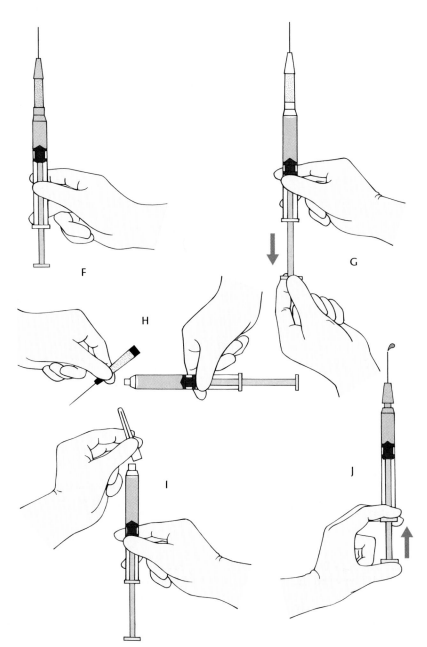

Figure 9-19, cont'd **F,** *Remove the filter needle from ampule and point needle vertically.* **G,** *Pull plunger downward to remove drug from needle.* **H,** *Remove filter needle.* **I,** *Replace filter needle with correct size needle for administering medication.* **J,** *Slowly push plunger until a drop of medication appears at needle tip. Recheck medication prepared against drug order.*

- Check the insulin order and calculations of the preparation with another qualified nurse, in accordance with hospital policy.
- Cleanse the top of BOTH vials with separate antiseptic swabs (Figure 9-22, *A*).
- Pull back the plunger on the syringe to an amount equal to the volume of the longer-acting insulin ordered (Figure 9-22, *B*).
- Insert the needle through the rubber seal of the longer-acting insulin bottle; inject air (Figure 9-22, *C*). (Do not inject air into the insulin solution because it may break up insulin particles.)
- Remove the needle and syringe. (Do not withdraw insulin at this time.)

- Pull back the plunger on the syringe to an amount equal to the volume of the shorter-acting insulin ordered (Figure 9-22, *D*).
- Insert the needle through the rubber seal of the second bottle; inject air (Figure 9-22, *E*). Invert the bottle and withdraw the volume of shorter-acting insulin ordered (Figure 9-22, *F*). *Note:* Check for bubbles in the insulin, flick the side of the syringe with the fingers to displace the bubbles, and then recheck the amount in the syringe.
- Check the medication order against the label of the container and the amount in the syringe.
- Rewipe the lid of the longer-acting insulin container (Figure 9-22, *G*); recheck the drug order against this

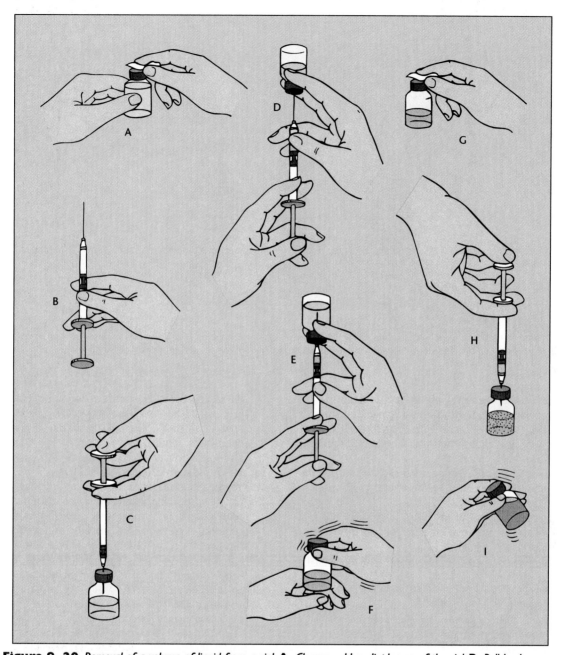

Figure 9-20 *Removal of a volume of liquid from a vial.* **A,** *Cleanse rubber diaphragm of the vial.* **B,** *Pull back on plunger of syringe to fill with an amount of air equal to the volume of solution to be withdrawn.* **C,** *Insert the needle through the rubber diaphragm; inject air with vial setting in downward position.* **D,** *Withdraw the volume of diluent required to reconstitute the drug.* **E,** *Move needle downward to facilitate removal of diluent.* **F,** *Tap the container with the powdered drug to break up the caked powder.* **G,** *Wipe the rubber diaphragm of the vial of powdered drug with a new antiseptic swab.* **H,** *Insert the needle in the rubber diaphragm and inject the diluent into the powdered drug.* **I,** *Mix thoroughly to ensure that the powdered drug is dissolved before withdrawing the prescribed dose. Change the needle before administering to the patient using the technique illustrated in Figure 9-19, H, I, and J.*

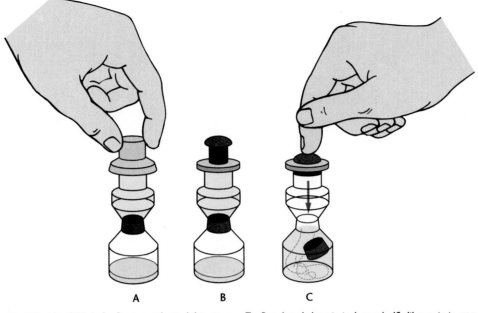

Figure 9-21 *Mix-O-Vial.* **A,** *Remove plastic lid protector.* **B,** *Powdered drug is in lower half; diluent is in upper half.* **C,** *Push firmly on the diaphragm-plunger. Downward pressure dislodges the divider between the two chambers.*

container; insert the needle of the syringe containing the shorter-acting insulin and withdraw the specified amount of longer-acting insulin (Figure 9-22, *H*). Be careful NOT to inject any of the first type of insulin already in the syringe into the vial.

- Remove the needle and syringe; recheck the drug order against the label on the insulin container and the amount in the syringe (Figure 9-22, *I*).
- Withdraw a small amount of air into the syringe and mix the two medications. Remove air carefully so that part of the medication is not displaced.
- Change needles and proceed to administer subcutaneously.

Preparing Medications for Use in the Sterile Field during an Operative Procedure

The following principles apply to the operating room:
1. All medications used during an operative procedure must remain sterile.
2. All medication containers (ampules, vials, piggyback, and blood bags) used during the operative procedure should remain in the operating room until the entire procedure is completed. (In case a question arises, the container is available.)
3. Do not save an unused portion of medication for use in another operative procedure. Discard at the end of the operative procedure or send the patient's medication to the patient care unit with the patient, if appropriate (for example, antibiotic ointment for a patient having ophthalmic surgery).
4. Adhere to hospital policies concerning handling and storage of medications in the operating room.
5. ALWAYS tell the surgeon the name and dosage or concentration of the medication or solution being handed to him or her.

6. ALWAYS repeat the entire medication order back to the surgeon at the time the request is made to verify all aspects of the order. If in doubt, repeat again until accuracy is certain.

The following technique is used to prepare medications for use in the sterile operative field:
1. Prepare the drug prescribed according to the directions.
2. Always check the accuracy of the drug order against the medication being prepared at least three times during the preparation phase: (1) when first removed from the drug storage area; (2) immediately before removing the solution for use on the sterile field; (3) immediately after completing the transfer of the medication or solution to the sterile field. ALWAYS tell the surgeon the name and dose or concentration of the medication or solution when passing it to him or her for use.
3. The circulating (nonsterile) nurse retrieves the medication from storage, reconstitutes as needed, and turns the medication container so the scrubbed (sterile) nurse can read the label. It is best to read the label aloud to ensure that both individuals are verifying the contents against the verbal order from the surgeon.

The following two methods may be used.

Method I
1. The circulating (nonsterile) nurse cleanses the top of the vial or breaks off the top of the ampule, as described earlier.
2. The scrubbed (sterile) person chooses a syringe of the correct volume for the medication to be withdrawn and attaches a large-bore needle to facilitate removal of the solution from the container.
3. The circulating (nonsterile) nurse holds the ampule or vial in such a way that the scrubbed (sterile) person can easily

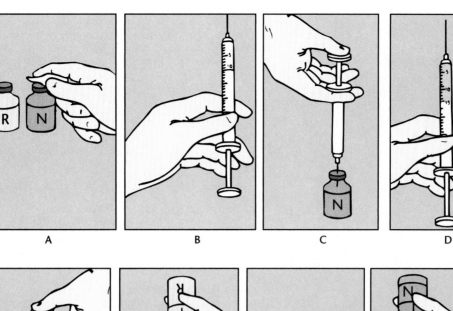

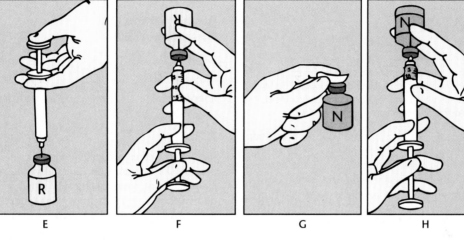

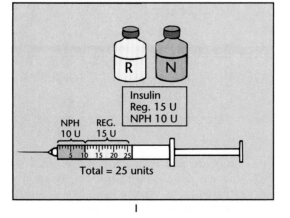

Figure 9-22 *Preparing two drugs in one syringe.* **A,** *Check insulin order; cleanse top of both vials with an antiseptic swab.* **B,** *Pull back on plunger to an amount equal to the volume of longer-acting insulin.* **C,** *Insert needle through the rubber diaphragm of the longer-acting insulin; inject air. Remove needle and syringe; do not remove insulin.* **D,** *Pull back the plunger on the syringe to a point equal to the volume of the shorter-acting insulin ordered.* **E,** *Insert needle through the rubber diaphragm; inject air.* **F,** *Invert the bottle and withdraw the volume of shorter-acting insulin ordered. Check amount withdrawn against amount ordered.* **G,** *Rewipe the lid of the longer-acting insulin.* **H,** *Insert needle; withdraw the specified amount of longer-acting insulin.* **I,** *Remove the needle and syringe; recheck the drug order against the labels on the insulin containers and the amount in the syringe. Pull plunger back slightly and proceed to mix two insulins (tilt syringe back and forth gently); change needle.*

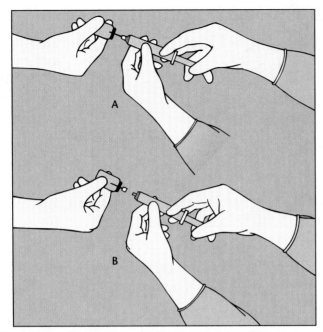

Figure 9-23 *Preparing a medication in the operating room.* **A,** *Circulating (unsterile) nurse holds vial to facilitate the "scrubbed" (sterile) person to insert the sterile needle tip into the medication container.* **B,** *The needle is disconnected from the syringe and left in the vial.*

insert the sterile needle tip into the medication container (Figure 9-23, *A*).

4. The scrubbed person pulls back the plunger on the syringe until all the medication prescribed has been withdrawn from the container and from the needle used to withdraw the medication.

5. The needle is disconnected from the syringe and left in the vial or ampule (Figure 9-23, *B*).

6. The medication container is again shown to the scrubbed person and read aloud to verify all components of the drug prepared against the medication or solution requested.

Method 2

1. The circulating (nonsterile) nurse removes the entire lid of the vial with a bottle opener, cleanses the rim of the vial, and pours the medication directly into a sterile medicine cup held by the scrubbed nurse.

2. The scrubbed person continues drug preparation on the sterile field in accordance with the intended use (such as irrigation or injection).

Regardless of the method used to transfer the medication to the sterile field, both the sterile scrubbed person and the nonsterile circulating nurse should know the location and exact disposition of each medication on the sterile field.

ADMINISTRATION OF MEDICATION BY THE INTRADERMAL ROUTE

Objective

1. Identify the equipment needed and describe the technique used to administer a medication via the intradermal route.

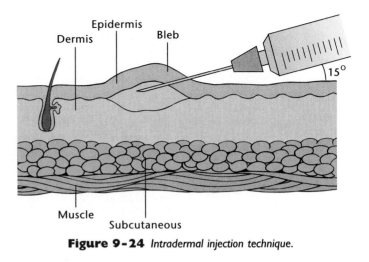

Figure 9-24 *Intradermal injection technique.*

Key Words

wheal	erythema
intradermal	papules
anergic	vesicles

Intradermal injections are made into the dermal layer of skin just below the epidermis (Figure 9-24). Small volumes, usually 0.1 ml, are injected to produce a **wheal.** The absorption from intradermal sites is slow, making it the route of choice for allergy sensitivity tests, desensitization injections, local anesthetics, and vaccinations.

Equipment

Medication to be injected
Tuberculin syringe with 26-gauge, ¼-, ⅜-, or ½-inch needle, OR a special needle and syringe for allergens
Metric ruler, if skin-testing procedure
Gloves
Antiseptic pledget

Sites

Intradermal injections may be made on any skin surface, but the site should be hairless and receive little friction from clothing. The upper chest, scapular areas of the back, and the inner aspect of the forearms are most commonly used (Figure 9-25, *A* and *B*).

Technique

The example of technique uses allergy sensitivity testing. CAUTION: Do not start any type of allergy testing unless emergency equipment is available in the immediate area in case of an anaphylactic response. Personnel should be familiar with the procedure to follow if an emergency does arise.

1. Check with the patient before starting the testing to be sure that he or she has not taken any antihistamines or

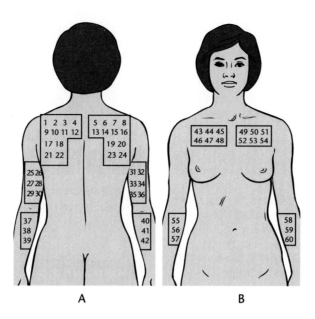

A   B

Reading Chart for Intradermal Testing

Patient Name: _____

Identification Number: _____

Physician Name: _____

DATE:	TIME:	AGENT	CONCENTRATION	DOSAGE	SITE NUMBER*	Reading Time in Hours or Minutes, i.e., 30 min. or 24, 48, or 72 hours		

*Refer to diagram of sites, Figure 9-25, *A, B.*
- Follow directions for the "reading" of the skin testing performed.
- Inspect sites in a good light
- Record reaction in upper half of box using the following guidelines, i.e., [2+]
    +   (1+) Redness of skin present (erythema)
    ++   (2+) Redness and solid elevated lesion up to 5 mm in diameter (erythema and papules)
    +++   (3+) Erythema, papules, and vesicles (blisterlike areas 5 mm or less in diameter)
    ++++   (4+) Generalized fusing of blisters
- Record measurement of induration (process of hardening) in mm. in lower half of box, i.e., [5mm]

Figure 9-25 *Intradermal sites.* **A,** *Posterior view.* **B,** *Anterior view.* **C,** *Reading chart for intradermal testing.*

antiinflammatory agents (such as aspirin, ibuprofen, corticosteroids) for 24 to 48 hours preceding the tests. If the patient has taken antihistamines or antiinflammatory agents, check with the physician before proceeding with the testing.
2. Cleanse the selected area thoroughly with an antiseptic pledget. Use circular motions starting at the planned site of injection, continuing outward in ever widening circular motions to the periphery. Allow the area to air-dry.
3. Prepare the designated solutions for injection using aseptic technique. Usual volumes to be injected range between 0.01 and 0.05 ml. A control injection of normal saline or diluent is also administered. Don gloves.
4. Insert the needle at a 15-degree angle with the needle bevel upward. The solution being injected is deposited in the space immediately below the skin; remove the needle quickly. A small *bleb* will appear on the surface of the skin as the solution enters the intradermal area (see Figure 9-24). Be careful not to inject into the subcutaneous space and do not wipe the site with alcohol after injection.
5. Do NOT recap any needles that have been used. Dispose of used needles and syringes in a puncture-resistant

container according to the policy of the employing institution (see Figure 9-10).

6. Remove gloves and dispose of them according to agency policy. Thoroughly wash hands.
7. Chart the times, agents, concentrations, and amounts injected (Figure 9-25, *C*). Make a diagram in the patient's chart numbering each location. Record what agent and concentration was injected at each site. (Subsequent "readings" of each area are then performed and charted on this record.)
8. Follow directions for the time of the reading of the skin testing being performed. Inspection of the injection sites should be performed in good light. Generally, a positive reaction (development of a wheal) to a dilute strength of suspected allergen is considered clinically significant. Measure the diameter in millimeters of erythema, and palpate and measure the size of any induration. No reaction to the allergens is known as an **anergic** reaction. *Anergy* is associated with immunodeficiency disorders. Record this information in the patient's chart. No reaction should be noted at the control site.

The technique can easily be modified for desensitization injections and vaccinations.

Patient Teaching

Tell the patient the time, date, and place to return to have the test sites read. Tell the patient not to wash or scrub the area until the injections have been read.

If the patient develops an area of severe burning or itching, he or she should try not to scratch. Tell the patient to report immediately the development of any breathing difficulty, severe hives, or rashes. He or she should go to the nearest emergency room if unable to reach the physician who prescribed the skin tests.

Documentation, the Sixth Right

Provide the RIGHT DOCUMENTATION of the medication administration and responses to drug therapy.

1. Chart the date, time, drug name (agent, concentration, amount), dosage, and site of administration (see Figure 9-25, *C*).
2. Perform a reading of each site after the application, as directed by the physician or the policy of the health care agency.
3. Chart and report any signs and symptoms of adverse drug effects.
4. Perform and validate essential patient education about the drug therapy and other essential aspects of intervention for the disease process affecting the individual.

The following is a list of commonly used readings of reactions and appropriate symbols:

+	(1+)	Redness of skin present (erythema)
++	(2+)	Redness and solid elevated lesions up to 5 mm in diameter (erythema and papules)
+++	(3+)	**Erythema, papules,** and **vesicles** (blisterlike areas 5 mm or less in diameter)
++++	(4+)	Generalized fusing of blistered areas

Generally, a positive reaction to *delayed hypersensitivity* skin testing (to evaluate in vivo cell-mediated immunity) requires an *induration* of at least 5 mm in diameter.

ADMINISTRATION OF MEDICATION BY THE SUBCUTANEOUS ROUTE

Objective

1. Identify the equipment needed and describe the technique used to administer a medication via the subcutaneous route.

Key Word

subcutaneous

Subcutaneous injections are made into the loose connective tissue between the dermis and muscle layer (Figure 9-26). Absorption is slower and drug action is generally longer with subcutaneous injections than with intramuscular or intravenous injections. If the circulation is adequate, the drug is completely absorbed from the tissue.

Many drugs cannot be administered by this route because no more than 2 ml can ordinarily be deposited at a subcutaneous site. The drugs must be soluble and potent enough to be effective in small volume, without causing significant tissue irritation. Drugs commonly injected into the subcutaneous tissue are heparin and insulin.

Equipment
Syringe Size
Choose a syringe that corresponds to the volume of drug to be injected at one site. The usual amount injected subcutane-

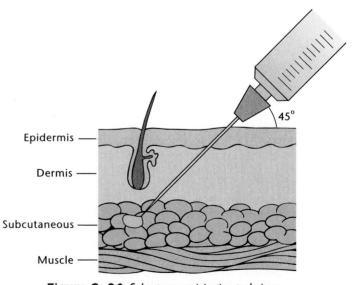

Figure 9-26 *Subcutaneous injection technique.*

ously at one site is 0.5 to 2 ml. Correlate syringe size with the size of the patient and the tissue mass.

Needle Length

Assess each patient so that the needle length selected will deposit the medication into the subcutaneous tissue, not muscle tissue. Needle lengths of ⅜, ½, and ⅝ inch are routinely used. It is prudent to leave an extra ¼ inch of needle extending above the skin surface in case the needle breaks.

Needle Gauge

Commonly used gauges for subcutaneous injections are 25 to 29 gauge.

Sites

Common sites used for the subcutaneous administration of medications include upper arms, anterior thighs, and abdomen (Figure 9-27, *A* and *B*). Less common areas are the buttocks and upper back or scapular region.

A plan for rotating injection sites should be developed for all patients who require repeated injections (Figure 9-27, *A* and *B*). The anterior view (Figure 9-27, *B*) illustrates areas easily used for self-administration. The posterior view (Figure 9-27, *A*) illustrates less commonly used areas that may be used by other persons injecting the medication.

When administering insulin subcutaneously it is important to rotate injection sites to prevent lipohypertrophy and lipoatrophy, which slow the absorption rate of insulin. The

American Diabetes Association Clinical Practice Recommendation of 1995 recommends that insulin injection sites be rotated systematically within one area before progressing to a new site for injection (see Figure 9-27). It is felt this will decrease variations in insulin absorption. Absorption is known to be fastest in the abdomen, followed by the arms, thighs, and buttocks. Because exercise is also known to affect the rate of insulin absorption, site selection should take this into consideration.

Technique

1. Prepare the medication as described earlier.
2. Check the accuracy of the drug order against the medication being prepared at least three times during the preparation phase: when first removing the drug from the storage area, immediately after preparation, and immediately before administration.
3. Check your hospital policy regarding whether 1 to 2 minims of air are added to the syringe AFTER accurately measuring the prescribed volume of drug for administration. (*Note:* The rationale for adding the air is that it will result in the needle being completely cleared of all medication at the time of injection. Conversely, if the volume of medication is completely drawn into the syringe before changing the needle, the drug volume ordered will still be administered as long as the same size needle is used for drawing up and injection. Thus the needle should not have to be completely cleared of medication by air during administration. This issue can be critical when small volumes of potent drugs are administered to infants.)
4. Consult the master rotation schedule for the patient so that the drug is administered at the correct site.
5. Identify the patient before administration of the medication by checking the bracelet.
6. Explain what you are going to do.
7. Position the patient appropriately.
8. Expose the selected site and locate the landmarks. Don gloves.
9. Cleanse the skin surface with an antiseptic pledget starting at the injection site and working outward in a circular motion toward the periphery.
10. Let the area air-dry.
11. Consult the institution's policy regarding which of the following methods to use.
    - **Method 1:** Grasp the skin area of the site selected, spread, hold firmly, and insert the needle quickly at a 45-degree angle; aspirate (DO NOT ASPIRATE FOR HEPARIN) and slowly inject the medication. If the aspiration draws blood, withdraw the needle and prepare an entirely new medication for administration (new syringe, needle, and drug).
    - **Method 2:** Grasp the skin area of the site selected and create a small roll, or "bunch." Insert the needle quickly at a 90-degree angle, aspirate (DO NOT ASPIRATE FOR HEPARIN), and slowly inject the medication. If the aspiration draws blood, withdraw the needle and prepare an entirely new medication for administration (new syringe, needle, and drug).
12. As the needle is withdrawn, apply gentle pressure to the site with an antiseptic pledget.

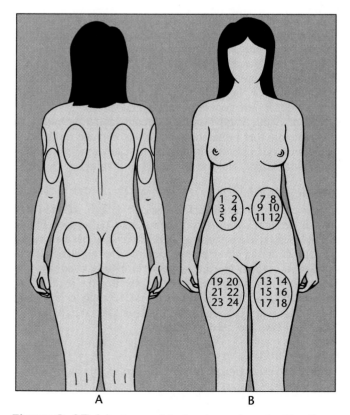

Figure 9-27 *Subcutaneous injection sites and rotation plan.* **A,** *Posterior view.* **B,** *Anterior view. Illustrates commonly used subcutaneous sites for self-administration and shows an example of a rotation schedule for insulin injection using one site systematically before proceeding to the next site of administration.*

13. Do NOT recap any needles that have been used. Dispose of used needles and syringes in a puncture-resistant container according to the policy of the employing institution.
14. Remove gloves and dispose of them according to agency policy. Thoroughly wash hands.
15. Provide emotional support for the patient.

Documentation, the Sixth Right

Provide the RIGHT DOCUMENTATION of the medication administration and response to drug therapy:
1. Chart the date, time, drug name, dosage, and route of administration.
2. Perform and record regular patient assessments for the evaluation of the therapeutic effectiveness (blood pressure, pulse, output, improvement or quality of cough and productivity, degree and duration of pain relief, and so on).
3. Chart and report any signs and symptoms of adverse drug effects.
4. Perform and validate essential patient education about the drug therapy and other essential aspects of intervention for the disease process affecting the individual.

ADMINISTRATION OF MEDICATION BY THE INTRAMUSCULAR ROUTE

Objectives

1. Identify the equipment needed and describe the technique used to administer medications in the vastus lateralis muscle, rectus femoris muscle, ventrogluteal area, dorsogluteal area, or the deltoid muscle.

2. For each anatomic site studied, describe the landmarks used to identify the site before administration of the medication.

3. Identify good sites for intramuscular administration of medication in an infant, a child, an adult, and an elderly person.

Key Words

intramuscular	dorsogluteal
vastus lateralis	deltoid
rectus femoris	Z-track method
ventrogluteal	

Intramuscular (IM) injections are made by penetrating a needle through the dermis and subcutaneous tissue into the muscle layer. The injection deposits the medication deep within the muscle mass (Figure 9-28). Absorption is more rapid than from subcutaneous injections because muscle tissue has a greater blood supply. Site selection is especially important with intramuscular injections because incorrect

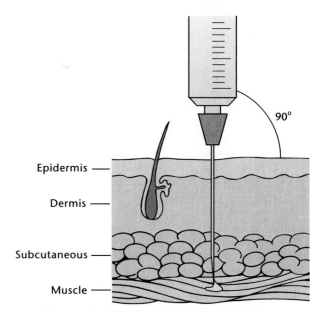

Figure 9-28 *Intramuscular injection technique.*

placement of the needle may cause damage to nerves or blood vessels. A large, healthy muscle free of infection or wounds should be used.

Equipment

Syringe Size

Choose a syringe that corresponds to the volume of drug to be injected at one site. The usual amount injected intramuscularly at one site is 0.5 to 2 ml. In infants and children, the amount should not exceed 0.5 to 1 ml. Correlate syringe size with the size of the patient and the tissue mass. In adults, divided doses are generally recommended for amounts in excess of 3 ml; 1 ml may be injected in the deltoid area. Other factors that influence syringe size include the type of medication and site of administration, thickness of subcutaneous fatty tissue, and the age of the individual.

Needle Length

Assess each patient so that the needle length selected will deposit the medication into the muscular tissue (see Figure 9-13). There is a significant difference among needle lengths appropriate for an obese patient, an infant, or an emaciated or debilitated patient. Needle lengths commonly used are 1 to 1½ inches long, although longer lengths may be required for an obese person. When estimating needle length, it is prudent to leave an extra ¼ inch of needle extending above the skin surface in case the needle breaks.

Needle Gauge

Commonly used gauges for intramuscular injections are 20 to 22 gauge.

Sites

Common sites used for the intramuscular administration of medication include the following.

Vastus Lateralis Muscle

The **vastus lateralis** muscle is located on the anterior lateral thigh away from nerves and blood vessels. The midportion is one handbreadth below the greater trochanter and one handbreadth above the knee (Figure 9-29, *A* and *B*). It is generally the preferred site for IM injections in infants because it has the largest muscle mass for that age group. The vastus lateralis muscle is also a good choice for an injection site in healthy, ambulatory adults (Figure 9-29, *B*). It accommodates a large volume of medication and permits good drug absorption. In the elderly, debilitated, or nonambulatory adult, the muscle should be carefully assessed before injection because significantly less muscle mass may be present. If muscle mass is insufficient, an alternative site should be selected.

LIFE SPAN ISSUES

INJECTION SITES

This vastus lateralis injection site is preferred in infants. In the elderly, debilitated, or nonambulatory adult, carefully assess the sufficiency of the muscle mass before using the site for injection. The gluteal site must not be used in children under 3 years of age because the muscle is not well developed yet.

Rectus Femoris Muscle

The **rectus femoris** muscle lies just medial (Figure 9-30, *A* and *B*) to the vastus lateralis muscle but does not cross the midline of the anterior thigh. The injection site is located in the same manner as the vastus lateralis muscle. It may be used in both children and adults when other sites are unavailable. A primary advantage to its use is that it may be used more easily by patients for self-administration. A disadvantage is that the medial border is close to the sciatic nerve and major blood vessels (see Figure 9-30, *A* and *B*). If the muscle is not well developed, injections in this site may cause considerable discomfort.

Gluteal Area

The gluteal area is a commonly used site of injection because it is free of major nerves and blood vessels. *It must not be used in children under 3 years of age because the muscle is not yet well developed from walking.* The area may be divided into two distinct injection sites: the **ventrogluteal** area and the **dorsogluteal** area.

Ventrogluteal Area

This site is easily accessible when the patient is in a prone, supine, or side-lying position. It is located by placing the palm of the hand on the lateral portion of the greater trochanter, the index finger on the anterior superior iliac spine, and the middle finger extended to the iliac crest. The injection is made into the center of the V formed between the

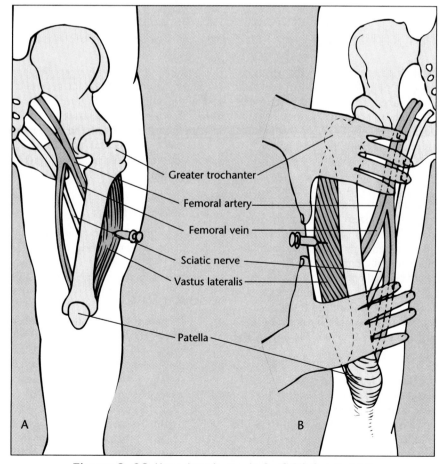

Greater trochanter
Femoral artery
Femoral vein
Sciatic nerve
Vastus lateralis
Patella

A   B

Figure 9-29 *Vastus lateralis muscle.* **A,** *Child/infant.* **B,** *Adult.*

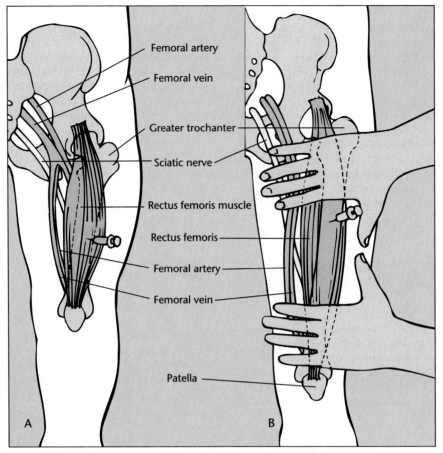

Figure 9-30 *Rectus femoris muscle.* **A,** *Child/infant.* **B,** *Adult.*

index and middle fingers with the needle directed slightly upward toward the crest of the ilium (Figure 9-31, *A* and *B*). Pain on injection can be minimized if the muscle is relaxed. The patient can aid in relaxation by pointing the toes inward while lying in a prone position (Figure 9-32) or by flexing the upper leg if lying on the side (Figure 9-33).

Dorsogluteal Area

To use this injection site (Figure 9-34, *A* and *B*), the patient must be placed in a prone position on a flat table surface. The site is identified by drawing an imaginary line from the posterior superior iliac spine to the greater trochanter of the femur. The injection should be given at any point between the imaginary straight line and below the curve of the iliac crest (hipbone). The syringe should be held perpendicular to the flat table surface with the needle directed on a straight back-to-front course. Pain on injection can be minimized if the muscle is relaxed. The patient can aid in relaxation by pointing the toes inward while lying in a prone position (see Figure 9-32).

Deltoid Muscle

The **deltoid** muscle is frequently used because of ease of access in the standing, sitting, or prone positions. However, it should be used in infants only when the volume to be injected is small, the drug is nonirritating, and the dose will be quickly absorbed. In adults, the volume should be limited to 2 cc or less and the substance must not cause irritation.

Caution must also be exercised to avoid the clavicle, humerus, acromion, brachial vein and artery, and radial nerve. The injection site (Figure 9-35, *A* and *B*) of the deltoid muscle is located by drawing an imaginary line across the armpit at the level of the axilla and the lower edge of the acromion. The lateral borders of the rectangle are vertical lines parallel to the area one third and two thirds of the way around the outer lateral aspect of the arm.

Site Rotation

A master plan for site rotation should be developed and used for all patients requiring repeated injections (Figure 9-36 *A* and *B*).

Technique

1. Prepare the medication as described earlier.
2. Check the accuracy of the drug order against the medication being prepared at least three times during the preparation phase: when first removing the drug from the storage area, immediately after preparation, and immediately before administration.
3. Check your hospital policy regarding whether 1 to 2 minims of air should be added to the syringe AFTER accurately measuring the prescribed volume of drug for administration. (*Note:* The rationale for adding the air is

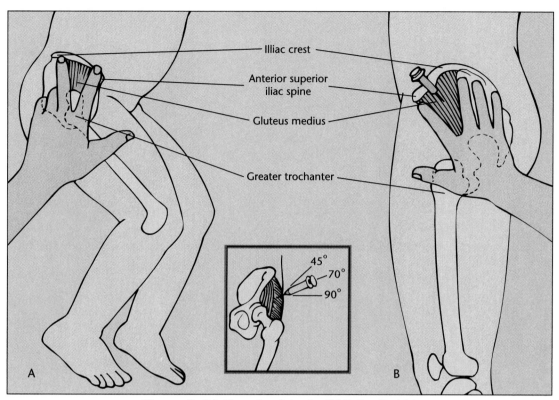

Figure 9-31 *Ventrogluteal site.* **A,** *Child/infant.* **B,** *Adult.*

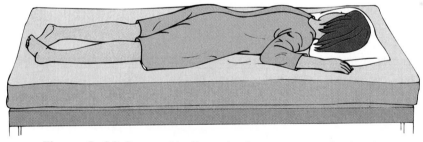

Figure 9-32 *Prone position. Toes pointed to promote muscle relaxation.*

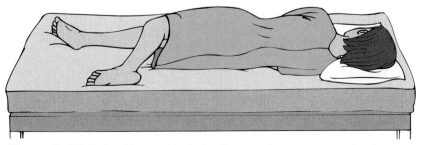

Figure 9-33 *Patient lying on side. Flexing the upper leg promotes muscle relaxation.*

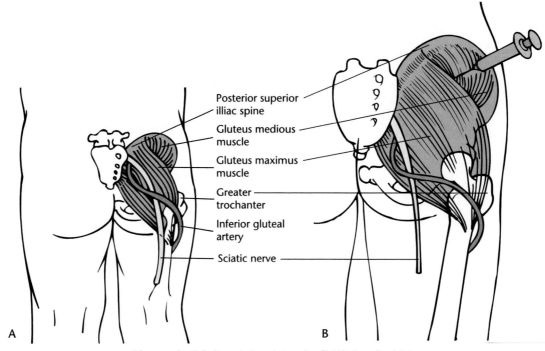

Figure 9-34 *Dorsal gluteal site.* **A,** *Child/infant.* **B,** *Adult.*

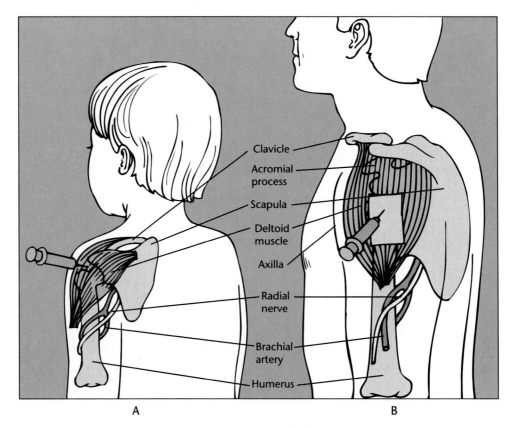

Figure 9-35 *Deltoid muscle site.* **A,** *Child/infant.* **B,** *Adult.*

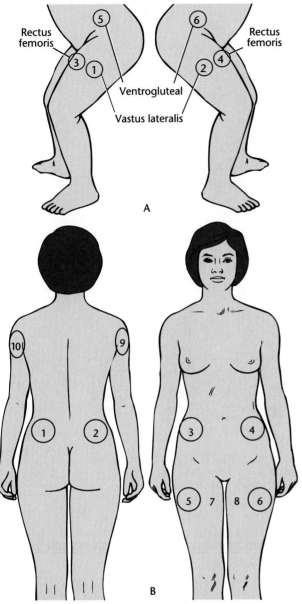

Figure 9-36 *Intramuscular master rotation plan.* **A,** *Infant/child. Note that the deltoid site may also be used in an infant or child; however, the volume of medication must be small and the drug nonirritating.* **B,** *Adult. In an adult, avoid the use of the rectus femoris (numbers 7 and 8) unless other sites are not available because of the pain produced when this site is used and the location of the sciatic nerve, femoral artery, and vein. If used, be certain to insert the needle lateral to the midline.*

that it will result in the needle being completely cleared of all medication at the time of injection. Conversely, if the volume is completely drawn into the syringe before changing the needle, the drug volume ordered will still be administered as long as the same size needle is used for drawing up and injection. Thus the needle should not have to be completely cleared of medication by air during administration. This issue can be critical when small volumes of potent drugs are administered repeatedly to infants.)

4. Consult the master rotation schedule for the patient so that the drug is administered at the correct site (see Figure 9-36).
5. Identify the patient before administration of the medication by checking the bracelet.
6. Explain what you are going to do.
7. Position the patient appropriately (see Figures 9-32 and 9-33 for relaxation techniques).
8. Expose the selected site and locate the landmarks. Don gloves.
9. Cleanse the skin surface with an antiseptic pledget starting at the injection site and working outward in a circular motion toward the periphery.
10. Let the area air-dry.
11. Insert the needle at the correct angle and depth for the site being used.
12. Aspirate. If no blood returns, slowly inject the medication using gentle, steady pressure on the plunger. If blood does return, place an antiseptic pledget over the injection site as the needle is withdrawn. Start the procedure over with a new syringe, needle, and medication.
13. After removing the needle, apply gentle pressure to the site. Massage can increase the pain if the muscle mass is stressed by the amount of medication given.
14. Do NOT recap any needles that have been used. Dispose of used needles and syringes in a puncture-resistant container according to the policy of the employing institution.
15. Remove gloves and dispose of them according to agency policy. Thoroughly wash hands.
16. Apply a small bandage to the site.
17. Provide emotional support to the patient. Children should be given comfort during and after the injection. Sometimes letting a child hold your hand or say "ouch" helps. Praise the patient for assistance and cooperation.

The Z-track Method

The use of a **Z-track method** (Figure 9-37) may be appropriate for medications that are particularly irritating or that stain the tissue. Check the hospital policy concerning which personnel may administer this method.

1. Expose the dorsogluteal site (Figure 9-37, *A*). Calculate and prepare the medication, and add 0.5 cc of air to ensure that the drug will clear the needle. Position the patient and cleanse the area for injection as previously described. Never inject into the arm or other exposed site. Don gloves.
2. Stretch the skin approximately 1 inch to one side (Figure 9-37, *B*).
3. Insert the needle. Choose a needle of sufficient length to ensure *deep* muscle penetration.
4. Aspirate and follow previous guidelines for use of the dorsogluteal site.
5. Gently inject the medication and wait approximately 10 seconds (Figure 9-37, *C*).
6. Remove the needle and allow the skin to return to the normal position (Figure 9-37, *D*).
7. Do NOT massage the injection site.
8. If further injections are to be made, alternate between dorsogluteal sites.

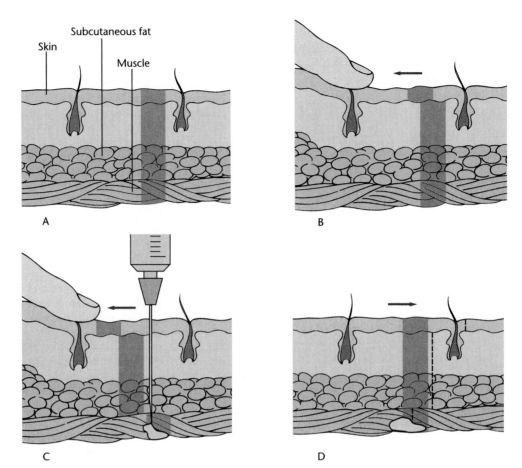

Figure 9-37 *Z-track method of intramuscular injection.* **A,** *Before starting Z tracking.* **B,** *Stretch skin slightly to one side, approximately 1 inch.* **C,** *Inject the medication; wait approximately 10 seconds.* **D,** *Remove needle and allow skin to return to normal position. Do not massage injection site.*

9. Do NOT recap any needles that have been used. Dispose of used needles and syringes in a puncture-resistant container according to the policy of the employing institution.
10. Remove gloves and dispose of them according to agency policy. Thoroughly wash hands.
11. Walking will help absorption. Vigorous exercise or pressure on the injection site (such as a tight girdle) should be temporarily avoided.

ADMINISTRATION OF MEDICATION BY THE INTRAVENOUS ROUTE

Objectives

1. Identify the dosage forms available, sites of administration, and general principles of administering medications via the IV route.

2. Describe the precautions needed to prevent the transmission of human immunodeficiency virus (HIV) that should be implemented for all patients requiring venipuncture.

3. Describe the correct techniques for administering medications by means of an established peripheral or central IV line, a vascular access device, a heparin lock, an IV bag, a bottle or volume-control device, or through a secondary piggyback set.

4. Describe the recommended guidelines and procedures for IV catheter care (including proper maintenance of patency of IV lines and implanted access device), IV line dressing changes, and for peripheral and central venous IV needle or catheter changes.

5. Discuss the proper baseline patient assessments needed to evaluate the IV therapy (such as phlebitis, extravasation, air in tubing).

6. Review the policies and procedures used at the practice setting to ensure that persons performing venipunctures and IV therapy have the required proficiency.

Key Words

intravenous	infiltration
venipuncture	pulmonary edema
phlebitis	pulmonary embolus

Intravenous administration of medication places the drug directly into the bloodstream, bypassing all barriers to drug absorption. Large volumes of medications can be administered into the vein, there is usually less irritation, and the onset of action is the most rapid of all parenteral routes. Drugs may be given by direct injection with a needle and syringe, but more commonly drugs are given intermittently or by continuous infusion through an established peripheral or central venous line or via an implantable venous access device also referred to as an implantable subcutaneous port.

Intravenous drug administration is usually more comfortable for the patient, especially when several doses of medication must be administered daily. However, use of the IV route requires time and skill to establish and maintain an IV site, the patient tends to be less mobile, and there is an increased possibility of infection and severe adverse reactions from the drug.

Dosage Forms

Medications for IV administration are available in ampules, vials, and prefilled syringes. Be certain that the label specifically states that the medication is "for IV use."

Intravenous physiologic solutions come in a variety of volumes and concentrations in glass or plastic containers (see Table 9-2).

Equipment

Gloves
Tourniquet
Administration set with appropriate needle, drip chamber, and filter
Medication
Physiologic solution ordered
Sterile dressing materials
Antiseptic solution
Syringe and needle (if by bolus)
Armboard
Tape
Standard IV pole or rod
Heparin lock, piggyback, and additional solutions, as appropriate

Additional supplies may be required to access, flush, or change IV administration sets, in-line filters, or dressings, depending on the type of peripheral, central, or implantable device being used.

Sites

Peripheral Access

When selecting an IV site consider length of time the IV will be required; condition and location of veins; purpose of infusion (for example, rehydration, delivery of nutritional needs [total parenteral nutrition, or TPN], chemotherapy, antibiotics); and patient status, cooperation, and preference for and amount of self-care of the injection site (if appropriate).

Peripheral IV devices include winged-tipped needle (see Figure 9-11), over-the-needle catheter (see Figure 9-12, *A*), and inside-the-needle catheter (see Figure 9-12, *B*).

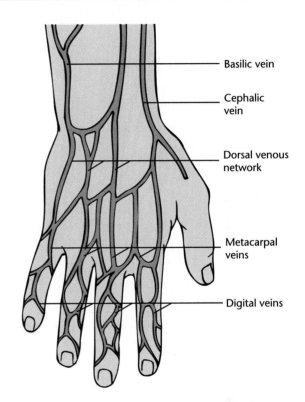

LIFE SPAN ISSUES

INTRAVENOUS SITES

The most commonly used veins for intravenous administration in infants and children are in the temporal region of the scalp, back of the hand, and dorsum of the foot.

— Basilic vein

— Cephalic vein

— Dorsal venous network

— Metacarpal veins

— Digital veins

Figure 9-38 *Intravenous sites on the hand.*

If a prolonged course of treatment is anticipated, start the first IV in the hand (Figure 9-38). The metacarpal veins, dorsal vein network, cephalic and basilic veins are commonly used. To avoid irritation and leakage from a previous puncture site, the subsequent venipuncture sites should be made above the earlier site. Refer to Figure 9-39 for the veins of the forearm area that could be used for additional venipuncture sites.

- Avoid the use of vessels over bony prominences or joints unless absolutely necessary.
- In the elderly, the use of the veins in the hand area may be a poor choice because of the fragility of the skin and veins in this area.
- Veins commonly used in infants and children for intravenous administration are on the back of the hand, dorsum of the foot, or the temporal region of the scalp (Figure 9-40).
- If possible, do not use the veins of the lower extremities because of the danger of developing thrombi and emboli.
- Do not use veins with varicosities or an extremity with impaired blood flow (for example, the affected side after a mastectomy and lymph node dissection).
- Whenever possible, initiate the IV in the nondominant arm.

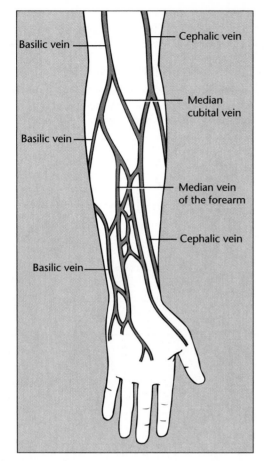

Figure 9-39 *Veins in the forearm used as intravenous sites.*

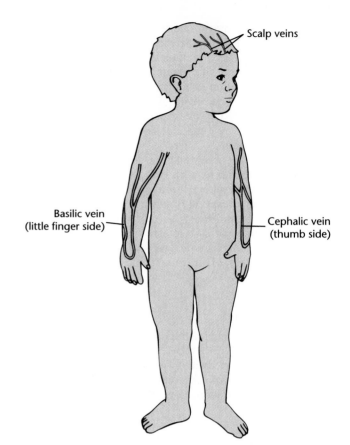

Figure 9-40 *Veins in infants and children used as intravenous sites.*

- Do not initiate an IV in an arm with compromised lymphatic or venous flow.
- *Never start an IV in an artery!*

Central Access

Central IV devices are used when the purpose of therapy dictates (for example, large volume, high concentration, or hypertonic solutions are to be infused); when peripheral sites have been exhausted because of repeated use or when condition of veins for access is poor; when long-term or home therapy is required; and when emergency condition mandates adequate vascular access.

The central venous sites most commonly used for inside-the-needle catheters (see Figure 9-12) are the subclavian, jugular, or femoral veins. A physician can also elect to perform a venisection, or "cutdown," to insert this type of catheter into the basilic or cephalic veins in the antecubital fossa.

Central sites commonly used for long-term silastic catheters (for example, Hickman, Broviac, or Groshong catheter, Figure 9-41) are the jugular, subclavian, or cephalic veins. The distal end of the silastic catheter is positioned in the superior vena cava to allow maximal dilution of the IV fluid with blood. The proximal end of the catheter is tunneled in subcutaneous tissue that acts as a barrier to pathogens that may later attach to the catheter line and migrate to the vein, causing an infection.

Implantable Vascular Access Devices

Vascular access devices, also known as implantable infusion ports (for example, Infus-A-Port, Port-A-Cath, Mediport, Chemoport) are used when long-term therapy is required and repeated accessing of the vein is required. Vascular access devices and ports (Figure 9-42) are implanted into a subcutaneous pocket in the chest area and are sutured in place. The distal end of the silicone catheter is threaded via the jugular, subclavian, or cephalic vein to the superior vena cava. The proximal end of the catheter is attached to the implanted port. The port itself contains a self-sealing silicone rubber septum specifically designed for repeated injections over an extended time period. A special noncoring Huber needle is used to penetrate the skin and the septum of the implanted device to minimize damage to the self-sealing septum.

General Principles of Intravenous Medication Administration

- Use appropriate barrier precautions (universal blood and body fluid precautions) to prevent the transmission of any infectious diseases, including HIV, as recommended by the Centers for Disease Control (CDC).
- Gloves should be worn throughout the venipuncture procedure. Care should be taken to wash the skin surface if the area is contaminated with blood.
- When the procedure is complete, remove the gloves and dispose of them in accordance with the policies of the

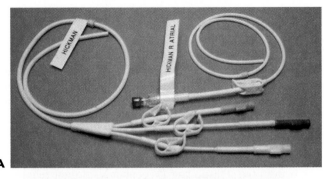

A

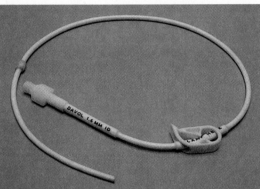

B

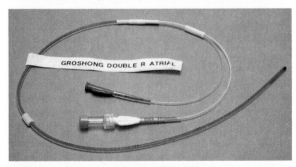

C

Figure 9-41 A, *Hickman catheter;* **B,** *Broviac catheter;* **C,**
Groshong catheter. Courtesy Chuck Dresner.

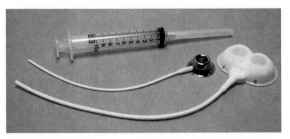

Figure 9-42 *Silicone venous catheters with infusion ports.* (From
Potter PA, Perry, AG: *Basic nursing: theory and practice,* ed 3, 1995, St. Louis,
Mosby.)

practice setting. WASH hands thoroughly as soon as the
gloves are removed. Care should be taken not to contaminate the IV tubing and rate regulator.
• Any used needles, syringes, venipuncture catheters, or
vascular access devices should be placed in a puncture-
resistant container in the immediate vicinity for disposal
according to the policies of the practice setting.

• Never recap, bend, or break used needles because of the
danger of inadvertently puncturing the skin.
• Whenever possible, use needle protector systems such as
blunt needles and injection ports, needle sheaths, and
needleless systems to prevent inadvertent needle sticks and
risk of introducing pathogens into oneself.
• Be certain medications to be administered IV are thoroughly dissolved in the correct volume and type of solution. *Always* follow the manufacturer's recommendations.
• Most clinical practice sites now use transparent dressings
over the IV insertion site that are changed in accordance
with hospital policies, generally every 48 hours. Some
clinical practice sites still use gauze dressings. When gauze
is used, the four edges of the dressing should be sealed
using tape. To prevent skin irritation, place tincture of
benzoin on the skin directly under the edge of the gauze
and allow it to dry before applying the dressing tape.
Always check the specific policies of the employing
institution as well as the physician's orders for frequency
of dressing changes.
• At the time of the dressing change on any type of IV site,
the area should be thoroughly inspected for any drainage,
redness, tenderness, irritation, or swelling. The presence of
any of these symptoms should be charted and reported to
the physician immediately. (Also take the patient's vital
signs and report these at the same time.)
• Use in-line filters as recommended by the manufacturer of
the drug to be delivered.
• Do NOT administer any drug or IV solution that is hazy or
cloudy or has foreign particles or a precipitate in it.
• Do NOT mix any other drugs with blood or blood products
(such as albumin).
• Do NOT administer a drug in an IV solution if the
compatibility is not known.
• Drugs must be entirely infused through the IV line before
adding a second medication to the IV line.
• Drugs given by IV push or bolus generally are given
following the SASH guideline:
    Saline flush first
    Administer the prescribed drug
    Saline flush following the drug
    Heparin flush line, depending on type of line, such as
Hickman (check policy of institution)
• Once mixed, know the length of time an agent remains
stable; all unused IV solutions should be returned to the
pharmacy if not used within 24 hours.
• Check the hospital policy for the definition of TKO (to
keep open). It is usually interpreted as "an infusion rate of
10 ml/hr" and should infuse less than 500 ml/24 hr.
• Shade IV solutions that contain drugs that should be
protected from light (such as hyperalimentation solutions,
nitrofurantoin, amphotericin B, nitroprusside).
• All IV solution bags and bottles should be changed every
24 hours (check hospital policy) to minimize the development of new infections. Label all IV solutions with the date
and time initiated and the nurse's initials. Do NOT use
marking pens directly on plastic IV containers because the
ink may permeate through the plastic into the IV solution.
• Administration sets should be changed every 24 to 48
hours (check hospital policy). The sets and tubing must be

labeled with the date and time initiated, the date to change the set, and the nurse's initials.

• Whenever a patient is receiving IV fluids, monitor intake and output accurately. Report declining hourly outputs and those of less than 30 to 40 ml/hr.

• Never "speed up" an IV flow rate to "catch up" when the volume to be infused has fallen behind. In certain cases, this could be dangerous. The physician should be consulted, particularly with patients who have cardiac, renal, or circulatory impairment.

Preparing an Intravenous Solution for Infusion

Dosage Form

Check the physician's order for the specific IV solution ordered and for any medication to be added. If not already prepared by the pharmacy, check the accuracy of the drug order against the medication or solution being prepared at least three times during the preparation phase: when first removing the drug or solution from the storage area, immediately after preparation, and immediately before administration. Check the expiration date on any additives and the primary solution.

Equipment

Administration set with appropriate drip chamber (microdrop or macrodrop), needle, IV catheter, and in-line filter (if used). The primary line administration set is usually labeled universal or continue flow.

Label for IV tubing
Medications for IV delivery and label
Physiologic solution ordered
Antiseptic pads
IV pole
Emesis basin

Technique

1. Assemble equipment and thoroughly wash hands.
2. Check the size and type of needle or catheter needed to access the vein selected for the IV or to access an implanted access device for the delivery of the IV solution or medication.

LIFE SPAN ISSUES

INTRAVENOUS FLUID MONITORING

The infusion of intravenous fluids necessitates careful monitoring for patients of all ages. The microdrip chamber, which delivers 60 drops (gtts)/ml, is used whenever a small volume of intravenous solution is ordered to be infused over a specific time. Many clinical sites interpret a small volume as below 100 ml/hr. In pediatric units controlled-volume chamber devices, such as Buretrol or Solu-set, and syringe pump infusers are commonly used to control the amount of fluid that is infused.

3. Check the physician's order against the physiologic solution chosen for administration.
4. Inspect the IV container for cloudiness, discoloration, or the presence of any precipitate.
5. Remove the plastic cover from the IV container and inspect the plastic IV bag to be certain it is intact; squeeze gently to detect any punctures. Inspect a glass container of IV solution for any cracks.
6. Choose the administration set appropriate for the type of solution ordered, the rate of delivery requested (microdrop or macrodrop), and for the type of IV container being used. Plastic bag IV containers do not require an air vent in the administration set. Glass containers for IV delivery must be vented or have an administration set with a vent in it. Remove the administration set from its container and inspect to ensure its sterility.
7. Move the roller or slide clamp to the upper portion of the IV line 6 to 8 inches from the drip chamber; close the clamp.
8. *Plastic IV bags:* Remove the tab from the spike receiver port; remove the tab from the administration set spike; insert the spike firmly into the bag port. Maintain sterility of port and spike throughout the process.

   Glass IV bottle: Peel back the metal tab and lift the protective metal disk from the container; remove the latex-type covering (if present) from the top of the rubber stopper. As the latex diaphragm is removed, a sudden noise should be heard as the vacuum within the glass container is released. If the noise is not heard, the contents of the IV container may not be sterile and should be discarded. Remove the tab from the administration set spike; insert the spike firmly into the port in the rubber stopper. Maintain sterility of the port and spike throughout the process.

   Note: When additive medications are ordered, they should be added to the large-volume container before tubing is attached to help ensure a uniform mixing of the medication and the physiologic solution. If medication is added to an existing IV solution, clamp the line before adding the medication to the container and make sure adequate mixing takes place before the infusion is started again. (See technique used for adding a medication to an IV solution.)

9. Hang the solution on an IV pole; squeeze the drip chamber and fill halfway; prime the IV line by removing the protective tab from the distal end of the IV line; invert the back-check valve, open the roller or slide clamp, and allow the solution to run until all the air is removed from the line. Cover the end of the IV tubing with a sterile cap. Inspect entire length of tubing to be certain all air is removed from line. Place an IV measuring device or tape strip on the plastic bag or glass IV container. Label the container with the patient's name and date and time of preparation. If medication has been added, all details of the medication must be marked on the label of the container: drug name, dose, rate of administration requested in physician's order, and the nurse's name who prepared IV. The IV tubing is labeled with the date and time it is opened and the date and time to be changed. The CDC recommends IV tubing be changed every 48 to 72 hours. Follow institutional policies where practicing.

Note: It may be necessary to add in-line filters to the setup if recommended for the administration of the medication ordered.

10. The IV solution can now be taken to the bedside for attachment after a venipuncture is performed or for addition to an existing IV system. For safety, all aspects of the IV order should be checked again immediately before attaching the IV for infusion.

Always identify the patient by checking the bracelet before initiating any intravenous procedure.

Intravenous Medication Administration

Researching the medication ordered as an IV additive (procedure also applies for direct push or bolus administration):
1. Name of drug.
2. Usual dose (take into consideration patient's age, weight, and hydration state).
3. Compatibility of drug with existing IVs and drugs infusing.
4. For IV push or bolus, does the drug need to be diluted, or can it be given undiluted (IV push)? If diluted, what types and amounts of solution can be used? If being added to an IV, what types of solution is the drug compatible with?
5. Recommended rate of infusion.

Premedication Assessment
1. Know basic patient data, diagnosis, symptoms of disorder or disease process for which the medication is ordered, and the desired action of the drug for this specific individual.
2. Obtain baseline vital signs.
3. Check for any drug allergies or prior drug reactions.
4. Review individual drug monograph to identify laboratory studies recommended before or intermittently during therapy, side effects to expect and side effects to report, monitoring parameters recommended for the specific drug prescribed, and so on.

Technique for Adding Medication to an Existing IV Solution
1. Prepare the medication as described previously.
2. Check the accuracy of the drug order against the medication or solution being prepared at least three times during the preparation phase: when first removing the drug or solution from the storage area, immediately after preparation, and immediately before administration. Check the expiration date on the solution.
3. Research drug, obtain patient data, and calculate dosage.

LIFE SPAN ISSUES

BENZYL ALCOHOL PRESERVATIVE

Do not use bacteriostatic water or saline containing the benzyl alcohol preservative to reconstitute or dilute medications or to flush IV catheters of newborns because the preservative is toxic to these patients.

4. Recheck that the drug being added to an existing IV line is compatible with the physiologic solution in the line by reviewing hospital policies or by consulting the pharmacist.
5. *Go to the bedside and identify the patient by checking the bracelet before initiating any intravenous procedure.*
6. Explain what you are going to do.
7. *Plastic IV container:* Clamp the IV tubing, wipe the injection port with an antiseptic pledget, and then insert the needle a short distance and inject the prescribed medication into the IV bag; agitate the bag to thoroughly disperse the IV medication throughout the IV bag. (Use a short needle to prevent inadvertently puncturing the back of the container.) Add a label showing the type and amount of medication added, time and date added, and initials of the preparer. Dispose of needle and syringe in a puncture-resistant container (see Figure 9-10).

   Glass IV container: Clamp the IV tubing, remove the protective cover from the air vent, remove needle from syringe, attach syringe to air vent port, and insert the medication; replace the air vent cover; gently rotate the glass container to thoroughly disperse the IV medication throughout the bottle. Add a label containing the type and amount of medication added, the time and date added, and the initials of the preparer. Adjust rate of IV flow.

   Note: Before adding a drug to an existing IV solution, dose must be adjusted to the amount of solution remaining.

Venipuncture

Follow these steps in performing **venipuncture.**
1. Wash hands thoroughly.
2. Position the patient appropriately. Immobilize an infant or child for patient safety, if necessary.
3. Cut tape for stabilizing the IV needle or catheter before starting the procedure. Turn the ends of the tape back on itself to form a tab that will not adhere to a glove when the tape is to be applied or removed. The nurse must consider his or her gloves to be contaminated when they come in contact with blood. If the gloves then contact the tape and dressing materials used at the venipuncture site, the outside of the dressings and tape are then potentially contaminated. Therefore during the procedure the nurse must focus on allowing contamination only of the dominant gloved hand; the nondominant hand must be maintained as noncontaminated to handle the taping and stabilization of the needle or IV catheter. Once the needle or catheter is stabilized, the gloves can be removed; wash hands thoroughly and apply the gauze or occlusive type of dressing materials according to the practice-setting policies.
4. Apply the tourniquet using a slip knot 2 to 6 inches above the site chosen (shaded area in Figure 9-43, *A*). Inspect the area to identify a vein of sufficient size to accommodate the needle and provide adequate anchorage. Palpate the vein to feel the depth and direction (Figure 9-43, *B* and *C*). To dilate the vein, it may be necessary to place the extremity in a dependent position; massage the vein against the direction of blood flow; have the patient open and close the hand repeatedly; lightly thump the vein with your fingertips; or remove the tourniquet and apply a heating pad or warm, wet towels to the extremity for 15 to 20 minutes, and then start the process all over.

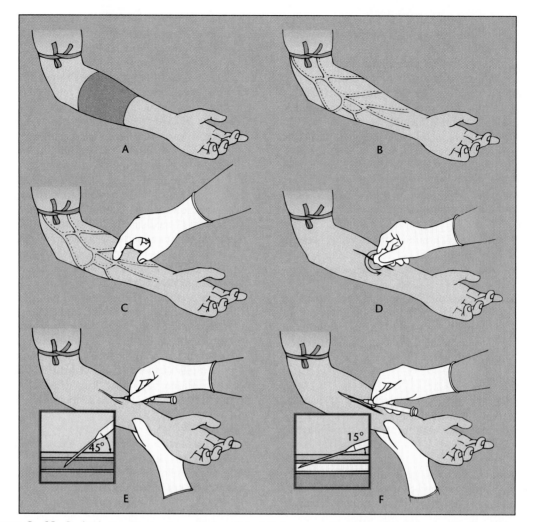

Figure 9-43 **A,** *Apply tourniquet using a slip knot 2 to 6 inches above the chosen (shaded) area.* **B,** *Allow veins to dilate.* **C,** *Palpate the vein to feel the depth and direction.* **D,** *Cleanse the skin surface with an antiseptic, starting at the anticipated site of entry, working outward in a circular motion to the periphery.* **E,** *Hold the needle (bevel up) at an angle slightly less than 45 degrees to penetrate the skin surface.* **F,** *Decrease the angle to 15 degrees and slowly advance the needle along the course of the vein.*

5. Cleanse the skin surface with the antiseptic starting at the site of entry and working outward in a circular motion toward the periphery (Figure 9-43, *D*).
6. Let the area air-dry.
7. Put on gloves.
8. Provide tension on the skin surface to stretch the skin and stabilize the vein.

When using an *administration set* or a *needle and syringe:* (1) Hold the needle (bevel up) at an angle slightly less than 45 degrees (Figure 9-43, *E*) and penetrate the skin surface approximately one-half inch below the intended entry site into the vein; decrease the angle to 15 degrees (Figure 9-43, *F*), and slowly advance the needle along the course of the vein. (2) When blood flow is established, connect the tubing to the needle, release the tourniquet, cleanse the area to eliminate any blood that may have contacted the skin or IV tubing, remove gloves, and anchor the needle and tubing to the arm or hand with tape (Figure 9-44) and dressing as prescribed in the practice-setting policy. (Because it is difficult to handle tape with gloves on, it is helpful to have a second person anchor the needle and tubing and adjust the

flow rate. The individual performing the venipuncture can then remove gloves and wash hands thoroughly.) (3) Adjust the rate of flow of the solution:

$$\frac{\text{ml of solution} \times \text{number of drops/ml}}{\text{hrs of administration} \times 60 \text{ min/hr}} = \text{drops/min}$$

(4) Regulate the flow by counting the drops for 15 seconds, multiply by 4, and adjust clamp on tubing for the appropriate rate.

When using a *plastic needle* (Figure 9-45): (1) Proceed as noted until blood flow is established (Figure 9-45, *A*). (2) Remove the inner needle (Figure 9-45, *B*), connect the tubing to the plastic needle (Figure 9-45, *C*), release the tourniquet, cleanse the area to eliminate any blood that may have contacted the skin or IV tubing, remove gloves, and anchor the needle and tubing to the arm or hand with tape (see Figure 9-44) and dressing as prescribed in the practice-setting policy. (Because it is difficult to handle tape with gloves on, it is helpful to have a second person anchor the needle and tubing and adjust the flow rate. The individual performing the venipuncture can dispose of all soiled dress-

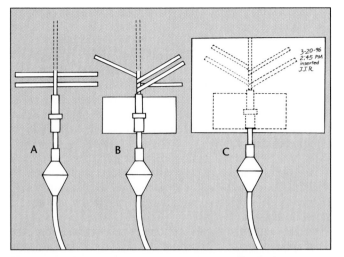

Figure 9-44 *Taping a plastic catheter or needle.* **A,** *Place two small adhesive strips under the needle or plastic catheter with the adhesive side up.* **B,** *Cross adhesive tapes one at a time to secure the plastic catheter or needle. The larger piece of tape is placed under the hub with adhesive side up. (It will adhere to larger tape to be applied later.)* **C,** *A larger piece of tape completes the stabilization of the plastic needle or catheter. Mark the date and time of insertion and the nurse's initials or signature.* **Note:** *There are several other methods for taping intravenous catheters or needles. Consult the procedure manual of the practice setting for the preferred method.*

ings or contaminated supplies according to the practice-setting policy. Remove gloves and wash hands thoroughly.) (3) Adjust the rate of flow solution:

$$\frac{\text{ml of solution} \times \text{number of drops/ml}}{\text{hrs of administration} \times 60 \text{ min ml}} = \text{drops/min}$$

(4) Regulate the flow by counting the drops for 15 seconds, multiply by 4, and adjust clamp on tubing for the appropriate rate.

Regardless of the apparatus used, mark the tape with the date and time of insertion and the initials of the nurse who started it (see Figure 9-44, *C*).

Many types of infusion pumps are available. The nurse should become familiar with the type used in his or her practice setting. Remember that the use of any type of equipment does not remove responsibility for visible monitoring of the rate of infusion and the infusion site at regularly scheduled intervals. Whenever an infusion pump is used, the danger of infiltration is increased.

Documentation, the Sixth Right

Provide the RIGHT DOCUMENTATION of the venipuncture, medication administration, and response to drug therapy:
1. Chart the date and time the venipuncture was performed.
2. Chart the site used and the type and size of needle or catheter inserted.

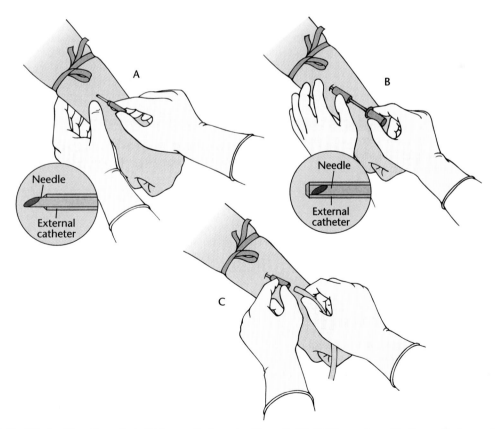

Figure 9-45 **A,** *"Over-the-catheter" type needle (see also Figure 9-12, A). When using a plastic needle, proceed as described in Figure 9-44, A-E, until blood flow is established.* **B,** *After the catheter has been advanced into the vein, remove the inner needle by withdrawing from the plastic needle.* **C,** *Connect the tubing to the plastic needle hub; release tourniquet.*

3. Chart the type and amount of IV solution started or added to an existing line.
4. If a medication was added, chart the drug name and amount added, as well as the date and time of the addition.
5. Perform and record regular patient assessments for the evaluation of the therapeutic effectiveness (blood pressure, pulse, output, lung field sounds, degree and duration of pain relief, and so on).
6. Chart and report any signs and symptoms of adverse effects.
7. Perform and validate essential patient education about the drug therapy and other essential aspects of intervention for the disease process affecting the individual.

Administration of Medication into an Established IV Line

1. Research and then prepare the medication as described earlier.
2. Identify the patient using the bracelet, and explain what you are going to do.
3. Put on gloves. It is helpful to keep one gloved hand uncontaminated.
4. Swab the self-sealing portal of the injection site with an antiseptic sponge.
5. Using a short needle on the syringe, puncture the portal site. (The short needle reduces the possibility of penetrating the opposite wall of the portal.)
6. Draw back the plunger of the syringe until blood flow is seen in the tubing at the venipuncture site to establish that the line is open into the vein.
7. While pinching the IV tubing *above* the portal to stop flow (use the uncontaminated gloved hand) inject the prescribed medication into the IV line at a rate recommended by the manufacturer.
8. When all the medication is administered, withdraw the needle from the portal, dispose of the syringe and needle in a puncture-resistant container using the contaminated gloved hand, and readjust the flow rate using the uncontaminated gloved hand. Cleanse the area of the skin and tubing contaminated by blood or fluid according to the policy of the practice setting. Remove gloves and wash hands thoroughly. (Flushing the IV line is not recommended because the medication still in the line would be administered as a bolus. This is contrary to the manufacturer's safety recommendation. Sudden boluses of certain medications may also cause severe hypotension or other signs of toxicity.)

Administration of Medication by a Heparin Lock (see Figure 9-11)

1. Select a syringe several cc larger than that required by the volume of the drug. This allows room for aspiration of blood to ensure placement of the needle and to allow blood to mix with the drug solution.
2. Research and then prepare the medication as described earlier. Prepare saline and/or heparin in syringes to flush before and after medication administration in accordance with hospital policy.

3. Identify the patient using the armband, and explain what you are going to do.
4. Put on gloves.
5. Swab the self-sealing rubber diaphragm with an antiseptic sponge and hold the sides of the injection port with your free hand.
6. Using a short, small-gauge needle, puncture the rubber diaphragm and gently pull back on the plunger for blood return, or use a blunt needle to access the diaphragm on a needleless setup.
7. If blood return is established, inject saline for flush or the medication at the rate specified by the manufacturer.
8. Periodically pull back on the plunger to mix blood with the saline or drug solution and to ensure that the needle is in the vein.
9. After administration, withdraw the needle from the diaphragm and dispose of it in a puncture-resistant container.
10. Remove the syringe and insert another syringe containing (usually) 1 to 2 ml of normal saline to flush the remaining drug from the butterfly line.
11. Flush the lock with 1 ml of heparin (10 U/ml to 100 U/ml as directed by hospital policy) (see Figure 9-11). Maintain constant pressure on the plunger of the syringe while simultaneously withdrawing the needle from the diaphragm to prevent backflow of blood. *Always* verify heparin dosage with another qualified nurse.
12. Cleanse the site of any blood or fluids. Remove gloves and dispose of properly. Wash hands thoroughly.

The heparin in the lock should be replaced when initially placed, after administering medications, after withdrawing blood samples, or every 8 hours if medications are not administered more frequently.

Check the hospital policy to determine how long a heparin lock may remain in place before changing it. Monitor the lock venipuncture site as you would any other venipuncture site.

Adding a Medication to an Intravenous Bag, Bottle, or Volume Control

1. Prepare and research the medication as described earlier.
2. Identify the patient using the bracelet, and explain what you are going to do.
3. Identify the injection port on the specific type of IV container or volume control set to be used; cleanse the portal with an antiseptic swab.
4. Clamp IV tubing.
5. Insert the sterile needle into the correct injection port and slowly add the prescribed medication to the IV solution. Always check to be certain the medication is being added to a compatible solution of sufficient volume to ensure proper dilution of the medication as specified by the manufacturer. Agitate the bag, bottle, or volume controller to thoroughly disperse the medication in the fluid.
6. For a volume-control apparatus, fill the volume chamber with the specified amount of IV solution; clamp the tubing between the IV bottle or bag and the volume control chamber.

7. Add the medication as described earlier via the cleansed injection port. Be sure medication is dispersed in the solution; adjust the rate of flow solution:

$$\frac{\text{ml of solution} \times \text{number of drops/ml}}{\text{hrs of administration} \times 60 \text{ min/ml}} = \text{drops/min}$$

8. Regulate the flow by counting the drops for 15 seconds, multiply by 4, and adjust clamp on tubing for the appropriate rate. *Note:* When IV medications are administered by a volume-control apparatus, calculation of the rate of infusion to administer the drug over the proper time must include an allowance for the volume of the fluid in the IV tubing *and* the volume of medication.
9. Affix a label to the container. Indicate the medication name, dosage, date and time prepared, rate of infusion, length of infusion time, and the nurse's signature.

Adding a Medication with a Piggyback or Secondary Set

1. Research and then prepare the medication as described earlier and add to an IV bag or bottle.
2. Identify the patient using the bracelet, and explain what you are going to do.
3. Insert the administration set into the container, attach a short sterile needle, clear the line of air, and clamp the tubing.
4. Connect to the primary IV tubing in one of the following ways:
   • *Piggyback:* Arrange the piggyback container so that it is *elevated higher* than the primary container (see Figure 9-18). Cleanse the secondary portal with an antiseptic swab and insert the needle, thereby connecting the piggyback tubing to the port of the tubing of the primary solution. Use a needleless system whenever possible. Secure in place.
   • *Secondary set:* Arrange both the primary and secondary containers at the same height, and connect the secondary tubing to the port of the tubing of the primary solution in the same manner as described for piggybacks.
5. Always check specific orders for the infusion rate and sequence of solution or medication administration. Clamp the tubing of the primary solution if ordered to do so.
6. Affix a label to the container. Indicate the medication name, dosage, date and time prepared, rate of infusion, length of infusion time, and the nurse's signature.

Changing to the Next Container of IV Solution

1. Monitor the rate of infusion at least once per hour. When the container nears completion, notify the nurse responsible for adding the next container.
2. Slow the rate to keep the vein open if the level of solution in the container is low.
3. Using aseptic technique, clamp the tubing and quickly exchange the new container for the empty one. Fill the chamber at least half full; then unclamp.
4. Adjust the flow rate as previously described, and inspect the injection site.

Administering Medication by a Venous Access Device

Equipment
Two pair sterile gloves
Antiseptic pledgets
0.9% normal saline in vial
Sterile 10 ml syringe
18- to 22-gauge, ⅝-inch needle
Antiseptic solution or swabsticks
Huber point access needle
Extension tubing

Technique
1. Research and prepare the medication as described earlier; then add to an IV bag or bottle or leave in a sterile syringe.
2. Insert the administration set into the IV container, prime the IV line to remove all air, and cover the end of the IV line with a sterile cap.
3. Take all supplies and IV medication to the patient's bedside.
4. Identify the patient using the bracelet, and explain what you are going to do.
5. Palpate the site where the venous access device is to be implanted.
6. Open the sterile gloves, using the package as a sterile field; drop the sterile syringe, Huber needle, and extension tubing on the sterile field.
7. Don sterile gloves and assemble the 10-ml syringe and 18-gauge needle; withdraw 10 ml of normal saline from the vial (the hand touching the saline vial is CONTAMINATED); maintain sterility of the saline-filled syringe while dropping it onto the sterile field; remove and discard gloves.
8. Reglove; assemble saline syringe and extension tubing; prime the extension tubing line; clamp the tubing; attach to Huber needle.
9. Use the nondominant gloved hand to cleanse the site of the venous access device; cleanse from intended site of insertion outward in ever-widening circles. Repeat cleansing process two more times. Allow antiseptic to dry, then repeat cleansing process using isopropyl alcohol.
10. Using the sterile gloved hand, grasp the Huber needle by the winged flanges and insert the needle perpendicular to the patient's skin until the needle tip comes in contact with the bottom of the port.
11. Unclamp the extension tubing and withdraw the plunger of the saline syringe slightly until blood returns; inject normal saline to flush port of heparin; attach syringe with medication or IV infusion of medication using a piggyback container. Administer medication as prescribed by the bolus technique, or provide support for the IV line that is attached to the Huber needle and tape it in place. After completion of the administration of the medication, flush the line and refill the port with heparinized solution according to the practice-setting policy. Maintain steady pressure on the plunger of the syringe as the needle is withdrawn from the access device to prevent the backflow of blood. Cleanse injection site with an antiseptic pledget after removal of the Huber needle.

12. Dispose of used needles in a puncture-resistant container. Dispose of used extension tubing and other supplies according to institution policy. Remove gloves and dispose according to policy. Wash hands thoroughly.

13. Document in the patient's record the medication administered and how well the procedure was tolerated.

Central Venous Catheter Care

Equipment

Clean gloves
Sterile gloves
Bag to discard old dressing
Antiseptic solution or swabsticks (for example, povidone iodine, alcohol, chlorhexidine)
Dressing change kit or dressing supplies
Mask or cap
Antibiotic ointment

Technique

1. Assemble needed supplies; wash hands thoroughly; don clean gloves.

2. Explain procedure to the patient; position patient appropriately for access.

3. Remove old dressing; discard dressing and gloves used to remove the dressing into an impenetrable bag.

4. Inspect the catheter site thoroughly; record and report any signs of infection.

5. Open a sterile dressing tray and use this as a sterile field; put on a mask and don sterile gloves.

6. Clean the skin around the catheter site by starting at the catheter and wiping outward in ever-widening circles. Repeat this cleansing process three times using a new sterile antiseptic swab each time.

7. Cleanse the outside of the catheter with a new sterile antiseptic swab. Start at the insertion site and cleanse distally along the catheter.

8. Apply antiseptic ointment (such as povidone iodine) to the catheter insertion site.

9. Apply the dressing (occlusive or gauze), being careful not to contaminate the outside of the dressing. Remove gloves and dispose of them. Cleanse the exposed portion of the catheter with alcohol; secure catheter. Wash hands thoroughly.

10. Label dressing with date and time changed and initials of nurse performing the procedure.

11. Document procedure in chart.

Discontinuing an Intravenous Infusion

Equipment

Tourniquet
Sterile sponges
Gloves
Dressing materials
Tape
Puncture-resistant container for needles, butterfly, or other types of IV catheter

Technique

1. Check the physician's orders. Verify that all IV solutions and medications have been completed.

2. Check the patient's identity using the bracelet before discontinuing the IV solutions.

3. Explain what you are going to do.

4. Adequately expose the IV site.

5. Clamp the IV tubing; turn off the electronic controller or infuser.

6. Loosen the tape at the venipuncture site while simultaneously stabilizing the needle to prevent venous damage. If the IV site is contaminated by blood or drainage, don gloves before handling the tape.

7. Review hospital policy regarding the placement of a tourniquet. (Some health care agencies state that a tourniquet should be applied before removal of the needle or IV catheter in case the tip breaks during removal. Other agencies state that the tourniquet should be loosely attached to the limb, but not tightened unless necessary.)

8. Put on gloves.

9. Using a gauze pad, gently apply pressure with the nondominant hand to the venipuncture site. Withdraw the needle, pulling out parallel to the skin surface. Inspect the tip of the needle or catheter to be sure it is intact. Release the tourniquet, if in place. Place the needle in the puncture-resistant container.

10. Cleanse the area if contaminated with any blood or fluid.

11. Continue to hold the IV site firmly until all bleeding ceases. If the venipuncture site was in the antecubital fossa, have the patient flex the elbow to hold the gauze in place.

12. Check for bleeding after 1 to 2 minutes. Remove gauze and discard with other contaminated dressings. Cleanse the area as appropriate.

13. Remove and discard gloves according to policy and wash hands thoroughly.

14. Apply a small dressing or bandage as stated by policy.

15. Provide patient comfort.

16. Dispose of IV catheter in a puncture-resistant container. Dispose of remainder of used supplies appropriately.

Documentation, the Sixth Right

Provide the RIGHT DOCUMENTATION of termination of IV therapy.

1. Chart the date and time of termination.

2. Perform and record regular patient assessments (site data, size of site, and color of skin at injection site).

3. Chart and report any signs of adverse effects (redness, warmth, swelling, or pain at the IV site).

4. Record total amount infused on intake and output record.

Monitoring Intravenous Therapy

Before initiating therapy, perform baseline patient assessments to evaluate the patient's current status. Report at appropriate intervals throughout the course of treatment.

The patient and the IV site should be checked at least every hour for flow rate, infiltration (tenderness, redness, puffiness), and adverse effects. If the flow rate is falling behind schedule:

1. Check for mechanical obstruction of the tubing (closed clamp, kinking) or filter and either irrigate or change the tubing.
2. Check the drip chamber. If less than half full, squeeze it to fill more completely. (Do not overfill.)
3. Check to make sure that the IV container is not empty. Also check to make sure the container is higher than 3 feet above the venipuncture site. The incorrect height may inadvertently occur if the patient is repositioned or the bed height is readjusted.
4. Check for tubing that has fallen below the venipuncture site. If a significant amount has fallen, elevate and carefully coil the tubing near the site of venipuncture.
5. Don gloves to inspect the IV site. Check the transparent dressing for date the infusion device was started; palpate gently around catheter or needle to elicit if edema, coolness, or pain is present, indicating infiltration. Check for any signs of redness or heat, indicating an inflammatory process. Check to determine whether the bevel of the needle is pushing against the wall of the vein. Do this by CAUTIOUSLY raising or lowering the angle of the needle slightly to see if flow is restored. If so, reposition slightly using a gauze pad in the most appropriate location.
6. Check the temperature of the solution being infused. Cold solutions can cause spasms in the vein.
7. Check to ensure that a restraint or blood pressure cuff applied to the arm has not interfered with the flow.
8. If it appears that the site is clotted, DO NOT attempt to clear the needle by flushing with fluid. This will dislodge the clot and may cause a thromboembolus. *Aspirate* the needle with a syringe to dislodge the clot.
9. Check medication administration record (MAR) or Kardex for IV medication and IV infusion orders for the patients assigned. During shift report, identify the exact volume of IV solution or medication that has been infused on the previous shift and the volume remaining to be infused during the next shift.
10. Immediately after receiving a report on your assigned patients make rounds to perform a baseline assessment. Data that should be analyzed with reference to IV therapy include the following:
    • Check that the ordered IV solution with or without medications is being administered to the correct patient at the correct rate of infusion.
    • Check the total amount infused against the amount that should have infused. Is the volume of infused IV solution or IV medication "on target," "ahead," or "behind"? Inspect the volume-infused strips attached to the infusing solution bag or bottle.
    • Calculate the drip rate. If the IV tubing is running by gravity, adjust it to the correct rate of infusion to deliver the milliliters per hour ordered. If an infusion pump is being used, check to be certain the drop sensor is positioned superior to fluid level in the drip chamber and inferior to port where the fluid drops from. Next be certain the infusion pump is set to deliver the prescribed volume (ml) per hour. There

are several models of infusion pumps available; become thoroughly versed in the operation of the type of infusion pump being used in the practice setting. If in doubt about any facet of its operation, request a service check on the equipment. In addition to being knowledgeable about IV medications and solutions, the nurse must have expertise in the operation of the delivery systems used within the practice setting. Computerized equipment is only as good as the individual's operating knowledge of the infusion pump.

• Check for in-line filters. If one is recommended for the medicine being infused, is it being used?
• Check the date and time the infusing IV solution or IV medication was hung. Identify when the IV solution infusing, administration set and tubing, and the IV site needles, IV catheters, or dressing are to be changed in accordance with policies of the practice setting.
• Check the date and time that procedures are ordered to maintain the patency of the established IV lines. Follow the practice-setting policies. The patency of all IV lines used for the *intermittent* delivery of IV medications must be maintained. The following are general guidelines:
• Peripheral intermittent IV lines are usually flushed every 8 hours or as stated in institution policy, using 1 to 2 ml of 10 or 100 U/ml heparinized saline solution or saline. Use positive pressure to prevent backflow of blood and possible occlusion.
• Central venous IV lines are usually flushed with 1 to 5 ml of 10 or 100 U/ml of heparinized saline solution; however, the intervals for flushing vary (once every 12 hours to one time per week). Always check specific policy of the institution where practicing.
• Groshong catheters have a two-way valve that prevents backflow; therefore, these catheters do not require heparin. Groshong catheters are flushed with 5 cc normal saline weekly or at an interval determined by institutional policy.
• The amount of solution used to flush a Hickman, Broviac, or Groshong catheter varies and must be sufficient to equal two times the volume required to fill the catheter lumen plus the volume of any extension tubing being used.
• Implantable vascular access devices and ports (for example, Port-a-Cath, Mediport) require that the port be filled with sterile heparinized solution, usually 100 U/ml, after each use. If not accessed regularly, flushes may be performed only once each month or at an interval determined by the employing institution. REMEMBER THAT ONLY A HUBER NEEDLE IS USED TO ACCESS AN IMPLANTABLE VASCULAR ACCESS DEVICE OR PORT.
• Whenever flushing a peripheral, central venous, or implantable vascular access device, the nurse should maintain positive pressure on the syringe barrel while simultaneously withdrawing the needle from the site. This will prevent backflow of blood and thus prevent occlusion.

- Prevent damage to any and all short- or long-term central venous catheters by only clamping the catheter with a padded hemostat or a smooth-edged clamp.
- Change the injection caps for lumen hubs on single- or multiple-lumen central venous catheters every 72 hours or as stated in the institutional policy.
- Check the IV tubing for any obstructions or air in the line. If running by gravity, be sure the tubing is not hanging below the level of the insertion site.
- Check the IV infusion site to ensure that the IV is infusing properly into the arterial, peripheral, central venous, or implanted access device. Report and take immediate action if the infusion is infiltrated, improperly infusing, or if signs of infection exist.
- Remain alert at all times for complications associated with IV therapy of any type (for example, phlebitis, infection, air in the tubing, circulatory overload, pulmonary edema, pyogenic reaction, pulmonary embolism, or drug reactions from the IV medications).
- Document all findings and procedures performed in association with IV therapy.

Phlebitis or Infection

If signs of redness, warmth, swelling, and burning pain along the course of the vein are present, infection or **phlebitis** may be developing. Confirm the presence of these signs with the supervising nurse; then discontinue the IV. Insert a new IV using all new equipment at a different site. Many hospitals also require that the infection control nurse be notified and that the site of phlebitis or infection be treated with hot or cold compresses. If purulent drainage is present, obtain a sample of the drainage for culture and sensitivity. If a fever and chills accompany these symptoms, a blood culture may also be indicated. Check practice setting policies about whether a physician's order is necessary to do this or whether standing orders exist as part of the infection control procedures that mandate these actions. Generally, follow-up treatment includes the application of warm, moist compresses to the site with elevation of the site.

Infiltration

Inspect the IV site at regular intervals for **infiltration.** Whenever a change in the limb's color, size, or skin integrity is observed, compare with the opposite limb. Apply a tourniquet *proximal* to the infusion site to constrict the flow. Continued flow with the tourniquet in place confirms infiltration. DO NOT rely on blood backflow into the tubing when the container is lowered. The venipuncture site could still be patent, but a laceration in the vessel may allow infiltration. Know the policies of your institution concerning the treatment of extravasation. Here are some general guidelines:
1. Stop the infusion.
2. Elevate the affected limb.
3. Remove the needle as described earlier.
4. Apply heat to the site of infiltration to produce vasodilation and drug absorption.
5. Contact the physician for the possible use of antidotes to minimize tissue damage.

Air in Tubing

If an air bubble is found in IV tubing, clamp the tubing immediately. Swab either the injection site in the rubber hub near the needle or the piggyback portal (whichever is closest to the air bubble) with an antiseptic sponge. Using sterile technique, insert a needle and syringe into the entry site below the air bubble and withdraw the air pocket.

If air has actually entered the patient via the IV tubing, turn the patient on the left side with the head in a dependent position. Administer oxygen and notify the physician immediately.

Circulatory Overload and Pulmonary Edema

Signs of circulatory overload caused by excessive volumes of fluid are engorged neck veins, dyspnea, reduced urine output, edema, bounding pulse, and shallow, rapid respirations. The signs of **pulmonary edema** are dyspnea, cough, anxiety, rales, rhonchi, and frothy sputum. When these symptoms develop, slow the IV immediately to a "keep open" rate. Place the patient in a sitting position, start oxygen, collect vital signs, lung sounds, and summon the physician immediately. Gather equipment for application of rotating tourniquets, but do not apply until an order is received.

Pyrogenic Reaction

A pyrogenic reaction should be suspected if the patient develops sudden onset of chills, fever, headache, nausea, and vomiting. Check the patient's vital signs, stop the IV, and notify the physician of the findings immediately.

Save the unused portion of solution. Return it to the pharmacy or laboratory for testing as specified by hospital policy.

Pulmonary Embolism

A **pulmonary embolus** may occur from foreign materials injected into the vein or from a blood clot that breaks loose. Emboli can be prevented by using an in-line filter, completely dissolving any medications added to a solution, using proper diluents for reconstitution, using IV solutions that are clear and have no visible signs of foreign matter or precipitate, and avoiding the use of veins in the lower extremities.

Documentation, the Sixth Right

Provide the RIGHT DOCUMENTATION of the medication administration and responses to drug therapy:
1. Chart the date, time, drug name, dosage, and route of administration.
2. Perform and record regular patient assessments for the evaluation of the therapeutic effectiveness (blood pressure, pulse, intake and output, lung-field sounds, respiratory rate, pain at infusion site, and so on).
3. Chart and report any signs and symptoms of adverse drug effects.
4. Perform and validate essential patient education about the drug therapy and other essential aspects of intervention for the disease process affecting the individual.
5. Chart dressing changes performed and cite any signs and symptoms of complications at the needle or central venous catheter site (for example, redness, tenderness, swelling, drainage).
6. Chart date and times that procedures are performed to maintain the patency of the IV needle, central venous

catheter, or port (for example, heparinized flush or, for Groshong catheter, the saline flush).

7. Perform and validate essential patient education about the drug therapy, site or central venous catheter care, dressing care, or flushing of the IV system being used to administer medication. Always teach the patient (and significant others) signs and symptoms of complications that should be reported immediately to the physician. Depending on the type of IV delivery system being used to administer the medication, instruct persons being treated on an outpatient or home health setting when to return for the next visit to the physician or clinic.

CHAPTER 10

Percutaneous Administration

CHAPTER CONTENT

ADMINISTRATION OF TOPICAL MEDICATIONS TO THE SKIN

Absorption of topical medications can be influenced by the drug concentration, the length of time the medication is in contact with the skin, the size of the affected area, the thickness of the skin, the hydration of tissues, and the degree of skin disruption.

Percutaneous administration refers to application of medications to the skin or mucous membranes for absorption. Methods of percutaneous administration include topical application of ointments, creams, powders, or lotions to the skin; instillation of solutions onto the mucous membranes of the mouth, eye, ear, nose, or vagina; and inhalation of aerosolized liquids or gases for absorption through the lungs. The primary advantage of the percutaneous route is that the action of the drug, in general, is localized to the site of application, which reduces the incidence of systemic side effects. Unfortunately, the medications are sometimes messy and difficult to apply, and they usually have a short duration of action and therefore require more frequent reapplication.

LIFE SPAN ISSUES

TOPICAL ADMINISTRATION

Topical administration with percutaneous absorption is usually effective in infants because the outer layer of skin is not fully developed. This skin is also more fully hydrated at this age, making water-soluble medicines more readily absorbed. Wearing a plastic-coated diaper forms a type of occlusive dressing that increases hydration of the skin and significantly increases medicine absorption. An inflammation such as a diaper rash also increases the amount of drug absorbed. Transdermal drug administration in the elderly results in erratic absorption of medicines because of the physiologic changes of aging (for example, decreased dermal thickness with drying and wrinkling, decreased cardiac output, and diminished tissue perfusion).

ADMINISTRATION OF CREAMS, LOTIONS, AND OINTMENTS

Objectives

1. Describe the topical forms of medications used on the skin.
2. Cite the equipment needed and techniques used to apply each of the topical forms of medications to the skin surface.

Key Words

creams

lotions

ointments

wet dressings

Dosage Forms

Creams

Creams are semisolid emulsions containing medicinal agents for external application. The cream base is generally non-greasy and can be removed with water. Many over-the-counter creams are used as moisturizing agents.

Lotions

Lotions are usually aqueous preparations that contain suspended materials. They are commonly used as soothing agents to protect the skin and relieve rashes and itching. Some lotions have a cleansing action, whereas others have an astringent or drawing effect. To prevent increased circulation and itching, lotions should be gently but firmly patted on the skin rather than rubbed in. Shake all lotions thoroughly immediately before application and use sparingly to avoid waste.

Ointments

Ointments are semisolid preparations of medicinal substances in an oily base such as lanolin or petrolatum. This type of preparation can be applied directly to the skin or mucous membrane and generally cannot be removed easily with water. The base helps keep the medicinal substance in prolonged contact with the skin.

Wet Dressings

Solutions frequently used for **wet dressings** include potassium permanganate, silver nitrate, and Burrow's solution. These substances are added to plain water or physiologic saline at room temperature. If making the potassium permanganate from tablets, always strain the solution *before* use. Potassium permanganate and silver nitrate *stain everything*. Use measures to prevent unnecessary staining.

Equipment

Prescribed cream, lotion, or ointment
2 × 2–inch gauze sponges
Cotton-tipped applicators
Tongue blade
Gloves

Sites

Sites are skin surfaces affected by the disorder being treated.

Technique

1. Wash hands and assemble the equipment.
2. Use the FIVE RIGHTS of medication preparation and administration throughout the procedure:
   RIGHT PATIENT
   RIGHT DRUG
   RIGHT ROUTE OF ADMINISTRATION
   RIGHT DOSAGE
   RIGHT TIME OF ADMINISTRATION
3. Provide privacy for the patient and give a thorough explanation of the procedure.
4. Place the patient in a position such that the surface on which the topical materials are to be applied is exposed. Assess current status of symptoms. Provide for patient comfort before starting therapy.

5. *Cleansing:* Follow the specific orders of the physician for cleansing of the site of application. *Oil-based* products may be removed with cottonseed oil and gauze. *Coal tar* products may be removed with corn oil and gauze. *Water-* or *alcohol-based* products may be removed with soap and water or water alone.
6. *Application:* Use gloves during the application process. Many of the agents used may be absorbed through the skin of both the patient and the person applying the medication. *Lotions:* Shake well until a uniform appearance of the solution is obtained. *Ointments* or *creams:* Use a tongue blade to remove the desired amount from a wide-mouth container; squeeze the amount needed onto a tongue blade or cotton-tipped applicator from a tube-type container. Apply lotions firmly but gently by dabbing the surface. Apply ointments and creams with a gloved hand using firm but gentle strokes. Creams are gently rubbed into the area.
7. *Dressings:* Check specific orders regarding the type of dressing to be used. If a dressing is to be applied, spread the prescribed amount of ointment directly on the dressing material with a tongue blade; the impregnated dressing material can then be applied to the affected skin surface. Secure the dressing in place.
8. *Wet dressings:* Wring out wet dressings to prevent dripping. Always completely remove and reapply potassium permanganate or silver nitrate dressings to prevent excessive chemical irritation from buildup of residue at the site of application. Secure the dressing in place. A binder or Montgomery tapes may be needed for dressings requiring frequent changes.
9. Clean up the area and equipment used and make sure the patient is comfortable after the application procedure.
10. Wash hands.

Patient Teaching

1. If appropriate, teach the patient to apply the medication and dressings.
2. Teach personal hygiene measures appropriate to the underlying cause of the skin condition (for example, acne, contact dermatitis, infection).
3. When dressings are ordered, discuss materials readily available at home, such as clean, old muslin sheets or cloth diapers with no cotton filling. You may also suggest the purchase of gauze and other necessary supplies.
4. Stress gentleness and moderation in the amount of medication to be applied.
5. Emphasize that the patient must avoid touching or scratching the affected area.
6. Tell the patient to wash hands before and after touching the affected area or applying the medication. Stress the prevention of spread of infection, when present.

Documentation, the Sixth Right

Provide the RIGHT DOCUMENTATION of the medication administration and responses to drug therapy.

1. Chart the date, time, drug name, dosage, and site and route of administration.
2. Perform and record regular patient assessments for the evaluation of the therapeutic effectiveness (change in size

of affected area, reduced drainage, decreased itching, lowered temperature with an infection, and so on).

3. Chart and report any signs or symptoms of adverse drug effects, and provide a narrative description of the area being treated.
4. Develop a written record for the patient to use in charting progress for evaluation of the effectiveness of the treatments being used. List the patient symptoms (such as rash on lower leg with redness and vesicles present; decubitus ulcer on the sacrum). List the data to be collected regarding the medication prescribed and the effectiveness (such as vesicles now crusted, weeping, or appear to be drying; redness in lower leg is lessening; area of decubitus is extending, remaining the same, or shrinking).
5. Perform and validate essential patient education about the drug therapy and other essential aspects of intervention for the disease process affecting the individual.

PATCH TESTING FOR ALLERGENS

Objectives

1. Describe the procedure used and purpose of performing patch testing.
2. Describe specific charting methods used with allergy testing.

Key Words

patch testing   antigen
allergen

Patch testing is a method used to identify a patient's sensitivity to contact materials (such as soaps, pollens, and dyes). The suspected **allergens (antigens)** are placed in direct contact with the skin surface and covered with nonsensitizing, nonabsorbent tape. Unless pronounced irritation appears, the patch is usually left in place for 48 hours and then removed. The site is left open to air for 15 minutes and then "read." A positive reaction is noted by the presence of redness and swelling and indicates allergy to the specific antigen. It may be necessary to read the areas in 3 days and again in 7 days to detect delayed reactions.

Intradermal tests may also be used to determine allergenicity to specific antigens.

Equipment

Alcohol for cleansing the area
Solutions of suspected antigens
2 × 2–inch pieces of typewriter paper
1 × 1–inch gauze pads
Droppers
Mineral or olive oil
Water
Hypoallergenic tape
Record for charting data on substances applied and responses

Sites

The back, arms, or thighs are commonly used. (Do NOT use the face or areas receiving friction from clothing.) Selected areas are spaced 2 to 3 inches apart. The type of allergen applied and the site of application are documented on the patient's chart (Figure 10-1). Hair is shaved from sites to ensure that the antigen is kept in close contact with the skin surface, thereby preventing a false-negative reaction.

Technique

CAUTION: Do NOT start any type of allergy testing unless emergency equipment is available in the immediate area in case of an anaphylactic response. Personnel should be familiar with the procedure to follow if an emergency arises.

1. Check with the patient before starting the testing to be sure that no antihistamines or antiinflammatory agents (such as aspirin, ibuprofen, corticosteroids) have been taken for 24 to 48 hours preceding the tests. If the patient has taken an antihistamine or antiinflammatory agent, consult the physician before proceeding with the testing.
2. Wash hands and assemble the equipment.
3. Use the FIVE RIGHTS of medication preparation and administration throughout the procedure:
   RIGHT PATIENT
   RIGHT DRUG
   RIGHT ROUTE OF ADMINISTRATION
   RIGHT DOSAGE
   RIGHT TIME OF ADMINISTRATION
4. Provide privacy for the patient and give a thorough explanation of the procedure.
5. Place the patient in a position such that the surface on which the test materials are to be applied is horizontal. Provide patient comfort before starting testing.
6. Cleanse the selected area thoroughly using an alcohol pledget. Use circular motions starting at the planned site of injection, continuing outward in ever-widening circular motions to the periphery. Allow the area to air-dry.
7. Prepare the designated solutions using aseptic technique.
8. Follow specific directions of the employing health care agency for the application of liquid and solid forms of suspected allergens. Usually a dropper is used to apply suspected liquid contact-type materials; solid materials are applied directly to the skin surface and then moistened with mineral or olive oil.
9. Any of the following methods can be used:
   - After application, each area used should be covered first with a 1 × 1 gauze followed by a 2 × 2 piece of typewriter paper; secure with hypoallergenic tape. (If the patient is known to be allergic to all types of tape, consider the use of a binder.)
   - Designated amounts of standardized-strength chemical solutions are arranged in metal receptacles that are backed with hypoallergenic adhesive. These are applied to the selected site. It is important to identify the contents of each receptacle correctly.
   - Patches impregnated with designated antigens are available for direct application to the prepared sites.
   - A patch test series kit with allergens of nonirritating concentration packaged in syringes for dispersement is available. Although the kit contains 20 allergens, any

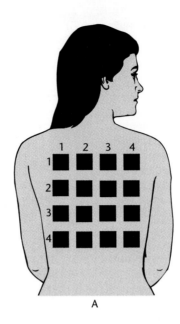

A

Reading Chart for Intradermal Testing

Patient Name: _____

Identification Number: _____

Physician Name: _____

DATE:	TIME:	AGENT	CONCENTRATION	DOSAGE	SITE NUMBER*	Reading Time in Hours or Minutes, i.e., 30 min. or 24, 48, or 72 hours		

*Refer to diagram of sites, Figure 9-25, *A, B.*
- Follow directions for the "reading" of the skin testing performed.
- Inspect sites in a good light
- Record reaction in upper half of box using the following guidelines, i.e., $\boxed{2+}$
  - +   (1+) Redness of skin present (erythema)
  - ++   (2+) Redness and solid elevated lesion up to 5 mm in diameter (erythema and papules)
  - +++   (3+) Erythema, papules, and vesicles (blisterlike areas 5 mm or less in diameter)
  - ++++   (4+) Generalized fusing of blisters
- Record measurement of induration (process of hardening) in mm. in lower half of box, i.e., $\boxed{5mm}$

Figure 10-1 *Patch test for contact dermatitis.* **A,** *Patch testing sites.* **B,** *Reading chart, patch testing.*

number of them may be applied to individual patches or holding devices and then applied to the patient's skin.

10. Chart the times, agents, concentrations, and amounts applied. Make a diagram in the patient's chart numbering each location. Record what agent and concentration was placed at each site. Subsequent readings of each area are then performed and charted on this record.

11. Follow directions for the time of the reading of the skin testing being performed. Inspection of the testing sites should be performed in good light. Generally, a positive reaction (development of a wheal) to a dilute strength of suspected allergen is considered clinically significant. Measure the diameter of erythema in millimeters and palpate and measure the size of any induration. Record this information in the patient's chart. No reaction should be noted at the control site.

Patient Teaching

1. Tell the patient the time, date, and place of the return visit to have the test sites read.

2. Tell the patient not to bathe or shower until the patches are read and removed. Explain the need to avoid activities that could cause excessive perspiration.

3. If the patient develops an area of severe burning or itching, lift the patch and gently wash the area. Tell the patient to report immediately the development of any breathing difficulty, severe hives, or rashes. The patient should be told to go to the nearest emergency room if unable to reach the physician who prescribed the skin tests.

Documentation, the Sixth Right

Provide the RIGHT DOCUMENTATION of the medication administration and responses to drug therapy.
1. Chart the date, time, drug name, dosage, and site of administration (see Figure 10-1).
2. Read each site 24, 48, and 72 hours after the application as directed by the physician or policy of the health care agency. Additional readings may be required up to 7 days after application.
3. Chart and report any signs or symptoms of adverse drug effects.
4. Perform and validate essential patient education about the testing and other essential aspects of intervention for the disease process affecting the individual.

Commonly used readings of reactions and appropriate symbols include the following:

+	(1+)	Redness of skin present (erythema)
++	(2+)	Redness and solid elevated lesions up to 5 mm in diameter (erythema and papules)
+++	(3+)	Erythema, papules, and vesicles (blisterlike areas 5 mm or less in diameter)
++++	(4+)	Generalized fusing of blistered areas

ADMINISTRATION OF NITROGLYCERIN OINTMENT

Objectives

1. Identify the equipment needed, sites used, techniques used, and patient education required when nitroglycerin ointment is prescribed.
2. Describe specific documentation methods used to record the therapeutic effectiveness of nitroglycerin ointment therapy.

Dosage Form

Nitroglycerin ointment (Nitro-Bid, Nitrol) provides relief of anginal pain for several hours longer than sublingual preparations. When properly applied, nitroglycerin ointment is particularly effective against nocturnal attacks of anginal pain. Specific instructions for nitroglycerin ointment are reviewed in this text because it is the only ointment currently available for which dosage is critical to the success of use. (See Chapter 23.)

Equipment

Nitroglycerin ointment
Applicator paper
Clear plastic wrap
Nonallergenic adhesive tape

Sites

Any area without hair may be used. Most people prefer the chest, flank, or upper arm areas (Figure 10-2). (Do NOT shave an area to apply the ointment; shaving may cause skin irritation.)

Technique

1. Wash hands and assemble the equipment.
2. Use the FIVE RIGHTS of medication preparation and administration throughout the procedure:
   RIGHT PATIENT
   RIGHT DRUG
   RIGHT ROUTE OF ADMINISTRATION
   RIGHT DOSAGE
   RIGHT TIME OF ADMINISTRATION
3. Provide privacy for the patient and give a thorough explanation of what you are going to do.
4. Place the patient in a position such that the surface on which the topical materials are to be applied is exposed. Provide patient comfort before starting therapy. *Note:* When reapplying ointment, remove plastic wrap, remove dose-measuring applicator paper from previous dose, and cleanse the area of remaining ointment on the skin surface. Select a new site for application of the medication, and then proceed with steps 5 through 9.
5. Place the dose-measuring applicator paper with the print side DOWN on the site (Figure 10-3, *A*). (The ointment will smear the print.)
6. Squeeze a ribbon of ointment of the proper length onto the applicator paper.

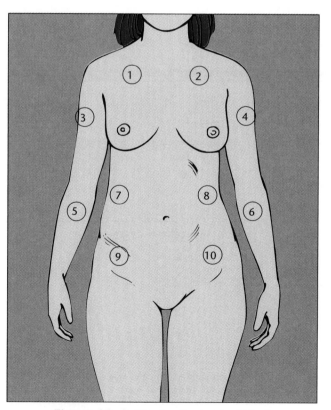

Figure 10-2 *Sites for nitroglycerin application.*

LIFE SPAN ISSUES

APPLYING NITROGLYCERIN

To promote personal safety when applying nitroglycerin to geriatric patients the nurse should always wear gloves when applying nitroglycerin ointment paper or handling transdermal patches. When nitroglycerin transdermal patches are applied, chart the specific site of application. Occasionally, patients move the transdermal patch themselves because of convenience, skin irritation, or confusion. If the patch is not found at the original location at the scheduled time of removal, examine other areas of the body to find it; do not assume that the patch fell off or was removed. Tolerance and loss of antianginal response could also develop if another patch is placed on the patient at the next scheduled time while the first patch is still on at the new location.

Always dispose of used nitroglycerin paper or transdermal patches in a receptacle to which the patient, children, and pets will not have access. A substantial amount of nitroglycerin remains on the patch and could be toxic.

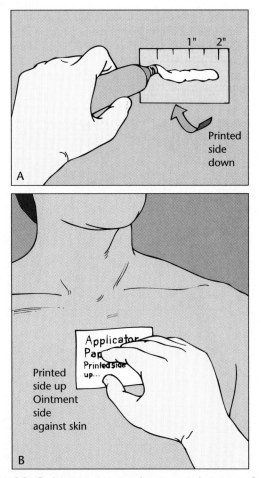

Figure 10-3 *Administering nitroglycerin topical ointment.* **A,** *Lay applicator paper printed side down and measure ribbon of ointment.* **B,** *Apply applicator to skin site, ointment side down. Spread in a uniform layer under applicator; leave paper in place.*

7. Place the measuring applicator on the skin surface at the site chosen on the rotation schedule, ointment side DOWN. Spread in a thin, uniform layer under the applicator. DO NOT RUB IN. Leave the paper in place. *Note:* Use of the applicator paper allows you to measure the prescribed dose and prevents absorption through the fingertips as you apply the medication (Figure 10-3, *B*).
8. Cover the area on which the paper is placed with plastic wrap and tape it in place.
9. Wash hands after applying the ointment.

Patient Teaching

1. Guide the patient in learning how to apply the ointment.
2. Tell the patient that the medication may discolor clothing. Use of clear plastic wrap protects clothing.
3. When the dose is regulated properly, the ointment may be used every 3 to 4 hours and at bedtime.
4. Tell the patient to wash hands after application to remove any nitroglycerin that came in contact with the fingers.
5. When terminating the use of this topical ointment, the dose and frequency of application should be gradually reduced over a 4- to 6-week period. Tell the patient to contact the physician if dosage adjustment is felt to be necessary. Encourage the patient not to discontinue the medication abruptly. (See Chapter 23.)

Documentation, the Sixth Right

Provide the RIGHT DOCUMENTATION of the medication administration and responses to drug therapy.
1. Chart the date, time, drug name, dosage, and site, and route of administration.
2. Perform and record regular patient assessment for the evaluation of therapeutic effectiveness (blood pressure, pulse, output, degree and duration of pain relief, and so on).
3. Chart and report any signs or symptoms of adverse drug effects.
4. Perform and validate essential patient education about the drug therapy and other essential aspects of intervention for the disease process affecting the individual.

ADMINISTRATION OF TRANSDERMAL DRUG DELIVERY SYSTEMS

Objectives

1. Identify the equipment needed, sites used, techniques used, and patient education required when transdermal medication systems are prescribed.
2. Describe specific documentation methods used to record the therapeutic effectiveness of medications administered by means of a transdermal delivery system.

Key Word

transdermal disk

Dosage Form

The **transdermal disk** provides controlled release of a prescribed medication (for example, nitroglycerin, clonidine, estrogen, nicotine, scopolamine) through a semipermeable membrane for 24 hours when applied to intact skin. The dosage released depends on the surface area of the disk in contact with the skin surface and the individual drug. See specific monographs for onset and duration of action of drugs using this delivery system.

Equipment

Transdermal disk
Shaving equipment as appropriate for the site and skin condition

Sites

Any area without hair may be used. Most people prefer the chest, flank, or upper arm areas. Develop a rotation schedule for use (see Figure 10-2).

Technique

1. Wash hands and assemble the equipment.
2. Use the FIVE RIGHTS of medication preparation and administration throughout the procedure:
   RIGHT PATIENT
   RIGHT DRUG
   RIGHT ROUTE OF ADMINISTRATION
   RIGHT DOSAGE
   RIGHT TIME OF ADMINISTRATION
3. Provide for patient privacy and give a thorough explanation of what is to be done.
4. Place the patient in a position such that the surface on which the topical materials are to be applied is exposed. Provide for patient comfort. *Note:* When reapplying a transdermal disk, remove the old disk and cleanse thoroughly. Select a new site for application. It is especially important in the elderly or confused patient to look for the old disk if it is not at the site at which the previous application is charted. The confused patient may actually have moved it elsewhere on the body or removed it. The old disk can be encased in the glove as the nurse removes it and should be disposed of in a receptacle on the medication cart not in the patient's room.
5. Apply the small adhesive topical disk. Figure 10-4, *A* to *D*, illustrates nitroglycerin being applied to one of the sites recommended by the rotation schedule. The frequency of application depends on the specific medication being applied in the transdermal disk and the duration of action of the prescribed medication. Nitroglycerin is applied once daily, whereas clonidine is applied once every 7 days.
6. Wash hands after application.

Patient Teaching

1. Guide the patient in learning how and when to apply the disks. *Note:* Transderm-Nitro and Nitro-dur may be

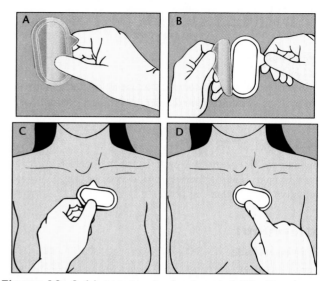

Figure 10-4 *Administering nitroglycerin topical disks (Transderm-Nitro).* **A,** *Carefully pick up the system lengthwise, with the tab up.* **B,** *Remove clear plastic backing from system at the tab. Do not touch inside of exposed system.* **C,** *Place the exposed adhesive side of the system on the chosen skin site; press firmly with the palm of the hand.* **D,** *Circle the outside edge of the system with one or two fingers.* Courtesy of CIBA Pharmaceutical Co., Summit, NJ.

worn while showering; Nitrodisc should be replaced after bathing or showering. Scopolamine, used for motion sickness, must be applied at least 4 hours before travel. Clonidine transdermal systems are applied once every 7 days.
2. If a disk becomes partially dislodged, the recommendations of the product should be followed. Nitroglycerin disks are removed and a new one is applied. Clonidine transdermal disks, on the other hand, come with a protective adhesive overlay to be applied over the patch to ensure skin contact of the transdermal system should the disk become loosened.
3. Patients receiving nitroglycerin transdermally may require sublingual nitroglycerin for anginal attacks, especially while the dosage is being adjusted.

Documentation, the Sixth Right

Provide the RIGHT DOCUMENTATION of the medication administration and the responses to drug therapy.
1. Chart the date, time, drug name, dosage, and site and route of administration.
2. Perform and record regular patient assessments for the evaluation of therapeutic effectiveness (blood pressure, pulse, degree and duration of pain relief, and so on).
3. Chart and report any signs or symptoms of adverse drug effects.
4. Perform and validate essential patient education about the drug therapy and other essential aspects of intervention for the disease process affecting the individual.

ADMINISTRATION OF TOPICAL POWDERS

1. Describe the dosage form, sites used, and techniques employed to administer medications in topical powder form.

Dosage Form

Powders are finely ground particles of medication contained in a talc base. They generally produce a cooling, drying, or protective effect where applied.

Equipment

Prescribed powder

Site

Site is to the skin surface of the body, as prescribed.

Technique

1. Wash hands.
2. Use the FIVE RIGHTS of medication preparation and administration throughout the procedure:
   RIGHT PATIENT
   RIGHT DRUG
   RIGHT ROUTE OF ADMINISTRATION
   RIGHT DOSAGE
   RIGHT TIME OF ADMINISTRATION
3. Provide privacy for the patient and give a thorough explanation of the procedure.
4. Place the patient in a position such that the surface on which the topical materials are to be applied is exposed. Provide patient comfort before starting therapy.
5. Wash and thoroughly dry the affected area before applying the powder.
6. Apply powder by gently shaking the container. This distributes the powder evenly over the area. Gently smooth over the area for even coverage.

Patient Teaching

Tell the patient to cleanse area of administration and reapply powder to external surface as directed by the physician. The patient should avoid inhaling the powder during application.

Documentation, the Sixth Right

Provide the RIGHT DOCUMENTATION of the medication administration and the responses to drug therapy.

1. Chart the date, time, drug name, dosage, and site and route of administration.
2. Perform and record regular patient assessments for the evaluation of therapeutic effectiveness.
3. Chart and report any signs or symptoms of adverse drug effects.
4. Perform and validate essential patient education about the drug therapy and other essential aspects of intervention for the disease process affecting the individual.

ADMINISTRATION OF MEDICATIONS TO MUCOUS MEMBRANES

1. Describe the dosage forms, sites, equipment used, and techniques for administration of medications to the mucous membranes.
2. Identify the dosage forms safe for administration to the eye.
3. Describe patient education necessary for patients requiring ophthalmic medications.
4. Compare the techniques used to administer ear drops in a child under 3 years of age and in patients over 3 years old.
5. Describe the purpose, precautions necessary, and patient education required for persons requiring medications by inhalation.
6. Describe the dosage forms available for vaginal administration of medications.
7. Identify the equipment needed, site, and specific techniques required to administer vaginal medications or douches.
8. State the rationale and procedure used for cleansing vaginal applicators or douche tips after use.
9. Develop a plan for patient education of persons receiving medications via the percutaneous routes.

buccal	nebulae
ophthalmic	aerosols
otic	metered-dose inhalers

Drugs are well absorbed across mucosal surfaces, and it is easy to obtain therapeutic effects. However, mucous membranes are highly selective in absorptive activity and differ in sensitivity. In general, aqueous solutions are quickly absorbed from mucous membranes, whereas oily liquids are not. Drugs in suppository form can be used for local effects on the mucous membranes of the vagina, urethra, or rectum. A drug may be inhaled and absorbed through the mucous membranes of the nose and lungs. It may be dissolved and absorbed by the mucous membranes of the mouth or applied to the eyes or ears for local action. It may be painted, swabbed, or irrigated on a mucosal surface.

Administration of Sublingual and Buccal Tablets

Dosage Forms

Sublingual tablets are designed to be placed under the tongue for dissolution and absorption through the vast network of blood vessels in this area. **Buccal** tablets are designed to be held in the buccal cavity (between the cheek and molar teeth) for absorption from the blood vessels of the cheek. The primary advantage of these routes of administration is the rapid absorption and onset of action—the drug passes directly into systemic circulation with no immediate pass through the liver, where extensive metabolism usually takes place. Contrary to most other forms of administration to mucous membranes, the action from these dosage forms is usually systemic rather than localized to the mouth.

Equipment

Prescribed medication. *Note:* The medications available to be administered by this route are forms of nitroglycerin. Once the self-administration technique is taught, the patient should carry the medication or keep it readily available at bedside for use as needed.

Sites

Sublingual area (under tongue) (Figure 10-5, *A*) or buccal pouch (between molar teeth and cheek) (Figure 10-5, *B*).

Technique

For Administration by the Nurse

Refer to Chapter 7 for correct technique with either the medication card system or the unit dose system.
1. Wash hands and assemble the equipment.
2. Use the FIVE RIGHTS of medication preparation and administration throughout the procedure:
   RIGHT PATIENT
   RIGHT DRUG
   RIGHT ROUTE OF ADMINISTRATION
   RIGHT DOSAGE
   RIGHT TIME OF ADMINISTRATION
3. Provide privacy for the patient and give a thorough explanation of the procedure.
4. Put on a glove and place the medication under the tongue (sublingual) (see Figure 10-5, *A*) or between the upper molar teeth and the cheek (buccal) (see Figure 10-5, *B*). The tablet is meant to dissolve in these locations. Do not administer with water. Encourage the patient to allow the drug to dissolve where placed.
5. Remove glove and dispose of it according to policy.
6. Wash hands thoroughly.

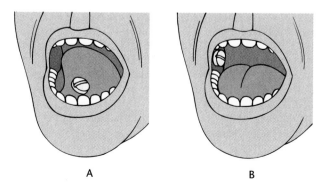

Figure 10-5 *Placing medication in the mouth.* **A,** *Under the tongue (sublingual).* **B,** *In the buccal pouch.*

Patient Teaching

Explain the exact placement of the medication and the dosage and frequency of doses. The patient should be told what side effects to expect, what adverse effects to report, where to carry the medication, how to store the medication, and how to refill the prescription when needed.

Documentation, the Sixth Right

Provide the RIGHT DOCUMENTATION of the medication administration and responses to drug therapy.
1. Chart the date, time, drug name, dosage, and site and route of administration.
2. Perform and record regular patient assessments for the evaluation of therapeutic effectiveness (blood pressure, pulse, degree and duration of pain relief, number of doses taken, and so on).
3. Chart and report any signs or symptoms of adverse drug effects.
4. Perform and validate essential patient education about the drug therapy and other essential aspects of intervention for the disease process affecting the individual.
   Note: When the patient is self-administering a medication, the nurse is still responsible for all aspects of the charting and monitoring parameters to document the drug therapy and response achieved.

Administration of Eye Drops and Ointment

Dosage Form

Medications for use in the eye should be labeled **ophthalmic.** If not labeled as such, do not administer to the eye. Ocular solutions are sterile, easily administered, and usually do not interfere with vision when instilled. Allow eye medication to warm to room temperature before administration.

Ocular ointments cause alterations in visual acuity. However, they have a longer duration of action than solutions.

Always use a separate bottle or tube of eye medication for each patient.

Equipment

Gloves
Eye drops or ointment prescribed (check strength carefully)
Dropper (use only the dropper supplied by the manufacturer)
Paper tissues or sterile cotton balls
Sterile eye dressing (pad), as appropriate
Normal saline solution, if needed for cleaning off exudate

Site

Eyes. OD is the Latin abbreviation for right eye; OS is the Latin abbreviation for left eye; OU is the Latin abbreviation for both eyes.

Technique

1. Wash hands and assemble *ophthalmic* medication.
2. Use the FIVE RIGHTS of medication preparation and administration throughout the procedure:
   RIGHT PATIENT
   RIGHT DRUG
   RIGHT ROUTE OF ADMINISTRATION
   RIGHT DOSAGE
   RIGHT TIME OF ADMINISTRATION

3. Provide privacy for the patient and give a thorough explanation of the procedure:

4. Position the patient such that that the back of the head is firmly supported on a pillow and the face is directed toward the ceiling. With children, restraints may be necessary if the child is too young to cooperate voluntarily. Always ensure patient safety.

5. Check to be certain that you have the correct medication according to the FIVE RIGHTS. Put on gloves. Inspect the affected eye to determine the current status. As appropriate, remove exudate from the eyelid and eyelashes using sterile saline solution. Always use a separate cotton ball for each wiping motion. Start at the inner canthus and wipe outward.

6. Expose the lower conjunctival sac by applying gentle traction to the lower lid at the bony rim of the orbit.

7. Approach the eye from above with the medication dropper or tube of ointment. (Never touch the eye dropper or ointment tip against the eye or face.)

8. At conclusion of either procedure remove the gloves and discard them according to the policy of the practice setting.

9. Wash hands thoroughly.

Drops (Figure 10-6)

• Have the patient look upward over your head.

• Drop the specified number of drops into the conjunctival sac. Never drop directly onto the eyeball.

• After instilling the drops, apply gentle pressure, using a cotton ball, to the inner corner of the eyelid on the bone for approximately 1 to 2 minutes. This prevents the medication from entering the canal, where it would be absorbed in the vascular mucosa of the nose and produce systemic effects. It also ensures an adequate concentration of medication in the eye.

• When more than one type of eye drop is ordered for the same eye, wait 1 to 5 minutes between instillation of the different medications. Use only the dropper provided by the manufacturer. Apply a sterile dressing as ordered.

Ointment

• Gently squeeze the ointment in a strip fashion into the conjunctival sac (Figure 10-7). Do not allow the tip to touch the patient.

• Tell the patient to close the eyes gently and move the eyes with the lid shut, as if looking around the room, to spread the medication. Apply a sterile dressing as ordered.

Patient Teaching

1. Guide the patient in learning self-administration of ophthalmic medication.

2. Tell the patient to wipe the eyes gently from the nose outward to prevent contamination between the eyes and possible spread of infection and to use a separate tissue to wipe each eye.

3. Instruct the patient to wash hands frequently and avoid touching the eye or immediate areas surrounding it, especially when an infection is present. Dispose of tissues in a manner that prevents spread of an infection.

4. Stress punctuality in administration of eye medications, especially when used for treating infections or increased intraocular pressure.

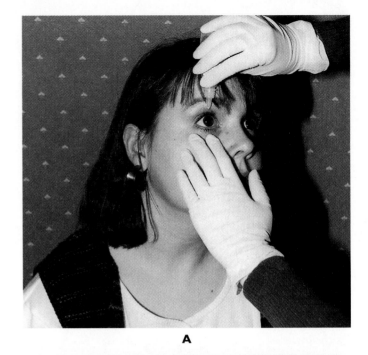

A

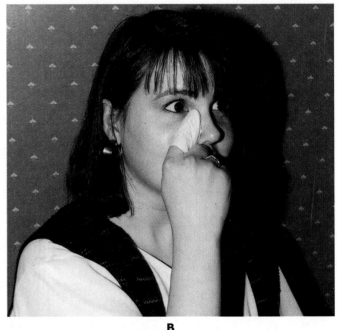

B

Figure 10-6 *Administering ophthalmic drops.* **A,** *Have the patient look upward; apply gentle traction to lower lid to expose conjunctival sac. Instill drops into sac.* **B,** *Using a tissue, apply gentle pressure to the inner corner of eyelid on bone for 1 to 2 minutes.* Courtesy Oscar H. Allison, Jr.

5. Tell the patient to discard eye medications that have changed color, have become cloudy, or contain particles. (If the patient's visual acuity is reduced, someone else should check clarity.)

6. The patient must not use over-the-counter eye washes without first consulting the physician managing the eye disorder.

7. Emphasize the need for careful follow-up of any eye disorder until the physician releases the patient from further care.

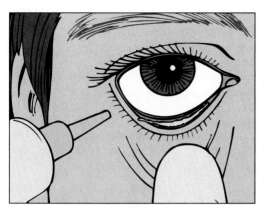

Figure 10-7 *Administering ophthalmic ointment. To instill the ointment, gently pull the lower lid down as patient looks upward. Squeeze ophthalmic ointment into lower sac. Avoid touching tube to eyelid.*

Documentation, the Sixth Right

Provide the RIGHT DOCUMENTATION of the medication administration and responses to drug therapy:
1. Chart the date, time, drug name, dosage, and site and route of administration.
2. Perform and record regular patient assessments for the evaluation of therapeutic effectiveness (redness, discomfort, visual activity, changes in infection or inflammatory reaction, degree and duration of pain relief, and so on).
3. Chart and report any signs or symptoms of adverse drug effects.
4. Perform and validate essential patient education about the drug therapy and other essential aspects of intervention for the disease process affecting the individual.

Administration of Ear Drops

Dosage Form

Ear drops are a solution containing a medication that is used for the treatment of localized infection or inflammation of the ear. Medications for use in the ear should be labeled **otic.** If not labeled as such, do not administer to the ear. Ear drops should be warmed to room temperature before use, and separate bottles of ear drops should be used for each patient.

Equipment

Gloves
Otic solution prescribed
Dropper provided by the manufacturer

Site

Ears

Technique

1. Review the policy of the practice setting and follow guidelines regarding whether gloves are to be worn during instillation of ear medications.
2. Wash hands and assemble the equipment.
3. Use the FIVE RIGHTS of medication preparation and administration throughout the procedure:
   RIGHT PATIENT
   RIGHT DRUG
   RIGHT ROUTE OF ADMINISTRATION
   RIGHT DOSAGE
   RIGHT TIME OF ADMINISTRATION
4. Provide privacy for the patient and give a thorough explanation of the procedure.
5. Place the patient in a position such that the affected ear is directed upward; put on gloves (according to policy).
6. Assess the ear canal for wax accumulation. If wax is present, obtain an order to irrigate the canal before instilling the ear drops.
7. Allow the medication to warm to room temperature, shake well, and draw up into the dropper.
8. *Administration:* For children under 3 years of age, restrain the child, turn the head to the appropriate side, and gently pull the earlobe *downward* and *back* (Figure 10-8, *A*). Instill the prescribed number of drops into the

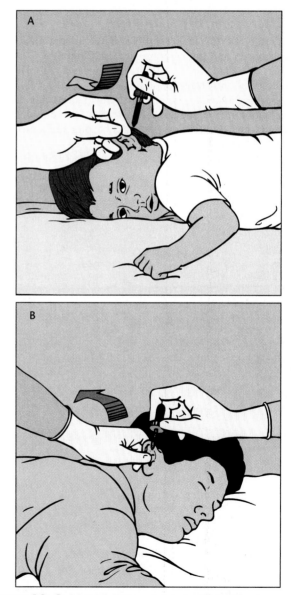

Figure 10-8 *Administering ear drops.* **A,** *Pull earlobe downward and back in children under 3 years of age.* **B,** *Pull earlobe upward and back in patients over 3 years of age.*

canal. Do not allow the dropper tip to touch any part of the ear. For children over 3 years of age and for adults, enlist cooperation or restrain as necessary, turn the head to the appropriate side, and gently pull the earlobe *upward* and *back* (Figure 10-8, *B*) to straighten the external auditory canal. Instill the prescribed number of drops into the canal. Do not allow the dropper tip to touch any part of the ear.

9. Instruct the patient to remain on the side for a few minutes following instillation; insert a cotton plug *loosely* if ordered.
10. Repeat the procedure if ear drops are ordered for both ears.
11. Remove gloves and dispose of them according to policy.

Patient Teaching

1. Explain the importance of administering the medication as prescribed.
2. Teach self-administration to the patient or administration to another person as appropriate.

Documentation, the Sixth Right

Provide the RIGHT DOCUMENTATION of the medication administration and the responses to drug therapy:
1. Chart the date, time, drug name, dosage, and site and route of administration.
2. Perform and record regular patient assessments for the evaluation of therapeutic effectiveness (redness, pressure, degree, and duration of pain relief, color and amount of drainage, and so on).
3. Chart and report any signs and symptoms of adverse drug effects.
4. Perform and validate essential patient education about the drug therapy and other essential aspects of intervention for the disease process affecting the individual.

Administration of Nose Drops

Nasal solutions are used to treat temporary disorders affecting the nasal mucous membrane. Always use the dropper provided by the manufacturer, and provide each patient with a separate bottle of nose drops.

Equipment

Gloves
Nose drops prescribed
Dropper supplied by the manufacturer
Tissue to blow the nose

Site

Nostrils

Technique

1. Review the practice setting policy and follow guidelines regarding whether gloves are to be used during the instillation of nose drops to prevent possible contact with body fluid secretions.
2. Wash hands and assemble the equipment.
3. Use the FIVE RIGHTS of medication preparation and administration throughout the procedure:
RIGHT PATIENT
RIGHT DRUG
RIGHT ROUTE OF ADMINISTRATION

RIGHT DOSAGE
RIGHT TIME OF ADMINISTRATION
4. Provide privacy for the patient and give a thorough explanation of the procedure.
5. *Administration* (Figure 10-9): For adults and older children:
   • Instruct the patient to blow the nose gently.
   • Have the patient lie down and hang the head backward over the edge of the bed.
   • Draw the medication into the dropper. Hold the dropper just above the nostril and instill the medication.

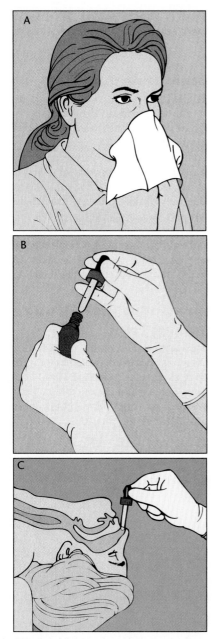

Figure 10-9 *Administering nose drops.* **A,** *Gently blow nose.* **B,** *Open medication and draw up to calibration on dropper.* **C,** *Instill medication. Have patient remain in position for 2 to 3 minutes. Repeat on other side if necessary.*

- After a brief time, instruct the patient to turn the head to the other side and repeat the administration process in the second nostril, if needed.
- Have the patient remain in this position for 2 to 3 minutes to allow the drops to remain in contact with the nasal mucosa.

For infants and young children:

- Position the infant or small child with the head over the edge of the bed or pillow, or use the "football" hold to immobilize the infant.
- Administer nose drops in the same manner as that for the adult.
- For the child who is cooperative, offer praise. Provide appropriate comforting and personal contact for all children or infants.

6. Have paper tissues available for use if absolutely necessary to blow the nose.

Patient Teaching

Guide the patient in learning self-administration of nose drops if necessary. Tell the patient that overuse of the nose drops can cause a "rebound effect," which causes the symptoms to become worse. If symptoms have not resolved after a week of nasal drop therapy, the physician should be consulted again.

Documentation, the Sixth Right

Provide the RIGHT DOCUMENTATION of the medication administration and responses to drug therapy:

1. Chart the date, time, drug name, dosage, and site and route of administration.
2. Perform and record regular patient assessments for the evaluation of the therapeutic effectiveness (nasal congestion, degree and duration of relief achieved, improvement in overall status, and so on).
3. Chart and report any signs or symptoms of adverse drug effects.
4. Perform and validate essential patient education about the drug therapy and other essential aspects of intervention for the disease process affecting the individual.

Administration of Nasal Spray

The mucous membranes of the nose absorb aqueous solutions well. When applied as a spray, the small droplets of solution containing medication coat the membrane and are rapidly absorbed. The advantage of spray over drops is less waste of medication because some of the drops often run down the back of the throat before absorption can take place. As with drops, each patient should have a personal container of spray.

Equipment

Gloves
Nasal spray prescribed
Paper tissues to blow the nose

Site

Nostrils

Technique

1. Review the policy of the practice setting and follow guidelines regarding whether gloves are to be used during the instillation of nasal sprays.
2. Wash hands and assemble the equipment.
3. Use the FIVE RIGHTS of medication preparation and administration throughout the procedure:
   RIGHT PATIENT
   RIGHT DRUG
   RIGHT ROUTE OF ADMINISTRATION
   RIGHT DOSAGE
   RIGHT TIME OF ADMINISTRATION
4. Provide privacy for the patient and give a thorough explanation of the procedure.
5. Instruct the patient to gently blow the nose (Figure 10-10, A to C).
6. Sit the patient upright.
7. Block one nostril.
8. Holding the spray bottle upright, shake the bottle.
9. Immediately after shaking, insert the tip into the nostril. Ask the patient to inhale through the open nostril and squeeze a puff of spray into the nostril at the same time.
10. Have paper tissues available for use if necessary to blow the nose.

Patient Teaching

Guide the patient in learning self-administration of nose drops if necessary. Tell the patient that overuse of nasal spray can cause a rebound effect, which causes the

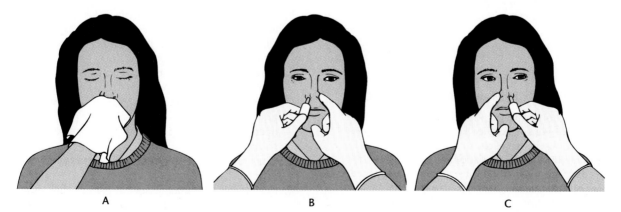

A   B   C

Figure 10-10 *Administering nasal spray.* **A,** *Gently blow nose.* **B,** *Block one nostril; shake bottle, insert tip into nostril and squeeze a puff of spray while patient is inhaling through the open nostril.* **C,** *Repeat step shown in* **B,** *blocking other nostril.*

symptoms to become worse. If symptoms have not resolved after a week of nasal spray therapy, the physician should be consulted again.

Documentation, the Sixth Right

Provide the RIGHT DOCUMENTATION of the medication administration and responses to drug therapy:

1. Chart the date, time, drug name, dosage, and site and route of administration.
2. Perform and record regular patient assessments for the evaluation of therapeutic effectiveness (nasal congestion, degree and duration of relief achieved, improvement in overall status, and so on).
3. Chart and report any signs or symptoms of adverse drug effects.
4. Perform and validate essential patient education about the drug therapy and other essential aspects of intervention for the patient's disease process.

Administration of Medications by Inhalation

The respiratory mucosa may be medicated by means of inhalation of sprays (**nebulae**) or aerosols. Nebulae are sprayed into the throat by a nebulizer. **Aerosols** use a flow of air or oxygen under pressure to disperse the drug throughout the respiratory tract. Oily preparations should not be applied to the respiratory mucosa because the oil droplets may be carried to the lung and cause lipid pneumonia. Although saliva as a body fluid has not been implicated in the transmission of the human immunodeficiency virus (HIV) at the time of this writing, the practice-setting policy manual should reflect current standards of universal precautions for all patients and health care personnel. Follow these procedures faithfully to prevent the transmission of this disease.

Equipment

Gloves
Liquid aerosol or spray forms of medications

Site

Respiratory tract

LIFE SPAN ISSUES

MEDICINES ADMINISTERED BY INHALATION

When muscle coordination is not fully developed, as in a younger child, or when dexterity has diminished in a geriatric patient, it may be beneficial to use a spacer device for medicines administered by inhalation.

When administering medicines by aerosol therapy to the elderly, make sure that they have the strength and dexterity to operate the equipment themselves before discharge.

Technique

1. Wash hands and assemble the equipment.
2. Use the FIVE RIGHTS of medication preparation and administration throughout the procedure:
   RIGHT PATIENT
   RIGHT DRUG
   RIGHT ROUTE OF ADMINISTRATION
   RIGHT DOSAGE
   RIGHT TIME OF ADMINISTRATION
3. Provide privacy for the patient and give a thorough explanation of the procedure.
4. Place the patient in a sitting position. This allows maximum lung expansion. Put on gloves (according to policy).
5. Prepare the medication according to the prescribed directions and fill the nebulizer with diluent. (This may be done before sitting the patient up if time is a factor to the patient's well-being.)
6. Direct the patient to exhale through pursed lips.
7. Put the nebulizer mouthpiece in the mouth. Do NOT seal the lips completely.
8. Activate the inhalation equipment and instruct the patient to inhale and breathe to full capacity simultaneously.
9. Direct the patient to exhale *slowly* through pursed lips.
10. WAIT approximately 1 minute and repeat the sequence according to the physician's directions or until all of the medication in the nebulizer is used.
11. Clean the equipment according to the manufacturer's directions.
12. Assist the patient to a comfortable position.
13. Remove gloves and wash hands.

Patient Teaching

1. As appropriate to the circumstances, teach the patient or significant others to operate the nebulizer to be used at home.
2. Explain the operation and cleansing of the equipment.
3. Before discharge have the patient or significant others administer the treatment using the equipment and medications prescribed for at-home use.
4. Stress the need to perform the procedure exactly as prescribed and to report any difficulties experienced after discharge for physician evaluation.

Documentation, the Sixth Right

Provide the RIGHT DOCUMENTATION of the medication administration and responses to drug therapy:

1. Chart the date, time, drug name, dosage, and site and route of administration.
2. Perform and record regular patient assessments for the evaluation of therapeutic effectiveness (blood pressure, pulse, improvement or quality of breathing, cough and productivity, degree and duration of pain relief, ability to operate the nebulizer, activity and exercise restrictions, and so on).
3. Chart and report any signs or symptoms of adverse drug effects.
4. Perform and validate essential patient education about the drug therapy and other essential aspects of intervention for the disease process affecting the individual.

Administration of Medications by Metered-Dose Inhalers

Dosage Forms

Bronchodilator and corticosteroid may be administered by inhalation through the mouth using an aerosolized, pressurized **metered-dose inhaler.** The primary advantage of the aerosolized inhalers is that the medication is applied directly to the site of action—the bronchial smooth muscle. Smaller doses are used, with rapid absorption and onset of action. The valve of the pressurized container also helps ensure that the same dose of medication is administered with each inhalation.

Approximately 25% of patients do not use metered-dose inhalers properly and therefore do not receive the maximal benefit of the medication. Devices known as extenders or spacers have been designed for patients who cannot coordinate the release of the medication with inhalation. The extender devices can be adapted to most pressurized canisters of metered-dose inhalers. These devices trap the aerosolized medication in a chamber through which the patient inhales within a few seconds after releasing the medication into the chamber.

Equipment

Gloves
Prescribed medication packaged in a metered-dose inhaler

Site

Respiratory tract

Technique

1. Wash hands and assemble the equipment.
2. Use the FIVE RIGHTS of medication preparation and administration throughout the procedure:
   RIGHT PATIENT
   RIGHT DRUG
   RIGHT ROUTE OF ADMINISTRATION
   RIGHT DOSAGE
   RIGHT TIME OF ADMINISTRATION
3. Provide privacy for the patient and give a thorough explanation of the procedure; put on gloves.
4. The following principles apply to all metered-dose inhalers. Read and adapt the technique to directions provided by the manufacturer for a specific inhaler and extender if needed.
   * If the medication is a suspension, shake the canister. This disperses and mixes the active bronchodilator and propellant together.
   * Open the mouth and place the canister outlet 2 to 4 inches in front of the mouth or use an extender. This space allows the propellant to evaporate and prevents large particles from settling in the mouth.
   * Activate the metered-dose inhaler and instruct patient to inhale deeply over 10 seconds to ensure that airways are open and that the drug is dispersed as deeply as possible.
   * Have patient hold breath, then exhale slowly to permit the drug to settle into pulmonary tissue.
   * If prescribed, repeat in 2 to 3 minutes. Using small doses with 2 to 3 inhalations enhances deposition of the drug in the smaller, peripheral airways for longer therapeutic effect.
   * Cleanse the apparatus according to the manufacturer's recommendations; remove gloves and dispose of them according to hospital policy.
   * The patient should not wait until the canister is empty before refilling the prescription. The last few doses in a canister are often subtherapeutic because of an imbalance in the remaining amounts of medication and propellant.

Patient Teaching

Explain the procedure and allow the patient to demonstrate the technique. Metered-dose inhalers without active ingredients are available from the pharmacy department to encourage patients to practice the technique before medication administration. In addition to technique, the patient should be told what side effects to expect, what adverse effects to report, how to carry the medication, how to store it, and how to have it refilled when needed.

Documentation, the Sixth Right

Provide the RIGHT DOCUMENTATION of the medication administration and responses to drug therapy:
1. Chart the date, time, drug name, dosage, and site and route of administration.
2. Perform and record regular patient assessments for the evaluation of therapeutic effectiveness (blood pressure, pulse, improvement or quality of breathing, cough and productivity, degree and duration of pain relief, ability to operate the metered-dose inhaler, activity and exercise restrictions, and so on).
3. Chart and report any signs or symptoms of adverse drug effects.
4. Perform and validate essential patient education about the drug therapy and other essential aspects of intervention for the disease process affecting the patient.

Administration of Vaginal Medications

Women with gynecologic disorders may require the administration of a medication intravaginally, usually for localized action. Vaginal medications may be creams, jellies, tablets, foams, suppositories, or irrigations (douches). The creams, jellies, tablets, and foams are inserted by means of special applicators provided by the manufacturer; suppositories are usually inserted with a gloved index finger. (See Administration of Vaginal Douche, p. 148.)

Equipment

Prescribed medication
Vaginal applicator
Perineal pad
Water-soluble lubricant (for suppository)
Gloves
Paper towel

Site

Vagina

Technique

1. Wash hands and assemble the equipment.
2. Use the FIVE RIGHTS of medication preparation and administration throughout the procedure:
   RIGHT PATIENT
   RIGHT DRUG
   RIGHT ROUTE OF ADMINISTRATION
   RIGHT DOSAGE
   RIGHT TIME OF ADMINISTRATION
3. Provide privacy for the patient and give a thorough explanation of the procedure. Have the patient void to ensure that the bladder is empty. Put on gloves.
4. Fill the applicator with the prescribed tablet, jelly, cream, or foam.
5. Place the patient in the lithotomy position and elevate the hips with a pillow. Drape the patient to prevent unnecessary exposure.
6. *Administration:* For creams, foams, and jellies, use the gloved, nondominant hand to spread the labia and expose the vagina. Assess the status of symptoms (such as color of discharge, volume, odor, level of discomfort). Gently insert the vaginal applicator as far as possible into the vagina and push the plunger to deposit the medication (Figure 10-11). Remove the applicator and wrap it in a paper towel for cleaning later. For suppositories, unwrap a vaginal suppository that has warmed to room temperature and lubricate with a water-soluble

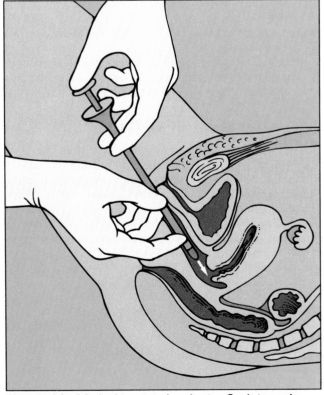

Figure I0-II *Applying vaginal medication. Gently insert the vaginal applicator as far as possible into the vagina and push plunger to deposit the medication.*

lubricant. Lubricate the gloved, dominant index finger. With the gloved, nondominant hand, spread the labia to expose the vagina. Insert the suppository (rounded end first) as far into the vagina as possible with the dominant index finger.
7. Remove glove by turning inside out; place on paper towel for later disposal.
8. Apply a perineal pad to prevent drainage onto the patient's clothing or bed.
9. Instruct the patient to remain in a supine position with hips elevated for 5 to 10 minutes to allow melting and spreading of the medication.
10. Dispose of all waste and wash hands.

Patient Teaching

1. Guide the patient in learning how to administer the medication correctly.
2. The applicator should be washed in warm soapy water after *each* use.
3. Review personal hygiene measures such as wiping from the front to the back after voiding or defecating.
4. Tell the patient not to douche and to abstain from sexual intercourse after inserting the medication.
5. With most types of infection, both the male and female partners require treatment. Partners should abstain from sexual intercourse until both partners are cured to prevent reinfections.

Documentation, the Sixth Right

Provide the RIGHT DOCUMENTATION of the medication administration and responses to drug therapy:
1. Chart the date, time, drug name, dosage, and site and route of administration.
2. Perform and record regular patient assessments for the evaluation of the therapeutic effectiveness (type of discharge present, irritation of labia, discomfort, degree and duration of pain relief, and so on).
3. Chart and report any signs or symptoms of adverse drug effects.
4. Perform and validate essential patient education about the drug therapy and other essential aspects of intervention for the disease process affecting the patient.

Administration of Vaginal Douche

Douches (irrigants) are used for washing the vagina. This procedure is not necessary for normal female hygiene but may be required if a vaginal infection and discharge are present. It should also be noted that douches are not effective methods of birth control.

Equipment

Intravenous (IV) pole
Gloves
Water-soluble lubricant
Douche bag with tubing and nozzle
Douche solution

Site

Vagina

Technique

1. Wash hands and assemble the equipment.
2. Use the FIVE RIGHTS of medication preparation and administration throughout the procedure:
   RIGHT PATIENT
   RIGHT DRUG
   RIGHT ROUTE OF ADMINISTRATION
   RIGHT DOSAGE
   RIGHT TIME OF ADMINISTRATION
3. Provide privacy for the patient and provide a thorough explanation of the procedure.
4. Ask the patient to void before the procedure.
5. If teaching this procedure to a patient for home use, the patient would customarily recline in a bathtub. Depending on the patient's condition in the hospital, this could occur there as well. However, it may be necessary to place the patient on a bedpan and drape for privacy.
6. Hang the douche bag on an IV pole, about 12 inches above the vagina; put on gloves; apply water-soluble lubricant to plastic vaginal tip.
7. Cleanse the vulva by allowing a small amount of solution to flow over the vulva and between the labia.
8. Gently insert the nozzle, directing the tip backward and downward 2 to 3 inches.
9. Hold the labia together to facilitate filling the vagina with solution. Rotate nozzle periodically to help irrigate all parts of the vagina.
10. Intermittently release the labia to allow the solution to flow out.
11. When all of the solution has been used, remove the nozzle. Have the patient sit up and lean forward to thoroughly empty the vagina.
12. Pat the external area dry.
13. Clean all equipment with warm soapy water after *every* use; rinse with clear water and allow to dry.
14. Thoroughly clean and disinfect the bathtub, if used. Remove gloves and dispose of them according to hospital policy.
15. Wash hands.

Patient Teaching

1. Guide the patient in learning how to correctly administer the douche.
2. Explain that the bag and tubing should be washed in warm soapy water after each use so that they will not become a source of reinfection.
3. Review personal hygiene measures such as wiping from the front to the back after voiding or defecating.
4. Explain that douching is not recommended during pregnancy.
5. With most types of infection, both the male and female partners require treatment. Partners should abstain from sexual intercourse until both partners are cured to prevent reinfections.

Documentation, the Sixth Right

Provide the RIGHT DOCUMENTATION of the medication administration and responses to drug therapy:

1. Chart the date, time, drug name, dosage, and site and route of administration.
2. Perform and record regular patient assessments for the evaluation of therapeutic effectiveness (type of discharge present, irritation of labia, discomfort, degree and duration of pain relief, and so on).
3. Chart and report any signs and symptoms of adverse drug effects.
4. Perform and validate essential patient education about the drug therapy and other essential aspects of intervention for patient's disease process.

PART TWO

APPLICATION OF THE NURSING PROCESS TO PHARMACOLOGY

CHAPTER

11

Drugs Affecting the Autonomic Nervous System

Objectives

1. Differentiate between afferent and efferent nerve conduction within the central nervous system.

2. Explain the role of neurotransmitters at synaptic junctions.

3. Name the most common neurotransmitters known to affect central nervous system function.

4. Identify the two major neurotransmitters of the autonomic nervous system.

5. Cite the names of nerve endings liberating acetylcholine and those liberating norepinephrine.

6. Explain the action of drugs that inhibit the actions of the cholinergic and adrenergic fibers.

7. Identify two broad classes of drugs used to stimulate the adrenergic nervous system.

8. Name the neurotransmitters called catecholamines.

9. Review the actions of adrenergic agents to identify conditions that would be affected favorably and unfavorably by these medications.

10. Explain the rationale for use of adrenergic blocking agents for conditions that have vasoconstriction as part of the disease pathophysiology.

11. Describe the benefits of using beta-adrenergic blocking agents for hypertension, angina pectoris, cardiac arrhythmias, and hyperthyroidism.

12. Identify disease conditions that would preclude the use of beta-adrenergic blocking agents.

13. List the neurotransmitters responsible for cholinergic activity.

14. List the predictable side effects of cholinergic agents.

15. List the predictable side effects of anticholinergic agents.

16. Describe the clinical uses of anticholinergic agents.

Key Words

central nervous system

afferent nerves

efferent nerves

peripheral nervous system

motor nervous system

autonomic nervous system

neuron

synapse

neurotransmitters

norepinephrine

acetylcholine

cholinergic fiber

adrenergic fiber

anticholinergic agent

adrenergic blocking agent

catecholamine

alpha receptor

beta receptor

dopaminergic receptors

CENTRAL AND AUTONOMIC NERVOUS SYSTEMS

Control of the human body as a living organism comes primarily from two major systems: the nervous system and the endocrine system. In general, the endocrine system controls the metabolism of the body. The nervous system regulates the ongoing activities of the body (for example, heart and respiratory muscle contractions), rapid response to sudden changes in the environment, and the rates of secretions of some glands.

The brain and the spinal cord make up the **central nervous system** (CNS). The CNS receives signals from sensory receptors (for example, vision, pressure, pain, cold, warmth, touch, smell) throughout the body that are transmitted to the spinal cord and brain by way of **afferent nerves.** The CNS processes these signals and controls body response by sending signals through **efferent nerves,** which leave the CNS to carry impulses to other parts of the body. The efferent and afferent nerves are known collectively as the **peripheral nervous system.** The efferent nerves transmit signals that control contractions of smooth and skeletal muscle and some glandular secretions.

The efferent system is subdivided into the **motor nervous system,** which controls skeletal muscle contractions, and the **autonomic nervous system.** The autonomic nervous system helps regulate such bodily functions as heart rate, blood pressure, thermal control, light regulation by the eyes, and many other activities.

Each nerve of the central and peripheral nervous systems is actually composed of a series of segments called **neurons.** The junction between one neuron and the next is called a **synapse.** The transmission of nerve signals or impulses occurs because of the activity of chemical substances called **neurotransmitters** (transmitters of nerve impulses). A neurotransmitter is released into the synapse at the end of one neuron, activating receptors on the next neuron in the chain or at the end of the nerve chain, stimulating the end organ (the heart, smooth muscle, or gland). Neurotransmitters can be either excitatory, stimulating the next neuron, or inhibitory, inhibiting the neuron. Because a single neuron releases only one type of neurotransmitter, the CNS is composed of systems of different types of neurons that secrete separate neurotransmitters. Research indicates that there are over 30 different types of neurotransmitters. The more common neurotransmitters throughout the CNS are acetylcholine, norepinephrine, epinephrine, dopamine, glycine, gamma-aminobutyric acid (GABA), and glutamic acid. Substance P and the enkephalins and endorphins regulate the sensation of pain, and serotonin regulates mood. Other neurotransmitters include the prostaglandins, histamine, cyclic adenosine monophosphate (AMP), and amino acids and peptides. Regulation of neurotransmitters by pharmacologic agents (medicines) is a major mechanism by which we can control diseases that are caused by either an excess or deficiency of these neurotransmitters. In Unit Three, utilization of inhibitory and excitatory neurotransmitters to control illnesses is explained.

AUTONOMIC NERVOUS SYSTEM

With the exception of skeletal muscle the autonomic nervous system controls the function of most tissues. This nervous system helps control blood pressure, gastrointestinal secretion and motility, urinary bladder function, sweating, and body temperature. In general, it maintains a constant, internal environment (homeostasis) and responds to emergency situations. The word *autonomic* means "self-governing" or "automatic"; because of this the autonomic nervous system has also been called the involuntary nervous system because we have little or no control over it. The motor nervous system controls skeletal muscle; we can exercise control over much of it.

The two major neurotransmitters of the autonomic nervous system are **norepinephrine** and **acetylcholine.** The nerve endings that liberate acetylcholine are called **cholinergic fibers;** those that secrete norepinephrine are called **adrenergic fibers.** Most organs are innervated by both adrenergic and cholinergic fibers, but they produce opposite responses. Examples of these opposing actions are in the heart, where adrenergic agents increase the heart rate and cholinergic agents slow the heart rate, and in the eyes, where adrenergic agents cause pupillary dilation and cholinergic agents cause pupillary constriction (Table 11-1).

Drugs that cause effects in the body similar to those produced by acetylcholine are called *cholinergic* or parasympathomimetic drugs because they mimic the action produced by stimulation of the parasympathetic division of the autonomic nervous system. Drugs that cause effects similar to those produced by the adrenergic neurotransmitter are called *adrenergic,* or sympathomimetic, drugs. Agents that block or inhibit cholinergic activity are called **anticholinergic agents,** and agents that inhibit the adrenergic system are referred to as **adrenergic blocking agents.** See Figure 11-1 for a diagram of the autonomic system and representative stimulants and inhibitors.

Drug Class: Adrenergic Agents
Actions

The adrenergic nervous system may be stimulated by two broad classes of drugs: **catecholamines** and noncatecholamines. The naturally-occurring catecholamines that are neurotransmitters in the human body are norepinephrine, epinephrine, and dopamine. Norepinephrine is secreted primarily from nerve terminals, epinephrine primarily from the adrenal medulla, and dopamine at selected sites within the brain, kidneys, and gastrointestinal tract. All three agents are also synthetically manufactured and may be administered to produce the same effects as naturally secreted neurotransmitters. The noncatecholamines have actions that are somewhat similar to those of the catecholamines but are more selective for certain types of receptors, are not quite as fast acting, and have a longer duration of action.

As illustrated in Figure 11-1, the autonomic nervous system can be subdivided into the **alpha, beta,** and **dopaminergic receptors.** These are specific types of receptors that, when stimulated by chemicals of certain shapes, produce a specific action on that tissue. In general, stimulation of the alpha-1 receptors causes vasoconstriction of blood vessels. The alpha-2 receptors appear to serve as mediators of negative feedback preventing further release of norepinephrine. Stimulation of beta-1 receptors causes an increase in the heart rate, and stimulation of beta-2 receptors causes relaxation of smooth muscle in the bronchi (bronchodilation), uterus (relaxation), and peripheral arterial blood vessels

Table 11-1

Actions of Autonomic Nerve Impulses on Specific Tissues

TISSUE	RECEPTOR TYPE*	ADRENERGIC RECEPTORS (SYMPATHETIC)	CHOLINERGIC RECEPTORS (PARASYMPATHETIC)
Blood vessels			
Arterioles			
Coronary	α; β_2	Constriction; dilation	Dilation
Skin	α	Constriction	Dilation
Renal	α_1; β_1 and β_2	Constriction; dilation	—
Skeletal muscle	α; β_2	Constriction; dilation	Dilation
Veins (systemic)	α_1; β_2	Constriction; dilation	—
Eye			
Radial muscle, iris	α_1	Contraction (mydriasis)	—
Sphincter muscle, iris	—	—	Contraction (miosis)
Ciliary muscle	β	Relaxation for far vision	Contraction for near vision
Gastrointestinal tract			
Smooth muscle	α; β_1 and β_2	Relaxation	Contraction
Sphincters	α	Contraction	Relaxation
Heart	β_1	Increased heart rate, force of contraction	Decreased heart rate
Kidney	Dopamine	Dilates renal vasculature, increasing renal perfusion	—
Lung			
Bronchial muscle	β_2	Smooth muscle relaxation (opens airways)	Smooth muscle contraction (closes airways)
Bronchial glands	α_1; β_2	Decreased secretions; increased secretions	Stimulation
Metabolism	β_2	Glycogenolysis (increases blood glucose)	—
Urinary bladder			
Fundus (detrusor)	β	Relaxation	Contraction
Trigone and sphincter	α	Contraction	Relaxation
Uterus	α; β_2	Pregnant: contraction (α); relaxation (β_2)	Variable

*α, Alpha receptors; β_1, beta-1 receptors; β_2, beta-2 receptors.

(vasodilation). Stimulation of the dopaminergic receptors improves the symptoms associated with Parkinson's disease and increases urine output because of stimulation of specific receptors in the kidneys that results in better renal perfusion.

Uses

As noted in Table 11-2, many drugs act on more than one type of adrenergic receptor. Fortunately each agent acts to varying degrees, allowing a certain agent to be used for a specific purpose without many adverse effects. If recommended dosages are exceeded, however, certain receptors may be stimulated excessively, causing serious adverse effects. An example of this is terbutaline, which is primarily a beta stimulant. With normal doses, terbutaline is an effective bronchodilator. In addition to bronchodilation, higher doses of terbutaline cause central nervous system stimulation, resulting in insomnia and wakefulness. See Table 11-2 for clinical uses of the adrenergic agents.

Nursing Process for Adrenergic Agents

See also nursing process for respiratory tract disease, bronchodilators, and decongestants (see Chapters 27 and 28).

Premedication Assessment

1. Take baseline vital signs of heart rate and blood pressure.
2. See also premedication assessment for respiratory tract disease, bronchodilators, and decongestants (see Chapters 27 and 28).

Planning

Availability. See Table 11-2.

Implementation

Dosage and administration. See Table 11-2.

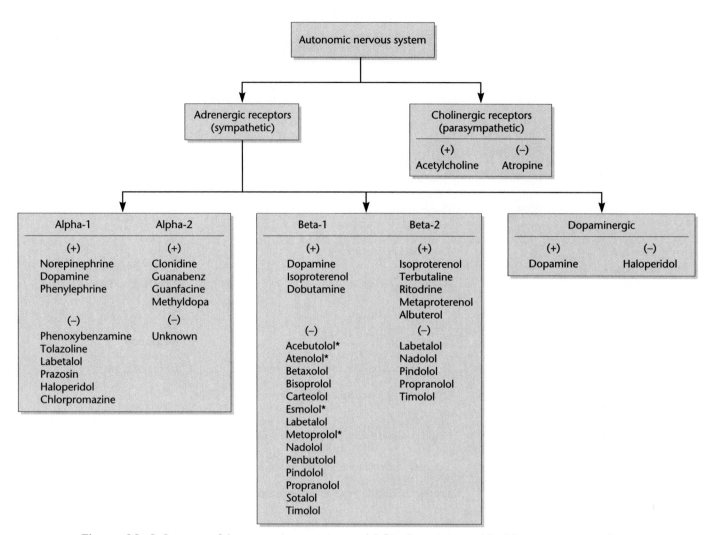

Figure 11-1 *Receptors of the autonomic nervous system. (+) Stimulates receptors; (−) inhibits receptors; asterisks indicate representative examples of selective beta-1 antagonists only.*

Evaluation

Side effects associated with the use of adrenergic agents are usually dosage related and resolve when the dosage is reduced or discontinued. Patients who are potentially more sensitive to adrenergic agents are those with impaired hepatic function, thyroid disease, hypertension, and heart disease. Patients with diabetes mellitus may also have increased frequency of episodes of hyperglycemia.

Side effects to expect

PALPITATIONS, TACHYCARDIA, SKIN FLUSHING, DIZZINESS, TREMORS. These side effects are usually mild and tend to resolve with continued therapy. Encourage the patient not to discontinue therapy without first consulting the physician.

ORTHOSTATIC HYPOTENSION. Although infrequent and generally mild, adrenergic agents may cause some degree of orthostatic hypotension manifested by dizziness and weakness, particularly when therapy is being initiated.

Monitor the blood pressure daily in both the supine and standing positions.

Anticipate the development of postural hypotension and take measures to prevent an occurrence. Teach the patient to rise slowly from a supine or sitting position; encourage the patient to sit or lie down if feeling faint.

Side effects to report

ARRHYTHMIAS, CHEST PAIN, SEVERE HYPOTENSION, HYPERTENSION, ANGINAL PAIN, NAUSEA, AND VOMITING. Discontinue therapy immediately and notify the physician.

Drug interactions

AGENTS THAT MAY INCREASE THERAPEUTIC AND TOXIC EFFECTS. Monoamine oxidase inhibitors (pargyline, tranylcypromine); tricyclic antidepressants (amitriptyline, imipramine, others); guanethidine, atropine, and cyclopropane or halothane anesthesia.

Monitor patients for tachycardia, serious arrhythmias, hypotension, hypertension, chest pain.

AGENTS THAT INHIBIT THERAPEUTIC ACTIVITY. Beta-adrenergic blocking agents (propranolol, nadolol, timolol, pindolol, atenolol, metoprolol, others); alpha-adrenergic blocking agents (phenoxybenzamine, phentolamine, tolazoline); guanethidine, reserpine, bretylium tosylate.

Concurrent use of these agents with adrenergic agents is not recommended.

Table 11-2

Adrenergic Agents

GENERIC NAME	BRAND NAME	AVAILABILITY	ADRENERGIC RECEPTOR	ACTION	CLINICAL USE
Albuterol*	Proventil, Ventolin Volmax	Aerosol: 90 mcg per puff Tablets: 2, 4 mg Syrup: 2 mg/5 ml Tablets: extended-release 4, 8 mg	Beta-2	Bronchodilator	Asthma, emphysema
Dopamine	Intropin, ♣ Revimine	IV: 40, 80, 160 mg/ml in 5 ml ampules	Alpha, beta-1, dopaminergic	Vasopressor	Shock, hypotension, inotropic agent
Dobutamine	Dobutrex	IV: 250 mg/20 ml vials	Beta-1	Cardiac stimulant	Inotropic agent
Ephedrine*	Ephedrine	SC, IM, IV: 25, 50 mg/ml in 1 ml ampules Tablets: 25, 50 mg Syrup: 20 mg/5 ml	Alpha, beta	Bronchodilator, vasoconstrictor	Nasal decongestant, hypotension
Epinephrine*	Adrenalin	IV: 1:1000 in 1 and 2 ml ampules: 1:10,000 in 3, 10 ml vials	Alpha, beta	Allergic reactions, vasoconstrictor, bronchodilator, cardiac stimulant	Anaphylaxis, cardiac arrest, topical vasoconstrictor
Isoetharine*	Bronkosol	Nebulization: 0.062, 0.08, 0.1, 0.125, 0.167, 0.2, 0.25, 0.5, 1% solutions	Beta-2	Bronchodilator	Inhalation therapy in bronchospasm, asthma
Isoproterenol	Isuprel	SC, IM, IV: 1:5000 solution, 1, 5, 10 ml vials Nebulization: 0.031, 0.065, 0.25, 0.5, 1% solution Aerosol: 0.2, 0.25% solution Sublingual tablets: 10, 15 mg	Beta	Bronchodilator, cardiac stimulant	Shock, digitalis toxicity, bronchospasm
Metaproterenol	Alupent, Metaprel	Aerosol: 5, 10 ml vial Nebulization: 0.4, 0.6, 5% solution Tablets: 10, 20 mg Syrup: 2 mg/ml	Beta-2	Bronchodilator	Bronchospasm
Metaraminol	Aramine	SC, IM, IV: 10 mg/ml in 10 ml vials	Alpha-1	Vasoconstrictor	Shock, hypotension
Norepinephrine (Levarterenol)	Levophed	IV: 1 mg/ml in 4 ml ampules	Alpha-1	Vasoconstrictor	Shock, hypotension
Phenylephrine†	Neo-Synephrine	SC, IM, IV: 1% in 1 ml ampules Ophthalmic drops: 0.12, 2.5, 10%	Alpha-1	Vasoconstrictor	Shock, hypotension, nasal decongestant, ophthalmic vasoconstrictor, mydriatic
Phenylpropanolamine†		Tablets: 25 mg Capsules: 37.5 mg Timed-release capsules and tablets: 25, 75 mg	Alpha-1	Vasoconstrictor	Nasal decongestant, anorectic
Ritodrine	Yutopar	Tablets: 10 mg IV: 10, 15 mg/ml in 5 and 10 ml vials	Beta-2	Uterine relaxant	Premature labor
Terbutaline*	Brethine, Bricanyl, Brethaire	Tablets: 2.5, 5 mg SC: 1 mg/ml in 1 ml ampules Aerosol: 0.2 mg/puff	Beta-2	Bronchodilator, uterine relaxant	Emphysema, asthma, premature labor

♣ Available in Canada only.
*See also Bronchodilators.
†See also Decongestants.

Drug Class: Alpha- and Beta-Adrenergic Blocking Agents

Actions

The alpha- and beta-adrenergic blocking agents act by plugging the alpha or beta receptors, which prevents other agents, usually the naturally occurring catecholamines, from stimulating the specific receptors.

The beta blockers can be subdivided into nonselective and selective beta antagonists. The nonselective blocking agents have an equal affinity for beta-1 and beta-2 receptors and inhibit both. These agents are propranolol, nadolol, pindolol, penbutolol, carteolol, sotalol, and timolol. The selective beta-1 blocking agents exhibit action against the beta-1 receptors of the heart (cardioselective) and do not readily affect the beta-2 receptors of the bronchi. Selective beta-1 antagonists available are esmolol, metoprolol, acebutolol, betaxolol, bisoprolol, and atenolol. This selective action is beneficial in patients, such as those with asthma, in whom nonselective beta blockers may induce bronchospasm. It is important to note, however, that the selectivity of these agents is only relative. In larger doses, these agents will also inhibit the beta-2 receptors. There are no selective beta-2 blockers available. Labetalol exhibits both selective alpha-1 and nonselective beta-adrenergic blocking activity.

Uses

Because a primary action of the alpha receptor stimulants is vasoconstriction, we would expect that alpha blocking agents would be indicated in patients with diseases associated with vasoconstriction. In fact, phenoxybenzamine and tolazoline are used as vasodilators in peripheral vascular diseases such as Raynaud's phenomenon and Buerger's disease. (See Chapter 24 for the clinical use of these agents.) Phentolamine is used in the diagnosis and treatment of pheochromocytoma, a tumor that secretes epinephrine.

The beta-adrenergic blocking agents (beta blockers) are used extensively in the treatment of hypertension, angina pectoris, cardiac arrhythmias, symptoms of hyperthyroidism, and "stage fright."

Beta blockers must be used with extreme caution in patients with respiratory conditions such as bronchitis, emphysema, asthma, or allergic rhinitis. Beta blockage produces severe bronchoconstriction and may aggravate wheezing, especially during the pollen season.

Use beta blockers with caution in diabetic patients and patients susceptible to hypoglycemia. The beta blockers further induce the hypoglycemic effects of insulin and reduce the release of insulin in response to hyperglycemia. All beta blockers mask most of the signs and symptoms of acute hypoglycemia.

Beta-adrenergic blocking agents should be used only in patients with controlled congestive heart failure. Further hypotension, bradycardia, or congestive heart failure may develop.

Nursing Process

See also nursing process for patients with antiarrhythmic therapy (p. 289) and for patients with hypertension (p. 261).

Premedication Assessment

1. Take baseline vital signs of heart rate and blood pressure.
2. See also premedication assessment for patients with antiarrhythmic therapy (p. 289) and for patients with hypertension (p. 261).

Planning

Availability. See Table 11-3.

Implementation

Dosage and administration. See Table 11-3.

Individualization of dosage. Although the onset of activity is fairly rapid, it may often take several days to weeks for a patient to show optimal improvement and become stabilized on an adequate maintenance dosage. Patients must be periodically reevaluated to determine the lowest effective dosage necessary to control the disorder being treated.

Sudden discontinuation. Patients must be counseled against poor compliance or sudden discontinuation of therapy without a physician's advice. Sudden discontinuation of therapy has resulted in an exacerbation of anginal symptoms followed in some cases by myocardial infarction. When discontinuing chronically administered beta blockers, the dosage should be gradually reduced over a period of 1 to 2 weeks with careful monitoring of the patient. If anginal symptoms develop or become more frequent, beta blocker therapy should be restarted at least temporarily.

Evaluation

Most of the adverse effects associated with beta-adrenergic blocking agents are dosage related. Response by individual patients is highly variable. Many of these side effects may occur but be transient. Strongly encourage patients to see their physician before discontinuing therapy. Minor dosage adjustment may be all that is required for the elimination of most side effects.

Side effects to expect and report

BRADYCARDIA, PERIPHERAL VASOCONSTRICTION (PURPLE, MOTTLED SKIN). Discontinue further dosages until the patient is evaluated by a physician.

BRONCHOSPASM, WHEEZING. Withhold additional doses until the patient has been evaluated by a physician.

DIABETIC PATIENTS. Monitor for hypoglycemia: headache, weakness, decreased coordination, general apprehension, diaphoresis, hunger, or blurred or double vision. Many of these symptoms may be masked by the beta-adrenergic blocking agents. Notify the physician if you suspect that any of the symptoms described are appearing intermittently.

HEART FAILURE. Monitor patients for an increase in edema, dyspnea, rales, bradycardia, and orthopnea. Notify the physician if these symptoms are developing.

Drug interactions

ANTIHYPERTENSIVE AGENTS. All the beta blocking agents have hypotensive properties that are additive with antihypertensive agents (guanethidine, methyldopa, hydralazine, clonidine, prazosin, minoxidil, captopril, and reserpine).

If it is decided to discontinue therapy in patients receiving beta blockers and clonidine concurrently, the beta blocker should be withdrawn gradually and discontinued several days before the gradual withdrawal of the clonidine.

Table 11-3

Beta-Adrenergic Blocking Agents

GENERIC NAME	BRAND NAME	AVAILABILITY	CLINICAL USE	DOSAGE RANGE
Acebutolol	Sectral ✽ Monitan	Capsules: 200, 400 mg	Hypertension, ventricular arrhythmias, angina	PO: Initial—400 mg daily Maintenance—800-1200 mg daily
Atenolol	Tenormin ✽ Nu-Atenol	Tablets: 25, 50, 100 mg Inj: 0.5 mg/ml in 10 ml amps	Hypertension, angina pectoris, after myocardial infarction	PO: Initial—50 mg daily Maintenance—Up to 200 mg daily
Betaxolol	Kerlone	Tablets: 10, 20 mg	Hypertension	PO: Initial—10 mg daily Maintenance—20 mg daily
Bisoprolol	Zebeta	Tablets: 5, 10 mg	Hypertension	PO: Initial—5 mg daily Maintenance—10-20 mg daily
Carteolol	Cartrol	Tablets: 2.5, 5 mg	Hypertension	PO: Initial—2, 5 mg daily Maintenance—2.5-10 mg daily
Carvedilol	Coreg	Tablets: 6.25, 12.5, 25 mg	Hypertension	PO: Initial—6.25 mg twice daily Maintenance—Up to 50 mg daily
Esmolol	Brevibloc	Inj: 10, 250 mg/ml in 10 ml amps	Supraventricular tachycardia, Hypertension	IV: Initial—500 μg/kg/min for 1 min, followed by 50 μg/kg/min for 4 min; then adjust to patient's needs
Labetalol	Normodyne, Trandate	Tablets: 100, 200, 300 mg Inj: 5 mg/ml in 20, 40, 60 ml vials	Hypertension	PO: Initial—100 mg two times daily Maintenance—up to 2400 mg daily
Metoprolol	Lopressor, Toprol XL ✽ Betaloc	Tablets: 50, 100 mg Inj: 1 mg/ml in 5 ml amps	Hypertension, myocardial infarction, arrhythmias, angina pectoris	PO: Initial—100 mg daily Maintenance—100-450 mg daily
Nadolol	Corgard ✽ Apo-Nadol	Tablets: 20, 40, 80, 120, 160 mg	Angina pectoris, hypertension, prophylaxis of migraine headaches	PO: Initial—40 mg once daily Maintenance—80-320 mg daily Maximum—640 mg/day
Penbutolol	Levatol	Tablets: 20 mg	Hypertension	PO: Initial—20 mg daily Maintenance—20 mg daily
Pindolol	Visken ✽ Apo-Pindol	Tablets: 5, 10 mg	Hypertension	PO: Initial—5 mg twice daily Maximum—60 mg/day
Propranolol	Inderal Inderal LA ✽ Detensol	Tablets: 10, 20, 40, 60, 80, 90 mg Solution 4, 8, 80 mg/ml Sustained release capsules: 60, 80, 120, 160 mg IV: 1 mg/ml in 1 ml ampules	Arrhythmias, hypertension, angina pectoris, myocardial infarction, migraine, tremor	PO: Initial—40 mg 2 times daily Maintenance—120-640 mg daily IV: 1-3 mg under close ECG monitoring
Sotalol	Betapace ✽ Sotacar	Tablets: 2.5, 5 mg	Hypertension	PO: Initial—2.5 mg once daily Maintenance—Up to 10 mg daily
Timolol	Blocadren	Tablets: 5, 10, 20 mg	Hypertension, myocardial infarction, migraine, angina pectoris	PO: Initial—10 mg twice daily Maintenance—Up to 30 mg twice daily

✽ Available in Canada only.

BETA-ADRENERGIC AGENTS. Depending on the dosages used, the beta stimulants (isoproterenol, metaproterenol, terbutaline, albuterol, and ritodrine) may inhibit the action of the beta blocking agents, and vice versa.

LIDOCAINE, PROCAINAMIDE, PHENYTOIN, DISOPYRAMIDE, DIGITALIS GLYCOSIDES. Although these drugs are occasionally used concurrently, monitor patients carefully for additional arrhythmias, bradycardia, and signs of congestive heart failure.

ENZYME-INDUCING AGENTS. Enzyme-inducing agents such as cimetidine, phenobarbital, nembutal, and phenytoin enhance the metabolism of propranolol, metoprolol, pindolol, and timolol. This reaction probably does not occur with nadolol or atenolol because they are not metabolized but excreted unchanged. The dosage of the beta blocker may have to be increased to provide therapeutic activity. If the enzyme-inducing agent is discontinued, the dosage of the beta blocking agent will also require reduction.

INDOMETHACIN AND SALICYLATES. Indomethacin and possibly other prostaglandin inhibitors inhibit the antihypertensive activity of propranolol and pindolol. This results in loss of hypertensive control.

The dosage of the beta blocker may have to be increased to compensate for the antihypertensive inhibitory effect of indomethacin and perhaps other prostaglandin inhibitors.

Drug Class: Cholinergic Agents

Actions

Cholinergic agents, also known as parasympathomimetic agents, produce effects that are similar to those of acetylcholine. Some cholinergic agents act by directly stimulating the parasympathetic nervous system, whereas other agents act by inhibiting *acetylcholinesterase,* the enzyme that metabolizes acetylcholine once it is released by the nerve ending. These latter agents are known as *indirect-acting cholinergic agents.* Some of the cholinergic actions observed are slowing of the heart; increased gastrointestinal motility and secretions; increased contractions of the urinary bladder, with relaxation of muscle sphincter; increased secretions and contractility of bronchial smooth muscle; sweating; miosis of the eye, which reduces intraocular pressure; increased force of contraction of skeletal muscle; and sometimes a decrease in blood pressure.

Uses

See Table 11-4.

Nursing Process

See also nursing process for patients with disorders of the eyes (see Chapter 40), for patients with glaucoma (see Chapter 40), for patients with urinary system disease (see Chapter 39), and for patients with respiratory tract disease (see Chapters 27 and 28).

Premedication Assessment

1. Take baseline vital signs of heart rate and blood pressure.
2. See also premedication assessment for patients with disorders of the eyes (see Chapter 40), for patients with glaucoma (see Chapter 40), for patients with urinary system disease (see Chapter 39), and for patients with respiratory tract disease (see Chapters 27 and 28).

Planning

Availability. See Table 11-4.

Evaluation

Because cholinergic fibers innervate the entire body, effects in most systems of the body can be expected. Fortunately, because all receptors do not respond to the same dosage, all adverse effects are not seen at all times. The higher the dosages used, however, the greater the likelihood for more adverse effects.

Side effects to expect

NAUSEA, VOMITING, DIARRHEA, ABDOMINAL CRAMPING. These symptoms are extensions of the pharmacologic effects of the medication and are dose related. Reduction in dosage may be effective in controlling adverse effects without eliminating the desired pharmacologic effect.

DIZZINESS, HYPOTENSION. Monitor blood pressure and pulse. To minimize hypotensive episodes instruct the patient to rise slowly from a supine or sitting position and perform exercises to prevent blood pooling while standing or sitting

Table 11-4

Cholinergic Agents

GENERIC NAME	BRAND NAME	AVAILABILITY	CLINICAL USE
Ambenonium	Mytelase	Tablets: 10 mg	Treatment of myasthenia gravis
Bethanechol	Urecholine		See Chapter 39
Edrophonium	Tensilon, Enlon	Inj: 10 mg/ml in 1, 10, 15 ml vials	Diagnosis of myasthenia gravis Reverse nondepolarizing muscle relaxants such as tubocurarine
Guanidine	Guanidine	Tablets: 125 mg	Treatment of myasthenia gravis
Neostigmine	Prostigmin	Tablets: 15 mg Inj: 0.25, 0.5, 1 mg/ml	Treatment of myasthenia gravis Reverse nondepolarizing muscle relaxants such as tubocurarine
Physostigmine	Antilirium	Inj: 1 mg/ml in 2 ml amp	Reverse toxicity of overdoses of anticholinergic agents (such as pesticides, insecticides)
Pilocarpine	IsoptoCarpine, Pilocar, Adsorbocarpine		See Chapter 40
Pyridostigmine	Mestinon, Regonol	Tablets: 60 mg Syrup: 60 mg/5 ml Sustained release tablets: 180 mg Inj: 5 mg/ml in 2, 5 ml ampules	Treatment of myasthenia gravis Reverse nondepolarizing muscle relaxants such as tubocurarine Reverse toxicity of overdoses of anticholinergic agents (such as pesticides, insecticides)

in one position for prolonged periods. Teach the patient to sit or lie down if feeling faint.

Side effects to report
BRONCHOSPASM, WHEEZING, BRADYCARDIA. Withhold the next dose until the patient is evaluated by a physician.

Drug interactions
ATROPINE, ANTIHISTAMINES. Atropine, other anticholinergic agents, and most antihistamines antagonize the effects of the cholinergic agents.

Drug Class: Anticholinergic Agents

Actions

Anticholinergic agents, also known as cholinergic blocking agents or parasympatholytic agents, block the action of acetylcholine in the parasympathetic nervous system. These drugs act by occupying receptor sites at parasympathetic nerve endings, which prevents the action of acetylcholine. The parasympathetic response is reduced depending on the amount of anticholinergic drug blocking the receptors. Inhibition of cholinergic activity (anticholinergic effects) includes mydriasis of the pupil with increased intraocular pressure in patients with glaucoma; dry, tenacious secretions of the mouth, nose, throat, and bronchi; decreased secretions and motility of the gastrointestinal tract; increased heart rate; and decreased sweating.

Uses

The anticholinergic agents are used clinically in the treatment of gastrointestinal and ophthalmic disorders, bradycardia, Parkinson's disease, and genitourinary disorders; as a preoperative drying agent; and to prevent vagal stimulation from skeletal muscle relaxants or placement of an endotracheal tube (Table 11-5).

Nursing Process

See also nursing process for patients with Parkinson's disease (see Chapter 13), for patients with disorders of the eyes (see Chapter 40), and for antihistamines (see Chapter 28).

Premedication Assessment
1. All patients should be screened for the presence of closed-angle glaucoma. Anticholinergic agents may precipitate an acute attack of angle-closure glaucoma. Patients with open-angle glaucoma can safely use anticholinergic agents in conjunction with miotic therapy.
2. Take baseline vital signs of heart rate and blood pressure.
3. See also premedication assessment for patients with Parkinson's disease (see Chapter 13), for patients with disorders of the eyes (see Chapter 40), and for antihistamines (see Chapter 28).

Planning
Availability. See Table 11-5.

Evaluation
Because cholinergic fibers innervate the entire body, we can expect to see effects from blocking this system throughout most systems in the body. Fortunately, because all receptors do not respond to the same dosage, all adverse effects are not seen to the same degree with all cholinergic blocking agents. The higher the dosages, however, the greater the likelihood for more adverse effects.

Table 11-5
Anticholinergic Agents

GENERIC NAME	BRAND NAME	AVAILABILITY	CLINICAL USE
Atropine	Atropine Sulfate	Inj: 0.1, 0.3, 0.4, 0.5, 0.8, 1.0 mg/ml Tablets: 0.4, 0.6 mg	Presurgery—reduce salivation and bronchial secretions; minimize bradycardia during intubation Treatment of pylorospasm and spastic conditions of the GI tract Treatment of urethral and biliary colic
Belladonna	Belladonna Tincture	Tincture: 30 mg/100 ml	Indigestion, peptic ulcer Nocturnal enuresis Parkinsonism
Clidinium bromide	Quarzan	Capsules: 2.5, 5 mg	Peptic ulcer diseases
Dicyclomine	Bentyl, Antispas, Dibent, ✱Bentylol	Tablets: 20 mg Capsules: 10, 20 mg Syrup: 10 mg/5 ml Inj: 10 mg/ml	Irritable bowel syndrome Infant colic
Glycopyrrolate	Robinul	Tablets: 1, 2 mg Inj: 0.2 mg/ml	Peptic ulcer disease Presurgery—reduce salivation and bronchial secretions; minimize bradycardia during intubation
Mepenzolate	Cantil	Tablets: 25 mg	Peptic ulcer disease
Propantheline	Pro-Banthine	Tablets: 7.5, 15 mg	Peptic ulcer disease

✱ Available in Canada only.

Side effects to expect

BLURRED VISION, CONSTIPATION, URINARY RETENTION, DRYNESS OF THE MUCOSA OF THE MOUTH, NOSE, AND THROAT. These symptoms are the anticholinergic effects produced by these agents. Patients taking these medications should be monitored for the development of these side effects.

Dryness of the mucosa may be alleviated by sucking hard candy or ice chips or by chewing gum.

If patients develop urinary hesitancy, assess for distention of the bladder. Report to the physician for further evaluation.

Give stool softeners as prescribed. Encourage adequate fluid intake and foods that provide sufficient bulk.

Caution the patient that blurred vision may occur, and make appropriate suggestions for personal safety of the individual.

Side effects to report

CONFUSION, DEPRESSION, NIGHTMARES, HALLUCINATIONS. Perform a baseline assessment of the patient's degree of alertness and orientation to name, place, and time before initiating therapy. Make regularly scheduled subsequent evaluations of mental status and compare findings. Report development of alterations.

Provide for patient safety during these episodes.

Reduction in the daily dosage may control these adverse effects.

ORTHOSTATIC HYPOTENSION. Although this occurs infrequently and is generally mild, all anticholinergic agents may cause some degree of orthostatic hypotension manifested by dizziness and weakness, particularly when therapy is being initiated.

Monitor the blood pressure daily in both the supine and standing positions.

Anticipate the development of postural hypotension, and take measures to prevent an occurrence. Teach the patient to rise slowly from a supine or sitting position, and encourage the patient to sit or lie down if feeling faint.

PALPITATIONS, ARRHYTHMIAS. Report for further evaluation.

GLAUCOMA. All patients should be screened for the presence of angle-closure glaucoma *before* initiating therapy.

Patients with open-angle glaucoma can safely use anticholinergic agents. Monitoring of intraocular pressures should be performed on a regular basis.

Drug interactions

AMANTADINE, TRICYCLIC ANTIDEPRESSANTS, PHENOTHIAZINES. These agents may potentiate anticholinergic side effects. Development of confusion and hallucinations are characteristic of excessive anticholinergic activity.

CHAPTER REVIEW

The nervous system is one of two primary regulators of body homeostasis and defense. The central nervous system is composed of the brain and spinal cord. The efferent nervous system is subdivided into the motor nervous system, which controls skeletal muscle, and the autonomic nervous system, which regulates smooth muscle and heart muscle and controls secretions from certain glands. Nerve impulses are passed between neurons and from neurons to end organs by neurotransmitters. Control of neurotransmitters is a primary way to alleviate symptoms associated with many diseases.

MATH REVIEW

1. Order: Benadryl 40 mg PO tid. Benadryl 12.5 mg/5 ml is available. Give _____.

2. Order: Propranolol 60 mg PO tid. Propranolol 40 mg tablets is available. Give _____.

3. Order: Dilantin suspension 150 mg q8h. Dilantin suspension 125 mg/5 ml is available. Give _____.

CRITICAL THINKING QUESTIONS

1. Based on a review of this chapter related to the actions, uses, and side effects of the primary drug classifications (adrenergic, adrenergic blocking agents, cholinergic, anticholinergic agents), develop a list of premedication assessments that should be made before use of these drugs.

2. Summarize the actions of the cholinergic and anticholinergic agents. Arrange the summaries in columns to compare cholinergic and anticholinergic actions.

3. Examine the drug actions listed for adrenergic blocking agents. Explain the mechanisms by which these drugs are beneficial for the treatment of angina pectoris, cardiac arrhythmias, and hypertension.

4. Explain the effect of vasoconstriction and vasodilation of blood vessels on blood pressure.

5. What type of autonomic system drugs should not be used in persons with pulmonary disorders?

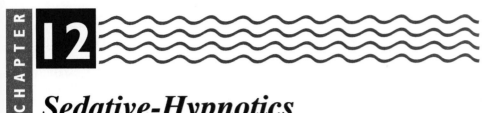

Sedative-Hypnotics

Objectives

1. Differentiate between the terms *sedative* and *hypnotic*; *initial, intermittent,* and *terminal insomnia*; and *rebound sleep* and *paradoxic excitement.*

2. Identify alterations found in the sleep pattern when hypnotics are discontinued.

3. Cite nursing interventions that can be implemented as an alternative to administering a sedative-hypnotic.

4. Compare the effects of barbiturates and benzodiazepines on the central nervous system.

5. Explain the major benefits of administering benzodiazepines rather than barbiturates.

6. Identify laboratory tests that should be monitored when benzodiazepines or barbiturates are administered over an extended period of time.

7. Develop a plan for patient education for a patient receiving a hypnotic.

Key Words

paradoxic sleep   hypnotic
REM sleep   sedative
insomnia   rebound sleep

SLEEP AND SLEEP PATTERN DISTURBANCE

Sleep is a state of unconsciousness from which a person can be aroused by appropriate stimulus. It is a naturally occurring phenomenon that occupies about one third of an adult's life. It is a different state of unconsciousness from that produced by deep anesthesia or coma.

Adequate sleep that progresses through the normal stages of sleep is important for maintainance of body function. Natural sleep is a rhythmic progression through four stages that provide physical and mental rest. Stages I and II are light sleep periods that allow easy arousal. Stage III is a transition from the lighter to the deeper state of sleep, stage IV. Each stage is characterized by a specific set of brain wave activities. Stage IV sleep is called deep sleep and is dreamless, restful, and associated with a 10% to 30% decrease in blood pressure, respiratory rate, and basal metabolic rate.

In a normal night of sleep, a person rhythmically cycles through the four stages of sleep. Approximately every 90 minutes or so, a person develops a sleep pattern called **paradoxic sleep**, or rapid eye movement sleep. It is superimposed on stages I and II of sleep. This type of sleep represents 20% to 25% of sleep time and is characterized by rapid eye movement, dreaming, increased heart rate, irregular breathing, secretion of stomach acids, and some muscular activity. **Rapid eye movement** (REM) **sleep** appears to be an important time for our subconscious minds to release anxiety and tension and reestablish a psychic equilibrium. The elderly take longer to move through the relaxation stages of non-REM sleep. There is an increased frequency and duration of awakenings. It is not necessarily true that the elderly require more sleep. In fact, they often sleep less but more frequently take naps during the day. Consequently, the geriatric patient may have difficulty sleeping through the night.

Insomnia is the most common sleep disorder known. Ninety-five percent of all adults experience insomnia at least once during their lives, and up to 35% of adults have insomnia in a given year. **Insomnia** is defined as the inability to sleep. Insomnia is not a disease but a symptom of physical or mental stress. It is usually mild and lasts for only a few nights. Common causes are changes in lifestyle or environment (such as hospitalization), pain, illness, excess consumption of products containing caffeine, eating large or "rich" meals shortly before bedtime, or anxiety. *Initial* insomnia is the inability to fall asleep when desired, *intermittent* insomnia is the inability to stay asleep, and *terminal* insomnia is characterized by early awakening with the inability to fall asleep again.

Sedative-Hypnotic Therapy

Drugs used in conjunction with altered patterns of sleep are known as sedative-hypnotics. A **hypnotic** is a drug that produces sleep. A **sedative** quiets the patient and gives a feeling of relaxation and rest, not necessarily accompanied by sleep. A good hypnotic should provide the following action within a short period: a restful natural sleep, a duration of action that allows the patient to awaken at the usual time, a natural awakening with no "hangover" effects, and no danger of habit formation. Unfortunately, the ideal hypnotic is not available. For short-term use, the benzodiazepines come the closest to ideal of those medicines available. The most frequently used sedative-hypnotics increase total sleeping time, especially in stages II (light sleep) and IV (deep sleep); however, they also decrease the number of REM periods and the total time in REM sleep. REM sleep is needed to help an individual maintain a mental balance during daytime activities. When REM sleep is decreased, there is a strong physiologic tendency to "make it up." Compensatory, or **rebound**, REM sleep seems to occur even when hypnotics are used for only 3 or 4 days. After chronic administration of sedative-hypnotic agents, REM rebound may be severe, accompanied by restlessness and vivid nightmares. Depending on the frequency of hypnotic administration, normal sleep patterns may not be restored for weeks. It is suspected that the effects of REM rebound may enhance chronic use of and dependence on these agents to avoid the unpleasant consequences of rebound. Because of this a vicious cycle occurs as the normal physiologic need for sleep is not met and the body attempts to compensate for it.

Actions

Sedatives, used to produce relaxation and rest, and hypnotics, used to produce sleep, are not always different drugs. Their effects may depend on the dose and the condition of the patient. A small dose of a drug may act as a sedative, whereas a larger dose of the same drug may act as a hypnotic and produce sleep.

The sedative-hypnotics may be classified into three groups: the barbiturates, the benzodiazepines, and the miscellaneous agents.

Uses

The primary uses for sedative-hypnotics are to improve sleep patterns for the temporary treatment of insomnia and to decrease the level of anxiety and increase relaxation or sleep before diagnostic or operative procedures.

Nursing Process for Sedative-Hypnotic Therapy

Assessment

Central nervous system (CNS) function. Because sedative-hypnotics depress overall CNS function, identify the patient's level of alertness and orientation and ability to perform motor functions.

Vital signs. Obtain current blood pressure, pulse, and respirations before initiation of drug therapy.

Sleep pattern. Assess the patient's usual pattern of sleep and obtain information on the pattern of sleep disruption (such as difficulty in falling asleep, inability to sleep the entire night, or awakening in the early morning hours unable to return to a restful sleep).

Ask the patient about the amount of sleep (hours) considered normal and how insomnia is managed at home. Does the patient have a regular time to go to bed and a regular time to wake up? If the patient is taking medications, determine the drug, dose, and frequency of administration and whether this may be contributing to sleeplessness.

Patients with persistent insomnia should be carefully monitored for the number of naps taken during the day. Investigate the type of activities performed immediately before retiring for sleep.

Anxiety level. Assess the patient's exhibited degree of anxiety. Is it really a sedative-hypnotic the patient needs as a therapeutic intervention or someone to *listen*? Ask what stressors the patient has been experiencing in both personal and work environments.

Environmental control. Obtain data relating to the possible disturbance present in the individual's sleeping environment that could potentially interfere with sleeping (for example, room temperature, lights, noise, traffic, restlessness, or snoring of sleeping partner).

Nutritional needs. Obtain a dietary history to identify sources of caffeinated products that may act as stimulants.

Exercise. Obtain data relating to the patient's usual degree and time of physical activity during the day.

Respiratory status. Persons with respiratory disorders and those who snore heavily may have low respiratory reserve and should not receive hypnotics because of the potential for causing respiratory depression.

Nursing Diagnosis
* Sleep pattern disturbances (indications)
* Injury, risk for (side effects)
* Knowledge deficit related to medication regimen

Planning

Planning for patient care should be based on the assessment data, and interventions should be individualized to meet patient needs.

Central nervous system function. Schedule CNS assessments and monitoring of vital signs at least every 8 hours.

Sleep pattern. • Routine orders: Many physicians order a sedative-hypnotic on an as required (prn) basis. Do not offer it unless the patient is having difficulty sleeping and other measures to meet comfort and psychologic needs have failed to produce the desired effect. • Never leave a medication at the bedside in case it is needed later. • Reassess the underlying cause of sleeplessness. Is it really pain control that is needed? If so, repeating the order for a hypnotic will not meet the patient's needs because these medicines have no analgesic value.

Anxiety level. Be aware of the possibility of a paradoxic response to sedative-hypnotic medicine, particularly in the elderly. If the patient is showing increasing signs of excitement, restlessness, euphoria, or confusion, it would be harmful to repeat the medication.

Environmental control. • Plan for the safety needs of the patient and protect from potential injury. Make sure that the call light is within reach and place the bed in the low position with side rails up. Leave a night light on. • Organize nursing activities so that the patient is disturbed as infrequently as possible while maintaining safe patient care.

LIFE SPAN ISSUES

SEDATIVE-HYPNOTIC THERAPY

The habitual use of sedative-hypnotic agents may result in psychologic and physical dependence, especially in geriatric patients. These medicines should be prescribed only for short-term use. Persons who have been taking sedative-hypnotics for several weeks should be gradually withdrawn from the medicine to prevent anxiety, insomnia, and nightmares.

Barbiturates may produce a paradoxic response in older patients shown by restlessness, excitement, euphoria, and confusion. Provide for the individual's safety and seek changes in the medication order.

Nutritional needs. Offer protein foods and dairy products at a specific time before sleep.

Exercise. Encourage adequate exercise during the day so the individual will be tired before trying to sleep.

Implementation

Vital signs. Obtain vital signs periodically as the situation indicates.

Preoperative medication. Give preoperative medications at the specified time.

Monitoring effects. When a medication is administered, carefully assess the patient at regular intervals for therapeutic and adverse effects.

PRN. If giving prn medications, assess the record for the effectiveness of previously administered therapy. It is sometimes necessary to repeat a medication if an order permits doing so. This is at the nurse's discretion based on the evaluation of a particular patient's needs.

Patient Education and Health Promotion

Bedtime. Encourage a standard time to go to bed to help the body establish a bedtime rhythm and routine.

Nutrition. • Teach appropriate nutrition information concerning the food pyramid, adequate intake of fluids, and use of vitamins. Communicate the information at the educational level of the patient. • Avoid heavy meals late in the evening. • Caffeine consumption should be reduced or discontinued, especially within several hours before bedtime. Introduce the patient to decaffeinated or herbal products that can be substituted for previously used foods containing caffeine. • Help the patient avoid products containing caffeine, such as coffee, tea, soft drinks, and chocolate. Limit the total daily intake of these items and give warm milk and crackers as a bedtime snack. Protein foods and dairy products contain an amino acid that synthesizes serotonin, a neurotransmitter that is found to increase sleep time and decrease the time required to fall asleep. • For insomnia, suggest warm milk about 30 minutes before bedtime.

Personal comfort. Position the patient for maximum comfort, provide a back rub, encourage the patient to empty the bladder, and be certain that bedding is clean and dry. Take time to meet patient's individual needs and calm fears. Foster a trusting relationship.

Environmental control. • Encourage the patient to provide for insomnia relief by attempting to sleep in the proper environment—a quiet, darkened room free from distractions. Avoid using the bedroom for watching television, preparing work for the following day, eating snacks, and paying bills. Provide for adequate ventilation, subdued lighting, correct room temperature, and control of traffic in and out of the patient's room. • Instruct the patient to provide for personal safety by leaving a night-light on and not smoking in bed after taking medication.

Activity and exercise. Suggest the inclusion of exercise in daily activities so that the patient obtains sufficient exercise and is tired enough to sleep. For some individuals, plan a quiet "unwinding" time before retiring for the night. For children, try a bedtime story that is pleasant and soothing, not one that will cause anxiety or fear.

Stress management. • Explore personal and work stressors that may have a bearing on the insomnia. Some stressors that create insomnia may be within the work environment; therefore involvement of the industrial nurse, along with a thorough exploration of work factors, may be appropriate. Stress produced within the dynamics of the family may require professional counseling. • Teach the patient relaxation techniques and personal comfort measures, such as a warm bath, to relieve stress. Playing soft music may also promote relaxation. • Make referrals for mastery of biofeedback, meditation, or other techniques to reduce stress levels. • Encourage the patient to express *feelings* openly with regard to stress and insomnia. The adjustment to this situation involves working through great personal fears, frustrations, hostilities, and resentments. • Explore coping mechanisms the person uses in response to stress and identify methods of channeling these toward positive realistic goals and alternatives to the use of medication.

Fostering health maintenance. • Throughout the course of treatment, discuss medication information and how it will benefit the patient. Stress the importance of the nonpharmacologic interventions and the long-term effects that compliance with the treatment regimen can provide. • Provide the patient or significant others with important information contained in the specific drug monograph for the medicines prescribed. Additional health teaching and nursing interventions for the side effects to expect and report are described in the following drug monographs.

Written record. Enlist the patient's aid in developing and maintaining a written record of monitoring parameters (such as extent of insomnia, frequency; see box on p. 164) and response to prescribed therapies for discussion with the physician. The patient should be encouraged to bring this record on follow-up visits.

Drug Class: Barbiturates

The first barbiturate was placed on the market as a sedative-hypnotic in 1903. It became so successful that chemists identified some 2500 barbiturate compounds, of which more than 50 were distributed commercially. Barbiturates became such a mainstay of therapy that fewer than a dozen other sedative-hypnotic agents were successfully marketed through 1960. The release of the first benzodiazepine (chlordiazepoxide) in 1961 started the decline in the use of barbiturates.

PATIENT EDUCATION & MONITORING FORM Sleeping Pills

MEDICATIONS	COLOR	TO BE TAKEN

Name _____

Physician _____

Physician's phone _____

Next appt.* _____

PARAMETERS		DAY OF DISCHARGE							COMMENTS
Time	Arising								
	Bedtime								
	Last cup of coffee								
Sleep pattern	Took ____ hr. or min. to get to sleep								
	Awaken during night; takes ____ hr. or min. to get back to sleep								
	Slept all night								
	Couldn't sleep								
	Went right to sleep								
Dreams	Dreamed all night								
	No. of dreams								
	Did not dream								
Feelings the next morning?	Very tired when I woke up								
	Awoke refreshed								
Exercise	No desire to exercise								
	Usual routine including work								
	Unable to work								
Stress level No time to relax Time to relax ┠0 ─── 5 ─── ┨									
Medication	Took ____ sleeping pills								

*Please bring this record with you to your next appointment.
Use the back of this sheet for additional information.

Table 12-1

Barbiturates

GENERIC NAME	BRAND NAME	AVAILABILITY	ADULT ORAL DOSE	COMMENTS
Amobarbital	Amytal	Inj: 500 mg vials	Sedation: 30-50 mg IM 2-3 times daily Hypnosis: 100-200 mg IM 30 min before bedtime	Intermediate acting; Schedule II Used primarily as a sedative before anesthesia or during labor
Butabarbital	Butisol, Busodium	Tablets: 15, 30, 100 mg Elixir: 30, 33.3 mg/5 ml	Sedation: 15-30 mg 3-4 times daily Hypnosis: 50-100 mg at bedtime	Elixir contains 7.5% alcohol; Intermediate acting; Schedule III Used primarily as a daytime sedative and bedtime hypnotic
Mephobarbital	Mebaral	Tablets: 32, 50, 100 mg	Sedation: 32-100 mg 3-4 times daily Anticonvulsant: 400-600 mg daily	Long acting; Schedule IV Used primarily as an anticonvulsant; may also be used as a daytime sedative
Pentobarbital	Nembutal	Capsules: 100 mg Elixir: 18.2 mg/5 ml Supp: 30, 60, 100, 200 mg Inj: 50 mg/ml	Sedation: 30 mg 3-4 times daily Hypnosis: 100 mg at bedtime	Short acting; Schedule II Used primarily as a daytime sedative and bedtime hypnotic; may also be used as a preanesthetic sedative Elixir contains 18% alcohol Also available for IM and IV use
Phenobarbital	Luminal, Solfoton, ✳ Barbilixir	Tablets: 15, 16, 30, 100 mg Capsules: 16 mg Elixir: 15, 20 mg/5 ml	Sedation: 8-30 mg 2-3 times daily Hypnosis: 100-320 mg Anticonvulsant: 50-100 mg 2-3 times daily	Long-acting; Schedule IV Used most commonly now as an anticonvulsant; may also be used as a daytime sedative, preanesthetic, or hypnotic agent Also available for IM and IV use Elixir contains 13.5% alcohol
Secobarbital	Seconal	Capsules: 100 mg Inj: 50 mg/ml in 2 ml Tubex	Hypnosis: 100-200 mg at bedtime	Short acting; Schedule II Used primarily as a daytime sedative or bedtime hypnotic Therapy is not recommended for longer than 14 days Also available for IM and IV use

✳ Available in Canada only.

However, several barbiturate compounds are still prescribed today (Table 12-1).

Actions

Barbiturates can reversibly depress the activity of all excitable tissues. The CNS is particularly sensitive, but the degrees of depression (ranging from mild sedation to deep coma and death) depend on the dosage, route of administration, tolerance from previous use, degree of excitability of the CNS at the time of administration, and condition of the patient.

Uses

Barbiturates are used primarily for their sedative and hypnotic effects. The long-acting barbiturate phenobarbital is also used as an anticonvulsant. The ultrashort-acting agents (methohexital, thiopental) may be administered intravenously as general anesthetics.

Nursing Process

Premedication Assessment

1. Seek information regarding prior use of sedative-hypnotic medications.
2. Obtain information relating to baseline neurologic function (for example, degree of alertness)

Planning

Availability. See Table 12-1.

Implementation

Dosage and administration. See Table 12-1. Rapidly discontinuing barbiturates after long-term use of high dosages may result in symptoms similar to those of alcohol withdrawal. These may vary from weakness and anxiety to delirium and grand mal seizures. Treatment consists of cautious and gradual withdrawal over a 2- to 4-week period.

Evaluation
General adverse effects of barbiturates include drowsiness, lethargy, headache, muscle or joint pain, and mental depression.

Side effects to expect
HANGOVER, SEDATION, LETHARGY. Patients may complain of morning hangover, blurred vision, and transient hypotension on arising. Hangover frequently occurs after administration of hypnotic doses of long-acting barbiturates. Patients may display a dulled affect, subtle distortion of mood, and impaired coordination. Explain to the patient the need for arising first to a sitting position, equilibrating, and then standing. Assistance with ambulation may be required.

If hangover becomes troublesome, there should be a reduction in the dosage, a change in the medication, or both.

People working around machinery, driving a car, pouring and giving medicines, or performing other duties in which they must remain mentally alert should not take these medications while working.

Side effects to report
EXCESSIVE USE OR ABUSE. Habitual use of barbiturates may result in physical dependence. Discuss the case with the physician and make plans to cooperatively approach gradual withdrawal of the medications being abused. Assist the patient to recognize the abuse problem. Identify underlying needs and plan for more appropriate management of those needs. Provide for emotional support of the individual; display an accepting attitude—be kind but firm.

PARADOXIC RESPONSE. Elderly patients and those in severe pain may respond paradoxically to barbiturates with excitement, euphoria, restlessness, and confusion. Provide supportive physical care and safety during these responses. Assess the level of excitement and deal calmly with the individual. During periods of excitement, protect the patient from harm and provide for physical channeling of energy (for example, walking). Seek change in the medication order.

HYPERSENSITIVITY. Reactions to barbiturates are infrequent but may be serious. Report symptoms of hives, pruritus, rash, high fever, or inflammation of mucous membranes for evaluation by the physician. Withhold further barbiturate administration until physician's approval has been granted.

BLOOD DYSCRASIAS. Blood dyscrasias are rare. However, routine laboratory studies (red blood cell count, white blood cell count, and differential counts) should be scheduled when symptoms indicate the need. Stress to the patient the importance of returning for this laboratory work. Monitor for the development of sore throat, fever, purpura, jaundice, or excessive and progressive weakness.

Drug interactions
DRUGS THAT INCREASE TOXIC EFFECTS. Antihistamines, alcohol, analgesics, anesthetics, tranquilizers, valproic acid, chloramphenicol, monoamine oxidase inhibitors, and other sedative-hypnotics: Monitor the patient for excessive sedation and reduce the dosage of the barbiturate if necessary.

PHENYTOIN. The effects of barbiturates on phenytoin are variable. Serum levels may be ordered, and a change in phenytoin dosage may be required. Observe patients for increased seizure activity and for signs of phenytoin toxicity, such as nystagmus, sedation, and lethargy.

BARBITURATES DECREASE THE EFFECTS OF. Warfarin: Monitor the prothrombin time and increase the dosage of warfarin if necessary.

Digitoxin: Monitor the digitoxin serum levels for signs of increased heart failure: dyspnea, orthopnea, edema. The dosage of digitoxin may have to be increased.

Estrogens: This drug interaction may be critical in patients receiving oral contraceptives containing estrogen. If patients develop spotting and breakthrough bleeding, a change in oral contraceptives and the use of alternative forms of contraception should be considered.

Corticosteroids, propranolol, doxycycline, antidepressants, quinidine, and chlorpromazine: The patient should be monitored for signs of increased activity of the illness for which the medication was prescribed. Dosage increases may be necessary or the barbiturate may have to be discontinued.

Drug Class: Benzodiazepines

Benzodiazepines have been extremely successful products from a therapeutic and safety standpoint. A major advantage over the barbiturate and nonbarbiturate sedative-hypnotics is the wide safety margin between therapeutic and lethal dosages. Intentional and unintentional overdoses of several hundred times the normal therapeutic doses are well tolerated and are not fatal.

More than 2000 benzodiazepine derivatives have been identified, and more than 100 have been tested for sedative-hypnotic or other activity. Although there are many similarities among the benzodiazepines, they are difficult to characterize as a class because certain benzodiazepines are effective anticonvulsants, others serve as antianxiety agents, and still others are used as sedative-hypnotics.

Actions
It is thought that the benzodiazepines have mechanisms of action similar to those of CNS depressants but that individual drugs within the benzodiazepine family act more selectively at specific sites, allowing for a variety of uses (for example, sedative-hypnotic, muscle relaxant, antianxiety, and anticonvulsant).

Uses
Benzodiazepines are the most commonly used sedative-hypnotics. When benzodiazepine therapy is started, patients feel a sense of deep or refreshing sleep. However, benzodiazepine-induced sleep varies from normal sleep in that there is less REM sleep. With long-term administration, the amount of REM sleep gradually increases as tolerance develops to the REM-suppressant effects. When benzodiazepines are discontinued, a rebound increase in REM sleep may occur despite the tolerance. During the rebound period, the number of dreams stays about the same, but many of the dreams are reported to be bizarre in nature. After long-term use of most benzodiazepines, there is also a rebound in insomnia. Consequently it is important to use these agents only for short courses of therapy.

The short-acting benzodiazepines (for example, midazolam) are used intramuscularly as a preoperative sedative and intravenously for conscious sedation before brief diagnostic procedures or for induction of general anesthesia. It has a more rapid onset of action then diazepam and a much shorter duration. It also produces a greater degree of amnesia than diazepam, which makes it beneficial for short diagnostic and operative procedures.

Therapeutic Outcomes

The primary therapeutic outcomes sought from benzodiazepine therapy are as follows:
- To produce mild sedation
- For short-term use to produce sleep
- Preoperative sedation with amnesia

Nursing Process

Premedication Assessment
1. Record baseline vital signs, particularly blood pressure, in sitting and lying positions.
2. Check for history of blood dyscrasias or hepatic disease.

Planning
Availability. See Table 12-2.
Pregnancy and lactation. • It is generally recommended that benzodiazepines not be administered during at least the first trimester of pregnancy. There may be an increased incidence of birth defects because these agents readily cross the placenta and enter fetal circulation. • Mothers who are breast-feeding should not receive benzodiazepines regularly. Benzodiazepines readily cross into breast milk and exert a pharmacologic effect on the infant.

Implementation
Dosage and administration. See Table 12-2. The habitual use of benzodiazepines may result in physical and psychologic dependence. Rapid discontinuance of benzodiazepines after long-term use may result in symptoms similar to those of alcohol withdrawal. These may vary from weakness and anxiety to delirium and grand mal seizures. The symptoms may not appear for several days after discontinuation. Treatment consists of gradual withdrawal of benzodiazepines over a 2- to 4-week period.

Evaluation
Side effects to expect
DROWSINESS, HANGOVER, SEDATION, LETHARGY. Patients may complain of morning hangover, blurred vision, and transient hypotension on arising. Explain to the patient the need for arising first to a sitting position, equilibrating, and then standing. Assistance with ambulation may be required.

If hangover becomes troublesome there should be a reduction in the dosage, a change in the medication, or both.

Persons who are working with machinery, driving a car, pouring and giving medicines, or performing other duties in which they must remain mentally alert should not take these medications while working.

Side effects to report
EXCESSIVE USE OR ABUSE. Habitual use of benzodiazepines may result in physical dependence. Discuss the case with the physician and make plans to cooperatively approach gradual withdrawal of the medications being abused. Assist the patient in recognition of the abuse problem. Identify underlying needs and plan for more appropriate management of those needs. Provide for

emotional support of the individual; display an accepting attitude—be kind but firm.

BLOOD DYSCRASIAS. Routine laboratory studies (red blood cell count, white blood cell count, and differential counts) should be scheduled. Stress to the patient the need to return for these tests. Monitor for the development of sore throat, fever, purpura, jaundice, or excessive and progressive weakness.

HEPATOTOXICITY. The symptoms of hepatotoxicity are anorexia, nausea, vomiting, jaundice, hepatomegaly, splenomegaly, and abnormal liver function tests (elevated bilirubin, aspartate transaminase [AST], alanine aminotransferase [ALT], gamma glutamyltransferase [GGT], alkaline phosphatase, prothrombin time).

Drug interactions
DRUGS THAT INCREASE TOXIC EFFECTS. Antihistamines, alcohol, analgesics, anesthetics, tranquilizers, narcotics, cimetidine, and other sedative-hypnotics.

SMOKING. Smoking enhances the metabolism of the benzodiazepines. Larger doses may be necessary to maintain sedative effects in patients who smoke.

Drug Class: Miscellaneous Sedative-Hypnotic Agents

The nonbarbiturate, nonbenzodiazepine sedative-hypnotics are listed in Table 12-3. They represent a variety of chemical classes, all of which cause CNS depression.

Actions
All have somewhat variable effects on REM sleep, development of tolerance, and rebound REM sleep and insomnia. Because of the safety factor, the use of these agents is diminishing in favor of the benzodiazepines.

Uses
These agents are used as sedative-hypnotics to produce sleep. Chloral hydrate is also used as a sedative for diagnostic procedures.

Therapeutic Outcomes
The primary therapeutic outcomes sought from miscellaneous sedative-hypnotic agents are as follows:
- To produce mild sedation
- For short-term use to produce sleep

Nursing Process

Premedication Assessment
1. Record baseline vital signs, particularly blood pressure, in sitting and lying positions.
2. Check for history of blood dyscrasias or hepatic disease.

Planning
Availability. See Table 12-3.
Implementation
Dosage and administration. See Table 12-3. The habitual use of these sedative-hypnotic agents may result in physical dependence. Rapid discontinuance after long-term use may result in symptoms similar to those of alcohol withdrawal. These may vary from weakness and anxiety to delirium and

Table 12-2

Benzodiazepines Used for Sedation-Hypnosis

GENERIC NAME	BRAND NAME	AVAILABILITY	ADULT ORAL DOSE	COMMENTS
Estrazolam	ProSom	Tablets: 1, 2 mg	Hypnosis: 1-2 mg at bedtime	Intermediate acting; Schedule IV Used for insomnia Tapering therapy recommended to reduce rebound insomnia Minimal morning hangover
Flurazepam	Dalmane, ✤ Novoflupam	Capsules: 15, 30 mg	Hypnosis: 15-30 mg at bedtime	Long acting; Schedule IV Used for short-term treatment of insomnia, up to 4 wk Morning hangover may be significant Rebound insomnia and REM sleep occur less frequently
Lorazepam	Ativan, ✤ Novolorazepam	Tablets: 0.5, 1, 2 mg Inj: 2 mg and 4 mg/ml in 1, 10 ml vials, 4 mg prefilled syringes	Hypnosis: 2-4 mg at bedtime	Used primarily for insomnia but may also be used for preoperative anxiety IM, IV administration also available
Midazolam	Versed	Inj: 1, 5 mg/ml in 1, 2, 5, 10 ml vials; 2 ml prefilled syringes	Preop: IM—0.07-0.08 mg/kg 1 hr before surgery Induction of anesthesia: IV—0.2-0.3 mg/kg Endoscopy: IV—0.1-0.15 mg/kg	Short acting; Schedule IV Onset: IM—15 minutes IV—3-5 min Duration: IM—30-60 min IV—2-6 hr Causes amnesia in most patients Lower doses in patients over age 55
Quazepam	Doral	Tablets: 7.5, 15 mg	Hypnosis: 7.5-15 mg at bedtime	Long acting; Schedule IV Used for insomnia Tapering therapy recommended to reduce rebound insomnia Morning hangover may be significant
Temazepam	Restoril	Capsules: 15, 30 mg	Hypnosis: 15-30 mg at bedtime	Intermediate acting; Schedule IV Used for insomnia Minimal if any morning hangover Rebound insomnia may occur
Triazolam	Halcion ✤ Novo-Triolam	Tablets: 0.125, 0.25 mg	Hypnosis: 0.25-0.5 mg at bedtime	Short acting; Schedule IV Used for insomnia but tends to lose effectiveness within 2 wk Tapering therapy is recommended to reduce rebound insomnia Rapid onset of action No morning hangover

✤ Available in Canada only.

grand mal seizures. Treatment consists of gradual withdrawal over a 2- to 4-week period.

PARALDEHYDE. Dilute oral form in milk or iced fruit juice to mask the taste and odor. Dispense only in glass container; do not use a plastic spoon or container.

Evaluation

General adverse effects include drowsiness, lethargy, headache, muscle or joint pain, and mental depression. Morning hangover frequently occurs after administration of hypnotic doses. Patients may display dulled effect, subtle distortion of mood, and impaired coordination. Some patients experience transient restlessness and anxiety before falling asleep.

Side effects to expect

HANGOVER, SEDATION, LETHARGY. Patients may complain of morning hangover, blurred vision, and transient hypotension on arising. Explain to the patient the need for arising first to a sitting position, equilibrating, and then standing. Assistance with ambulation may be required. If hangover becomes troublesome, there should be a reduction in the dosage, a change in medication, or both.

Table 12-3
Miscellaneous Sedative-Hypnotic Agents

GENERIC NAME	BRAND NAME	AVAILABILITY	ADULT ORAL DOSE	COMMENTS
Chloral hydrate	Noctec, Aquachloral, ✶ Novochlorhydrate	Capsules: 250, 500 mg Syrup: 250, 500 mg/5 ml Suppositories: 325, 500, 650 mg	Sedation: 250 mg 3 times daily after meals Hypnosis: 500 mg to 1 g 15-30 min before bedtime	The original "Mickey Finn"; Schedule IV Used primarily as a bedtime hypnotic, but also is used as a preoperative sedative because it does not depress respirations or cough reflex May cause nausea; administer with full glass of water; do not chew capsules See Drug Interactions
Ethchlorvynol	Placidyl	Capsules: 200, 500, 750 mg	Hypnosis: —Usual dose 500 mg at bedtime —100-200 mg may be administered if patient wakes up after 500-750 mg	Short acting: Schedule IV Used for short-term insomnia Therapy is not recommended beyond 1 wk
Glutethimide	N/A	Tablets: 500 mg	Hypnosis: 250-500 mg at bedtime	Short acting; Schedule II Used for short-term insomnia; not recommended for use beyond 3-7 days See Drug Interactions
Paraldehyde	Paral	Liquid: 30 ml (for oral or rectal use)	Sedation: 4-8 ml	Bitter tasting, unpleasant odor; administer in milk or iced fruit juice to mask taste and odor Dispense only in a glass container; do not use a plastic spoon or container Used predominantly as a sedative in treating delirium tremens This agent imparts a strong, foul odor to the breath for up to 24 hr after administration; the patient is often unaware of the foul smell Schedule IV
Zolpidem	Ambien	Tablets: 5, 10 mg	Hypnosis: 10 mg at bedtime	Elderly patients should start with 5 mg Short acting; Schedule IV

✶ Available in Canada only.

Persons who are working with machinery, driving a car, pouring and giving medicines, or performing other duties in which they must remain mentally alert should not take these medications while working.

RESTLESSNESS, ANXIETY. These side effects are usually mild and do not warrant discontinuation of the medication. Encourage the patient to try to relax and let the sedative effect take over.

Elderly patients and those in severe pain may respond paradoxically with excitement, euphoria, restlessness, and confusion.

Safety measures such as maintenance of bed rest, side rails, and observation should be used during this period.

Drug interactions
CENTRAL NERVOUS SYSTEM DEPRESSANTS. CNS depressants, including sleeping aids, analgesics, anesthetics, narcotics, tranquilizers, and alcohol, increase the sedative effects of the sedative-hypnotics.

WARFARIN. Glutethimide and ethchlorvynol may diminish the anticoagulant effects of warfarin. Monitor the prothrombin time and increase the dosage of warfarin if necessary.

Chloral hydrate may enhance the anticoagulant effects of warfarin. Observe for the development of petechiae, ecchymoses, nosebleeds, bleeding gums, dark tarry stools, and bright red or "coffee-ground" emesis. Monitor the prothrombin time and reduce the dosage of warfarin if necessary.

DISULFIRAM. Disulfiram may prolong the activity of paraldehyde. Monitor the patient for excessive sedation.

CLINITEST. Chloral hydrate may produce false-positive Clinitest results. Use Clinistix or Tes-tape to measure urine glucose.

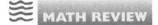

CHAPTER REVIEW

There are many types of sleep disorders, but by far the most common is insomnia. Most cases of insomnia are short lived and can be most effectively treated by nonpharmacologic methods such as a back rub, eating a lighter meal in the evening, elimination of naps, and reduction of stimulants such as caffeine. A variety of sedative-hypnotics are available for pharmacologic treatment; the drugs of choice are the benzodiazepines because of their wide margin of safety.

MATH REVIEW

1. Dr. Smith wrote orders to start Mrs. Haggerty on Triazolam 0.5 mg at bedtime for 4 days only. Triazolam is available in 0.125 and 0.25 mg tablets. What will you administer to Mrs. Haggerty?

2. Dr. Jones wrote orders for Mr. Smith to receive 400 mg of chloral hydrate 1 hour before a computed tomography scan. Chloral hydrate is available in 250 and 500 mg capsules and 250 and 500 mg/5 ml syrup. What will you administer to Mr. Smith?

3. Mr. Haig is scheduled for an endoscopy at 9 AM tomorrow morning. He weighs 60 kg. A dose of midazolam 7.5 mg IV is scheduled to be administered a few minutes before the endoscopy. The normal midazolam dose is 0.1 to 0.15 mg/kg. Is the 7.5 mg dose a reasonable dose for this patient?

CRITICAL THINKING QUESTIONS

1. Three hours after being given a hypnotic, Mrs. Grimes is still awake. She is having major surgery in the morning. Describe the actions you should initiate and the rationale for performing each.

2. Why should patients be cautioned against the use of alcohol when taking sedative-hypnotics?

3. Describe situations in which repeating a dose of a sedative-hypnotic would be appropriate.

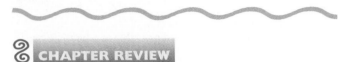

Drugs Used for Parkinson's Disease

CHAPTER CONTENT

Objectives

1. Prepare a list of signs and symptoms of Parkinson's disease and accurately define the vocabulary used for the pharmacologic agents prescribed and the disease state.

2. Name the neurotransmitter that is found in excess and the neurotransmitter that is deficient in persons with parkinsonism.

3. Describe reasonable expectations of medications prescribed for treatment of Parkinson's disease.

4. Identify the period of time necessary for a therapeutic response to be observed when drugs used to treat parkinsonism are initiated.

5. List symptoms that can be attributed to the cholinergic activity of pharmacologic agents.

6. Name the action of bromocriptine mesylate, carbidopa, and levodopa on neurotransmitters involved in Parkinson's disease.

7. Cite the specific symptoms that should show improvement when anticholinergic agents are administered to the patient with Parkinson's disease.

8. Develop a health teaching plan for an individual being treated with levodopa.

Key Words

Parkinson's disease	dyskinesia
dopamine	propulsive movements
neurotransmitter	livido reticularis
acetycholine	anticholinergic agents
tremor	

PARKINSON'S DISEASE

Parkinson's disease is a chronic, progressive disorder of the central nervous system. Approximately 1% of the U.S. population over the age of 50 is afflicted by this disorder. Thirty percent of patients report onset of symptoms before age 50, 40% report onset between 50 and 60 years of age, and the remainder report onset after the age of 60. Characteristic symptoms are muscle tremors, slowness of movement (*bradykinesia*), muscle weakness with rigidity, and alterations in posture and equilibrium. The symptoms associated with parkinsonism are caused by a dopamine deficiency in the extrapyramidal system within the basal ganglia of the brain. The extrapyramidal system is responsible for maintenance of posture and muscle tone and the regulation of voluntary smooth muscle activity. Normally a balance exists between **dopamine**, an inhibitory **neurotransmitter**, and **acetylcholine**, an excitatory neurotransmitter. With a deficiency of dopamine, a relative increase in acetylcholine activity occurs, causing excitation and the symptoms of parkinsonism. Approximately 80% of the dopamine must be depleted for symptoms to develop.

There are two types of parkinsonism. Primary or idiopathic parkinsonism is caused by reduction in dopamine-producing cells in the basal ganglia. The cause is not yet known, but environmental toxins such as pesticides are suspected. Heredity is no longer considered a factor in the development of the disease. Secondary parkinsonism is caused by head trauma, intracranial infections, tumors, and drug exposure. Medicines that deplete dopamine causing secondary parkinsonism include the phenothiazines, reserpine, methyldopa, and metoclopramide. In most cases of drug-induced parkinsonism, recovery is complete if the chemical is removed.

The symptoms of parkinsonism start insidiously and almost imperceptibly at first, with weakness and tremors, gradually progressing to involve movement disorders throughout the body. The symptoms usually begin on one side of the body, such as a tremor of a finger or hand, and progress to become bilateral. The upper part of the body is usually affected first. Eventually the individual has postural and gait alterations that result in the need for assistance with total care needs. Dementia, resembling that with Alzheimer's disease, occurs in a significant number of patients, but there is continuing debate as to whether it is part of the Parkinson's disease process or caused by concurrent drug therapy, Alzheimer's disease, or other factors.

The patient and family need assistance to learn the medical regimen used to control the symptoms and maintain the patient at an optimal level of participation in the activities of daily living. The drug therapy presents the potential for many side effects that all involved parties must understand.

Nurses can have a major influence in the positive use of coping mechanisms as the patient and family express varying degrees of anxiety, frustration, hostility, conflict, and fear. The primary goal of nursing intervention should be to keep the patient socially interactive and participatory in daily activities. This can be accomplished through the use of physical therapy, adherence to the drug regimen, and management of the course of treatment.

Drug Therapy for Treatment of Parkinson's Disease

Actions

The goal of treatment of parkinsonism is minimizing the symptoms because there is no cure for the disease. Goals are to relieve symptoms and restore dopaminergic activity and neurotransmitter function as close to normal as possible. Drug therapy includes the use of selegiline to protect dopaminergic nerve cells from further deterioration; levodopa, carbidopa, bromocriptine, pergolide, or amantadine to enhance dopaminergic activity; and anticholinergic agents to inhibit the relative excess in cholinergic activity. Therapy must be individualized, and realistic goals must be set for each patient. It is not possible to eliminate all

LIFE SPAN ISSUES

PARKINSON'S DISEASE

Parkinson's disease, which is most often seen in geriatric patients, causes a relative excess of acetylcholine because of a deficiency of dopamine. Drug therapy with dopaminergic agents increases dopamine availability while anticholinergic medicines are taken to counterbalance the availability of acetylcholine. Approximately 40% of patients with parkinsonism have some degree of clinical depression because of reduced availability of active metabolites of dopamine in the brain.

All drugs prescribed for Parkinson's disease produce a pharmacologic effect on the central nervous system. An assessment of the patient's mental status and physical functioning before therapy is initiated is essential to serve as a baseline so that comparisons can be made with subsequent evaluations.

Parkinson's disease is, at present, progressive and incurable. The goal of treatment is to moderate the symptoms and slow the progression of the disease. It is important to encourage the patient to take medications as scheduled and stay as active and involved in daily activities as possible.

Orthostatic hypotension is common with most of the medicines used to treat Parkinson's disease. In providing for patient safety, teach the patient to rise slowly from a supine or sitting position; encourage the patient to sit or lie down if feeling faint.

Constipation is a frequent problem with patients with Parkinson's disease. Instruct the patient to drink six to eight 8 oz glasses of liquid daily and increase bulk in the diet to prevent constipation. Bulk-forming laxatives may also need to be added to the daily regimen.

symptoms of the disease because the side effects of the medicines would not be tolerated. The trend is to use the lowest possible dosage of medicines so that, as the disease progresses, dosages can be increased and other medicines added to obtain a combined effect from therapy.

Uses

Selegiline is used to slow the course of Parkinson's disease by slowing the progression of deterioration of dopaminergic nerve cells. Levodopa, carbidopa, bromocriptine, pergolide, or amantadine replace deficient dopamine to the basal ganglia of the brain, and anticholinergic agents provide symptomatic relief from excessive acetylcholine. These agents are often used in combination to promote optimal levels of motor function (for example, improved gait, posture, and speech) and decrease disease symptoms (for example, tremors, rigidity, and drooling).

Nursing Process for Parkinson's Disease

Premedication Assessment

History of parkinsonism. Obtain data to classify the extent of parkinsonism that the patient is exhibiting. A rating scale may be used to assess the severity of Parkinson's disease based on the degree of disability exhibited by the patient (Figure 13-1):

Stage 1: involvement of one limb; mild disease
Stage 2: involvement of two limbs
Stage 3: significant gait alterations and moderate generalized disability
Stage 4: akinesia (abnormal state of motor and psychic hypoactivity or muscle paralysis), rigidity, and severe disability
Stage 5: unable to perform all activities of daily living

Motor function. Patients with Parkinson's disease progress through the following symptoms:

Tremor. **Tremors** are often observed in the hands and may involve the jaw, lips, and tongue. A "pill-rolling" motion in the fingers and thumbs is a characteristic movement. Tremors are usually reduced with voluntary movement. Emotional stress and fatigue may increase the frequency of tremors.

Assess the degree of tremor involvement and specific limitations in activities being affected by the tremors.

Dyskinesia. **Dyskinesia** is the impairment of the individual's ability to perform voluntary movements. This symptom commonly starts in one arm or hand. It is usually most noticeable because the patient ceases to swing the arm on the affected side while walking.

As the dyskinesia progresses, movement, especially in small muscle groups, becomes slow and jerky. This motion is often referred to as cogwheel rigidity. Muscle soreness, fatigue, and pain are associated with the prolonged muscle contractibility. The patient develops a shuffling gait, and once-automatic movements such as getting out of a chair or walking require a concentrated effort to be accomplished.

Along with the shuffling gait, the head and spine flex forward and the shoulders become rounded and stooped.

As mobility deteriorates, steps quicken and become shorter. **Propulsive, uncontrolled movement** forward or backward is evident. Patient safety becomes a primary consideration.

Bradykinesia. Bradykinesia is extremely slow body movement, which may eventually progress to akinesia, or lack of movement.

Facial appearance. The patient typically appears expressionless, as if wearing a mask; eyes are wide open and fixed in position. Some patients have almost total eyelid closure.

Salivation. As a result of excessive cholinergic activity, patients salivate excessively. As the disease progresses, patients may be unable to swallow all secretions and will frequently drool. If pharyngeal muscles are involved, the patient will have difficulty chewing and swallowing.

Emotional lability. The disease does *not* affect the intellectual capacity of the patient. The chronic nature of the disease and physical impairment produce mood swings and serious depression. Patients commonly display a delayed reaction time. The individual should be observed for the development of signs of dementia, which may be associated with the disease, may be a result of medications, or may be a new medical diagnosis.

Stress. Obtain a detailed history of the manner in which the patient has controlled physical and mental stress in the past.

Safety. Assess the level of assistance needed for mobility and performance of activities of daily living and self-care.

Family resources. Determine what family resources are available and the closeness of the family during daily as well as stress-producing events.

Nursing Diagnosis
- Constipation, risk for (side effect)
- Knowledge deficit related to medication regimen
- Injury, risk for (indications)
- Noncompliance, risk for related to drug side effects or lack of understanding of response time required for therapeutic response (side effects)

Planning

History of parkinsonism. Schedule a meeting to plan needed baseline assessments of the patient's functional abilities, including mental status, before initiating therapy and periodically throughout therapy to differentiate disease symptoms from drug-induced side effects.

Safety. Provide for patient safety on a continuum. Obtain antislip pads for chair and other positioning devices.

Care needs. Coordinate care needs with other departments, for example, physical therapy and dietary and social services. Parkinson's disease is a progressive disorder, and it is important to plan for periodic evaluation of the patient's status on a continuum. Plan with the patient and family how the patient's daily care needs will be accomplished.

Medication therapy. Schedule determination of vital signs on a routine basis, especially blood pressure monitoring. This is particularly important during initiation of therapy and when dosage adjustments or medication changes are made. Plan to stress that the effectiveness of medication therapy may take several weeks to be achieved. Schedule monitoring of behav-

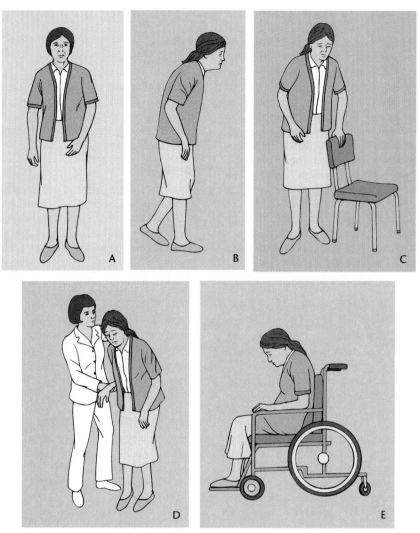

Figure 13-1 *Stages of parkinsonism.* **A,** *Flexion of affected arm. Patient leans toward the unaffected side.* **B,** *Slow shuffling gait.* **C,** *Patient has increased difficulty walking and looks for sources of support to prevent falls.* **D,** *Further progression of weakness. Patient requires assistance from another person for ambulation.* **E,** *Profound disability. Patient may be confined to a wheelchair because of increasing weakness.*

ioral changes on a continuum consistent with the clinical practice setting.

Implementation

- Implement planned interventions consistent with assessment data and identified individual needs of the patient.
- Monitor and record vital signs, especially blood pressure, during the course of therapy. Report significant changes in blood pressure. These are most likely to occur during dosage adjustments. Emphasize measures to prevent orthostatic hypotension.
- Monitor for degree of therapeutic response and side effects using forms provided by the clinical site to document changes in function. (See written record p. 175.)
- Monitor bowel function and implement measures to prevent constipation (for example, adequate fluid intake, bulk in diet, use of stool softeners).
- Support the patient's efforts to remain mobile. Provide a safe environment by removing clutter and throw rugs; use correct equipment and supportive devices.

- Minimize deformities by encouraging erect posture. Maintain joint mobility through the use of active and passive exercises.
- Reinforce the principles taught for gait training.
- Nutritional needs must be carefully assessed because dietary modifications will be required as the disease progresses. Be vigilant for difficulty in swallowing, and realize that the patient may be prone to aspiration of food or water. Weigh the patient weekly; evaluate and report fluctuations in body weight to the dietitian or physician.
- Encourage self-maintenance and social involvement.
- Provide a restful environment and attempt to keep stressors at a minimum.
- Monitor mood and affect. Be alert for signs of depression. Mood alterations and depression are secondary to disease progression (for example, lack of ability to participate in sex, immobility, incontinence) and may be expected but should not be ignored.
- Provide for patient safety during ambulation and delivery of care.

Patient Education and Health Promotion

Nutrition. • Instruct the patient to drink at least 6 to 8 glasses of water or fluid per day to maintain adequate hydration. Because constipation is frequently a problem, instruct the patient to include bulk in the diet and use stool softeners as needed. As the disease progresses, the type and consistency of the foods eaten will need to be adjusted to meet the individual's needs. Because of fatigue and difficulty in eating, assistance appropriate to the degree of impairment should be given. Do not rush the individual when eating; cut foods into bite-sized pieces. Plan six smaller meals daily rather than three larger meals. • Instruct the patient to weigh weekly. Ask the patient to state the guidelines for weight loss or gain that should be reported to the physician. • Stress that vitamins should not be taken unless prescribed by the physician. Pyridoxine (B_6) reduces the therapeutic effect of levodopa.

Stress management. Explain to the patient and caregivers the importance of maintaining an environment that is as stress free as possible. Explain that symptoms such as tremors are enhanced by anxiety.

Self-reliance. Encourage patients to perform as many activities of daily living as possible. Explain to caregivers that it is important not to "take over"; encourage self-maintenance, continued social involvement, and participation in activities such as hobbies.

Exercise. Instruct the patient and caregiver about the importance of maintaining correct body alignment, walking as erect as possible, and practicing the gait training taught by the physical therapy department. Gait training is essential if the patient is to delay the onset of shuffling and propulsion of the gait. Exercises to maintain the strength of facial muscles and the tongue will maintain speech clarity and the ability to swallow. Active and passive range-of-motion exercises to all joints will help minimize deformities. Explain that maintenance of the exercise program will increase the long-term well-being of the patient.

Mood alterations. Explain to the patient and caregiver that depression and mood alterations are secondary to disease progression (for example, inability to participate in sex, immobility, incontinence) and may be expected. Changes in mental outlook should be discussed with the physician.

Fostering health maintenance. • Provide the patient and significant others with important information contained in the specific drug monograph for the medicines prescribed. Stress the importance of nonpharmacologic interventions and the long-term effects that compliance with the treatment regimen can provide. Additional health teaching and nursing interventions for the side effects to expect and report are described in the drug monographs that follow. • Seek cooperation and understanding of the following points so that medication compliance is increased: name of medication, dosage, route and times of administration, side effects to expect, and side effects to report. • Written record: Enlist the patient's aid in developing and maintaining a written record. (See Patient Education and Monitoring box on p.175.) of monitoring parameters (such as degree of tremor relief, stability, changes in mobility and rigidity, sedation, constipation, drowsiness, mental alertness, or deviations) and response to prescribed therapies for discussion with the physician. Patients should be encouraged to bring this record to follow-up visits.

Drug Class: Dopamine Agonists

amantadine hydrochloride (a-man'ta-deen)
Symmetrel (sim'eh-trel)

Amantadine is a compound developed originally to treat viral infections. It was administered to a patient with parkinsonism who also had the Asian flu. During the course of therapy for the flu, the patient showed definite improvement in the parkinsonian symptoms.

Actions

The exact mechanism of action is unknown but appears to be unrelated to the drug's antiviral activity. Amantadine seems to slow the destruction of dopamine, which makes the small amount present more effective. It may also aid in the release of dopamine from its storage sites. Unfortunately, approximately half of the patients who benefit from amantadine therapy will begin to notice a reduction in benefit after 2 or 3 months. An increase in dosage or temporary discontinuation followed by a reinitiation of therapy several weeks later may restore the therapeutic benefits.

Uses

Amantadine is used for the relief of symptoms associated with Parkinson's disease and for the treatment of susceptible strains of viral influenza.

Therapeutic Outcomes

The primary therapeutic outcome sought from amantadine in treating parkinsonism is to establish a balance of dopamine and acetylcholine in the basal ganglia of the brain by enhancing delivery of dopamine to brain cells.

Nursing Process

Premedication Assessment

1. Perform baseline assessment of parkinsonism.
2. Amantadine should be used with caution in patients with a history of seizure activity, liver disease, uncontrolled psychosis, or congestive heart failure. Amantadine may cause an exacerbation of these disorders.
3. Take baseline blood pressures in supine and standing positions.

Planning

Availability. PO—100 mg capsules, 50 mg per 5 ml syrup.

Implementation

Dosage and administration. Adult: PO—Initially 100 mg twice daily. Maximum daily dose is 400 mg.

Because of the possibility of insomnia, plan the last dose to be administered in the afternoon rather than at bedtime.

Evaluation

Most of the adverse effects of amantadine therapy are dose related and reversible.

Side effects to expect

CONFUSION, DISORIENTATION, MENTAL DEPRESSION. Perform a baseline assessment of the patient's degree of alert-

PATIENT EDUCATION AND MONITORING FORM   Antiparkinson Agents

MEDICATIONS	COLOR	TO BE TAKEN

Name _____

Physician _____

Physician's phone _____

Next appt.* _____

PARAMETERS		DAY OF DISCHARGE								COMMENTS
Weight										
Blood Pressure										
Pulse										
Tremor relief or pain relief Little relief — 10 / Moderate relief — 5 / Good relief — 1										
Mobility and rigidity–gait training, working or not? No improvement — 10 / 5 / Less rigidity — 1										
Control of secretions? Worse — 10 / Improved — 5 / No problem — 1										
Alertness and orientation to time, person, and place (T.P.P.). Poor — 10 / 5 / Good — 1										
Exercise: Note present level of activity: Walking, getting out, performing range of motion (R.O.M.) exercises.										
Bowel and Bladder	Constipated = C Normal = N (Check one)	C ____ N ____	C ____ N ____	C ____ N ____	C ____ N ____	C ____ N ____	C ____ N ____	C ____ N ____		
	Difficulty urinating = D									
	Occasional problem urinating									
Dietary needs	No problem eating or drinking.									
	Drinks (____) glasses fluid per day.									
	Needs frequent small meals.									
	Needs a lot of time to eat.									
Socialization Withdrawn — 10 / 5 / Active involved — 1										

*Please bring this record with you to your next appointment.
Use the back of this sheet for additional information.

ness and orientation to name, place, and time before initiating therapy. Make regularly scheduled subsequent evaluations of mental status and compare findings. Report development of alterations.

DIZZINESS, LIGHT-HEADEDNESS, ANOREXIA, NAUSEA, ABDOMINAL DISCOMFORT. These side effects are usually mild and tend to resolve with continued therapy. Encourage the patient not to discontinue therapy without first consulting the physician. Provide for patient safety during periods of dizziness or light-headedness.

LIVIDO RETICULARIS (SKIN MOTTLING). A dermatologic condition known as **livido reticularis** is frequently observed in conjunction with amantadine therapy. It is characterized by diffuse, rose-colored mottling of the skin, often accompanied by pedal edema, predominantly in the extremities. It is more noticeable when the patient is standing or exposed to cold. It is reversible within 2 to 6 weeks after discontinuation of amantadine. However, discontinuation of therapy is not usually necessary.

These side effects are usually mild and tend to resolve with continued therapy. Symptoms are enhanced by exposure to cold or by prolonged standing. Encourage the patient not to discontinue therapy without first consulting the physician.

Side effects to report

LIVER DISEASE. The symptoms of liver disease are anorexia, nausea, vomiting, jaundice, hepatomegaly, splenomegaly, and abnormal liver function tests (elevated bilirubin, aspartate aminotransaminase [AST], alanine aminotransferase [ALT], gamma glulamyltransferase [GGT], alkaline phosphatase, prothrombin time).

SEIZURE DISORDERS, PSYCHOSIS. Provide for patient safety during episodes of dizziness; report symptoms for further evaluation.

DYSPNEA/EDEMA. If amantadine is used for a patient who has a history of congestive heart failure, assess lung sounds, additional edema, and weight gain on a regular basis.

Drug interactions

ANTICHOLINERGIC AGENTS (TRIHEXYPHENIDYL BENZTROPINE, PROCYLIDINE, DIPHENHYDRAMINE). Amantadine may exacerbate the side effects of **anticholinergic agents** that may also be used to control the symptoms of parkinsonism. Confusion and hallucinations may gradually develop. The dosage of amantadine or the anticholinergic agent should be reduced.

bromocriptine mesylate (broe-moe-krip′teen)
Parlodel (par-lo′del)

Actions

Bromocriptine stimulates dopamine receptors in the basal ganglia of the brain.

Uses

Because parkinsonian patients are deficient in dopamine in basal ganglia, there is pronounced improvement in the symptoms of the disease with bromocriptine therapy. Bromocriptine appears to be nearly as effective as levodopa in treating parkinsonism and is occasionally useful in patients who are no longer benefiting from levodopa therapy.

Therapeutic Outcomes

The primary therapeutic outcome sought from bromocriptine in treating parkinsonism is to stimulate dopaminergic neurotransmission to counterbalance acetylcholine action in the basal ganglia of the brain.

Nursing Process

Premedication Assessment

1. Perform baseline neurologic assessment so that symptoms of disease and drug side effects can be more effectively differentiated.
2. Take baseline blood pressures in supine and standing positions.

Planning

Availability. PO—2.5 mg tablets and 5 mg capsules.

Implementation

Dosage and administration. Adult: PO—Initially 1.25 mg 2 times daily with meals. Increase the dosage by 2.5 mg per day every 2 to 4 weeks. The dosage must be adjusted according to the patient's response and tolerance. Dosages in the range of 50 to 100 mg daily are not uncommon for maximal therapeutic benefit.

If severe side effects do appear, they can also be minimized by reducing the dosage for a few days, then increasing the dosage more gradually.

Side effects can be minimized by starting with small doses and then increasing the dosage gradually and by administering medication with food in the evening.

Evaluation

Side effects to expect

GASTROINTESTINAL EFFECTS. Most of these effects may be minimized by temporary reduction in dosage, administration with food, and use of stool softeners for constipation.

OTHER SIDE EFFECTS. Dryness of the mouth, double vision, nasal congestion, and metallic taste may also occur.

Side effects to report

NEUROLOGIC. Neurologic effects often occur with higher dosages.

Perform a baseline assessment of the patient's degree of alertness and orientation to name, place, and time before initiating therapy. Make regularly scheduled subsequent evaluations of mental status and compare findings. Report development of alterations.

Provide for patient safety, be emotionally supportive, and assure the patient that these adverse effects dissipate within 2 to 3 weeks of discontinuing therapy.

ORTHOSTATIC HYPOTENSION. Monitor the blood pressure daily in both the supine and standing positions.

Anticipate the development of postural hypotension and take measures to prevent an occurrence. Teach the patient to rise slowly from a supine or sitting position; encourage the patient to sit or lie down if feeling faint.

HYPERTENSION. Although hypotension at the start of therapy is not uncommon, hypertension may begin to develop in the first or second week of therapy. Monitor carefully and report if a trend in higher blood pressures develops. If the patient begins complaining of headaches and the blood pressure is higher than the patient's normal blood pressure, report to the physician immediately.

Drug interactions

LEVODOPA. Bromocriptine and levodopa have additive neurologic effects. This interaction may be advantageous because it often allows a reduction in dosage of the levodopa.

ANTIHYPERTENSIVE AGENTS. Dosage adjustment of the antihypertensive agent is frequently necessary because of excessive orthostatic hypotension.

carbidopa (kar bi-doe'-pa), levodopa
Sinemet (sin'eh-met)

Actions

Sinemet is a combination of carbidopa and levodopa used for treatment of the symptoms of Parkinson's disease. Carbidopa is an enzyme inhibitor that reduces the metabolism of levodopa, allowing a greater portion of the administered levodopa to reach the desired receptor sites in the basal ganglia. Carbidopa has no effect when used alone; it must be used in combination with levodopa.

Uses

Carbidopa is used to reduce the dose of levodopa required by approximately 75%. When administered with levodopa, carbidopa increases both plasma levels and the plasma half-life of levodopa.

Therapeutic Outcomes

The primary therapeutic outcome sought from Sinemet in treating parkinsonism is to establish a balance of dopamine and acetylcholine in the basal ganglia of the brain by enhancing delivery of dopamine to brain cells.

Nursing Process

Premedication Assessment

1. Review medicines prescribed that may need dosage adjustments. Plan to perform focused assessments to detect responses to therapy that would need to be reported to the physician.
2. Review the symptoms manifested by the patient. Patients with irregular "on-and-off" responses to levodopa do not show benefit from Sinemet.

Planning

Availability. PO—Sinemet is a combination product containing both carbidopa and levodopa. The combination product is available in ratios of 10/100, 25/100, and 25/250 mg of carbidopa and levodopa, respectively. There is also a sustained-release product, Sinemet CR, which contains 50 mg per 200 mg of carbidopa/levodopa.

Implementation

Dosage and administration. Adult: PO—Patients not currently receiving levodopa: Initially Sinemet 10/100 or 25/100 3 times daily, increasing by 1 tablet every other day until a dosage of 6 tablets daily is attained. As therapy progresses and patient shows indications of requiring more levodopa, substitute Sinemet 25/250, 1 tablet 3 to 4 times daily. Increase by 1 tablet every other day to a maximum of 8 tablets daily.

Evaluation

Side effects to expect. Carbidopa has no effect when used alone; it must be used in combination with levodopa. The side effects seen with combined therapy are actually an enhancement of the effects of levodopa because the carbidopa is allowing more levodopa to reach the brain. See also "Levodopa."

Drug interactions. Sinemet may be used to treat parkinsonism in conjunction with amantadine or anticholinergic agents. The dosages of all medications may need to be reduced because of combined therapy. See also "Levodopa."

levodopa (lee-voe-doe'pa),
Larodopa (lar-oh-do'pah), Dopar (do'par)

Actions

Dopamine, when administered orally, does not enter the brain. Levodopa crosses into the brain, is metabolized to dopamine, and replaces the dopamine deficiency in the basal ganglia.

Uses

About 75% of patients with parkinsonism respond favorably to levodopa therapy, but after a few years the response diminishes, becomes more uneven, and is accompanied by many more side effects. This loss of therapeutic effect reflects the progression of the underlying disease process.

Therapeutic Outcomes

The primary therapeutic outcome sought from levodopa in treating parkinsonism is to establish a balance of dopamine and acetylcholine in the basal ganglia of the brain by enhancing delivery of dopamine to brain cells.

Nursing Process

Premedication Assessment

1. Obtain a history of gastrointestinal and cardiovascular symptoms, including baseline vital signs (for example, blood pressure, pulse).
2. Ask specifically about any symptoms of hallucinations, nightmares, dementia, or anxiety.
3. Inquire about any urine testing being done.
4. All patients should be screened for the presence of angle-closure glaucoma before the initiating therapy. Patients with open-angle glaucoma can safely use levodopa. Do not administer the medicine to a person with a history of glaucoma unless specifically approved by the physician.

Planning

Availability. PO— 100, 250, and 500 mg tablets and capsules.

Implementation

Dosage and administration. Adult: PO—Initially 0.5 to 1 g daily in divided doses, administered with food. Do not exceed 8 g per day. Administer medication with food or milk to reduce gastric irritation. Therapy for at least 6 months may be necessary to determine full therapeutic benefits.

Evaluation

Levodopa causes many side effects but most are dose related and reversible. Side effects vary greatly, depending on the stage of the disease.

Side effects to expect

NAUSEA, VOMITING, ANOREXIA. These effects can be reduced by slowly increasing the dose, dividing the total daily dose into 4 to 6 doses, and administering the medication with food or antacids.

ORTHOSTATIC HYPOTENSION. Although generally mild, levodopa may cause some degree of orthostatic hypotension manifested by dizziness and weakness, particularly when therapy is being initiated. Tolerance usually develops after a few weeks of therapy.

Monitor the blood pressure daily in both the supine and standing positions.

Anticipate the development of postural hypotension and take measures to prevent an occurrence. Teach patients to rise slowly from a supine or sitting position; encourage them to sit or lie down if feeling faint.

Side effects to report

CHEWING MOTIONS, BOBBING, FACIAL GRIMACING, ROCKING MOVEMENTS. These involuntary movements occur in approximately half of the patients taking levodopa for more than 6 months. A reduction in dosage may be beneficial.

NIGHTMARES, DEPRESSION, CONFUSION, HALLUCINATIONS. Perform a baseline assessment of the patient's degree of alertness and orientation to name, place, and time before initiating therapy. Make regularly scheduled subsequent evaluations of mental status and compare findings. Report development of alterations.

Provide for patient safety during these episodes.

Reduction in the daily dosage may control these adverse effects.

TACHYCARDIA, PALPITATIONS. Take the pulse at regularly scheduled intervals. Report for further evaluation.

Drug interactions

PHENELZINE, ISOCARBOXAZID. These agents unpredictably exaggerate the effects of levodopa. They should be discontinued at least 14 days before the administration of levodopa.

ISONIAZID. Use with caution in conjunction with levodopa. Discontinue isoniazid if patients taking levodopa develop hypertension, flushing, palpitations, and tremor.

PYRIDOXINE: Pyridoxine (vitamin B_6) in oral doses of 5 to 10 mg reverses the toxic and therapeutic effects of levodopa. Normal diets contain less than 1 mg of pyridoxine, therefore dietary restrictions are not necessary. However, the ingredients of multiple vitamins should be considered.

There is a pyridoxine-free multiple vitamin (Larobec) made specifically for patients taking levodopa.

DIAZEPAM, CHLORDIAZEPOXIDE, PAPAVERINE, PHENYLBUTAZONE, CLONIDINE, PHENYTOIN. These agents appear to cause a deterioration in the therapeutic effects of levodopa.

Use with caution in patients with parkinsonism, and discontinue if the patient's clinical status deteriorates.

PHENOTHIAZINES, RESERPINE, HALOPERIDOL, METHYLDOPA. A side effect associated with these agents is a Parkinson-like syndrome. Because this will nullify the therapeutic effects of levodopa, do not use concurrently.

EPHEDRINE, EPINEPHRINE, ISOPROTERENOL, AMPHETAMINES. Levodopa may increase the therapeutic and toxic effects of these agents. Monitor for tachycardia, arrhythmias, and hypertension. Reduce the dose of these agents if necessary.

ANTIHYPERTENSIVE AGENTS. Dosage adjustment of the antihypertensive agent is frequently necessary because of excessive orthostatic hypotension.

KETOSTIX, LABSTIX. Levodopa may produce false-positive urine ketone results with these products. Use Acetest tablets.

CLINITEST. Levodopa may produce a false-positive trace of urinary glucose.

TES-TAPE, CLINISTIX. Levodopa may produce false-negative urine glucose results with these products.

BOWL CLEANERS. The metabolites of Levodopa react with toilet-bowl cleaners to turn the urine a red to black color. This may also occur if the urine is exposed to air for long periods of time. Inform the patient that there is no cause for alarm.

pergolide mesylate (pur-go′lid)
Permax (pĕr′m•aks)

Actions

Pergolide is a potent dopamine receptor stimulant. It is thought to exert its therapeutic effect in patients with Parkinson's disease by directly stimulating postsynaptic dopamine receptors in the nigrostriatal system of the brain.

Uses

Pergolide is used in combination with levodopa/carbidopa in the management of Parkinson's disease.

Therapeutic Outcomes

The primary therapeutic outcome sought from pergolide in treating Parkinsonism is to stimulate dopaminergic neurotransmission to counterbalance acetylcholine action in the basal ganglia of the brain.

Nursing Process

Premedication Assessment

1. Obtain a history of cardiovascular symptoms, including baseline vital signs (for example, blood pressure, pulse)
2. Perform a baseline assessment of the patient's degree of alertness and orientation to name, place, and time before initiating therapy. Make regularly scheduled subsequent evaluations of mental status and compare findings. Report development of alterations.

Planning

Availability. PO—0.05, 0.25, and 1 mg tablets.

Implementation

Dosage and administration. Adult: Dosage must be adjusted according to the patient's response and tolerance. Side effects can be minimized by starting with small doses, then increasing the dosage gradually. PO—Initiate with a daily dose of 0.05 mg for the first 2 days. Gradually increase the dosage by 0.1 or 0.15 mg per day every third day over the 12 days of therapy. The dosage may then be increased by 0.25 mg per day every third day until an optimal dose is achieved. Pergolide is usually administered in divided doses 3 times daily. During dosage titration, the dosage of concurrent carbidopa/levodopa should be cautiously decreased. The usual total daily dose of pergolide is 3 mg.

Evaluation

Side effects with pergolide are fairly common. Approximately 25% of patients receiving pergolide must discontinue therapy because of side effects.

Side effects to expect

GASTROINTESTINAL EFFECTS. Gastrointestinal effects include nausea, constipation, diarrhea, and upset stomach. Most of these effects may be minimized by temporary reduction in dosage, administration with food, and use of stool softeners for constipation.

Side effects to report

NEUROLOGIC. Approximately 14% of patients develop hallucinations. Provide for patient safety, be emotionally supportive, and assure the patient that these adverse effects usually dissipate as tolerance to the adverse effects develops in a few weeks.

ORTHOSTATIC HYPOTENSION. Monitor the blood pressure daily in both the supine and standing positions.

Anticipate the development of postural hypotension and take measures to prevent an occurrence. Teach the patient to rise slowly from a supine or sitting position; encourage the patient to sit or lie down if feeling faint.

Drug interactions

LEVODOPA. Pergolide and levodopa have additive neurologic effects. This interaction may be beneficial because it often allows a reduction in dosage of the levodopa.

DOPAMINE ANTAGONISTS. Dopamine antagonists include phenothiazines, butyrophenones, thioxanthenes, and metoclopramide. These agents diminish the effectiveness of pergolide, a dopaminergic agonist.

ANTIHYPERTENSIVE AGENTS. Dosage adjustment of the antihypertensive agent is frequently necessary because of excessive orthostatic hypotension.

Drug Class: Miscellaneous Antiparkinson Agent

selegiline (sel-ee-igill′-ene)
Eldepryl (el-deh-pril′)

Actions

The mechanism of antiparkinsonian action of selegiline is unknown. It is known to be a potent monoamine oxidase–type B inhibitor, but this does not explain all of its actions.

Uses

Levodopa and carbidopa are the current drugs of choice for the treatment of Parkinson's disease. Unfortunately, these agents lose effectiveness (on-off phenomenon) and cause

more adverse effects (dyskinesias) over time. It is often necessary to add other dopamine receptor agonists such as bromocriptine and pergolide to improve the patient response and tolerance. Selegiline has been found to have similar adjunctive activity to levodopa/carbidopa in the treatment of Parkinson's disease. The combination of selegiline and levodopa/carbidopa improves memory and motor speed and may increase life expectancy.

Selegiline has also been found to have a "neuroprotective" effect by interfering with the degeneration of striated dopaminergic neurons. It is now also being used early in the treatment of Parkinson's disease to slow the progression of symptoms.

Therapeutic Outcomes

The primary therapeutic outcomes sought from use of selegiline in treating parkinsonism are as follows:
1. Slow the development of symptoms and progression of the disease
2. Establish a balance of dopamine and acetylcholine in the basal ganglia of the brain by enhancing delivery of dopamine to brain cells

Nursing Process

Premedication Assessment

1. Obtain a history of gastrointestinal symptoms.
2. Perform a baseline assessment of the patient's degree of alertness and orientation to name, place, and time before initiating therapy.
3. Check for any antihypertensive therapy currently prescribed. Monitor blood pressure daily in both the supine and standing positions. If antihypertensive medications are being taken, report this to the physician for possible dosage adjustment.
4. Check other medications prescribed. Do not administer selegiline with meperidine.

Planning

Availability. PO—5 mg tablets.

Implementation

Dosage and administration. Dosage must be adjusted according to the patient's response and tolerance. Adult: PO—5 mg at breakfast and lunch. Do not exceed 10 mg daily. After 2 to 3 days of treatment, the dose of levodopa/carbidopa should start being titrated downward.

It may be possible to reduce levodopa/carbidopa dosages by 10% to 30%.

Evaluation

Selegiline causes relatively few adverse effects. It may increase the adverse dopaminergic effects of levodopa such as chorea, confusion, or hallucinations, but these can be controlled by reducing the dose of levodopa.

Side effects to expect

GASTROINTESTINAL EFFECTS. Most of these effects may be minimized by temporary reduction in dosage, administration with food, and use of stool softeners for constipation.

Side effects to report

NEUROLOGIC. Selegiline may increase the adverse dopaminergic effects of levodopa, such as chorea, confusion, and hallucinations. Make regularly scheduled subsequent evaluations of mental status and compare findings. Report development of alterations.

Provide for patient safety, be emotionally supportive, and assure the patient that these adverse effects usually dissipate as tolerance to the adverse effects develops over a few weeks.

ORTHOSTATIC HYPOTENSION. Monitor blood pressure daily in both the supine and standing positions.

Anticipate the development of postural hypotension and take measures to prevent an occurrence. Teach the patient to rise slowly from a supine or sitting position; encourage the patient to sit or lie down if feeling faint.

Drug interactions

LEVODOPA. Selegiline and levodopa have additive neurologic effects. This interaction may be beneficial because it often allows a reduction in dosage of the levodopa.

MEPERIDINE. Fatal drug interactions have been reported between monoamine oxidase inhibitors and meperidine. Although this interaction has not been reported with selegiline, it is recommended that the two agents not be given concurrently.

ANTIHYPERTENSIVE AGENTS. Dosage adjustment of the antihypertensive agent is frequently necessary because of excessive orthostatic hypotension.

Drug Class: Anticholinergic Agents

Actions

Parkinsonism is induced by an imbalance of neurotransmitters in the basal ganglia of the brain. The primary imbalance appears to be a deficiency of dopamine, with a relative excess of the cholinergic neurotransmitter acetylcholine. Therefore *anticholinergic agents* are used to reduce hyperstimulation caused by excessive acetylcholine.

Uses

The anticholinergic agents reduce the severity of the rigidity, sweating, drooling, depression, and tremor that characterize parkinsonism. Anticholinergic agents may be useful for patients with minimal symptoms, for those unable to tolerate the side effects of levodopa, and for those who have not benefited from levodopa therapy. Combination therapy with levodopa and anticholinergic agents is also successful in controlling symptoms of the disease more completely in approximately half of the patients already stabilized on levodopa therapy.

Therapeutic Outcomes

The primary therapeutic outcome sought from anticholinergic agents in treating parkinsonism is reduction in the severity of the rigidity, sweating, drooling, depression, and tremor that are caused by a relative excess of acetylcholine in the basal ganglia.

_____

Nursing Process

Premedication Assessment

1. Obtain baseline data relating to patterns of urinary and bowel elimination.

2. Perform a baseline assessment of the patient's degree of alertness and orientation to name, place, and time before initiating therapy.

3. Take blood pressure in both the supine and standing positions. Record pulse rate, rhythm, and regularity.

4. All patients should be screened for the presence of angle-closure glaucoma before initiating therapy. Anticholinergic agents may precipitate an acute attack of angle-closure glaucoma. Patients with open-angle glaucoma can safely use anticholinergic agents. Monitoring of intraocular pressure should be performed on a regular basis.

Planning
Availability. See Table 13-1.

Implementation
Dosage and administration. Adult: PO—See Table 13-1. Administer medication with food or milk to reduce gastric irritation.

Evaluation
Most side effects observed with anticholinergic agents are direct extensions of their pharmacologic properties.
Side effects to expect

BLURRED VISION, CONSTIPATION, URINARY RETENTION, DRYNESS OF MUCOSA OF THE MOUTH, THROAT, AND NOSE. These symptoms are the anticholinergic effects produced by these agents. Patients taking these medications should be monitored for the development of these side effects.

Dryness of the mucosa may be relieved by sucking hard candy or ice chips or by chewing gum.

If patients develop urinary hesitancy, assess for distention of the bladder. Report to the physician for further evaluation.

Give stool softeners as prescribed. Encourage adequate fluid intake and foods to provide sufficient bulk.

Caution the patient that blurred vision may occur and make appropriate suggestions for personal safety of the individual.
Side effects to report

NIGHTMARES, DEPRESSION, CONFUSION, HALLUCINATIONS. Make regularly scheduled subsequent evaluations of mental status and compare findings. Report development of alterations.

Provide for patient safety during these episodes.

Reduction in the daily dosage may control these adverse effects.

ORTHOSTATIC HYPOTENSION. Although the instance is infrequent and generally mild, all anticholinergic agents may cause some degree of orthostatic hypotension manifested by dizziness and weakness, particularly when therapy is being initiated.

Monitor blood pressure daily in both the supine and standing positions.

Anticipate the development of postural hypotension and take measures to prevent an occurrence. Teach the patient to rise slowly from a supine or sitting position; encourage the patient to sit or lie down if feeling faint.

PALPITATIONS, ARRHYTHMIAS. Report for further evaluation.

Drug interactions

AMANTADINE, TRICYCLIC ANTIDEPRESSANTS, PHENOTHIAZINES. These agents may enhance the anticholinergic side

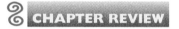

Table 13-1

Agents with Anticholinergic Properties Used to Treat Parkinsonism

GENERIC NAME	BRAND NAME	AVAILABILITY	INITIAL DOSE (PO)	MAXIMUM DAILY DOSE (MG)
Benztropine mesylate	Cogentin	Tablets: 0.5, 1, 2 mg Inj: 1 mg/ml in 2 ml amps	0.5 - 1 mg at bedtime	6
Biperiden hydrochloride	Akineton	Tablets: 2 mg	2 mg 1-3 times daily	10
Diphenhydramine hydrochloride	Benadryl, ✤ Allerdryl	Tablets: 25, 50 mg Capsules: 25, 50 mg Elixir: 12.5 mg/5ml Syrup: 12.5 mg/5 ml		
Orphenadrine hydrochloride	Banflex, Norflex	Sustained-release tablets: 100 mg Inj: 30 mg/ml in 2, 10 ml vials	50 mg 3 times daily	150-250
Procyclidine hydrochloride	Kemadrin, ✤ Procyclid	Tablets: 5 mg	2 mg 3 times daily	15-20
Trihexyphenidyl hydrochloride	Artane, Trihexane ✤ Aparkane	Tablets: 2, 5 mg Elixir: 2 mg/5 ml	1 mg daily	12-15

✤ Available in Canada only.

effects. Developing confusion and hallucinations are characteristic of excessive anticholinergic activity. Dosage reduction may be required.

LEVODOPA. Large doses of anticholinergic agents may slow gastric emptying and inhibit absorption of levodopa. An increase in the dosage of levodopa may be required.

CHAPTER REVIEW

Parkinson's disease is a progressive neurologic disorder caused by deterioration of dopamine-producing cells in the portion of the brain responsible for maintenance of posture and muscle tone and the regulation of voluntary smooth muscles. Normally, a balance exists between dopamine, an inhibitory neurotransmitter, and acetylcholine, an excitatory neurotransmitter. The symptoms associated with Parkinson's disease develop because of a relative excess of acetylcholine in the brain. The goal of treatment of parkinsonism is to restore dopamine neurotransmitter function as close to normal as possible and relieve symptoms caused by "excessive" acetylcholine. Therapy must be individualized, but selegiline therapy is often started first to slow the development of symptoms. As selegiline becomes less effective, levodopa is started, with or without selegiline. Later, dopamine agonists (amantadine, bromocriptine, pergolide) may be added to directly stimulate dopamine receptors. Anticholinergic agents may be added at any time to reduce the effects of the "excessive" acetylcholine. Nonpharmacologic treatment (for example, diet, exercise,

physical therapy) of Parkinson's disease is equally important in maintaining the long-term well-being of the patient.

MATH REVIEW

1. Dr. Jones wrote orders to start Mr. Lienemann on Sinemet 25/100 at an initial dose of one tablet 3 times daily. Sinemet is available in ratios of 10/100, 25/100, 25/250, and 50/200 mg strengths. Which strength should be used and how many tablets should be administered for each individual dose?

2. Dr. Jones wrote orders to start Mr. James on levodopa 0.25 g 4 times daily. Levodopa is available in 100, 250, and 500 mg strengths. Which strength should be used and how many tablets should be administered at one time?

3. Dr. Jones wrote orders to start Mrs. Smith on bromocriptine at an initial dose of 1.25 mg 2 times daily with meals. Bromocriptine is available in 2.5 mg tablets and 5 mg capsules. What will you administer to Mrs. Smith?

CRITICAL THINKING QUESTIONS

1. What physiologic effect does stimulation of dopamine receptors have?

2. Mrs. Hanegan's family asks you to explain the basic underlying problem that is causing the symptoms of Parkinson's disease in their mother. Give a simple explanation of the symptoms, appropriate for use with a

lay person. Include an explanation of what a neurotransmitter is and the basic imbalances found with Parkinson's disease.

3. Discuss the normal course of progression of Parkinson's disease and include the rationale for drug therapy to alleviate the symptoms.

4. Develop a teaching plan to be used with the patient and family of an individual being started on Sinemet for the treatment of Parkinson's disease.

5. Explain why baseline assessment of an individual's mental status and physical symptoms are important before and periodically throughout the course of treatment of Parkinson's disease.

6. Mr. Janna is being started on an anticholinergic drug as part of the treatment plan for Parkinson's disease. What symptoms could you anticipate improvement in and, conversely, what problems could also arise from starting this medication?

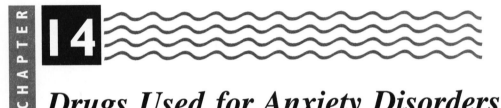

CHAPTER 14

Drugs Used for Anxiety Disorders

CHAPTER CONTENT

Objectives

1. Define terminology associated with anxiety states.

2. Describe the essential components of a baseline assessment of a patient's mental status.

3. Cite the side effects of hydroxyzine therapy and identify those effects requiring close monitoring when used preoperatively.

4. Develop a teaching plan for patient education of persons taking antianxiety medications.

5. Describe signs and symptoms the patient will display when a positive therapeutic outcome is being seen for the treatment of a high-anxiety state.

6. Discuss psychologic and physiologic drug dependence.

Key Words

anxiety

panic disorder

phobias

obsession

compulsion

anxiolytics

tranquilizers

ANXIETY DISORDERS

Anxiety is a normal human emotion, similar to fear. It is an unpleasant feeling of apprehension or nervousness caused by the perception of potential or actual danger threatening the security of the person. *Mild anxiety* is a state of heightened awareness of the surroundings and is seen in response to day-to-day circumstances. This type of anxiety can be beneficial as a motivator for the individual to take action in a reasonable and adaptive manner. It is sometimes said that we "rise to the occasion." Patients are said to suffer from *anxiety disorder* when their responses to stressful situations are abnormal, irrational, and impair normal daily functioning. The National Institute of Mental Health identifies anxiety disorders as the most frequently encountered mental disorder in clinical practice. Sixteen percent of the general population will experience an anxiety disorder during their lifetime. Anxiety disorders usually begin before the age of 30 and are more common in women than men. The most common types of anxiety disorders are generalized anxiety disorder, panic disorder, social phobia, simple phobia, and obsessive compulsive disorder.

Generalized anxiety disorder is described as excessive and unrealistic worry about two or more life circumstances (for example, finances, illness, misfortune) for 6 months or more. Symptoms are both psychologic (tension, fear, difficulty concentrating, and apprehension) and physical (tachycardia, palpitations, tremor, sweating, and gastrointestinal upset). The disease has a gradual onset, usually in the 20 to 30 year age group, and is equally common in men and women. This illness usually follows a chronic fluctuating course of exacerbations and remissions triggered by stressful events in the person's life.

Panic disorder is recognized as a separate disease and not a more severe form of chronic generalized anxiety disorder. The average age of onset is in the late twenties. It is often relapsing and may require lifetime treatment. Genetic factors appear to play a significant role in the disease because 15% to 20% of patients have a close relative with a similar illness. Panic disorder begins as a series of acute or unprovoked anxiety (panic) attacks involving an intense, terrifying fear. The attacks do not occur on exposure to an anxiety-causing situation as phobias do. Initially the panic attacks are spontaneous, but later in the course of the illness they may be associated with certain actions (for example, driving a car, being in a crowded place). Symptoms include dyspnea, dizziness, palpitations, trembling, choking, sweating, numbness, and chest pain. There are usually feelings of impending doom or a fear of losing control.

Phobias are irrational fears of a specific object, activity, or situation. Unlike other anxiety disorders, the object or activity that creates the feeling of fear is recognized by the patient, who also realizes that the fear is unreasonable. The fear persists, however, and the patient seeks to avoid the situation. *Social phobia* is described as a fear of certain social situations in which the person is exposed to scrutiny by others and fears doing something embarassing. A social phobia toward public speaking is common and is usually avoided by the individual. If the speaking is unavoidable, it is done, but with intense anxiety. Social phobias are rarely incapacitating but do cause some interference with social or occupational functioning. *Simple phobia* is an irrational fear of a specific object or situation such as heights (acrophobia), closed spaces (claustrophobia), air travel, or driving. Phobias to animals, such as spiders, snakes, and mice, are particularly common. If the person is exposed to the object, there is an immediate feeling of panic, sweating, and tachycardia. Persons are aware of the phobia and simply avoid the feared object.

Obsessive-compulsive disorder is the most disabling of the anxiety disorders, although it is responsive to treatment. The primary features of the illness are recurrent obsessions or compulsions that cause significant distress and interfere with normal occupational responsibilities, social activities, and relationships. The average age of onset of symptoms of obsessive compulsive disorder is late adolescence to early twenties. It occurs with equal frequency in men and women. There also appears to be a genetic component to the disease. An **obsession** is an unwanted thought, idea, image, or urge that the patient recognizes as time consuming and senseless but that repeatedly intrudes into the consciousness despite attempts to ignore, prevent, or counteract it. Examples of obsessions are recurrent thoughts of dirt or germ contamination, fear of losing things, need to know or remember, need to count or check, blasphemous thoughts, or concerns about something happening to oneself or others. An obsession produces a tremendous sense of anxiety in the person. **Compulsions** are repetitive, intentional, purposeful behaviors performed to decrease the anxiety associated with an obsession. The act is done to prevent a vague, dreaded event, but the person does not derive pleasure from the act. Common compulsions deal with cleanliness, grooming, and counting. When patients are prevented from performing a compulsion, there is a sense of mounting anxiety. In some individuals, the compulsion can become the person's lifetime activity. Obsessive-compulsive disorder is a complex condition that requires a highly individualized, integrated approach to treatment with pharmacologic, behavioral, and psychosocial components.

Drug Therapy for Anxiety Disorders

Anxiety is a component of many medical illnesses involving the cardiovascular, pulmonary, digestive, or endocrine systems. It is also a primary symptom of many psychiatric disorders such as schizophrenia, mania, depression, dementia, and substance abuse. Therefore evaluation of the anxious patient requires a thorough history and physical and psychiatric examination to determine whether the anxiety is a primary condition or secondary to another illness. Persistent irrational anxiety or episodic anxiety usually requires medical and psychiatric treatment. Treatment of anxiety disorders usually requires a combination of nonpharmacologic and pharmacologic therapies. When it is decided to treat the anxiety in addition to the other medical or psychiatric diagnoses, *antianxiety* medications, also known as **anxiolytics** or **tranquilizers**, are prescribed.

Actions

A great many medications have been used to treat anxiety. They range from the purely sedative effects of ethanol, bromides, chloral hydrate, and barbiturates to drugs with more specific antianxiety and less sedative activity, such as the benzodiazepines, buspirone, meprobamate, and hydroxyzine. More recently, tricyclic antidepressants (for example, imipramine), propranolol (a beta-adrenergic antagonist), and fluoxetine and fluoxamine (serotonin agonists) have been successful in treating anxiety disorders. See individual monographs for mechanisms of action.

Uses

Generalized anxiety disorder is treated with psychotherapy and the short-term use of antianxiety agents. The benzodiazepines, buspirone, and to some extent the beta-adrenergic blocking agents (See Chapter 11) are used. Barbiturates, meprobamate, and antihistamines such as hydroxyzine are infrequently prescribed. Panic disorders may be treated with a variety of agents in addition to behavioral therapy. Alprazolam (a benzodiazepine) is approved by the Food and Drug Administration (FDA) for treatment of panic disorder. Other agents that have been beneficial are the tricyclic antidepressants imipramine, desipramine, and clomipramine (See

Chapter 15), the serotonin agonist fluoxetine (See Chapter 15), and the monoamine oxidase inhibitor phenelzine (See Chapter 15). Phobias are treated with behavior therapy and beta-adrenergic blockers such as propranolol or atenolol or the monoamine oxidase inhibitor phenelzine. Obsessive-compulsive disorder is treated with behavioral and psycho-social therapy in addition to clomipramine, fluoxetine, or fluvoxamine.

Nursing Process for Anxiety Disorders

Assessment

History of behavior. • Obtain a history of the precipitating factors that may have triggered or contributed to the individual's current anxiety. Has the individual been using alcohol or drugs? Has the patient had a recent loss, for example job, relationship, death of loved one, divorce? Has the individual witnessed or survived a traumatic event? Does the individual have any medical problems that could be attributed to these symptoms, for example, hyperthyroidism? Are there symptoms present that could be attributed to a panic attack, for example, feeling of choking, palpitations, sweating, chest pain or discomfort, nausea or abdominal distress, fear of losing control or going crazy, fear of dying? Does the individual have symptoms of obsessions or compulsions? Does the individual have a history of agoraphobia (situations in which the individual feels trapped or unable to escape)? Did the attack occur in response to a social or performance situation? Is the patient also depressed? What specific fears does the individual have? • Take a detailed history of all medications the individual is taking. Is there any use of central nervous system stimulants, for example, cocaine or amphetamines, or central nervous system depressants, for example, alcohol or barbiturates? • Ask details regarding the length of time the individual has been exhibiting anxiety. Has the person been treated for anxiety previously? When did the symptoms start? Did the symptoms start during intoxication or during withdrawal from a substance?

Basic mental status. • Note general appearance and appropriateness of attire. Is the individual clean and neat? Is the posture stooped, erect, or slumped? Is the person oriented to date, time, place, and person? • What coping mechanisms has the individual been using to deal with the situation? Are they adaptive or maladaptive? • Assess the relationships that provide the individual with support. Identify persons that are supportive.

Mood/affect. • Is the individual tearful, excessively excited, angry, hostile, or apathetic? Is the facial expression tense, fearful, sad, angry, or blank? Ask the person to describe his or her feelings. Is there worry over real-life problems? Are the person's responses displayed as an intense fear, detachment, or an absence of emotions? If the patient is a child, are there episodes of tantrums or clinging? • Patients experiencing altered thinking, behavior, or feelings need careful evaluation of both verbal and nonverbal actions. Many times, the thoughts, feelings, and behaviors displayed are inconsistent with the so-called normal responses of individuals in similar circumstances. • Assess whether the mood being described is consistent with the circumstances being described; for example, is the person speaking of death, yet smiling?

Clarity of thought. Evaluate the coherency, relevancy, and organization of thoughts. Ask specific questions regarding the individual's ability to make judgments and decisions. Is there any memory impairment?

Psychomotor functions. Ask specific questions regarding the activity level the patient has maintained. Is the person able to work or go to school? Is the person able to fulfill responsibilities at work, socially, or within the family? How have the person's normal responses to daily activities been altered? Is the individual irritable, angry, easily startled, or hypervigilant? Observe for gestures, gait, hand tremors, voice quivering, and level of activity, for example, pacing or inability to sit still.

Obsessions or compulsions. Does the individual have persistent thoughts, images, or ideas that are inappropriate and cause increased anxiety? Are there repetitive physical or mental behaviors, for example, hand washing, need to arrange things in perfect symmetric order, praying, silently repeating words? If obsessions or compulsions are present, how often do these occur? Do the obsessions or compulsions impair the person's social or occupational functioning?

Sleep pattern. What is the person's normal sleep pattern and how has it varied since the onset of the symptoms? Ask specifically whether insomnia is present. Ask the individual to describe the amount and quality of sleep. What is the degree of fatigue present? Is the individual having recurrent, distressful dreams (after a traumatic event)? Is there difficulty falling or staying asleep?

Dietary history. Ask questions relating to appetite and note weight gains or losses not associated with intentional dieting.

Nursing Diagnosis
- Anxiety, acute, chronic, panic (indication)
- Individual coping, ineffective (indication)
- Posttraumatic response (indication)
- Injury, risk for (side effects)

Planning

History of behavior. • Review data collected to identify individual's ability to understand new information, follow directions, and provide self-care. • Review medications being taken to specifically identify any that are central nervous system stimulants or depressants.

Basic mental status. • Plan to perform a baseline assessment of the individual's mental status at specific intervals throughout the course of treatment to identify the level of anxiety present and response to therapeutic interventions (including medication therapy). • Identify events that trigger anxiety. • Review coping mechanisms being used and plan to discuss those that are maladaptive. Initiate changes by guiding the individual in the use of more effective coping strategies to deal with the threatening stimuli. • Schedule specific times to discuss the patient's behavior and thoughts and foster understanding of it with family members. Involve family or significant others in the discussion of the anxiety-producing events or circumstances and ways that they can be helpful to the patient in reducing the anxiety or coping more adaptively with stressors.

Mood/affect. Review assessment data to plan strategies to assist the individual to decrease the level of anxiety and to identify management techniques to handle anxiety-producing situations effectively.

Clarity of thought. • Identify areas in which the patient is capable of input to set goals and make decisions. (This will aid the individual to overcome a sense of powerlessness over life situations.) Provide an opportunity to plan for self-care. When the patient is unable to make decisions, plan to make them and set goals to involve the patient to the degree of capability as abilities change with treatment. • Identify signs of escalating anxiety; plan interventions to decrease escalation of anxiety.

Psychomotor function. • Review activities offered within the clinical setting and plan for the individual to participate in those that will provide distraction and relaxation and decrease the level of anxiety exhibited. • Provide a structured, safe environment in which the individual can function. • During severe or panic anxiety, provide a safe place for the release of energy.

Sleep pattern. Plan for providing a nonstimulating environment (dim lighting, quiet area) that will encourage drowsiness and sleep.

Dietary needs. Provide an opportunity for the individual to be involved in selecting foods appropriate to needs (to lose or gain weight).

Implementation

- Deal with problems as they present themselves; practice reality orientation.
- Provide a safe, structured environment; set limits on aggressive and destructive behaviors.
- Establish a trusting relationship with the patient by providing support and reassurance.
- Reduce stimulation by having interactions with the patient in a quiet, calm environment.
- Provide an opportunity for the individual to express feelings. Use active listening and therapeutic communication techniques. Be especially aware of cues that would indicate the patient may be considering self-harm. (If suspecting suicidal ideas, ask the patient directly if suicide is being considered and intervene to provide for safety.)
- Allow patients to make decisions of which they are capable, make decisions when the patient is not capable, and provide a reward for progress when decisions are initiated appropriately. Involve the patient in self-care activities. During periods of severe anxiety or during escalating anxiety the individual may be unable to have insight and make decisions appropriately.
- Encourage the individual to develop coping skills through the use of various techniques, for example, rehearsing or role-playing responses to threatening stressors. Have the individual practice problem solving; discuss possible consequences of the solutions offered by the patient.

Patient Education and Health Promotion

- Orient the individual to the unit, explaining rules and the process of "privileges" and how they are obtained or lost. (The extent of the orientation and explanations given will depend on the individual's orientation to date, time, and place and abilities.)
- Explain the activity groups available and how and when the individual will participate in these. A variety of group process activities (for example, social skills group, self-esteem groups, work-related groups, and physical exercise groups) exist within particular therapeutic settings. Meditation, biofeedback, and relaxation therapy may also be beneficial.
- Involve the patient and family in goal setting and integrate into the available group processes to develop positive experiences for the individual to enhance coping skills.
- Patient education will be individualized and based on assessment data to provide the individual with a structured environment in which to grow and enhance self-esteem. Initially, the individual may not be capable of understanding lengthy explanations, therefore the approaches used will be based on the patient's capabilities.
- Explore coping mechanisms the person uses in response to stressors, and identify methods of channeling these toward positive realistic goals as an alternative to the use of medications.

Fostering health maintenance. • Throughout the course of treatment, discuss medication information and how it will benefit the patient. Stress the importance of the nonpharmacologic interventions and the long-term effects that compliance with the treatment regimen can provide. • Provide the patient and significant others with important information contained in the specific drug monograph for the medicines prescribed. Additional health teaching and nursing interventions for the side effects to expect and report are described in the drug monographs that follow. • Seek cooperation and understanding of the following points so that medication compliance is increased: name of medication, dosage, route and times of administration, side effects to expect, and side effects to report. • Written record: Enlist the patient's aid in developing and maintaining a written record of monitoring parameters (See Patient Education and Monitoring box on p. 186.) Instruct the patient to bring the written record to follow-up visits.

Drug Class: Benzodiazepines

Benzodiazepines are most commonly used because they are more consistently effective, less likely to interact with other drugs, less likely to cause overdose, and have less potential for abuse than barbiturates and other antianxiety agents. They now account for perhaps 75% of the 100 million prescriptions written annually for anxiety. More than 2000 benzodiazepine derivatives have been identified, and more than 100 have been tested for sedative-hypnotic or other activity. Eight benzodiazepine derivatives are used as antianxiety agents (Table 14-1).

Actions

It is thought that the benzodiazepines have mechanisms of action similar to those of central nervous system depressants but that individual drugs within the benzodiazepine family act more selectively at specific sites, which allows for a variety of uses (for example, sedative-hypnotic, muscle relaxant, antianxiety, and anticonvulsant). The benzodiazepines reduce anxiety by stimulating the action of an inhibitory neurotransmitter, gamma-aminobutyric acid (GABA).

In patients with reduced hepatic function or in the elderly, alprazolam, lorazepam, or oxazepam may be most appropri-

PATIENT EDUCATION AND MONITORING Antianxiety Medication

MEDICATIONS	COLOR	TO BE TAKEN

Name _____

Physician _____

Physician's phone _____

Next appt.* _____

PARAMETERS	DAY OF DISCHARGE							COMMENTS
Weight								
Blood Pressure	AM / PM	AM / PM	AM / PM	AM / PM	AM / PM	AM / PM	AM / PM	
Resting pulse rate								
I would like to be alone? All the time 10 Some of the time 5 Not really 1								
How I feel about my children? Too much work 10 5 Fun to be with 1								
How I feel today? Poor 10 Fair 5 Okay 1								
Appetite? Poor 10 Fair 5 Good 1 (B L D SNACK)								
Has family noted any problems: Judgment? Socialization?								
Does patient dress daily (Yes/No)?								
Does patient take pride in appearance (Yes/No)?								
Use of alcohol (Yes/No)? Amount (e.g., one drink)?								
General Mood: Tearful, excessively excited, angry, hostile, happy or apathetic.								
Sleep pattern: Amount of sleep per night: _____ hrs. Degree of fatigue: rested, slightly fatigued, exhausted. Insomnia: Yes or No								

*Please bring this record with you to your next appointment.
Use the back of this sheet for additional information.

Table 14-1

Benzodiazepines Used to Treat Anxiety

GENERIC NAME	BRAND NAME	AVAILABILITY	INITIAL DOSE (PO)	MAXIMUM DAILY DOSE (MG)
Alprazolam	Xanax	Tablets: 0.25, 0.5, 1, 2 mg Solution: 0.5 mg/5 ml, 1 mg/ml	0.25-0.5 mg 3 times daily	4
Chlordiazepoxide	Librium, Mitran	Tablets: 5, 25 mg Capsules: 5, 10, 25 mg Inj: 100 mg	5-10 mg 3-4 times daily	300
Clorazepate	Tranxene ✲ Novo-Clopate	Tablets: 3.75, 7.5, 11.25, 15, 22.5 mg	10 mg 1-3 times daily	60
Diazepam	Valium ✲ Meval	Tablets: 2, 5, 10 mg Caps, Extended Release: 15 mg Liquid: 5 mg/5 ml Inj.: 5 mg/ml in 1, 2, 10 ml vials	2-10 mg 2-4 times daily	—
Halazepam	Paxipam	Tablets: 20, 40 mg	20 mg 1-2 times daily	160
Lorazepam	Ativan ✲ Nu-Loraz	Inj.: 2, 4 mg/ml in 1, 10 ml vials; Liquid: 2 mg/ml Tablets: 0.5, 1, 2 mg	2-3 mg 2-3 times daily	10
Oxazepam	Serax ✲ Oxpam	Tablets: 15 mg Capsules: 10, 15, 30 mg	10-15 mg 3-4 times daily	120

✲ Available in Canada only.

ate because they have a relatively short duration of action and have no active metabolites. Oxazepam has been the most thoroughly investigated. The other benzodiazepines all have active metabolites that significantly prolong the duration of action and may accumulate to the point of excessive side effects with long-term administration. The primary active ingredient of both prazepam and clorazepate is desmethyldiazepam; therefore similar activity and patient response should be expected. Halazepam and diazepam are therapeutically active, but their major metabolite is also desmethyldiazepam; therefore similar responses should be expected with long-term administration. Oxazepam, lorazepam, chlordiazepoxide, diazepam, and clorazepate are all approved for use in treating the anxiety associated with alcohol withdrawal. Oxazepam is the drug of choice because it has no active metabolites. However, its use is somewhat limited in patients who cannot tolerate oral administration because it causes nausea and vomiting. Chlordiazepoxide, diazepam, or lorazepam may be administered intramuscularly in this case.

Uses

Patients with anxiety reactions to recent events and patients with a treatable medical illness that induces anxiety respond most readily to benzodiazepine therapy. Because all the benzodiazepines have similar mechanisms of action, selection of the appropriate derivative depends on how the benzodiazepine is metabolized. See under Actions. Oxazepam, lorazepam, chlordiazepoxide, diazepam, and clo-

razepate are all approved for use in treating the anxiety associated with alcohol withdrawal.

Therapeutic Outcomes

The primary therapeutic outcome expected from the benzodiazepine antianxiety agents is a decrease in the level of anxiety to a manageable level (for example, coping is improved; physical signs of anxiety, such as look of anxiety, tremor, and pacing, are reduced).

Nursing Process

Premedication Assessment

1. Record baseline data on level of anxiety present.
2. Record baseline vital signs, particularly blood pressure, in sitting and supine positions.
3. Check for history of blood dyscrasias or hepatic disease.
4. Determine whether the individual is pregnant or breastfeeding.

Planning

Availability. See Table 14-1.

Pregnancy and lactation. It is generally recommended that benzodiazepines not be administered during at least the first trimester of pregnancy. There may be an increased incidence of birth defects because these agents readily cross the placenta and enter fetal circulation. Mothers who are breastfeeding should not receive benzodiazepines regularly. The benzodiazepines readily cross into breast milk and exert a pharmacologic effect on the infant.

Implementation

Dosage and administration. See Table 14-1. The habitual use of benzodiazepines may result in physical and psychologic dependence. Rapid discontinuance of benzodiazepines after long-term use may result in symptoms similar to those of alcohol withdrawal. These may vary from weakness and anxiety to delirium and grand mal seizures. The symptoms may not appear for several days after discontinuation. Treatment consists of gradual withdrawal of benzodiazepines over a 2- to 4-week period.

Evaluation

Side effects to expect

DROWSINESS, "HANGOVER," SEDATION, LETHARGY. Patients may complain of "morning hangover," blurred vision, and transient hypotension on arising. Explain to the patient the need for rising first to a sitting position, equilibrating, and then standing. Assistance with ambulation may be required.

If hangover becomes troublesome there should be a reduction in the dosage, a change in the medication, or both.

Persons who are working with machinery, driving a car, pouring and giving medicines, or performing other duties in which they must remain mentally alert should not take these medications while working.

Side effects to report

EXCESSIVE USE OR ABUSE. Habitual use of barbiturates may result in physical dependence. Discuss the case with the physician and make plans to cooperatively approach gradual withdrawal of the medications being abused. Assist the patient in recognizing the abuse problem. Identify underlying needs and plan for more appropriate management of those needs. Provide for emotional support of the individual; display an accepting attitude—be kind but firm.

BLOOD DYSCRASIAS. Routine laboratory studies (red blood cell count [RBC], white blood cell [WBC], and differential counts) should be scheduled. Stress the patient's need to return for these tests. Monitor for the development of sore throat, fever, purpura, jaundice, or excessive and progressive weakness.

HEPATOTOXICITY. The symptoms of hepatotoxicity are anorexia, nausea, vomiting, jaundice, hepatomegaly, splenomegaly, and abnormal liver function tests (elevated bilirubin, aspartate transaminase [AST], alanine aminotransferose [ALT], gamma glutalnufitransferase [GGT], alkaline phosphatase, prothrombin time).

Drug interactions

DRUGS THAT INCREASE TOXIC EFFECTS. Antihistamines, alcohol, analgesics, anesthetics, tranquilizers, narcotics, cimetidine, and other sedative-hypnotics increase toxic effects.

SMOKING. Smoking enhances the metabolism of the benzodiazepines. Larger doses may be necessary to maintain sedative effects in patients who smoke.

Drug Class: Azapirones

 buspirone (byoo-spye′rown)
BuSpar (byoo-spar′)

Actions

Buspirone is an antianxiety agent from the chemical class known as the azapirones. They are chemically unrelated to the barbiturates, benzodiazepines, or other anxiolytic agents. The mechanism of action of buspirone is not fully understood. It is a serotonin partial agonist and interacts in several ways with nerve systems in the midbrain; therefore it is sometimes called a midbrain modulator. Its advantage over other antianxiety agents is that it has lower sedative properties. It requires 7 to 10 days of treatment before initial signs of improvement are evident and 3 to 4 weeks of therapy for optimal effects.

Uses

It is approved for use in the treatment of anxiety disorders and for the short-term relief of the symptoms of anxiety. Buspirone has no antipsychotic activity and should not be used in place of appropriate psychiatric treatment. Because there is minimal potential for abuse with buspirone, it is not a controlled substance.

Therapeutic Outcomes

The primary therapeutic outcome expected from buspirone is a decrease in the level of anxiety to a manageable level (for example, coping is improved; physical signs of anxiety, such as look of anxiety, tremor, and pacing, are reduced).

Nursing Process

Premedication Assessment

Record baseline data on the level of anxiety present.

Planning

Availability. PO—5 and 10 mg tablets. Schedule assessments periodically throughout therapy for development of slurred speech or dizziness, which are signs of excessive dosage.

Implementation

Dosage and administration. Adult: PO—Initially 5 mg 3 times daily. Doses may be increased by 5 mg every 2 to 3 days. Maintenance therapy often requires 20 to 30 mg daily in divided dosages. Do not exceed 60 mg daily.

Evaluation

Side effects to expect

SEDATION, LETHARGY. The most common adverse effects of buspirone therapy are central nervous system disturbances (3.4%), which include dizziness, insomnia, nervousness, drowsiness, and light-headedness.

Persons who are working around machinery or performing other duties in which they must remain mentally alert should not take this medication while working.

Side effects to report

SLURRED SPEECH, DIZZINESS. These are signs of excessive dosage. Report to the physician for further evaluation. Provide for patient safety during these episodes.

Drug interactions

ALCOHOL. Buspirone and alcohol generally do not have additive central nervous system depressant effects, but individual patients may be susceptible to impairment. Use with extreme caution.

Drug Class: Selective Serotonin Reuptake Inhibitors (SSRI)

fluvoxamine (floo-vox′a-meen)
Luvox (loo-vox′)

Action

Fluvoxamine inhibits the reuptake of serotonin at nerve endings, which prolongs serotonin activity.

Uses

Fluvoxamine is used in the treatment of obsessive-compulsive disorder when obsessions or compulsions cause marked distress, are time consuming, or interfere substantially with social or occupational responsibilities. Fluvoxamine reduces the symptoms of this disorder but does not prevent obsessions and compulsions. However, patients indicate that the obsessions are less intrusive and they have more control over them.

Therapeutic Outcomes

The primary therapeutic outcome expected from fluvoxamine is a decrease in the level of anxiety to a manageable level (for example, coping with obsession is improved, frequency of compulsive activity is reduced).

Nursing Process

See "Selective Serotonin Reuptake Inhibitors" above.

Drug Class: Miscellaneous Antianxiety Agents

hydroxyzine (hye-drox′ee-zeen)
Vistaril (vĭs′-tăr′ĭl), **Atarax** (ăt′-ā-raks″)

Actions

Defined strictly by chemical structure, hydroxyzine is an antihistamine. However, it acts within the central nervous system to produce sedation and antiemetic, anticholinergic, antihistaminic, antianxiety, and antispasmodic activity. This variety of actions makes it a somewhat multipurpose agent.

Uses

Hydroxyzine is used as a mild tranquilizer in psychiatric conditions characterized by anxiety, tension, and agitation. It is also routinely used as a preoperative or postoperative sedative to control vomiting, diminish anxiety, and reduce the amount of narcotics needed for analgesia. Hydroxyzine may also be used as an antipruritic agent to relieve the itching associated with allergic reactions.

Therapeutic Outcomes

The primary therapeutic outcomes expected from hydroxyzine are as follows:

- A decrease in the level of anxiety to a manageable level (for example, coping is improved; physical signs of anxiety, such as look of anxiety, tremor, and pacing, are reduced)
- Sedation, relaxation, and reduced requirements for analgesics before and after surgery
- Absence of vomiting when used as an antiemetic
- Itching controlled in allergic reactions

Nursing Process

Premedication Assessment

1. Perform baseline assessment of anxiety symptoms.
2. Determine level of anxiety present before and after surgical intervention; record and intervene appropriately.
3. For nausea and vomiting, administer when nausea first starts and determine effectiveness of control of nausea before giving subsequent doses.
4. For allergic reactions, perform baseline assessment of physical symptoms before administering dose; repeat before administration of subsequent doses to determine effectiveness.
5. Monitor for level of sedation present, slurred speech, and dizziness; report to physician if excessive before administering repeat doses.

Planning

Availability. PO—10, 25, 50, and 100 mg tablets and capsules, 10 mg per 5 ml syrup, 25 mg per 5 ml suspension. IM—25 and 50 mg per ml.

Implementation

Dosage and administration
Antianxiety. Adult: PO—25 to 100 mg 3 to 4 times daily. IM—50 to 100 mg every 4 to 6 hours.
Preoperative and Postoperative. Adult: IM—25 to 100 mg.
Antiemetic. Adult: IM—25 to 100 mg.

Evaluation

Side effects to expect
BLURRED VISION, CONSTIPATION, DRYNESS OF MUCOSA OF THE MOUTH, THROAT, AND NOSE. These symptoms are the anticholinergic effects produced by hydroxyzine. Patients taking these medications should be monitored for the development of these side effects.

Dryness of the mucosa may be relieved by sucking hard candy or ice chips or by chewing gum.

The use of stool softeners such as docusate may be required for constipation.

Caution the patient that blurred vision may occur, and make appropriate suggestions for personal safety.

SEDATION. Persons who are working with machinery, driving a car, pouring and giving medicines, or performing other duties in which they must remain mentally alert should not take these medications while working.

Side effects to report
SLURRED SPEECH, DIZZINESS. These are signs of excessive dosage. Report to the physician for further evaluation. Provide for patient safety during these episodes.

Drug interactions
DRUGS THAT INCREASE TOXIC EFFECTS. Antihistamines, alcohol, analgesics, anesthetics, tranquilizers, barbiturates,

narcotics, and other sedative-hypnotics. Monitor the patient for excessive sedation, and reduce the dosage of the hydroxyzine if necessary.

meprobamate (me-proe-ba′mate)
Equanil (ek′wah′-nil), **Miltown** (mil′-taün)

Actions

Meprobamate acts on multiple sites within the central nervous system to produce mild sedation, antianxiety, and muscle relaxation. The mechanism of action is unknown.

Uses

Meprobamate is used as an antianxiety agent and mild skeletal muscle relaxant for the short-term relief (less than 4 months) of anxiety and tension. It is of little use in the treatment of psychoses.

Therapeutic Outcomes

The primary therapeutic outcome expected from meprobamate is a decrease in the level of anxiety to a manageable level (for example, coping is improved; physical signs of anxiety, such as look of anxiety, tremor, and pacing, are reduced).

Nursing Process

Premedication Assessment

Record baseline data on the level of anxiety present.

Planning

Availability. PO—200, 400, and 600 mg tablets; 200 and 400 mg extended-release capsules. Schedule assessments periodically throughout therapy for development of slurred speech or dizziness, which are signs of excessive dosage, use, or abuse.

Implementation

Dosage and administration. Adult: PO—400 mg 3 to 4 times daily. Smaller doses may work well in elderly and debilitated patients. Maximum daily doses should not exceed 2400 mg.

Evaluation

Side effects to expect

SEDATION. Persons who are working with machinery, driving a car, pouring and giving medicines, or performing other duties in which they must remain mentally alert should not take these medications while working.

Side effects to report

SLURRED SPEECH, DIZZINESS. These are signs of excessive dosage. Report to the physician for further evaluation. Provide for patient safety during these episodes.

EXCESSIVE USE OR ABUSE. Psychologic and physiologic dependence may occur in patients taking doses of 3.3 to 6.4 g per day for 40 or more days. Symptoms of chronic use and abuse of high doses include ataxia, slurred speech, and dizziness. Withdrawal reactions such as vomiting, tremors, confusion, hallucinations, and grand mal seizures may develop within 12 to 48 hours after abrupt discontinuation. Symptoms usually decline within the next 12 to 48 hours.

Withdrawal from high and prolonged dosages should be completed gradually over 1 to 2 weeks.

Discuss the case with the physician and make plans to cooperatively approach gradual withdrawal of the medications being abused. Assist the patient in recognizing the abuse problem. Identify underlying needs and plan for more appropriate management of those needs. Provide for emotional support of the individual; display an accepting attitude—be kind but firm.

ORTHOSTATIC HYPOTENSION (DIZZINESS, WEAKNESS, FAINTNESS). Although this effect is infrequent and generally mild, meprobamate may cause some degree of orthostatic hypotension manifested by dizziness and weakness, particularly when therapy is being initiated.

Anticipate the development of postural hypotension and take measures to prevent an occurrence. Teach the patient to rise slowly from a supine or sitting position; encourage the patient to sit or lie down if feeling faint.

Monitor the blood pressure daily in both the supine and standing positions.

PARADOXIC EXCITEMENT, ARRHYTHMIAS. Withhold further doses, report for further evaluation.

HIVES, PRURITUS, RASH. Report symptoms for further evaluation by the physician. Pruritus may be relieved by adding baking soda to the bath water.

Drug interactions

DRUGS THAT INCREASE TOXIC EFFECTS. Antihistamines, alcohol, analgesics, tranquilizers, narcotics, and other sedative-hypnotics. Monitor the patient for excessive sedation, and reduce the dosage of the meprobamate if necessary.

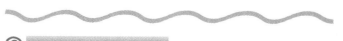

CHAPTER REVIEW

Anxiety is an unpleasant feeling of apprehension or nervousness caused by the perception of danger threatening the security of the person. In most cases, it is a normal human emotion. When a person's response to anxiety is irrational and impairs daily functioning, patients are said to suffer from an anxiety disorder. Approximately 16% of the general population will experience an anxiety disorder during their lifetime. The most common types of anxiety disorders are generalized anxiety disorder, panic disorder, social phobia, simple phobia, and obsessive-compulsive disorder.

Anxiety is a component of many medical illnesses involving the cardiovascular, pulmonary, digestive, or endocrine systems. It is also a primary symptom of many psychiatric disorders. Therefore evaluation of the anxious patient requires a thorough history and physical and psychiatric examination to determine whether the anxiety is a primary condition or secondary to another illness. Persistent irrational anxiety or episodic anxiety usually requires medical and psychiatric treatment. Treatment of anxiety disorders usually requires a combination of nonpharmacologic and pharmacologic therapies. It is the responsibility of the nurse to educate patients about their therapy, monitoring for therapeutic benefit, and side effects to expect and to report, intervening whenever possible to optimize therapeutic outcomes.

MATH REVIEW

1. Ordered: Hydroxyzine (Vistaril) 20 mg, IM, stat.
   On hand: Hydroxyzine (Vistaril) 25 mg per ml.
   Give: _____ml.

2. Ordered: Meprobamate (Equanil) 1600 mg PO daily in 4 divided doses.
   How many mg per dose will be administered?

3. Ordered: Loprazepam (Ativan) 2.5 mg, IM, stat.
   On hand: Lorazepam (Ativan) 4 mg per ml.
   Give: _____ml.

CRITICAL THINKING QUESTIONS

Mrs. Higginbaum is admitted to the unit with symptoms of generalized anxiety disorder. During the admission interview the following information was obtained.

She is so fearful of losing her job that she discusses it several times a day as a possibility. This has been an increasing concern to her over the past 8 months. Her work performance was regarded as above average; however, over the past 2 months she has had increasing difficulty concentrating and completing her responsibilities. Finally, last week her employer suggested she take a brief vacation to "get it together." Since then the symptoms have escalated significantly.

She is having difficulty falling asleep and frequently awakens with palpitations and clammy hands.

When asked to describe her feelings she says, "I'm out of control, I'm going to lose my job. What am I ever going to do?"

1. What additional nursing assessments must be made? Research a typical data intake assessment sheet used with anxiety disorders.

2. Her admission orders include administering alprazolam 0.25 mg, tid. What time schedule would be used to administer these doses?

3. Describe premedication assessment data needed and what additional assessments should be made after initiation of drug therapy using benzodiazepines.

4. How soon after initiation of drug therapy is it reasonable to expect a therapeutic response from the antianxiety medication?

5. Describe the behavior monitoring system and intervention flow records used in the clinical setting that were assigned to detect the side effects of anxiolytic drugs.

6. What assessments and nursing interventions (including health teaching) should be performed to deal with the possible physical dependence or tolerance known to occur with benzodiazepine therapy?

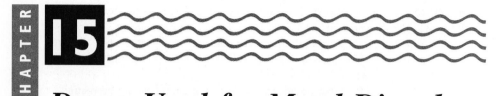

Drugs Used for Mood Disorders

CHAPTER CONTENT

Key Words

mood	mania
mood disorder	euphoria
depression	labile mood
neurotransmitter	grandiose
cognitive symptoms	suicide
psychomotor symptoms	antidepressant
bipolar disorder	

Objectives

1. Describe the essential components of a baseline assessment of a patient with depression or bipolar disorder.

2. Discuss the mood swings associated with bipolar disorder.

3. Compare drug therapy used during the treatment of the manic phase and depressive phase of bipolar disorder.

4. Cite monitoring parameters used for persons taking monoamine oxidase inhibitors (MAOIs), selective serotonin reuptake inhibitors (SSRIs), or tricyclic antidepressants.

5. Prepare a teaching plan for an individual receiving tricyclic antidepressants.

6. Differentiate between the physiologic and psychologic therapeutic responses seen with antidepressant therapy.

7. Identify the premedication assessments necessary before administration of MAOIs, SSRIs, tricyclic antidepressants, and antimanic agents.

8. Compare the mechanism of action of SSRIs to that of other antidepressant agents.

9. Cite the advantages of SSRIs over other antidepressant agents.

10. Examine the drug monograph for SSRIs to identify significant drug interactions.

MOOD DISORDERS

Mood is a sustained emotional feeling perceived along a normal continuum of sad to happy. Mood is our perception of our surroundings. **Mood disorders** (affective disorders) are said to be present when certain symptoms impair a person's ability to function for a duration of time. Mood disorders are characterized by abnormal feelings of **depression** or euphoria. They involve prolonged, inappropriate expression of emotion that go beyond brief emotional upset from negative life experiences. In severe cases, other psychotic features may also be present. At least 10% of persons in the United States suffer from a diagnosable mood disorder in their lifetime. Mood disorders are divided into depressive (unipolar) and bipolar disorders.

The underlying causes of mood disorders are still unknown. The disorders are too complex to be completely explained by a single social, developmental, or biologic theory. A variety of factors appear to work together to cause depressive disorders. It is known that patients with depression have changes in the brain **neurotransmitters** norepinephrine, serotonin and dopamine, but other unexpected negative life events (for example, sudden death of a loved one, unemployment, medical illness, other stressful events) also play a major role. Endocrine abnormalities such as excessive secretion of cortisol and abnormal thyroid-stimulating hormone (TSH) have been found to be present in 45% to 60% of patients with depression. Genetic factors also predispose patients to the development of depression. Depressive disorders and suicide tend to cluster in families, and relatives of patients with depression are two to three times more likely to develop depression.

The onset of depression tends to be in the late twenties. The lifetime frequency of depressive symptoms appears to be as high as 26% for women and 12% for men. Risk factors for depression include a personal or family history of depression, prior suicide attempts, female gender, lack of social support, stressful life events, substance abuse (especially alcohol and cocaine abuse), and medical illnesses. The American Psychiatric Association classifies episodes of depression into mild, moderate, and severe. *Mild depression* causes only minor functional impairment. Patients with *severe depression* have several symptoms that exceed the minimum diagnostic criteria, and daily functioning is greatly impaired. Hospitalization may be required. *Moderate depression* is intermediate between mild and severe conditions for both symptomatology and functional impairment.

Patients experiencing *depression* display varying degrees of emotional, physical, cognitive, and psychomotor symptoms. *Emotionally*, the depression is characterized by a persistent, reduced ability to experience pleasure in life's usual activities, such as hobbies, family, and work. Patients frequently appear sad, and a change in personality is common. They may describe mood as sad, hopeless, or blue. Patients often feel that they have let others down, although these guilt feelings are unrealistic. Anxiety symptoms (see Chapter 14) are present in almost 90% of depressed patients. *Physical* symptoms often motivate the person to seek medical attention. Chronic fatigue, sleep disturbances such as frequent early-morning awakening (terminal insomnia), appetite disturbances (weight loss or gain), and other symptoms, such as stomach complaints or heart palpitations, are common. **Cognitive symptoms** such as inability to concentrate, slowed thinking, confusion, and poor memory of recent events are particularly common in elderly patients suffering from depression. **Psychomotor symptoms** of depression include slowed or retarded movements, thought processes, and speech, or, conversely, agitation manifesting as purposeless, restless motion (for example, pacing, wringing of hands, and outbursts of shouting).

Bipolar disorder (formerly known as manic depression) is another of several mood disorders. It is characterized by distinct episodes of mania (elation, euphoria) and depression separated by intervals without mood disturbances. The patient displays extreme changes in mood, cognition, behavior, perception, and sensory experiences. At any one time, a patient with bipolar disorder may be manic or depressed, may exhibit symptoms of both mania and depression (mixed), or may be between episodes.

The depressive state has been previously described. Symptoms of acute **mania** usually begin abruptly and escalate over several days. These symptoms are a heightened mood (**euphoria**), quicker thoughts (flight of ideas), more and faster speech (pressured speech), increased energy, increased physical and mental activities (psychomotor excitement), decreased need for sleep, irritability, heightened perceptual acuity, paranoia, increased sexual activity, and impulsivity. The patient's mood is often **labile**, with rapid shifts toward anger and irritability. The attention span is short, resulting in an inability to concentrate. Anything in the environment may change the topic of discussion, leading to flight of ideas. Social inhibitions are lost and the patient may become interruptive and loud, departing suddenly from the social interaction, leaving everything in disarray. As the manic phase progresses, approximately two thirds of patients with bipolar disorder develop psychotic symptoms (see Chapter 16), primarily paranoid or **grandiose** delusions, if

treatment interventions have not been initiated. Unfortunately, most manic patients do not recognize the symptoms of illness in themselves and resist treatment.

Bipolar disorder occurs equally between men and women and has a prevalence rate of 0.6% to 0.9% of the adult population. The onset of bipolar disorder is usually in late adolescence or early twenties. It is rare in preadolescence and may occur as late as 50 years of age. Approximately 60% to 80% of patients with bipolar disease begin with a manic episode. Without treatment, episodes last 6 months to 1 year for depression and 4 months for mania.

Patients with mood disorders have a high incidence of attempting **suicide**. The frequency of successful suicide is 15%, 30 times higher than that in the general population. All patients with depressive symptoms should be assessed for the presence of suicidal thoughts. Factors that increase the risk of suicide include increasing age, being widowed, being unmarried, unemployment, living alone, substance abuse, previous psychiatric admission, and feelings of hopelessness. The presence of a detailed plan with intention and ability to carry it out indicates strong intent and a high risk of suicide. Other hints of potential suicidal intent include changes in personality, a sudden decision to make a will or give away possessions, and a recent purchase of a gun or hoarding a large supply of medication, including antidepressants, tranquilizers, or other toxic substances.

The prognosis for mood disorders is highly variable. From 20% to 30% of patients with major depression recover fully and do not experience another bout of depression. Another 50% have recurring episodes, often with a year

LIFE SPAN ISSUES

DEPRESSION

The patient and caregivers must understand the importance of continuing to take the prescribed antidepressant medication despite minimal initial response. The lag time of 1 to 4 weeks between initiation of therapy and therapeutic response must be emphasized. In most cases the symptoms of depression may improve within a few days (e.g., improved appetite, sleep, and psychomotor activity). The depression, however, still exists, and monitoring should be continued for negative thoughts, feelings, and behaviors. Suicide precautions should be maintained until assessment indicates that suicidal ideation is no longer present.

Suicide statistics are varied and not well documented. However, older people with depressions are more likely to commit suicide than are depressed persons of other age groups. It appears that the elder suicide victim is serious when attempting suicide because one of two attempts by elders is successful.

Suicide is the third-leading cause of death in adolescents; the incidence may be even higher because of underreporting. Suicide is a "call for help"; however, it is permanent when successfully completed. All comments of suicide or suicide gestures should be taken seriously.

or more seperating the events. The remaining 20% of patients have a chronic course with persistent symptoms and social impairment. Most treated episodes of depression last approximately 3 months, and those untreated last 6 to 12 months. Patients with bipolar illness are more likely to have multiple subsequent episodes of symptoms.

Treatment

Treatment of mood disorders requires both nonpharmacologic and pharmacologic therapy. Cognitive, behavioral, and interpersonal psychotherapy and pharmacologic treatment have been shown to be more successful than either treatment alone. Psychotherapy improves psychosocial function, interpersonal relationships, and day-to-day coping. Patients and family should be educated about recognizing the signs and symptoms of mania and depression and the importance of treatment compliance to minimize recurrence of the illness. Patients should be encouraged to target symptoms to help them recognize mood changes and to seek treatment as soon as possible.

Another form of nonpharmacologic treatment for depression and bipolar illness is electroconvulsive therapy (ECT). Under guidelines provided by the American Psychiatric Association, ECT is safe and effective for all subtypes of major depression and bipolar disorders. It is more effective, more rapid in onset of effect, and safer in patients with cardiovascular disease than many drug therapies. A course of ECT usually consists of 6 to 12 treatments, but the number is individualized to the needs of the patient. Patients are now premedicated with anesthetics and neuromuscular blocking agents to prevent many of the adverse effects previously associated with ECT. Although it has been misused in the past, ECT should be viewed as a treatment option that can be life saving for patients who otherwise would not recover from depressive illnesses. It is usually followed by drug therapy to minimize the rate of relapse.

Drug Therapy for Mood Disorders

Actions

Pharmacologic treatment of depression is recommended for patients with symptoms of moderate to severe depression and should be considered for patients who do not respond well to psychotherapy. The treatment is accomplished with several classes of drugs collectively known as **antidepressants**. The antidepressants can be subdivided into the monamine oxidase inhibitors (MAOIs), tricyclic antidepressants, selective serotonin reuptake inhibitors (SSRIs), and a miscellaneous group of monocyclic and tetracyclic agents. All of these agents have varying degrees of effect on norepinephrine, dopamine, and serotonin, blocking reuptake and destruction of these neurotransmitters, thereby prolonging their action. They also have an effect on neurotransmitter receptors that requires 2 to 4 weeks of therapy at adequate dosages. This coincides with the time necessary for development of clinical antidepressant response. Although much is known about the pharmacologic actions of the antidepressants, the exact mechanism of action of these agents in treating depression is still unknown. It is now understood, however, that depression is not simply a deficiency of neurotransmitters.

Uses

Two factors are important in selecting an antidepressant drug: the patient's past history of response to previously prescribed antidepressants and the potential for adverse effects associated with different classes of antidepressants. Contrary to marketing claims, there are no differences among antidepressant drugs (with the exception of the MAOIs) in relative overall therapeutic efficacy and onset caused by full therapeutic effect. There are, however, substantial differences in the adverse effects caused by different agents. It is not possible to predict which drug will be most effective in an individual patient, but patients do show a better response to a specific drug. Approximately 30% of patients do not show appreciable therapeutic benefit with the first agent used but have a high degree of success with a change in medication. The history of previous treatment is helpful in selection of new treatment if illness returns. Approximately 65% to 70% of patients respond to antidepressant therapy, and 30% to 40% of patients respond to placebo treatment. Therapeutic success can be improved by monitoring serum levels and adjusting doses to maintain therapeutic serum levels. Certain types of mood disorders respond more readily than others.

Patients must be counseled on expected therapeutic benefits and adverse effects to be tolerated from antidepressant therapy. The physiologic manifestations of depression (for example, sleep disturbance, change in appetite, loss of energy, fatigue, palpitations) will begin to be alleviated within the first week of therapy. The psychologic symptoms (for example, depressed mood, lack of interest, social withdrawal) will improve after 2 to 4 weeks of therapy at an effective dosage. Therefore it may take 4 to 6 weeks to adjust the dosage to optimize therapy and minimize side effects. Unfortunately, some adverse effects develop early in therapy, and patients, who are already pessimistic because of their illness, have a tendency to be noncompliant.

The pharmacologic treatment of bipolar disorder must be individualized because the clinical presentation, severity, and frequency of episodes vary widely among patients. Acute mania is initially treated with lithium in conjunction with benzodiazepines (see Chapter 14) or antipsychotics (see Chapter 16) for sedation. Once the patient is stabilized, most patients are placed on long-term lithium therapy to minimize future episodes. Therapy with carbamazepine or valproic acid may be used for patients who do not adequately respond to lithium.

Nursing Process for Mood Disorders

Assessment

History of mood disorder. • Obtain a history of the mood disorder. Is it depressive only, or are there both manic and depressive phases interspersed with periods of normalcy? What precipitating factors contribute to the changes in mood? How frequently do the depressive, normal, and manic moods persist? Are there better or worse times of the day? Has the patient been treated previously for a mood disorder? What is the patient's current status? Has the individual been using alcohol or drugs? Has there been a recent loss, for example, job, relationship, death of loved one? • Take a detailed history of all medications the individual is taking and those taken within the last 2 months. How compliant has the patient been with the treatment regimen?

Basic mental status. • Note general appearance and appropriateness of attire. Is the individual clean and neat? Is the posture erect, stooped, or slumped? Is the individual oriented to date, time, place, and person? • What coping mechanisms has the individual been using to deal with the mood disorder? How adaptive are the coping mechanisms?

Interpersonal relationships. • Assess the individual's interpersonal relationships. Identify persons that are supportive. • Identify whether interpersonal relationships have declined between the patient and persons in the family and at work or in social settings.

Mood/affect • Is the individual elated, overjoyed, angry, irritable, crying, tearful, or sad? Is the facial expression tense, worried, sad, angry, or blank? Tell the person to describe feelings. Be alert for expressions of loneliness, apathy, worthlessness, or hopelessness. Moods may change suddenly. • Patients experiencing altered thinking, behavior, or feelings must be carefully evaluated for both verbal and nonverbal actions. Many times, the thoughts, feelings, and behaviors displayed are inconsistent with the so-called normal responses of individuals in similar circumstances. • Assess whether the mood being described is consistent with the circumstances being described; for example, is the person speaking of death, yet smiling?

Clarity of thought. Evaluate the coherency, relevancy, and organization of thoughts—observe for flight of ideas, hallucinations, delusions, paranoia, or grandiose ideation. Ask specific questions regarding the individual's ability to make judgments and decisions. Is there evidence of memory impairment?

Thoughts of death. If the individual is suspected of being suicidal, ask the patient if there have ever been thoughts about suicide. If the response is yes, get more details. Is a specific plan formulated? How often do these thoughts occur? Does the individual make direct or indirect statements regarding death, for example, things would be better at death.

Psychomotor function. Ask specific questions regarding the activity level the patient has maintained. Is the person able to work or go to school? Is the person able to fulfill responsibilities at work, socially, and within the family? How have the person's normal responses to daily activities been altered? Is the individual withdrawn and isolated or still involved in social interactions? Check gestures, gait, pacing, presence or absence of tremors, and ability to perform gross or fine motor movements. Is the patient hyperactive or impulsive? Note the speech pattern. Are there prolonged pauses before answers are given or altered levels of volume and inflection?

Sleep pattern. What is the person's normal sleep pattern and how does it vary with mood swings? Ask specifically whether insomnia is present and whether it is initial or terminal in nature. Ask the individual to describe the perception of the amount and quality of the sleep nightly. Are naps taken regularly?

Dietary history. Ask questions relating to appetite and note weight gains or losses not associated with intentional dieting. During the manic phase the individual may be anorexic. Is the person able to sit down to eat a meal or eat only small amounts while pacing?

Nursing Diagnosis
- Risk for violence: self-directed (indication)
- Hopelessness (indication)
- Dysfunctional grieving (indication)
- Ineffective individual coping (indication)
- Social isolation (indication)
- Sensory-perceptual alterations (indications)

Planning
History of mood disorder. • Review data collected to identify individual's strengths and weaknesses. • Review medications being taken to specifically identify any that are known to cause depression.

Basic mental status. • Plan to perform a baseline assessment of the individual's mental status at specific intervals throughout the course of treatment. • Review coping mechanisms being used. Plan to discuss those that are maladaptive. Plan to initiate changes by guiding the individual in the use of more adaptive coping strategies. • Schedule specific times to discuss the patient's behavior and foster understanding of it with family members.

Mood/affect. • Review assessment data to develop strategies to assist the individual to cope more effectively with exhibited behaviors. Reward positive accomplishments for progress made. • It is difficult to plan activities with a patient in a manic phase because the patient's mood may be argumentative and aggressive and tend toward self-injury. Be brief, direct, and to the point with these individuals. Setting of limits will be necessary. Plan to approach the individual in a quiet, safe environment with other staff available in case the person is aggressive or threatens personal harm or harm to others.

Clarity of thought. • Identify areas in which the patient is capable of input to set goals and make decisions. (This will aid the individual to overcome a sense of powerlessness over life situations.) When the patient is unable to make decisions, plan to make them. Set goals to involve the patient as abilities change with treatment. Provide an opportunity to plan for self-care. • Manic patients are frequently manipulative and argumentative, seek less vulnerable individuals with whom to pick fights, and project blame on others. The nursing staff must plan collaboratively for these possible behaviors, and interventions must be consistent between all caregivers.

Thoughts of death. Provide for a safe environment for the individual. Search the surroundings for objects that could be used to inflict self-harm. Because the manic patient may also be harmful to others, a safe, structured environment must be maintained.

Psychomotor function. Review activities offered within the clinical setting and plan for the individual to participate in those that will be beneficial and foster success, for example, channeling for hyperactivity yet being safe for the patient and others. During initiation of therapy the individual may not be capable of participating in group activities.

Sleep pattern. • For the depressed patient, provide specific parameters in which the patient can function that do not allow the individual to continually sleep. Design activities during the day that stimulate the individual and promote sleep at night. Plan to use relaxation techniques. • For patients in the manic phase, plan activities that channel excessive energy. Recognize that sleep deprivation is a possibility with manic patients and can be life threatening. Select a quiet, nonstimulating environment in which to sleep. Plan to schedule specific rounds to evaluate the individual's sleep and safety.

Dietary needs. • Provide an opportunity for the individual to be involved in selecting foods appropriate to needs (to lose or gain weight). • Request a nutritional assessment by a dietitian to identify foods the person may eat (finger foods may work best). Supplemental feedings with nutritional preparations such as special high-calorie shakes may be needed. Obtain weights weekly or more frequently, and monitor intake and output.

Implementation

- Nursing interventions must be individualized and based on patient assessment data.
- Provide an environment of acceptance that focuses on the individual's strengths while minimizing the weaknesses.
- Provide an opportunity for the individual to express feelings. Use active listening and therapeutic communication techniques. Provide an opportunity for the person to express feelings in nonverbal ways, for example, involvment in physical activities or occupational therapy. Recognize that patients are hyperactive and talkative during the manic phase; it may be necessary to interrupt talking and to give concise, simple directions.
- Remain calm, direct, and firm in providing care. Because patients in the manic phase tend to be argumentative, avoid getting involved in an argument. State the unit rules in a matter-of-fact manner and enforce them.
- Allow the patient to make decisions if capable; make those the patient is not capable of making. Provide a reward for progress when decisions are initiated appropriately. Involve the patient in self-care activities. If suicidal, ask for details of the plan being formulated. Follow up on details obtained with appropriate family members or significant others, for example, have guns removed from home if this is part of the plan. Provide for patient safety and supervision, and record observations at specified intervals consistent with severity of the suicide threat and policies of the practice site.
- Manic patients may be harmful to others; it may be necessary to limit interactions with other patients. Patients in the manic phase may require the use of a quiet room.
- Stay with patients who are highly agitated.
- Administer prn drugs ordered for hyperactivity. Make necessary observations for response to medications administered.
- Use physical restraints within the guidelines of the clinical setting as appropriate to the behaviors being exhibited. Use the least restrictive alternative possible for the circumstances. Have sufficient staff available to assist with violent behavior to demonstrate ability to control the situation while providing for the safety and well-being of the patient and fellow staff members.
- Provide for nutritional needs by having high-protein, high-calorie foods appropriate for the individual to eat while pacing or highly active. Have nutritious snacks the patient is known to like available on the unit. Offer these at specific intervals throughout the day. Administer vitamins and liquid supplemental feedings as ordered.

- Manipulative behavior must be handled in a consistent manner by all staff members. Use limit setting and consequences that are agreed to in advance by all staff members. When the patient attempts to blame others, refocus on the patient's responsibilities. Give positive reinforcement for nonmanipulative behaviors when they occur.

Patient Education and Health Promotion

- Orient the individual to the unit, explaining rules and the process of privileges and how they are obtained or lost. (The extent of the orientation and explanations given will depend on the individual's orientation to date, time, and place and abilities.)
- Explain unit rules and therapeutic rules.
- Explain the activity groups available and how and when the individual will participate in these. A variety of group process activities (for example, social skills group, self-esteem groups, and physical exercise groups) are available within particular therapeutic settings.
- The patient and family must be involved in goal setting and integrated into the appropriate group processes to develop positive experiences for the patient to enhance coping skills.
- Patient education must be based on assessment data and individualized to provide the patient with a structured environment in which to grow and enhance self-esteem.
- Before discharge the patient and family must understand the goals of treatment and the entire follow-up plan (for example, frequency of therapy sessions, doctor visits, return to work goals).

Fostering health maintenance. • Throughout the course of treatment, discuss medication information and how it will benefit the patient. • Drug therapy is not immediately effective for the treatment of depression. Therefore the patient and significant others must understand the importance of continuing to take the prescribed medications despite minimal initial response. The lag time of 1 to 4 weeks between initiation of drug therapy and therapeutic response must be stressed. • Emphasize the need for lithium blood levels to be taken at specified intervals. Give details of date, time, and place for these to be done. Stress the importance of adequate hydration (6 to 8 glasses of water per day) and sodium intake when receiving lithium therapy. Instruct the patient to weigh daily. • Provide the patient or significant others with important information contained in the specific drug monograph for the medicines prescribed. Additional health teaching and nursing interventions for the side effects to expect and report are described in the drug monographs that follow. • Seek cooperation and understanding of the following points so that medication compliance is increased: name of medication, dosage, route and times of administration, side effects to expect, and side effects to report.

Written record. Enlist the patient's aid in developing and maintaining a written record of monitoring parameters. (See Patient Education and Monitoring box on p. 197.) Instruct the patient to bring the written record to follow-up visits.

Drug Class: Monoamine Oxidase Inhibitors

In the early 1950s, isoniazid and iproniazid were released for the treatment of tuberculosis. It was soon reported that

PATIENT EDUCATION AND MONITORING FORM Antidepressants

MEDICATIONS	COLOR	TO BE TAKEN

Name _____

Physician _____

Physician's phone _____

Next appt.* _____

PARAMETERS	DAY OF DISCHARGE							COMMENTS
Weight								
Blood pressure	AM / PM	AM / PM	AM / PM	AM / PM	AM / PM	AM / PM	AM / PM	
Resting pulse rate								
I would like to be alone? (All the time 10 / Some of the time 5 / Not really 1)								
How I feel about my children? (Too much work 10 / 5 / Fun to be with 1)								
How I feel today? (Poor 10 / Fair 5 / Okay 1)								
Appetite? (Poor 10 / Fair 5 / Good 1) [B L D SNACK]								
Has family noted any problems: Judgment? Socialization?								
Does patient dress daily (Yes/No)?								
Does patient take pride in appearance (Yes/No)?								
Use of alcohol (Yes/No)? Amount (e.g., one drink)?								
General Mood: Briefly describe whether tearful, excessively excited, happy, angry, hostile, depressed, sad, or having suicidal thoughts								
Anxiety level: Pacing, tremors, hyperactivity, or slow, retarded movements								

*Please bring this record with you to your next appointment.
Use the back of this sheet for additional information.

iproniazid had mood-elevating properties in tuberculosis patients. It was discovered in further investigation that iproniazid, in addition to its antitubercular properties, inhibited monoamine oxidase, whereas isoniazid did not. Other MAOIs were synthesized and used extensively to treat mental depression until the 1960s, when the tricyclic antidepressants became available.

Actions

The MAOIs act by blocking the metabolic destruction of norepinephrine, dopamine, and serotonin neurotransmitters by the enzyme monoamine oxidase in the presynaptic neurons of the brain. They prevent the degradation of these central nervous system neurotransmitters so that the concentration is increased. Although MAO inhibition starts within a few days of initiating therapy, the antidepressant effects require 2 to 4 weeks to become evident. Approximately 60% of the clinical improvement of symptoms of depression occurs in 2 weeks, and maximum improvement is usually attained within 4 weeks.

Uses

The MAOIs used today are phenelzine and tranylcypromine (Table 15-1). They are equally effective and have similar side effects. They are most effective in atypical depression, panic disorder, obsessive-compulsive disorder, and some phobic disorders. They are also used when tricyclic antidepressant therapy is unsatisfactory and when ECT is inappropriate or refused.

Therapeutic Outcomes

The primary therapeutic outcome expected from the monoamine oxidase inhibitors is elevated mood and reduction of symptoms of depression.

Nursing Process

Premedication Assessment

1. Obtain blood pressure and pulse rate before and at regular intervals after initiation of therapy.
2. If the patient is diabetic, monitor blood glucose to establish baseline values and assess periodically during therapy. Because MAOIs cause hypoglycemia, a dosage adjustment in insulin or oral hyperglycemic therapy may be required. If the patient has a history of severe renal disease, liver disease, cerebral vascular disease, or congestive heart failure, do not give medication. Consult with prescribing physician.
3. Complete a diet history to ensure that the patient has not ingested meals with a high tyramine content in the last few days.
4. Complete a medication history to ensure that the patient has not taken any of the following medicines in the last few days before therapy: ephedrine, phenylpropanolamine, amphetamine, methylphenidate, levodopa, or meperidine.

Planning

Availability. See Table 15-1.

Implementation

1. Instruct the patient on how to eliminate tyramine-containing foods that may cause a life-threatening hypertensive crisis if ingested concurrently with MAOIs.
2. The dosage should be taken in divided doses, with the last dose administered no later than 6 PM to prevent drug-induced insomnia. Caution the patient not to abruptly discontinue the medicine. If dosage is missed, take immediately and space the remainder of the daily dose throughout the rest of the day.
3. Check to be certain the patient is not receiving meperidine.

Evaluation

Side effects to expect

ORTHOSTATIC HYPOTENSION. The most common side effect of MAOIs is hypotension; it is more significant with phenelzine than tranylcypromine. Although generally mild, orthostatic hypotension manifested by dizziness and weakness is more common when therapy is being started. Daily divided dosages help minimize the hypotension. Tolerance usually develops after a few weeks of therapy.

Monitor the blood pressure daily in both the supine and standing positions.

Anticipate the development of postural hypotension and take measures to prevent an occurrence. Teach patients to rise slowly from a supine or sitting position; encourage them to sit or lie down if feeling faint.

DROWSINESS, SEDATION. Phenelzine has mild to moderate sedating effects. These symptoms tend to disappear with continued therapy and possible readjustment of the dosage.

Inform the patient of possible sedative effects. The patient should use caution while driving or performing other tasks that require alertness. Consult with the physician to consider moving the daily dosage to bedtime if sedation continues to be a problem.

RESTLESSNESS, AGITATION, INSOMNIA. These effects are more common with tranylcypromine and are transient as the dosage is being adjusted. Take the last dose before 6 PM to minimize insomnia.

BLURRED VISION, CONSTIPATION, URINARY RETENTION, DRYNESS OF MUCOSA OF THE MOUTH, THROAT, AND NOSE. These symptoms are the anticholinergic effects produced by these agents. Patients taking these medications should be monitored for the development of these side effects.

Dryness of the mucosa may be relieved by sucking hard candy or ice chips or by chewing gum.

If the patient develops urinary hesitancy, assess for distention of the bladder. Report to the physician for further evaluation.

Give stool softeners as prescribed. Encourage adequate fluid intake and foods to provide sufficient bulk.

Caution the patient that blurred vision may occur, and make appropriate suggestions for personal safety of the individual.

Side effects to report

HYPERTENSION. A major potential complication with MAOI therapy is that of hypertensive crisis, particularly with tranylcypromine. Because MAOIs block amine metabolism in tissues outside the brain, patients who consume foods or medications (see Drug interactions) containing indirect sympathomimetic amines are at considerable risk for a hypertensive crisis. Foods containing significant quantities of tyramine include well-ripened cheeses (Camembert, Edam, Roquefort, Parmesan, mozzarella, cheddar); yeast extract; red wines; pickled herring; sauerkraut; overripe bananas, figs, or avocadoes; chicken livers; and beer. Foods containing other vasopressors include fava beans, chocolate, coffee, tea, and colas. Common prodromal symptoms of hypertensive crisis include severe occipital headache, stiff neck, sweating, nausea, vomiting, and sharply elevated blood pressure.

Drug interactions

DRUGS THAT INCREASE TOXIC EFFECTS: The following drugs potentiate the toxicity of MAOIs by raising neurotransmitter levels: amphetamines, ephedrine, methyldopa, mazindol, phenylpropanolamine, levodopa, epinephrine, and norepinephrine.

TRICYCLIC ANTIDEPRESSANTS. The MAOIs and tricyclic antidepressants (especially imipramine and desipramine) should not be administered concurrently. It is recommended that at least 14 days elapse between the discontinuation of MAOIs and the initiation of another antidepressant.

SELECTIVE SEROTONIN REUPTAKE INHIBITORS. Severe reactions, including convulsions, hyperpyrexia, and death, have been reported with concurrent use. It is recommended that at least 14 days lapse between discontinuance of an MAOI and starting fluoxetine therapy.

GENERAL ANESTHESIA, DIURETICS, AND ANTIHYPERTENSIVE AGENTS. The MAOIs may potentiate the hypotensive effects of general anesthesia, diuretics, and antihypertensive agents.

INSULIN, ORAL HYPOGLYCEMIC AGENTS. The MAOIs have an additive hypoglycemic effect in combination with insulin and oral sulfonylureas. Monitor blood glucose; lower hypoglycemic doses if necessary.

MEPERIDINE. When used concurrently, meperidine and MAOIs may cause hyperpyrexia, restlessness, hypertension, hypotension, convulsions, and coma. The effects of this interaction may occur for several weeks after the discontinuation of an MAOI. Use morphine instead of meperidine.

Drug Class: Selective Serotonin Reuptake Inhibitors (SSRI)

Actions

The SSRIs (Table 15-1) are a newer class of antidepressant chemically unrelated to other antidepressants. They act by inhibiting the reuptake and destruction of serotonin from the synaptic cleft, thereby prolonging the action of the neurotransmitter.

Uses

The SSRIs have become the most widely used class of antidepressants. They have been shown to be equally effective in treating depression as the tricyclic antidepressants. A particular advantage of the SSRIs is that they do not have the anticholinergic and cardiovascular side effects that often limit the use of the tricyclic antidepressants. As with other antidepressants, it takes a full 2 to 4 weeks of therapy to obtain the full therapeutic benefit in treating depression. The SSRIs are also being studied for the treatment of obsessive-

compulsive disorder, obesity, eating disorders (anorexia nervosa, bulimia nervosa), bipolar disorder, and several other disorders. Fluvoxamine and fluoxetine are approved for use in obsessive-compulsive disorder.

Therapeutic Outcomes

The primary therapeutic outcome expected from the SSRIs is elevated mood and reduction of symptoms of depression.

Nursing Process

Premedication Assessment

1. Obtain baseline blood pressures in supine, sitting, and standing positions; record and report significant lowering to physician before administering drug.
2. Obtain baseline weight; schedule weekly weights.
3. Note any gastrointestinal symptoms present before start of therapy.
4. Monitor central nervous system symptoms present, for example, insomnia or nervousness.
5. Check hepatic studies before initiation and periodically throughout course of administration.
6. Perform DISCUS or AIMS (see p. 212) at specified intervals to detect or check on extrapyramidal symptoms; record and report according to policy. (See Appendixes G and H.)

Planning

Availability. See Table 15-1.

Implementation

Dosage and administration. See Table 15-1.

OBSERVATION. Symptoms of depression may improve within a few days (for example, improved appetite, sleep, and psychomotor activity). The depression still exists, however, and it usually takes several weeks of the therapeutic doses before improvement is noted. Suicide precautions should be maintained during this time.

Evaluation

Side effects to report

RESTLESSNESS, AGITATION, ANXIETY, INSOMNIA. This usually occurs early in therapy and may require short-term treatment with sedative-hypnotic agents. Avoiding bedtime doses may also help decrease the incidence of insomnia.

SEDATIVE EFFECTS. Tell the patient of possible sedative effects. The patient should use caution while driving or performing other tasks that require alertness. Consult with the physician to consider moving the daily dosage to bedtime if sedation continues to be a problem.

GASTROINTESTINAL EFFECTS. Most of these effects may be minimized by temporary reduction in dosage and administration with food. Encourage the patient not to discontinue therapy without consulting the physician first.

SUICIDAL ACTIONS. Monitor the patient for changes in thoughts, feelings, and behaviors during the initial stages of therapy.

Drug interactions

TRICYCLIC ANTIDEPRESSANTS. The interaction between SSRIs and tricyclic antidepressants is complex. The net

Table 15-1

Antidepressants

GENERIC NAME	BRAND NAME	AVAILABILITY	INITIAL DOSE (PO)	DAILY MAINTENANCE DOSE (MG)	MAXIMUM DAILY DOSE (MG)
Monoamine oxidase inhibitors (MAOIs)					
Phenelzine	Nardil	Tablets: 15 mg	15 mg 3 times daily	15-60	90
Tranylcypromine	Parnate	Tablets: 10 mg	10 mg 2 times daily	30	60
Tricyclic antidepressants					
Amitriptyline	Elavil, Endep	Tablets: 10, 25, 50, 75, 100, 150 mg IM: 10 mg/ml in 10 ml vials	25 mg 3 times daily	150-250	300
Amoxapine	Asendin	Tablets: 25, 50, 100, 150 mg	50 mg 3 times daily	200-300	400 (outpatients) 600 (inpatients)
Clomipramine	Anafranil	Capsules: 25, 50, 75 mg	25 mg 3 times daily	100-150	250
Desipramine	Norpramin, Pertofrane	Tablets: 10, 25, 50, 75, 100, 150 mg Capsules: 25, 50 mg	25 mg 3 times daily	75-200	300
Doxepin	Adapin, Sinequan, ✤Triadapin	Capsules: 10, 25, 50, 75, 100, 150 mg Oral concentrate 10 mg/ml	25 mg 3 times daily	at least 150	300
Imipramine	Tofranil, Janimine, ✤Impril	Tablets: 10, 25, 50 mg IM: 25 mg/2 ml	30-75 mg daily at bedtime	150-250	300
Nortriptyline	Aventyl, Pamelor	Capsules: 10, 25, 75 mg	25 mg 3-4 times daily	50-75	100
Protriptyline	Vivactil, ✤Triptil	Tablets: 5, 10 mg	5-10 mg 3-4 times daily	20-40	60
Trimipramine	Surmontil	Capsules: 25, 50, 100 mg	25 mg 3 times daily	50-150	200 (outpatients) 300 (inpatients)
Selective Serotonin Reuptake Inhibitors (SSRIs)					
Fluoxetine	Prozac	Capsules: 10, 20 mg	20 mg in morning	20-60	80
Fluvoxamine	Luvox	Tablets: 50, 100 mg	50 mg at bedtime	100-300	300
Paroxetine	Paxil	Tablets: 20, 30 mg	20 mg daily	20-50	50
Sertraline	Zoloft	Tablets: 50, 100 mg	50 mg daily	50-200	200

✤ Available in Canada only.

result is that there is an increased toxicity from the tricyclic antidepressants. Observe patients for signs of toxicity, including arrhythmias, seizure activity, and central nervous system stimulation.

LITHIUM. Fluoxetine has been reported to reduce lithium levels and to increase levels to induce lithium toxicity. Monitor for lithium toxicity manifested by nausea, anorexia, fine tremors, persistent vomiting, profuse diarrhea, hyperreflexia, lethargy, and weakness.

MONOAMINE OXIDASE INHIBITORS. Severe reactions, including excitement, diaphoresis, rigidity, convulsions, hyperpyrexia, and death, have been reported with concurrent use of MAOIs and SSRIs. It is recommended that at least 14 days lapse between discontinuance of an MAOI and starting SSRI therapy and vice versa. It is further recommended that there be a 5-week stop interval between discontinuing fluoxetine and starting MAOIs.

HALOPERIDOL. Fluoxetine increases haloperidol levels and increases the frequency of extrapyramidal symptoms. If used concurrently, the dosage of haloperidol may need to be decreased.

PHENYTOIN, PHENOBARBITAL. Complex interactions occur in which phenobarbital and phenytoin enhance the metabolism of paroxetine, requiring a dosage increase in paroxetine for therapeutic effect. In a similar fashion, paroxetine increases the metabolism of phenytoin and phenobarbital, thus requiring an increase in dosage of these two agents for maintaining therapeutic effect. Conversely, fluoxetine may diminish the metabolism of phenytoin, resulting in potential phenytoin toxicity.

CARBAMAZEPINE. Fluoxetine can increase carbamazepine concentrations, resulting in signs of toxicity: vertigo, tremor, headache, drowsiness, nausea, and vomiting. The dosage of carbamazepine may need to be reduced.

DIAZEPAM. Fluoxetine and sertraline prolong the activity of diazepam, resulting in excessive sedation and impaired motor skills.

CIMETIDINE. Cimetidine inhibits the metabolism of paroxetine and sertraline. Patients should be closely monitored when cimetidine is added to paroxetine or sertraline therapy.

WARFARIN. Fluoxetine, paroxetine, sertraline, and fluvoxamine may enhance the anticoagulant effects of warfarin. Observe for the development of petechiae, ecchymoses, nosebleeds, bleeding gums, dark tarry stools, and bright red "coffee-ground" emesis. Monitor the prothrombin time and reduce the dosage of warfarin if necessary.

Drug Class: Tricyclic Antidepressants

Actions

Until recently, the tricyclic antidepressants (see Table 15-1) have been the most widely used medications in the treatment of depression. The serotonin agonists (SSRIs) now have that distinction, but long-term outcome is yet to be determined. The tricyclic antidepressants prolong the action of norepinephrine, dopamine, and serotonin to varying degrees by blocking the reuptake of these neurotransmitters in the synaptic cleft between neurons. The exact mechanism of action when used as antidepressants is unknown.

Uses

The tricyclic antidepressants produce antidepressant and mild tranquilizing effects. After 2 to 4 weeks of therapy, the tricyclic antidepressants elevate mood, improve appetite, and increase alertness in approximately 80% of patients with endogenous depression. Combination therapy with phenothiazine derivatives may be beneficial in the treatment of the depression of schizophrenia or moderate to severe anxiety and depression observed with psychosis.

The tricyclic antidepressants are equally effective in treating depression, assuming that appropriate dosages are used for an adequate duration of time. Consequently the selection of an antidepressant is based primarily on the characteristics of each individual agent. Sedation is more notable with amitriptyline, doxepin, and trimipramine. Protriptyline has no sedative properties and may actually produce mild stimulation in some patients. All tricyclic compounds display anticholinergic activity, with amitriptyline displaying the most and desipramine the least. This factor should be considered in patients with cardiac disease, prostatic hypertrophy, or glaucoma. Other factors to consider are that men tend to respond better to imipramine than do women, and the elderly tend to respond better to amitriptyline than do younger patients.

Therapeutic Outcomes

The primary therapeutic outcome expected from the tricyclic antidepressants is elevated mood and reduction of symptoms of depression.

Nursing Process

Premedication Assessment

1. Note consistency of bowel movements; constipation is common when taking tricyclics.
2. Obtain baseline blood pressures in supine and standing positions; record and report significant hypotension to physician before administering drug.
3. Check history for symptoms of arrhythmias, tachycardia, or congestive heart failure; if present consult physician before starting therapy. (May require electrocardiogram [ECG] before starting therapy.)
4. If history of seizures exists, check with the physician to see if a dosage adjustment is to be made in anticonvulsant therapy medications.

Planning
Availability. See Table 15-1

Implementation
Dosage and administration. Adult: PO—See Table 15-1. Dosage should be initiated at a low level and increased gradually, particularly in elderly or debilitated patients. Increases in dosage should be made in the evening because increased sedation is often present.

OBSERVATION. Symptoms of depression may improve within a few days (for example, improved appetite, sleep, and psychomotor activity). The depression still exists, however, and it usually takes several weeks of the therapeutic doses before improvement is noted. Suicide precautions should be maintained during this time.

Evaluation
Side effects to expect

BLURRED VISION, CONSTIPATION, URINARY RETENTION, DRYNESS OF MUCOSA OF THE MOUTH, THROAT, AND NOSE. These symptoms are the anticholinergic effects produced by these agents. Patients taking these medications should be monitored for the development of these side effects.

Dryness of the mucosa may be relieved by sucking hard candy or ice chips or by chewing gum.

The use of stool softeners such as docusate or the occasional use of a potent laxative such as bisacodyl may be required for constipation.

Caution the patient that blurred vision may occur, and make appropriate suggestions for personal safety of the individual.

ORTHOSTATIC HYPOTENSION. All tricyclic antidepressants may cause some degree of orthostatic hypotension manifested by dizziness and weakness, particularly when therapy is being initiated.

Monitor the blood pressure daily in both the supine and standing positions.

Anticipate the development of postural hypotension and take measures to prevent an occurrence. Teach the patient to rise slowly from a supine or sitting position; encourage the patient to sit or lie down if feeling faint.

SEDATIVE EFFECTS. Tell the patient of sedative effects, especially during the onset of therapy. Single doses at bedtime may diminish or relieve the sedative effects.

Side effects to report

TREMOR. Approximately 10% of patients develop this adverse effect. The tremor can be controlled with small doses of propranolol.

NUMBNESS, TINGLING. Report for further evaluation.

PARKINSONIAN SYMPTOMS. If these symptoms develop, the tricyclic antidepressant dosage must be reduced or discontinued.

Antiparkinsonian medications will not control symptoms induced by tricyclic antidepressants.

ARRHYTHMIAS, TACHYCARDIA, HEART FAILURE. Report for further evaluation.

SEIZURE ACTIVITY. High doses of antidepressants lower the seizure threshold. Adjustment of anticonvulsant therapy may be required, especially in seizure-prone patients.

SUICIDAL ACTIONS. Monitor the patient for changes in thoughts, feelings, and behaviors during the initial stages of therapy.

Drug interactions

ENHANCED ANTICHOLINERGIC ACTIVITY. The following drugs enhance the anticholinergic activity associated with tricyclic antidepressant therapy: antihistamines, phenothiazines, trihexyphenidyl, benztropine, and meperidine. The side effects are usually not severe enough to cause discontinuation of therapy, but stool softeners may be required.

ENHANCED SEDATIVE ACTIVITY. The following drugs enhance the sedative activity associated with tricyclic antidepressant therapy: ethanol, barbiturates, narcotics, tranquilizers, antihistamines, anesthetics, and sedative-hypnotics. Concurrent therapy is not recommended.

BARBITURATES. Barbiturates may stimulate the metabolism of tricyclic antidepressants. Dosage adjustments of the antidepressant may be necessary.

METHYLPHENIDATE, THYROID HORMONES. These agents may increase serum levels of the tricyclic antidepressants. This reaction has been advantageous in attempts to gain a faster onset of antidepressant activity, but an increased incidence of arrhythmias also has been reported.

GUANETHIDINE, CLONIDINE. Tricyclic antidepressants inhibit the antihypertensive effects of these agents. Concurrent therapy is not recommended.

MONOAMINE OXIDASE INHIBITORS. Severe reactions, including convulsions, hyperpyrexia, and death, have been reported with concurrent use. It is recommended that 2 weeks lapse between discontinuance of an MAOI and starting tricyclic antidepressants.

PHENOTHIAZINES. Concurrent therapy may increase serum levels of both drugs, causing an increase in anticholinergic and sedative activity. Dosages of both agents may be reduced.

SELECTIVE SEROTONIN REUPTAKE INHIBITORS. The interaction between SSRIs and tricyclic antidepressants is complex. The net result is that there is an increased toxicity from the tricyclic antidepressants. Observe patients for signs of toxicity, for example, arrhythmias, seizure activity, central nervous system stimulation.

Drug Class: Miscellaneous Agents

bupropion hydrochloride (byoo-pro′ pee-on)
Wellbutrin (wel′ byü′-trin)

Actions

Bupropion is a monocyclic antidepressant chemically related to phenylethylamine antidepressants. Its mechanism of action is unknown. Compared with the tricyclic antidepressants, it is a weak inhibitor of the reuptake and inactivation of the neurotransmitters serotonin, norephinephrine, and dopamine.

Uses

It is approved for use in patients unresponsive to the tricyclic antidepressants and in patients who cannot tolerate the adverse effects of the tricyclic antidepressants. Disadvantages include seizure activity and the requirement of multiple dosages daily. It must not be used in patients with psychotic disorders because its dopamine agonist activity causes increased pyschotic symptoms.

Therapeutic Outcomes

The primary therapeutic outcome expected from bupropion therapy is elevated mood and reduction of symptoms of depression.

Nursing Process

Premedication Assessment

1. Obtain baseline weight.
2. Perform DISCUS or AIMS (see p. 212) at specified intervals to detect or check on extrapyramidal symptoms; record and report according to policy. (See Appendixes G and H.)

Planning

Availability. PO—75 and 100 mg tablets.

Implementation

Dosage and administration. Adult: PO—Initially, 100 mg twice daily. This may be increased to 100 mg 3 times daily (at least every 6 hours) after several days of therapy. No single dose of bupropion should exceed 150 mg; do not exceed 450 mg daily. Avoid a dosage shortly before bedtime.

OBSERVATION. Symptoms of depression may improve within a few days (for example, improved appetite, sleep, and psychomotor activity). The depression still exists, however, and it usually takes several weeks of the therapeutic doses before improvement is noted. Suicide precautions should be maintained during this time.

Evaluation

Side effects to expect.

GASTROINTESTINAL EFFECTS. Most of these effects may be minimized by temporary reduction in dosage, administration with food, and use of stool softeners for constipation.

RESTLESSNESS, AGITATION, ANXIETY, INSOMNIA. This usually occurs early in therapy and may require short-term treatment with sedative-hypnotic agents. Avoiding bedtime doses may also help decrease the incidence of insomnia.

Side effects to report

SEIZURES. See Nursing Assessments for patients with seizure disorders (p. 219).

SUICIDAL ACTIONS. Monitor the patient for changes in thoughts, feelings, and behaviors during the initial stages of therapy.

Drug interactions

CARBAMAZEPINE, CIMETIDINE, PHENOBARBITAL, PHENYTOIN. Bupropion may be an inducer of hepatic enzymes that may metabolize these agents more quickly. The dosage of these medications may need to be increased if taken concurrently with bupropion.

LEVODOPA. Bupropion has some mild dopaminergic activity and may cause an increase in adverse effects from levodopa. If bupropion is to be added to levodopa therapy, it should be initiated in small doses with small increases in the dosage of bupropion.

maprotiline hydrochloride (ma-proe′ ti-leen)
Ludiomil (loo-dee′-oh-mill)

Actions

Maprotiline was the first of the tetracyclic antidepressants to be released for clinical use. The mechanism of action is unknown, but pharmacologic response is similar to that with tricyclic antidepressants. The frequency and severity of anticholinergic effects, cardiac arrhythmias, and orthostatic hypotension are reported to be lower with maprotiline when compared with the tricyclic antidepressants. There is a threefold higher incidence of seizure activity and delirium associated with maprotiline therapy.

Uses

Maprotiline is used in the treatment of depression and the depressive phase of bipolar disorder and for the relief of anxiety associated with depression.

Therapeutic Outcomes

The primary therapeutic outcome expected from maprotiline therapy is elevated mood and reduction of symptoms of depression.

Nursing Process

Premedication Assessment

1. Obtain baseline blood pressures in supine, sitting, and standing positions; record and report significant hypotension to physician before administering drug.
2. Obtain baseline weight; schedule weekly weights.
3. Check for history of seizures. If present, notify physician before starting therapy.
4. Check hepatic studies before initiation and periodically throughout course of administration.
5. Perform DISCUS or AIMS at specified intervals to detect or check on extrapyramidal symptoms; record and report according to policy.

Planning

Availability. PO—25, 50, and 75 mg tablets.

Implementation

Dosage and administration. Adult: PO—Initially, 75 mg daily. Increase in increments of 25 to 50 mg daily as needed and tolerated. The usual maintenance dose is 150 mg daily. The maximum dose is 225 mg daily. Therapeutic blood levels are 50 to 200 ng per ml. Increases in dosage should be made in the evening because increased sedation is often present.

OBSERVATION. Symptoms of depression may improve (for example, improved appetite, sleep, and psychomotor activity) within a few days. The depression still exists, however, and it usually takes several weeks of therapeutic doses before improvement in the depression is noted. Suicide precautions should be maintained during this time.

Evaluation

See Tricyclic Antidepressants (p. 201).

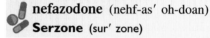
nefazodone (nehf-as′ oh-doan)
Serzone (sur′ zone)

Actions

Nefazodone is an antidepressant similar in chemical structure to trazodone. It inhibits serotonin reuptake from the neuronal cleft, prolonging its action. It also blocks serotonin-2 receptors. Its mechanism of action as an antidepressant is unknown.

Use

Nefazodone is used to treat depression. This agent appears to have less anticholinergic, hypotensive, and sedative activity relative to the tricyclic antidepressants.

Therapeutic Outcomes

The primary therapeutic outcome expected from nefazodone therapy is elevated mood and reduction of symptoms of depression.

Nursing Process

Assessment

1. Obtain blood pressures in the supine, sitting, and standing positions; report significant lowering to the physician before administering the medicine.
2. Obtain heart rate before and at regular intervals following initiation of therapy. An ECG may be required for baseline information before start of therapy. Report significant lowering of blood pressure to the physician before administering the medicine.
3. Note any gastrointestinal symptoms present before start of therapy.
4. Monitor central nervous system symptoms present (for example, insomnia or nervousness).

Planning

Availability. PO-100, 150, 200, 250 mg tablets

Implementation

Dosage and administration. Adult: PO-Initially, 100 mg 2 times daily. At no less than weekly intervals, increase the dosage by 100 to 200 mg, again on a twice-daily schedule as tolerated. Several weeks of adjustment may be required for optimization of therapy. The normal dosage range is 300 to 600 mg daily.

OBSERVATION. Symptoms of depression (for example, improved appetite, sleep, and psychomotor activity) may improve within a few days. The depression still exists, however, and it usually takes several weeks of therapeutic doses before improvement is noted. Suicide precautions should be maintained during this time.

Evaluation
Side effects to expect
DROWSINESS, SEDATION. Phenelzine has mild to moderate sedating effects. These symptoms tend to disappear with continued therapy and possible readjustment of the dosage.

Inform the patient of possible sedative effects. The patient should use caution while driving or performing other tasks that require alertness. Consult with the physician to consider moving the daily dosage to bedtime if sedation continues to be a problem.

BLURRED VISION, CONSTIPATION, URINARY RETENTION, DRYNESS OF MUCOSA OF THE MOUTH, THROAT, AND NOSE. These symptoms are the anticholinergic effects produced by these agents. Patients taking these medications should be monitored for the development of these side effects.

Dryness of the mucosa may be relieved by sucking hard candy or ice chips or by chewing gum.

The use of stool softeners such as docusate or the occasional use of a potent laxative such as bisacodyl may be required for constipation.

Caution the patient that blurred vision may occur, and make appropriate suggestions for personal safety of the individual.

ORTHOSTATIC HYPOTENSION. Nefazodone may cause some degree of orthostatic hypotension manifested by dizziness and weakness, particularly when therapy is being initiated.

Monitor the blood pressure daily in both the supine and standing positions.

Anticipate the development of postural hypotension and take measures to prevent an occurrence. Teach the patient to rise slowly from a supine or sitting position; encourage the patient to sit or lie down if feeling faint.

SEDATIVE EFFECTS. Tell the patient of sedative effects, especially during the onset of therapy. Single doses at bedtime may diminish or relieve the sedative effects.

Side effects to report
BRADYCARDIA. Monitor heart rate as therapy is initiated and the dosage is adjusted. Bradycardias with a drop in 15 beats per minute and rates below 50 beats per minute have been reported. Notify the physician immediately. Withhold the next dosage until specifically approved.

SUICIDAL ACTIONS. Monitor the patient for changes in thoughts, feelings, and behaviors during the initial stages of therapy.

Drug interactions
TERFENADINE, ASTEMIZOLE. These antihistamines should not be administered concurrently with nefazodone. Nefazodone significantly increases serum levels of these agents, which causes cardiac toxicity that has been fatal in several cases.

MONOAMINE OXIDASE INHIBITORS. Severe reactions, including excitement, diaphoresis, rigidity, convulsions, hyperpyrexia, and death, have been reported with concurrent use of MAOIs and nefazodone. It is recommended that at least 14 days lapse between discontinuance of an MAOI and starting nefazodone. It is further recommended that there be a 1-week stop interval between discontinuing nefazodone and starting MAOI therapy.

HALOPERIDOL. Nefazodone inhibits the metabolism of haloperidol. It does not apparently increase the serum levels but does prolong the action of haloperidol. Dosage may have to be given less frequently to prevent potential toxicity.

ALPRAZOLAM, TRIAZOLAM. Nefazodone significantly increases serum levels of these benzodiazepines. Monitor closely for excessive sedation and impaired motor skills.

DIGOXIN. Nefazodone significantly increases serum levels of digoxin. Monitor serum levels and signs of toxicity, for example, arrhythmias, bradycardia.

trazodone hydrochloride (tray′ zoe-done)
Desyrel (dez-er′ el)

Actions
Trazodone was the first of the triazolopyridine antidepressants to be released for clinical use. The triazolopyridines are chemically unrelated to the other classes of antidepressants. The exact mechanisms of action of trazodone are unknown. The actions are complex and in some ways resemble those of the tricyclic antidepressants, benzodiazepines, and phenothiazines; however, the overall activity of trazodone is different from that of each of these classes of drugs.

Uses
Trazodone has been shown to be as effective in treating depression, depression associated with schizophrenia, and depression, tremor, and anxiety associated with alcohol dependence. Compared with other antidepressants, it has a low incidence of anticholinergic side effects, which makes trazodone particularly useful in patients whose antidepressant dosages are limited by anticholinergic side effects and in patients with severe angle-closure glaucoma, prostatic hypertrophy, organic mental disorders, and cardiac arrhythmias.

Therapeutic Outcomes
The primary therapeutic outcome expected from trazodone therapy is elevated mood and reduction of symptoms of depression.

Nursing Process

Premedication Assessment
Obtain baseline blood pressures in supine, sitting, and standing positions; record and report significant hypotension to physician before administering drug.

Planning
Availability. PO—50, 100, 150, and 300 mg tablets.

Implementation

Dosage and administration. • Adult: PO—Initially, 150 mg in 3 divided doses. Increase in increments of 50 mg daily every 3 to 4 days while monitoring clinical response. Do not exceed 400 mg daily in outpatients or 600 mg daily in hospitalized patients. • Dosage should be initiated at a low level and increased gradually, particularly in elderly or debilitated patients. • Increases in dosage should be made in the evening because increased sedation is often present. • Administer medication shortly after a meal or with a light snack to reduce adverse effects.

OBSERVATION. Symptoms of depression may improve (for example, improved appetite, sleep, and psychomotor activity) within a few days. The depression still exists, however, and it usually requires several weeks of therapeutic doses before improvement is noted. Suicide precautions should be maintained during this time.

Evaluation

Side effects to expect and report

CONFUSION. Perform a baseline assessment of the patient's degree of alertness and orientation to name, place, and time before start of therapy. Make regularly scheduled subsequent evaluations of mental status and compare findings. Report development of alterations.

DIZZINESS, LIGHT-HEADEDNESS. Provide for patient safety during episodes of dizziness; report for further evaluation.

DROWSINESS. Persons who are working with machinery, driving a car, pouring and giving medicines, or performing other duties in which they must remain mentally alert should not take these medications while working.

ORTHOSTATIC HYPOTENSION. Although episodes are infrequent and generally mild, trazodone may cause some degree of orthostatic hypotension manifested by dizziness and weakness, particularly when therapy is being initiated.

Monitor blood pressure daily in both the supine and standing positions.

Anticipate the development of postural hypotension and take measures to prevent an occurrence. Teach the patient to rise slowly from a supine or sitting position; encourage the patient to sit or lie down if feeling faint.

ARRHYTHMIAS, TACHYCARDIA. Report for further evaluation.

Drug interactions

ENHANCED SEDATIVE ACTIVITY. The following drugs enhance the sedative effects associated with trazodone therapy: ethanol, barbiturates, narcotics, tranquilizers, antihistamines, anesthetics, and sedative-hypnotics. Concurrent therapy is not recommended.

GUANETHIDINE, CLONIDINE. Trazodone inhibits the antihypertensive effects of these agents. Concurrent therapy is not recommended.

venlafaxine (vehn-lah-fax′ een)
Effexor (eef′ ex-ohr)

Action

Venlafaxine is a phenethylamine derivative antidepressant structurally related to bupropion. Although its antidepressant action is unknown, it is a potent inhibitor of reuptake of serotonin and norepinephrine and a weak inhibitor of dopamine reuptake in the neuronal cleft.

Uses

Venlafaxine is approved for use in patients for the treatment of depression. A disadvantage is the requirement of multiple dosages daily.

Therapeutic Outcomes

The primary therapeutic outcome expected from venlafaxine therapy is elevated mood and reduction of symptoms of depression.

Nursing Process

Premedication Assessment
1. Obtain baseline weight.
2. Note any gastrointestinal symptoms present before start of therapy.
3. Monitor central nervous system symptoms present, for example, insomnia, nervousness.

Planning
Availability. PO—25, 37.5, 50, 75, and 100 mg tablets.

Implementation
Dosage and administration. Adult: PO-75 mg daily, taken with food in 2 or 3 doses. Dosages may be increased by 75 mg daily at intervals greater than every 4 days. The maximum recommended dosage is 375 mg daily, generally in 3 divided doses.

Discontinuation of therapy. If the patient has taken the medicine for more than 1 week, the dosage should be tapered over the next few days. If venlafaxine has been taken for longer than 6 weeks, the dosage should gradually be tapered over the next 2 weeks.

OBSERVATION. Symptoms of depression may improve within a few days (for example, improved appetite, sleep, and psychomotor activity). The depression still exists, however, and it usually requires several weeks of the therapeutic doses before improvement is noted. Suicide precautions should be maintained during this time.

Evaluation
Side effects to expect

DIZZINESS, DROWSINESS. Persons should be warned not to work with machinery, drive a car, pour or give medicines, or perform other duties in which mental alertness is required until they are sure that these side effects are not impairing actions and judgment.

NAUSEA, ANOREXIA. Most of these effects may be minimized by temporary reduction in dosage and administration with food.

RESTLESSNESS, AGITATION, ANXIETY, INSOMNIA. This usually occurs early in therapy, and the patient may require short-term treatment with sedative-hypnotic agents. Avoiding bedtime doses may help decrease the incidence of insomnia.

Side effects to report

SUICIDAL ACTIONS. Monitor the patient for changes in thoughts, feelings, and behaviors during the initial stages of therapy.

Drug interactions

MONOAMINE OXIDASE INHIBITORS. Severe reactions, including excitement, diaphoresis, rigidity, convulsions, hyperpyrexia, and death, have been reported with concurrent use of MAOIs and venlafaxine. It is recommended that at least 14 days lapse between discontinuance of an MAOI and start of venlafaxine therapy and vice versa.

CIMETIDINE. Cimetidine inhibits the metabolism of venlafaxine. Patients should be closely monitored for excessive effects of venlafaxine when cimetidine is added to the therapeutic regimen.

Drug Class: Antimanic Agent

lithium carbonate (li th-ee'-um)
Eskalith (esk-ah' lith), **Lithane** (lith' ahn)

Actions

Lithium is a monovalent cation that competes with other monovalent and divalent cations (potassium, sodium, calcium, magnesium) at cellular binding sites that are sensitive to changes in cation concentration. Lithium replaces intracellular and intraneuronal sodium, stabilizing the neuronal membrane. It also reduces the release of norepinephrine and increases the uptake of tryptophan, the precursor to serotonin. It also interacts with second-messenger cellular processes to inhibit intracellular concentrations of cyclic adenosine monophosphate. Because of the complexity of the central nervous system, the exact mechanisms of action of lithium in treating mood disorders are unknown. It has no sedative, depressant, or euphoric properties, differentiating it from all other psychotropic agents.

Uses

Lithium is used to treat acute mania and for the prophylaxis of recurrent manic and depressive episodes in bipolar disorder. In patients with bipolar disorder, it is more effective in preventing signs and symptoms of mania than those of depression. It is also effective in some patients in reducing the recurrence of depressive episodes in unipolar disorder.

Therapeutic Outcome

The primary therapeutic outcome expected from lithium therapy is maintaining the individual at an optimal level of functioning with minimal exacerbations of mood swings.

Nursing Process

Premedication Assessment

1. Before the initiation of lithium therapy, the following laboratory tests should be completed for baseline information: electrolytes, fasting blood glucose, blood-urea-nitrogen (BUN), serum creatinine, creatinine clearance, urinalysis, and thyroid function tests.

2. Obtain baseline blood pressures in supine, sitting, and standing positions; record and report significant hypotension to physician before administering drug.
3. Weigh daily; check hydration of patient (moistness of mucous membrane, skin turgor, firmness of eyeball); monitor urine specific gravity.
4. Lithium may enhance sodium depletion, which enhances lithium toxicity. Assess for early signs of lithium toxicity before giving medication.

Planning

Availability

PO—150, 300, 600 mg capsules and tablets, 300 and 450 mg slow-release tablets, and 300 mg per 5 ml syrup.

SERUM LITHIUM LEVELS. Levels are monitored once or twice weekly during initiation of therapy and monthly while on maintenance dose. Blood should be drawn approximately 12 hours after the last dose was administered. The normal serum level is 0.4 to 1.5 mEq per L. Report serum levels above these values to the physician promptly.

GOOD NUTRITION. Lithium may enhance sodium depletion, which enhances lithium toxicity. It is important that patients maintain a normal dietary intake of sodium with adequate maintenance fluids (10 to 12 8-ounce glasses of water daily), especially during the initiation of therapy, to prevent toxicity.

Implementation

Dosage and administration. Adult: PO—300 to 600 mg 3 to 4 times daily. Administer with food or milk. Adequate diet is important to maintain normal serum sodium levels and prevent the development of toxicity. Onset of the acute antimanic effect of lithium usually occurs within 5 to 7 days; full therapeutic effect often requires 10 to 21 days.

Evaluation

Side effects to expect

NAUSEA, VOMITING, ANOREXIA, ABDOMINAL CRAMPS. These side effects are usually mild and tend to resolve with continued therapy. Encourage the patient not to discontinue therapy without first consulting the physician.

If gastric irritation occurs, administer medication with food or milk. If symptoms persist or increase in severity, report for physician evaluation. These may also be early signs of toxicity.

EXCESSIVE THIRST AND URINATION, FINE HAND TREMOR. These side effects are usually mild and tend to resolve within a week with continued therapy. Encourage the patient not to discontinue therapy without first consulting the physician.

If these symptoms persist or become severe, the patient should consult the physician.

Side effects to report

PERSISTENT VOMITING, PROFUSE DIARRHEA, HYPERREFLEXIA, LETHARGY, AND WEAKNESS. These are all signs of impending serious toxicity. Report immediately and do not administer the next dosage until reconfirmed by the physician.

PROGRESSIVE FATIGUE, WEIGHT GAIN. These may be early signs of hypothyroidism. Report for further evaluation.

PRURITUS, ANKLE EDEMA, METALLIC TASTE, HYPERGLYCEMIA. These are all rare side effects from lithium therapy. Report for further evaluation.

NEPHROTOXICITY. Monitor urinalysis and kidney function tests for abnormal results. Report an increasing BUN and creatinine, increasing or decreasing urine output or decreasing specific gravity (despite amount of fluid intake), and casts or protein in the urine.

Drug interactions

REDUCED SERUM SODIUM LEVELS. Therapeutic activity and toxicity of lithium are highly dependent on sodium concentrations. Decreased sodium levels significantly enhance the toxicity of lithium.

Patients who are to begin diuretic therapy, a low-sodium diet, or activities that produce excessive and prolonged sweating should be observed particularly closely.

METHYLDOPA. Monitor patients on concurrent, long-term therapy for signs (nausea, vomiting, abdominal pain, diarrhea, lethargy, speech difficulty, mild dizziness, and tremor) of the development of lithium toxicity.

INDOMETHACIN, PIROXICAM. Indomethacin reduces the renal excretion of lithium, allowing it to accumulate to potentially toxic levels.

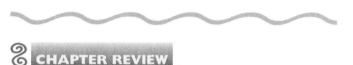

CHAPTER REVIEW

Mood disorders (affective disorders) are said to be present when certain symptoms impair the person's ability to function for a duration of time. At least 10% of persons in the United States suffer from a diagnosable mood disorder in their lifetime. Mood disorders are divided into depressive (unipolar) and bipolar disorders. Treatment of mood disorders requires both nonpharmacologic and pharmacologic therapy. Simultaneous psychotherapy and pharmacologic treatment have been shown to be more successful than either treatment alone. Antidepressant medications act on a variety of receptors both in the central nervous system and in the peripheral tissues and are associated with many side effects and drug interactions. It is a responsibility of the nurse to educate patients about therapy, monitoring for therapeutic benefit, and side effects to expect and report, intervening whenever possible to optimize therapeutic outcomes.

MATH REVIEW

1. Ordered: Lithium carbonate 300 mg PO twice daily
   On hand: Lithium carbonate 150 mg tablets
   Give: _____ tablets

2. Ordered: Maprotiline 100 mg PO this AM
   On hand: None found in medication container; consult

drug monograph for dosage availability. What strength tablets would most likely be dispensed, and how would you administer the dose?

CRITICAL THINKING QUESTIONS

1. During her clinic visit Mrs. Smalley complains to the nurse that since she started taking amitriptyline (Elavil) for depression, she has had a "terrible dry mouth" and she feels "sleepy all the time." What additional information would you elicit? What interventions to alleviate these symptoms could be suggested?

2. The next patient at the clinic is taking fluoxetine (Prozac). He is 5' 6" tall, weighs 120 lb, and has been receiving the medication for 6 weeks. He reports that he feels like a "cloud has been lifted from my mind." What additional data would be appropriate to collect during this visit?

3. When a patient is starting therapy with an MAOI, what health teaching would be important?

4. When looking at the drug monograph for MAOI therapy it states that one major potential complication of this therapy is a hypertensive crisis. Discuss what this is, how to recognize it, and the interventions that should be anticipated if it occurred.

5. Discuss the behavioral monitoring sheets used in the clinical settings where practicing to assess for the development of extrapyramidal symptoms. How often are the assessments made, how are they recorded, and when is the physician notified of changes in the patient's behavior?

   Clinical Case
   Martha Halleran, age 34, is being treated for bipolar disorder with lithium 300 mg PO, 4 times daily. She is being seen today in the clinic. During the intake interview she tells the nurse that her medicine "never works." Further exploration reveals that she has not taken the medication for the past 4 days.

6. As the nurse in this situation, how would you proceed? When reviewing Martha's history, the nurse reads that her lithium level taken the month before was 2.0 mEq per L.

7. What symptoms might be seen with this lithium level?

8. The history also notes that the importance of adequate intake of water and sodium was discussed with Martha. How does the sodium level within the body influence the metabolism of lithium?

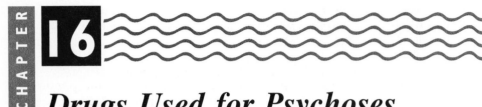

CHAPTER **16**

Drugs Used for Psychoses

CHAPTER CONTENT

Objectives

1. Identify signs and symptoms of psychotic behavior.
2. Describe major indications for the use of antipsychotic agents.
3. Identify common adverse effects observed with antipsychotic medications.
4. Develop a teaching plan for a patient taking haloperidol and for a person receiving clozapine.

Key Words

psychosis

delusions

hallucinations

disorganized thinking

loosening of associations

disorganized behavior

changes in affect

target symptoms

typical and atypical antipsychotic agents

equipotent doses

extrapyramidal symptoms

dystonia

pseudoparkinsonian symptoms

akathisia

tardive dyskinesia

abnormal involuntary movement scale

dyskinesia identification systems: condensed user scale

neuroleptic malignant syndrome

depot antipsychotic medicine

PSYCHOSIS

Psychosis does not have a single definition but is a clinical descriptor that means being out of touch with reality. Psychotic symptoms can be associated with many illnesses, including dementias and delirium, that may have metabolic, infectious, or endocrine causes. Psychotic symptoms are also common in mood disorders such as major depression and bipolar disorder. Psychosis can also be caused by many drugs (for example, phencyclidine, opiates, amphetamines, cocaine, hallucinogens, anticholinergic agents, and alcohol). Psychotic disorders are characterized by loss of reality, perceptual deficits such as hallucinations and delusions, and deterioration in social functioning. Of the several psychotic disorders defined by the American Psychiatric Association in the *Diagnostic and Statisical Manual of Mental Disorders,* ed. 4, schizophrenia is the most common.

Psychotic disorders are extremely complex illnesses that are influenced by biologic, psychosocial, and environmental circumstances. Some of the disorders require several months of observation and testing before a final diagnosis can be determined. It is beyond the scope of this text to discuss psychotic disorders in detail, but general types of symptoms associated with psychotic disorders are described.

A **delusion** is a false or irrational belief that is firmly held despite obvious evidence to the contrary. Delusions may be persecutory, grandiose, religious, sexual, or hypochondriac. Delusions of reference, in which the patient attributes a special, irrational, and usually negative significance to other people, objects, or events, such as song lyrics or newspaper articles, in relation to self are common. Delusions may be defined as bizarre if they are clearly irrational and do not derive from ordinary life experiences. A common bizarre delusion is the patient's belief that the thinking processes, parts of the body, or actions or impulses are controlled or dictated by some external force.

Hallucinations are false sensory perceptions that are experienced without an external stimulus but that nevertheless seem real to the patient. Auditory hallucinations, experienced as "voices" characteristically heard commenting negatively about the patient in the third person, are prominent in schizophrenia. Hallucinations of touch, sight, taste, smell, and bodily sensation also occur.

Disorganized thinking is commonly associated with psychoses. The thought disorders may consist of a **loosening of associations,** so that the speaker jumps from one idea or topic to another unrelated one (derailment) in an illogical, inappropriate, or disorganized way. Answers to questions may be obliquely related or completely unrelated (tangentiality). At its most serious, this incoherence of thought extends into pronunciation itself, and the speaker's words become garbled or unrecognizable. Speech may also be overly concrete (loss of ability to think in abstract terms) and inexpressive; it may be repetitive, or, though voluble, it may convey little or no real information.

Disorganized behavior is another common characteristic of psychoses. Problems may be noted in any form of goal-directed behavior, leading to difficulties in performing activities of daily living such as organizing meals or maintaining hygiene. The patient may appear disheveled, may dress in an unusual manner (for example, wearing several layers of clothing, scarves, and gloves on a hot day), or may display clearly inappropriate sexual behavior (for example, public masterbation) or unpredictable and untriggered agitation (for example, shouting or swearing). Disorganized behavior must be distinguished from behavior that is merely aimless or generally unpurposeful and from organized behavior that is motivated by delusional beliefs.

Changes in affect may also be symptoms of psychosis. Emotional expressiveness is diminished; there is poor eye contact and reduced spontaneous movement. Patients appear to be withdrawn from others; the face appears immobile and unresponsive. Speech is often minimal with only brief, slow, monotone replies to questions. There is a withdrawal from areas of functioning in interpersonal relationships, work, education, and self-care.

Treatment

The importance of initial assessment for accurate diagnosis cannot be underestimated in a patient with acute psychosis. A thorough physical and neurologic examination, a mental status examination, a complete family and social history, and a laboratory workup must be performed to exclude other causes of psychoses, such as substance abuse. Both drug and nondrug therapies are critical to the treatment of most psychoses. Long-term outcome is improved in patients with an integrated drug and nondrug treatment regimen. Nonpharmacologic interventions such as individual psychotherapy to improve insight into the illness and to assist the patient in coping with stress, group therapy to enhance socialization skills, and behavioral or cognitive therapy and vocational training are of benefit to patients.

Before initiation of therapy, the treatment goals and baseline level of functioning must be established and documented. **Target symptoms** must also be identified and documented. Target symptoms are critical monitoring parameters that are used to assess change in clinical status and response to medications. Examples of target symptoms include frequency and type of agitation, degree of suspiciousness, delusions, hallucinations, loose associations, grooming habits and hygiene, sleep patterns, speech patterns, social skills, and judgment. The ultimate goal is to restore behavioral, cognitive, and psychosocial process and skills to as near baseline levels as possible so that the patient is reintegrated into the community. Realistically, unless the psychosis is part of another medical diagnosis such as substance abuse, most patients will have recurring symptoms of their mental disorder most of their lives. Treatment is therefore focused at decreased severity of target symptoms that most interfere with functioning.

Drug Therapy for Psychoses

Pharmacologic treatment of psychoses is accomplished with several classes of drugs. The most specific are the antipsy-chotic agents, but benzodiazepines (p. 185) are often used for control of acute psychotic symptoms. The beta-adrenergic blocking agents (p. 156), antiparkinson agents (p. 179), and anticholinergic agents (p. 180) occasionally play a role in controlling adverse effects of antipsychotic therapy.

Antipsychotic agents can be classified in several ways. Traditionally, they have been divided into the phenothiazines and the nonphenothiazines (see Table 16-1). Antipsychotic agents can also be classified as low-potency or high-potency drugs. The terminology of low and high potency refers only to the milligram doses used for these medicines and does not suggest any difference in effectiveness (for example, 100 mg of chlorpromazine, a low-potency agent, is equivalent in antipsychotic activity to 2 mg of haloperidol, a high-potency agent). Chlorpromazine and thioridazine are considered low-potency agents. Trifluoperazine, fluphenazine, thiothixene, haloperidol, loxapine, and molindone are considered high-potency agents. Since 1990 antipsychotic agents have also been classified as *typical* or *atypical* based on mechanism of action. The **atypical antipsychotic agents** are clozapine and risperidone. All of the remaining antipsychotic agents in Table 16-1 are considered to be **typical antipsychotic agents.**

Actions

All antipsychotic agents antagonize the neurotransmitter dopamine in the central nervous system. However, the exact mechanisms by which this prohibits psychotic symptoms is unknown. There is substantially more to the development of psychotic symptoms than elevated dopamine levels. It is known that there are at least five types of dopamine receptors in various areas of the central nervous system. The typical antipsychotic agents specifically block D1 and D2 receptors. It is thought that antagonism of the D2 receptors in the mesolimbic area of the brain reduces psychotic symptoms. Antipsychotic agents also block cholinergic, histaminic, serotonergic, and adrenergic neurotransmitter receptors to varying degrees, accounting for many of the adverse effects of therapy. Clozapine and risperidone are atypical in their actions in that clozepine activity appears to be more specific for blocking D1 and D4 receptors, whereas risperidone, in addition to D2 blocking activity, also blocks serotonin receptors.

Uses

All antipsychotic agents are equal in efficacy when used in **equipotent doses.** There is some unpredictable interpatient variation, however, and individual patients do sometimes show a better response to particular drugs. In general, selection of medication should be based on the need to avoid certain side effects in concurrent medical or psychiatric disorders. Despite practice trends, no proof exists that agitation responds best to sedating drugs or that withdrawn patients respond best to nonsedating drugs. Medication history should be a major factor in drug selection. The final important factors in drug selection are the clinically important differences in frequency of adverse effects. No one drug is least likely to cause all adverse effects; thus individual response will be the best determinant of which drug should be used.

The initial goal of antipsychotic therapy is to both calm the agitated patient who may be a physical threat to self or

Table 16-1

Antipsychotic Agents

GENERIC NAME	BRAND NAME	AVAILABILITY	ADULT DOSAGE RANGE (MG)	SEDATION	EPS*	HYPOTENSION	ACE†
Phenothiazines							
Chlorpromazine	Thorazine, ✸ Largactil	Tablets: 10, 25, 50, 100, 200 mg Sustained release capsules: 30, 75, 150 mg Syrup: 10 mg/5ml; 30, 100 mg/ml Injection: 25 mg/ml Suppository: 25, 100 mg	30-1000	+++	++	+++	++
Fluphenazine	Prolixin, Permitil ✸ Moditen	Tablets: 1, 2.5, 5, 10 mg Elixir: 2.5 mg/5 ml; 5 mg/ml Injection: 25 mg/ml	0.5-20	+	+++	+	+
Mesoridazine	Serentil	Tablets: 10, 25, 50, 100 mg Concentrate: 25 mg/ml Injection: 25 mg/ml	30-400	+++	+	++	++
Perphenazine	Trilafon	Tablets: 2, 4, 8, 16 mg Concentrate: 16 mg/5 ml	12-64	+	+++	+	++
Prochlorperazine	Compazine ✸ Stemetil	Tablets: 5, 10, 25 mg Sustained release capsules: 10, 15 mg Syrup: 5 mg/5 ml Injection: 5 mg/ml Suppository: 2.5, 5, 25 mg	15-150	+	+++	+	+
Promazine	Sparine	Tablets: 25, 50 mg Injection: 25, 50 mg/ml	40-1000	++	++	++	+++
Thioridazine	Mellaril, ✸ Novoridazine	Tablets: 10, 15, 25, 50, 100, 150, 200 mg Suspension: 25, 100 mg/5 ml Concentrate: 30, 100 mg/ml	150-800	+++	+	++	++
Trifluoperazine	Stelazine, ✸ Terfluzine	Tablets: 1, 2, 5, 10 mg Concentrate: 10 mg/ml Injection: 2 mg/ml	2-40	+	+++	+	+
Triflupromazine	Vesprin	Injection: 10, 20 mg/ml	60-150	+++	++	+++	++
Thioxanthenes							
Thiothixene	Navane	Capsules: 1, 2, 5, 10, 20 mg	6-60	+	+++	+	+
Nonphenothiazines							
Clozapine	Clozaril	Tablets: 25, 100 mg	300-900	+++	+	+++	++
Haloperidol	Haldol ✸ Peridol	Tablets: 0.5, 1, 2, 5, 10, 20 mg Concentrate: 2 mg/ml Injection: 5, 50, 100 mg/ml	1-15	+	+++	+	+
Loxapine	Loxitane, ✸ Loxapac	Capsules: 5, 10, 25, 50 mg Concentrate: 25 mg/ml Injection: 50 mg/ml	20-250	++	+++	++	+
Molindone	Moban	Tablets: 5, 10, 25, 50, 100 mg Concentrate: 20 mg/ml	15-225	++	++	++	+
Risperidone	Risperdal	Tablets: 1, 2, 3, 4 mg	4-16	+	+	−	−

Key to symbols: (+) low; (++) moderate; (+++) high.
*Extrapyramidal symptoms (EPS).
†Anticholinergic effects (ACE).
✸ Available in Canada only.

Antipsychotic Medicines

Patients starting to take antipsychotic medicine can expect some therapeutic effect such as reduced psychomotor agitation and insomnia within 1 week of therapy, but reduction in hallucinations, delusions, and thought disorders often requires 6 to 8 weeks for full therapeutic response. Rapid increases in dosages of antipsychotic medication will not reduce the antipsychotic response time but will increase the frequency of adverse effects.

Antipsychotic medicines may produce extrapyramidal effects. Tardive dyskinesia may be reversible in the early stages, but it becomes irreversible with continued use of the antipsychotic medication. Regular assessment for tardive dyskinesia should be completed for all patients receiving antipsychotic agents.

others and to begin treatment of the psychosis and thought disorder. Combined therapy with benzodiazepines (often lorazepam) and antipsychotic agents allows lower doses of the antipsychotic agent to be used, reducing the risk of serious adverse effects more commonly seen with higher-dose therapy. Some therapeutic effect such as reduced psychomotor agitation and insomnia are observed within 1 week of therapy, but reductions in hallucinations, delusions, and thought disorder often require 6 to 8 weeks for full therapeutic effect. Rapid increases in the dosages of antipsychotic medicines will not reduce the antipsychotic response time. Patients, families, and the health care team must be educated to give antipsychotic agents an adequate chance to work before unnecessarily escalating the dosage and increasing the risk of adverse effects.

After an acute psychotic episode has resolved and the patient is free from overt psychotic symptoms, a decision must be made as to whether maintenance therapy is necessary. This will depend on the diagnosed psychotic disorder and the tolerance of the adverse effects of the medicine by the patient. However, most psychotic disorders are treated with lower maintenance doses to minimize the risk of recurrence of the disorder.

Adverse Effects

Many of the serious adverse effects of the antipsychotic agents can be attributed to the pharmacologic effect of blocking dopaminergic, cholinergic, histaminic, serotonergic, and adrenergic neurotransmitter receptors. Whereas these agents block D2 receptors in the mesolimbic area of the brain to stop psychotic symptoms, blockade of the D2 receptors in other areas of the brain explains the occurrence of extrapyramidal effects.

The extrapyramidal effects are the most troublesome side effects and the most frequent cause of noncompliance associated with antipsychotic therapy. There are four categories of **extrapyramidal symptoms** (EPS): dystonic reactions,

pseudoparkinsonism, akathisas, and tardive dyskinesia. Neuroleptic malignant syndrome is a potentially fatal adverse effect of antipsychotic therapy in which the patient displays extrapyramidal manifestations as part of the symptoms of the disorder.

Acute **dystonia** has the earliest onset of all the EPSs. Dystonias are spasmodic movements (prolonged tonic contractions) of muscle groups, such as tongue protrusion, rolling back of the eyes (oculogyric crisis), spasm of the jaw (trismus), or torsion of the neck (torticollis). These symptoms are often frightening and painful for the patient. Approximately 90% of all dystonic reactions occur in the first 72 hours of therapy. Dystonic reactions are most frequent in younger patients, males, and patients receiving high-potency medicines such as haloperidol. Dystonic reactions are generally brief and are most responsive of the EPSs to treatment. Acute dystonic reactions may be controlled by intramuscular injections of diphenhydramine, benztropine, diazepam, or lorazepam.

Pseudoparkinsonian symptoms of tremor, muscular rigidity, masklike expression, shuffling gait, and loss or weakness of motor function typically begin after 2 to 3 weeks of antipsychotic drug therapy but may occur up to 3 months after starting therapy. They are more commonly seen in the elderly. The cause of these symptoms is a relative deficiency of dopamine with cholinergic excess caused by the antipsychotic agents. These symptoms are well controlled by anticholinergic antiparkinsonian agents (e.g., benztropine, diphenhydramine, trihexyphenidyl).

Akathisia is a syndrome consisting of subjective feelings of anxiety and restlessness and objective signs of pacing, rocking, and inability to sit or stand in one place for extended periods of time. Akathisia can increase aggression and is a frequent cause of noncompliance. It occurs more commonly when high-potency antipsychotic agents are used. The mechanism of action is not understood. Reduction of the dosage of the antipsychotic agent or switching to a low-potency agent should be considered. Treatment with anticholinergic agents, benzodiazepines (diazepam or lorazepam), beta-adrenergic blocking agents (propranolol), and clonidine has been successful to varying degrees.

With the possible exception of clozepine, all antipsychotic agents have the potential to produce **tardive dyskinesia.** Tardive dyskinesia is a syndrome of persistent and involuntary hyperkinetic abnormal movements. This drug-induced, late-appearing neurologic disorder is noted for such symptoms as bucco-lingual-masticatory (BLM) syndrome, or orofacial movements. The BLM movements begin with mild forward, backward, or lateral movement of the tongue. As the disorder progresses, more obvious movements appear, including tongue thrusting, rolling, or fly-catching movement and chewing or lateral jaw movements producing smacking noises. Symptoms may interfere with the patient's ability to chew, speak, or swallow. Facial movements include frequent blinking, brow arching, grimacing, and upward deviation of the eyes. The severity of symptoms of tardive dyskinesia can fluctuate daily, and symptoms often will remit during sleep. The clinical manifestations of tardive dyskinesia are similar to those of EPS, but there are some significant differences as well. Tardive dyskinesia typically appears after antipsychotic dose reduction or discontinuation, improves when the antipsychotic dose is increased, worsens with administration of anticholinergic agents, and may persist for months or years after antipsychotic medicines are discontinued. The exact cause of tardive dyskinesia is unknown. Early signs of tardive dyskinesia may be reversible but over time may become irreversible, even with discontinuation of the antipsychotic medicine.

The best treatment approach to tardive dyskinesia is prevention. Patients who receive maintenance antipsychotic drug therapy should be assessed for early signs of tardive dyskinesia at least semiannually and preferably quarterly. Findings should be documented in patient records to ensure continuity of care and medicolegal protection. Because of the variabiity in severity and presentation, rating scales have been developed to standardize assessments and diagnoses. The **abnormal involuntary movement scale** (AIMS) rates dyskinetic movements but is not exclusively diagnostic for tardive dyskinesia. The **dyskinesia identification system: condensed user scale** (DISCUS) rates the presence and severity of abnormal movements and considers other variables when formulating a conclusion. The DISCUS evaluation specifically describes the type of tardive dyskinesia and allows diagnoses to change over time. (See Appendix G.)

Treatment of tardive dyskinesia is not particularly successful. The most beneficial treatments are anticholinergic withdrawal, adrenergic blocking agents (for example, beta blockers, clonidine), and benzodiazepines. Antipsychotic dosages may be increased, but this only masks symptoms and eventually will worsen tardive dyskinesia. Clozepine is the antipsychotic agent least likely to cause tardive dyskinesia. Patients with severe symptoms of tardive dyskinesia who must be maintained on antipsychotic therapy may be candidates for clozepine therapy.

Neuroleptic malignant syndrome (NMS) occurs in 0.5% to 1.4% of patients receiving antipsychotic therapy. It has been most frequently reported with high-potency antipsychotic agents given intramuscularly. It typically occurs after 3 to 9 days of treatment with antipsychotic agents and is not related to dose or previous drug exposure. Once NMS begins, symptoms rapidly progress over 24 to 72 hours. Symptoms usually last 5 to 10 days after discontinuing oral medications and 13 to 30 days with **depot antipsychotic medicine** (depot = injectible, slow-release dosage form). Most cases of NMS occur in patients under 40 years of age, and it occurs twice as frequently in males. The syndrome is characterized by fever, severe extrapyramidal symptoms such as lead-pipe rigidity, trismus, choreiform movements, and opisthotonus; autonomic instability such as tachycardia, labile hypertension, diaphoresis, and incontinence; and alterations in consciousness such as stupor, mutism, and coma. Mortality rates have been as high as 20% to 30%, but prompt recognition of the symptoms has reduced the mortality rate to 4% in recent years. It is hypothesized that the cause of the symptoms is excessive dopamine depletion. Treatment includes bromocriptine or amantadine as dopamine agonists and dantrolene as a muscle relaxant. Fever is treated by using cooling blankets, adequate hydration, and antipyretics. Once the patient's condition is stabilized, a thorough evaluation of the medications being prescribed is made. Resumption of the antipsychotic agent may result in a recurrence of NMS; therefore the lowest dosage possible of the antipsychotic agent is prescribed, and close observation of the patient's response is required.

Other adverse effects of antipsychotic therapy can also be predicted based on the receptor-blocking activity of the agents.

Blocking of the *cholinergic (acetylcholine) receptors* explains the anticholinergic effects (dry mouth, constipation, sinus tachycardia, blurred vision, inhibition or impairment of ejaculation, and urinary retention) associated with antipsychotic agents.

Blocking *histamine-1 receptors* causes sedation, drowsiness, and appetite stimulation and contributes to the hypotensive effects as well as potentiation of central nervous system (CNS) depressant drugs. Molindone has no histamine-1 blocking effect and therefore causes no weight gain when compared with other antipsychotic agents.

Antipsychotic agents also block α_1 and α_2 *adrenergic receptors,* causing postural hypotension, reflex tachycardia, and potentiation of antihypertensive agents. The most potent α_1 blockers are mesoridazine, chlorpromazine, and thioridazine; molindone and haloperidol have virtually no effect on α_1 receptors.

Antipsychotic agents may lower the seizure threshold in patients with seizure disorders and may produce a myriad of side effects other than those already listed. These include hepatotoxicity, blood dyscrasias, allergic reactions, endocrine disorders, skin pigmentation, and reversible effects in the eyes. Patients receiving clozapine are particularly susceptible to developing agranulocytosis. Regularly scheduled white blood cell (WBC) counts are mandatory.

Nursing Process for Psychoses

Assessment

History of behavior. • Gather information from the patient and other historians relating to the onset, duration, and progression of the patient's symptoms. Has the patient previously been treated for this or other mental disorders? Does the patient have any coexisting health conditions? • Take a detailed history of all medications the individual is taking or has taken in the last 3 months. • Inquire about the use of substances.

Basic mental status. • Note general appearance and appropriateness of attire. Is the individual clean and neat? Is the posture erect, stooped, or slumped? Is the patient oriented to date, time, place, and person? • What coping mechanisms has the individual been using to deal with the situation? How adaptive are the coping mechanisms? • Has the patient been able to carry out self-care activities and social and work obligations? • Are symptoms of depression present? Symptoms may not be evident during the acute phase of schizophrenia.

Interpersonal relationships. Assess the quality of relationships in which the individual is involved. Identify persons that are supportive. Ask the family and significant others to describe the relationships they have with the patient. Has there been a deterioration in their closeness and ability to interrelate effectively?

Mood/affect. • Patients experiencing altered thinking, behavior, or feelings require careful evaluation of both verbal and nonverbal actions. Often the thoughts, feelings, and behaviors displayed are inconsistent with the so-called normal responses of individuals in similar circumstances. Is the facial expression worried, sad, angry, or blank? • Is the individual displaying behaviors that are inappropriate, blunted, or have a flattened affect? Is the patient apathetic to normal situations? • Is there consistency in the verbal and nonverbal expression of feelings? • Does the patient overreact to situations at times?

Clarity of thoughts/perception. • Does the patient suffer from delusions, disorganized speech pattern, flight of ideas, autism, grandiose ideas, or mutism? Ask about the presence of hallucinations (auditory, visual, tactile). • Does the patient talk about unrelated topics (loose association) as though they are connected and related? • Is the patient self-absorbed and not in contact with reality? • Does the patient display interruption of thoughts? • Does the patient display paranoid behavior?

Thoughts of death. If the individual is suspected of being suicidal, ask if there have ever been thoughts about suicide. If the response is yes, get more details. Is a specific plan formulated? How often do these thoughts occur? Does the individual make direct or indirect statements regarding death, for example, things would be better after death?

Psychomotor function. What is the patient's activity level? Is the individual unable to sit still or pacing continually? Or is the patient catatonic (immobile because of psychologic functioning, nonphysiologic).

Sleep pattern. What is the person's normal sleep pattern, and how has it varied since the onset of the psychotic symptoms? Ask specifically whether insomnia is present. Ask the individual to describe the perception of the amount and quality of sleep nightly. What is the level of fatigue? Are naps taken regularly?

Dietary history. Ask questions relating to appetite, and note weight gains or losses not associated with intentional dieting.

Nursing Diagnosis
* Adjustment, impaired (indication)
* Communication, impaired (indication)
* Coping, ineffective individual (indication)
* Role performance, altered (indication)
* Thought process, altered (indication)
* Injury, risk for (side effects)

Planning

History of psychotic behavior. • Review data collected to identify individual's strengths and weaknesses. • Review medications being taken to identify any that are known to cause any of the symptoms being exhibited.

Basic mental status. • Plan to perform a baseline assessment of the individual's mental status at specific intervals throughout the course of treatment. • Review coping mechanisms being used. Plan to discuss those that are maladaptive. Plan to initiate changes by guiding the individual in the use of more adaptive coping strategies. • Schedule specific times to discuss the patient's behavior with family members to foster understanding.

Mood/affect. Review assessment data to develop strategies to assist the individual to cope more effectively with exhibited behaviors. Reward positive accomplishments for progress made.

Clarity of thought/perception. • Plan to monitor the patient carefully for altered thoughts and perceptions. Develop approaches that could be tried when the individual is having delusions or hallucinations. Decrease the stimuli within the patient's immediate environment. • Identify areas in which the patient is capable of input to set goals and make decisions. When the patient is unable to make decisions, plan to make them. Set goals to involve the patient as abilities change with treatment. Provide an opportunity to plan for self-care.

Thoughts of death. Provide for a safe environment for the individual. Search the surroundings for objects that could be used to inflict self-harm.

Psychomotor function. Review activities offered within the clinical setting, and plan for the individual to participate in those that will be beneficial and nonthreatening.

Sleep pattern. Provide specific parameters in which the patient can function that allow the individual's need for sleep to be met.

Dietary needs. Provide an opportunity for the individual to be involved in selecting foods appropriate to needs (to lose or gain weight). If the person is paranoid and suspects being poisoned, plan for the individual to self-serve food, open canned food, and so on, as appropriate within the setting.

Implementation
* Nursing interventions must be individualized and based on patient assessment data.
* Provide the individual with a structured environment that is safe and decreases external stimuli.
* Provide an environment of acceptance that focuses on the individual's strengths while minimizing weaknesses.
* Provide an opportunity for the individual to express feelings. Use active listening and therapeutic communication techniques. Provide an opportunity for the person to express feelings in nonverbal ways (for example, involve in physical activities, occupational therapy).
* Allow the patient to make decisions if capable; make those the patient is not capable of making. Provide a reward for progress when decisions are initiated appropriately.
* Involve the patient in self-care activities. Assist with personal grooming, as needed. Ensure that the patient is dressed appropriately to prevent embarrassment.
* Set limits and enforce them in a kind, firm manner to handle inappropriate behaviors.
* Once you know the content, do not reinforce hallucinations or delusions.
* When the person has altered perceptions, provide diversional activities and minimize interactions such as television programs watched that may reinforce the distorted perceptions.

- Be open and direct in handling patients who are highly suspicious. Speak distinctly so they can hear you; do not whisper or laugh in circumstances the patients could misconstrue.
- If the patient is suicidal, ask for details of the plan being formulated. Follow up on details obtained with appropriate family members or significant others, for example, have guns removed from home if this is part of the plan. Provide for patient safety and supervision and record observations at specified intervals consistent with severity of the suicide threat and policies of the practice site.
- Use physical restraints within the guidelines of the clinical setting as appropriate to the behaviors being exhibited. Use the least restrictive alternative possible for the circumstances. Have sufficient staff available to assist with violent behavior to demonstrate ability to control the situation while providing for the safety and well-being of the patient and fellow staff members.
- Provide for nutritional needs by having high-protein, high-calorie foods appropriate for the individual to eat while pacing or highly active. Have nutritious snacks the patient is known to like available on the unit. Offer these at specific intervals throughout the day. Administer vitamins and liquid supplemental feedings as ordered.
- Manipulative behavior must be handled in a consistent manner by all staff members. Use limit setting and consequences that are agreed to in advance by all staff members. When the patient attempts to blame others, refocus on the patient's responsibilities. Give positive reinforcement for nonmanipulative behaviors when they occur.

Patient Education and Health Promotion

- Orient the individual to the unit, explaining rules and the process of privileges and how they are obtained or lost. (The extent of the orientation and explanations given will depend on the individual's orientation to date, time, and place and abilities.)
- Explain unit rules and therapeutic rules. Keep explanations clear and concise.
- Patient education must be based on assessment data and individualized to provide the patient with a structured environment in which to grow and enhance self-esteem.
- Explain the activity groups available and how and when the individual will participate in these. A variety of group process activities, for example, social skills group, self-esteem groups, and physical exercise groups, are available within particular therapeutic settings.
- The patient and family must be involved in goal setting and integrated into the appropriate group processes to develop positive experiences for the patient to enhance coping skills. Those patients who are disruptive, withdrawn, or who have impaired communication need individualized approaches to improve patient education.
- Before discharge the patient and family must understand the goals of treatment and the entire follow-up plan, for example, frequency of therapy sessions, doctor visits, and return to work goals.

Fostering health maintenance. Throughout the course of treatment, discuss medication information and how it will benefit the patient's symptoms and circumstances. Drug therapy is a major portion of antipsychotic therapy. Although symptoms may improve they may not be totally eliminated. The onset of the drug's effectiveness varies widely depending on the drug administered and the route of administration. Noncompliance is a major problem in this group of patients, therefore tracking of the medications being taken needs careful scrutiny. On an outpatient basis, many of these patients require administration of their medication by another responsible individual. (The patient may find this stressful.) Noncompliance is thought to be a major cause of rehospitalization in this group of patients. Long-acting injections may be used on some patients in an attempt to overcome this problem. On an inpatient basis the nurse must always check to be sure the patient is actually swallowing the medication because there is a high incidence of "cheeking" the medication.

Today, mandatory periodic assessments for the development of extrapyramidal symptoms are required. The DISCUS or AIMS behavior-monitoring parameters are completed at prescribed intervals and information is recorded on a behavior-monitoring flow sheet.

Provide the patient and significant others with important information contained in the specific drug monograph for the medicines prescribed. Additional health teaching and nursing interventions for the side effects to expect and report are described in the drug monographs that follow.

Seek cooperation and understanding of the following points so that medication compliance is increased: name of medication, dosage, route and times of administration, side effects to expect, and side effects to report.

Written record: Enlist the patient's aid in developing and maintaining a written record of monitoring parameters. Instruct the patient to bring the written record to follow-up visits. Because there are a number of side effects that are considered debilitating by the patient and others are life threatening if not acted on correctly, it is important that open communication with the physician, nurses, therapist, and pharmacist be encouraged throughout the course of therapy.

Drug Class: Antipsychotic Agents

Phenothiazines, thioxanthenes, haloperidol, molindone, loxapine, clozapine, and risperidone

Actions

Although the antipsychotic agents are from distinctly different chemical classes, all antipsychotic agents are similar in that they act by blocking the action of dopamine in the brain. Because they work at different sites within the brain, the side effects are observed on different systems throughout the body.

Uses

Antipsychotic agents, also known as neuroleptic agents, are used to treat psychoses associated with mental illnesses such as schizophrenia, mania, psychotic depression, and psychotic organic brain syndrome. Medications used to treat these disorders are grouped into two broad categories:

the phenothiazines and the nonphenothiazines (thioxanthenes, haloperidol, molindone, loxapine, clozapine, and risperidone).

Therapeutic Outcomes

The primary therapeutic outcome from antipsychotic therapy is maintaining the individual at an optimal level of functioning with minimal exacerbations of psychotic symptoms.

Nursing Process

Premedication Assessment

1. Obtain baseline blood pressures in supine, sitting, and standing positions; record and report significant lowering to physician before administering drug.
2. Check electrolytes, hepatic function, renal function, cardiac function, and thyroid function before initiation and periodically throughout course of administration.
3. Perform DISCUS or AIMS at specified intervals to detect or check on extrapyramidal symptoms; record and report according to agency policy.
4. Use of clozapine requires baseline and weekly WBC counts because of the high incidence of agranulocytosis.

Planning

Availability. See Table 16-1.

Implementation

Dosage and Administration. See Table 16-1. Dosages must be individualized according to the degree of mental and emotional disturbance. It will often take several weeks for a patient to show optimal improvement and become stabilized on an adequate maintenance dosage. As a result of the cumulative effects of antipsychotic agents, patients must be reevaluated periodically to determine the lowest effective dosage necessary to control psychiatric symptoms. Sedative effects associated with antipsychotic therapy can be minimized by giving the dose of medication at bedtime.

Evaluation

Side effects to expect

CHRONIC FATIGUE, DROWSINESS. Persons who are working around machinery, driving a car, pouring and giving medicines, or performing other duties in which they must remain mentally alert should not take these medications while working.

ORTHOSTATIC HYPOTENSION. All antipsychotic agents may cause some degree of orthostatic hypotension manifested by dizziness and weakness, particularly when therapy is being initiated.

Monitor the blood pressure daily in the supine, sitting, and standing positions.

Anticipate the development of postural hypotension, and take measures to prevent an occurrence. Teach the patient to rise slowly from a supine or sitting position; encourage the patient to sit or lie down if feeling faint.

BLURRED VISION, CONSTIPATION, URINARY RETENTION, DRYNESS OF THE MUCOSA OF THE MOUTH, THROAT, AND NOSE. These symptoms are the anticholinergic effects produced by these agents. Patients taking these medications

should be monitored for the development of these side effects.

Dryness of the mucosa may be relieved by sucking hard candy or ice chips or by chewing gum.

The use of stool softeners such as docusate or the occasional use of a potent laxative such as bisacodyl may be required for constipation.

Caution the patient that blurred vision may occur, and make appropriate suggestions for personal safety of the individual.

Side effects to report

SEIZURE ACTIVITY. Provide for patient safety during episodes of seizures; report for further evaluation. Adjustment of anticonvulsant therapy may be required, especially in seizure-prone patients.

PARKINSONIAN SYMPTOMS. Report the development of drooling, cogwheel rigidity, shuffling gait, masklike expression, or tremors. Anticholinergic agents may be used to control these symptoms.

TARDIVE DYSKINESIA. Report the development of fine tremors of the tongue, "fly catching" tongue movements, and lip smacking. This is particularly important in patients who have been receiving antipsychotic agents and anticholinergic agents for several years.

HEPATOTOXICITY. The symptoms of hepatotoxicity are anorexia, nausea, vomiting, jaundice, hepatomegaly, splenomegaly, and abnormal liver function tests (elevated bilirubin, aspartate transaminase [AST], alanine aminotransferase [ALT], gamma glutamyltransferase [GGT], alkaline phosphatase, prothrombin time).

BLOOD DYSCRASIAS. Routine laboratory studies (red blood cell [RBC], white blood cell [WBC], and differential counts) should be scheduled. This is particularly important for patients receiving clozapine.

Monitor for the development of sore throat, fever, purpura, jaundice, or excessive and progressive weakness.

HIVES, PRURITUS, RASH. Report symptoms for further evaluation by the physician.

PHOTOSENSITIVITY. The patient should be cautioned to avoid exposure to sunlight and ultraviolet light. Suggest wearing long-sleeved clothing, a hat, and sunglasses when exposed to sunlight. Advise against using artificial tanning lamps. Notify the physician for the advisability of discontinuing therapy.

Drug interactions

DRUGS THAT INCREASE TOXIC EFFECTS. Antihistamines, alcohol, analgesics, anesthetics, tranquilizers, barbiturates, narcotics, and sedative-hypnotics. Monitor the patient for excessive sedation and reduce the dosage of the above-mentioned agents if necessary.

GUANETHIDINE. Antipsychotic agents may inhibit the antihypertensive effect of guanethidine. Concurrent therapy is not recommended.

BETA-ADRENERGIC BLOCKERS. Beta-adrenergic blocking agents (propanolol, timolol, nadolol, pindolol, and others) significantly enhance the hypotensive effects of antipsychotic agents. Concurrent therapy is not recommended unless used to treat adverse effects of antipsychotic agents.

BARBITURATES. Barbiturates may stimulate the rate of metabolism of phenothiazines. Dosage adjustments of the antipsychotic agent may be necessary.

INSULIN, ORAL HYPOGLYCEMIC AGENTS. Diabetic or pre-diabetic patients must be monitored for the development of hyperglycemia, particularly during the early weeks of therapy.

Assess regularly for glycosuria and report if it occurs with any frequency.

Patients receiving oral hypoglycemic agents or insulin may require an adjustment in dosage.

CHAPTER REVIEW

Psychoses are symptoms of psychotic disorders, that is, illnesses in which the patient has lost touch with reality. The underlying illness must be treated—not just the psychosis. A combination of nonpharmacologic and pharmacologic therapies provides the most successful outcomes to therapy. The emphasis on community treatment and the closing of many state mental hospitals has ensured that virtually all health care settings treat patients with psychotic symptoms. Community hospitals and health maintenance organizations now provide care to many psychiatric patients, and nurses increasingly serve residential care facilities. Many patients require years of antipsychotic drug treatment to to prevent exacerbations of illness. Although antipsychotic agents cause many adverse effects, most can be minimized by patient education, manipulation of doses and schedule, and sometimes adjunctive drug treatments. These patients require careful monitoring of target symptoms to maximize response and minimize adverse effects.

MATH REVIEW

1. The doctor orders chlorpromazine (Thorazine) 125 mg PO. On hand is chlorpromazine 100 mg per 5 ml. Give _____ ml.

2. The physician orders benztropine mesylate (Cogentin) 1 mg PO at bedtime daily. Available is benztropine mesylate 0.5 mg tablets. Give _____ tablets.

3. The physician orders trifluoperazine (Stelazine) 12 mg IM. On hand is trifluoperazine 10 mg per ml and 20 mg per ml. Which concentration would you use, and what volume should be injected?

CRITICAL THINKING QUESTIONS

Jessica Smith is taking a high-potency antipsychotic medication.

1. What is meant by the term *high-potency antipsychotics,* and what drugs are included in this category?

2. What is meant by extrapyramidal side effects? How often should the patient be monitored for these symptoms? When found, what nursing actions are appropriate?

3. It is decided that Jessica should receive clozapine. What are the side effects to expect and those to report with this medication?
Discuss monitoring for agranulocytosis.

4. Why is an anticholinergic agent frequently given in addition to haloperidol? What is its action?

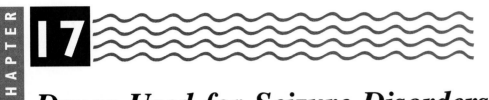

Drugs Used for Seizure Disorders

Key Words

seizures	atonic seizure
epilepsy	myoclonic seizures
partial seizures	absence (petit mal) epilepsy
anticonvulsants	seizure threshold
tonic phase	GABA
clonic phase	gingival hyperplasia
postictal state	nystagmus
status epilepticus	urticaria

Objectives

1. Prepare a chart to be used as a study guide that includes the following information:
   Name of seizure type
   Description of seizure
   Medications used to treat each type of seizure
   Nursing interventions and monitoring parameters for seizures

2. Describe the effects of the hydantoins on patients with diabetes and on persons receiving oral contraceptives, theophylline, folic acid, or antacids.

3. Cite precautions needed when administering phenytoin or diazepam intravenously.

4. Explain the rationale for proper dental care for persons receiving hydantoin therapy.

5. Develop a teaching plan for patient education for persons diagnosed with a seizure disorder.

6. Cite the desired therapeutic outcomes for seizure disorders.

7. Identify the mechanisms of action thought to control seizure activity when anticonvulsants are administered.

8. Discuss the basic classification systems used for epilepsy.

SEIZURE DISORDERS

Seizures are symptoms of an abnormality in the nerve centers of the brain. They are brief periods of abnormal electrical activity in the brain. Seizures may be convulsive (that is, accompanied by violent, involuntary muscle contractions) or nonconvulsive. During periods of seizure activity, there is often a change in the person's consciousness, sensory and motor systems, subjective well-being, and objective behavior. Seizures may result from fever, head injury, brain tumor, meningitis, hypoglycemia, drug overdose or withdrawal, or poisoning. It is estimated that 8% to 10% of all people will have a seizure during their lifetime. If the seizures are chronic and recurrent, the patient is diagnosed as having **epilepsy.** Epilepsy is the most common of all neurologic disorders. It is not a single disease but several different diseases that have one common characteristic: a sudden discharge of excessive electrical energy from nerve cells in the brain. An estimated 2 million Americans suffer from this disorder; an estimated 100,000 new cases are diagnosed annually. The cause of epilepsy may be unknown (idiopathic epilepsy), or it may be the result of a head injury, a brain tumor, meningitis, or a stroke.

Epilepsy has been classified in several different ways. Traditionally, the most important subdivisions have been *grand mal, petit mal, psychomotor,* and *jacksonian* types. An international commission has reclassified epilepsies into two broad categories based on clinical and electroencephalographic (EEG) patterns: generalized and partial (localized).

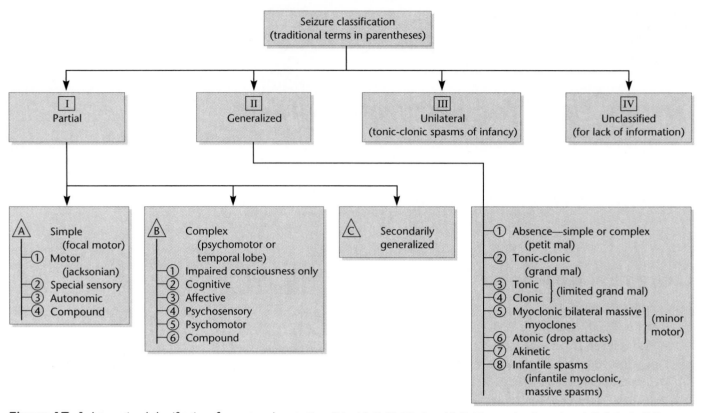

Figure 17-1 *International classification of common seizures.* (From Hahn AG, Barkin RL, Oestreich SJ: *Pharmacology in nursing,* ed 15, St Louis, 1982, Mosby.)

Generalized seizures affect both hemispheres of the brain, are accompanied by loss of consciousness, and may be subdivided into convulsive and nonconvulsive types. **Partial seizures** may be subdivided into simple and complex symptom types; with complex seizures there is a change in consciousness. Partial seizures begin in a localized area in one hemisphere of the brain. Both simple and complex partial seizures can evolve into generalized seizures, a process referred to as *secondary generalization.* See Figure 17-1 for a classification of epilepsies. Because the traditional terms are still frequently used, they have been included in the figure in parentheses. Epilepsy is treated almost exclusively with medications (**anticonvulsants**).

Descriptions of Seizures

Generalized Convulsive Seizures

The most common generalized convulsive seizures are the tonic-clonic, atonic, and myoclonic seizures.

Tonic-Clonic (Grand Mal) Seizures

Tonic-clonic (grand mal) seizures are the most common type of seizure. In the **tonic phase,** patients suddenly develop intense muscular contractions that cause the patient to fall to the ground, lose consciousness, and lie rigid. There may be arching of the back, flexion of the arms, extension of the legs, and clenching of the teeth. Air is forced up the larynx, extruding saliva as foam and producing an audible crylike sound. Respirations stop, and the patient may become cyanotic. The tonic phase usually lasts 20 to 60 seconds before a

diffuse trembling sets in. The **clonic phase,** manifested by bilaterally symmetric jerks alternating with relaxation of extremities, then begins. The clonic phase starts slightly and then gradually becomes more violent and involves the whole body. Patients often bite their tongues and become incontinent of urine or feces. Usually within 60 seconds this phase proceeds to a resting, recovery phase of flaccid paralysis and sleep lasting 2 to 3 hours (**postictal state**). The patient has no recollection of the attack after awakening. The severity, frequency, and duration of attacks are highly variable. They may last from 1 to 30 minutes and occur as frequently as daily or as infrequently as every few years. **Status epilepticus** is a rapidly recurring generalized seizure that does not allow the individual to regain normal function between seizures. It is a medical emergency that requires prompt treatment to minimize permanent nerve damage and death.

Atonic or Akinetic Seizures

A sudden loss of muscle tone is known as an **atonic seizure,** or *drop attack.* This may be described as a head drop, the dropping of a limb, or a slumping to the ground. There is a sudden loss of consciousness and muscle tone that results in a dramatic fall. Seated patients may slump forward violently. The attacks are short, but there is frequent injury from the uncontrolled falls. These patients often wear protective headgear to minimize the trauma.

Myoclonic Seizures

Myoclonic seizures involve lightning-like repetitive contractions of the voluntary muscles of the face, trunk, and extremities. The jerks may be isolated events or rapidly repetitive. It is not uncommon for patients to lose balance and fall to the floor. These attacks occur most frequently at night as the patient enters sleep.

Generalized Nonconvulsive Seizures

By far the most common generalized nonconvulsive seizure disorder is **absence (petit mal) epilepsy.** These seizures occur primarily in children and usually disappear at puberty, although the patient may develop a second type of seizure activity. Attacks consist of paroxysmal episodes of altered consciousness lasting for 5 to 20 seconds. There are no prodromal or postictal phases. Patients appear to be staring into space and may exhibit a few rhythmic movements of the eyes or head, lip smacking, mumbling, chewing, or swallowing movements. Falling does not occur, patients do not convulse, and they have no memory of events occurring during the seizures.

Partial (Localized) Seizures

The most common types of nongeneralized seizures are unilateral seizures and partial seizures.

Unilateral Seizures

Unilateral seizures involve seizure activity confined to one side of the brain. The seizures, which may last from several minutes to hours, are manifested by one-sided clonus with or without loss of consciousness. After an attack, the patient's affected side is usually left with postictal paralysis that recedes over time.

Partial Seizures

Partial seizures are subdivided into partial simple motor seizures and partial complex seizures. *Partial simple motor (jacksonian) seizures* involve localized convulsions of voluntary muscles. A single body part, such as a finger or an extremity, may start jerking. The muscle spasm may end spontaneously or spread over the whole body. The patient does not lose consciousness unless the seizure develops into a generalized convulsion. *Partial seizures with complex symptoms (psychomotor seizures)* are manifested by a vast array of possible symptoms. The patient's outward appearance may be normal or there may be aimless wandering, unusual and repeated chewing, lip smacking, or swallowing movements. The person is conscious but may be in a confused, dreamlike state. The attacks, which may occur several times daily and last for several minutes, commonly end in sleep or with a clouded sensorium with no recollection of the events of the attack.

Anticonvulsant Therapy

Identification of the cause of seizure activity is important in determining the type of therapy required. Contributing factors (for example, head injury, fever, hypoglycemia, drug overdose) must be specifically treated to correct the underlying cause before chronic anticonvulsant therapy is started. Once the underlying cause is treated, it is rare that chronic antiepileptic therapy is needed. When seizure activity continues, drug therapy is the primary form of treatment. The goals of therapy are to reduce the frequency of seizure activity and minimize the adverse effects of the medicine. Therapeutic goals must be individualized for each patient. The selection of the medicine depends on the type of seizure, the age and sex of the patient, other medical conditions present, and the potential adverse effects of the individual medicines.

In general, anticonvulsant therapy should start with the use of a single, preferably nonsedating, agent. The benzodiazepine anticonvulsants and phenobarbital are sedating; phenytoin, carbamazepine, valproate, and ethosuximide are nonsedating. Occasionally, some patients will require multiple drug therapy with a combination of sedating and nonsedating agents and will still not be completely seizure free.

Actions

Unfortunately, the mechanisms of seizure activity are extremely complex and not well understood. In general, anticonvulsants increase the **seizure threshold** and regulate neuronal firing by either inhibiting excitatory processes or enhancing inhibitory processes. The medicines can also prevent the seizure from spreading to adjacent neurons. Phenytoin, carbamazepine, lamotrigine, and valproic acid act on sodium channels to stabilize the neuronal membrane and may decrease the release of excitatory neurotransmitters. Barbiturates and benzodiazepines enhance the inhibitory effect of gamma aminobutyric acid (**GABA**), an inhibitory neurotransmitter that counterbalances the effect of excitatory neurotransmitters.

Uses

Anticonvulsants are used to reduce the frequency of seizures.

Nursing Process for Patients with Seizure Disorders

Nurses may play an important role in the correct diagnosis of seizure disorders. Accurate seizure diagnosis is crucial

---

LIFE SPAN ISSUES

ANTICONVULSANT THERAPY

In children, anticonvulsant therapy may cause a change in personality and possible indifference to school activities and family activities. Behavioral differences must be discussed with the physician, family, and teachers. The school nurse must be informed of medications prescribed.

Liquid dosage forms of anticonvulsants must be measured accurately to help maintain seizure control. It is extremely important to shake the liquid first to disperse the medicine uniformly in the suspension. The dosage should then be measured with an oral syringe to help ensure accuracy before administration.

Medicines should be taken at the same time daily to maintain a constant blood level. Dosages should not be self-adjusted, and drugs should not be suddenly discontinued.

Monitoring response to anticonvulsant therapy is essential. Dosages may need to be adjusted weekly, especially during initiation of therapy.

to the selection of the most appropriate medications for each individual patient. Because physicians are not always able to observe patient seizures directly, nurses should learn to observe and record these events objectively.

Assessment

History of seizure activity. • What activities was the individual engaging in immediately before the seizure? • Has the individual noticed any particular activity that usually precedes attacks? • When was the last seizure before the current one? • Did the individual experience any changes in behavior before the onset of the seizure (for example, increasing anxiety or depression)? • Is the individual aware of a preseizure "aura" (a particular feeling or odor that occurs before a seizure onset)? • Was there an epileptic cry?

Seizure description. • Record the exact time of seizure onset and duration of each phase, a description of the specific body parts involved, and any progression of the affected body parts. • Did the patient lose consciousness? • Was stiffening and jerking present? • Describe autonomic responses usually seen during the clonic phase—altered, jerky respirations or frothy salivation, dilated pupils and any eye movements, cyanosis, diaphoresis, incontinence.

Postictal behavior. • Record the level of consciousness—orientation to time, place, and person. • Assess the degree of alertness, fatigue, or headache present. • Evaluate the degree of weakness, alterations in speech, and memory loss. • Patients frequently experience muscle soreness and extreme need for sleep. Record the duration of sleep. • Evaluate any bodily harm that occurred during the seizure—bruises, cuts, lacerations.

Nursing Diagnosis

• Injury, risk for (indication)
• Body-image disturbance (indication, side effects)
• Impaired gas exchange (indication)
• Sensory/perceptual alteration: visual, tactile (indication)

Planning

Seizure activity. • Identify the need for seizure precautions on Kardex/care plan. • Have equipment and supplies needed for care of patient during seizure available in immediate area. • Order periodic laboratory studies to detect adverse effects (for example, blood dyscrasias, hepatotoxicity, and anticonvulsant serum levels) at intervals specified by the physician.

Psychosocial. • Plan specific times to discuss the concerns of the patient, family, or significant others with regard to the seizure disorder. Set specific goals for health teaching needed. • Arrange for a social worker to intervene with care needs in the school or work setting.

Implementation

Management of seizure activity. Assist the patient during a seizure by doing the following:

• Protect the patient from further injury. Place padding around or under the head; do not try to restrain; loosen tight clothing. If in a standing position initially, lower the patient to a horizontal position.

• If possible, place a soft object such as a face cloth between the patient's teeth to prevent accidental biting of the tongue or breakage of the teeth.

• Once the patient enters into the relaxation stage, turn slightly on the side to allow secretions to drain out of the mouth.

• Remain calm and quiet and give reassurance to the patient when the seizure is over.

• Provide a place for the patient to rest immediately after a seizure. Summon appropriate assistance so that the individual can get home.

• If the patient has another seizure or if a seizure lasts longer than 4 minutes, immediately summon assistance; the patient may be going into status epilepticus.

Psychologic implications

Lifestyle. Encourage maintenance of a normal lifestyle. Provide for appropriate limitations (such as limits on operating power equipment or a motor vehicle, limits on swimming) to ensure patient safety. The Epilepsy Foundation of America and State Vocational Rehabilitation Agencies can provide the patient with information about vocational rehabilitation and employment.

Expression of feelings. Allow for ventilation of feelings. Seizures may occur in public and may be accompanied by incontinence. Patients are usually embarrassed about having a seizure in front of others. Provide for ventilation of any discrimination the patient feels at the workplace.

School-age children. Acceptance by peers can present a problem to the patient. The school nurse can help teachers and other children to understand seizures.

Denial. Be alert for signs of denial of the disease. An indication of this is increased seizure activity in a previously well-controlled patient. Question compliance with the drug regimen.

Compliance. Determine the patient's current medication schedule: name of medication, dosage, when last dose was taken; have any doses been skipped, and if so, how many? If compliance appears to be a problem, try to determine the reasons for patient noncompliance so appropriate interventions can be implemented.

Status epilepticus

1. Provide for patient protection and summon assistance for transportation of the patient to an emergency facility.
2. Administer oxygen; have suction and resuscitation equipment available.
3. Establish an IV and have available drugs for treatment (such as diazepam, phenytoin, phenobarbital).
4. Monitor vital signs and neurologic status.
5. Insert a nasogastric tube if vomiting is present.

Patient Education and Health Promotion

Exercise and activity. Encourage maintenance of a regular lifestyle with moderate activity. Avoid excessive exercise that would lead to excessive fatigue.

Nutrition. Avoid excessive use of stimulants (for example, caffeine-containing products). Seizures are also known to follow the significant intake of alcoholic beverages; therefore ingestion should be avoided or limited.

Safety. • Teach the patient to avoid operating power equipment or machinery. Driving may be minimized or prohibited.

Check state laws regarding how or if an individual with a history of seizure activity may qualify for a driver's license.
• In the elderly, be especially alert to signs of confusion and impaired coordination. Provide for safety.

Stress. Reduction of tension and stress within the individual's environment may reduce seizure activity in some patients.

Oral hygiene. Encourage maintenance of daily oral hygiene practices and scheduling of regular dental exams. **Gingival hyperplasia,** gum overgrowth associated with hydantoins (phenytoin, ethotoin, and mephenytoin), can be reduced by good oral hygiene, frequent gum massage, regular brushing, and proper dental care.

Medication considerations. • If pregnancy is suspected, consult an obstetrician as soon as possible. Inform the physician of seizure medications. Do not discontinue medications unless told to do so by the physician. • The patient should carry an identification card or bracelet.

Expectations of therapy. • Discuss the expectations of therapy (for example, level of seizure control, degree of lethargy, sedation, frequency of use of therapy, relief of symptoms, sexual activity, maintenance of mobility, ability to maintain activities of daily living or work, and limitations in operating power equipment or a motor vehicle). • Assess changes in expectations as therapy progresses and the patient gains understanding and skill in the management of the diagnosis.

Fostering health maintenance. Throughout the course of treatment, discuss medication information and how it will benefit the patient. Recognize that noncompliance may be a means of denial. Explore underlying problems in acceptance of disease and the need for strict compliance for maximum seizure control. Provide the patient and significant others with important information contained in the specific drug monograph for the medicines prescribed. Additional health teaching and nursing interventions for the side effects to expect and report are described in the drug monographs that follow.

Seek cooperation and understanding of the following points so that medication compliance is increased: name of medication, dosage, route and times of administration, side effects to expect, and side effects to report. Enlist the patient's aid in developing and maintaining a written record (Patient Education and Monitoring Form on p. 222) of monitoring parameters (such as degree of lethargy; sedation; oral hygiene for gum disorders; degree of seizure relief; nausea, vomiting, or anorexia present) and response to prescribed therapies for discussion with the physician.

Have others record the date, time, duration, and frequency of any seizure episodes. Also record the behavior immediately before and after seizures.

Patients should be encouraged to bring this record with them on follow-up visits.

Difficulty in comprehension: If it is evident that the patient or family does not understand all aspects of continuing therapy being prescribed (such as administration and monitoring of medications, management of seizure activity when present, diets, follow-up appointments, and the need for lifelong management), consider use of social service or visiting nurse agencies.

Drug Class: Barbiturates

Actions

The barbiturates elevate the seizure threshold and prevent the spread of electrical seizure activity by enhancing the inhibitory effect of GABA. The exact mechanism is unknown.

Uses

The long-acting barbiturates (phenobarbital, mephobarbital) are effective anticonvulsants. Because of their sedative effects, however, they are now used primarily as an alternative when single nonsedating anticonvulsants are unsuccessful in controlling seizures. The barbiturates are most useful in the treatment of partial and generalized tonic-clonic seizures, usually in combination with other anticonvulsants (Table 17-1). Barbiturates are discussed in greater detail in Chapter 12.

Therapeutic Outcomes

The primary therapeutic outcomes expected from the barbiturates are as follows:
• Reduced frequency of seizures and reduced injury from seizure activity
• Minimal adverse effects from therapy

Drug Class: Benzodiazepines

Actions

The mechanism of action for benzodiazepines is not fully understood, but it is thought that the benzodiazepines inhibit neurotransmission by enhancing the effects of GABA in postsynaptic clefts between nerve cells.

Uses

The three benzodiazepines approved for use as anticonvulsants are diazepam, clonazepam, and clorazepate. Clonazepam is useful in the oral treatment of absence, akinetic, and myoclonic seizures in children. Diazepam must be administered intravenously to control seizures but is the drug of choice for treatment of status epilepticus. Clorazepate is used with other antiepileptic agents to control partial seizures.

Therapeutic Outcomes

The primary therapeutic outcomes expected from the benzodiazepines are as follows:
• Reduced frequency of seizures and reduced injury from seizure activity
• Minimal adverse effects from therapy

Nursing Process

Premedication Assessment

1. Review routine blood studies to detect blood dyscrasias and hepatotoxicity.
2. Monitor behavioral responses to therapy.

Planning

Availability. See Table 17-1.

PATIENT EDUCATION & MONITORING FORM   Anticonvulsants

MEDICATIONS	COLOR	TO BE TAKEN

Name _____

Physician _____

Physician's phone _____

Next appt.* _____

PARAMETERS		DAY OF DISCHARGE							COMMENTS
Previous seizure activity	Number / day?								
	Lasted how long?								
	Type, describe								
Present seizure activity	Number / day?								
	Lasted how long?								
	Type, describe								
	Slept after?								
Compliance	I take my medication as ordered.								
	Sometimes I forget.								
	I don't like to take medication.								
Drowsiness: Feel like sleeping all day — Feel like being active 10 5 1									
Disease acceptance: I don't want people to know I have epilepsy — I have epilepsy and take medication 10 5 1									
Oral hygiene: brushing and flossing teeth	3 times a day								
	2 times a day								
	1 time a day								
	I forgot								
Condition of gums?	No bleeding								
	Some bleeding (___) times / day								
	Bleeding every time I brush								
Nausea and vomiting	All day								
	Sometimes (when?)								

*Please bring this record with you to your next appointment.
Use the back of this sheet for additional information.

Table 17-1
Anticonvulsants

GENERIC NAME	BRAND NAME	AVAILABILITY	ADULT DOSAGE RANGE	USE IN SEIZURES
Barbiturates				
Mephobarbital	Mebaral	Tablets: 32, 50, 100 mg	400-600 mg/day	Grand mal, petit mal
Phenobarbital	Luminal, Solfoton	Tablets: 16, 30, 65, 100 mg Capsules: 16 mg Elixir: 20 mg/5ml	100-300 mg/day	All forms of epilepsy
Benzodiazepines				
Clonazepam	Klonopin, *Rivotril	Tablets: 0.5, 1, 2 mg	Up to 20 mg/day	Petit mal, myoclonic seizures
Clorazepate	Tranxene, *Novo clopate	Tablets: 3.75, 7.5, 11.25, 15, 22.5 mg	Up to 90 mg/day	Focal seizures
Diazepam	Valium, *Meval	Tablets: 2.5, 5, 10 mg IV: 5 mg/ml Liquid: 1, 5 mg/ml	Initially 5-10 mg, up to 30 mg	All forms of epilepsy; used in conjunction with other agents
Hydantoins				
Ethotoin	Peganone	Tablets: 250, 500 mg	2-3 g/day	Grand mal, psychomotor seizures
Mephenytoin	Mesantoin	Tablets: 100 mg	200-600 mg/day	Grand mal, psychomotor seizures, focal seizures, jacksonian seizures
Phenytoin	Dilantin	Tablets: 50 mg Capsules: 30, 100 mg Suspension: 30, 125 mg/5 ml Inj: 50 mg/ml in 2 and 5 ml amps	300-600 mg/day	Grand mal, psychomotor seizures
Succinimides				
Ethosuximide	Zarontin	Capsules: 250 mg Syrup: 250 mg/5 ml	1000-1250 mg/day	Petit mal
Methsuximide	Celontin	Capsules: 300 mg	900-1200 mg/day	Petit mal
Phensuximide	Milontin	Capsules: 500 mg	1-2 g/day	Petit mal

*Available in Canada only.

Implementation
Dosage and administration. See Table 17-1. *Note:* Rapid discontinuance of benzodiazepines after long-term use may result in symptoms similar to those of alcohol withdrawal. These may vary from weakness and anxiety to delirium and grand mal seizures. The symptoms may not appear for several days after discontinuation. Treatment consists of gradual withdrawal of benzodiazepines over a 2- to 4-week period.

IV: Do not mix parenteral diazepam in the same syringe with other medications; do not add to other IV solutions because of precipitate formation. Administer slowly at a rate of no more than 5 mg per minute. If at all possible, give under electrocardiogram (ECG) monitoring and observe closely for bradycardia. Stop boluses until the heart rate returns to normal.

Evaluation
Side effects to expect
SEDATION, DROWSINESS, DIZZINESS, BLURRED VISION, FATIGUE, LETHARGY. The more common side effects of benzodiazepines are extensions of their pharmacologic properties.

These symptoms tend to disappear with continued therapy and possible readjustment of the dosage. Encourage the patient not to discontinue therapy without first consulting the physician.

Persons who are working around machinery, driving a car, or performing other duties in which they must remain mentally alert should be particularly cautious. Provide for patient safety during episodes of dizziness and ataxia; report for further evaluation.

Caution the patient that blurred vision may occur, and make appropriate suggestions for personal safety of the individual.
Side effects to report
BEHAVIORAL DISTURBANCES. Behavioral disturbances such as aggressiveness and agitation have been reported, especially in patients who are mentally retarded or have psychiatric disturbances. Provide supportive physical care and safety during these responses.

Assess the level of excitement and deal calmly with the individual. During periods of excitement, protect persons from harm and provide for physical channeling of energy (for example, walk with them).

Seek change in the medication order.

BLOOD DYSCRASIAS. Routine laboratory studies (red blood cell count [RBC], white blood cell count [WBC], and differential counts) should be scheduled. Monitor for the development of sore throat, fever, purpura, jaundice, or excessive and progressive weakness.

HEPATOTOXICITY. The symptoms of hepatotoxicity are anorexia, nausea, vomiting, jaundice, hepatomegaly, splenomegaly, and abnormal liver function tests (elevated bilirubin, aspartate transaminase [AST], alanine aminotransferase [ALT], gamma glutamyltransferase [GGT], alkaline phosphatase [ALP], prothrombin time [PT]).

Drug interactions

DRUGS THAT INCREASE TOXIC EFFECTS. Antihistamines, alcohol, analgesics, anesthetics, tranquilizers, narcotics, cimetidine, sedative-hypnotics, and other anticonvulsants.

Monitor the patient for excessive sedation, and eliminate the nonanticonvulsants if possible.

SMOKING. Smoking enhances the metabolism of the benzodiazepines. Larger dosages may be necessary to maintain effects in patients who smoke.

Drug Class: Hydantoins

Actions

The mechanism of action of the hydantoins is unknown.

Uses

Hydantoins (phenytoin, ethotoin, and mephenytoin) are anticonvulsants used to control partial and generalized tonic-clonic seizures. Mephenytoin may also be used to treat partial seizures when less toxic anticonvulsants are unsuccessful. Phenytoin is by far the most commonly used anticonvulsant of the hydantoins.

Therapeutic Outcomes

The primary therapeutic outcomes expected from the hydantoins are as follows:
• Reduced frequency of seizures and reduced injury from seizure activity
• Minimal adverse effects from therapy

Nursing Process

Premedication Assessment

1. Review routine blood studies to detect blood dyscrasias and hepatotoxicity.
2. Obtain baseline blood sugar levels in diabetic patients, and monitor periodically at specified intervals because hyperglycemia may be caused by hydantoin therapy.
3. Monitor behavioral responses to therapy.

Planning

Availability. See Table 17-1.

Implementation

Dosage and administration. See Table 17-1. PO—Administer medication with food or milk to reduce gastric irritation. If an oral suspension is used, shake well first. Encourage the use of an oral syringe for accurate measurement. IM—If at all possible, avoid IM administration. Absorption is slow and

painful. IV—Do not mix parenteral phenytoin in the same syringe with other medications; because of precipitate formation, do not add to other IV solutions. Administer slowly at a rate of 25 to 50 mg per minute. If at all possible, give under ECG monitoring and observe closely for bradycardia. Stop boluses until the heart rate returns to normal. Therapeutic blood levels for phenytoin are 10 to 20 mg/L.

Evaluation

Side effects to expect

NAUSEA, VOMITING, INDIGESTION. These effects are common during initiation of therapy. Gradual increases in dosage and administration with food or milk will reduce gastric irritation.

SEDATION, DROWSINESS, DIZZINESS, BLURRED VISION, FATIGUE, LETHARGY. These symptoms tend to disappear with continued therapy and possible adjustment of dosage. Encourage the patient not to discontinue therapy without first consulting the physician.

Persons who are working around machinery, driving a car, or performing other duties in which they must remain mentally alert, should be particularly cautious.

Provide for patient safety during episodes of dizziness; report for further evaluation.

Caution the patient that blurred vision may occur, and make appropriate suggestions for personal safety of the individual.

CONFUSION. Perform a baseline assessment of the patient's degree of alertness and orientation to name, place, and time before initiating therapy. Make regularly scheduled subsequent evaluations of mental status and compare findings. Report development of alterations.

GINGIVAL HYPERPLASIA. The frequency of gum overgrowth may be reduced by good oral hygiene, including gum massage, frequent brushing, and proper dental care.

Side effects to report

HYPERGLYCEMIA. Hydantoins may elevate blood sugar levels, especially if higher doses are used; patients with diabetes mellitus are more susceptible to hyperglycemia. Particularly during the early weeks of therapy, diabetic or prediabetic patients must be monitored for the development of hyperglycemia.

Assess regularly for glycosuria and report if it occurs with any frequency.

Patients receiving oral hypoglycemic agents or insulin may require an adjustment in dosage.

BLOOD DYSCRASIAS. Routine laboratory studies (RBC, WBC, and differential counts) should be scheduled. Monitor for the development of sore throat, fever, purpura, jaundice, or excessive and progressive weakness.

HEPATOTOXICITY. The symptoms of hepatotoxicity are anorexia, nausea, vomiting, jaundice, hepatomegaly, splenomegaly, and abnormal liver function tests (elevated bilirubin, AST, ALT, GGT, alkaline phosphatase, prothrombin time).

DERMATOLOGIC REACTIONS. Report a rash or pruritus immediately, and withhold additional doses pending approval by the physician.

Drug interactions

DRUGS THAT ENHANCE THERAPEUTIC AND TOXIC EFFECTS. Warfarin, carbamazepine, disulfiram, phenylbutazone, amiodarone, isoniazid, chloramphenicol, cimetidine, and sulfonamides. Monitor patients with concurrent therapy for signs of phenytoin toxicity—**nystagmus,** sedation, lethargy. Serum levels may be ordered, and a reduced dosage of phenytoin may be required.

DRUGS THAT DECREASE THERAPEUTIC EFFECTS. Barbiturates, folic acid, and antacids. Monitor patients with concurrent therapy for increased seizure activity. Monitoring changes in serum levels should help warn of possible increased seizure activity.

DISOPYRAMIDE, QUINIDINE, MEXILETINE. Phenytoin decreases serum levels of these agents. Monitor patients for redevelopment of arrhythmias.

PREDNISOLONE, DEXAMETHASONE. Phenytoin decreases serum levels of these agents. Monitor patients for reduced antiinflammatory activity.

ORAL CONTRACEPTIVES. Spotting or bleeding may be an indication of reduced contraceptive activity. Use of alternative forms of birth control is recommended.

THEOPHYLLINE. Phenytoin decreases serum levels of theophylline derivatives. Monitor patients for a greater frequency of respiratory difficulty. The theophylline dose may need to be increased 50% to 100% to maintain the same therapeutic response.

VALPROIC ACID. This agent may increase or decrease the activity of phenytoin. Monitor for increased frequency of seizure activity. Monitoring changes in serum levels should help warn of possible increased seizure activity. Monitor patients with concurrent therapy for signs of phenytoin toxicity: nystagmus, sedation, lethargy. Serum levels may be ordered, and a reduced dosage of phenytoin may be required.

KETOCONAZOLE. Concurrent administration with ketoconazole may alter the metabolism of one or both drugs. Monitoring for both is recommended.

CYCLOSPORINE. Phenytoin enhances the metabolism of cyclosporine. Increased doses of cyclosporine may be necessary in patients receiving concomitant therapy.

Drug Class: Succinimides

Actions

The mechanism of action of the succinimides is unknown.

Uses

Succinimides (ethosuximide, methsuximide, and phensuximide) are used for the control of absence (petit mal) seizures.

Therapeutic Outcomes

The primary therapeutic outcomes expected from the succinimides are as follows:
- Reduced frequency of seizures and reduced injury from seizure activity
- Minimal adverse effects from therapy

Nursing Process

Premedication Assessment
1. Review routine blood studies to detect blood dyscrasias and hepatotoxicity.
2. Monitor behavioral responses to therapy.

Planning
Availability. See Table 17-1.

Implementation
Dosage and administration. See Table 17-1.

Evaluation
Side effects to expect
NAUSEA, VOMITING, INDIGESTION. These effects are common during initiation of therapy. Gradual increases in dosage and administration with food or milk will reduce gastric irritation.

SEDATION, DROWSINESS, DIZZINESS, FATIGUE, LETHARGY. These symptoms tend to disappear with continued therapy and possible adjustment of dosage. Encourage the patient not to discontinue therapy without first consulting the physician.

Persons who are working around machinery, driving a car, or performing other duties in which they must remain mentally alert should be particularly cautious.

Provide for patient safety during episodes of dizziness; report for further evaluation.
Drug interactions
DRUGS THAT ENHANCE TOXIC EFFECTS. Antihistamines, alcohol, analgesics, anesthetics, tranquilizers, other anticonvulsants, and sedative-hypnotics.

Drug Class: Miscellaneous Anticonvulsants

carbamazepine (kar-ba-maz′e-peen)
Tegretol (teg′reh-tol)

Actions

Carbamazepine blocks the reuptake of norepinephrine, decreases the release of norepinephrine, and decreases the rate of dopamine and GABA turnover. Despite knowing these pharmacologic effects, the mechanisms of action as an anticonvulsant, selective analgesic, and antimanic agent are unknown. Carbamazepine is structurally related to the tricyclic antidepressants.

Uses

Carbamazepine is an anticonvulsant frequently used in combination with other anticonvulsants to control generalized tonic-clonic and partial seizures. It is not effective in the control of myoclonic or absence seizures. Carbamazepine has also been used successfully to treat the pain associated with trigeminal neuralgia (tic douloureux). It may also be used to treat manic-depressive disorders when lithium therapy has not been optimal.

Therapeutic Outcomes

The primary therapeutic outcomes expected from carbamazepine are as follows:
- Reduced frequency of seizures and reduced injury from seizure activity
- Minimal adverse effects from therapy

Nursing Process

Premedication Assessment
1. As a result of serious adverse reactions, the manufacturer recommends that the following baseline studies be

repeated at regular intervals: complete blood count, liver function tests, urinalysis, blood urea nitrogen (BUN), serum creatinine, and ophthalmologic examination.

2. Monitor behavioral responses to therapy.

Planning

Availability. PO—100 and 200 mg tablets; 100 mg per 5 ml suspension.

Implementation

Dosage and administration. Adult: PO—Initial dose is 200 mg 2 times daily in the first day. Increase gradually by 200 mg per day in divided doses at 6- to 8-hour intervals. Do not exceed 1200 mg daily. Therapeutic plasma levels for carbamazepine are 4 to 10 mg/ L.

Evaluation

Side effects to expect

NAUSEA, VOMITING, DROWSINESS, DIZZINESS. These effects can be reduced by slowly increasing the dose. These effects are usually mild and tend to resolve with continued therapy. Encourage the patient not to discontinue therapy without first consulting the physician.

Provide for patient safety during episodes of dizziness.

Persons who are working around machinery, driving a car, or performing other duties in which they must remain mentally alert should not take these medications while working.

Side effects to report

ORTHOSTATIC HYPOTENSION, HYPERTENSION. Monitor the blood pressure daily in both the supine and standing positions. Anticipate the development of postural hypotension, and take measures to prevent an occurrence. Teach the patient to rise slowly from a supine or sitting position; encourage the patient to sit or lie down if feeling faint.

DYSPNEA, EDEMA. If carbamazepine is used in patients with a history of congestive heart failure, monitor daily weights, lung sounds, and accumulation of edema.

NEUROLOGIC. Perform a baseline assessment of the patient's speech patterns and degree of alertness and orientation to name, place, and time before initiating therapy. Make regularly scheduled subsequent evaluations of mental status and compare findings. Report development of alterations.

NEPHROTOXICITY. Monitor urinalysis and kidney function tests for abnormal results. Report increasing BUN and creatinine, decreasing urine output or decreasing specific gravity (despite amount of fluid intake), casts or protein in the urine, frank blood or smoky-colored urine, or RBC in excess of 0 to 3 on the urinalysis report.

HEPATOTOXICITY. The symptoms of hepatotoxicity are anorexia, nausea, vomiting, jaundice, hepatomegaly, splenomegaly, and abnormal liver function tests (elevated bilirubin, AST, ALT, GGT, alkaline phosphatase, and prothrombin time).

BLOOD DYSCRASIAS. Routine laboratory studies (RBC, WBC, and differential counts) should be scheduled. Monitor for the development of sore throat, fever, purpura, jaundice, or excessive and progressive weakness.

DERMATOLOGIC REACTIONS. Report a rash or pruritus immediately, and withhold additional doses pending approval by the physician.

Drug interactions

ISONIAZID, FLUOXETINE. Isoniazid and fluoxetine inhibit the metabolism of carbamazepine. Monitor for signs of toxicity: disorientation, ataxia, lethargy, headache, drowsiness, nausea, and vomiting. Dosage reductions in carbamazepine may be necessary.

PROPOXYPHENE, VERAPAMIL, DILTIAZEM. Propoxyphene, verapamil, and diltiazem increase serum levels of carbamazepine. Monitor for signs of toxicity: disorientation, ataxia, lethargy, headache, drowsiness, nausea, and vomiting. A 40% to 50% decrease in carbamazepine dosage may be necessary.

WARFARIN. Carbamazepine may diminish the anticoagulant effects of warfarin. Monitor the prothrombin time and increase the dosage of warfarin if necessary.

PHENOBARBITAL, PHENYTOIN, VALPROIC ACID, PRIMIDONE. Carbamazepine enhances the metabolism of these agents. Monitor for increased frequency of seizure activity. Monitoring changes in serum levels should help warn of possible increased seizure activity.

DOXYCYCLINE. Carbamazepine enhances the metabolism of this antibiotic. Monitor patients for signs of continued infection.

ORAL CONTRACEPTIVES. Carbamazepine enhances the metabolism of estrogens. Spotting or bleeding may be an indication of reduced contraceptive activity. Use of other forms of birth control is recommended.

gabapentin (gab′ə-pen-tin)
Neurontin (nuhr′on-tin)

Actions

The mechanism of action of gabapentin is unknown. It does not appear to enhance GABA.

Uses

Gabapentin is an anticonvulsant usually used in combination with other anticonvulsants to control partial seizures.

Therapeutic Outcomes

The primary therapeutic outcomes expected from gabapentin are as follows:
- Reduced frequency of seizures and reduced injury from seizure activity
- Minimal adverse effects from therapy

Nursing Process

Premedication Assessment
Monitor behavioral responses to therapy.

Planning
Availability. PO—100, 300, and 400 mg capsules.

Implementation
Dosage and administration. Adult: PO—900 to 1800 mg daily. Initially, administer 300 mg at bedtime on day 1, 300 mg 2 times daily on day 2, then 300 mg 3 times daily on day 3. Adjust the dosage upward to a maximum of 1800 mg daily in 3 divided doses using a combination of 300 and 400 mg

capsules. The maximum time between doses in the 3-times-daily schedule should not exceed 12 hours.

If the patient also uses antacids, administer gabapentin at least 2 hours after the last dose of antacid. Antacids reduce the absorption of gabapentin.

Evaluation
Side effects to expect
SEDATION, DROWSINESS, DIZZINESS, BLURRED VISION. These symptoms tend to disappear with continued therapy and possible adjustment of dosage. Encourage the patient not to discontinue therapy without first consulting the physician.

Persons who are working around machinery, driving a car, or performing other duties in which they must remain mentally alert should be particularly cautious while working.

Provide for patient safety during episodes of dizziness; report for further evaluation.

Caution the patient that blurred vision may occur, and make appropriate suggestions for personal safety of the individual.
Side effects to report
NEUROLOGIC. Perform a baseline assessment of the patient's speech patterns and degree of alertness and orientation to name, place, and time *before* initiating therapy. Make regularly scheduled subsequent evaluations of mental status and compare findings. Report development of alterations.
Drug interactions
ENHANCED SEDATION. Central nervous system (CNS) depressants, including sleeping aids, analgesics, tranquilizers, and alcohol, will enhance the sedative effects of gabapentin. Persons who are working around machinery, driving a car, or performing other duties in which they must remain mentally alert should not take these medications while working.

URINE PROTEIN. False-positive readings for protein in the urine have been reported by patients taking gabapentin when using the Ames N-Multistix SG dipstick test. The manufacturer recommends that the more specific sulfosalicylic acid precipitation procedure be used to determine the presence of urine protein.

lamotrigine (lah-mot' rah-geen)
Lamictal (lah-mik' tahl)

Actions
Lamotrigine is a new anticonvulsant chemically unrelated to other agents. It is thought to act by blocking voltage-sensitive sodium channels in neuronal membranes. This stabilizes the neuronal membranes and inhibits the release of excitatory neurotransmitters such as glutamate that may induce seizure activity.

Uses
Lamotrigine is used in combination with other anticonvulsants to treat partial seizures.

Therapeutic Outcomes
The primary therapeutic outcomes expected from lamotrigine are as follows:
• Reduced frequency of seizures and reduced injury from seizure activity
• Minimal adverse effects from therapy

Nursing Process
Premedication Assessment
1. Monitor behavioral responses to therapy.
2. Review the medication history to determine whether the patient is already taking valproic acid for seizure control.

Planning
Availability. PO—25, 100, 150, and 200 mg tablets.

Implementation
Dosage and administration. Adult: PO—If not already taking valproic acid for seizure control, initiate therapy at 50 mg once a day for 2 weeks, followed by 100 mg per day given in 2 divided doses for 2 weeks. Thereafter, the usual maintenance dose is 300 to 500 mg per day in 2 divided doses. If the patient is already receiving valproic acid for seizure control, the dosage of lamotrigine is less than half these dosages.

Evaluation
Side effects to expect
NAUSEA, VOMITING, INDIGESTION. These effects are common during initiation of therapy. Gradual increases in dosage and administration with food or milk will reduce gastric irritation.

SEDATION, DROWSINESS, DIZZINESS, BLURRED VISION. These symptoms tend to disappear with continued therapy and possible adjustment of dosage. Encourage the patient not to discontinue therapy without first consulting the physician.

Persons who are working around machinery, driving a car, or performing other duties in which they must remain mentally alert should be particularly cautious while working.

Provide for patient safety during episodes of dizziness; report for further evaluation.

Caution the patient that blurred vision may occur, and make appropriate suggestions for personal safety of the individual.
Side effects to report
SKIN RASH. Approximately 10% of patients receiving lamotrigine develop a skin rash and **urticaria** in the first 4 to 6 weeks of therapy. Slower increases in the dosage are thought to decrease the incidence of rash. In most cases, the rash resolves with continued therapy; however, the physician should be promptly informed because the rash could also be an early indicator of a more serious condition. Combination therapy with valproic acid appears to be more likely to precipitate a serious rash.

Encourage the patient not to discontinue the lamotrigine until alternative anticonvulsant therapy can be considered to prevent renewed seizure activity.
Drug interactions
ENHANCED SEDATION. CNS depressants, including sleeping aids, analgesics, tranquilizers, and alcohol, will enhance the sedative effects of lamotrigine. Persons who are working around machinery, driving a car, or performing other duties in which they must remain mentally alert should not take these medications while working.

VALPROIC ACID. Valproic acid reduces the metabolism of lamotrigine by as much as 50%. Significant lamotrigine dosage reductions may be required.

PHENOBARBITAL, PHENYTOIN, CARBAMAZEPINE. These agents may enhance the metabolism of lamotrigine. Monitor for increased frequency of seizure activity. Monitoring changes in serum levels should help warn of possible increased seizure activity.

primidone (pri′mi-done)
Mysoline (my′so-leen)

Actions

Primidone is structurally related to the barbiturates. It is metabolized into phenobarbital and phenylethylmalonamide (PEMA), both of which are active anticonvulsants. The exact mechanism of anticonvulsant action is unknown.

Uses

Primidone is used in combination with other anticonvulsants to treat partial and generalized tonic-clonic seizures.

Therapeutic Outcomes

The primary therapeutic outcomes expected from primidone are as follows:
• Reduced frequency of seizures and reduced injury from seizure activity
• Minimal adverse effects from therapy

Nursing Process

Premedication Assessment
1. Review routine blood studies to detect blood dyscrasias.
2. Monitor behavioral responses to therapy. In children, assess degree of excitability present.

Planning
Availability. PO—50 and 250 mg tablets and 250 mg per 5 ml oral suspension.

Implementation
Dosage and administration. Adult: PO—250 mg daily, with weekly increases of 250 mg until therapeutic response or intolerance develops. Usual dose is 750 to 1500 mg daily. Do not exceed 2000 mg daily.

Evaluation
Side effects to expect
SEDATION, DROWSINESS, DIZZINESS, BLURRED VISION. These symptoms tend to disappear with continued therapy and possible adjustment of dosage. Encourage the patient not to discontinue therapy without first consulting the physician.

Persons who are working around machinery, driving a car, or performing other duties in which they must remain mentally alert should be particularly cautious while working.

Provide for patient safety during episodes of dizziness; report for further evaluation.

Caution the patient that blurred vision may occur, and make appropriate suggestions for personal safety of the individual.
Side effects to report
BLOOD DYSCRASIAS. Routine laboratory studies (RBC, WBC, and differential counts) should be scheduled. Monitor for the development of sore throat, fever, purpura, jaundice, or excessive and progressive weakness.

PARADOXIC EXCITABILITY. Primidone may cause paradoxic excitability in children. Blood dyscrasias have rarely been reported with the use of primidone. During a period of excitement, protect persons from harm and provide for physical channeling of energy (for example, walk with them). Notify the physician for a possible change in medication.
Drug interactions
ORAL CONTRACEPTIVES. Spotting or bleeding may be an indication of reduced contraceptive activity. Use of alternative forms of birth control is recommended.

PHENYTOIN. Phenytoin may increase the phenobarbital serum levels when taken concurrently with primidone. Monitor patients for increased sedation.

valproic acid (val-proe′ik)
Depakene (dep′ah-keen)

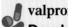

Actions

Valproic acid is an anticonvulsant structurally unrelated to any other agent used to treat seizure disorders. Its mechanism of action is unknown; however, it appears to support GABA activity as an inhibitory neurotransmitter.

Uses

Valproic acid has broad activity against both partial and generalized tonic-clonic seizures. It is the only available agent that can be used as single-drug therapy for treating patients with a combination of generalized tonic-clonic and absence of myoclonic seizures. Valproic acid is also being tested to be used either alone or in combination with lithium or carbamazepine for the treatment of acute mania of bipolar disorder in patients who do not respond to lithium therapy alone.

Therapeutic Outcomes

The primary therapeutic outcomes expected from valproic acid are as follows:
• Reduced frequency of seizures and reduced injury from seizure activity
• Minimal adverse effects from therapy

Nursing Process

Premedication Assessment
1. The manufacturer recommends that the following baseline studies be completed before therapy is initiated and at regular intervals thereafter: liver function tests, bleeding time determination, and platelet count.
2. PATIENTS WITH DIABETES: One of the metabolites of valproic acid is a ketone. It is excreted in the urine and may produce a false-positive test (Ketostix, Acetest) for urine ketones.
3. Review routine blood studies to detect blood dyscrasias and hepatotoxity.
4. Monitor behavioral responses to therapy.

Planning
Availability. PO—250 mg capsules; 125 mg capsules containing coated particles; 125, 250, and 500 mg sustained-release tablets; 250 mg per 5 ml syrup.

Implementation

Dosage and administration. Adult: PO—5 mg/kg every 8 hours. Administer medication with food or milk to reduce gastric irritation. Increase by 5 to 10 mg/kg per day at weekly intervals. The maximum daily dosage is 30 mg/kg. Therapeutic blood levels are 50 to 100 mg/L. A capsule containing enteric-coated particles is available for those patients having persistent difficulty with nausea and vomiting.

Evaluation

Side effects to expect

NAUSEA, VOMITING, INDIGESTION. These effects are common during initiation of therapy. Gradual increases in dosage and administration with food or milk will reduce gastric irritation.

SEDATION, DROWSINESS, DIZZINESS, BLURRED VISION. These symptoms tend to disappear with continued therapy and possible adjustment of dosage. Encourage the patient not to discontinue therapy without first consulting the physician.

Persons who are working around machinery, driving a car, or performing other duties in which they must remain mentally alert should not take these medications while working.

Provide for patient safety during episodes of dizziness; report for further evaluation.

Caution the patient that blurred vision may occur, and make appropriate suggestions for personal safety of the individual.

Side effects to report

BLOOD DYSCRASIAS. Routine laboratory studies (RBC, WBC, and differential counts) should be scheduled. Monitor for the development of sore throat, fever, purpura, jaundice, or excessive and progressive weakness.

HEPATOTOXICITY. The symptoms of hepatotoxicity are anorexia, nausea, vomiting, jaundice, hepatomegaly, splenomegaly, and abnormal liver function tests (elevated bilirubin, AST, ALT, GGT, alkaline phosphatase, and prothrombin time).

Drug interactions

ENHANCED SEDATION. CNS depressants, including sleeping aids, analgesics, tranquilizers, and alcohol, will enhance the sedative effects of valproic acid. Persons who are working around machinery, driving a car, or performing other duties in which they must remain mentally alert should not take these medications while working.

PHENOBARBITAL, PHENYTOIN, CARBAMAZEPINE. Monitor for increased frequency of seizure activity. Monitoring changes in serum levels should help warn of possible increased seizure activity.

CHAPTER REVIEW

Seizures are the result of the sudden, excessive firing of a small number of neurons and the spread of electrical activity to adjacent neurons. There are several types of seizures and many causes of seizures. If the seizures are chronic and recurrent, the patient is diagnosed as having epilepsy. Epilepsy is treated almost exclusively with anticonvulsant medications. The effective treatment of epilepsy requires the cooperation of the patient and the health care provider. The goal of treatment is to reduce the frequency of seizures while minimizing adverse effects of drug therapy. To attain this goal, therapy must be individualized to consider the type of seizure activity and the age, sex, and concurrent medical condition of the patient. Patients and their families also require education and support regarding their responsibilities in the management of epilepsy.

MATH REVIEW

1. Dr. Frye wrote orders to start Mrs. Boeckermann on Dilantin 100 mg PO TID and hs. What is your interpretation of the order, and how will you administer it to Mrs. Boeckermann?

2. Dr. Haycock wrote orders to start Belinda Smith, a 10-year-old patient, on Tegretol suspension 50 mg PO QID. The suspension is 100 mg per 5 ml. How will you administer this dose?

3. Dr. Tindall wrote orders for Jimmy Smith, a 12-year-old, 110 lb newly diagnosed epileptic patient, to be started on Depakene syrup, 5 ml PO TID. The normal starting dose is 15 mg/kg daily. Is Dr. Tindall's order reasonable, and if so how would you administer it?

CRITICAL THINKING QUESTIONS

1. Both Valium and Dilantin have specific administration precautions when these agents are administered intravenously. What are these precautions?

2. Mr. Callihan suddenly has a tonic-clonic seizure while attending a class at college. When his family is notified of this and his need for transportation home, his wife tells you that he has not been taking his medications regularly. Describe how you as a nurse would address this situation.

3. While working in the emergency department (ED), the rescue squad notifies the ED desk that a patient is being transported who is in status epilepticus. What medicines and equipment would you have ready for the patient's arrival?

4. What health teaching should be done for individuals recently diagnosed with epilepsy?

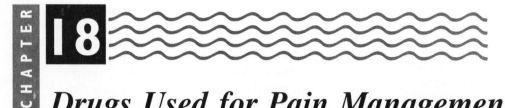

Drugs Used for Pain Management

Key Words

pain experience

pain perception

pain threshold

pain tolerance

analgesics

opiate agonists

opiate partial agonists

opiate antagonists

nonsteroidal
antiinflammatory agents

nociceptors

opiate receptors

addiction

drug tolerance

ceiling effect

salicylates

Objectives

1. Differentiate among opiate agonists, opiate partial agonists, and opiate antagonists.

2. Describe monitoring parameters necessary for patients receiving opiate agonists.

3. Cite the side effects to expect when opiate agonists are administered.

4. Compare the analgesic effectiveness of opiate partial agonists when administered before or after opiate agonists.

5. Explain when naloxone can be used effectively to treat respiratory depression.

6. State the three pharmacologic effects of salicylates.

7. Prepare a list of side effects to expect, side effects to report, and drug interactions that are associated with salicylates.

8. Explain why synthetic nonopiate analgesics are not used for inflammatory disorders.

9. Prepare a patient education plan for a person being discharged with a continuing prescription for an analgesic.

10. Examine Table 18-4 and identify the active ingredients in commonly prescribed analgesic combination products. Identify products containing aspirin and compare the analgesic properties of agents available in different strengths.

PAIN

Pain is an unpleasant sensation that is part of a larger situation called **pain experience.** The pain experience includes all the emotional sensations (attention, anxiety, fatigue, suggestion, prior conditioning) for a particular person under a certain set of circumstances. This accounts for the wide variation in individual responses to the sensation of pain.

Three terms used in relationship to the pain experience are **pain perception, pain threshold,** and **pain tolerance.** *Pain perception* is the individual's awareness of the feeling or sensation of pain. *Pain threshold* is the point at which an individual first acknowledges or interprets a sensation as being painful. *Pain tolerance* is the individual's ability to endure the pain being experienced.

Pain has both a physical and an emotional component. Factors that decrease an individual's tolerance to pain include prolonged pain that is insufficiently relieved, fatigue accompanied by the inability to sleep, an increase in anxiety or fear, unresolved anger, depression, and isolation. Patients with severe, intractable pain fear that the pain cannot be relieved, and patients with cancer fear that new or increasing pain means that the cancer is spreading to a new site or that a reoccurrence is present.

Pain is usually described as acute or short term and as chronic or long term. Initially, with acute pain, the sympathetic nervous system is activated resulting in an increase in the heart rate, pulse, respirations, and blood pressure. This also causes nausea, diaphoresis, dilated pupils, and an elevation in glucose. Over time and with the recurrence of pain, the parasympathetic nervous system reverses these findings and the pulse, respiration, and blood pressure decrease. In chronic, poorly controlled pain, these symptoms are generally absent, and the predominant descriptors parallel those of depression.

Drug Therapy for Pain Management

Analgesics are drugs that relieve pain without producing loss of consciousness or reflex activity. The search for an ideal analgesic continues, but it is difficult to find one that does all that is desired of it. It should be potent, so that it will afford maximum relief of pain; it should not cause dependence; it should exhibit a minimum of side effects such as constipation, hallucinations, respiratory depression, nausea, and vomiting; it should not cause tolerance to develop; it should act promptly and over a long period of time with a minimum amount of sedation so that the patient is able to remain conscious and responsive; and it should be relatively inexpensive. Needless to say, no present-day analgesic has all these qualifications, so the search must continue.

There is at present no completely satisfactory classification of analgesics. Historically, they have been categorized based on potency (mild, moderate, and strong analgesics), origin (opium, semisynthetic, synthetic, coal-tar derivatives), or addictive properties (narcotic and nonnarcotic agents).

Research into the control of pain over the past decade has given new insight into pathways of pain within the nervous system and a better understanding of precise mechanisms of action of analgesic agents. The current nomenclature for analgesics stems from these recent discoveries into mechanisms of actions. In this section the medications have been divided into **opiate agonists, opiate partial agonists, opiate antagonists, nonsteroidal antiinflammatory agents,** and miscellaneous analgesic agents.

Actions

The pathways to pain transmission from the site of injury to the brain for processing and reflexive action have not been fully identified. It is known that the first step leading to the sensation of pain is the stimulation of receptors known as **nociceptors.** These nerve endings are found in skin, blood vessels, joints, subcutaneous tissues, periosteum, viscera, and other tissues. The exact mechanism that causes stimulation of nociceptors is not understood; however, bradykinins, prostaglandins, leukotrienes, histamine, and serotonin sensitize these receptors. Receptor activation leads to action potentials that are transmitted along afferent nerve fibers to the spinal cord. A series of neurotransmitters (somatostatin, cholecystokinin, and substance P) play roles in the transmission of nerve impulses from the site of damage to the spinal cord. Within the central nervous system (CNS), there may be at least four pain-transmitting pathways up the spinal cord to various areas of the brain for response.

Within the CNS is a series of receptors that control pain. These are known as **opiate receptors** because stimulation of these receptors by the opiates block the pain sensation. These receptors are subdivided into four types: the mu (μ), delta (δ), kappa (κ), and sigma (σ) receptors. The receptors are located in different areas of the CNS. κ-Receptors are found in greatest concentration in the cerebral cortex and in the substantia gelatinosa of the dorsal horn of the spinal cord and are responsible for analgesia at the levels of the spinal cord and the brain. Stimulation of κ-receptors also produces

sedation and miosis. μ-Receptors are located in the pain-modulating centers of the CNS and induce central analgesia, euphoria, physical dependence, and respiratory depression. δ-Receptors are located in the limbic area of the brain and in the spinal cord and may play a role in the euphoria that selected opiates produce. σ-Receptors are thought to produce the autonomic stimulation and psychotomimetic (for example, hallucinations) and dysphoric effects of some opiate agonists and partial agonists. Research is now focusing on building synthetic chemicals that are selective for specific receptors to maximize analgesia but minimize the potential for adverse effects such as **addiction.**

As described, other chemicals released during trauma also contribute to pain. Histamine, prostaglandins, serotonin, leukotrienes, substance P, and bradykinins all contribute to the pain sensation. Developing pharmaceuticals that block these chemicals is another effective way of stopping pain. Antihistamines (for example, diphenhydramine), prostaglandin inhibitors, substance P antagonists (for example, capsaicin), and selective serotonin reuptake inhibitors (for example, fluoxetine) all have analgesic properties.

Other pharmacologic agents can be used as adjuncts to pain suppression by a variety of mechanisms. Adrenergic agents such as norepinephrine and clonidine and gamma-aminobutyric acid (GABA) receptor stimulants (for example, baclofen) produce significant analgesia by blocking nociceptor activity. Valproic acid and carbamazepine act as analgesics by suppression of spontaneous neuronal firing, as occurs in trigeminal neuralgia. Tricyclic antidepressants inhibit the reuptake of serotonin and norepinephrine, causing the onset of analgesia to be more rapid, as well as improving the outlook of the person who is suffering from chronic pain. Some antidepressants (for example, amitriptyline) also block pain by antihistaminic and anticholinergic activity.

Uses

Mild, acute pain is effectively treated with analgesics such as aspirin or acetaminophen. Pain associated with inflammation responds well to the nonsteroidal antiinflammatory agents. Moderate pain is generally treated with a moderate potency opiate such as codeine or oxycodone. These two agents are often used in combination with acetaminophen or aspirin (for example, Empirin with codeine no. 3, Tylenol no. 3, Percodan). Severe, acute pain is treated with the opiate partial agonists (for example, buprenorphine, butorphanol) or the opiate agonists (for example, morphine, meperidine, methadone). Morphine sulfate is usually the drug of choice for the treatment of severe, chronic pain. Other agents may be used as adjunctive therapy with analgesics, such as antidepressants.

Nursing Process for Pain Management

Nurses must assist the patient in the management of pain. The first vital step in this process is to believe the patient's description of the pain being experienced. Pain brings with it a variety of feelings, such as anxiety, anger, loneliness, frustration, and depression. Part of the patient's response is tied to past experiences, sociocultural factors, current emotional state, and beliefs regarding pain.

Psychologic, physical, and environmental factors all must be considered in the management of the pain. Never overlook the value of general comfort measures such as a back rub, repositioning, and the use of hot or cold applications. A variety of relaxation techniques, as well as diversional activities, may prove psychologically beneficial. Measures to decrease environmental stimuli and thereby provide for successful periods of rest are essential.

It is important to evaluate the pain being experienced in a consistent manner. Therefore several assessment tools have been developed in an attempt to gain some degree of uniformity in interpreting and recording the patient's description of the pain experience.

Pain assessment tools such as The McGill-Melzack Pain Questionnaire may be used to assist the patient in describing subjective pain experience (Figure 18-1). This tool uses descriptive words or phrases to identify the pain being experienced. It is especially useful for individuals who have chronic pain. When possible, chart the description in the patient's exact words. It may be necessary to seek additional data from significant others.

Scales (Figure 18-2) are frequently used to assess acute pain. The most common scale used has the patient rate the pain being experienced on a scale of 0 (no pain) to 10 (intense or excruciating). The degree of relief for the pain after an analgesic is given is again rated using the same 0 to 10 scale. When different potencies of analgesic agents are ordered for the same patient, the nurse can use this numeric rating data in combination with the other data gathered to determine whether a more-potent or less-potent analgesic agent should be administered. Other scales sometimes used include faces depicting facial grimacing, smiles, and so forth. This approach is useful with children or persons with a language barrier. Another scale that shows an intense color that gradually fades from a deep shade (intense pain) to a lighter shade (less pain) may be used to evaluate the degree of pain present. This color scale is similar to a slide rule. The patient selects the hue or depth of color that corresponds with the pain being experienced. The nurse turns the slide rule scale over, and a numeric value is identified that can be used to consistently record the patient's response.

Effective pain control must depend on the degree of pain being experienced. The use of the previously described scale of 0 (no pain) to 10 (intense/unbearable pain) can prove useful. For a patient with mild to moderate acute pain, a nonnarcotic agent may be successful in pain control. With severe, chronic pain, a potent analgesic such as morphine may be necessary. The route of administration chosen must be based on several factors. One major consideration is how soon the action of the drug is needed. The oral and rectal routes have a longer onset of action than the parenteral route. It is sometimes erroneously felt that the oral route of administration is inadequate to treat pain. In truth, oral medications can provide adequate pain relief if adequate dosages are provided. Generally, the oral route is used initially to treat pain if no nausea and vomiting are present. Patients may initially be treated effectively with administration via the oral route; however, the rectal, transdermal, subcutaneous, intramuscular, intraspinal, epidural, and intravenous routes may be required depending on the patient and the course of the underlying disease.

Nurses must evaluate and document in the patient's chart the effectiveness of the pain medications given. This requires careful assessments at intervals following the administration of the analgesics that will validate the duration and degree of pain relief attained from the analgesic. Recording the patient's rating of the degree of pain relief at 1-, 2-, and 3-hour intervals after administration will provide useful information for evaluating future analgesic needs for the individual. Record and report all complaints of pain for analysis by the physician. The pattern of pain, particularly an increase in frequency or severity, may indicate new causes of pain. Major reasons for increased frequency or intensity of pain are pain from long-term immobility; pain from the treatment modalities used—surgery, chemotherapy, or radiation therapy; pain from direct extension of a tumor or metastases into bone, nerve, or viscera; and pain unrelated to the original cause or the therapeutic modalities being used.

Assessment

History of pain experience. Medication history: What medications are being prescribed, and how effective have they been? What dosage has been required for adequate comfort to be achieved? Is the patient suffering from any side effects to the medications? If yes, get details of side effects and measures taken for management. What is the patient's attitude toward the use of pain medications (opioids, anxiolytics, and so on)? What are the family's or significant others' attitudes toward the use of medications to control the pain? Is there any history of substance abuse?

The patient's perception of pain: Identify the causes of the patient's pain by having the patient describe the perception of the pain experienced.

Listen to the patient and *believe the pain experience* being described regardless of whether the physical data substantiate the degree of discomfort described. *Do not* let personal biases or values interfere with establishing interventions that provide for maximum pain relief for the individual.

Onset: When was the pain first noticed? When was the most recent attack? Is the onset slow or abrupt? Is there any particular activity that starts the pain?

Location: What is the exact location of the pain being experienced? Having the patient shade in a human figure with the areas where the pain is felt may be helpful, especially with pediatric patients, who can be given different-color crayons as a means of identifying different intensities in addition to the location. With acute pain the site of the pain can be more easily identified; however, with chronic pain this may be more difficult because the normal physiologic responses of the sympathetic nervous system are no longer present.

Depth: What is the depth of the pain? Does the pain radiate, having the sensation of spreading out or diffusing over an area, or is it localized in a specific site? It is important to recognize that the lack of physical symptoms comparable with the pain described *does not* mean that the patient's complaints should be ignored.

Quality: What is the actual sensation felt when the pain is present—stabbing, dull, cramping, sore, burning, other? Is the pain always in the same place and of the same intensity?

Duration: Is the pain continuous or intermittent? How often does it occur, and once felt how long does it persist? Is there a cyclic pattern to the pain?

McGill-Melzack
Pain Questionnaire

Patient's name _____ Age _____
File No. _____ Date _____
Clinical category (e.g., cardiac, neurologic)
Diagnosis:_____
_____
_____

Analgesic (if already administered):
1. Type _____
2. Dosage_____
3. Time given in relation to this test_____
Patient's intelligence: circle number that represents best estimate.

1 (low)   2   3   4   5 (high)

This questionnaire has been designed to tell us more about your pain. Four major questions we ask are:

1. Where is your pain?
2. What does it feel like?
3. How does it change with time?
4. How strong is it?

It is important that you tell us how your pain feels now. Please follow the instructions at the beginning of each part.

Part 1. Where Is Your Pain?

Please mark on the drawing below the areas where you feel pain. Put E if external, or I if internal, near the areas you mark. Put EI if both external and internal.

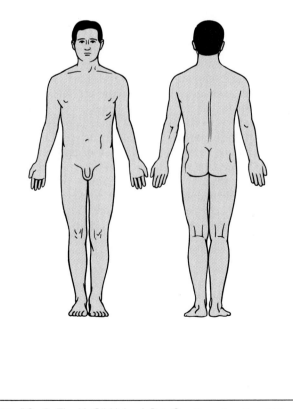

Part 2. What Does Your Pain Feel Like?

Some of the words below describe your present pain. Circle *ONLY* those words that best describe it. Leave out any category that is not suitable. Use only a single word in each appropriate category—the one that best applies.

1	6	11	16
Flickering	Tugging	Tiring	Annoying
Quivering	Pulling	Exhausting	Troublesome
Pulsing	Wrenching	12	Miserable
Throbbing	7	Sickening	Intense
Beating	Hot	Suffocating	Unbearable
Pounding	Burning	13	17
2	Scalding	Fearful	Spreading
Jumping	Searing	Frightful	Radiating
Flashing	8	Terrifying	Penetrating
Shooting	Tingling	14	Piercing
3	Itchy	Punishing	18
Pricking	Smarting	Grueling	Tight
Boring	Stinging	Cruel	Numb
Drilling	9	Vicious	Drawing
Stabbing	Dull	Killing	Squeezing
Lancinating	Sore	15	Tearing
4	Hurting	Wretched	19
Sharp	Aching	Blinding	Cool
Cutting	Heavy		Cold
Lacerating	10		Freezing
5	Tender		20
Pinching	Taut		Nagging
Pressing	Rasping		Nauseating
Gnawing	Splitting		Agonizing
Cramping			Dreadful
Crushing			Torturing

Part 3. How Does Your Pain Change with Time?

1. Which word or words would you use to describe the *pattern* of your pain?

1	2	3
Continuous	Rhythmic	Brief
Steady	Periodic	Momentary
Constant	Intermittent	Transient

2. What kind of things *relieve* your pain?

3. What kind of things *increase* your pain?

Part 4. How Strong Is Your Pain?

People agree that the following 5 words represent pain of increasing intensity. They are:

1	2	3	4	5
Mild	Discomforting	Distressing	Horrible	Excruciating

To answer each question below, write the number of the most appropriate word in the space beside the question.

1. Which word describes your pain right now? _____
2. Which word describes it at its worst? _____
3 Which word describes it when it is least? _____
4. Which word describes the worst toothache you ever had? _____
5. Which word describes the worst headache you ever had? _____
6. Which word describes the worst stomachache you ever had? _____

Figure 18-1 *The McGill-Melzack Pain Questionnaire.* (From Melzack R: The McGill Pain Questionnaire: major properties and scoring methods, *Pain* 1:277, 1975.)

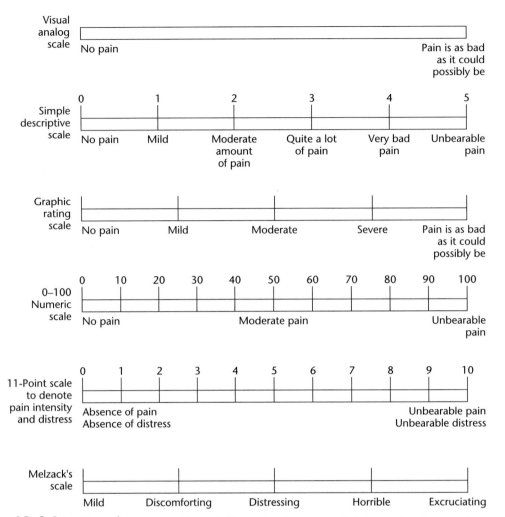

Figure 18-2 *Pain-rating scales.* (From Ignativicius DD, Workman ML, Mishler MA: *Medical-surgical nursing: a nursing process approach,* Philadelphia, 1995, Saunders.)

LIFE SPAN ISSUES

PAIN IN THE ELDERLY PATIENT

Pain assessment in the geriatric patient must include more than a simple rating of pain using a pain scale. Because many elders suffer from more than one chronic illness, a nursing history and a physical and functional assessment must be performed to understand the impact of pain on the patient's ability to meet self-care needs.

Severity: Have the patient rate the pain being experienced using the pain scale methodology that is standard for the clinical setting.

Nonverbal observations. Note the patient's general body position during an episode of pain. Be particularly observant about subtle clues such as facial grimaces, immobility of a particular part, and holding or resisting movement of an extremity.

Pain relief. What specific measures relieve the pain? What has already been tried for pain relief, and what if anything has been beneficial?

Physical data. In the presence of pain, always examine the affected part for any alterations in appearance, change in sensation, or limitation in mobility or range of motion.

Behavioral responses. What coping mechanisms does the patient use to handle the pain experience—crying, anger, withdrawal, depression, anxiety, fear, hopelessness? Is the individual introspective and self-focusing? Does the individual continue to perform activities of daily living despite the pain? Does the individual alter lifestyle patterns appropriately to enhance pain relief measures prescribed? Is the individual able to continue to work? Is the individual socially withdrawn? Is the person seeing more than one physician in hope of obtaining an answer to the origin of the pain?

Nursing Diagnosis
- Pain, acute or chronic (indication)
- Altered bowel elimination, risk for (side effect)
- Impaired gas exchange, risk for (side effect)
- Altered pattern of urine elimination, risk for retention (side effect)

Planning
History of pain experience. • Plan to evaluate the pain being experienced on a continuum, for example, location,

depth, quality, duration, and severity. • Perform baseline vital signs at least every shift or more frequently as dictated by patient's condition and type of medications being administered.

Pain relief. • Update the Kardex and care plan with details of nursing interventions that are successful in reducing the pain being experienced. This will allow all staff to intervene more knowledgeably. • Plan to implement nonpharmacologic as well as pharmacologic measures for the control of pain. • Develop goals cooperatively with the patient to make lifestyle changes necessary.

Environmental control. • Provide for a quiet environment with as little distraction as possible during periods of rest. Modify hospital schedules such as routine testing of vital signs and specimen collection so that the individual is not disturbed once asleep. Establish a schedule that provides for sufficient rest. (Fatigue and anxiety may increase the perception of pain.) • Schedule diversional activities through the appropriate use of television, visitors, card games, and other patients to take the patient's mind off the pain.

Psychologic interventions. During the planning process it is important to stress to support persons that they can be involved in a positive way by expressing understanding, helping to provide diversional activities, and encouraging frequent rest periods, especially after the administration of analgesics, antidepressants, and antianxiety medications.

Medication administration. • Plan to check frequently on the degree of pain relief being achieved and to administer medications as scheduled around the clock to achieve a steady blood level and consistent control of the pain. Have orders available to deal with breakthrough pain on an as-needed (prn) basis. • Keep an adequate supply of pain medication available for immediate use on the unit so that the patient is not kept waiting because the drug has not "come up from pharmacy."

Implementation

Comfort measures. • Provide for the patient's basic hygiene and comfort. Use such techniques as back rubs, massage, hot and cold applications, or warm baths, as ordered. • Ask the patient what measures have been successful in the past in providing pain relief. • Relieve pain by doing any or all of the following, as appropriate: support an affected part during movement; provide appropriate assistance during movement or activities; apply binders or splint an incisional area before initiating activities such as deep breathing and coughing; give analgesics in advance of undertaking painful activities, and plan for the activity to take place during the peak action of the medication given; or use hot or cold applications, massage, warm baths, pressure, and vibration as interventions for pain relief.

Exercise and activity. Unless contraindicated, moderate exercise should be encouraged. Many times, pain causes the individual not to move the affected part or to position it in a manner that provides relief. Stress the need to prevent complications by using a passive range of motion.

Nonpharmacologic approaches. • Use nonpharmacologic strategies to enhance the effects of the medication therapy, such as relaxation techniques, visualization, meditation, biofeedback, and transcutaneous electrical nerve stimulation (TENS) units. (The patient will require education for utilization of each of these prescribed techniques.) • Assist with

referral to pain clinic for management of pain, especially chronic pain.

Medication. Encourage the patient to request pain medication before the pain escalates and becomes severe. Encourage open communication between the patient and health care team regarding the effectiveness of the medications being used. Although the smallest dose possible to control the pain is the goal of therapy, it is also important that the dose be sufficient to provide adequate relief. Therefore the patient must understand the importance of expressing the degree of relief being obtained so that appropriate adjustments in dosage and analgesics can be made.

The medication administration record (MAR) may list more than one analgesic order for the same patient. This requires the nurse to use judgment in choosing the correct medication for the patient based on pain assessment data collected.

The nurse must identify when the last dose of pain medication was administered by checking both the patient's MAR and the narcotic control record. It is common practice for analgesics to be ordered intermittently on a prn basis every 3 to 4 hours. However, in the case of chronic pain or intractable pain, it has been found that giving analgesics to persons on a scheduled basis every 3 to 4 hours will maintain a more constant plasma level of the drug, providing more effective analgesia. This approach can result in better control of the pain while using less of the analgesic ordered.

Patient-controlled analgesia (PCA) is gaining acceptance in both the inpatient and ambulatory settings. This method of administration allows the patient to control a small syringe pump containing an opiate agonist, usually morphine, which is connected to an intravenous (iv) indwelling catheter. When initiating the PCA pump procedure, a loading dose is frequently given to gain rapid blood plasma levels necessary for analgesia. The patient then receives a slow, continuous infusion from the syringe pump. Depending on the activity level and the level of analgesia needed, the patient may push a button, self-administering a small bolus of analgesic to meet the immediate need. A timing device on the pump limits the amount and frequency of the dose that can be self-administered per hour. Additional adjustments in the dosing and frequency may be required as therapy continues. This approach allows the patient to have some control over the pain relief being provided and eliminates the need for the patient to wait for a nurse to answer the call light, check the last dosage of analgesics given, and prepare and administer the medication. After discharge from the hospital, this method of administration also allows significantly more freedom of movement for the patient and care giver.

When PCA is used, the nurse should explain the use of the PCA pump to the patient and observe the patient using it to validate understanding. (It also should be explained to the family and significant others.) Record the amount used every shift and the amount remaining in the syringe at the end of the shift, and notify the pharmacy well in advance of the need for more medication so that additional medication is available when needed. The degree of pain relief being achieved should always be recorded. When pain relief is inadequate, assess for other causes and contact the physician and discuss a modification of the regimen.

Pain control. Some patients will not ask for pain medication; therefore it is important to anticipate their needs and intervene for individuals who hold this belief. Whenever pain is being treated it is important not to make the patient wait unnecessarily for the pain medication.

Nutritional aspects. The patient should eat a diet that is well balanced and high in B-complex vitamins; should limit or eliminate sugar, nicotine, caffeine, and alcoholic intake; and should drink 8 to 10 8-ounce glasses of water per day and maintain normal elimination patterns. To minimize or avoid the constipating effects of opiates, increase intake of fiber and fluids. If long-term use of opiates is planned, stool softeners may be necessary.

Patient Education and Health Promotion

Orient the patient, family, and significant others to the benefits of adequate pain control. Work with the patient, family, and significant others to determine their perception of pain management and the use of drug therapy and nonpharmacologic approaches to pain management. If the patient is hesitant about these approaches, determine why. Stress that addiction is not a major factor with short-term use of analgesics and that during long-term use, such as with cancer, it is not the primary concern.

With long-term use of analgesics the major issues are obtaining sufficient pain control to ensure comfort, ensuring that the patient has ample rest, and enhancing the quality of life to an optimal level for the individual.

Teach the patient what medications are available for pain control and when and how to request them. Discuss the patient's expectations of pain management and how to rate the severity of pain honestly so that expectations for pain control can be met. Ask what level of exercise is attainable without severe pain. Is the pain control adequate for the individual to maintain activities of daily living or work?

Assess changes in expectations as therapy progresses and the patient gains understanding and skill in the management of the diagnosis.

In terminal illnesses, increasing pain necessitates careful management. The duration and intensity of the pain should be constantly reported to the physician for appropriate modifications of the medication regimen.

Assist the patient in learning to cope effectively with the pain. Discuss changes in lifestyle needed to support adequate pain control. Include family members in discussion of pain management. Give praise when techniques are tried whether or not success is achieved.

Teach the patient how to self-administer the analgesics ordered on an outpatient basis. This will include such routes of administration as transdermal, transmucosal, oral, and rectal, and will include care of infusion ports and central lines. (Be sure to validate and record the degree of understanding of the prescribed pain regimen.)

Include social services in the patient education process especially to connect with community resources available for the patient and family. Remember, not everyone has the financial resources to obtain the medicine prescribed. The degree of support by professionals needed to implement the planned pain control regimen at home must be carefully evaluated.

Make sure the patient and family understand how to obtain assistance with pain medication administration and patient care needs (for example, visiting nurse, hospice).

Fostering Health Maintenance. Throughout the course of treatment, discuss medication information and how it will benefit the patient. Drug therapy for the management of pain should be coupled with comfort measures, relaxation techniques, meditation, stress management, and meeting the total care needs of the individual to ensure maintenance of activities of daily living. Provide the patient and significant others with important information contained in the specific drug monograph for the medicines prescribed. Additional health teaching and nursing interventions for the side effects to expect and report are described in the drug monographs that follow.

Seek cooperation and understanding of the following points so that medication compliance is increased: name of medications, dosage, route and times of administration, side effects to expect, and side effects to report.

Written record. Enlist the patient's aid in developing and maintaining a written record (see the Patient Education and Monitoring Form on p. 237) of monitoring parameters (such as frequency of pain attacks, activity being performed when pain occurs, techniques being used to control pain, degree of pain relief, exercise tolerance) and response to prescribed therapies for discussion with the physician. Patients should be encouraged to bring this record with them on follow-up visits.

Drug Class: Opiate Agonists

The term *opiate* was once used to refer to drugs derived from opium, such as heroin and morphine. It has been found that many other analgesics not related to morphine act at the same sites within the brain. It is now understood that when we refer to opiate agonists or opiate antagonists, we are referring to drugs that act at the same site as morphine either to stimulate analgesic effects (opiate agonists) or block the effects of opiate agonists (opiate antagonists).

Another outdated word is *narcotic*. Originally it referred to medications that induced a stupor or sleep. Over the past 80 years it has gradually come to refer to addictive, morphine-like analgesics. The Harrison Narcotic Act of 1914, which placed morphine-like products under governmental control, helped foster this association. With the development in recent years of analgesics that are as potent as morphine but that do not have the sedative or addictive properties of morphine, the term *narcotic* should be abandoned in exchange for *opiate agonists* and *opiate partial agonists*.

Actions

Opiate agonists are a group of naturally occurring, semisynthetic, and synthetic drugs that have the capability to relieve severe pain without the loss of consciousness. The opiate agonists act by stimulation of the opiate receptors in the CNS. Most of these agents also have the ability to produce physical dependence and are thus considered controlled substances under the Federal Controlled Substances Act of 1970.

These agents can be subdivided into three groups: the morphine-like derivatives, the meperidine-like derivatives, and the methadone-like derivatives. (See Table 18-1.) Administration of these agents causes primary effects on the CNS (analgesia, suppression of the cough reflex, respiratory depression, drowsiness, sedation, mental clouding, euphoria, nausea, and vomiting); there are also significant effects on the cardiovascular, gastrointestinal, and urinary tracts.

PATIENT EDUCATION & MONITORING FORM | Analgesics

MEDICATIONS	COLOR	TO BE TAKEN

Name _____

Physician _____

Physician's phone _____

Next appt.* _____

PARAMETERS		DAY OF DISCHARGE												COMMENTS
Pain: onset	Example: 8 AM | 3 PM / 9 PM													
duration	Before taking medication													
relief	Example: 6 hrs | 3 hrs													
Describe pain	Location													
	Check one: C = Constant I = Intermittent	C___ I___	C___ I___	C___ I___	C___ I___	C___ I___	C___ I___	C___ I___						
	Record: Sharp, dull, throbbing													
Pain before medication Intense 10 / Moderate 5 / Low 1	Time: e.g., 8 AM = 9													
Pain after medication Intense 10 / Moderate 5 / Low 1 / None 0	Time: e.g., 9 AM = 5													
	9 PM = 8													
	2 AM = 1													
Sleep No Sleep 10 / Fair 5 / Sleep well 1														
Appetite Poor 10 / Decreased 5 / Normal 1														
I enjoy life? Yes 10 / Only when not in pain 5 / No 1														
Activities of daily living: Check one: Perform without difficulty Perform with difficulty Unable to function adequately														

*Please bring this record with you to your next appointment.
Use the back of this sheet for additional information.

Table 18-1

Opiate Agonists

GENERIC NAME	BRAND NAME	AVAILABILITY	INITIAL ADULT DOSE	DURATION (HOURS)	DOSE EQUAL TO MORPHINE (10 MG)	
					IM (MG)	ORAL (MG)
Morphine and morphine-like derivatives						
Codeine	Codeine Sulfate Codeine Phosphate ♣Paveral	Tablets: 15, 30, 60 mg Inj: 30, 60 mg Oral solution: 15 mg/5 ml	PO, SC, IM, IV: Analgesic: 15-60 mg every 4-6 hr Antitussive: 10-20 mg every 4-6 hr	4-6	130	200
Hydromorphone	Dilaudid, Dilaudid-HP	Tablets: 1, 2, 4, 8 mg Liquid: 1 mg/ml Suppositories: 3 mg Inj: 1, 2, 3, 4, 10 mg/ml	PO: 2 mg every 4-6 hr SC, IM 2 mg every 4-6 hr Rectal: 3 mg every 6-8 hr	4-5	1.5	7.5
Levorphanol	Levo-Dromoran	Tablets: 2 mg Inj: 2 mg/ml	PO: 2 mg SC, IM, IV: 2 mg	4-8	2	4
Morphine	Roxanol, Morphine Sulfate, Duramorph, MS Contin	Tablets: 15, 30 mg Capsules: 15, 30 mg Sustained-release tablets: 15, 30, 60, 100, 200 mg Solution: 10, 20, mg/5 ml; 20 mg/ml Suppositories: 5, 10, 20, 30 mg Inj: 0.5, 1, 2, 4, 5, 8, 10, 15, 25, 50 mg/ml	PO: 10-30 mg every 4 hr SC, IM: 10 mg/70 kg IV: 4-10 mg slowly Rectal: 10-20 mg every 4 hr	up to 7	10	60
Oxycodone	Roxicodone	Tablets: 5 mg Oral solution: 5 mg/5 ml; 20 mg/ml	PO: 5 mg every 6 hr	4-5	15	30
Oxycodone	Percodan (with aspirin)	Tablets: 5 mg Solution: 5 mg/ml	PO: 5 mg every 6 hr	4-5	15	30
Oxymorphone	Numorphan	Inj: 1, 1.5 mg/ml Suppositories: 5 mg	IV: 0.5 mg SC, IM: 1-1.5 mg every 4-6 hr Rectal: 5 mg every 4-6 hr	3-6	1	6

continued

With continued, prolonged use the opiate agonists may produce **drug tolerance** or psychologic and physical dependence (addiction). Tolerance occurs when a patient requires increases in dosages to receive the same analgesic relief. Development of tolerance seems to depend on the extent and duration of CNS depression. Patients who have prolonged depression by the continued use of opiate agonists have a higher incidence of developing tolerance. Patients who have developed tolerance to one opiate agonist usually require increased doses of all opiate agonists.

Patients who are physically dependent on opiate agonists remain asymptomatic as long as they are able to maintain their daily opiate agonist requirement. Addiction may develop after 3 to 6 weeks of continuous use of the opiate agonists. Early signs of withdrawal are restlessness, perspiration, gooseflesh, lacrimation, runny nose, and mydriasis. Over the next 24 hours these symptoms intensify, and the patient develops muscular spasms; severe aches in the back, abdomen, and legs; abdominal and muscle cramps; hot and cold flashes; insomnia; nausea, vomiting, and diarrhea; se-

Table 18-1

Opiate Agonists—cont'd

					DOSE EQUAL TO MORPHINE (10 MG)	
GENERIC NAME	BRAND NAME	AVAILABILITY	INITIAL ADULT DOSE	DURATION (HOURS)	IM (MG)	ORAL (MG)
Meperidine-like derivatives						
Alfentanil	Alfenta	Inj: 500 µg/ml in 2, 5, 10, 20 ml capsules	IV: variable	>45 min	—	—
Fentanyl	Sublimaze	Inj: 0.05, 1.5, 2.5 mg/ml Lozenges: 200, 300, 400 mcg	IM: 0.05-0.1 mg	1-2	0.1	—
Meperidine	Demerol	Tablets: 50, 100 mg Syrup: 50 mg/5 ml Inj: 10, 25, 50, 75, 100 mg/l ml	PO, SC, IM: 50-150 mg every 3-4 hr IV: 25-100 mg very slowly	2-4	75	300
Sufentanil	Sufenta	Inj: 50 µg/ml in 1, 2, 5 ml ampules	IV: variable	2-3	—	—
Methadone-like derivatives						
Methadone	Methadone, Dolophine	Tablets: 5, 10, 40 mg Solution: 5, 10 mg/5 ml Inj: 10 mg/ml Oral concentrate: 10 mg/ml	Analgesia: PO, SC, IM: 2.5-10 mg every 3-4 hr Maintenance: PO: 20-40 mg; up to 120 mg daily	4-6	10	20
Other opiate agonists						
Tramadol	Ultram	Tablets: 50 mg	PO: 50-100 mg	4-6	—	100

✦ Available in Canada only.

vere sneezing; and increases in body temperature, blood pressure, respiratory rate, and heart rate. These symptoms reach a peak at 36 to 72 hours after discontinuation of the medication and disappear over the next 5 to 14 days.

Uses

The opiate agonists are used to relieve acute or chronic moderate to severe pain such as that associated with acute injury, postoperative pain, renal or biliary colic, myocardial infarction, or terminal cancer. These agents may be used to provide preoperative sedation and supplement anesthesia. In patients with acute pulmonary edema, small doses of the opiate agonists are used to reduce anxiety and produce positive cardiovascular effects to control edema.

Tramadol is a new synthetic opiate agonist that acts as an analgesic by selectively binding to the µ-receptors and inhibiting the reuptake of norepinephrine and serotonin. Because of this selective activity, it is anticipated that physical addiction will not occur.

Therapeutic Outcomes

The primary therapeutic outcomes from opiate agonist therapy are as follows:
• Relief of pain to a level of comfort the patient deems appropriate

• Control of side effects from the use of analgesics, for example, constipation, nausea, vomiting

Nursing Process

Premedication Assessment

1. Perform baseline neurologic assessment, for example, orientation to date, time, and place, mental alertness, bilateral hand grip, and motor functioning.
2. Take vital signs; hold medication if respirations are below 12 per minute and consult with physician. Check bowel sounds and note consistency of stools. Review voiding pattern and urine output.
3. Check prior use of analgesics.
4. Perform pain assessment before administration of an opiate agonist and at appropriate intervals during therapy. Report poor pain control promptly and obtain modification in orders.

Planning
Availability. See Table 18-1.
Antidotes. Naloxone, Naltrexone.

Implementation
Dosage and administration. See Table 18-1.

ANALGESICS

It is important to maintain a relatively steady blood level of analgesic to gain the best control of pain. However, drug absorption, metabolism, and excretion are affected by age. Dosages and frequency of administration of analgesics may have to be increased in children, especially teenagers, because many medicines are more rapidly metabolized and excreted in this age group. Conversely, the elderly may need a somewhat lower dose of an analgesic less frequently because of slower metabolism and excretion. In either situation, it is imperative that the nurse make regular assessments of the patient's pain level and contact the physician for adjustments in dosages and frequency based on the response to the analgesic.

Before initiating a pain assessment, assess the patient for hearing and visual impairment. Data collected may be invalidated by the person's inability to hear the questions or see the visual aids used to assess pain.

Evaluation

Side effects to expect

LIGHT-HEADEDNESS, DIZZINESS, SEDATION, NAUSEA, VOMITING, SWEATING. These effects tend to occur most frequently with the initial dosage. Symptoms can be reduced by keeping the patient supine. Provide for patient safety, assurance, and comfort.

CONFUSION, DISORIENTATION. Perform a baseline assessment of the patient's degree of alertness and orientation to name, place, and time *before* initiating therapy. Make regularly scheduled subsequent evaluations of mental status and compare findings. Report development of alterations. Provide for patient safety during these episodes.

ORTHOSTATIC HYPOTENSION. Orthostatic hypotension, manifested by dizziness and weakness, occurs particularly when therapy is being initiated in a patient who is not in a supine position. Monitor blood pressure closely, especially if the patient complains of dizziness or faintness. Do not allow the patient to sit up.

CONSTIPATION. Continued use may cause constipation. Maintain the patient's state of hydration and obtain an order for stool softeners or bulk-forming laxatives if necessary. Encourage the inclusion of sufficient roughage, fresh fruits, vegetables, and whole-grain products in the diet.

Side effects to report

RESPIRATORY DEPRESSION. Opiate agonists make the respiratory centers less sensitive to carbon dioxide, causing respiratory depression. This may occur before either the reduction in respiratory rate or tidal volume is noticeable. Check the respiratory rate and depth frequently. Have equipment for respiratory assistance available.

URINARY RETENTION. Opiate agonists may produce spasms of the ureters and bladder, causing urinary retention. Patients may also have difficulty in starting the stream for urination. If the patient develops urinary hesitancy, assess for distention of the bladder. Report to the physician for further evaluation. Try to stimulate urination by running water or placing the patient's hands in water; if permitted, have male patients stand to void; female patients should sit on a bedpan or toilet with receptacle.

EXCESSIVE USE OR ABUSE. Evaluate the patient's response to the analgesic. Identify underlying needs and plan for more appropriate management of those needs. Discuss the case with the physician and make plans to cooperatively approach gradual withdrawal of the medications being abused. Suggest a change to a milder analgesic when indicated.

Patients do not have to undergo the symptoms of withdrawal to be treated for addiction. Patients may be treated by gradual reduction of daily opiate agonist dosages. If withdrawal symptoms become severe, the patient may receive methadone. Temporary administration of tranquilizers and sedatives may aid in reducing patient anxiety and craving for the opiate agonist.

Assist the patient in recognizing the abuse problem. Provide for emotional support of the individual; display an accepting attitude—be kind but firm.

Drug interactions

CNS DEPRESSANTS. The following drugs may enhance the depressant effects of the opiate agonists: general anesthetics, phenothiazines, tranquilizers, sedative-hypnotics, tricyclic antidepressants, antihistamines, and alcohol.

Respiratory depression, hypotension, and profound sedation or coma may result from this interaction unless the dose of the opiate agonist has been reduced appropriately (usually by one third to one half the normal dose).

PHENOBARBITAL, PHENYTOIN, RIFAMPIN, CHLORPROMAZINE. These enzyme-inducing agents may enhance the metabolism of meperidine to normeperidine. Patients receiving long-term, large oral doses of meperidine, those with renal impairment, and those with highly acidic urine are predisposed to accumulating normeperidine. Evidence of toxic levels of normeperidine are seizures, tremors, and excitation.

Drug Class: Opiate Partial Agonists

Actions

Opiate partial agonists (buprenorphine, butorphanol, dezocine, nalbuphine, and pentazocine) are an interesting class of drugs in that their pharmacologic actions depend on whether an opiate agonist has been administered previously and the extent to which physical dependence has developed to that opiate agonist. When used without prior administration of opiate agonists, the opiate partial agonists are effective analgesics. Their potency with the first few weeks of therapy is similar to that of morphine; however, after prolonged use, tolerance may develop. Increasing the dosage does not significantly increase the analgesia but definitely increases the incidence of side effects. This is called a **ceiling effect** in that, contrary to the action of the opiate agonists, a larger dose does not produce a significantly higher analgesic effect.

If an opiate partial agonist is administered to a patient addicted to an opiate agonist such as morphine or meperidine, the opiate partial agonist will induce withdrawal symptoms from the opiate agonist. If the patient is not addicted to the opiate agonist, there is no interaction and the patient will be relieved of pain.

Uses

Opiate partial agonists may be used for the short-term relief (up to 3 weeks) of moderate to severe pain associated with cancer, burns, renal colic, preoperative analgesia, and obstetric and surgical analgesia. Butorphanol, nalbuphine, and dezocine have minimal addiction liability and are not controlled substances.

Therapeutic Outcomes

The primary therapeutic outcomes from opiate agonist therapy are as follows:
- Relief of pain to a level of comfort that the patient deems appropriate
- Control of side effects from the use of analgesics, for example, constipation, nausea, vomiting

Nursing Process

Premedication Assessment

1. Perform baseline neurologic assessment, for example, orientation to date, time, and place, mental alertness, bilateral hand grip, motor functioning.
2. Take vital signs; hold medication if respirations are below 12 and consult with physician.
3. Check bowel sound and note consistency of stools. Review voiding pattern and urine output.
4. Check previous use of opiate agonists.
5. Perform pain assessment before administration of opiate agonist and at appropriate intervals during therapy. Report poor pain control promptly and obtain modification in orders.

Planning

Availability. See Table 18-2.
Antidotes. Naloxone, naltrexone.

Implementation

Dosage and administration. See Table 18-2.

Evaluation

Side effects to expect

CLAMMINESS, DIZZINESS, SEDATION, NAUSEA, VOMITING, DRY MOUTH, SWEATING. These effects tend to occur most frequently with the initial dosage. Symptoms can be reduced by keeping the patient supine. Provide for patient safety, assurance, and comfort.

CONSTIPATION. Continued use may cause constipation. Maintain the patient's state of hydration and obtain an order for stool softeners or bulk-forming laxatives if necessary. Encourage the inclusion of sufficient roughage, fresh fruits, vegetables, and whole-grain products in the diet.

Side effects to report

CONFUSION, DISORIENTATION, HALLUCINATIONS. Butorphanol and pentazocine, and to a lesser degree nalbuphine, may produce hallucinations. Patients may complain of seeing

Table 18-2

Opiate Partial Agonists

GENERIC NAME	BRAND NAME	AVAILABILITY	ADULT DOSAGE	DURATION (HOURS)	DOSE EQUAL TO MORPHINE (10 MG)
Buprenorphine	Buprenex	Inj: 0.3 mg/ml in 1 ml ampules	0.3-0.6 mg repeated in 5-6 hr	6	0.3 mg
Butorphanol	Stadol	Inj: 1, 2 mg in 1, 2, 10 ml vials	IM: 2 mg, repeated in 3-4 hr; do not exceed single doses of 4 mg IV: 1 mg, repeated in 3-4 hr	(IM) 3-4	(IM) 2-3 mg
	Stadol NS	Nasal Spray: 10 mg/ml	Nasal: 1 spray in each nostril repeated in 3-4 hr		
Dezocine	Dalgan	Inj: 5, 10, 15 mg/ml in 2 ml ampules	IM: 5-20 mg (usual, 10 mg) every 3-6 hr IV: 2.5-10 mg every 2-4 hr	3-4	20 mg
Nalbuphine	Nubain	Inj: 10, 20 mg/ml in 1, 2, 10 ml vials	SC, IM, IV: 10 mg/70 kg, repeat every 3-6 hr; do not exceed 160 mg daily	3-6	10 mg
Pentazocine	Talwin, Talwin NX*	Inj: 30 mg/ml in 1, 2, 10 ml vials Tablets: 50 mg	PO: 50-100 mg every 3-4 hr; do not exceed 600 mg daily SC, IM, IV: 30 mg every 3-4 hr; do not exceed 360 mg daily	2-3	30-60 mg

*Tablets contain naloxone to prevent abuse.

multicolored flashing patterns or animals, with and without sound, or may have vivid dreams. These adverse effects have been reported after only one or two doses of medication and may occur in as many as one third of patients taking butorphanol or pentazocine.

Perform a baseline assessment of the patient's degree of alertness and orientation to name, place, and time before initiating therapy. Make regularly scheduled subsequent evaluations of mental status and compare findings. Report development of alterations. Provide for patient safety during these episodes. If recurring, seek a change in the medication order.

RESPIRATORY DEPRESSION. Opiate partial agonists make the respiratory centers less sensitive to carbon dioxide, causing respiratory depression. This may occur before either the reduction in respiratory rate or tidal volume is noticeable. Check the respiratory rate and depth frequently.

EXCESSIVE USE OR ABUSE. Repeated use may lead to tolerance, dependence, and addiction. Evaluate the patient's response to the analgesic. Identify underlying needs and plan for more appropriate management of those needs. Discuss the case with the physician and make plans to cooperatively approach gradual withdrawal of the medications being abused. Suggest a change to a milder analgesic when indicated.

Patients do not have to experience the symptoms of withdrawal to be treated for addiction. Patients may be treated by gradual reduction of daily opiate agonist dosages. If withdrawal symptoms become severe, the patient may receive methadone. Temporary administration of tranquilizers and sedatives may aid in reducing patient anxiety and craving for the opiate agonist.

Assist the patient in recognizing the abuse problem. Provide for emotional support of the individual; display an accepting attitude—be kind but firm.

Drug interactions

CNS DEPRESSANTS. The following drugs may enhance the depressant effects of the opiate partial agonists: general anesthetics, phenothiazines, tranquilizers, sedative-hypnotics, tricyclic antidepressants, antihistamines, and alcohol.

Respiratory depression, hypotension, and profound sedation or coma may result from this interaction unless the dose of the opiate partial agonist has been reduced appropriately (usually by one third to one half the normal dose).

OPIATE AGONISTS. Opiate partial agonists have weak antagonist activity. When administered to patients who have been receiving opiate agonists such as morphine or meperidine on a regular basis, it may precipitate withdrawal symptoms.

Drug Class: Opiate Antagonists

naloxone (nal-oks-one)
Narcan (nar-can)

Actions

Naloxone is a so-called pure opiate antagonist because it has no effect of its own other than its ability to reverse the CNS depressant effects of opiate agonists, opiate partial agonists, and propoxyphene. When administered to patients who have not recently received opiates, there is no respiratory depression,

psychomimetic effect, circulatory changes, or other pharmacologic activity. If administered to a person addicted to the opiate agonists or the opiate partial agonists, withdrawal symptoms may be precipitated. Naloxone is not effective in CNS depression induced by tranquilizers or sedative-hypnotics.

Uses

Naloxone is a drug of choice for treatment of respiratory depression when excessive doses of opiate agonists, opiate partial agonists, or propoxyphene have been administered or when the causative agent is unknown.

Therapeutic Outcomes

The primary therapeutic outcome expected from naloxone is reversal of respiratory depression.

Nursing Process

Premedication Assessment

1. Perform baseline neurologic assessment, for example, orientation to date, time, and place, mental alertness, bilateral hand grip, and motor functioning.
2. Take vital signs—blood pressure, pulse, and respirations should be taken at frequent intervals until resolution of CNS depression. Then schedule vital signs to be taken at appropriate intervals because the duration of action of naloxone is short.
3. Check prior use or dependence on opiate agonists or opiate partial agonists. Diagnostic tests for narcotic dependence may be performed in accordance with policies of the clinical site. Inform patient of risks involved.
4. Have supportive equipment available in immediate area to maintain respirations.
5. Check bowel sounds. Review voiding pattern and urine output.

Planning

Availability. Injection—0.02 mg/ml (for neonatal use); 0.4 mg/ml and 1 mg/ml.

Implementation

Dosage and administration. Adult: IV—Postoperative opiate depression: 0.1 to 0.2 mg every 2 to 3 minutes until the desired response is achieved. Opiate overdose: 0.4 to 2 mg every 2 to 3 minutes. If no response is seen after 10 minutes, the depressive condition may be caused by a drug or disease process not responsive to naloxone.

Evaluation

Side effects to expect

MENTAL DEPRESSION, APATHY, NAUSEA, AND VOMITING. Naloxone rarely causes any side effects. The following adverse effects have been reported rarely when extremely high doses have been used: mental depression, apathy, inability to concentrate, sleepiness, irritability, anorexia, nausea, and vomiting. These adverse effects usually occurred in the first few days of treatment and dissipate rapidly with continued therapy.

Naloxone should be used with caution after the use of opiates during surgery because it may result in excitement, an increase in blood pressure, and clinically important reversal of analgesia. The early reversal of opiate effects may induce nausea, vomiting, sweating, and tachycardia.

Naloxone should be given with caution to patients known or suspected to be physically dependent on opiates (including neonates born to women who are opiate dependent) because the drug may precipitate severe withdrawal symptoms. The severity of the symptoms depends on the dose of the naloxone and the degree of dependence.

Drug interactions. There are no drug interactions other than that of the antagonist activity toward opiate agonists, opiate partial agonists, and propoxyphene.

naltrexone (nal-trex-one)
ReVia (rhe-vee' ah)

Actions

Naltrexone is a pure opioid antagonist that is closely related to naloxone. It differs, however, in that it is active after oral administration and has a considerably longer duration of action. Naltrexone blocks the effects of opioids by competitive binding at opioid receptors. The mechanism of action of naltrexone in alcoholism is not known.

Uses

Naltrexone is used clinically to block the pharmacologic effects of exogenously administered opiates in patients who are enrolled in drug abuse treatment programs. The rationale for using naltrexone as an adjunct in treatment is that naltrexone may diminish or eliminate opiate-seeking behavior by blocking the euphoric reinforcement produced by self-administration of opiates and by preventing the conditioned abstinence syndrome (that is, opiate craving) that occurs after opiate withdrawal. Naltrexone has been added to pentazocine formulations (Talwin NX) to reduce abuse of pentazocine by blocking the euphoric high associated with pentazocine.

Naltrexone has also been approved as an adjunct in the treatment of alcoholism to support abstinence and reduce relapse rates and alcohol consumption. It must be used with other treatment modalities; the expected effect of the drug treatment is a modest improvement in the outcome of conventional treatment.

Therapeutic Outcomes

The primary therapeutic outcomes expected from naloxone are as follows:
- Improved compliance with a substance abuse program because of reduced craving of opioids
- Improved compliance with an alcohol treatment program by diminishing craving for alcohol

Nursing Process

Premedication Assessment

1. Perform baseline neurologic assessment, for example, orientation to date, time, and place, mental alertness, bilateral hand grip, and motor functioning.
2. Take vital signs—temperature, blood pressure, pulse, and respirations.

3. Check laboratory values for hepatotoxicity; urine screen for opiate use.
4. Monitor for gastrointestinal symptoms before and during therapy.
5. The manufacturer recommends that baseline determinations of liver function should be performed in all patients before initiation of therapy and repeated monthly for the next 6 months.
6. The manufacturer recommends a minimum of 7 to 10 days of abstinence from all opiates, a urinalysis to confirm the absence of opiates, and the use of a naloxone challenge test to ensure that the patient will not develop withdrawal symptoms.

Planning
Availability. PO—50 mg tablets.

Implementation
Dosage and administration. Behavior modification: Naltrexone therapy in combination with behavioral therapy has been shown to be more effective than naltrexone or behavioral therapy alone in prolonging opiate or alcohol cessation in patients formerly physically dependent on opiates or alcohol.

Treatment of narcotic dependence: PO—Induction regimen, 25 mg. Observe for development of withdrawal symptoms. If none occur, administer 50 mg the next day. Maintenance regimen—50 mg daily. Alternative regimens of 100 mg every other day or 150 mg every third day have been used to improve compliance during a behavior modification program.

Withdrawal symptoms: Naltrexone may precipitate acute and severe withdrawal symptoms in patients who are physically dependent on opioids. Addicts must be completely detoxified and opioid free before taking naltrexone. The manufacturer recommends a minimum of 7 to 10 days of abstinence from all opiates, a urinalysis to confirm the absence of opiates, and the use of a naloxone challenge test to ensure that the patient will not develop withdrawal symptoms.

Patients undergoing naltrexone therapy must be carefully instructed about the expectations of behavioral modification associated with therapy. They should also be advised that self-administration of small doses of opiates (such as heroin) during naltrexone therapy will not result in any pharmacologic effect and that large doses may result in serious pharmacologic effects, including coma and death. Patients should also be given identification to notify medical personnel that they are taking a long-acting opiate antagonist.

Treatment of alcoholism: PO—50 mg once daily.

Evaluation
Many adverse effects have been associated with naltrexone therapy, but it is difficult to know exactly which adverse effects are secondary to naltrexone alone because some patients may have been experiencing mild opiate withdrawal symptoms as well. The adverse effects of drug and alcohol abuse and poor nutritional states may also contribute to the patient's discomfort.

Side effects to expect

NAUSEA, VOMITING, HEADACHE, ANOREXIA, ABDOMINAL CRAMPS. These side effects are usually mild and tend to resolve with continued therapy. Encourage the patient not to discontinue therapy without first consulting the physician and treatment program.

Side effects to report

HEPATOTOXICITY. A major adverse effect is hepatotoxicity after doses of 300 mg daily for 3 to 8 weeks. The symptoms of hepatotoxicity are jaundice, nausea, vomiting, anorexia, hepatomegaly, splenomegaly, and abnormal liver functions tests (elevated bilirubin, aspartate transaminase [AST], alanine aminotransferase [ALT], alkaline phosphatase, prothrombin time). Because many of these patients do not develop clinical symptoms but do develop abnormal liver function tests, strongly encourage patients to report for blood tests as scheduled. Report abnormal values to the appropriate physician.

Drug interactions

OPIATE-CONTAINING PRODUCTS. Patients taking naltrexone will probably not benefit from opioid-containing medicines such as analgesics, cough and cold preparations, and antidiarrheal preparations. Use of these products should be avoided during naltrexone therapy when nonopiate therapy is available.

CLONIDINE. Clonidine may be administered in patients to reduce the severity of withdrawal symptoms precipitated or exacerbated by naltrexone.

Drug Class: Antiinflammatory Agents

salicylates (sahl-ihs-il' ate)

Actions

The **salicylates** are the most common analgesics used for the relief of slight to moderate pain. The salicylates were introduced into medicine in the late nineteenth century because of their three primary pharmacologic effects as analgesic, antipyretic, and antiinflammatory agents. Although the mechanisms of action are not fully known, most of the activity of the salicylates comes from inhibition of prostaglandin synthesis. Salicylates inhibit the formation of prostaglandins that sensitize pain receptors to stimulation causing pain (analgesia); they inhibit the prostaglandins that produce the signs and symptoms of inflammation (redness, swelling, warmth); and they inhibit the synthesis and release of prostaglandins in the brain that cause the elevation of body temperature (antipyresis). A major benefit of the salicylates is that they do not dull the consciousness level and do not cause mental sluggishness, memory disturbances, hallucinations, euphoria, or sedation.

A unique property of aspirin, compared with other salicylates, is inhibition of platelet aggregation and enhancement of bleeding time. The platelet loses its ability to aggregate and form clots for the duration of its lifetime (7 to 10 days). The mechanism of action is inhibition of the synthesis of thromboxane A2, a potent vasoconstrictor and inducer of platelet aggregation.

Uses

The combination of pharmacologic effects makes the salicylates the drugs of choice for symptomatic relief of discomfort, pain, inflammation, or fever associated with bacterial and viral infections, headache, muscle aches, and rheumatoid arthritis. Salicylates can be taken to relieve pain on a long-term basis without causing drug dependence.

Because of its antiplatelet activity, aspirin is also indicated for reducing the risk of recurrent transient ischemic attack (TIA) or stroke in men. Aspirin is also used to reduce the risk of myocardial infarction in patients with previous myocardial infarction or unstable angina pectoris.

Therapeutic Outcomes

The primary therapeutic outcomes expected from nonsteroidal antiinflammatory agents are reduced pain, reduced inflammation, and elimination of body fever. The primary therapeutic outcomes expected from aspirin when used for antiplatelet therapy are reduced frequency of TIA or stroke in men and reduced frequency of myocardial infarction.

Nursing Process

Premedication Assessment

1. Perform baseline neurologic assessment, for example, orientation to date, time, and place, mental alertness, bilateral hand grip, motor functioning, balance, and hearing.
2. Take vital signs—temperature, blood pressure, pulse, and respirations.
3. Check laboratory values for hepatotoxicity and renal impairment; clotting time.
4. Monitor for gastrointestinal symptoms before and during therapy; stool guiaic if suspecting gastrointestinal (GI) tract bleeding.
5. Check for concurrent use of anticoagulant agents.
6. If on oral hypoglycemics, review baseline serum glucose level.
7. When used as analgesic, perform pain assessment before administration of salicylate and at appropriate intervals during therapy. Report poor pain control promptly and obtain modification in orders.

Planning

Availability. See Tables 18-3 and 18-4.

Implementation

Dosage and administration. For treatment of pain: see Tables 18-3 and 18-4. For prevention of blood clots: PO—80 to 1300 mg daily. The dosage depends on whether the patient has a previous history of clot formation and other medications the patient may be receiving. The larger doses are usually subdivided into 325 mg 2 to 4 times daily.

Evaluation

As beneficial as the salicylates are, they are not without adverse effects. In normal therapeutic doses, salicylates may produce gastrointestinal irritation, occasional nausea, and gastric hemorrhage. Extreme caution should be used with

Table 18-3

Nonsteroidal Antiinflammatory Agents

GENERIC NAME	BRAND NAME	AVAILABILITY	USES AND DOSAGES	MAXIMUM DAILY DOSE (MG)
Salicylates				
Aspirin	Easprin, Zorprin, A.S.A., Bayer, Empirin	Tablets: 65, 81, 325, 487.5, 650 mg Capsules: 325, 500 mg Suppositories: 60, 130, 195, 300, 325, 600, 625, 1200 mg	Minor aches and pains: 325-600 mg every 4 hr Arthritis: 2.6-5.2 g/day in divided doses Acute rheumatic fever: 7.8 g/day	—
Choline salicylate	Arthropan	Liquid: 870 mg/5 ml	Mild pain: 870 mg every 3-4 hr (fewer GI side effects)	7000
Diflunisal	Dolobid	Tablets: 250, 500 mg	Mild to moderate pain: Initially, 1000 mg, then 500 mg every 8 hr Osteoarthritis: 250-500 mg 2 times daily	1500
Magnesium salicylate	Magan, Mobidin	Tablets: 325, 500, 545, 600 mg	Mild aches and pains: 500-650 mg 3 or 4 times daily	9600
Salicylamide	Uromide, Salicylamide	Tablets: 325, 667 mg	Minor aches and pains: 325-667 mg 3 or 4 times daily (less effective than equal doses of aspirin)	4000
Salsalate	Disalcid Artha-G	Tablets: 500, 750 mg Capsules: 500 mg	Mild pain: 500-750 mg 4-6 times daily	3000
Sodium salicylate	Uracel 5, Sodium Salicylate, ✽S-60	Tablets: 325, 650 mg Enteric-coated tablets: 325, 650 mg	Mild analgesia: 325-650 mg every 4-8 hr (less effective than equal doses of aspirin)	3900
Sodium thiosalicylate	Asproject, Tusal	Inj: 50 mg/ml in 2 and 30 ml vials	Acute gout: IM: 100 mg every 3-4 hr for 2 days, then 100 mg/day Rheumatic fever: IM: 100-150 mg every 4-6 hr for 3 days, then 100 mg twice daily	—
Nonsteroidal antiinflammatory agents				
Diclofenac	Cataflam, Voltaren	Tablets: 50 mg Tablets delayed release: 25, 50, 75 mg	Rheumatoid and osteoarthritis, ankylosing spondylitis: 25-75 mg 2-3 times daily	200
Etodolac	Lodine	Capsules: 200, 300 mg	Osteoarthritis, pain: 300-400 mg 3-4 times daily	1200
Fenoprofen	Nalfon	Capsules: 200, 300 mg Tablets: 600 mg	Rheumatoid and osteoarthritis: 300-600 mg 3 or 4 times daily Mild to moderate pain: 200 mg every 4-6 hr	3200
Flurbiprofen	Ansaid	Tablets: 50, 100 mg	Rheumatoid and osteoarthritis: 50-100 mg 2-3 times daily	300
Ibuprofen	Motrin, Rufen, ✽Novoprofen	Tablets: 200, 300, 400, 600, 800 mg Suspension: 100 mg/5 ml	Rheumatoid and osteoarthritis: 300-600 mg 3-4 times daily Mild to moderate pain: 400 mg every 4-6 hr Primary dysmenorrhea: 400 mg every 4 hr	2400

continued

Table 18-3

Nonsteroidal Antiinflammatory Agents—cont'd

GENERIC NAME	BRAND NAME	AVAILABILITY	USES AND DOSAGES	MAXIMUM DAILY DOSE (MG)
Nonsteroidal antiinflammatory agents—cont'd				
Indomethacin	Indocin, ❋Indocid	Capsules: 25, 50, 75 mg Sustained release capsules: 75 mg Oral suspension: 25 mg/5 ml Suppository: 50 mg	Rheumatoid and osteoarthritis, ankylosing spondylitis: 25-50 mg 3-4 times daily Acute painful shoulder: 25-50 mg 2-3 times daily Acute gouty arthritis: 50 mg 3 times daily Closure of patent ductus arteriosus: IV—1-3 IV doses given at 12-24 hr intervals	200
Ketoprofen	Orudis ❋Rhodis ❋Oruvail	Capsules: 25, 50, 75 mg Extended-release capsules: 100, 150, 200 mg	Rheumatoid and osteoarthritis: Initially, 75 mg 3 times daily or 50 mg 4 times daily; reduce initial dose by 1/2 to 1/3 in elderly patients or those with impaired renal function	300
Ketorolac	Toradol, ❋Acular	Tablets: 10 mg Injection: 15, 30 mg/ml in 1, 2 ml prefilled syringes	Injectable analgesic, antiinflammatory, antipyretic used for acute, short-term pain management; 30-60 mg IM initially, 15-30 mg every 6 hr prn pain; then PO ≤ 40 mg/24 hr	120-150
Meclofenamate	Meclomen	Capsules: 50, 100 mg	Rheumatoid and osteoarthritis: 200-400 mg daily in 3-4 equal doses. Mild to moderate pain: 50-100 mg 3-4 times daily; Primary dysmenorrhea: 100 mg 3 times daily	400
Mefenamic acid	Ponstel, ❋Ponstan	Capsules: 250 mg	Moderate pain or primary dysmenorrhea: Initially 500 mg, then 250 mg every 6 hr	1000
Nabumetone	Relafen	Tablets: 500, 750 mg	Rheumatoid and osteoarthritis: 1000-1500 mg daily in one or two doses	2000
Naproxen	Naprosyn	Tablets: 200, 250, 375, 500 mg Oral suspension: 125 mg/ml	Rheumatoid and osteoarthritis, ankylosing spondylitis: 250-375 mg 2 times daily	1000
Naproxen sodium	Anaprox, Anaprox DS	Tablets: 275 mg Tablets: 550 mg	Acute gout: 750-825 mg initially, followed by 250-275 mg every 8 hr Moderate pain, primary dysmenorrhea, acute tendonitis, bursitis: 500-550 mg followed by 250-275 mg	1100
Oxaprozin	Daypro	Caplets: 600 mg	Rheumatoid arthritis, osteoarthritis: 1200 mg once daily	1800
Phenylbutazone	Cotylbutazone, ❋Nova-Butazone	Tablets: 100 mg Capsules: 100 mg	Rheumatoid and osteoarthritis, ankylosing spondylitis: 100 mg 4 times daily	600
Piroxicam	Feldene, ❋Nu-pirox	Capsules: 10, 20 mg	Rheumatoid and osteoarthritis: 20 mg 1 time daily	20

continued

Table 18-3

Nonsteroidal Antiinflammatory Agents—cont'd

GENERIC NAME	BRAND NAME	AVAILABILITY	USES AND DOSAGES	MAXIMUM DAILY DOSE (MG)
Nonsteroidal antiinflammatory agents—cont'd				
Sulindac	Clinoril ✹Apo-Sulin	Tablets: 150, 200 mg	Rheumatoid and osteoarthritis, ankylosing spondylitis: 150 mg 2 times daily Acute painful shoulder: 200 mg 2 times daily	400
Tolmetin	Tolectin	Tablets: 200, 600 mg Capsules: 400 mg	Rheumatoid and osteoarthritis: 400-600 mg 3 times daily	2000

GI, Gastrointestinal.
✹Available in Canada only.

administration to those patients with a history of peptic ulcer, liver disease, or coagulation disorders.

Side effects to expect

GASTRIC IRRITATION. If gastric irritation occurs, administer medication with food, milk, antacids (1 hour later), or large amounts of water. If symptoms persist or increase in severity, report for physician evaluation. Aspirin is available in enteric-coated form to reduce gastric irritation.

Side effects to report

GASTROINTESTINAL BLEEDING. Dark tarry stools and bright red or "coffee-ground" emesis. Test any suspicious stools or emesis for presence of occult blood.

SALICYLISM. Patients receiving higher dosages on a continuing basis are susceptible to developing salicylate intoxication (salicylism). Symptoms include tinnitus (ringing in the ears), impaired hearing, dimness of vision, sweating, fever, lethargy, dizziness, mental confusion, nausea, and vomiting. This condition is reversible on reduction of the dosage. Massive overdoses may lead to respiratory depression and coma. There is no antidote; primary treatment is discontinuation of the drug, gastric lavage, forced IV fluids, and alkalinization of the urine with IV sodium bicarbonate.

Patients who develop signs of salicylate toxicity should be reevaluated for other underlying disease and the possibility that other medication would be more effective.

Drug interactions

SULFINPYRAZONE, PROBENECID. Salicylates inhibit the excretion of uric acid by these agents. Although an occasional aspirin will not be sufficient to interfere with the effectiveness of these agents, regular use of salicylates or products containing salicylate should be discouraged. If analgesia is required, suggest acetaminophen.

WARFARIN. The salicylates may enhance the anticoagulant effects of warfarin. Observe for the development of petechiae, ecchymoses, nosebleeds, bleeding gums, dark tarry stools, and bright red or coffee-ground emesis. Monitor the prothrombin time and reduce the dosage of warfarin if necessary.

PHENYTOIN. Monitor patients with concurrent therapy for signs of phenytoin toxicity: nystagmus, sedation, lethargy. Serum levels may be ordered, and a reduced dosage of phenytoin may be required.

ORAL HYPOGLYCEMIC AGENTS. The salicylates may enhance the hypoglycemic effects of these agents. Monitor for hypoglycemia: headache, weakness, decreased coordination,

general apprehension, diaphoresis, hunger, blurred or double vision. The dosage of the hypoglycemic agent may need to be reduced. Notify the physician if any of the above-mentioned symptoms appear.

METHOTREXATE. Monitor for methotrexate toxicity: bone marrow suppression, decreased white blood cell count (WBC) or red blood cell count (RBC), sore throat, fever, lethargy.

CORTICOSTEROIDS. Although frequently used together, salicylates and corticosteroids may produce GI ulceration. Monitor for signs of GI bleeding: observe for the development of dark tarry stools and bright red or coffee-ground emesis.

ETHANOL. Patients should avoid aspirin within 8 to 10 hours of heavy alcohol use. Small amounts of GI bleeding often occur. If aspirin therapy is absolutely necessary, an enteric-coated product should be used.

CLINITEST. Ingestion of 8 to 18 of the 325 mg tablets of aspirin daily may result in false-positive Clinitest and false-negative Tes-Tape urine glucose determinations. Blood glucose measurements may be required for an accurate reading.

Drug Class: Nonsteroidal Antiinflammatory Agents

Actions

The nonsteroidal antiinflammatory drugs (NSAIDs) are also known as aspirin-like drugs. They are chemically unrelated to the salicylates but are prostaglandin inhibitors and share many of the same therapeutic actions and side effects. They all have varying degrees of analgesic, antipyretic, and antiinflammatory activity.

Uses

In clinical studies, all of these agents (see Table 18-3) are superior to placebos and approach aspirin in effectiveness, but none is superior to aspirin. Depending on the agent used, the dosage, and the patient, the side effects of therapy tend to be somewhat less than those associated with salicylate therapy. The cost of therapy with NSAIDs is considerably higher than that with aspirin treatment. Thus these agents are most effectively used as alternatives for patients who do not tolerate aspirin. These agents are used to relieve the pain and inflammation of rheumatoid arthritis, osteoarthritis, ankylosing

Table 18-4
Ingredients of Selected Analgesic Combination Products

Product	NONCONTROLLED SUBSTANCE			CONTROLLED SUBSTANCE	
	Aspirin (mg)	Acetaminophen (mg)	Other (mg)	Codeine (mg)	Other (mg)
Anacin Tablets	400		Caffeine 32		
Anacin Maximum Strength	500		Caffeine 32		
Buffets II Tablets	227	162	Caffeine 32.4 Aluminum Hydroxide 50		
BC Powder	650		Caffeine 32 Salacylamide 145		
Darvocet N 50		325			Propoxyphene napsylate 50
Darvocet N 100		650			Propoxyphene napsylate 100
Darvon					Propoxyphene HCl 65
Darvon-N					Propoxyphene napsylate 100*
Darvon Compound 65	389		Caffeine 32		Propoxyphene HCl 65
Empirin					
Codeine #3	325			30	
Codeine #4	325			60	
Excedrin	250	250	Caffeine 65		
Fioricet		325	Caffeine 40		Butalbital 50
Fiorinal	325		Caffeine 40		Butalbital 50
Fiorinal w/Codeine	325		Caffeine 40	30	Butalbital 50
Percocet		325			Oxycodone 5
Percodan	325				Oxycodone 5
Percogesic		325	Phenyltoloxamine 30		
Talwin Compound Caplets	325				Pentazocine 12.5
Tylenol		325			
Tylenol					
Codeine #2		300		15	
Codeine #3		300		30	
Codeine #4		300		60	

*Propoxyphene napsylate 100 mg is equipotent to propoxyphene HCl 65 mg.

spondylitis, and gout. Certain agents are also approved for use to control the discomfort of primary dysmenorrhea. Ibuprofen and naproxen are available on a nonprescription basis to be used for the temporary relief of minor aches and pains associated with colds, headaches, toothaches, muscular aches, backaches, arthritis, and menstrual cramps, and for reduction of fever.

Therapeutic Outcomes
The primary therapeutic outcomes expected from NSAIDS are reduced pain, reduced inflammation, and elimination of body fever.

Nursing Process

Premedication Assessment
1. Perform baseline neurologic assessment, for example, orientation to date, time, and place, mental alertness, bilateral hand grip, motor functioning, peripheral sensations, and vision and hearing.
2. Take vital signs—temperature, blood pressure, pulse, and respirations.
3. Check laboratory values for hepatotoxicity, nephrotoxicity, bleeding time, and blood dyscrasias.

4. Monitor for GI symptoms before and during therapy; stool guaiac if suspecting GI tract bleeding.
5. Check bowel sounds and note consistency of stools. Review voiding pattern and urine output.
6. Check for concurrent use of anticoagulant agents.
7. When used as analgesic, perform pain assessment before administration of NSAIDS and at appropriate intervals during therapy. Report poor pain control promptly and obtain modification in orders.

Planning
Availability. See Table 18-3.

Implementation
Dosage and administration. See Table 18-3. *Note:* Do not administer to patients who are allergic to aspirin.

Evaluation
Side effects to expect
GASTRIC IRRITATION. If gastric irritation occurs, administer medication with food, milk, antacids, or large amounts of water. If symptoms persist or increase in severity, report for physician evaluation.

CONSTIPATION. The use of stool softeners or bulk-forming laxatives may be necessary. Maintain the patient's state of hydration. Encourage the inclusion of sufficient roughage, fresh fruits, vegetables, and whole-grain products in the diet.

DIZZINESS. Provide for patient safety during episodes of dizziness.

DROWSINESS. Persons who are working around machinery, driving a car, or performing other duties in which they must remain mentally alert should not take these medications while working.

Side effects to report
GASTROINTESTINAL BLEEDING. Observe for the development of dark tarry stools and bright red or coffee-ground emesis.

CONFUSION. Perform a baseline assessment of the patient's degree of alertness and orientation to name, place, and time before initiating therapy. Make regularly scheduled subsequent evaluations of mental status and compare findings. Report development of alterations.

HIVES, PRURITUS, RASH. Report symptoms for further evaluation by the physician.

NEPHROTOXICITY. Monitor urinalysis and kidney function tests for abnormal results. Report an increasing blood urea nitrogen (BUN) and creatinine, decreasing urine output or decreasing urine specific gravity despite amount of fluid intake, casts or protein in the urine, frank blood or smoky-colored urine, or RBC in excess of 0 to 3 on the urinalysis report.

HEPATOTOXICITY. The symptoms of hepatotoxicity are anorexia, nausea, vomiting, jaundice, hepatomegaly, splenomegaly, and abnormal liver function tests (elevated bilirubin, AST, ALT, alkaline phosphatase, prothrombin time).

BLOOD DYSCRASIAS. Routine laboratory studies (RBC, WBC, and differential counts) should be scheduled. Monitor for the development of sore throat, fever, purpura, jaundice, or excessive and progressive weakness.

Drug interactions
WARFARIN. The NSAIDs may enhance the anticoagulant effects of warfarin. Observe for the development of pete-chiae, ecchymoses, nosebleeds, bleeding gums, dark tarry stools, and bright red or coffee-ground emesis. Monitor the prothrombin time and reduce the dosage of warfarin if necessary.

PHENYTOIN. Monitor patients with concurrent therapy for signs of phenytoin toxicity: nystagmus, sedation, lethargy. Serum levels may be ordered, and a reduced dosage of phenytoin may be required.

VALPROIC ACID. Aspirin inhibits valproic acid metabolism, increasing valproic acid blood levels. Monitor for valproic acid toxicity: sedation, drowsiness, dizziness, blurred vision. Serum levels may be ordered, and a reduced dosage of valproic acid may be required.

ORAL HYPOGLYCEMIC AGENTS. Monitor for hypoglycemia: headache, weakness, decreased coordination, general apprehension, diaphoresis, hunger, blurred or double vision. The dosage of the hypoglycemic agent may need to be reduced. Notify the physician if any of the above-mentioned symptoms appear.

FUROSEMIDE, THIAZIDE DIURETICS. Indomethacin inhibits the diuretic activity of this agent. The dose of the diuretic agents may need to be increased or indomethacin discontinued. Maintain accurate intake and output and blood pressure records, and monitor for a decrease in diuretic and antihypertensive activity.

PROBENECID. Probenecid inhibits the excretion of NSAIDs. Monitor patients for signs of indomethacin toxicity: headache, drowsiness, mental confusion.

LITHIUM. NSAIDs (except possibly sulindac and aspirin) may induce lithium toxicity. Monitor patients for lithium toxicity manifested by nausea, anorexia, fine tremors, persistent vomiting, profuse diarrhea, hyperreflexia, lethargy, and weakness.

CHOLESTYRAMINE. Cholestyramine resins bind to NSAIDs in the gut, inhibiting absorption. Separate dosing administration by 2 hours. The dose of NSAID may need to be increased.

Drug Class: Miscellaneous Analgesics

acetaminophen (a-seat-a-mee-noe-fen)
Tylenol (ty-le-nol), **Datril** (day-tril), **Tempra** (tem-prah)

Actions
Acetaminophen is a synthetic nonopiate analgesic. The site and mechanism of action is unknown. Its antipyretic effectiveness and analgesic potency are similar to those of aspirin in equal doses.

Uses
Acetaminophen is an effective analgesic-antipyretic for fever and discomfort associated with bacterial and viral infections, headache, and conditions involving musculoskeletal pain. It is a good substitute for patients who cannot take products containing aspirin because of allergic reactions, hypersensitivities, anticoagulant therapy, or possible bleeding problems from gastric or duodenal ulcers, gastritis, and hiatus hernia. This drug has no antiinflammatory activity and is therefore ineffective (other than as an analgesic) in the relief of symptoms of rheumatoid arthritis or other inflammation.

Therapeutic Outcomes

The primary therapeutic outcomes expected from acetaminophen are reduced pain and body fever.

Nursing Process

Premedication Assessment

1. Take vital signs—temperature, blood pressure, pulse, and respirations.
2. Check laboratory values for hepatotoxicity, nephrotoxicity.
3. Monitor for GI symptoms before and during therapy.
4. Check bowel sounds and review voiding pattern and urine output.
5. When used as analgesic, perform pain assessment before administration of acetaminophen and at appropriate intervals during therapy. Report poor pain control promptly and obtain modification in orders.
6. When used as antipyretic, take baseline temperature and continue monitoring temperature at appropriate intervals (for example, every 2 or 4 hours) depending on severity of temperature elevation.

Planning

Availability. PO—80, 160, 325, 500, and 650 mg tablets; 500 mg capsules; 120 mg per 5 ml, 160 mg per 5 ml, 325 mg per 5 ml elixir; 100 mg per ml, 120 mg per 2.5 ml solution; 165 mg per 5 ml liquid. Rectal—120, 125, 300, 325, 650 mg suppositories.

Implementation

Dosage and administration. Adult: PO—300 to 650 mg every 4 hours. Doses up to 100 mg may be given 4 times daily for short-term therapy. Do not exceed 2.6 g daily. Pediatric: PO—0 to 3 months, 40 mg; 4 to 11 months, 80 mg; 12 to 24 months, 120 mg; 2 to 3 years, 160 mg; 4 to 5 years, 240 mg; 6 to 8 years, 320 mg; 9 to 10 years, 400 mg; 11 to 12 years, 480 mg. Rectal—as for oral doses.
Antidote. Acetylcysteine.

Evaluation

When used as directed, acetaminophen is essentially free of side effects.
Side effects to expect
    GASTRIC IRRITATION. If gastric irritation occurs, administer medication with food, milk, antacids, or large amounts of water. If symptoms persist or increase in severity, report for physician evaluation.
Side effects to report
    OVERDOSAGE, HEPATOTOXICITY. Overdosage because of acute and chronic ingestion has risen dramatically in the last few years. Severe, life-threatening hepatotoxicity has been reported in patients who either ingest 5 to 8 g daily for several weeks or attempt suicide by consuming large quantities at one time.
    Early indications of toxicity include anorexia, nausea, vomiting, low blood pressure, drowsiness, confusion, and abdominal pain—symptoms often attributed to other causes. Within the next 2 to 4 days, symptoms of hepatotoxicity develop (jaundice and a rise in the AST and ALT levels and prothrombin time).

If acetaminophen toxicity is suspected, consult the manufacturer, a university drug information center, or a poison-control center for the most current recommendations for therapy.
Drug interactions
    BARBITURATES, CARBAMAZEPINE, PHENYTOIN, RIFAMPIN, SULFINPYRAZONE. If acetaminophen is taken in large doses or long term, these agents may enhance hepatotoxicity.
    ALCOHOL. Chronic, excessive ingestion may increase the potential for hepatotoxicity of larger therapeutic doses or overdoses of acetaminophen.

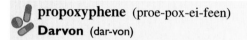

propoxyphene (proe-pox-ei-feen)
Darvon (dar-von)

Actions

Propoxyphene is an effective, well-tolerated, synthetic opiate agonist analgesic structurally related to methadone. It is one third to one half as potent as codeine. It is similar to aspirin in potency and duration of analgesic effect.

Uses

Propoxyphene is used for the relief of mild to moderate pain associated with muscular spasms, premenstrual cramps, bursitis, minor surgery and trauma, headache, and labor and delivery. Greater pain relief may be attained when used in combination with aspirin or acetaminophen.

Therapeutic Outcomes

The primary therapeutic outcome expected from propoxyphene is reduced pain.

Nursing Process

Premedication Assessment

1. Perform baseline neurologic assessment, for example, orientation to date, time, and place, mental alertness, and balance.
2. Take vital signs—temperature, blood pressure, pulse, and respirations.
3. Monitor urine pattern and amount.
4. Monitor for GI symptoms before and during therapy; monitor stools for consistency and number.
5. When used as analgesic, perform pain assessment before administration of propoxyphene and at appropriate intervals during therapy. Report poor pain control promptly and obtain modification in orders.

Planning

Availability. PO—65 mg capsules, 50 and 100 mg tablets, and 10 mg/ml suspension. (The 65 mg capsules and the 100 mg tablets are equal in analgesic potency.) Propoxyphene is also available in combination: Darvocet (propoxyphene, acetaminophen), Darvon Compound (propoxyphene, aspirin, caffeine).

Implementation

Dosage and administration. Adult: PO—65 mg capsules or 100 mg tablets every 4 hours as needed. Do not exceed 390 mg (capsules) or 600 mg (tablets) daily. If gastric irritation occurs, administer medication with food or milk.

Antidotes. Naloxone, naltrexone. Symptoms of acute overdose are coma, respiratory depression, pulmonary edema, and seizures. Symptoms of propoxyphene overdose may be complicated by salicylism, which may also develop as a result of an overdose of combination products containing both propoxyphene and aspirin.

Evaluation

Side effects to expect

GASTRIC IRRITATION. If gastric irritation occurs, administer medication with food or milk. If symptoms persist or increase in severity, report for physician evaluation.

SEDATION. This side effect is usually mild and tends to resolve with continued therapy.

DIZZINESS. Provide for patient safety during episodes of dizziness.

Side effects to report

EXCESSIVE USE OR ABUSE. Habitual use of propoxyphene may result in physical dependence. Discuss the case with the physician and make plans to cooperatively approach gradual withdrawal of the medications being abused. Assist the patient in recognizing the abuse problem. Identify underlying needs and plan for more appropriate management of those needs. Provide for emotional support of the individual; display an accepting attitude—be kind but firm.

SKIN RASHES. Report for further evaluation.

Drug interactions

ORPHENADRINE. Combined use with propoxyphene is not recommended. Cases of mental confusion, anxiety, and tremors have been reported.

CARBAMAZEPINE. Propoxyphene inhibits the metabolism of carbamazepine. Monitor patients for signs of carbamazepine toxicity: dizziness, nausea, drowsiness, headache. Carbamazepine dosages usually need to be reduced.

CHAPTER REVIEW

Pain management has made significant progress over the past 15 years, primarily because of better understanding of the pain experience. However, there is still a great deal to do in educating patients, family, and some health care practitioners about appropriate pain management. Nurses can play an important role in providing counseling and guidance to these groups in understanding pain and how to maintain an appropriate balance between daily activities and timing of analgesics to optimize quality of life.

MATH REVIEW

1. Ordered: aspirin 650 mg PO QID.
   On hand: aspirin 325 mg tablets.
   Give _____ tablets for each dose.

2. The pediatrician orders a 75 mg PO dose of ibuprofen suspension for a child. On hand is 100 mg per 5 ml. Give _____ ml.

3. Morphine, 15 mg IV q6h, has been ordered. Concentrations of 3, 4, 5, 8, 10, and 15 mg per ml are available. Which concentration would you use, and what volume should be injected?

4. Dr. Sandmann wrote orders to start Mrs. Phillips on codeine 30 mg QID after her wisdom tooth extraction. What is your interpretation of the order, and how will you administer it to Mrs. Phillips?

CRITICAL THINKING QUESTIONS

1. Mr. Cantazoni, a terminal cancer patient, returns to the unit with a morphine PCA. His daughter comes to you alarmed that her father may "overuse" the morphine and become addicted. How would you, as the nurse, respond to her? (Support your answer with rationale.)

2. What is the difference between an order for morphine sulfate immediate release (MSIR) and an order for MS Contin?

3. Mrs. Tantillian, age 86, is taking enteric-coated aspirin for arthritis. She reports to the nurse that she thinks she saw a "whole tablet" in her stools. What follow-up would you do? She has been on continuous aspirin therapy for two years. Explain appropriate assessments that must be made.

4. The head nurse sends the student nurse to evaluate Mandi Sue's postoperative pain. After entering the patient's room, the student observes Mandi Sue conversing and joking with her friends. The student decides not to further investigate the question of postoperative pain. Evaluate the correctness of the student's decision, and give underlying rationale for the views expressed.

Unit Four
DRUGS AFFECTING THE CARDIOVASCULAR SYSTEM

Drugs Used to Treat Hyperlipidemias

Objectives

1. Identify the four major types of lipoproteins.
2. Describe the primary treatment modalities for lipid disorders.
3. State specific oral administration instructions needed with antilipemic agents.
4. Analyze Table 19-1 to identify the specific agents used to treat type II and type IV forms of hyperlipidemia.

Key Words

atherosclerosis   lipoproteins
hyperlipidemia   chylomicrons
triglycerides

ATHEROSCLEROSIS

Coronary heart disease (CHD) is a major cause of premature death in the United States and in most other industrialized nations. Major treatable causes of CHD are hypertension, cigarette smoking, and atherosclerosis. **Atherosclerosis** is characterized by the accumulation of fatty deposits on the inner walls of arteries and arterioles throughout the body that reduces the blood supply to vital organs resulting in stroke, angina pectoris, myocardial infarction, and peripheral vascular disease. A primary cause of atherosclerosis is the abnormal elevation of cholesterol and triglycerides in the blood in a disease known as **hyperlipidemia**. Hyperlipidemia can be caused by genetic abnormalities, secondary causes (for example, lifestyle, drugs, or underlying diseases), or both. A diet high in saturated fats, cholesterol, carbohydrates, total calories, and alcohol and a sedentary lifestyle contribute significantly to hyperlipidemia.

Cholesterol is a naturally occurring substance that is essential for synthesizing body steroids used by the endocrine system, for synthesizing bile acids needed for food absorption, and for cell wall synthesis. The body is able to manufacture enough cholesterol to meet metabolic needs. However, the body also converts excess dietary carbohydrates into **triglycerides** (a precursor of cholesterol) and dietary fat into cholesterol. Once absorbed from the gastrointestinal tract, the fats (lipids), triglycerides, and cholesterol are bound to circulating proteins called **lipoproteins** for transport through the body. Lipoproteins are subdivided into five categories based on composition: chylomicrons, very-low-density lipoproteins (VLDL), intermediate-density lipoproteins (IDL), low-density lipoproteins (LDL), and high-density lipoproteins (HDL). The five types differ in concentration of triglycerides, cholesterol, and proteins. **Chylomicrons** consist of about 90% triglycerides and 5% cholesterol; VLDL represents about 10% to 15% of total serum cholesterol, and HDLs contain about 20% to 30% cholesterol and 1% to 7% triglycerides. The purpose of HDLs appears to be to transport cholesterol from peripheral cells to the liver for metabolism. High-density lipoproteins are sometimes referred to as "good" lipoproteins because high levels indicate that cholesterol is being removed from vascular tissue where it may participate in the development of CHD. Low levels of HDL are considered a positive risk factor in the development of CHD; high levels of HDL are a negative factor in CHD. Low-density lipoprotein accounts for 60% to 70% of total serum cholesterol and is the major contributor to atherosclerosis. The probability that atherosclerosis will develop is related directly to the concentration of LDL-cholesterol (LDL-C) in the blood circulation. Consequently, patient assessment and cholesterol-lowering treatment regimens are based on the LDL-C and HDL-C levels.

Treatment of Hyperlipidemias

The lipid disorders are classified into six types (Table 19-1). The most common hyperlipidemias are types II and IV. The National Cholesterol Education Program (NCEP) recommends that treatment regimens be based on whether CHD is present, the level of total cholesterol, level of HDL-C, and

the success of appropriate diet intervention. The primary treatment for hyperlipidemia is weight reduction, exercise, and a diet low in cholesterol and fat. Studies now show that with reduction in elevated cholesterol or triglycerides the frequency of heart attacks and strokes is substantially reduced. The American Heart Association and the NCEP recommend that total fat intake be reduced to less than 30% of calories, with a reduced cholesterol and saturated fat intake and increased polyunsaturated and monosaturated fats. Weight reduction can substantially reduce LDL-C while raising HDL levels. Regular exercise can also raise HDL levels, promote weight loss, lower blood pressure, reduce the risk of diabetes mellitus, and improve coronary blood flow. If a good trial of change in diet and exercise does not produce an acceptable decrease in blood lipid levels, an antilipemic agent may be added to the patient's regimen.

Table 19-1

Classification of Hyperlipidemias

Type	Generic Name	Elevated Lipoproteins Patterns	Elevated Cholesterol	Elevated Triglycerides	Incidence	Treatment Diet	Treatment Drugs
I	Exogenous hyperlipemia	Chylomicrons		↑	Rare	Very low fat: 25 to 35 g a day; high carbohydrate	None
IIa	Familial hypercholesterolemia	LDL (beta lipoproteins)	↑		Common	Low cholesterol (300 mg a day); low saturated fat; high unsaturated fat	Cholestyramine, colestipol, statin, nicotinic acid
IIb	Combined hyperlipoproteinemia	LDL + VLDL	↑	↑	Common	Low cholesterol; high unsaturated fat. Reduce obesity	Gemfibrozil, nicotinic acid, cholestyramine, statin
III	Broad-beta hyperlipidemia (familial dysbetalipoproteinemia)	IDL (broad-beta lipoproteins)	↑	↑	Rare	See II-b	Gemfibrozil, nicotinic acid
IV	Endogenous hyperlipemia	VLDL (prebeta lipoproteins)		↑	Common	Low carbohydrate: high unsaturated fat; low cholesterol and alcohol. Reduce obesity	Gemfibrozil, nicotinic acid, clofibrate
V	Mixed hyperlipemia	VLDL + chylomicrons		↑	Rare	Low fat and carbohydrate; high protein. Low alcohol	Gemfibrozil, nicotinic acid

IDL, Intermediate-density lipoprotein; *LDL,* low-density lipoprotein; *VLDL,* very low-density lipoprotein.
Modified from Hahn AB et al: *Mosby's pharmacology in nursing,* ed 16, St. Louis, 1986, Mosby.

Drug Therapy for Hyperlipidemias

Actions

Antilipemic agents may be used to treat hyperlipidemias only if diet, exercise, and weight reduction are not successful in adequately lowering LDL-C levels. (See individual monographs for mechanisms of action of antilipemic agents.)

Uses

The NCEP recognizes bile acid resins (cholestyramine, colestipol), niacin, and the HMG CoA reductase inhibitors (statins) (fluvastatin, lovastatin, pravastatin, simvistatin) as the primary drugs for lowering serum cholesterol levels. The fibric acids (clofibrate, gemfibrozil) are effective triglyceride-lowering agents but are not first-line drugs to treat hyperlipidemias because they do not usually produce substantial reductions in LDL-C.

Pharmacologic antilipemic therapy is often started with the bile acid resins because of their safety record and success in lowering cholesterol levels. Niacin is effective in lowering total cholesterol and triglyceride levels and raising HDL cholesterol levels. The statins are highly effective in lowering LDL-C and appear to be relatively safe. However, long-term safety has not yet been proved.

After starting drug therapy, the LDL-C level should be measured at 4 to 6 weeks and again at 3 months. If the response to initial drug therapy is inadequate, the patient should be switched to another drug or to a combination of two drugs. The combination of a bile acid resin with either niacin or a statin has the potential of lowering LDL-C levels by 40% to 50%. In rare cases of particularly high cholesterol levels, triple therapy with a bile acid–binding resin, niacin, and a statin may be required. Drug therapy is likely to continue for many years or a lifetime.

Nursing Process for Hyperlipidemia Therapy

Assessment

History of risk factors. Ask age, note gender and race, and take family history of incidence of elevated cholesterol and lipids.

Hypertension. Take blood pressure in supine and lying positions daily. Ask about medications that have been prescribed. Are the medications being taken regularly? If not, why not?

Smoking. Obtain a history of the number of cigarettes or cigars smoked daily. How long has the person smoked? Has the patient ever tried to stop smoking? Ask what effect smoking has on the vascular system. How does the individual feel about modifying the smoking habit?

Dietary habits. • Obtain a dietary history. Ask specific questions to obtain data relating to foods eaten that are high in fat, cholesterol, refined carbohydrates, and sodium. Using a calorie counter, ask the person to estimate the number of calories eaten per day. How much meat, fish, and poultry is eaten daily (size and number of servings)? Estimate the percent of total daily calories provided by fat. • Discuss food preparation— for example, baked, broiled, and fried foods. How many servings of fruits and vegetables are eaten daily? What types of oils or fats are used in food preparation? See a nutrition text for further dietary history questions. • What is the frequency and volume of alcoholic beverages consumed?

Glucose intolerance. Ask specific questions regarding whether the individual now has or ever had an elevated serum glucose (blood sugar). If yes, what dietary modifications have been made? How successful are they? What medications are being taken for the elevated serum glucose (for example, oral hypoglycemic agents or insulin)?

Elevated serum lipids. Find out whether the patient is aware of having elevated lipids, triglycerides, or cholesterol. If elevated, what measures has the patient tried for reduction and how much impact have the interventions had on the blood levels at subsequent examinations? Review laboratory data available (for example, LDL, VLDL).

Obesity. Weigh the patient. Ask about any recent weight gain or loss and whether it was intentional or unintentional.

Psychomotor functions. • Type of lifestyle: Ask the patient to describe the exercise level in terms of amount (for example, walking 3 miles), intensity (for example, walking 3 mph), and frequency (for example, walking every other day). Is the patient's job physically demanding or of a sedentary nature? • Psychologic stress: How much stress does the individual estimate having in life? How does the patient cope with stressful situations at home and in the work setting?

Nursing Diagnosis

• Tissue perfusion, alteration in (indication)
• Health maintenance, impaired (indication)
• Knowledge deficit (side effects)

Planning

History of risk factors. • Review the modifiable risk factors and plan interventions and health teaching needed for appropriate alterations in lifestyle. • Review ordered medications to be used concurrently with lifestyle modifications for health teaching needed regarding their use. • Order baseline laboratory studies (for example, lipid profile studies, liver function tests, clotting time).

Medication administration. Plan drug administration in accordance with recommendations in individual drug monographs to avoid possible interference with the absorption of other drugs ordered.

Implementation

Nursing interventions must be individualized and based on patient assessment data.

Patient Education and Health Promotion

Nutrition. • Patients who take bile acid–sequestering resins may require supplemental vitamins. (The fat-soluble [vitamins D, E, A, and K] may become deficient with long-term resin therapy.) • Encourage intake of high-bulk foods (for example, whole grains, raw fruits, and raw vegetables) and intake of 8 to 10 glasses of water per day to minimize constipating effects of resins. • Arrange a dietary consultation with the nutritionist to address dietary modifications needed, (for example, low fat, low cholesterol). Nurses should enhance and reinforce this teaching on a continuum.

Vitamin K deficiency. If the patient is receiving a prescription for a bile acid resin, teach the patient the signs and symptoms of vitamin K deficiency—bleeding gums, bruising, dark tarry stools, "coffee-ground" emesis. This interaction is rare, but if symptoms occur they should be reported immediately to the physician.

Follow-up care. Stress the need for long-term regular assessment of the required serum levels (for example, lipid profile values, liver studies, bleeding times) to track progress and to detect possible side effects from the medications. To do so, blood studies and regular visits to the physician will be necessary.

Relating to medication regimen. Examine the individual drug monographs for details on mixing and scheduling medication administration and techniques to improve compliance of these medications.

Fostering Health Maintenance. • Throughout the course of treatment, discuss medication information and how it will benefit the patient. • Drug therapy is one component in the management of hyperlipemia. Lifestyle changes are equally important to drug therapy; therefore the need to modify dietary habits and to control obesity, glucose levels, serum cholesterol, lipids, and hypertension must be greatly emphasized. Cessation of smoking is strongly recommended. • Provide the patient and significant others with important information contained in the specific drug monograph for the drugs prescribed. Additional health teaching and nursing interventions for side effects to expect and report are described in the drug monographs that follow. • Seek cooperation and understanding of the following points so that medication compliance is increased: name of medication, dosage, route and times of administration, side effects to expect, and side effects to report.

Written record. Enlist the patient's aid in developing and maintaining a written record of monitoring parameters such as daily serum glucose levels, blood pressure, and weight. An individualized nutritional diary should also be kept while instituting and learning the diet modifications (for example, reduction in fats, refined carbohydrates, low-cholesterol foods). Instruct the patient to bring the written record to follow-up visits.

Drug Class: Bile Acid–Binding Resins

Actions

Cholestyramine and colestipol are resins that bind bile acids in the intestine. After oral administration, the resin forms a non-absorbable complex with bile acids, preventing enterohepatic recirculation of the bile acids. Because of the removal of bile acids, liver cells compensate by increasing metabolism of cholesterol to produce more bile acids, resulting in a net reduction in total cholesterol levels. Bile acid–binding resins can reduce LDL-C by 15% to 30% and increase HDL up to 5%. Some patients also have a secondary increase in triglyceride levels.

Uses

Cholestyramine and colestipol are used in conjunction with dietary therapy to decrease elevated cholesterol concentrations in type II hyperlipidemia and to reduce the risks of atherosclerosis leading to coronary heart disease.

Other uses of the bile acid–binding resins include treatment of pruritus secondary to partial biliary stasis, treatment of diarrhea secondary to excess fecal bile acids or pseudomembranous colitis, and treatment of digitalis glycoside toxicity.

Therapeutic Outcomes

The primary therapeutic outcome expected from bile acid–binding resin therapy is reduction of LDL and total cholesterol levels.

Nursing Process

Premedication Assessment

1. Serum triglyceride and cholesterol levels should be determined before initiation of therapy and periodically thereafter.
2. Obtain data relating to any gastrointestinal alterations before initiation of therapy (for example, abdominal pain, nausea, flatus).

Planning

Availability. Cholestyramine: 1 g tablets; 4 g powder packets. Colestipol: 1 g tablets; granules in 5 g packets, 300 and 500 g containers.

Implementation

Dosage and administration. Cholestyramine: PO—4 g 1 to 6 times daily. Initial dose is 4 g daily. Maintenance dose is 8 to 16 g per day. Maximum daily dose is 24 g. Colestipol: PO—granules: 5 to 30 g of granules per day in divided doses; initial dose is 5 g 1 or 2 times daily. Tablets: 2 to 16 g tablets per day; initial dose 2 g 1 or 2 times daily.

• The powder resin must be mixed with 2 to 6 ounces of water, juice, soup, applesauce, or crushed pineapple and should be allowed to stand for a few minutes to allow absorption and dispersion. Do not attempt to swallow the dry powder. Follow administration with an additional glass of water.

• Recommended time of administration is with meals but may be modified to avoid interference with absorption of other medications.

• Tablets should be swallowed whole; do not crush, chew, or cut. Tablets should be taken with liquids.

• Taste may become a reason for noncompliance. Place the powder in a favorite beverage, or use the tablets to minimize objectionable taste.

Evaluation

Side effects to expect

CONSTIPATION, BLOATING, FULLNESS, NAUSEA, AND FLATULENCE. These adverse effects can be minimized by starting with low dosage, mixing the resin with noncarbonated, pulpy juices or sauces, and swallowing without gulping air. Maintain adequate fiber in the diet.

Drug interactions

DIGITOXIN, WARFARIN, THYROXINE, THIAZIDE DIURETICS, PHENOBARBITAL, NONSTEROIDAL ANTIINFLAMMATORY DRUGS, TETRACYCLINE, AMIODARONE, BETA-BLOCKERS. The resins may bind these medicines, which reduces absorption. The interaction can usually be minimized by administering these medicines 1 hour before or 4 hours after administration of resins.

FAT-SOLUBLE VITAMINS (D, E, A, K) AND FOLIC ACID. High doses of resins may reduce absorption of these agents, but this interaction is not usually significant in normally nourished patients.

Drug Class: Niacin

Actions

Niacin, also known as nicotinic acid, is a water-soluble B vitamin. The mechanisms of action as an antilipemic agent are not completely known but are not related to its effects as a vitamin. Niacin inhibits VLDL synthesis by liver cells, which causes a decrease in LDL and triglyceride production. Triglyceride levels are reduced by 30% to 60%, and total cholesterol and LDL-C can be reduced by 15% to 25%. Niacin may also reduce the metabolism of HDL, causing a 25% to 35% increase in HDL levels.

Uses

Niacin is used in conjunction with dietary therapy to decrease elevated cholesterol concentrations in types II, III, IV, and V hyperlipidemias and to reduce the risks of atherosclerosis leading to coronary heart disease. It can be used in combination with bile acid–binding resins or the statins for greater combined lowering of cholesterol levels. Another benefit to niacin therapy is its significantly lower cost in comparison with the other antilipemic agents.

Therapeutic Outcomes

The primary therapeutic outcomes expected from niacin are reduction of LDL and total cholesterol levels, reduction in triglyceride levels, and an increase in HDL levels.

Nursing Process

Premedication Assessment

1. Serum triglyceride and cholesterol levels should be determined before initiation of therapy and periodically thereafter.
2. Liver function tests, aspartate transferase (AST), alanine aminotransferase (ALT), alkaline phosphatase (ALP), and bilirubin should be determined before initiation of therapy and every 6 to 8 weeks during the first year of therapy.
3. Baseline uric acid and blood glucose levels should be determined before initiation of therapy. Niacin therapy may induce hyperuricemia, gout, and hyperglycemia in susceptible patients.
4. Baseline blood pressure and heart rate should be determined before initiation of therapy.
5. Obtain data relating to any gastrointestinal alterations before initiation of therapy (for example, abdominal pain, nausea, flatus).

Planning

Availability. PO—50, 100, 500 mg tablets; 100 mg capsules; 125, 250, 400, 500 mg timed-release capsules; 500, 750, 1000 mg timed-release tablets; 50 mg per 5 ml elixir.

Implementation

Dosage and administration. PO—initially, 100 g 3 times daily with meals. Increase by 300 mg weekly until the therapeutic level is achieved or the maximum level is attained. Usual daily dosages range from 3 to 6 g daily, but some patients require 9 g daily. Hepatotoxicity: There appears to be a higher incidence of hepatotoxicity associated with the extended-release products. Some clinicians recommend limiting the extended-release products to 1500 mg daily to reduce the risk of hepatotoxicity.

Evaluation

Side effects to expect

FLUSHING, ITCHING, RASH, TINGLING, HEADACHE. These symptoms are common at the beginning of therapy, but tolerance develops quickly. Administer niacin with food. Patients can also reduce symptoms by taking aspirin (325 mg) 30 minutes before each dose of niacin.

NAUSEA, GAS, ABDOMINAL DISCOMFORT AND PAIN. Gastrointestinal upset can be minimized by starting with low dosages and administering all dosages with food.

DIZZINESS, FAINTNESS, HYPOTENSION. Niacin is a vasodilator and may cause hypotension, especially if a patient is receiving other antihypertensive agents. Anticipate the development of hypotension and take measures to prevent an occurrence. Teach the patient to rise slowly from a supine or sitting position and to sit or lie down if feeling faint. Monitor blood pressures in both the supine and sitting positions.

Side effects to report

FATIGUE, ANOREXIA, NAUSEA, MALAISE, JAUNDICE. These are the early symptoms associated with hepatotoxicity. Report to the physician for further evaluation.

MYOPATHY. Symptoms of muscle aches, soreness, and weakness may be early signs of myopathy. Serum creatine phosphokinase levels more than 10 times the upper limit of normal confirm the diagnosis. The myopathy is most common with lovastatin and niacin (at <1%).

Drug interactions

LOVASTATIN. The potential of developing lovastatin-induced myopathy is increased when niacin is added to the treatment regimen.

Drug Class: HMG-CoA Reductase Inhibitors

Actions

The hydroxymethylglutaryl coenzyme A (HMG-CoA) reductase enzyme inhibitors (fluvastatin, lovastatin, pravastatin, simvastatin) are the newest antilipemic agents available. They are also known as the *statins*. The statins competitively inhibit the enzyme responsible for converting HMG-CoA to mevalonate in the biosynthetic pathway to cholesterol in the liver. The reduction in liver cholesterol increases the removal of LDL from the circulating blood. Levels of LDL-C may be reduced by 25% to 30%. The statins also cause a reduction in VLDL and triglyceride levels and mild increases in HDL. These agents are more effective if administered at night because of peak production of cholesterol at this time.

Uses

The statins are used in conjunction with dietary therapy to decrease elevated cholesterol concentrations in type II hyperlipidemia and to reduce the risks of atherosclerosis leading to coronary heart disease. The four statins listed are similar in effectiveness at recommended starting doses and times.

Therapeutic Outcomes

The primary therapeutic outcome expected from HMG-CoA reductase inhibitors is reduction of LDL and total cholesterol levels.

Nursing Process

Premedication Assessment

1. Serum triglyceride and cholesterol levels should be determined before initiation of therapy and periodically thereafter.
2. Liver function tests should be obtained before initiation of therapy, every 4 to 6 weeks during the first 3 months of therapy, every 6 to 12 months during the next 12 months or after dosage elevation, and every 6 months thereafter.
3. Obtain data relating to any gastrointestinal alterations before initiation of therapy (for example, abdominal pain, nausea, flatus).
4. Confirm that the patient is not pregnant before initiating a statin. Inform the patient to notify the physician should she be contemplating conception or should she become pregnant while receiving statin therapy.

Planning

Availability. See Table 19-2.

Implementation

Dosage and administration. See Table 19-2. Lovastatin should be administered with food to enhance absorption. The other statins may be administered without food.

Evaluation

Side effects to expect

HEADACHES, NAUSEA, ABDOMINAL BLOATING, GAS. These symptoms are usually mild and disappear with continued therapy.

Side effects to report

LIVER DYSFUNCTION. Liver function tests should be monitored as described previously. If the transaminases (AST, ALT) rise to 3 times the upper limit of normal and are persistent, the drug should be discontinued.

MYOPATHY. Symptoms of muscle aches, soreness, and weakness may be early signs of myopathy. Serum creatine phosphokinase levels more than 10 times the upper limit of normal confirm the diagnosis. Myopathy is most common with lovastatin (at <1%).

Drug interactions

CYCLOSPORINE, GEMFIBROZIL, NIACIN, ERYTHROMYCIN. The incidence of myopathy is increased when lovastatin is prescribed in conjunction with these medicines.

WARFARIN. When lovastatin and warfarin are prescribed together, the prothrombin time may be prolonged. Observe for possible overanticoagulation and bleeding.

Drug Class: Fibric Acids

Actions

The mechanism of action of the fibric acids (clofibrate, gemfibrozil) is unknown; however, they do lower triglyceride levels by 20% to 50%, and in patients with hypertriglyceridemia they raise HDL levels by 10% to 15%. They also reduce LDL-C by 10% to 15% in patients with elevated cholesterol. However, in patients with concurrent hypertriglyceridemia, gemfibrozil may have no effect on or may slightly increase LDL-C levels.

Uses

Clofibrate is used in conjunction with dietary therapy to decrease elevated triglyceride concentrations in type III hyperlipidemia. It may also be used in patients with types IV or V hyperlipidemia who are at risk of abdominal pain and pancreatitis. Gemfibrozil is used in conjunction with dietary therapy to decrease elevated triglyceride levels in types IV and V hyperlipidemia in patients who are at risk of pancreatitis. Gemfibrozil can also be used in patients with type IIb hyperlipidemia who have low HDL levels and elevated LDL-C and triglycerides and who have not responded to weight loss, dietary therapy, and other pharmacologic therapy such as resins, statins, or niacin.

Therapeutic Outcomes

The primary therapeutic outcome expected from fibric acid therapy is a 30% to 60% reduction in triglyceride levels and a 10% to 30% increase in HDL levels.

Nursing Process

Premedication Assessment

1. Serum triglyceride and cholesterol levels should be determined before initiation of therapy and periodically thereafter.

Table 19-2

HMG-CoA Reductase Inhibitors (Statins)

GENERIC NAME	BRAND NAME	AVAILABILITY	DAILY DOSE	MAXIMUM DAILY DOSE
Fluvastatin	Lescol	Capsules: 20, 40 mg	20 mg at bedtime	Up to 40 mg at bedtime
Lovastatin	Mevacor	Tablets: 10, 20, 40 mg	20-40 mg with evening meal	80 mg daily
Pravastatin	Pravachol	Tablets: 10, 20, 40 mg	10-20 mg at bedtime	Up to 40 mg at bedtime
Simvastatin	Zocor	Tablets: 5, 10, 20, 40 mg	5-20 mg at bedtime	Up to 40 mg at bedtime

2. Liver function tests should be obtained before initiation of therapy, and every 6 months thereafter.
3. Baseline blood glucose levels should be determined before gemfibrozil therapy. Gemfibrozil may cause moderate hyperglycemia.
4. Obtain data relating to any gastrointestinal alterations before initiation of therapy (for example, abdominal pain, nausea, flatus).

Planning

Availability. Clofibrate (Atromid-S): 500 mg capsules. Gemfibrozil (Lopid): 300 mg capsules; 600 mg tablets.

Implementation

Dosage and administration. Clofibrate: 500 mg 3 to 4 times daily. Gemfibrozil: 1200 mg per day in 2 divided doses, 30 minutes before the morning and evening meals.

Evaluation

Side effects to expect

NAUSEA, DIARRHEA, FLATULENCE, BLOATING, ABDOMINAL DISTRESS. These are relatively common adverse effects. Starting with a lower dosage taken between meals can help minimize these effects. If symptoms persist, notify the physician. Potentially more serious complications may be developing.

Side effects to report

FATIGUE, ANOREXIA, NAUSEA, MALAISE, JAUNDICE. These are the early symptoms associated with gall bladder disease and hepatotoxicity. Report to the physician for further evaluation.

MYOPATHY. Symptoms of muscle aches, soreness, and weakness may be early signs of myopathy. Serum creatine phosphokinase levels more than 10 times the upper limit of normal confirm the diagnosis. Myopathy is most common with lovastatin and gemfibrozil.

Drug interactions

WARFARIN. The fibric acids may enhance the pharmacologic effect of warfarin. Reduce the dosage of warfarin using the prothrombin time as an indicator to prevent bleeding.

INSULIN AND SULFONYLUREAS. Clofibrate may increase the pharmacologic effect of these agents. Monitor for signs of hypoglycemia and reduce the dose of the insulin or sulfonylurea as needed.

PROBENECID. Probenecid may increase the toxic effects of clofibrate by impairing its metabolism and excretion. A clofibrate dosage reduction may be necessary.

CHAPTER REVIEW

Coronary heart disease is a major cause of premature death in the United States. Major treatable causes of CHD are hypertension, cigarette smoking, and atherosclerosis. A primary cause of atherosclerosis is the abnormal elevation of cholesterol and triglycerides in the blood in a disease known as *hyperlipidemia*. A diet high in saturated fats, cholesterol, carbohydrates, total calories, and alcohol and a sedentary lifestyle are the most common and treatable causes of hyperlipidemia.

The most cost-effective and successful forms of treatment are smoking cessation, weight reduction, exercise, and dietary modification. If a good trial of change in diet and exercise does not produce an acceptable decrease in blood lipid levels, an antilipemic agent may be added to the patient's regimen. Patients should be fully informed of the significance of hyperlipidemias, the potential complications of not modifying lifestyles, and drug therapy. Drug therapy is likely to continue for many years or a lifetime.

MATH REVIEW

1. Ordered: Nicotinic acid (Niacin) 1.5 g, PO, in 3 divided doses, daily.
   On hand: Nicotinic acid (Niacin) 500 mg tablets.
   Give _____ tablets per dose.
   A total of _____ mg daily.
2. Ordered: Lovastatin (Mevacor) 80 mg, PO, daily.
   On hand: Lovastatin (Mevacor) 20 mg tablets.
   Give _____ tablets.

CRITICAL THINKING QUESTIONS

1. Why is it essential to monitor a patient taking a bile-sequestering medication for a fat-soluble vitamin deficiency?
2. Why would bleeding problems be a potential side effect of bile-sequestering hypolipemic drugs?
3. What effects do HMG-CoA reductase inhibitors have on LDL, HDL, VLDL cholesterol, and plasma triglycerides?

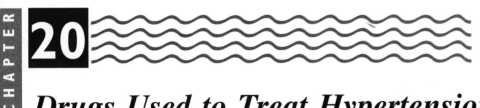

Drugs Used to Treat Hypertension

CHAPTER CONTENT

Objectives

1. Summarize nursing assessments and interventions used during the treatment of hypertension.

2. State lifestyle modifications that should be implemented when a diagnosis of hypertension is made.

3. Identify nine types of drugs used to treat hypertension.

4. Review Figure 20-1 to identify options and progression of treatment for hypertension.

5. Identify specific factors the hypertensive patient can use to assist in the management of the disease.

6. Develop objectives for patient education for patients with hypertension.

7. Summarize the mechanism of action of each drug class used to treat hypertension.

Key Words

arterial blood pressure
systolic blood pressure
diastolic blood pressure
pulse pressure
mean arterial pressure
cardiac output
hypertension
primary hypertension
secondary hypertension

HYPERTENSION

A primary function of the heart is to circulate blood to the organs and tissues of the body. When the heart contracts (systole), blood is pumped out of the pulmonary artery to the lungs and out of the aorta to the tissues. The pressure with which the blood is pushed from the heart is referred to as the **arterial blood pressure,** or **systolic blood pressure.** When the heart muscle relaxes (diastole) between contractions the blood pressure drops to a lower level, the **diastolic blood pressure.** When recorded in the patient's chart, the systolic pressure is recorded first, followed by the diastolic pressure (for example, 120/80 mm Hg). The difference between the systolic and diastolic pressure is called the **pulse pressure,** which is an indicator of the tone of the arterial blood vessel walls. The **mean arterial pressure** (MAP) is the average pressure throughout each cycle of the heartbeat and is significant because it is the pressure that actually pushes the blood through the circulatory system to perfuse tissue. It is calculated by adding one third of the pulse pressure to the diastolic pressure or using the following equation:

$$MAP = \frac{Systolic\ pressure - Diastolic\ pressure}{3} + Diastolic\ pressure$$

Under normal conditions, the arterial blood pressure stays within narrow limits. It reaches its peak during high physical or emotional activity and is usually at its lowest level during sleep.

Arterial blood pressure (BP) can be defined as the product of **cardiac output** (CO) and peripheral vascular resistance (PVR):

$$BP = CO \times PVR$$

Cardiac output is the primary determinant of systolic pressure: peripheral vascular resistance determines the diastolic pressure. Cardiac output is determined by the stroke volume (the volume of blood ejected in a single contraction of the left ventricle), heart rate (controlled by the autonomic nervous system), and venous capacitance (capability of veins to return blood to the heart). Systolic blood pressure is thus increased by factors that increase heart rate or stroke volume. Venous capacitance affects the volume of blood (or preload) that is returned to the heart through the central venous circulation. Venous constriction decreases venous capacitance, increasing preload and systolic pressure, and venous dilatation increases venous capacitance and decreases preload and systolic pressure. Peripheral vascular resistance is regulated primarily by contraction and dilatation of arterioles. Arteriolar constriction increases peripheral vascular resistance and thus diastolic blood pressure. Other factors that affect vascular resistance include the elasticity of the blood vessel walls and the viscosity of the blood.

Hypertension is a disease characterized by an elevation of either the systolic blood pressure, the diastolic blood pressure, or both. Statistics in North America show that blood pressures above 140/90 mm Hg are associated with premature death, which results from accelerated vascular disease of the brain, heart, and kidneys.

The Fifth Report of the Joint National Committee on Detection, Evaluation, and Treatment of High Blood Pressure (JNC V) has classified blood pressure into stages that represent the degree of risk of nonfatal and fatal cardiovascular disease events and renal disease (Table 20-1).

The category of "high normal" has been added to the classification system because patients with BP readings in this range are at an increased risk of developing definite high blood pressure and experiencing cardiovascular events (stroke, myocardial infarction) compared with otherwise similar persons with lower blood pressure. The JNC V guidelines consider an elevation in both systolic and diastolic blood pressure readings when making a diagnosis of hypertension. The individual must have two or more readings on two or more separate occasions after initial screening to be classified as having hypertension. When readings, systolic and diastolic, fall into two different stages, the higher of the two stages is used to classify the degree of hypertension present.

Primary hypertension accounts for 90% of all clinical cases of high blood pressure. The etiology of primary hypertension is unknown. It is incurable at present, but it is controllable. It is estimated that as many as 50 million people in the United States have hypertension. The prevalence increases steadily with advancing age. In every age group, the incidence of hypertension is higher for black persons than for white persons of both sexes. Other factors associated with high blood pressure are family history of hypertension, obesity, spikes of high blood pressure in young adult years, cigarette smoking, hyperglycemia, hypercholesterolemia, preexisting cardiovascular disease (angina, heart failure), abnormal renal function, retinopathies, and a history of a previous stroke. **Secondary hypertension** occurs after the development of another disorder within the body such as renal disease, head trauma, coarctation of the aorta, or Cushings's syndrome.

Treatment

The goal of antihypertensive therapy is to prolong useful life by preventing cardiovascular complications. To accomplish this goal, the blood pressure must be reduced and maintained below 140/90 mm Hg, if possible. Treatment schedules should interfere as little as possible with the patient's lifestyle; however, nonpharmacologic therapy must include elimination of smoking, weight control, routine activity, restriction of alcohol intake, stress reduction, and sodium control. If this therapy is successful in controlling high blood pressure, drug therapy is not necessary. Even if lifestyle changes are not adequate to control hypertension, they may reduce the number and doses of antihypertensive medications needed to manage the condition.

Patient education is vitally important in treating hypertension. This education should be emphasized and reiterated frequently by the physician, pharmacist, and nurse.

Drug Therapy

Actions

Many drugs are used in the treatment of hypertension, but, in general, they can be subdivided into several classes of therapeutic agents. The JNC V classifies antihypertensive agents into primary and supplementary agents. The primary

Table 20-1

Recommendations for Follow-up Based on Initial Set of Blood Pressure Measurements for Adults		
INITIAL SCREENING BLOOD PRESSURE (MM HG*)		
SYSTOLIC	**DIASTOLIC**	**FOLLOW-UP RECOMMENDED†**
<130	<85	Recheck in 2 yr
130-139	85-89	Recheck in 1 yr‡
140-159	90-99	Confirm with 2 mo
160-179	100-109	Evaluate or refer to source of care within 1 mo
180-209	110-119	Evaluate or refer to source of care within 1 wk
≥210	≥120	Evaluate or refer to source of care immediately

*If the systolic and diastolic categories are different, follow recommendation for the shorter-time follow-up (for example, 160/85 mm Hg should be evaluated or referred to source of care within 1 month).
†The scheduling of follow-up should be modified by reliable information about past blood pressure measurements, other cardiovascular risk factors, or target-organ disease.
‡Consider providing advice about lifestyle modifications.

antihypertensive agents are diuretics, beta-adrenergic blockers, alpha-1-adrenergic blockers, angiotensin-converting enzyme inhibitors, and calcium antagonists. The supplementary antihypertensive agents are centrally acting alpha-2 agonists, peripherally acting adrenergic antagonists, and direct vasodilators. All of these agents can effectively lower blood pressure, acting either directly or indirectly by reducing the peripheral vascular resistance, thereby lowering blood pressure. See individual monographs for mechanisms of action of each class of antihypertensive agent.

Uses

A key to long-term success with antihypertensive therapy is to individualize therapy for a patient based on demographic characteristics (age, gender, and race), coexisting diseases and risk factors (for example, migraine headaches, arrhythmias, angina, diabetes mellitus), previous therapy (what has or has not worked in the past), concurrent drug therapy for other illnesses, and cost. As outlined in Figure 20-1, the JNC V recommends that if lifestyle modifications do not lower blood pressure adequately for patients with stage 1 or stage 2 hypertension, a diuretic or a beta-adrenergic blocking agent should be the initial treatment of choice. A low dose should be selected to protect the patient from adverse effects, although it may not immediately control the blood pressure. It must be recognized that it may take months to control hypertension adequately while avoiding adverse effects of therapy. If after 1 to 3 months the first drug is not effective, the dosage may be increased, another agent from another class may be substituted, or a second drug from another class may be added. The JNC V also recommends that if the first drug started was not a diuretic, a diuretic should be initiated as the second drug, if needed, because the majority of patients will respond to a two-drug regimen if it includes a diuretic. Therefore by appropriate selection of agents most patients do not require more than two drugs for successful antihypertensive therapy. After blood pressure is reduced to the goal level and maintenance doses of medicines are stabilized, it may be appropriate to change a patient's medication to a combination antihypertensive product to simplify the regimen and enhance compliance. See Table 20-2 for a list of the ingredients of common antihypertensive combination products.

Patients with stages 3 or 4 hypertension may require more aggressive therapy with a second or third agent added if control is not achieved by monotherapy in a relatively short time. Patients with an average diastolic blood pressure of greater than 120 mm Hg require immediate therapy and, if significant organ damage is present, may require hospitalization for initial control.

Patients who have modified their lifestyles with appropriate exercise, diet, weight reduction, and control of hypertension for at least 1 year may be candidates for "step-down" therapy. The dosage of antihypertensive medications may be gradually reduced in a slow, deliberate manner. Most patients will still require some therapy, but occasionally the medicine can be discontinued. Patients whose drugs have been discontinued should have regular follow-up examination because blood pressure often rises again to hypertensive levels, sometimes months or years later, especially if lifestyle modifications are not continued.

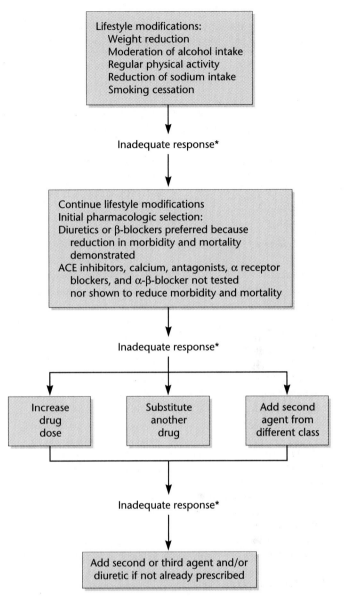

Figure 20-1 *Treatment algorithm. Asterisk indicates that response means the patient achieved goal blood pressure or the patient is making considerable progress toward this goal. ACE, Angiotensin-converting enzyme.* Joint National Committee on Detection, Evaluation and Treatment of High Blood Pressure: The fifth report of the National Committee on Detection, Evaluation and Treatment of High Blood Pressure (JNC V), *Arch Intern Med* 153: 154, 1993.

Nursing Process for Hypertensive Therapy

Assessment

History of risk factors. • Make note of patient's sex, age, and race. Persons who are older, male, and of the black race have higher incidences of hypertension. • Has the client been told previously about the elevated blood pressure readings? If so, under what circumstances were the blood pressure readings taken? • Is there is a family history of hypertension, coronary heart disease, stroke, diabetes mellitus, or hyperlipidemia?

Table 20-2

Ingredients of Common Antihypertensive Combination Products*

PRODUCT	DIURETIC (MG)	ANTIHYPERTENSIVE (MG)	OTHER (MG)
Aldoril-15	Hydrochlorothiazide (15)	Methyldopa (250)	
Apresazide 100/50	Hydrochlorothiazide (50)	Hydralazine (100)	
Capozide 25/25	Hydrochlorothiazide (25)	Captopril (25)	
Combipres 0.1	Chlorthalidone (15)	Clonidine (0.1)	
Combipres 0.2	Chlorthalidone (15)	Clonidine (0.2)	
Corzide 40/5	Bendroflumethiazide (5)	Nadolol (40)	
Diupres-250	Chlorothiazide (250)	Reserpine (0.125)	
Diutensen-R	Methyclothiazide (2.5)	Reserpine (0.1)	
Enduronyl	Methyclothiazide (5)	Deserpidine (0.25)	
Hydropres-25	Hydrochlorothiazide (25)	Reserpine (0.125)	
Hyzaar	Hydrochlorothiazide (12.5)	Losartan (50)	
Inderide LA 120/50	Hydrochlorothiazide (50)	Propranolol (120)	
Lopressor HCT 100/50	Hydrochlorothiazide (50)	Metoprolol (100)	
Minizide 1	Polythiazide (0.5)	Prazosin (1)	
Oreticyl 25	Hydrochlorothiazide (25)	Deserpidine (0.125)	
Regroton	Chlorthalidone (50)	Reserpine (0.25)	
Renese-R	Polythiazide (2)	Reserpine (0.25)	
Salutensin	Hydroflumethiazide (50)	Reserpine (0.125)	
Ser-Ap-Es	Hydrochlorothiazide (15)	Reserpine (0.1)	Hydralazine (25)
Tenoretic 50	Chlorthalidone (25)	Atenolol (50)	
Timolide 10-25	Hydrochlorothiazide (25)	Timolol (10)	
Vaseretic 10-25	Hydrochlorothiazide (25)	Enalapril (10)	
Zestoretic	Hydrochlorothiazide (25)	Lisinopril (20)	
Ziac	Hydrochlorothiazide (6.25)	Bisoprolol (5)	

*This is a representative listing. Other strengths of these products, as well as products not listed, are available.

Smoking. Obtain a history of the number of cigarettes or cigars smoked daily. How long has the person smoked? Has the person ever tried to stop smoking? Ask if the person knows what effect smoking has on the vascular system. How does the individual feel about modifying the smoking habit?

Dietary habits. • Obtain a dietary history. Ask specific questions to obtain data relating to the amount of salt used in cooking and at the table and foods eaten that are high in fat, cholesterol, refined carbohydrates, and sodium. Using a calorie counter, ask the person to estimate the number of calories eaten per day. How much meat, fish, and poultry is eaten daily (size and number of servings)? Estimate the percent of total daily calories provided by fats. • Discuss food preparation—for example, baked, broiled, or fried foods. How many servings of fruits and vegetables are eaten daily? What types of oils and fats are used in food preparation? See a nutrition text for further dietary history questions. • What is the frequency and volume of alcoholic beverages consumed?

Elevated serum lipids. Ask whether the patient is aware of having elevated lipids, triglycerides, or cholesterol. If elevated, what measures has the person tried for reduction and how much impact have the interventions had on the blood levels at subsequent examinations? Review laboratory data available.

Obesity. Weigh the patient. Ask about any recent weight gains or losses and whether intentional or unintentional.

Psychomotor functions. • Determine type of lifestyle. Ask the patient to describe exercise level in terms of amount (for example, walking 3 miles), intensity (for example, walking 3 mph) and frequency (walking every other day). Is the patient's job physically demanding or of a sedentary nature? • Determine psychologic stress. How much stress does the individual estimate having in life? How does the person cope with stressful situations at home and in the work setting? • Has the patient experienced any episodes of confusion, blurred vision, dizziness, or nosebleeds recently?

Medication history. • Has the patient ever taken or is the patient currently taking any medications for the treatment of high blood pressure? If blood pressure medications have been prescribed but are not being taken, why was the medicine discontinued? Were any side effects noticed while receiving the medications, and how did the patient manage them? • Obtain a listing of all medications being taken. Research these medications in the drug monographs to determine potential drug-drug interactions that may affect the individual's blood pressure or the effectiveness of the medicines prescribed. • If the patient is female, ask if she is now or has been taking oral contraceptives or is receiving estrogen replacement therapy.

Physical assessments. • *Blood pressure.* Obtain two or more blood pressure measurements separated by 2 minutes with the patient either supine or seated and after standing for at least 2 minutes. Verify the readings in the opposite arm. Be sure to use the correct technique for blood pressure measurement to ensure that the readings will be accurate (for example, correct-size cuff applied properly after ensuring that the patient has not just ingested caffeine). • *Height and weight.* Weigh and measure the patient. What has the person's weight been? Ask about any recent weight gains or losses and whether intentional or unintentional. • Bruits. Check neck, abdomen, and extremities for the prescence of bruits. • Peripheral pulses. Palpate and record femoral, popliteal, and pedal pulses bilaterally. • *Eyes.* As appropriate to the level of education, perform a funduscopic examination of interior eye, noting arteriovenous nicking, hemorrhages, exudates, or papilledema.

Nursing Diagnosis
- Knowledge deficit related to hypertension (indication)
- Noncompliance drug therapy (indication, side effects)
- Sexual dysfuntion (side effects)

Planning
History of risk factors. • Examine data to determine the individual's extent of understanding of hypertension and its control. • Analyze lifestyle elements of the history to determine health teaching needs of the individual and significant others.

Medication history. Plan patient education needed to implement or reinforce prescribed medication therapy.

Physical assessment. Schedule physical assessments at specific intervals as appropriate to the patient's status and clinical site policies (for example, vital signs taken every 4 or 8 hours).

Diagnostics. Review the chart and reports available used to build baseline information (for example, electrolytes, renal function studies).

Implementation
- Perform nursing assessments on a scheduled basis.
- Make referrals as indicated for stress management, smoking cessation, and dietary counseling.
- When initiating antihypertensive therapy in the hospitalized patient, protect from possible falls secondary to hypotension by assisting during ambulation and carefully assessing for faintness. Take blood pressure in supine, sitting, and standing positions to identify hypotensive responses.

Patient Education and Health Promotion
Smoking. Suggest that the patient stop smoking. Explain the increased risk of coronary artery disease if the habit is continued. It may be necessary to settle for a drastic decrease in smoking in some persons, although total abstinence should be the goal.

Nutritional status. Dietary counseling is essential in the treatment of hypertension. Control of obesity alone may be sufficient to alter the hypertensive condition. Most patients are placed on a reduced-sodium (2.3 g of sodium or less than 6 g of table salt per day), low-fat, and low-calorie diet. The goal of dietary therapy is a reduction of cholesterol, lipids, saturated fats, caffeine, and alcohol consumpton. Foods high in potassium and calcium are encouraged to decrease blood pressure.

Dietary planning should always involve the patient in menu planning so that personal preferences, availability of food products, and cost are discussed. Include the person who purchases as well as prepares the meals in the dietary counseling.

Show the patient various food labels and explain which words to watch for that would indicate a high sodium content (such as salt, sodium, sodium chloride, sodium bicarbonate, sodium aluminum sulfate). Suggest the use of a variety of spices as substitutes for sodium when cooking. Explain foods that should be avoided in large quantities (such as bacon, smoked meats, crabmeat, tuna, crackers, processed cheeses, ham).

Teach the individual to take and record weight in the same clothing, at the same time daily, using the same scale. Generally, a weight gain or loss of over 2 pounds is reported to the physician; however, specific parameters may vary and should be discussed during initiation of therapy.

Stress management. • Identify stress-producing situations in the patient's life and seek means to significantly reduce these factors. In some cases, referral for training in stress management, relaxation techniques, meditation, or biofeedback may be necessary. If stress is produced in the work setting, it may be appropriate to involve the industrial nurse. • Stress within the family is often significant and may require professional counseling for the family and patient.

Exercise and activity. Develop a plan for moderate exercise to improve the patient's general condition. Consult the physician for any individual modifications deemed appropriate. Suggest including activities that the patient finds helpful in reducing stress.

Blood pressure monitoring. Demonstrate the correct procedure for taking blood pressure. Validate the patient's and family's understanding by having them perform this task on several occasions under supervision.

Medication regimen. Caution the patient that for the first 2 weeks of antihypertensive therapy drowsiness often occurs. Patients should be told that this side effect is self-limiting. They should be cautious in operating power equipment and driving while this symptom exists.

A common side effect of antihypertensive medications is hypotension. Instruct the patient to rise slowly from a sitting or supine position. Tell the patient to avoid standing for long periods, especially within 2 hours of taking antihypertensive medication. Weakness, dizziness, or faintness can usually be relieved by increasing muscular activity or by sitting or lying down.

Teach the person to perform exercises that prevent blood pooling in the extremities when sitting or standing for long periods of time. These exercises include flexing the calf muscles, wiggling the toes, rising on the toes, and then returning to the feet in a flat position.

Teach the person and significant other how to take and record blood pressure at prescribed intervals.

The patient should always report a lack of response to the medication prescribed or a blood pressure that *continues to rise* after medications have been taken. (Ask the physician to state specific parameters.)

Fostering health maintenance. Throughout the course of treatment, discuss medication information and how it will benefit the patient.

Drug therapy is one component in the management of hypertension. Lifestyle changes are equally important to drug therapy; therefore the need to maintain an exercise program and modify dietary habits to control obesity and serum cholesterol is crucial. Cessation of smoking and minimal alcoholic intake is strongly recommended.

Provide the patient and significant others with the important information contained in the specific drug monograph for the drugs prescribed. Additional health teaching and nursing interventions for drug side effects to expect and report will be found in each drug monograph.

Seek cooperation and understanding of the following points so that medication compliance is increased: name of medication, dosage, route and times of administration, side effects to expect, and side effects to report. Enlist the patient's aid in developing and maintaining a written record of monitoring parameters such as blood pressures, weight, and exercise. (See Appendix I.) Instruct the patient to bring the written record to follow-up visits.

Drug Class: Diuretics

Actions

Diuretics act as antihypertensive agents by causing volume depletion, sodium excretion, and vasodilation of peripheral arterioles. The mechanism of peripheral arteriolar vasodilation is unknown.

Uses

There are four classes of diuretic agents: carbonic anhydrase inhibitors, thiazide and thiazide-like agents, loop diuretics, and potassium-sparing diuretics. (See Chapter 25.) The carbonic anhydrase inhibitors are weak antihypertensive agents and therefore are not used for this purpose. The potassium-sparing diuretics are rarely used alone but are commonly used in combination with the thiazide and loop diuretics for added antihypertensive effect and to counteract the potassium-excreting effects of these more potent diuretic-antihypertensive agents.

The diuretics are the most commonly prescribed antihypertensive agents because they are one of only two classes of agents that have been shown to reduce cardiovascular morbidity and mortality associated with hypertension. The thiazides are most effective if the renal creatinine clearance is above 30 ml per minute; however, as renal function deteriorates, the more potent loop diuretics are needed to continue excretion of sodium and water.

Diuretics are also frequently prescribed in combination therapy. They potentiate the hypotensive activity of the nondiuretic antihypertensive agents, have a low incidence of adverse effects, and are often the least expensive of the antihypertensive agents.

Diuretics are used (often with other classes of antihypertensive therapy) to treat all stages of hypertension. The agents are discussed more extensively in Chapter 25.

Nursing Process

Premedication Assessment

1. Obtain baseline blood pressure readings in supine and standing positions.
2. Obtain baseline weight.
3. Initiate laboratory studies requested by the physician (for example, electrolytes).
4. Obtain baseline assessments of patient's state of hydration.

Planning

Availability. See Chapter 25.

Implementation

Dosage and administration. See Chapter 25.

Evaluation

See Chapter 25.

Drug Class: Beta-Adrenergic Blocking Agents

Actions

The beta-adrenergic blocking agents (beta blockers) (see Table 11-3) inhibit cardiac response to sympathetic nerve stimulation by blocking the beta receptors. As a result, the heart rate, cardiac output, and renin released from the kidneys—and consequently the blood pressure—are reduced.

Uses

The beta-adrenergic blocking agents are agents of another class that have been shown to reduce morbidity and mortality associated with hypertension; therefore, they are widely used as antihypertensive agents. The clinical advantages of the beta-adrenergic blocking agents in treating hypertension include minimal postural or exercise hypotension, no effect on sexual function, blood pressure reduction in the supine position, and little or no slowing of the central nervous system.

The JNC V recommends beta blockers as initial therapy for stages 1 and 2 hypertension. However, beta blockers are not as effective in black patients and should be avoided in patients with asthma, type I diabetes mellitus, heart failure caused by systolic dysfunction, and peripheral vascular disease.

Nursing Process

Premedication Assessment

1. Check history for respiratory conditions that could be aggravated by bronchoconstriction, and for type I diabetes mellitus, heart failure, or peripheral vacular disease. If any of these conditions are present, contact the physician to discuss the situation before initiation of beta-adrenergic blocking agent therapy.
2. Obtain baseline blood pressure readings.

Planning

Availability. See Table 11-3.

Implementation

Dosage and administration. See Table 11-3.
Individualization of dosage. Although the onset of activity is rapid, it may often take several days to weeks for a patient to show optimal improvement and become stabilized on an adequate maintenance dosage. Patients must be periodically reevaluated to determine the lowest effective dosage necessary to control the disorder being treated.

Sudden discontinuation. Patients must be counseled against poor compliance or sudden discontinuation of therapy without a physician's advice. Sudden discontinuation of therapy has resulted in an exacerbation of anginal symptoms followed in some cases by myocardial infarction. When discontinuing long-term treatment with beta blockers, the dosage should be gradually reduced over a period of 1 to 2 weeks with careful monitoring of the patient. If anginal symptoms develop or become more frequent, beta-blocker therapy should be restarted at least temporarily.

Evaluation

Most of the adverse effects associated with beta-adrenergic blocking agents are dosage related. Response by individual patients is highly variable. Many of these side effects may occur but may be transient. Strongly encourage patients to see their physicians before discontinuing therapy. Minor dosage adjustment may be all that is required for most side effects.

Side effects to expect and report

BRADYCARDIA, PERIPHERAL VASOCONSTRICTION (PURPLE MOTTLED SKIN). Discontinue further dosages until the patient is evaluated by a physician.

BRONCHOSPASM, WHEEZING. Withhold additional doses until the patient has been evaluated by a physician.

DIABETIC PATIENTS. Monitor for hypoglycemia: headache, weakness, decreased coordination, general apprehension, diaphoresis, hunger, or blurred or double vision. Many of these symptoms may be masked by the beta-adrenergic blocking agents. Notify the physician if you suspect that any of the above-mentioned symptoms are appearing intermittently.

HEART FAILURE. Monitor patients for an increase in edema, dyspnea, rales, bradycardia, and orthopnea. Notify the physician if these symptoms are developing.

Drug interactions

ANTIHYPERTENSIVE AGENTS. All the beta-blocking agents have hypotensive properties that are additive with antihypertensive agents (guanethidine, methyldopa, hydralazine, clonidine, prazosin, minoxidil, captopril, saralasin, and reserpine).

If it is decided to discontinue therapy in patients receiving beta blockers and clonidine concurrently, the beta blocker should be withdrawn gradually and discontinued several days before the gradual withdrawal of the clonidine.

BETA-ADRENERGIC AGENTS. Depending on the dosages used, the beta stimulants (isoproterenol, metaproterenol, terbutaline, albuterol, and ritodrine) may inhibit the action of the beta-blocking agents, and vice versa.

LIDOCAINE, PROCAINAMIDE, PHENYTOIN, DISOPYRAMIDE, DIGITALIS GLYCOSIDES. Although these drugs are occasionally used concurrently, monitor patients carefully for additional arrhythmias, bradycardia, and signs of congestive heart failure.

ENZYME-INDUCING AGENTS. Enzyme-inducing agents such as cimetidine, phenobarbital, nembutal, and phenytoin enhance the metabolism of propranolol, metoprolol, pindolol, and timolol. This reaction probably does not occur with nadolol or atenolol because they are not metabolized but excreted unchanged. The dosage of the beta blocker may have to be increased to provide therapeutic activity. If the enzyme-inducing agent is discontinued, the dosage of the beta-blocking agent will also require reduction.

INDOMETHACIN AND SALICYLATES. Indomethacin and possibly other prostaglandin inhibitors inhibit the antihypertensive activity of propranolol and pindolol, resulting in loss of hypertensive control.

The dosage of the beta blocker may have to be increased to compensate for the antihypertensive inhibitory effect of indomethacin and perhaps other prostaglandin inhibitors.

Drug Class: Alpha-1 Adrenergic Blocking Agents

Actions

The alpha-1 blockers, doxazosin, prazosin, and terazosin, act by blocking postsynaptic alpha-1 adrenergic receptors to produce arteriolar and venous vasodilation, reducing peripheral vascular resistance without reducing cardiac output or inducing a reflex tachycardia. They produce a decrease in standing blood pressure slightly greater than that in supine blood pressure. These agents also have a modest positive effect on serum lipids, increasing high-density lipoprotein cholesterol and reducing low-density lipoprotein cholesterol, total cholesterol, and triglyceride concentrations.

The alpha-1 blockers do not increase catecholamines, therefore there is no increase in heart rate or myocardial oxygen consumption. They also have no effect on uric acid concentrations.

Because of the presence of alpha-1 receptors in the prostate gland and certain areas of the bladder, terazosin and doxazosin are also to able reduce urinary outflow resistance in men with enlarged prostate glands.

Uses

These agents may be used alone or in combination with other antihypertensive agents in the treatment of stages 1 to 4 hypertension. They have additive effects with beta blockers and diuretics. The JNC V lists these agents as alternatives if beta-blocker or diuretic therapy is not successful or not tolerated. Blood pressure response in alpha-1 blockers appears to be similar in white and black patients. They can be used safely in patients with angina, gout, and hyperlipidemia. The three alpha-1 blockers have similar antihypertensive effects and adverse effects. Doxazosin and terazosin have a longer duration of action and can be administered once daily. Prazosin is often used in combination with diuretic therapy because of its tendency to cause sodium and water retention.

Doxazosin and terazosin are also used to reduce mild to moderate urinary obstruction manifestations (hesitancy, terminal dribbling of urine, interrupted stream, impaired size and force of stream, and sensation of incomplete bladder emptying) in men with benign prostatic hypertrophy.

Therapeutic Outcomes

The primary therapeutic outcomes expected from alpha-1 adrenergic receptor blocker therapy are reduction of blood pressure and reduced symptoms and improvement in urine flow associated with prostatic enlargement.

Nursing Process

Premedication Assessment

1. Obtain baseline blood pressure readings in supine and standing positions.
2. Check if patient is pregnant or has a history of severe cerebral or coronary arteriosclerosis, gastritis, or peptic

ulcer disease. (Reduction of blood pressure may diminish blood flow to these regions, which causes therapy to worsen the condition.

Planning

Availability. See Table 20-3.

Implementation

Dosage and administration. See Table 20-3. *Note:* The initial doses of doxazosin, prazosin, and terazosin may cause hypotension with dizziness, tachycardia, and fainting; these adverse effects occur in less than 1% of patients starting therapy. Symptoms occur 15 to 90 minutes after initial dosages and occur most frequently in patients who are already receiving propranolol (and presumably other beta-adrenergic blocking agents). This effect may be minimized by giving the first doses with food and limiting the initial dose to 1 mg. Patients should be warned that this side effect may occur, that it is transient, and that they should lie down immediately if symptoms develop.

Evaluation

Side effects to expect

DROWSINESS, HEADACHE, DIZZINESS, WEAKNESS, LETHARGY. Tell the patient that these side effects may occur but that they tend to be self-limiting. Tell the patient not to stop taking the medication and to consult the physician if the problem becomes unacceptable.

DIZZINESS, TACHYCARDIA, FAINTING. These side effects occur in about 1% of patients when therapy is initiated. They develop 15 to 90 minutes after the first dosage is taken. To decrease the incidence, administer the first dose with food and limit the initial dose to 1 mg.

Instruct the patient to lie down immediately if these symptoms begin to occur.

Provide for the patient's safety.

Drug interactions

DRUGS THAT ENHANCE THERAPEUTIC AND TOXIC EFFECTS. Diuretics, verapamil, tranquilizers, alcohol, barbiturates, antihistamines, beta-adrenergic blocking agents (propranolol, atenolol, pindolol, others), and other antihypertensive agents.

Table 20-3
Alpha-1 Adrenergic Blocking Agents

GENERIC NAME	BRAND NAME	AVAILABILITY	DOSAGE RANGE
Doxazosin	Cardura	Tablets: 1, 2, 4, 8, mg	Hypertension: PO: Initial—1 mg daily AM or PM. Hypotensive effects are most likely with 2 to 6 hr. Monitor standing blood pressure Maintenance—Increase to 2 mg, then, if needed, 4, 8, and 16 mg to achieve desired reduction in blood pressure. Benign prostatic hypertrophy: PO: Initial—as for hypertension. Increase dose at weekly intervals to 2 mg, then 4 and 8 mg once daily. Maintenance—8 mg daily; monitor blood pressure.
Prazosin	Minipress	Capsules: 1, 2, 5, mg	Hypertension: PO: Initial—1 mg 2 or 3 times daily with first dose at bedtime to reduce syncopal episodes. Maintenance—6 to 15 mg/day in two to three divided doses. Maximum dose—20-40 mg/day.
Terazosin	Hytrin	Tablets: 1, 2, 5, 10 mg Capsules: 1, 2, 5, 10 mg	Hypertension: PO: Initial—1 mg at bedtime. Measure blood pressure 2 to 3 hr after dosing and evaluate for symptoms of dizziness or tachycardia; if response is substantially diminished at 24 hr, increase dose. Maintenance—1 to 5 mg daily Maximum dose—20 mg/day. Benign prostatic hypertrophy: PO: Initial—as for hypertension; gradually increase dose in stepwise fashion to 2, 5, or 10 mg daily for acceptable urinary output Maintenance—10 mg daily for 4 to 6 weeks to assess urinary response. Maximum dose—20 mg/day.

Monitor the blood pressure response to the cumulative effects of antihypertensive agents. Take the blood pressures in supine and erect positions.

Monitor for an increase in severity of side effects such as sedation, hypotension, and bradycardia or tachycardia.

Drug Class: Angiotensin-Converting Enzyme Inhibitors

Actions

Angiotensin-converting enzyme (ACE) inhibitors represent a major breakthrough in the treatment of hypertension. The renin-angiotensin-aldosterone system plays a major role in the regulation of blood pressure. When there is a reduction in blood pressure, sodium concentration, or renal blood flow, renin is secreted by the kidneys. The renin converts angiotensinogen, which is secreted by the liver, to angiotensin I. Angiotensin I is converted by angiotensin I–converting enzyme to angiotensin II. Angiotensin II produces potent vasoconstriction by acting on receptors within blood vessels. It also promotes aldosterone secretion, which causes sodium retention by stimulation of angiotensin receptors in the adrenal cortex. These actions result in increased blood pressure secondary to the vasoconstriction and enhanced cardiac output secondary to sodium retention. The ACE inhibitors inhibit angiotensin I–converting enzyme, the enzyme responsible for the conversion of angiotensin I to angiotensin II, thus reducing serum levels of this potent vasoconstrictor and aldosterone stimulant.

Uses

The ACE inhibitors reduce blood pressure, preserve cardiac output, and increase renal blood flow. They are effective as single therapy for stages 1 or 2 hypertension, severe accelerated hypertension, and renal hypertension. The JNC V considers them an alternative to diuretic or beta-blocker therapy. Although they may be used alone, they tend to be more effective when combined with diuretic therapy. They are not as effective in lowering blood pressure in blacks unless used with a diuretic. Advantages of ACE inhibitors are infrequency of orthostatic hypotension; lack of central nervous system (CNS) depression and sexual dysfunction side effects; lack of aggravation of asthma, obstructive pulmonary disease, gout, cholesterol levels, or diabetes; and an additive effect with diuretics. The ACE inhibitors are also effective in the treatment of heart failure and may also be used to slow the progression of diabetic nephropathy.

Therapeutic Outcomes

The primary therapeutic outcome expected from the ACE inhibitors is reduction in blood pressure.

Nursing Process

Premedication Assessment

1. Obtain baseline blood pressure readings in supine and standing positions.
2. Obtain a history of bowel elimination patterns.
3. Initiate laboratory studies as requested by the physician (for example, renal function tests—blood urea nitrogen [BUN] and serum creatinine, electrolytes, and complete blood count (CBC) to serve as a baseline for future comparison.
4. Ask whether the patient is pregnant or likely to become pregnant. If so, discuss with the physician before initiating ACE inhibitor therapy.

Planning

Availability. See Table 20-4.

Implementation

Dosage and administration. See Table 20-4. Captopril should be administered without food and requires twice-daily dosing. All of the other agents are administered once daily. NOTE: The initial doses of ACE inhibitors may cause hypotension with dizziness, tachycardia, and fainting; these adverse effects occur more commonly in patients also receiving diuretics. Symptoms occur within 3 hours after the first several dosages. This effect may be minimized by discontinuing the diuretic 1 week before initiating ACE inhibitor therapy. Patients should be warned that this side effect may occur, that it is transient, and that they should lie down immediately if symptoms develop.

Evaluation

Side effects to expect

NAUSEA, FATIGUE, HEADACHE, DIARRHEA. These side effects are usually mild and tend to resolve with continued therapy. Encourage the patient not to discontinue therapy without first consulting a physician.

ORTHOSTATIC HYPOTENSION (DIZZINESS, WEAKNESS, FAINTNESS). Although these side effects are infrequent and usually mild, certain patients, particularly those also receiving diuretics, may suffer some degree of orthostatic hypotension, particularly when therapy is initiated. Observe the patient closely for at least 2 hours after the initial dose and for at least an additional hour until blood pressure has stabilized.

Monitor the blood pressure in both the supine and standing positions.

Anticipate the development of postural hypotension and take measures to prevent an occurrence. Instruct the patient to rise slowly from a supine or sitting position and to sit or lie down if feeling faint.

Side effects to report

SWELLING OF THE FACE, EYES, LIPS, TONGUE; DIFFICULTY IN BREATHING. Angioedema has been reported to occur in a small number of patients, especially after the first dose. Patients should be cautioned to discontinue further therapy and seek medical attention immediately.

NEUTROPENIA. Neutropenia (300 neutrophils/mm^3) and agranulocytosis (drug-induced bone marrow suppression) have been observed in patients receiving ACE inhibitors. The neutropenia appears within the first 3 to 12 weeks of therapy and develops slowly; the white count falls to its nadir in 10 to 30 days. The white count returns to normal about 2 weeks after discontinuation of ACE inhibitor therapy.

The patients most susceptible are those receiving captopril who also have impaired renal function or serious autoimmune diseases (such as lupus erythematosus) or who are exposed to drugs known to affect the white cells or immune response (such as corticosteroids).

Table 20-4

Angiotensin-Converting Enzyme (ACE) Inhibitors

GENERIC NAME	BRAND NAME	AVAILABILITY	APPROVED USES	DOSAGE RANGE
Benazepril	Lotensin	Tablets: 5, 10, 20, 40 mg	Hypertension	PO: Initial—2.5-5 mg once daily Maintenance—20-40 mg daily
Captopril	Capoten	Tablets: 12.5, 25, 50, 100 mg	Hypertension; heart failure, diabetic nephropathy	PO: Initial—25 mg 2 to 3 × daily Maintenance—75-450 mg daily
Enalapril	Vasotec	Tablets: 2.5, 5, 10, 20 mg	Hypertension; heart failure	PO: Initial—2.5-5 mg once daily Maintenance—10-40 mg daily
Enalaprilat	Vasotec IV	Inj.: 1.25 mg/ml	Hypertension	IV: 1.25 mg every 6 hr over 5 min
Fosinopril	Monopril	Tablets: 10, 20 mg	Hypertension; heart failure	PO: Initial—10 mg once daily Maintenance—20-80 mg daily
Lisinopril	Prinivil, Zestril	Tablets: 2.5, 5, 10, 20, 40 mg	Hypertension; heart failure	PO: Initial—5-10 mg once daily Maintenance—20-40 mg daily
Moexipril	Univase	Tablets: 7.5, 15 mg	Hypertension	PO: Initial—with diuretic 3.75 mg; without diuretic, 7.5 mg Maintenance—7.5-30 mg in 1 or 2 divided doses 1 hr before meals
Quinapril	Accupril	Tablets: 5, 10, 20, 40 mg	Hypertension, heart failure, Raynaud's disease	PO: Initial—10 mg daily Maintenance—20-80 mg daily
Ramipril	Altace	Capsules: 1.25, 2.5, 5, 10 mg	Hypertension	PO: Initial—1.25-2.5 mg daily Maintenance—2.5-20 mg daily

LIFE SPAN ISSUES

ANTIHYPERTENSIVE THERAPY

The elderly are more likely to develop orthostatic hypotension with antihypertensive therapy. The nurse should initiate monitoring of the patient's blood pressure in a lying and sitting position during initiation of antihypertensive therapy or when drug dosages are adjusted. Safety precautions should be initiated to prevent accidental injury. Teach the patient to rise slowly from a supine to a sitting and then standing position.

Patients at risk should have differential and total white cell counts before initiation of therapy and then every 2 weeks thereafter for the first 3 months of therapy. Stress the importance of returning for this laboratory work. Patients should be told to notify their physicians promptly if any evidence of infection such as sore throat or fever (which may be an indicator of neutropenia) should develop.

NEPHROTOXICITY. A small number of hypertensive patients who are receiving ACE inhibitors, particularly those with preexisting renal impairment, have developed increases in BUN and serum creatinine. These elevations have usually been minor and transient, especially when the ACE inhibitor was administered concomitantly with a diuretic. Renal function should be monitored during the first few weeks of therapy. Report an increasing BUN and creatinine level. Dosage reduction of the ACE inhibitor or possible discontinuation of the diuretic may be required.

HYPERKALEMIA. Because ACE inhibitors inhibit aldosterone, patients may develop slight increases in serum potassium. Approximately 1% of patients may develop hyperkalemia (greater than 5.7 mEq/L). Most cases resolve without discontinuation of therapy. Patients most susceptible to the development of hyperkalemia are those with renal impairment or diabetes mellitus and those already receiving a potassium supplement. Many symptoms associated with altered fluid and electrolyte balance are subtle and interspersed with general symptoms of drug toxicity or the disease process itself.

Gather data relative to *changes* in the patient's mental status (such as alertness, orientation, and confusion), muscle strength, muscle cramps, tremors, nausea, and general appearance (drowsy, anxious, or lethargic).

Always check the electrolyte reports for early indications of electrolyte imbalance.

Keep accurate records of intake and output, daily weights, and vital signs.

CHRONIC COUGH. As many as one third of patients receiving ACE inhibitors may develop a chronic, dry, nonproductive, persistent cough. It may appear from 1 week to 6 months after initiation of ACE inhibitor therapy. Women appear to be more susceptible than men. Patients should be told to contact their physicians if the cough becomes troublesome. The cough resolves within 1 to 30 days after discontinuation of therapy.

PREGNANCY. Medicines that act directly on the renin-angiotensin system can cause fetal and neonatal harm. There is concern about the potential for birth defects in neonates whose mothers received ACE inhibitors, especially during the second and third trimesters of pregnancy. Women who wish to become pregnant who become pregnant while receiving ACE inhibitors should discuss alternative therapies with their physicians as soon as possible.

Drug interactions

DRUGS THAT ENHANCE THERAPEUTIC AND TOXIC EFFECTS. Diuretics, phenothiazines, alcohol, beta-adrenergic blocking agents (propranolol, atenolol, pindolol, and others), and other antihypertensive agents. Probenecid blocks the excretion of captopril, causing an increased antihypertensive effect. Monitor the blood pressure response to the cumulative effects of antihypertensive agents. Take the blood pressures in supine and erect positions.

DRUGS THAT REDUCE THERAPEUTIC EFFECTS. Antacids may diminish absorption of ACE inhibitors. Separate the administration times by 1 to 2 hours. Indomethacin may reduce the antihypertensive effects of the ACE inhibitors. Rifampin may decrease the antihypertensive effects of enalapril. Monitor carefully for poor blood pressure control or a gradually increasing blood pressure.

DIGOXIN. ACE inhibitors may increase the serum levels of digoxin. Monitor the patient for symptoms of anorexia, nausea, vomiting, headaches, blurred or colored vision, and bradycardia. A digoxin serum level may be ordered by the physician.

LITHIUM. ACE inhibitors may induce lithium toxicity. Monitor for lithium toxicity manifested by nausea, anorexia, fine tremors, persistent vomiting, profuse diarrhea, hyperreflexia, lethargy, and weakness.

HYPERKALEMIA. ACE inhibitors may cause small increases in potassium levels by inhibiting aldosterone secretion. Patients should not take dietary supplements of potassium or potassium-sparing diuretics (triamterene, spironolactone, or amiloride) without specific approval from the physician. If a patient has received spironolactone up to several months before ACE inhibitor therapy, the serum potassium level should be monitored closely, because the potassium-sparing effect of spironolactone persists.

CAPSAICIN. Capsaicin may cause or aggravate coughing associated with ACE inhibitor therapy. Monitor for increased frequency of dry, persistent cough. Report to the physician.

Drug Class: Angiotensin II Receptor Antagonists

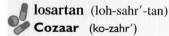

losartan (loh-sahr'-tan)
Cozaar (ko-zahr')

Actions

Losartan is the first of a new class of antihypertensive agents that act by binding to angiotensin II receptor sites, blocking the potent vasoconstrictor from binding to the receptor (also called AT$_1$ receptor) sites in the vascular smooth muscle and adrenal gland. The blood pressure–elevating and sodium-retaining effects of angiotensin II are thus antagonized. Losartan has no effect on renal function, prostaglandin levels, triglycerides, cholesterol, or blood glucose levels.

Uses

Losartan became available after the JNC V report was published, so it is not included in the recommendations. However, losartan has been found to be as effective in lowering blood pressure as the ACE inhibitors and beta blockers. Men and women and patients over and under age 65 usually have similar responses; however, black patients do not respond as well to monotherapy with losartan. Losartan is indicated for the treatment of hypertension and may be used alone or in combination with other antihypertensive agents. The blood pressure–lowering effect of losartan is seen within 1 week, but may take 3 to 6 weeks for full therapeutic effect. If the antihypertensive effect is not controlled by losartan alone, a low dose of a diuretic may be added. Hydrochlorothiazide has an additive effect.

Therapeutic Outcomes

The primary therapeutic outcome expected from losartan is reduction in blood pressure.

Nursing Process

Premedication Assessment

1. Obtain baseline blood pressure readings in supine and standing positions.
2. Initiate laboratory studies requested by the physician (for example, renal function tests—BUN and serum creatinine, electrolytes, and CBC) to serve as a baseline for future comparison.
3. Ask whether the patient is pregnant or likely to become pregnant. If so, discuss with the physician before initiating ACE inhibitor therapy.

Planning

Availability. 25 and 50 mg tablets.

Implementation

Dosage and administration. PO—initially, 50 mg once daily. Maintenance dose ranges from 25 to 100 mg daily in one or two doses. It may be administered with or without food.

Evaluation

Side effects to expect

DYSPEPSIA, CRAMPS, DIARRHEA. These side effects are usually mild and tend to resolve with continued therapy. Encourage the patient not to discontinue therapy without first consulting the physician.

ORTHOSTATIC HYPOTENSION (DIZZINESS, WEAKNESS, FAINTNESS). Although these side effects are infrequent and usually mild, certain patients, particularly those also receiving diuretics, may suffer some degree of orthostatic hypotension, particularly when therapy is initiated. Observe the patient closely for at least 2 hours after the initial dose and for at least an additional hour until blood pressure has stabilized.

Monitor the blood pressure in both the supine and standing positions.

Anticipate the development of postural hypotension and take measures to prevent an occurrence. Teach the patient to rise slowly from a supine or sitting position and to sit or lie down if feeling faint.

Side effects to report

PREGNANCY. Medicines that act directly on the renin-angiotensin system can cause fetal and neonatal harm. There is potential for birth defects in neonates whose mothers received ACE inhibitors, especially during the second and third trimesters of pregnancy. Women who wish to become pregnant or who become pregnant while receiving losartan should discuss alternative therapies with their physicians as soon as possible.

HYPERKALEMIA. Because losartan inhibits aldosterone secretion, patients may develop slight increases in serum potassium. Most cases resolve without discontinuation of therapy. Patients most susceptible to the development of hyperkalemia are those with renal impairment or diabetes mellitus and those already receiving a potassium supplement. Many symptoms associated with altered fluid and electrolyte balance are subtle and interspersed with general symptoms of drug toxicity or the disease process itself. Gather data relative to changes in the patient's mental status (such as alertness, orientation, and confusion), muscle strength, muscle cramps, tremors, nausea, and general appearance (drowsy, anxious, or lethargic).

Always check the electrolyte reports for early indications of electrolyte imbalance.

Keep accurate records of intake and output, daily weights, and vital signs.

Drug interactions

DRUGS THAT ENHANCE THERAPEUTIC AND TOXIC EFFECTS. Diuretics, phenothiazines, alcohol, beta-adrenergic blocking agents (propranolol, atenolol, pindolol, and others), and other antihypertensive agents. Cimetidine inhibits the metabolism of losartan, causing an increased antihypertensive effect. Monitor the blood pressure response to the cumulative effects of antihypertensive agents. Take blood pressure readings in supine and erect positions.

DRUGS THAT REDUCE THERAPEUTIC EFFECTS. Phenobarbital may decrease the antihypertensive effects of losartan. Monitor carefully for poor blood pressure control or a gradually increasing blood pressure.

HYPERKALEMIA. Losartan may cause small increases in potassium levels by reducing aldosterone secretion. Patients should not take dietary supplements of potassium or potassium-sparing diuretics (triamterene, spironolactone, or amiloride) without specific approval from the physician. If a patient has received spironolactone up to several months before losartan therapy, the serum potassium level should be monitored closely, because the potassium-sparing effect of spironolactone persists.

Drug Class: Calcium Ion Antagonists

Actions

Calcium ion antagonists are known variously as calcium antagonists, calcium channel blockers, slow channel blockers, and calcium ion influx inhibitors. These agents inhibit the movement of calcium ions across a cell membrane. This results in fewer arrhythmias, a slower rate of contraction of the heart, and

relaxation of smooth muscle of blood vessels, resulting in vasodilation and reduced blood pressure. The calcium ion antagonists are classified by structure: benzthiazepines—diltiazem, diaminopropanol ether—bepridil; diphenylalkylamines— verapamil; and dihydropyridines—amlodipine, felodipine, isradipine, nicardipine, nifedipine, and nimodipine.

Uses

Although each of these agents act by calcium ion inhibition, there are significant differences in clinical use because they act somewhat differently on coronary blood vessels, systemic blood vessels, the pacemaker cells of the heart, and the conducting tissue of the heart. Their clinical effects are also dependent on the type and severity of the patient's disease. All of the available calcium channel blockers are effective antihypertensive agents, but clinicians tend to use the dihydropyridine group more often because they have better peripheral vasodilating effects. Calcium channel blockers are more effective in patients with higher pretreatment blood pressures. They increase renal sodium excretion and are generally well tolerated. Calcium channel blockers are ideal as first- or second-line medicines in patients with hypertension and coexisting angina and are an alternative to the use of beta blockers in patients with asthma or diabetes mellitus. They are particularly effective in blacks and elderly hypertensive patients, who are more likely to have low-renin hypertension. The calcium channel blockers do not affect gout or peripheral vascular disease.

Therapeutic Outcomes

The primary therapeutic outcome expected from calcium ion antagonist therapy is reduction in blood pressure.

Nursing Process

Premedication Assessment

1. Obtain baseline blood pressure readings in the supine and standing positions.
2. Obtain baseline weight.
3. If the patient is taking digitalis glycosides concurrently, initiate close monitoring for potential digitalis toxicity.

Planning

Availabililty. See Table 20-5.

Implementation

Dosage and administration. See Table 20-5.
Dosage adjustments. See individual drugs for dosage parameters. Adjustments are made based on the individual patient's response to therapy.

Evaluation

Side effects to report

HYPOTENSION, SYNCOPY. Caution the patient that hypotension and syncopy may occur during the first week. These side effects decline once the dosage is stabilized.

Take blood pressure readings every shift in the hospitalized patient and stress the need for the patient to monitor blood pressure after discharge.

Prevent hypotensive episodes instructing the patient to rise slowly from a supine or sitting position and perform

Table 20-5

Calcium Ion Antagonists Used to Treat Hypertension

GENERIC NAME	BRAND NAME	AVAILABILITY	DOSAGE RANGE
Amlodipine	Norvasc	Tablets: 2.5, 5, 10 mg	PO: Initial—5 mg once daily; adjust over 7-14 days to a maximum of 10 mg/day
Diltiazem	Cardizem	Tablets: 30, 60, 90, 120 mg Sustained-release capsules: 60, 90, 120, 180, 240, 300 mg IV: 5 mg/ml in 5 and 10 ml vials	PO: Initial—60 to 120 mg sustained-release capsule twice daily; adjust as needed after 14 days Maintenance—240 to 360 mg daily
Felodipine	Plendil	Tablets: 5, 10 mg	PO: Initial—5 mg daily; adjust after 14 days Maintenance—5 to 10 mg daily Maximum—20 mg daily
Isradipine	DynaCirc	Capsules: 2.5, 5 mg	PO: Initial—2.5 mg two times daily; maximal response may require 2 to 4 weeks Maintenance—10 mg daily Maximum—20 mg daily
Nicardipine	Cardene	Capsules: 20, 30 mg Extended-release capsules: 30, 45, 60 mg IV: 2.5 mg/ml in 10 ml vials	PO: Initial—20 mg three times daily Maximal response may require 2 weeks of therapy; adjust dose by measuring blood pressure approximately 8 hr after last dose; peak effect determined by measuring blood pressure 1 to 2 hr after dosage administration Maintenance—20 to 40 mg three times daily
Nifedipine	Procardia	Capsules: 10, 20 mg Sustained-release tablets: 30, 60, 90 mg	PO: Initial—10 mg three times daily; adjust over 7-14 days to balance antianginal and hypotensive activity. Maintenance—10 to 20 mg three times daily Sustained-release tablets are administered once daily Maximum—capsules, 180 mg daily; sustained-release tablets, 120 mg daily
Verapamil	Calan, Isoptin	Tablets: 40, 80, 120 mg Sustained-release tablets: 180, 240 mg IV: 2.5 mg/ml in 2 and 4 ml ampules and syringes	PO: Initial—80 mg 3 to 4 times daily Sustained-release tablets: 120 to 240 mg once daily in the morning Maintenance—240-480 mg daily. Administer with food

exercises to prevent blood pooling when standing or sitting in one position for prolonged periods. If the patient feels faint, instruct to sit or lie down.

EDEMA. Assess the patient for development of edema. Perform daily weights at the same time, in similar clothing, and on the same scale. Report increases in weight to the physician for further evaluation.

Drug interactions

DRUGS THAT ENHANCE THERAPEUTIC AND TOXIC EFFECTS. Diuretics, phenothiazines, alcohol, beta-adrenergic blocking agents (propranolol, atenolol, pindolol, and others), histamine H_2 antagonists (cimetidine, ranitidine), and other antihypertensive agents. Monitor the blood pressure response to the cumulative effects of antihypertensive agents. Take the blood pressures in supine and erect positions. Assess the

patient for hypotension, light-headedness, dizziness, and bradycardia. Provide for patient safety; prevent falls.

DIGITALIS GLYCOSIDES. Calcium ion antagonists may increase serum levels of digitalis glycosides. Monitor the patient for symptoms of anorexia, nausea, vomiting, headaches, blurred or colored vision, and bradycardia. The physician may order a digitalis serum level.

GLUCOSE METABOLISM. The dosage of oral hypoglycemic agents may require adjustment in non–insulin-dependent diabetes mellitus (NIDDM) patients. Assess for signs of hyperglycemia. Perform blood glucose testing on a regular basis.

VERAPAMIL AND DISOPYRAMIDE. Do NOT administer disopyramide 48 hours before or 24 hours after the administration of verapamil.

Drug Class: Centrally Acting Alpha-2 Agonists

Actions

The centrally acting alpha-2 agonists (clonidine, guanabenz, guanfacine, and methyldopa) act by stimulating the alpha-adrenergic receptors in the brainstem, resulting in reduced sympathetic outflow from the CNS with a decrease in heart rate and peripheral vascular resistance, which causes a decrease in both systolic and diastolic blood pressures.

Uses

The JNC V now lists the alpha-2 agonists as supplemental antihypertensive agents. When used as monotherapy, the alpha-2 agonists are as effective as diuretics and beta blockers for controlling blood pressure. Clonidine is available as a transdermal therapeutic system (TTS) that is applied once weekly. These drugs cause more frequent side effects such as sedation, dizziness, dry mouth, fatigue, and sexual dysfunction. When used alone, methyldopa frequently causes fluid retention. They can safely be used in combination with other agents such as diuretics, vasodilators, and beta blockers.

Therapeutic Outcomes

The primary therapeutic outcome expected from the alpha-2 agonists is reduction in blood pressure.

Nursing Process

Premedication Assessment

1. Obtain baseline blood pressure readings in supine and standing positions.
2. Assess the patient's mental status—affective and cognitive behaviors should be used as a baseline for subsequent comparison. If depression is suspected, report to the physician.
3. Obtain baseline data relating to usual sleep pattern.

Planning

Availability. See Table 20-6.

Implementation

Dosage and administration. See Table 20-6.
Sudden discontinuation. Never suddenly discontinue clonidine or guanabenz because it may cause a rebound effect and a rapid increase in blood pressure, manifested by nervousness, agitation, restlessness, tremors, headache, nausea, and increased salivation. Rebound symptoms are most pronounced after 1 to 2 months of therapy and may begin to appear within a few hours of a missed dose. Within 8 to 24 hours, severe symptoms may develop. When therapy is to be discontinued, a gradual reduction in dosage is necessary over

Table 20-6

Centrally-Acting Alpha-2 Agonists

GENERIC NAME	BRAND NAME	AVAILABILITY	DOSAGE RANGE
Clonidine	Catapres Catapres-TTS	Tablets: 0.1, 0.2, 0.3 mg Transdermal patch: 2.5, 5, 7.5 mg	PO: Initial—0.1 mg twice daily Maintenance—0.2-0.8 mg daily in divided doses Maximum—2.4 mg daily Transdermal—Apply to a hairless area of intact skin on upper arm or torso once every 7 days; use a different site each week Initial—Start with 2.5 mg patch; after 2 wk add another 2.5 mg patch or use a larger system Maximum—two 7.5 mg patches per wk NOTE: Antihypertensive effect starts 2 to 3 days after initiation of therapy
Guanabenz	Wytensin	Tablets: 4, 8 mg	PO: Initial—4 mg twice daily; increase 4 to 8 mg daily every 1 to 2 wk Maximum—32 mg twice daily
Guanfacine	Tenex	Tablets: 1, 2 mg	PO: Initial—1 mg daily at bedtime Maintenance—1-2 mg Maximum—3 mg daily
Methyldopa	Aldomet	Tablets: 125, 250, 500 mg Suspension: 250 mg/5 ml IV: 250 mg/5 ml in 5 and 10 ml vials	PO: Initial—250 mg two or three times daily Maintenance—500 mg to 3 g daily in 2 to 4 doses

2 to 4 days, during which blood pressure must be carefully monitored. If the transdermal patch becomes loose, the adhesive overlay should be applied directly over the patch to ensure good adhesion.

Evaluation
Side effects to expect
DROWSINESS, DRY MOUTH, DIZZINESS. Tell the patient that these symptoms may occur but that they tend to be self-limiting. Tell the patient not to discontinue the medication and to consult the physician if the side effects become an unacceptable problem.

ALTERED URINE COLOR. Methyldopa or its metabolites may discolor the urine, causing it to darken on exposure to air. It is to be expected and is not harmful.

ALTERED TEST REACTIONS. A false-positive urine glucose test may occur when using Clinitest. Diastix and Tes-Tape are not affected by methyldopa.

Methyldopa may cause up to 20% of patients to develop a positive reaction to the direct Coombs' test. Fewer than 0.2% of these patients will develop hemolytic anemia, however. Blood counts should be determined annually during therapy to detect hemolytic anemia.

Side effects to report
DEPRESSION. Assess the patient's affective (loneliness, sadness, anxiety, and anger), cognitive (confusion, ambivalence, and loss of interest), and other behavioral responses (agitation, irritability, altered activity level, and withdrawal) before starting therapy. After starting therapy with clonidine, carefully monitor the patient for changes in usual response patterns. Assess otherwise normal emotions for an increase in duration or intensity.

Note the patient's degree of socialization, response to stimulation, and changes in interactions with others. All individuals taking this drug should be monitored for development of depression, especially those with a history of depression.

RASH. Approximately 10% to 15% of patients using the clonidine patch develop a contact dermatitis. Patients who develop moderate or severe erythema or vesicle formation at the site of application of clonidine transdermal patches should consult their physicians about the possible need to remove the patch and alternative therapy.

Drug interactions
DRUGS THAT ENHANCE THERAPEUTIC AND TOXIC EFFECTS. Guanethidine, digitalis glycosides, barbiturates, tranquilizers, antihistamines, alcohol, and beta-adrenergic blocking agents (such as propranolol, atenolol, pindolol, and others), and other antihypertensive agents. Monitor the blood pressure response to the cumulative effects of antihypertensive agents. Take the blood pressures in supine and erect positions.

Monitor for an increase in severity of side effects such as sedation, hypotension, and bradycardia or tachycardia.

DRUGS THAT REDUCE THERAPEUTIC EFFECTS. Tricyclic antidepressants (amitriptyline, imipramine, and desipramine) and trazodone. Monitor carefully for poor blood pressure control or a gradually increasing blood pressure.

SEDATIVE EFFECTS. Alcohol, barbiturates, phenothiazines, benzodiazepines, and antihistamines all potentiate the sedative effects of guanabenz. Patients should be warned that tolerance to alcohol and other depressants may be diminished.

HALOPERIDOL. Methyldopa used concurrently with haloperidol may produce irritability, aggressiveness, assaultiveness, and dementia. Concurrent use is usually not recommended.

Drug Class: Peripherally Acting Adrenergic Antagonists

guanadrel (gwan'a-drel)
Hylorel (hi-lor'el)

Actions
Guanadrel is similar to guanethidine as an antihypertensive agent in that it causes a release and subsequent depletion of norepinephrine from adrenergic nerve endings. This causes a relaxation of vascular smooth muscle, which decreases total peripheral resistance and venous return. A hypotensive effect results that is greater in the standing than in the supine position. Heart rate is slightly decreased, but there is no significant change in cardiac output. Fluid retention often occurs.

Uses
Guanadrel is recommended for use in refractory hypertension uncontrolled by other agents with fewer side effects. Guanadrel is used in combination with a thiazide diuretic.

Therapeutic Outcomes
The primary therapeutic outcome of guanadrel is reduction in blood pressure.

Nursing Process
Premedication Assessment
1. Obtain baseline blood pressure readings in the supine and standing positions.
2. Obtain baseline weight.

Planning
Availability. PO—10 and 25 mg tablets.

Implementation
Dosage and administration. Adult: PO—Initially 10 mg daily in two divided doses. Adjust the dosages weekly to monthly until the therapeutic goal has been attained. The usual dosage range is 20 to 75 mg divided into two to three daily doses.

Evaluation
Side effects to expect
ORTHOSTATIC HYPOTENSION. Orthostatic hypotension occurs frequently, especially with sudden changes in posture. Patients can generally avoid this complication by rising slowly from supine and sitting positions. Patients should also be cautioned not to stand in one position for prolonged periods. These orthostatic effects are increased with alcohol consumption or prolonged standing with little movement.

SEDATION. Sedation and lethargy commonly occur when guanadrel therapy is initiated or during adjustment to higher doses. These effects are most notable during the first few days and tend to subside with time.

Side effects to report

EDEMA. Some patients will develop significant salt and water retention, causing edema and congestive heart failure. Weigh patients daily, using the same scale, at the same time of day, in similar clothing. Report increases of 2 pounds or more per week.

Report edema of the extremities and increase in dyspnea, pallor, tachycardia, wheezing, and frothy or blood-tinged sputum.

Drug interactions

DRUGS THAT ENHANCE THERAPEUTIC AND TOXIC EFFECTS. Guanethidine, barbiturates, disopyramide, quinidine, diuretics, tranquilizers, antihistamines, alcohol, and beta-adrenergic blocking agents (such as propanolol, atenolol, pindolol, and others), diuretics, and other antihypertensive agents. Monitor the blood pressure response to the cumulative effects of antihypertensive agents. Take the blood pressures in supine and erect positions.

Monitor for an increase in severity of side effects such as sedation, hypotension, and bradycardia or tachycardia.

DRUGS THAT REDUCE THERAPEUTIC EFFECTS. Tricyclic antidepressants (amitriptyline, imipramine, and others), amphetamines, ephedrine, phenothiazines, monoamine oxidase inhibitors, and haloperidol. Monitor carefully for poor blood pressure control or a gradually increasing blood pressure.

guanethidine sulfate (gwan-eth′i-deen)
Ismelin (is′meh-lin)

Actions

Guanethidine depletes norephinephrine from postganglionic sympathetic nerve terminals. It also inhibits the release of norephinephrine in response to sympathetic nerve stimulation. Blood pressure decreases because of a reduction in cardiac output and peripheral vascular resistance. Because reflex-mediated vasoconstriction is blocked by guanethidine, a much greater hypotensive effect occurs when standing, and postural hypotension is common.

Uses

Guanethidine is recommended for use in refractory hypertension uncontrolled by other agents with fewer side effects. Guanethidine is used in combination with a diuretic.

Therapeutic Outcomes

The primary therapeutic outcome of guanethidine is reduction in blood pressure.

Nursing Process

Premedication Assessment
1. Obtain baseline blood pressure readings in the supine and standing positions.
2. Obtain baseline weight.

Planning
Availability. PO—10 and 25 mg tablets.

Implementation

Dosage and administration. Adult: PO—Initially 10 mg daily. Increase the dose 10 mg every 5 to 7 days, if the blood pressure measurements so indicate and side effects are tolerable. Maintenance doses range between 25 and 50 mg daily; however, much higher doses are occasionally required.

Evaluation
Side effects to expect

LIGHT-HEADEDNESS, WEAKNESS. Guanethidine causes arteriolar and venous dilatation that permits pools of blood to collect in the lower extremities, causing a reduction in cerebral blood flow. These symptoms often disappear during the day and can be lessened by rising slowly, sitting on the edge of the bed for a few minutes, and performing leg, foot, and toe exercises before standing.

These orthostatic effects are increased with alcohol consumption or prolonged standing with little movement.

Side effects to report

EDEMA. Some patients will develop significant salt and water retention, causing edema and heart failure. Weigh patients daily, using the same scale, at the same time of day, in similar clothing. Report increases of 2 pounds or more per week.

Report edema of the extremities and increase in dyspnea, pallor, tachycardia, wheezing, and frothy or blood-tinged sputum.

Drug interactions

DRUGS THAT ENHANCE THERAPEUTIC AND TOXIC EFFECTS. Barbiturates, disopyramide, quinidine, diuretics, tranquilizers, antihistamines, alcohol, and beta-adrenergic blocking agents (propranolol, atenolol, pindolol, and others), and other antihypertensive agents. Monitor the blood pressure response to the cumulative effects of antihypertensive agents. Take the blood pressure in supine and erect positions.

Monitor for an increase in severity of side effects, such as sedation, hypotension, and bradycardia or tachycardia.

DRUGS THAT REDUCE THERAPEUTIC EFFECTS. Tricyclic antidepressants (amitriptyline, imipramine, and others), amphetamines, ephedrine, phenothiazines, and haloperidol. Monitor carefully for poor blood pressure control or a gradually increasing blood pressure.

INSULIN AND ORAL HYPOGLYCEMIC AGENTS. Guanethidine may increase the hypoglycemic effects of insulin and oral hypoglycemic agents.

Monitor these patients for headache, weakness, decreasing muscle coordination, and diaphoresis. (Onset of hypoglycemic symptoms may be rapid.)

Give orange juice with two teaspoonfuls of sugar if the patient is still alert and responsive.

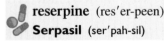

reserpine (res′er-peen)
Serpasil (ser′pah-sil)

Actions

Reserpine is an alkaloid obtained from the root of a species of *Rauwolfia*. It is one of the oldest antihypertensive agents available. Reserpine acts as an antihypertensive agent by reducing norepinephrine levels in peripheral nerve endings, which slows heart rate and reduces peripheral vascular resistance. It also stimulates the vagus nerve, causing a further reduction in heart rate. Reserpine also depletes norepinephrine from various other organs, including the brain. Brain depletion of norepinephrine and serotonin may be the cause of the sedative and depressive actions of reserpine. Reserpine's strong inhibition of sympathetic activity allows increased parasympatheitc activity to occur, which is responsible for some of its side effects, including nasal stuffiness, increased gastric acid secretion, diarrhea and bradycardia.

Uses

Reserpine has an extremely long duration of action; it may take 2 to 6 weeks before the maximal effect of the drug is seen. It is used to treat stage 1 hypertension. It is relatively inexpensive when compared with other antihypertensive agents and is thus preferred by funding agencies, but the side effects associated with therapy often lead to noncompliance.

Therapeutic Outcomes

The primary therapeutic outcome of reserpine is reduction in blood pressure.

Nursing Process

Premedication Assessment

1. Obtain baseline blood pressure readings in the supine and standing positions.
2. Obtain baseline weight.
3. Assess the patient's mental status—affective and cognitive behaviors should be used as a baseline for subsequent comparison. If depression is suspected, report to the physician.
4. Obtain baseline data relating to usual sleep pattern.

Planning
Availability. PO—0.1, 0.25, and 1 mg tablets.

Implementation
Dosage and administration. Adult: PO—Initially 0.5 mg daily for 1 to 2 weeks. Maintenance: 0.1 to 0.25 mg daily.

Evaluation
Side effects to expect

NASAL STUFFINESS. Encourage the patient not to treat this symptom with over-the-counter nasal decongestants because they aggravate the hypertension. Fortunately, this side effect tends to be self-limiting, but tell the patient to consult the physician if it becomes a serious problem.

DIARRHEA. Diarrhea and stomach cramps may be associated with depressed sympathetic activity. These side effects tend to be self-limiting, but if they persist or if there is an increase in abdominal pain the physician should be notified.

Side effects to report

DEPRESSION. Depression caused by this medication may progress to the point of the patient's becoming suicidal.

Assess the patient's affective (loneliness, sadness, anxiety, and anger), cognitive (confusion, ambivalence, and loss of interest), and other behavioral responses (agitation, irritability, altered activity level, and withdrawal) before starting therapy. After starting medication therapy with reserpine, carefully monitor the patient for changes in usual response

patterns. Assess otherwise normal emotions for an increase in duration or intensity.

Note the patient's degree of socialization, responses to stimulation, and changes in interactions with others. All individuals taking this drug should be monitored for development of depression, especially those with a history of depression.

NIGHTMARES, INSOMNIA. If these symptoms occur, report them to the physician for evaluation. Drug therapy may need to be changed.

GASTRIC SYMPTOMS. Patients experiencing gastric symptoms such as burning, pain, nausea, or vomiting should report them immediately because this medication can cause formation of new ulcers or exacerbation of old ulcers.

Drug interactions

DRUGS THAT ENHANCE THERAPEUTIC AND TOXIC EFFECTS. Phenothiazines, procainamide, disopyramide, thiothixene, quinidine, diuretics, tranquilizers, antihistamines, alcohol, beta-adrenergic blocking agents (propranolol, atenolol, pindolol, and others), and other antihypertensive agents. Monitor the blood pressure response to cumulative effects of antihypertensive agents. Take blood pressure readings in supine and erect positions.

Monitor for an increase in severity of side effects, such as sedation, hypotension, and bradycardia or tachycardia.

DRUGS THAT REDUCE THERAPEUTIC EFFECTS. Tricyclic antidepressants (amitriptyline, imipramine, doxepin, and others). Monitor carefully for poor blood pressure control or a gradually increasing blood pressure.

Drug Class: Direct Vasodilators

 hydralazine (hy-dral'ah-zeen)
Apresoline (ah-pres'o-leen)

Actions

Hydralazine causes direct arteriolar smooth muscle relaxation, resulting in reduced peripheral vascular resistance. The reduction in peripheral resistance causes a reflex increase in heart rate, cardiac output, and renin release with sodium and water retention. Consequently, the hypotensive effectiveness is reduced unless the patient is also taking a sympathetic inhibitor (for example, beta blockers) and a diuretic.

Uses

This antihypertensive agent is used to treat stages 3 and 4 hypertension and hypertension associated with renal disease and toxemia of pregnancy. It may also be used to provide symptomatic relief in patients with heart failure by reducing resistance (afterload) to left ventricular output.

Therapeutic Outcomes

The primary therapeutic outcome of hydralazine is reduction in blood pressure.

Nursing Process

Premedication Assessment
Obtain baseline blood pressure readings in the supine and standing positions.

Planning

Availability. PO—10, 25, 50, and 100 mg tablets; IV—20 mg/ml in 1 ml ampules.

Implementation

Dosage and administration. Adult: PO—Initially, 10 mg 4 times daily for the first 2 to 4 days, then 25 mg 4 times daily. The second week, increase the dosage to 50 mg 4 times daily as the patient tolerates the dosage and the blood pressure is brought under control. IM, IV—20 to 40 mg repeated as necessary. Monitor blood pressure frequently. Results usually become evident within 10 to 20 minutes.

Evaluation

Side effects to expect

NAUSEA, DIZZINESS, PALPITATIONS, TACHYCARDIA, NUMBNESS AND TINGLING IN THE LEGS, NASAL CONGESTION. Although these symptoms may be anticipated, they require monitoring. If severe, they should be reported so that the dosage can be adjusted appropriately. Nasal congestion can be treated with an antihistamine, such as chlorpheniramine.

ORTHOSTATIC HYPOTENSION. This may occur, particularly during initiation of therapy. Patients can generally avoid this complication by rising slowly from supine and sitting positions.

Side effects to report

FEVER, CHILLS, JOINT AND MUSCLE PAIN, SKIN ERUPTIONS. Tell patients to report the development of these symptoms. Monitor laboratory reports for leukocyte counts and the antinuclear antibody (ANA) titer.

Drug interactions

DRUGS THAT ENHANCE THERAPEUTIC AND TOXIC EFFECTS. Diuretics, alcohol, beta-adrenergic blocking agents (propranolol, atenolol, pindolol, and others), and other antihypertensive agents. Monitor the blood pressure response to the cumulative effects of antihypertensive agents. Take the blood pressures in supine and erect positions.

Monitor for an increase in severity of side effects, such as sedation, hypotension, and bradycardia or tachycardia.

minoxidil (min-ox′i-dil)

Loniten (lon′-i-ten) **Minodyl** (min-oh′dil)

Actions

Minoxidil acts by direct relaxation of the smooth muscle of arterioles, reducing peripheral vascular resistance. Because of the decrease in peripheral vascular resistance, there is a compensatory increase in heart rate and sodium and water retention. For this reason, minoxidil is usually administered in conjunction with a beta-adrenergic blocking agent and a potent diuretic such as furosemide or bumetanide.

Uses

Minoxidil is used only for severely hypertensive patients who do not respond adequately to maximum therapeutic doses of a diuretic and two other antihypertensive agents.

Therapeutic Outcomes

The primary therapeutic outcome of minoxidil is reduction in blood pressure.

Nursing Process

Premedication Assessment

1. Obtain baseline blood pressure readings in the supine and standing positions.
2. Obtain baseline weight.
3. Obtain resting pulse rate to serve as a baseline for subsequent comparisons.

Planning

Availability. PO—2.5 and 10 mg tablets.

Implementation

Dosage and administration. Adult: PO—Initially 5 mg daily. Dosage may be gradually increased after at least 3-day intervals to 10 mg, 20 mg, and then 40 mg daily in 1 to 2 doses. Maintenance dosage: 10 to 40 mg daily. Maximum dosage is 100 mg daily.

Evaluation

Side effects to expect

HAIR GROWTH. Within 3 to 6 weeks after start of therapy, about 80% of patients will start developing *hypertrichosis*—an elongation, thickening, and increased pigmentation of fine body hair. It is usually noticed first on the face and later extends to the back, arms, legs, and scalp.

Growth may be controlled by shaving or by depilatory creams. After discontinuation, new hair growth stops, but it may take up to 6 months for complete return to pretreatment appearance.

Side effects to report

GYNECOMASTIA. Swelling or tenderness of the breasts may develop in men.

SALT AND WATER RETENTION. This drug is usually administered with a diuretic and a beta-adrenergic blocking agent to reduce the incidence of fluid retention and for additive antihypertensive effects.

Perform daily weights using the same scale, in similar clothing, and at approximately the same time of day. Report gains of more than 2 pounds per week and swelling or puffiness of the face, ankles, or hands to the physician.

INCREASED RESTING PULSE. Instruct and validate the patient's ability to take own pulse.

A resting pulse that increases 20 or more beats per minute above normal should be reported.

LIGHT-HEADEDNESS, FAINTING, DIZZINESS. These symptoms should be reported to the physician. If possible, the patient's blood pressure during these episodes should be taken and reported.

ORTHOSTATIC HYPOTENSION. This may occur, particularly during initiation of therapy. Patients can generally avoid this complication by rising slowly from supine and sitting positions.

HEART FAILURE. Assess for development of dyspnea, orthopnea, edema, and weight gain.

Drug interactions

DRUGS THAT ENHANCE THERAPEUTIC AND TOXIC EFFECTS. Diuretics, alcohol, beta-adrenergic blocking agents (propanolol, atenolol, pindolol, and others), guanethidine, guanadrel, and other antihypertensive agents. Monitor the blood pressure response caused by the cumulative effects of anti-hypertensive agents. Take the blood pressures in supine and erect positions.

Monitor for increase in severity of side effects, such as sedation, hypotension, and bradycardia or tachycardia.

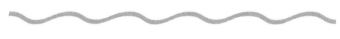

nitroprusside sodium (ny-tro-prus′ide)
Nipride (ny′pryd)

Actions

Nitroprusside is a potent vasodilator that acts directly on the smooth muscle of blood vessels. It produces both arterial and venous vasodilation, thus reducing both preload and after-load on the heart.

Uses

Nitroprusside is used in patients with sudden severe hypertensive crisis, and in those with refractory heart failure.

Therapeutic Outcomes

The primary therapeutic outcomes of nitroprusside are reduction in blood pressure and improvement is symptoms associated with heart failure.

Planning
Availability. IV—10 mg/ml in 5 ml vials.

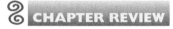

CHAPTER REVIEW

The public has made significant strides in the past two decades in recognizing the risk factors associated with cardiovascular disease. This awareness had led to reduction in the incidence of heart attacks and strokes. Hypertension, however, is still a national health problem. Nurses can play a significant role in public education efforts, monitor for noncompliance, monitor blood pressure response to therapy, and encourage patients to make changes in lifestyle to reduce the severity of hypertension.

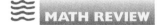

MATH REVIEW

1. Ordered: Clonidine hydrochloride (Catapres) 0.6 mg PO daily in two divided doses.
   On hand: Clonidine hydrochloride (Catapres) 0.1 and 0.2 mg tablets.

Give: _____tablets of _____mg and _____tablets of _____mg.
(Catapres is available in 0.3 mg tablets. What nursing action would be appropriate?)

2. Ordered: Methyldopa (Aldomet) 3 g PO daily in three divided doses.
   On hand: Methyldopa (Aldomet) 500 mg tablets.
   Give: _____tablets per dose.
   What time schedule could be established for this order?

CRITICAL THINKING QUESTIONS

1. Mr. Longsdanto is receiving 3 g per day of methyldopa. Sexual dysfunction is a possible nursing diagnosis related to methyldopa therapy manifested by impotence or failure to ejaculate. Address the health teaching needed and how the nurse could approach this subject.

2. Discuss the essential patient education needed regarding the initiation of therapy with prazosin.

3. State the nursing assessments needed to monitor therapeutic response and the development of side effects to expect or report from beta-adrenergic blocking agents and calcium antagonists.

4. Review beta-adrenergic blocking agent information in the monograph and develop patient education objectives for a patient receiving this class of drugs for treatment of hypertension.

5. Mrs. Janousek is being started on a drug regimen for hypertension that includes the use of reserpine. Initially her BP is 160/100, pulse is 64, respirations are 20 per minute and weight is 148 pounds. She seems quiet, introspective and contributes little information other than "yes" or "no" responses during an initial assessment. What further nursing actions would be appropriate?

6. Mr. Sanchez, age 56, is receiving quanethidine and a diuretic for treatment of hypertension that has not been controlled previously by other antihypertensive therapy. His weight is 168 pounds, BP is 190/110, pulse is 78, and respirations are 18 per minute. He has type I diabetes mellitus. Design a specific plan for nursing assessments needed for Mr. Sanchez before and after initiation of his antihypertensive regimen.

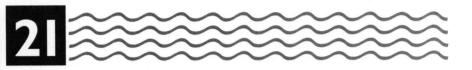

21

Drugs Used to Treat Heart Failure

CHAPTER CONTENT

Objectives

1. Summarize the pathophysiology of heart failure, including the body's compensatory mechanisms.

2. Identify the goals of treatment of heart failure.

3. Identify the similarity in spelling of the generic names of the major cardiac glycosides.

4. Explain the process of digitalizing a patient, including the initial dose, preparation and administration of the medication, and nursing assessments needed to monitor therapeutic response and digitalis toxicity.

5. Describe safety precautions associated with the preparation and administration of digitalis glycosides.

6. State the primary actions of digitalis glycosides, angiotensin-converting enzyme inhibitors, nitrates, and calcium channel blockers on cardiac output.

7. Identify essential assessment data, nursing interventions, and health teaching needed for a patient with heart failure.

Key Words

systolic dysfunction	positive inotropy
diastolic dysfunction	negative chronotropy
inotropic agents	digitalization
digitalis toxicity	

HEART FAILURE

Heart failure is a cluster of signs and symptoms that arise when the left or right ventricle or both ventricles lose the ability to pump enough blood to meet the body's circulatory needs. There are several causes of heart failure, the most common of which is **systolic dysfunction.** Normally the heart pumps with regularity to support the body's need for blood flow and oxygenation of the vital organs and muscles. Systolic heart failure results from the heart's inability to contract with sufficient force to pump all the blood (decreased cardiac output) with which it is presented to meet the body's oxygenation needs (decreased tissue perfusion). Early clinical symptoms are decreased exercise tolerance and poor perfusion to peripheral tissues. As the condition progresses, the left ventricle chamber enlarges (left ventricular hypertrophy) and an increase in blood volume is required to fill the expanding ventricle to maintain cardiac output. Causes of systolic dysfunction are those that cause damage to heart muscle itself. The most common is coronary artery disease leading to myocardial infarction. Other causes are arrhythmias, cardiomyopathies, and congenital heart disease. Usually the left ventricle fails first, but with progression of the disease the right ventricle also enlarges because of increased pulmonary resistance and eventually fails.

Diastolic dysfunction causes heart failure because the left ventricle develops a "stiffness," failing to relax enough between contractions to allow adequate filling before the next contraction. Symptoms of diastolic dysfunction are pulmonary congestion and peripheral edema. There are many causes for the development of diastolic dysfunction, such as constrictive pericarditis, ventricular muscle hypertrophy caused by chronic hypertension, valvular heart disease causing flow resistance, and aortic stenosis.

When the vital organs and peripheral tissues are not adequately perfused, compensatory mechanisms begin to overcome the inadequate heart output. The sympathetic nervous system releases epinephrine and norepinephrine, producing tachycardia and increasing contractility. The increased sympathetic stimulation also increases peripheral vasoconstriction, causing an increased afterload against which the heart must pump, resulting in a further decrease in cardiac output. The renin-angiotensin-aldosterone system stimulates renal distal tubule sodium and water retention in an effort to increase circulating blood volume, which increases preload to the heart. There is increased production of vasopressin (antidiuretic hormone) from the pituitary gland that increases water recovery from the kidneys and increases intravascular volume and preload. With decreased perfusion secondary to low cardiac output, the kidneys increase sodium reabsorption in the proximal tubules to help expand circulating blood volume. The increased intravascular volume initially improves tissue perfusion, but over time excessive amounts of sodium and water are retained, causing increased pressure within the capillaries and resulting in edema formation.

The early symptoms of heart failure are variable depending on the underlying etiology of the disease. Patients with long-standing bronchitis and chronic obstructive lung disease develop right-sided failure and have symptoms of gradual weight gain, peripheral edema, and diminishing exercise tolerance. Patients who develop left ventricular systolic failure secondary to a myocardial infarction have hypotension, acute shortness of breath, and shock, but little peripheral edema. Patients with long-term, poorly controlled hypertension often develop signs and symptoms of both right and left ventricular failure with tachycardia, dyspnea, orthopnea, paroxysmal nocturnal dyspnea, jugular venous distention, peripheral pitting edema, and diminished exercise tolerance.

Treatment

The goals of treatment of heart failure are reduction of signs and symptoms associated with fluid overload, increased exercise tolerance, and prolongation of life. If the heart failure is acute the patient must be hospitalized for a diagnostic workup to determine the underlying cause. Heart failure is treated by correction of the underlying disease (for example, coronary artery disease, hypertension, or thyroid disease), bed rest, sodium-restricted diet, and control of symptoms with a combination of pharmacologic agents.

Drug Therapy

Actions

Heart failure is treated with a combination of vasodilator, inotropic, and diuretic therapy. If the failure is acute, most therapy will be administered by intravenous (IV) routes in an intensive care unit. Vasodilators are used to reduce the strain on the left ventricle by reducing the systemic vascular resistance (afterload) against which the left ventricle is working. The reduced vascular resistance will also increase tissue perfusion to vital organs and muscles. The second goal of use of vasodilators is to reduce preload so that the high volume of blood returning to the heart is decreased. The reduction in preload decreases pulmonary congestion and allows the patient to breath more easily.

Inotropic agents stimulate the heart to increase the force of contractions, thus boosting cardiac output. This also helps reduce pulmonary congestion and improve tissue perfusion. As renal perfusion is improved, potent diuretics are administered to enhance sodium and water excretion. This provides substantial symptomatic relief to the patient, in addition to reducing the workload on the heart.

Uses

Intravenous nitroglycerin (see Chapter 23) and nitroprusside (see Chapter 20) are used as vasodilators to reduce preload and afterload in critically ill patients. Angiotensin-converting enzyme (ACE) inhibitors are the mainstay of oral vasodilator therapy for treating chronic heart failure. Other vasodilators used are minoxidil and hydralazine (see Chapter 20). The calcium ion antagonists (for example, nifedipine, amlodipine, and nicardipine) may be used to reduce afterload in patients with heart failure; however, the calcium ion antagonists also have negative inotropic properties that can aggravate heart failure in certain patients (see Chapters 20 and 23).

Inotropic agents used to treat acute failure are intravenous dobutamine or amrinone or milrinone. Digoxin, a digitalis glycoside, has been used for decades for treating heart conditions when an oral inotropic agent is needed. Most patients with heart failure require a loop diuretic such as furosemide or bumetanide (see Chapter 25) to assist in reduction of fluid and sodium overload.

Nursing Process for Heart Failure Therapy

Assessment

History of heart disease. Obtain a history of prior treatment for heart and related cardiovascular disease, for example, hypertension and hyperlipidemia.

Medication history. Obtain details of all medications prescribed. Tactfully determine if the prescribed medications are being taken regularly and if not, why.

History of six cardinal signs of heart disease

Dyspnea (difficulty breathing). Record if dyspnea occurs while resting, on exertion, or while asleep at night (paroxysmal nocturnal dyspnea). Are symptoms of dyspnea accompanied by a productive or nonproductive cough? Ask the patient to describe sputum. (With heart failure it is frothy and may be blood tinged.) How has the patient been coping with any orthopneic problems?

Chest pain. Because heart failure results in decreased cardiac output and lower oxygenation of tissue, the heart may experience inadequate tissue perfusion, resulting in chest pain. Record data as to the time of onset, frequency, duration, and quality of chest pain. Note any conditions the patient has found that either aggravate or relieve the chest pain.

Fatigue. Determine whether fatigue occurs only at specific times of the day, such as toward evening. Ask the patient if fatigue decreases in relation to a decrease in activity level or is present at about the same time daily.

Edema. Record the presence or absence of edema. If present, record location of edema, assessment data (for example, degree of pitting present; ankle, midcalf, or thigh circumference), degree of pitting present and appearance of the skin (for example, shiny or weeping with pressure), and any measures the patient has used to eliminate edema. Chart the time of day that the edema is present (for example, when arising in the morning; evening), and the specific parts on the body where present. When performing daily weights, use the same scale, at the same time of day, with the patient in a similar type of clothing.

Syncope. Ask the patient about conditions surrounding any episodes of syncope. Record the degree of symptoms, such as general muscle weakness, inability to stand upright, feeling faint, or loss of consciousness. Record what activities, if any, bring on these syncopal episodes.

Palpitations. Record the patient's description of palpitations, such as, "my heart skips some beats." Ask if these conditions are preceded by strenuous or mild exercise and how long the palpitations last.

Indications of altered cardiac function

Basic mental status. Identify the individual's level of consciousness (for example, drowsiness, lethargic, confused; orientation to date, time, and place). Assess the clarity of thought present. Both level of consciousness and clarity of thought are indicators of adequate cerebral perfusion.

Vital signs. Obtain vital signs as often as necessary to monitor the patient's status.

Blood pressure. Obtain baseline readings and a history of prior treatment for hypertension. Monitor at specific intervals and report a narrowing pulse pressure (difference between systolic and diastolic readings). With heart failure hypotension may be present.

Temperature. Record every 8 hours; monitor more frequently if elevated.

Pulse. Record the rate, quality, and rhythm of the pulse. With heart failure, tachycardia may represent an attempt by the body to compensate for decreased cardiac output.

Heart and lung sounds. Nurses with advanced skills can perform auscultation and percussion to note changes in heart size and heart and lung sounds. Lung fields are assessed in a sitting position to detect abnormal lung sounds, for example, wheezes or rales. (Refer to a medical-surgical nursing textbook for details of performing these skills.)

Skin color. Note the color of the skin, mucous membranes, tongue, earlobes, and nailbeds. Chart exact location of any pallor or cyanosis present.

Neck veins. Record any jugular vein distention.

Clubbing. Inspect the fingernails and toenails for clubbing. Perform the blanching test on fingernails and toenails.

Central venous pressure. If ordered, obtain baseline and subsequent readings at specified intervals. Report alterations within parameters indicated by the physician.

Abdomen. Inspect abdomen, noting size, shape, softness, or distention. Read history to obtain data relating to liver enlargement.

Fluid volume status. Continue to assess intake and output at intervals appropriate to the patient's condition (every hour during acute, severe status). Report intake that exceeds output. Ask about the frequency of nocturia. This often occurs with heart failure because renal perfusion is improved when the patient lies down and fluid moves from the interstitial spaces back into the general circulation.

Laboratory tests. Review laboratory tests and report abnormal results to the physician promptly. Tests include serum electrolytes, especially potassium, calcium, magnesium, and sodium; arterial blood gases; serum lipids; electrocardiogram (ECG); echocardiogram; chest x-ray; urinalysis and kidney function; and hemodynamic assessments.

Nutrition. Obtain a history of the diet that has been prescribed and assess compliance to the diet. Obtain data regarding appetite and the presence of nausea and vomiting.

Activity and exercise. Ask questions to gather information about the effect of exercise on the patient's functioning. Is the person normally sedentary or moderately or very active? Has there been a reduction in activity level to handle associated fatigue or dyspnea? Are the activities of daily living being performed by the person?

Anxiety level. Patients experiencing cardiac disorders exhibit varying degrees of anxiety. Note the level of anxiety or depression present.

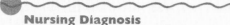

Nursing Diagnosis

- Cardiac output, decreased (indication)
- Gas exchange, impaired (indication)
- Activity intolerance (indication)
- Tissue perfusion, altered: decreased (indication)
- Fluid volume excess (indication)

Planning

Medication. Order medications prescribed and schedule these on the medication administration record (MAR). Perform focused assessments to determine effectiveness and side effects of pharmacologic interventions.

History of six cardinal signs of cardiovascular disease. Individualize the care plan to address the patient's degree of dyspnea, chest pain, fatigue, edema, syncope, and palpitations.

Altered cardiac functions. Plan interventions to address indicators of altered cardiac functions that will stabilize the patient's condition. Educate the patient with heart failure to the physiologic and psychologic changes that occur, and plan with the patient for the needed interventions and lifestyle changes.

Laboratory tests. Order stat and subsequent laboratory studies.

Implementation

- Obtain baseline arterial blood gases. Administer oxygen therapy as prescribed and periodically review results.
- Position the patient in Fowler's or semi-Fowler's position to maximize lung expansion and oxygenation. Reposition the patient at least every 2 hours; use alternate mattress and provide skin care to prevent breakdown.
- Auscultate lung sounds at specified intervals consistent with the patient's condition. Assess for neck vein distention.
- Perform daily weights using the same scale, in similar clothing, at the same time daily—usually before breakfast. Record and report significant weight changes. (Weight gains and losses are the best indicators of fluid gain or loss.) As appropriate to patient's condition, obtain and record abdominal girth measurements.
- When fluid restrictions are prescribed, one half of fluids is generally given with meals and the other half is given on a per shift basis.
- Maintain degree of dietary sodium restriction prescribed.
- Avoid use of salt substitutes when potassium-sparing diuretics are given.
- Administer medications prescribed (for example, bronchodilators, ACE inhibitors, nitrates, digitalis glycosides, diuretics, antianxiety agents) on schedule or as needed. Monitor degree of response achieved and report ineffectiveness.
- Pace nursing activities to avoid undue fatigue; implement exercise gradually while monitoring vital signs before and after ambulation. Assess for signs and symptoms of fatigue or poor oxygenation before, during, and after exercise.

- Do not plan exercise or ambulation within 1 hour after eating to avoid excessive oxygen depletion.
- Monitor vital signs and perform focused assessment of heart and respiratory functions at specified intervals.
- Perform neurologic assessment to determine changes in mental status.
- Deal calmly with an anxious patient; offer explanations of procedures being performed; listen to concerns and intervene appropriately.
- Monitor the rate of IV infusions carefully; contact physician regarding concentration of admixtures of drugs to IV infusion solution when limitation of fluids is indicated.
- Give stool softeners to avoid Valsalva maneuver.

Patient Education and Health Promotion

- Teach the patient and significant others the functional changes caused by heart failure. Emphasize the need for lifelong treatment and adherence to drug therapy, diet, and exercise regimens to obtain maximum control of the disease process.
- Assess understanding of symptoms that indicate when to call the doctor: dyspnea, a productive cough, worsening fatigue, edema in the feet, ankles, or legs, weight gain of 2 pounds or more in a 2-day period, and development of angina or chest pain, palpitation, or confusion.
- Provide instructions on taking blood pressure, pulse, and respirations and explain acceptable parameters for each, as prescribed by the physician.
- Explain oxygen therapy that is prescribed and, if being discharged on O2, where to obtain oxygen equipment and supplies, rate of administration, and the care and maintenance of the equipment.
- Demonstrate patient positioning in a semi-Fowler's or high-Fowler's position. Discuss adaptations needed at home to use these positions for relief of dyspnea. Explain that an upright position provides maximum oxygenation.
- Teach good skin care and the need to change positions at least every 2 hours, especially when edema is present. Have the patient inspect ankles, feet, and abdomen daily for edema. If using a recliner or bed, the sacral area should also be checked regularly for edema.
- Discuss the importance of spacing of activities of daily living to conserve energy and avoid fatigue. Review the prescribed activity level and stress monitoring pulse, dyspnea, and fatigue levels as a guide to when the patient is overexerting.
- Explore coping mechanisms the person uses in response to stress. Discuss how the patient is adapting to the needed changes in lifestyle to manage the disease process. Address depression issues if present.
- Diet therapy is an integral part of the treatment of heart failure. Schedule meetings with the nutritionist to learn how to manage specific dietary modifications prescribed (usually a low-sodium, high-potassium diet with weight reduction parameters for obese patients). If possible, have the patient practice food selections using the daily menus while still in the hospital. The nurse can then offer guidance. Teach about foods low in sodium and high in potassium. Potassium restrictions may be indicated if the patient is taking a potassium-sparing diuretic. Salt substitutes are high in potassium so use must be limited.
- Fluid restrictions may be imposed; discuss specific ways to manage these limitations.
- Teach the signs and symptoms of potassium deficiency or excess, depending on medications prescribed.

Medication regimen. Heart failure requires lifelong treatment, and adherence to prescribed therapy is imperative to gain control of the disease.

Teach the signs and symptoms of **digitalis toxicity** (anorexia, nausea, vomiting, bradycardia, visual disturbances, and psychiatric disturbances). Explain medication administration parameters: if the pulse is below 60 or above 100 do not administer digitalis until checking with the physician. (An antidote is available for digitalis toxicity.) Instruct the patient that it is important to report for blood draws to check serum levels of the drug at the specific times scheduled.

Diuretics should be taken in the morning to avoid a nighttime diuresis. Depending on the type of diuretic prescribed, potassium supplements may be necessary. However, if a potassium-sparing diuretic is ordered, limiting potassium intake may be appropriate. Salt substitutes should be avoided because they are high in potassium content.

Tell the patient to perform daily weights using the same scale, in similar clothing, at the same time daily—usually before breakfast. Record and report significant weight changes because weight gains and losses are the best indicators of fluid gain or loss. Usually a gain of 2 pounds in 2 days should be reported.

When ACE inhibitors are ordered, hypotension, hyperkalemia, and a persistent cough are possible. Discuss management of these side effects.

Fostering health maintenance. Throughout the course of treatment, discuss medication information and how it will benefit the patient.

Drug therapy is one component of the treatment of heart failure, and it is critical that the medications be taken as prescribed. Provide the patient and significant others with the important information contained in the specific drug monograph for the drug prescribed. Additional health teaching and nursing interventions for drug side effects to expect and report will be found in each drug monograph.

It is important to control the underlying condition causing the heart failure (for example, hypertension or hyperlipidemia). The patient and family must understand the importance of complying with diet, exercise, and other prescribed treatments designed to maximize the patient's degree of oxygenation.

Seek cooperation and understanding of the following points so that medication compliance is increased: name of medication, dosage, route and times of administration, side effects to expect, and side effects to report.

Enlist the patient's aid in developing and maintaining a written record of monitoring parameters (for example, pulse rate, blood pressure, degree of dyspnea and what precipitates it, chest pain, edema) (see the box on p. 282). Instruct the patient to bring the written record to follow-up visits.

PATIENT EDUCATION & MONITORING FORM — Cardiovascular Agents

MEDICATIONS	COLOR	TO BE TAKEN

Name _____

Physician _____

Physician's phone _____

Next appt.* _____

PARAMETERS		DAY OF DISCHARGE							COMMENTS
Weight	AM / PM								
Blood Pressure	AM / PM								
Pulse	AM / PM								
Chest pain	Activity Lasting how long? How many nitroglycerin taken?								
Bowel movements	Normal (times) Diarrhea (times) Constipation								
Fatigue All day 10 After exercise 5 Normal 1									
Edema	Morning								
	Evening								
	Other								
	Can wear shoes, slippers?								
Visual changes	Clear, hazy, blurred, colored halos?								
Fainting and dizziness	Standing, sitting, or lying								
Heart beat ("Skips a beat," "racing" feeling, or irregular)	Times per day At rest Activity Asleep								
Difficulty breathing	Times per day At rest Activity Asleep (___) of pillows?								
Exercise: Degree of tiredness: Extremely 10 Very 5 Normal 1	Walk across room Walk (___) stairs Walk (___) blocks								
Sexual activity (Note pain experienced in comments at right side.) Very tired 10 Tired 5 Normal 1									

*Please bring this record with you to your next appointment.
Use the back of this sheet for additional information.

Drug Class: Digitalis Glycosides

digoxin (di-joks'in)
Lanoxin (lah-noks'in)

Actions

The digitalis glycosides are among the oldest therapeutic agents for the treatment of heart failure. Their use in medicine dates to the eighteenth century. In 1785 William Withering, an English physician and botanist, published excellent observations on the treatment of various ailments with digitalis. Once derived naturally from the dried leaves of *Digitalis purpurea* (purple foxglove), the drug is now synthetically prepared.

Digitalis glycosides have two primary actions on the heart: digitalis increases the force of contraction (**positive inotropy**) and slows the heart rate (**negative chronotropy**), reducing the conduction velocity and prolonging the refractory period at the atrioventricular (AV) node. The exact mechanisms of these actions are unknown, but the net result is that the heart is able to fill and empty more completely, thus improving circulation. With improved circulation, there is a reduction in systemic and pulmonary congestion, a reduction in heart size toward normal, and a reduction in peripheral edema because of better perfusion of blood through the kidneys.

Uses

Digitalis glycosides (digoxin and digitoxin) are used to treat moderate to severe systolic heart failure not responding to diuretics and ACE inhibitors. Digitalis glycosides may also be used in the treatment of atrial fibrillation, atrial flutter, and paroxysmal tachycardia. The digitalis glycosides are generally not used in treating diastolic heart failure and may indeed worsen this condition.

The goal of treatment for heart failure is to give adequate doses of digitalis so that the most optimal cardiac effects are achieved and cardiac output is increased, pulse rate is slowed, and vasoconstriction decreases, resulting in the disappearance of many of the signs and symptoms of heart failure (that is, dyspnea, orthopnea, and edema). The patient is often given a loading dose of the drug over a period of hours or days necessary to produce the desired cardiac effect. This is known as **digitalization** of the patient. A maintenance dose is then given, usually once daily. Many patients must continue to take digitalis preparations for the remainder of their lives.

Digoxin is the most commonly used member of the digitalis glycoside family. It digitalizes more rapidly than digitoxin. Oral administrations may digitalize within a few hours and IV injections within a few minutes.

LIFE SPAN ISSUES

DIGOXIN AND DIGITOXIN

Pediatric dosages of digoxin and digitoxin are extremely small and should be measured in a tuberculin syringe using the metric scale. All dosage calculations should be checked with a second qualified nurse in accordance with institutional policy.

Therapeutic Outcomes

The primary therapeutic outcomes expected from digitalis glycoside therapy are improved cardiac output resulting in improved tissue perfusion and improved tolerance to activity as demonstrated by the ability to perform activities of daily living without supplemental oxygen therapy or fatigue.

Nursing Process

Premedication Assessment

1. Take *apical* pulse for *1 full minute*; follow institution guidelines for withholding drug, for example, pulse less than 60 or greater than 100 beats per minute. NOTE: In long-term care setting, radial pulse may be acceptable.
2. Obtain baseline data before initiation of therapy, such as vital signs, lung sounds, weight, laboratory studies (for example, serum electrolytes and liver and kidney function studies).
3. As therapy progresses, monitor for development of digitalis toxicity, hypokalemia, or sudden increase in pulse rate that previously has been normal or low.

Planning

Availability. PO—0.125, 0.25, and 0.5 mg tablets; 0.05, 0.1, and 0.2 mg Gelcaps; pediatric elixir, 0.05 mg/ml. IV—0.25 mg/ml in 1 and 2 ml vials and ampules and 0.1 mg/ml in 1 ml ampules.

Implementation

Digitalization. Digitalization is the administration of a larger dose of digoxin for an initial period of 24 to 48 hours. After this initial "loading" period, the patient is switched to a daily maintenance dose. Be sure to monitor the patient carefully for signs of digitalis toxicity.

Pulse variations. Always take the apical pulse 1 *full* minute *before* administering any digitalis preparation. Do not administer the drug when the pulse rate in an adult is below 60 beats per minute until the physician is consulted. In a child report findings below 90 beats per minute. The physician may decide to withhold the medication.

Accurate identification. Digitalis glycosides are frequently given in minute amounts. *Always* have mathematic computations checked by another professional nurse. Use the correct type of syringe to facilitate accuracy in dosage measurement.

Always question any order that is unusual *before* administration. Read the medication label carefully; *digoxin* and *digitoxin* are *not* the same.

Dosage and administration. Give digoxin after meals to minimize gastric irritation. NOTE: A baseline ECG is recommended before initiation of therapy. Assuming the patient has not ingested a digitalis preparation in the preceding 2 weeks, the following dosages apply.

Adult. PO—digitalizing: 0.25 to 0.50 mg initially followed by 0.125 mg every 6 hours until adequate digitalization is achieved; maintenance: 0.125 to 0.25 mg daily. Some patients may require 0.375 to 0.5 mg daily. IV—digitalizing: 0.25 to 0.5 mg initially followed by 0.125 mg every 6 hours until adequate digitalization is achieved. Administer at a rate of 0.5 to 1 ml per minute; maintenance: same as for PO administration. Adult therapeutic blood levels are 0.5 to 1.8 ng/ml.

Pediatric. Premature: IM or IV—digitalizing: 0.015 to 0.02 mg/kg initially followed by 0.01 mg every 6 to 8 hours for 2 doses (total digitalizing dose: 0.03 to 0.05 mg/kg); maintenance: 0.003 to 0.006 mg/kg every 12 hours.

Ages 2 weeks to 2 years: PO—digitalizing: 0.03 to 0.04 mg/kg initially followed by 0.02 mg/kg every 6 to 8 hours for 2 doses (total digitalizing dose: 0.06 to 0.08 mg/kg); maintenance: 0.006 to 0.01 mg/kg every 12 hours. IM or IV—digitalizing: 0.02 to 0.03 mg/kg initially, followed by 0.01 to 0.015 mg/kg every 6 to 8 hours for 2 doses (total digitalizing dose: 0.04 to 0.06 mg/kg); maintenance: 0.003 to 0.006 mg/kg every 12 hours.

Over 2 years of age: PO—digitalizing: 0.02 to 0.03 mg/kg initially, followed by 0.01 to 0.015 mg every 6 to 8 hours for 2 doses (total digitalizing dose: 0.04 to 0.06 mg/kg); maintenance: 0.004 to 0.009 mg/kg every 12 hours. IM or IV—digitalizing: 0.01 to 0.02 mg/kg initially, followed by 0.005 to 0.01 mg/kg every 6 to 8 hours for 2 doses (total digitalizing dose: 0.02 to 0.04 mg/kg); maintenance: 0.002 to 0.004 mg/kg every 12 hours.

Serum levels. Serum levels of digitalis are performed to measure the amount of digitalis in the bloodstream. Blood should be drawn before the daily dose of medication or at least 6 hours after administration. It is important to be consistent in the time of drawing the blood and administering the dose if more than one serum level is to be drawn in the same patient.

Treatment of digitalis toxicity. Basic treatment of digitalis-induced arrhythmias consists of stopping the digitalis and any potassium-depleting diuretics, checking the potassium level (administering potassium as indicated), and administering antiarrhythmics (for example, phenytoin and lidocaine). In some instances, atropine may be prescribed for sinus bradycardia. A pacemaker may be necessary for continuing bradycardia.

In cases of severe digitalis intoxication—as indicated by life-threatening arrhythmias such as ventricular tachycardia, fibrillation or severe sinus bradycardia, steady-state digoxin serum concentrations greater than 10 ng/ml, or a serum potassium concentration greater than 5mEq/L in a known case of digitalis ingestion—treatment with an antidote, digoxin immune Fab (ovine) (Digibind), is usually indicated. This product contains antigen-binding fragments from sheep that have been injected with a digoxin–human albumin complex, against which the sheep makes antibodies. The antibodies are harvested and purified into the antigen-binding fragments that have strong binding affinity for digoxin. When injected into humans who have received digoxin (or digitoxin), the fragments bind to molecules of digoxin, making them unavailable for binding at the site of action. The fragment-digoxin complex accumulates in the blood and is excreted by the kidneys. Improvement in signs and symptoms of digitalis intoxication begins less than 30 minutes after injection of the antigen-binding fragments.

Evaluation
Side effects to report

DIGITALIS TOXICITY. Cardiac effects: Always observe the patient for the development of a pulse deficit, bradycardia (heart rate below 60 beats per minute), tachycardia (heart rate over 100 beats per minute), or bigeminy. These may be signs of developing heart block. Whenever the individual is attached to a monitor, the pattern should be closely watched for any type of abnormal cardiac arrhythmia.

In children, digitalis toxicity is often first detected by the development of atrial arrhythmias.

Noncardiac effects: Noncardiac symptoms of digitalis toxicity are often vague and are difficult to separate from symptoms of heart disease. Any patient taking digitalis products who develops loss of appetite, nausea, vomiting, diarrhea, extreme fatigue, weakness of the arms and legs, psychiatric disturbances (nightmares, agitation, listlessness, or hallucinations), or visual disturbances (hazy or blurred vision, difficulty in reading, and difficulty in red-green color perception) should be evaluated for digitalis toxicity.

Other diseases: The patient's other clinical conditions may also induce digitalis intoxication. Patients who suffer from hypothyroidism, acute myocardial infarction, renal disease, severe respiratory disease, or far-advanced heart failure may require lower than normal doses of the digitalis glycosides. Monitor closely.

ELECTROLYTE BALANCE. Adverse effects of digitalis may also be induced by electrolyte imbalance, resulting in hypokalemia, hypomagnesemia, and hypocalcemia. (See Drug Interactions for agents that may induce electrolyte imbalance, p. 285.)

Monitor lab reports and notify the physician of deviations from the normal range of 4 to 5.4 mEq/L of potassium. Always monitor the pulse carefully if potassium level is abnormal. Hypokalemia is especially likely to occur when the patient exhibits nausea, vomiting, diarrhea, or heavy diuresis.

Drug interactions

DRUGS THAT ENHANCE THERAPEUTIC AND TOXIC EFFECTS. Nefazodone, quinidine, nifedipine, verapamil, antibiotics, propafenone, beta-adrenergic blocking agents (such as atenolol, esmolol, timolol, nadolol, propranolol, and others), succinylcholine, calcium gluconate, and calcium chloride. Monitor for signs and symptoms of digitalis toxicity.

DRUGS THAT REDUCE THERAPEUTIC EFFECTS. Cholestyramine, neomycin, and antacids. Monitor patient symptoms for response to therapy; recurrence or intensification of the patient's disease should be reported to the physician.

LIFE SPAN ISSUES

DIGITALIS TOXICITY

Digitalis toxicity frequently occurs in the elderly because digitalis has a long half-life. Early symptoms of toxicity are anorexia and mild nausea but are frequently overlooked by the elderly or are not associated with medicine toxicity. Any change in pulse rhythm and rate or central nervous systems signs (mental status, orientation, change in color vision, hallucinations, or behavioral changes) should be investigated and reported. In children, digitalis toxicity is often first detected by the development of atrial arrhythmias.

DRUGS THAT MAY ALTER ELECTROLYTE BALANCE, ALTERING DIGITALIS RESPONSE. Drugs that may alter digitalis response and the incidence of any of the side effects by alteration of electrolyte balance include the following. For hypokalemia:

- Amphotericin B (Fungizone)
- Bumetanide (Bumex)
- Chlorthalidone (Hygroton)
- Corticosteroids
- Ethacrynic acid (Edecrin)
- Furosemide (Lasix)
- Metolazone (Zaroxolyn)
- Thiazide diuretics

For hyperkalemia:

- Amiloride (Midamor)
- Beta-adrenergic blockers
- Heparin
- Mannitol infusions
- Potassium chloride
- Potassium gluconate
- Potassium penicillin G
- Potassium supplements (K-Lyte, Kaon, K-Lor, others)
- Salt substitutes
- Succinylcholine

For hypomagnesemia:

- Chlorthalidone (Hygroton)
- Ethacrynic acid (Edecrin)
- Ethanolamine
- Furosemide (Lasix)
- Metolazone (Zaroxolyn)
- Neomycin (Mycifradin)
- Thiazide diuretics

Drug Class: Phosphodiesterase Inhibitors

amrinone (am'rhin-own)
Inocor (aye'noh-cohr)

Actions

Amrinone is an inotropic agent that increases the force and velocity of myocardial contractions by inhibiting phosphodiesterase enzymes in heart muscle. It also is a vascular smooth muscle relaxant that causes vasodilation, reducing preload and afterload.

Uses

Amrinone is used for the short-term management of systolic dysfunction heart failure in patients who have not responded adequately to digitalis, diuretics, or vasodilator therapy. The inotropic effects of amrinone are additive to those of digitalis, and it can be used in fully digitalized patients. Amrinone is usually not used in treating diastolic heart failure and may indeed worsen this condition.

Therapeutic Outcomes

The primary therapeutic outcomes expected from amrinone therapy are improved cardiac output resulting in improved tissue perfusion and reduced dyspnea, orthopnea, and fatigue.

Premedication Assessment

1. Take baseline vital signs.
2. Obtain baseline laboratory studies ordered by the physician (for example, complete blood cell count [CBC], aspartate transaminase [AST], alanine aminotransferose [ALT]).
3. Record any gastrointestinal symptoms present before initiation of therapy.

Planning

Availability. IV—5 mg/ml in 20 ml ampules.

Implementation

Dosage and administration. Do *not* dilute amrinone with dextrose solutions. With time, the amrinone loses potency. Amrinone may be injected into running dextrose infusions through a Y connector or directly into the tubing.

Adult: IV—initiate therapy with a bolus of 0.75 mg/kg given slowly over 2 to 3 minutes. Continue therapy with a maintenance infusion between 5 and 10 µg/kg per minute. This should place the amrinone serum level approximately at the 3 µg/ml level. Based on clinical response, an additional bolus injection of 0.75 mg/kg may be given 30 minutes after the initial bolus. In general, the total daily dose should not exceed 18 mg/kg/24 hr.

Evaluation

Side effects to expect

NAUSEA, VOMITING, ABDOMINAL DISCOMFORT. These side effects are usually transient and subside with continued therapy. If discomfort becomes severe, reduce the dosage rate and call a physician immediately.

Side effects to report

ARRHYTHMIAS, HYPOTENSION. As would be expected, the cardiovascular side effects of arrhythmias (3%) and hypotension (1.3%) are the most commonly reported adverse effects. Monitor blood pressure and heart rate and rhythm closely during therapy. These adverse effects are often dose related and will respond to a reduction in infusion rate. Contact a physician immediately if arrhythmias or significant hypotension develops.

THROMBOCYTOPENIA. Thrombocytopenia with platelet counts of less than 100,000/mm^3 has been reported in 2.4% of patients. It appears to be dose dependent, occurring within 48 to 72 hours after initiation of therapy. It is more frequent with higher than recommended dosages. Platelet counts should be performed before and periodically during therapy. If thrombocytopenia does occur, discontinuation of therapy should be considered, especially when platelet counts decrease to fewer than 50,000/mm^3. The nadir in platelet count appears to be variable but occurs within 1 to 4 weeks.

HEPATOTOXICITY. Hepatotoxicity has been reported in approximately 0.2% of patients after IV therapy. The symptoms of hepatotoxicity are anorexia, nausea, vomiting, jaundice, hepatomegaly, splenomegaly, and abnormal liver function tests (elevated bilirubin, AST, ALT, alkaline phosphatase, and prothrombin time). If these symptoms appear, it is recommended that amrinone therapy be discontinued.

Drug interactions

DIGITALIS GLYCOSIDES. Concurrent administration of amrinone and digitalis glycosides produces additive inotropic effects.

FUROSEMIDE. Amrinone and furosemide are chemically incompatible. When furosemide is mixed with amrinone, a precipitate forms immediately. Do not infuse into the same intravenous line.

milrinone (mihl'rhin-own)
Primacor (pr-aye'mah-cohr)

Actions

Milrinone is an inotropic agent that increases the force and velocity of myocardial contractions by inhibiting phosphodiesterase enzymes in heart muscle. It also is a vascular smooth muscle relaxant that causes vasodilation, reducing preload and afterload.

Uses

Milrinone is used for the short-term management of severe systolic dysfunction heart failure in patients who have not responded adequately to digitalis, diuretics, or vasodilator therapy. It has the advantages of fewer gastrointestinal side effects and a substantially lower frequency of thrombocytopenia and hepatotoxicity when compared with amrinone. Milrinone does, however, cause a higher incidence of supraventricular and ventricular arrhythmias than does amrinone.

The inotropic effects of milrinone are additive to those of digitalis, and it can be used in fully digitalized patients. Milrinone is usually not used in treating diastolic heart failure and may indeed worsen this condition.

Therapeutic Outcomes

The primary therapeutic outcomes expected from milrinone therapy are improved cardiac output resulting in improved tissue perfusion and reduced dyspnea, orthopnea, and fatigue.

Nursing Process

Premedication Assessment
1. Take baseline vital signs.
2. Obtain baseline laboratory studies ordered by the physician (for example, CBC).

Planning
Availability. IV—1 mg/ml in 10 and 20 ml vials and 5 ml cartridge-needle injection units.

Implementation
Dosage and administration. Diluents: 0.45% or 0.9% sodium chloride or dextrose 5% for injection may be used to prepare dilutions of milrinone for IV infusion.

Adult: IV—Initiate therapy with a loading dose of 50 mg/kg given slowly over 10 minutes. Continue therapy with a maintenance infusion between 0.375 and 0.75 µg/kg per minute. In general, the total daily dose should not exceed 1.13 mg/kg .

Evaluation
Side effects to report

ARRHYTHMIAS, HYPOTENSION The cardiovascular side effects of arrhythmias (12%) and hypotension (1.3%) are the most commonly reported adverse effects. Monitor blood pressure and heart rate and rhythm closely during therapy. These adverse effects are often dose related and will respond to a reduction in infusion rate. Contact a physician immediately if arrhythmias or significant hypotension develops.

THROMBOCYTOPENIA. Thrombocytopenia with platelet counts of less than 100,000/mm³ has been reported in 0.4% of patients. See previous section on amrinone for additional information regarding thrombocytopenia.

Drug interactions

FUROSEMIDE. Milrinone and furosemide are chemically incompatible. When furosemide is mixed with amrinone, a precipitate forms immediately. Do not infuse into the same intravenous line.

Drug Class: Angiotensin-Converting Enzyme Inhibitors

Actions

Angiotensin-converting enzyme inhibitors represent a major breakthrough in the treatment of heart failure. The ACE inhibitors reduce afterload by blocking angiotensin II–mediated peripheral vasoconstriction and help reduce circulating blood volume by inhibiting the secretion of aldosterone. (See Chapter 20 for a more complete description of the mechanism of action of ACE inhibitors.)

Uses

The ACE inhibitors reduce blood pressure (afterload), preserve cardiac output, and increase renal blood flow. Captopril, enalapril, fosinopril, lisinopril, and quinapril are now recommended as the drugs of choice over digoxin for the treatment of mild to moderate systolic dysfunction heart failure.

Therapeutic Outcomes

The primary therapeutic outcomes expected from ACE inhibitors are improved cardiac output resulting in improved tissue perfusion and improved tolerance to activity as demonstrated by the ability to perform activities of daily living without supplemental oxygen therapy or fatigue.

Nursing Process

See Chapter 20 for a more complete description of the nursing process for ACE inhibitors.

CHAPTER REVIEW

Heart failure is a cluster of signs and symptoms that arise when the left or right ventricle or both ventricles lose the ability to pump enough blood to meet the body's circulatory needs. It is an illness that is growing in frequency as the general population ages. The morbidity and mortality associated with heart failure can be reduced through medication, diet, and activity and symptom monitoring. Nurses can play a significant role in discussion of treatment options, planning for lifestyle changes, counseling before discharge, and reinforcement of key points during office visits. Best results are attained when the patient, family, and nurse work together in developing the care plan.

MATH REVIEW

1. Mr. Arpostole, age 64, weight 165 pounds, is in the emergency room with stat orders:
   Ordered: digoxin 6 µg/kg , IV, stat.
   On hand: digoxin 0.1 mg/ml.
   165 pounds = _____ kg.
   Based on this order, what dose of digoxin would be given stat? _____ µg or _____ mg.
   Use any drug reference to determine the following:
   Is digoxin given IV diluted or undiluted?
   What rate of IV injection is recommended?
   With what IV solution(s) is digoxin compatible?

2. Mr. Arpostole is transferred from the emergency room to the coronary unit for 24 hours. The following orders exist for medications:

   Ordered: digoxin 0.125 mg IV every 6 hours after stat dose.
   On hand: digoxin 0.1 mg/ml and digoxin 0.25 mg/ml.
   Give: digoxin _____ ml of _____ mg/ml.

3. After digitalization Mr. Arpostole is placed on a maintenance dose as follows:
   Ordered: digoxin 0.375 mg PO daily.
   On hand: digoxin 0.125 mg and 0.25 mg tablets.
   Give: _____ tablets of _____ mg tablet(s).

CRITICAL THINKING QUESTIONS

1. During the digitalization process what assessments should be made on a continuum? Discuss the rationale for these observations.

2. In addition to the medications listed in the Math Review, Mr. Arpostole is started on furosemide 60 mg daily. What is the action of furosemide? Explain the nursing assessments that should be made to evaluate the effectiveness of the diuretic therapy.

3. Describe the purpose of drug therapy for heart failure when administering vasodilator drugs such as nitroprusside or nifedipine, a calcium channel blocker.

Drugs Used to Treat Arrhythmias

Objectives

1. Describe the therapeutic response that should be observable when an antiarrhythmic agent is administered.

2. Identify baseline nursing assessments that should be implemented during the treatment of arrhythmias.

3. List the dosage forms and precautions needed in the preparation of intravenous lidocaine for the treatment of arrhythmias.

4. Cite common side effects that may be observed with the administration of amiodarone, bretylium tosylate, disopyramide, lidocaine, flecainide, mexiletine, phenytoin, procainamide, quinidine, and tocainide.

5. Identify the potential effects of muscle relaxants used during surgical intervention when combined with antiarrhythmic therapy.

Key Words

electrical system
arrhythmia
atrial flutter
atrial fibrillation

paroxysmal supra-
   ventricular tachy-
   cardia
atrioventricular blocks
tinnitus

ARRHYTHMIAS

The function of the heart is to rhythmically pump blood to itself through the coronary arteries and to the rest of the body's tissues to sustain life. The **electrical system,** or conduction system, of the heart is the anatomic structure that controls the sequence of muscle contractions so that an optimal volume of blood is pumped from the heart with each beat (Figure 22-1). The electrical system is composed of nerve fibers that conduct electrical impulses to cardiac muscle, causing it to contract.

In the normal heart, a contraction of the heart muscle begins in the pacemaker cells of the sinoatrial (SA) node. The electrical wave passes through the electrical system in the atrial muscle and cause it to contract, forcing blood in the atrial chambers into the ventricles below. The electrical current then enters the atrioventricular (AV) node, which focuses and conducts an electrical current through the bundle of His and the Purkinje fibers to the ventricular muscle tissue. The muscle contracts from the apex upward, causing blood to be pumped from the ventricles into the pulmonary artery to the lungs and into the aorta to the rest of the body.

An **arrhythmia** occurs when there is a disturbance of the normal electrical conduction resulting in an abnormal heart muscle contraction or heart rate. All people have an occasional irregular contraction of the heart. The danger is the frequency with which the arrhythmia occurs because the heart muscle loses its efficiency in pumping an adequate volume of blood and certain types of arrhythmias can produce additional arrhythmias that can stop the heart from pumping even though it continues to beat for a short time (fibrillation). A person may "sense" an abnormal contraction (arrhythmia) because of a "flip-flop" or "racing" of the heart. Nurses may also suspect that a patient is having arrhythmias because of an irregular pulse. Arrhythmias, however, must be identified with the aid of an electrocardiogram (ECG), which provides a tracing of the electrical activity of the heart.

Arrhythmias are caused by the firing of abnormal pacemaker cells, the blockage of normal electrical pathways, or a combination of both. Normally, the rate and rhythm of electrical activity and muscle contraction are regulated by the pacemaker cells of the SA node. In times such as high emotional stress, ischemia (see Chapter 23), or fiber stretching (see Chapter 21), normally quiet pacemaker cells in areas of the heart other than the SA or AV nodes may fire. This sends an electrical impulse out of sequence with those from the normal pacemaker cells, causing an irregular muscular contraction, sometimes sensed as a flip-flop of the heart. The second cause of arrhythmias is a partial obstruction of the normal conduction pathway causing an irregular flow of electrical impulses resulting in an irregular pattern of muscle contractions. This is sometimes called a reentrant arrhythmia. Normally, healthy heart tissue has mechanisms that protect against reentrant arrhythmias. Various forms of heart disease result in changes in the conduction pathways that allow continuous reentrant arrhythmias.

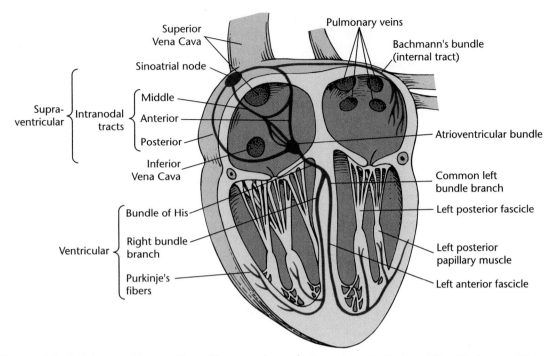

Figure 22-1 *Schematic diagram of heart illustrating the conduction system.* (Modified from Phipps WJ, Cassmeyer VL, Sands JK, Lehman MK: *Medical-surgical nursing,* ed 5, St Louis, 1995, Mosby.)

Arrhythmias are most commonly classified by origin within the heart tissues. Those that develop above the bundle of His (Figure 22-1) are called supraventricular. Examples of supraventricular arrhythmias are **atrial flutter, atrial fibrillation,** premature atrial contractions (PAC), sinus tachycardia, sinus bradycardia, and **paroxysmal supraventricular tachycardia.** Arrhythmias developing below the bundle of His are referred to as ventricular arrhythmias. These include premature ventricular contractions (PVCs), ventricular tachycardia (VT), and ventricular fibrillation (VF). Arrhythmias that result from obstruction of conduction pathways are described by location (for example, supraventricular or ventricular and left or right bundle branches). **Atrioventricular blocks** can be subclassified by degree of block: first degree—partial block, delayed AV conduction; second degree—partial block with occasional blocked beats; and third degree—complete block, the atria and ventricles function independently of each other.

The tissues of the electrical system can be classified into two types depending on whether calcium or sodium ions create the stimulus for muscle contraction. The SA and AV nodes depend on calcium ions for electrical conduction and are referred to as slow conduction fibers. The atrial muscle, His-Purkinje system, and the ventricular muscle depend on sodium for contraction and are sometimes referred to as fast conduction fibers.

Treatment

When an arrhythmia is suspected, a patient is frequently admitted to a coronary care unit where wire leads are placed in appropriate locations to provide continuous ECG monitoring. A combination of the physical examination, patient history, and ECG pattern is used to diagnose the underlying cause of the arrhythmia. The goal of treatment is to restore normal sinus rhythm and normal cardiac function and to prevent recurrence of life-threatening arrhythmias.

Drug Therapy
Actions

Antiarrhythmic agents are complex agents with multiple mechanisms of action. They are classified according to their effects on the electrical conduction system of the heart (Table 22-1). Class I agents act as myocardial depressants by inhibiting sodium ion movement. Class Ia agents prolong the duration of the electrical stimulation on cells and the refractory time between electrical impulses. Class Ib agents shorten the duration of the electrical stimulation and the time between the electrical impulses. Class Ic antiarrhythmics are the most potent myocardial depressants and slow conduction rate through the atria and the ventricles.

Class II agents are beta-adrenergic blocking agents. Many arrhythmias are caused by stimulation of the beta cells of the sympathetic nervous system of the heart. Class III agents slow the rate of electrical conduction and prolong the time interval between contractions. Class IV agents block calcium ion flow, prolonging duration of the electrical stimulation and slowing AV node conduction.

Uses

See individual monographs for uses of antiarrhythmic agents.

Nursing Process for Antiarrhythmic Drugs

The information nurses assess relative to the cardinal signs of cardiovascular disease can provide a basis for subsequent

Table 22-1

Classification of Antiarrhythmic Agents

CLASS	GENERIC NAME	BRAND NAME
I	Moricizine	Ethmozine
Ia	Disopyramide	Norpace
	Procainamide	Pronestyl, Procan SR
	Quinidine	Quinidex, Quinaglute
IIb	Lidocaine	Xylocaine
	Mexiletine	Mexitil
	Phenytoin	Dilantin
	Tocainide	Tonocard
Ic	Flecainide	Tambocor
	Propafenone	Rythmol
II	Acebutolol	Sectral
	Esmolol	Brevibloc
	Propranolol	Inderal
III	Amiodarone	Cordarone
	Bretylium	Bretylol
	Sotalol	Betapace
IV	Verapamil	Calan, Isoptin
—	Adenosine	Adenocard

evaluation of the patient's response to the therapeutic modalities prescribed.

Assessment

Arrhythmias are initially assessed by electrocardiographic monitoring. A 24-hour ambulatory electrocardiogram (Holter monitor), electrophysiologic studies (EPS), exercise electrocardiography, and laboratory values are used to analyze and diagnose the patient's myocardial status.

Patients are usually admitted to the coronary care unit, where specialized monitoring equipment is available for continuous surveillance of the patient. The nurses have advanced education in cardiac physiology and the nursing care of these individuals. (See a general medical-surgical nursing text for an in-depth explanation of care of the patient with arrhythmias.)

Medication history. Obtain details of all medications prescribed and being taken. Tactfully find out if the prescribed medications are being taken regularly and if not, why.

History of six cardinal signs of cardiovascular disease

Dyspnea (difficulty in breathing). Record if dyspnea occurs while resting or during exertion. How has the patient been coping with any orthopneic problems?

Chest pain. Record data as to the time of onset, frequency, duration, and quality of the chest pain. Note any conditions the patient has found that either aggravate or relieve the chest pain. (Not all patients with arrhythmias will suffer chest pain.)

Fatigue. Determine whether fatigue occurs only at specific times of the day, such as toward evening. Ask the patient if fatigue decreases in relation to a decrease in activity level or if it is present at about the same time daily.

Edema. Record the presence or absence of edema. If present, record location of edema, assessment data (for example, degree of pitting present; ankle, midcalf, or thigh

circumference), and any measures the patient has used to eliminate edema. Chart the time of day that the edema is present (for example, when arising in the morning; evening) and the specific parts on the body where present. When performing daily weights, use the same scale, at the same time of day, with the patient in a similar type of clothing.

Syncope. Ask the patient about conditions surrounding any episodes of syncope. Record the degree of symptoms such as general muscle weakness, inability to stand upright, feeling faint, or loss of consciousness. Record what activities, if any, bring on these syncopal episodes.

Palpitations. Record the patient's description of palpitations, such as "my heart skips some beats" or "it began to feel like it was racing." Ask if these conditions are preceded by mild or strenuous exercise and how long the palpitations last.

Basic mental status. Identify the person's level of consciousness and clarity of thought. Both of these factors are indicators of adequate or inadequate cerebral perfusion. Subsequent regular observations for these data should be made so that apparent improvement or deterioration can be assessed.

Vital signs. Vital signs should be taken as often as necessary to monitor the patient's status.

Blood pressure. Blood pressure readings should be performed at least two times daily in stable cardiac patients and more frequently if indicated by the patient's symptoms or the physician's orders. Be sure to use the proper-sized blood pressure cuff and place the patient's arm at heart level.

Record the blood pressure in both arms. A systolic pressure variance of 5 to 10 mm Hg is normal; readings reflecting a variance of more than 10 mm Hg should be reported for further evaluation. *Always report a narrowing pulse pressure* (difference between systolic and diastolic readings).

Pulse. Assess bilaterally the rhythm, quality, equality, and strength of the pulses (carotid, brachial, radial, femoral, popliteal, posterior tibial, and dorsalis pedis). If any pulse is diminished or absent, record the level at which initial changes are noted. The usual words to describe the pulse are "absent," "diminished" or "average," "full and brisk," or "full bounding, frequently visible." Check for delayed capillary refill.

Respirations. Observe and chart the rate and depth of respirations. Check breath sounds at least every shift, and make specific notations regarding the presence of abnormal breath sounds, for example, crackles, wheezes, rales. Observe the degree of dyspnea that occurs and whether it happens with or without exertion.

Temperature. Record temperature at least every shift.

Auscultation and percussion. Nurses with advanced skills can perform auscultation and percussion to note changes in heart size and heart and lung sounds. (See a medical-surgical nursing text for details of performing these advanced skills.) As appropriate to nursing skills, note changes in cardiac rhythm, heart rate, changes in heart sounds, or murmurs.

Laboratory tests. Review laboratory tests and report abnormal results to the physician promptly. Such tests may include serum electrolytes, especially potassium, calcium, magnesium, and sodium; arterial blood gases, such as pH, PO_2, PCO_2, and HCO_3; coagulation studies to evaluate the blood clotting; serum enzymes (aspartate serum transaminase [AST], creatine phosphokinase [CPK], lactic acid dehydrogenase [LDH]); serum lipids (cholesterol, triglycerides);

electrocardiogram; radiographic examinations; nuclear cardiography; and cardiac catheterization.

Examine urinalysis reports and perform hourly monitoring of intake and output (I&O) as ordered. Report output that is less than intake or is below 30 to 50 ml per hour. Monitor other renal function tests such as the blood urea nitrogen (BUN) and serum creatinine. Abnormalities of these tests or insufficient hourly output may indicate inadequate renal perfusion.

Nursing Diagnosis
- Cardiac output, decreased (indication)
- Activity intolerance (indication)
- Tissue perfusion altered (indication)

Planning
Medication. Order medications prescribed and schedule these on the medication administration record (MAR).
History of six cardinal signs of cardiovascular disease. Individualize the care plan to address the patient's degree of dyspnea, chest pain, fatigue, edema, syncope, and palpitations.
Basic mental status. Schedule basic neurologic checks at least once per shift.
Vital signs, auscultation, and percussion. Schedule measurement of vital signs and auscultation and percussion of the heart and chest in a manner consistent with the patient's status.
Laboratory tests. Order stat and subsequent laboratory studies.

Implementation
- Monitor electrocardiographic tracings on a continuum.
- Perform physical assessments of the patient in accordance with the clinical setting policies (for example, every 4 or 8 hours depending on the patient's status).
- Assist the patient, as needed, to perform activities of daily living. Make note of the degree of impairment or dyspnea seen with and without exertion.
- Administer oxygen as ordered and as necessary (prn).
- Administer prescribed medications and treatments that can best alleviate the patient's symptoms and provide maximum level of comfort.
- Encourage physical activity as prescribed. Do not allow the patient to overexert or become fatigued.
- Institute measures to reduce anxiety. Support the patient in a calm manner even if the response is hostile or confrontive.

Patient Education and Health Promotion
- Review the patient's history to identify modifiable coronary artery disease factors. Design an individualized approach to help the patient modify factors that are within the patient's control.
- Cooperatively discuss and practice using coping mechanisms to handle the individual's anxiety.
- Teach the patient to take own pulse and blood pressure, and stress signs and symptoms that should be reported.
Fostering health maintenance. Throughout the course of treatment, discuss medication information and how it will benefit the patient.

Drug therapy is one component of the treatment of arrhythmias, and it is critical that the medications be taken as prescribed. Provide the patient and significant others with the important information contained in the specific drug monograph for the drugs prescribed. Additional health teaching and nursing interventions for drug side effects to expect and report will be found in each drug monograph.

Seek cooperation and understanding of the following points so that medication compliance is increased: name of medication, dosage, route and times of administration, side effects to expect, and side effects to report.

Enlist the patient's aid in developing and maintaining a written record of monitoring parameters (pulse rate, blood pressure, degree of dyspnea and what precipates it, chest pain, edema, etc.). (See the Patient Education and Monitoring Form in Chapter 21, p. 282.) Instruct the patient to bring the written record to follow-up visits.

Antiarrhythmic Agents

adenosine (aden'oh-seen)
Adenocard (aden'oh-card)

Actions
Adenosine is a naturally occurring chemical found in every cell within the body. It is not related to other antiarrhythmic agents. It has a variety of physiologic roles, including energy transfer, promotion of prostaglandin release, inhibition of platelet aggregation, antiadrenergic effects, coronary vasodilation, and suppression of heart rate.

Uses
Because of its strong depressant effects on the SA and AV nodes, adenosine is recommended for the treatment of paroxysmal supraventricular tachycardia that involves conduction in the SA node, atrium, or AV node.

Therapeutic Outcomes
The primary therapeutic outcome expected from adenosine therapy is conversion of supraventricular tachycardias to normal sinus rhythm.

Nursing Process

Premedication Assessment
Obtain data relating to the six cardinal signs of cardiovascular disease to be used as a baseline for subsequent evaluation of response to therapy.

Planning
Availability. IV—3 mg/ml in 2 ml vials.

Implementation
Dosage and administration. IV—6 mg administered by rapid IV bolus injection (over 1 to 2 seconds) followed by a saline flush. A follow-up dose of 12 mg rapid IV bolus is recommended if the initial dose is unsuccessful in restoring a normal heart rate. The 12 mg dose may be repeated once if required.

Evaluation
Side effects to expect
The most commonly reported adverse reactions with adenosine include flushing of the face (18%), shortness of breath

(12%), chest pressure (7%), nausea (3%), and headache and light-headedness (2%). Because the half-life of adenosine is less than 10 seconds, adverse effects are short-lived. Treatment of any prolonged adverse effect would include oxygen and possibly other antiarrhythmic agents.

Drug interactions

DRUGS THAT ENHANCE THERAPEUTIC AND TOXIC EFFECTS. Dipyridamole and carbamazepine potentiate the effects of adenosine. Smaller doses of adenosine should be used if therapy is required.

DRUGS THAT REDUCE THERAPEUTIC EFFECTS. Theophylline, aminophylline, and caffeine competitively antagonize adenosine, thus larger doses of adenosine are required with concurrent use.

amiodarone hydrochloride (am e-o'dahr-own)
Cordarone (cor-dahr'own)

Actions

Amiodarone is a member of a chemical class of antiarrhythmic agents and is not related to any other available antiarrhythmic product. Although its mechanism of action is unknown, it is a class III agent that acts by prolonging the action potential of atrial and ventricular tissue and by increasing the refractory period without altering the resting membrane potential, thus delaying repolarization. In addition, amiodarone has been shown to antagonize noncompetitively both alpha- and beta-adrenergic receptors, causing systemic and coronary vasodilation.

Uses

Amiodarone is being used in the management of life-threatening supraventricular tachyarrhythmias, atrial fibrillation and flutter, bradycardia-tachycardia syndromes, ventricular tachycardia and fibrillation, and hypertrophic cardiomyopathy resistant to currently available therapy.

Side effects

Adverse reactions are common with the use of amiodarone, particularly in patients receiving more than 400 mg per day. Approximately 15% to 20% of patients discontinue therapy because of adverse effects.

Therapeutic Outcomes

The primary therapeutic outcome expected from amiodarone therapy is conversion to normal sinus rhythm.

Nursing Process

Premedication Assessment

1. Obtain data relating to the six cardinal signs of cardiovascular disease to be used as a baseline for subsequent evaluation of response to therapy.
2. Initiate requested laboratory tests to be used for evaluation of pulmonary, thyroid, and liver functions.
3. Record data relating to the patient's usual sleep pattern and any gastrointestinal symptoms present before initiation of therapy.

Planning

Availability. PO—200 mg tablets.

Implementation

Dosage and administration. Note: Amiodarone is contraindicated in patients with severe sinus-node dysfunction that causes sinus bradycardia, with second- and third-degree AV block, and when episodes of bradycardia have caused syncope (except in the presence of a pacemaker).

The difficulty of using amiodarone effectively and safely is that it poses a significant risk to patients. Patients must be hospitalized while the loading dose is given, and the response often requires 2 weeks or more. Because absorption and elimination are variable, maintenance-dose selection is difficult, and it is not unusual to require a reduction in dosage or a discontinuation of treatment. The time at which a previously controlled life-threatening arrhythmia will recur after discontinuation or dosage adjustment is unpredictable, ranging from weeks to months. Attempts to substitute other antiarrhythmic agents when amiodarone is discontinued are made difficult by the gradually but unpredictably changing amiodarone body store. A similar problem exists when amiodarone is not effective; it still poses the risk of a drug interaction with whatever subsequent treatment is tried.

PO: loading dose—800 to 1600 mg daily in divided doses for 1 to 3 weeks until an initial therapeutic response occurs. After the loading dose, a dosage of 600 to 800 mg daily is given for approximately 1 month. Maintenance—the lowest effective dose should be used, usually 400 mg daily.

Before start of therapy, baseline pulmonary, thyroid, and liver function tests should be completed. If gastric irritation occurs, administer with food or milk. If symptoms persist or increase in severity, report for physician evaluation.

Evaluation

Side effects to report

FATIGUE, TREMORS, INVOLUNTARY MOVEMENTS, SLEEP DISTURBANCES, NUMBNESS AND TINGLING, DIZZINESS, ATAXIA, CONFUSION. Many of these symptoms are dose related and resolve with reduction of dosage or discontinuation of therapy. Peripheral neuropathy may be associated with long-term therapy, although the onset and presentation of symptoms are variable. Symptoms usually resolve 1 to 4 months after the discontinuation of therapy.

Teach the patient to rise slowly from a supine or sitting position, and encourage the patient to sit or lie down if feeling faint.

Perform a baseline assessment of the patient's degree of alertness and orientation to name, place, and time before initiating therapy. Make regularly scheduled subsequent mental status evaluations and compare findings. Report development of alterations.

Provide for patient safety during episodes of dizziness.

EXERTIONAL DYSPNEA, NONPRODUCTIVE COUGH, PLEURITIC CHEST PAIN. Pulmonary interstitial pneumonitis/alveolitis has been reported in 10% to 15% of patients. Particular care should be taken not to assume that such symptoms are related to cardiac failure. Tests for diffusion capacity are most likely to show abnormality. Symptoms gradually resolve after discontinuation of therapy. Periodic chest x-rays and clinical evaluation are recommended every 3 to 6 months.

THYROID DISORDERS. Administration of amiodarone has been associated with the development of hypothyroidism (2% to 10%) and hyperthyroidism (1% to 3%). Patients with a history of thyroid disorders appear to be more susceptible to this complication. Baseline and periodic thyroid function tests should be completed in all patients.

YELLOW-BROWN PIGMENTATIONS IN THE CORNEA, BLURRED VISION, HALOS. Corneal microdeposits have been observed by slit-lamp examination as early as 2 weeks after the initiation of therapy. Symptoms of blurred vision or visual halos develop in about 10% of patients. This complication is reversible after drug withdrawal. Use of methylcellulose ophthalmic solution and a minimization of the maintenance doses may limit this complication. Provide for patient safety during temporary visual impairment. Instruct the patient not to rub the eyes with force when tearing.

NAUSEA, VOMITING, CONSTIPATION, ABDOMINAL PAIN, ANOREXIA. Gastrointestinal complaints occur in about 25% of patients but rarely require discontinuation of therapy. These adverse effects commonly occur during high-dosage administration and usually respond to dosage reduction or divided dosages.

ARRHYTHMIAS. Amiodarone can cause an exacerbation of the preexisting arrhythmias and in 2% to 4% of patients induce others as well.

PHOTOSENSITIVITY. Amiodarone has produced photosensitivity in approximately 10% of patients. The severity of the rash may depend on the degree of sun exposure. Symptoms such as burning, tingling, erythema, and blistering may occur as early as 2 hours after exposure to the sun. The use of sunscreens may minimize this adverse effect. Patients should be encouraged to wear long-sleeved shirts and to avoid wearing shorts outdoors. Photosensitivity may persist for up to 4 months after discontinuation of therapy. With long-term treatment, a blue-gray discoloration of the exposed skin may occur. The risk is increased in patients of fair complexion and those with excessive sun exposure and may be related to cumulative dose and duration of therapy. This effect gradually subsides after discontinuation of therapy. The patient should also be instructed not to use artificial tanning lamps.

HEPATOTOXICITY. Abnormal liver function tests (AST and alanine aminotransferase [ALT]) occur in 4% to 9% of patients. Liver enzymes in patients on relatively high maintenance doses should be monitored on a regular basis. Persistent significant elevations in the liver enzymes or hepatomegaly are indications for considering a reduction in dosage or discontinuation of therapy. Hepatitis and other liver abnormalities may develop in 1% to 3% of patients. The symptoms of hepatotoxicity are anorexia, nausea, vomiting, jaundice, hepatomegaly, splenomegaly, and abnormal liver function tests.

Drug interactions

DIGOXIN, DIGITOXIN. Administration of amiodarone to patients receiving digoxin or digitoxin therapy regularly results in an increase in the serum digitalis concentration. The dose of digitalis should be reduced by 50% or discontinued. Digitalis serum levels should be closely monitored and patients observed for clinical evidence of toxicity (anorexia, nausea, fatigue, blurred or colored vision, bradycardia, and arrhythmias).

WARFARIN. Potentiation of warfarin is almost always seen within 3 to 4 days in patients receiving concomitant therapy. The dose of the anticoagulant should be reduced by one-third to one-half, and prothrombin times should be monitored closely. Observe for the development of petechiae, ecchymoses, nosebleeds, bleeding gums, dark tarry stools, and bright red or "coffee-ground" emesis.

QUINIDINE. Elevation of quinidine serum levels (32% to 50%) is often observed within 2 to 3 days. The dose of quinidine should be reduced by one third to one half or discontinued.

PROCAINAMIDE. Elevation of procainamide serum levels (50%) is often observed in less than 7 days. The dose of procainamide should be reduced by one third or discontinued.

PHENYTOIN. Elevation of phenytoin levels (200% to 300%) is observed over several weeks. The dose of phenytoin must be gradually reduced based on patient response. Monitor patients with concurrent therapy for signs of phenytoin toxicity: nystagmus, sedation, and lethargy. Serum levels should be monitored periodically. Phenytoin may also reduce amiodarone levels. Monitor closely for loss of therapeutic effects.

BETA-BLOCKING AGENTS (PROPRANOLOL, TIMOLOL, NADOLOL, PINDOLOL, AND OTHERS), CALCIUM ANTAGONISTS (DILTIAZEM, VERAPAMIL, AND NIFEDIPINE). Amiodarone should be used with caution in patients receiving beta-adrenergic blocking agents or calcium antagonists because of the possible potentiation of bradycardia, sinus arrest, and AV block. If necessary, amiodarone can be used after insertion of a pacemaker in patients with severe bradycardia or sinus arrest.

THEOPHYLLINE. Amiodarone may increase theophylline levels, resulting in toxicity. Effects may not be observed until after least 1 week of concurrent therapy. Toxicity may persist for more than 1 week after amiodarone has been discontinued.

Drug Class: Beta-Adrenergic Blocking Agents

Actions

The beta-adrenergic blocking agents (acebutolol, esmolol, and propranolol) are widely used as antiarrhythmic agents. These agents inhibit cardiac response to sympathetic nerve stimulation by blocking the beta receptors. As a result, the heart rate, systolic blood pressure, and cardiac output are reduced.

Uses

These agents are effective in the treatment of various ventricular arrhythmias, sinus tachycardia, paroxysmal atrial tachycardia, premature ventricular contractions, and tachycardia associated with atrial flutter or fibrillation because atrioventricular conduction is diminished.

Therapeutic Outcomes

The primary therapeutic outcome expected from beta-blocker therapy is conversion to normal sinus rhythm.

Nursing Process

See Chapter 11 for further discussion of nursing process associated with beta-adrenergic inhibition.

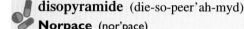

bretylium tosylate (bret-il'ee-um tahs'e-layt)
Bretylol (bret'il-ol)

Actions

Bretylium, an adrenergic blocking agent, inhibits the release of norepinephrine.

Uses

Bretylium is a class III antiarrhythmic agent used for short-term suppression of life-threatening ventricular arrhythmias, primarily tachycardia and fibrillation, that have not responded to other widely used antiarrhythmic drugs. Bretylium is not a cardiac depressant, so it is particularly useful in patients with poor myocardial contractility and low cardiac output.

Therapeutic Outcomes

The primary therapeutic outcome expected from bretylium therapy is conversion of arrhythmia to normal sinus rhythm.

Nursing Process

Premedication Assessment

1. Obtain data relating to the six cardinal signs of cardiovascular disease to be used as a baseline for subsequent evaluation of response to therapy.
2. Schedule blood pressure readings at intervals appropriate to the patient's status.

Planning

Availability. IV—50 mg/ml in 10 ml ampules.

Implementation

Dosage and administration. For ventricular fibrillation—after failure of electrical cardioversion, 5 mg/kg IV undiluted. Repeat cardioversion. If fibrillation persists, the dosage may be increased to 10 mg/kg and repeated every 15 to 30 minutes. Dosages up to 40 mg/kg per day have been reported. For other ventricular arrhythmias—administer 5 to 10 mg/kg IV over 8 to 10 minutes. The dose may be repeated in 1 to 2 hours if the arrhythmia persists. IV—continuous infusion: recommended dosage is 1 to 2 mg per minute. IM—5 to 10 mg/kg undiluted. Do not give more than 5 ml at one site. Dosage may be repeated in 1 to 2 hours if the arrhythmia persists. Thereafter repeat every 6 to 8 hours. Observe injection site for signs of inflammation and necrosis.

Evaluation

Side effects to expect

DIZZINESS, LIGHT-HEADEDNESS. These symptoms are transient and may be reduced by keeping the patient in a supine position. When changing positions, encourage the patient to move slowly and to lie down if feeling faint.

HYPERTENSION, HYPOTENSION. Transient hypertension followed by hypotension is frequently observed when therapy is initiated. Avoid the use of subtherapeutic doses (less than 5 mg/kg) because hypotension frequently occurs. Systolic blood pressures below 75 mm Hg may be treated with infusions of dopamine. Initiate dopamine at low doses and titrate as needed based on frequent blood pressure readings.

Drug interactions

DIGITALIS GLYCOSIDES. Bretylium is not recommended in the treatment of arrhythmias associated with digitalis toxicity. The sudden release of norepinephrine caused by the initiation of bretylium therapy may seriously aggravate the digitalis toxicity.

disopyramide (die-so-peer'ah-myd)
Norpace (nor'pace)

Actions

Disopyramide is a class Ia antiarrhythmic agent.

Uses

Disopyramide is used to treat atrial fibrillation, Wolff-Parkinson-White syndrome, paroxysmal supraventricular tachycardia, premature ventricular tachycardia, and ventricular tachycardia. It may be used in both digitalized and nondigitalized patients. It is usually a useful drug as an alternative to quinidine or procainamide when patients develop an intolerance to or serious side effects from these agents.

Therapeutic Outcomes

The primary therapeutic outcome expected from disopyramide therapy is conversion of arrhythmia to normal sinus rhythm.

Nursing Process

Premedication Assessment

1. Obtain data relating to the six cardinal signs of cardiovascular disease to be used as a baseline for subsequent evaluation of response to therapy.
2. Assess usual pattern of urination and defecation.

Planning

Availability. PO—100 and 150 mg capsules; 100 and 150 mg controlled-release capsules.

Implementation

Dosage and administration. PO—dosage is individualized. Recommended adult dosage schedule is 150 mg every 6 hours. If body weight is less than 110 pounds (50 kg), the recommended dose is 100 mg every 6 hours. Therapeutic blood level is 2 to 6 mg/L.

Evaluation

Side effects to expect

DRY MOUTH, NOSE, THROAT. Suggest frequent mouth rinses or sucking on ice chips or hard candy to relieve symptoms.

Side effects to report

MYOCARDIAL TOXICITY. Report bradycardia or increasing signs of heart failure. Monitoring of the ECG for various types of arrhythmias may be indicated as ordered by the physician.

URINARY HESITANCY. Tell the patient that hesitancy in starting to urinate may occur. Suggest running tap water or immersing hands in water as means to stimulate urination. Report decreased urinary output and bladder distention.

In the hospitalized patient, record I&O. Palpate the area of the symphysis pubis to assess for distention.

CONSTIPATION WITH DISTENTION AND FLATUS. Report difficulties in defecation to the physician. Assess distention by measuring abdominal girth, as appropriate. Assess ability to expel flatus.

Drug interactions

DRUGS THAT ENHANCE THERAPEUTIC AND TOXIC EFFECTS. Procainamide, quinidine, digitalis, and beta-adrenergic blocking agents (propranolol, atenolol, timolol, and others): Monitor for increases in severity of drug effects such as bradycardia and hypotension.

DRUGS THAT REDUCE THERAPEUTIC EFFECTS. Phenytoin, barbiturates, glutethimide, primidone, and rifampin. Monitor for an increase in frequency of the patient's arrhythmias.

DRUGS THAT INCREASE HYPOTENSIVE EFFECTS. Diuretics and antihypertensive agents. Instruct patients to rise slowly from a supine position. If symptoms become more severe, report to the physician.

flecainide acetate (fleh-kayn'ayd)
Tambocor (tam-boh'kor)

Actions

Flecainide acetate is a class Ic antiarrhythmic agent that may be taken orally.

Uses

Flecainide acetate may be used in the treatment of sustained ventricular tachycardia, nonsustained ventricular tachycardia, and frequent premature ventricular contractions. Flecainide is usually used for more serious ventricular arrhythmias that have not responded to more traditional therapy. In addition to its therapeutic activity, a particular advantage is its twice-daily dosing schedule. Flecainide has a negative inotropic effect and may cause or worsen heart failure, particularly in patients with preexisting severe heart failure. This adverse effect may take hours to months to develop. New or worsened heart failure occurs in approximately 5% of patients. Flecainide may also aggravate existing arrhythmias and precipitate new ones, especially in patients with underlying heart disease.

Therapeutic Outcomes

The primary therapeutic outcome expected from flecainide therapy is conversion of arrhythmias to normal sinus rhythm.

Nursing Process

Premedication Assessment

1. Obtain data relating to the six cardinal signs of cardiovascular disease to be used as a baseline for subsequent evaluation of response to therapy.
2. If any symptoms of heart failure are present, notify the physician before initiating therapy.

Planning

Availability. PO—100 mg tablets.

Implementation

Dosage and administration. Note: Flecainide should not be used in patients with second- or third-degree atrioventricular block in the absence of an artificial ventricular pacemaker and must be used with caution in patients with known heart failure. Monitor the ECG before and during initiation of therapy.

Adult: sustained ventricular tachycardia, PO—initially, 100 mg every 12 hours. Increase in 50 mg increments twice daily every 4 days. Most patients respond at 150 mg twice daily. Maximum daily dose is 400 mg.

Evaluation

Side effects to expect

The more frequent adverse effects that occur with flecainide therapy are dizziness, light-headedness, faintness, and unsteadiness (19%); visual disturbances such as blurred vision, difficulty in focusing, and spots before the eyes (16%); dyspnea (1%); headache (10%); nausea (9%); fatigue (8%); constipation (5%); edema (3%); and abdominal pain.

DIZZINESS, HEADACHE, CONSTIPATION, NAUSEA. These side effects are usually mild and tend to resolve with continued therapy. Encourage the patient not to discontinue therapy without first consulting a physician.

Side effects to report

VISUAL DISTURBANCES. Provide for patient safety during temporary visual impairment. Caution the patient to avoid temporarily tasks that require visual acuity, such as driving or operating power machinery. Instruct the patient not to rub the eyes with force when tearing. These side effects are usually mild and tend to resolve with continued therapy. Encourage the patient not to discontinue therapy without first consulting the physician.

INCREASING DYSPNEA, EXERCISE INTOLERANCE, EDEMA. Flecainide may induce or aggravate preexisting heart failure. If these symptoms become more pronounced, the patient should be instructed to contact the physician for further evaluation.

ARRHYTHMIAS. Flecainide may induce or aggravate preexisting arrhythmias. The patient should be instructed to contact the physician for further evaluation if sensations of a "jumping" or "racing" heart develop.

Drug interactions

DRUGS THAT ENHANCE THERAPEUTIC AND TOXIC EFFECTS. Amiodarone, cimetidine, and disopyramide: monitor for increases of drug effects such as arrhythmias, heart failure, and bradycardia.

DIGOXIN. When multiple doses of flecainide are administered to patients stabilized on a dose of digoxin, there is a 10% to 20% increase in serum digoxin concentrations. This increase may result in signs of digitalis toxicity, such as anorexia, nausea, fatigue, blurred or colored vision, bradycardia, and arrhythmias. Monitor serum digoxin levels, ECG readings, and the clinical course of the patient closely.

PROPRANOLOL. When flecainide and propranolol are administered concurrently, there is a 20% increase in serum flecainide levels and a 30% increase in propranolol levels, with additive pharmacologic effects. Monitor serum levels,

ECG readings, and the clinical course of the patient closely. Dosage reductions of either one or both agents may be required.

URINARY ACIDIFIERS. These agents may lower the urine pH, causing an increase in the urinary excretion of flecainide. Patients should be observed for redevelopment of arrhythmias, which may require an increase in dosage of flecainide.

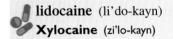 **lidocaine** (li'do-kayn)
Xylocaine (zi'lo-kayn)

Actions

Lidocaine is a class Ib agent.

Uses

Lidocaine has become one of the most frequently used drugs in the treatment of ventricular arrhythmias and the drug of choice for the treatment of ventricular arrhythmias associated with acute myocardial infarction and ventricular tachycardia.

Therapeutic Outcomes

The primary therapeutic outcome expected from lidocaine therapy is conversion of arrhythmia to normal sinus rhythm.

Nursing Process

Premedication Assessment

1. Obtain data relating to the six cardinal signs of cardiovascular disease to be used as a baseline for subsequent evaluation of response to therapy.
2. Assess and record data relating to the patient's basic mental status (for example, orientation, agitation, confusion).
3. Label the container for IV use: "lidocaine for arrhythmias."

Planning

Availability. IM—300 mg per 3 ml; 10% (100 mg/ml) in 5 ml ampules. Direct IV—1% (10 mg/ml) in five disposable syringes; 2% (20 mg/ml) in 5 ml disposable syringes and ampules. IV admixtures—4% (40 mg/ml) in 5 ml ampules and 25 and 50 ml vials and additive syringes; 20% (200 mg/ml) in 5 ml and 10 ml additive syringes. IV infusion—0.2% (2 mg/ml) in 500 and 1000 ml of 5% dextrose; 0.4% (4

mg/ml) in 250 and 500 ml of 5% dextrose; 0.8% (8 mg/ml) in 250 and 500 ml of 5% dextrose.

Implementation

Dosage and administration. Note: Lidocaine for IV use for arrhythmias is *different* from lidocaine used as a local anesthetic. For use with arrhythmias, check the label carefully to be certain it says "lidocaine for arrhythmias" or "lidocaine without preservatives." Severe arrhythmias could result if lidocaine with preservatives or lidocaine with epinephrine are administered to these patients. Lidocaine should *not* be used in patients with complete heart block.

Adult: IM—200 to 300 mg in the deltoid muscle. Intramuscular injections of lidocaine should be given in the deltoid. The IM route should be used only in emergency situations until an IV can be established. IV—initial dose (bolus) is 50 to 100 mg (1 mg/kg) at a rate of 25 to 50 mg per minute. Boluses of 50 to 100 mg may be given every 3 to 5 minutes until the desired effect is achieved or side effects appear. Do not exceed 300 mg by intermittent bolus. To maintain the antiarrhythmic effect, an IV infusion must be initiated. The usual rate of administration is 1 to 4 mg per minute. For routine lidocaine administration for cardiac arrhythmias, add 50 ml of 40 mg/ml (2 g) of lidocaine to dextrose 5%. Therapeutic blood levels are 1 to 5 mg/L.

Pediatric: IV—initial bolus: 1 mg/kg up to 15 mg if under 25 kg (55 pounds); up to 25 mg if over 25 kg (55 pounds). Continuous infusion: 20 to 40 µg/kg per minute (maximum total dose 5 mg/kg).

Evaluation

Side effects to report

LIGHT-HEADEDNESS, MUSCLE TWITCHING, HALLUCINATIONS, AGITATION, EUPHORIA. Monitor patients carefully for progressive symptoms of restlessness, agitation, anxiety, hallucinations, and euphoria.

Act calmly with the excited, anxious, or euphoric patient. Provide for safety and fulfillment of patient's needs. Report patient's alteration in response to the physician as soon as possible.

RESPIRATORY DEPRESSION. Observe the rate and depth of respiratory effort. Monitor for cyanosis and increasing frequency of arrhythmias.

Drug interactions

DRUGS THAT ENHANCE THERAPEUTIC AND TOXIC EFFECTS. Phenytoin, cimetidine, procainamide, tocainide, and beta-adrenergic blocking agents (nadolol, atenolol, timolol, propranolol, and others). Monitor for an increase in severity of side effects such as bradycardia and hypotension.

NEUROMUSCULAR BLOCKING ACTION. When lidocaine is administered in conjunction with succinylcholine, observe for respiratory depression. Patients who are on respirators may require additional time to be weaned off ventilatory assistance.

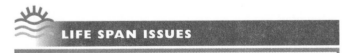 **mexiletine** (mehx-ihl'et-een)
Mexitil (mehx-it'ihl)

Actions

Mexiletine is a class Ib antiarrhythmic agent similar in many respects to lidocaine.

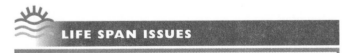

LIFE SPAN ISSUES

LIDOCAINE

Lidocaine for IV use for arrhythmias, often used for geriatric patients, is different from lidocaine used as a local anesthetic. For use with arrhythmias, check the label carefully to ensure that is says "lidocaine (or Xylocaine) for cardiac arrhythmias." Serious arrhythmias may result if lidocaine with preservatives or lidocaine with epinephrine are administered IV to the patient.

Uses

Mexiletine has the advantage of good oral absorption with minimal initial hepatic metabolism, thus allowing it to be administered orally. Mexiletine can be effective therapy in the treatment of unifocal and multifocal premature ventricular contractions, couplets, and ventricular tachycardia but is usually ineffective in the therapy of drug-resistant ventricular tachycardia. It is usually more effective against drug-resistant ventricular tachycardia when used in combination with other antiarrhythmic agents.

Therapeutic Outcomes

The primary therapeutic outcome expected from mexiletine therapy is conversion of arrhythmia to normal sinus rhythm.

Nursing Process

Premedication Assessment

1. Obtain data relating to the six cardinal signs of cardiovascular disease to be used as a baseline for subsequent evaluation of response to therapy.
2. Record data relating to any gastrointestinal symptoms present before initiation of therapy.
3. Assess and record data relating to the patient's mental status (for example, orientation, agitation, confusion).

Planning

Availability. PO—150, 200, and 250 mg capsules.

Implementation

Dosage and administration. PO—200 to 400 mg every 8 hours or 10 to 14 mg/kg per day.

Note: Mexiletine should not be used in patients with second- or third-degree heart block if a pacemaker is not present.

Dosage adjustment is necessary in patients with severe renal dysfunction (creatinine clearance less than 10 ml per minute) and in patients with severe congestive heart failure or acute myocardial infarction.

Administration with food or antacids may minimize gastric irritation without significantly inhibiting absorption. If symptoms persist or increase in severity, report for physician evaluation.

Evaluation

Side effects to expect

NAUSEA, VOMITING, DYSPEPSIA. Mexiletine may cause gastrointestinal adverse effects in approximately 40% of patients. These adverse effects are usually not serious and do not correlate well with high serum levels but are more prevalent with large orally administered doses.

Side effects to report

ARRHYTHMIAS. Mexiletine may induce or aggravate arrhythmias. This is uncommon in patients with less serious arrhythmias, such as frequent premature beats or nonsustained ventricular tachycardia. Patients with more serious arrhythmias, such as sustained ventricular tachycardia, are more susceptible to myocardial toxicity.

NEUROTOXICITY, SEIZURES. Mexiletine has dose-related effects on the central nervous system. At higher serum levels (greater than 2.0 µg/ml) mexiletine may precipitate neurologic toxicity and occasionally paradoxic seizure activity.

The initial manifestation of mexiletine neurotoxicity is usually a fine hand tremor, but ataxia, dizziness, lightheadedness, nystagmus, paresthesia, blurred vision, diplopia, dysarthria, confusion, and drowsiness are other signs of impending toxicity. Provide for patient safety during these episodes.

CONFUSION. Some patients have been reported to experience serious side effects such as seizures, severe ataxia, or mental confusion without manifestation of early warning signs. Perform a baseline assessment of the patient's degree of alertness and orientation to name, place, and time before initiating therapy. Make regularly scheduled subsequent mental status evaluations and compare findings. Report development of alterations.

Drug interactions

DRUGS THAT REDUCE THERAPEUTIC EFFECTS (PHENYTOIN, RIFAMPIN). The hepatic metabolism of mexiletine is enhanced by rifampin and phenytoin. Patients should be observed for redevelopment of arrhythmias, which may require an increase in dosage of mexiletine.

URINARY ACIDIFIERS. These agents may lower the urine pH, causing an increase in the urinary excretion of mexiletine. Patients should be observed for redevelopment of arrhythmias, which may require an increase in dosage of mexiletine.

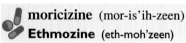 **moricizine** (mor-is'ih-zeen)
Ethmozine (eth-moh'zeen)

Actions

Moricizine is an antiarrhythmic agent chemically unrelated to other medicines used to treat arrhythmias. It acts by inhibition of influx of sodium ions into myocardial cells, making it a class I agent. It cannot be subclassified into the a, b, or c groups because it contains properties of each of the subcategories.

Uses

Moricizine is used for the treatment of life-threatening ventricular arrhythmias. Because of its ability to cause additional arrhythmias, its use is reserved for those patients in whom the benefits outweigh the potential risks.

Therapeutic Outcomes

The primary therapeutic outcome expected from moricizine therapy is conversion of arrhythmia to normal sinus rhythm.

Nursing Process

Premedication Assessment

1. Obtain data relating to the six cardinal signs of cardiovascular disease to be used as a baseline for subsequent evaluation of response to therapy.
2. Record data relating to any gastrointestinal symptoms present before initiation of therapy.
3. Assess and record data relating to the patient's mental status (for example, orientation, agitation, confusion).

Planning

Availability. PO—200, 250, and 300 mg tablets.

Implementation

Dosage and administration. PO—Initially, 200 mg every 8 hours. Dosages may be adjusted every 3 days in increments of 150 mg per day. The usual adult dosage is between 600 and 900 mg daily. Administer in divided dosages around the clock. If gastric irritation is a problem, administer with food or milk.

Evaluation

Side effects to expect

HYPOTENSION, DIZZINESS. These may occur, particularly during initiation of therapy. They usually subside within a few days. Instruct the patient to rise slowly from a supine position. Monitor the patient's blood pressure.

NAUSEA. Gastrointestinal complaints occur in about 10% of patients but discontinuation of therapy is rarely required. Administer with food or milk to alleviate nausea. Encourage the patient not to discontinue therapy without first consulting a physician.

Side effects to report

ARRHYTHMIAS. Moricizine may induce or aggravate arrhythmias. Patients with more serious arrhythmias, such as sustained ventricular tachycardia, are more susceptible to myocardial toxicity. The patient should be instructed to contact the physician for further evaluation if sensations of a jumping or racing heart develop.

EUPHORIA, CONFUSION. Perform a baseline assessment of the patient's degree of alertness and orientation to name, place, and time before initiating therapy. Make regularly scheduled subsequent mental status evaluations and compare findings. Report development of alterations. Provide for patient safety during episodes of dizziness. After discharge, caution the patient about operating machinery or driving if this is a recurrent problem.

Drug interactions

DRUGS THAT ENHANCE THERAPEUTIC AND TOXIC EFFECTS. Digoxin, cimetidine, and propranolol. Monitor for an increase in severity of side effects such as emesis, lethargy, hypotension, arrhythmias, and bradycardia.

THEOPHYLLINE. Moricizine, when given with theophylline, may result in theophylline toxicity. Observe for vomiting, dizziness, restlessness, and cardiac arrhythmias. Monitor theophylline serum levels. The dosage of theophylline may have to be reduced.

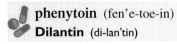

phenytoin (fen'e-toe-in)
Dilantin (di-lan'tin)

Actions

Phenytoin was introduced about 50 years ago for the treatment of epilepsy, but it is also effective in controlling arrhythmias. It is classified as a class Ib antiarrhythmic agent.

Uses

Phenytoin is used for paroxysmal atrial tachycardia and ventricular arrhythmias, particularly those induced by digitalis toxicity. (For use in seizure disorders, see p. 224.)

Side Effects

Phenytoin has a wide variety of side effects associated with therapy, but most occur after long-term use. Sedation, lethargy, dizziness, blurred vision, hypotension, and bradycardia are the most common adverse effects observed when phenytoin is used as a short-term antiarrhythmic agent. Occasionally, antiarrhythmic therapy may be continued on a long-term basis. Adverse effects and nursing interventions associated with long-term treatment with phenytoin are presented in the next section.

Therapeutic Outcomes

The primary therapeutic outcome expected from phenytoin therapy is conversion of arrhythmia to normal sinus rhythm.

Nursing Process

Premedication Assessment

1. Obtain data relating to the six cardinal signs of cardiovascular disease to be used as a baseline for subsequent evaluation of response to therapy.
2. Record data relating to any gastrointestinal symptoms present before initiation of therapy.
3. Assess and record data relating to the patient's mental status (for example, orientation, agitation, confusion).

Planning

Availability. PO—30 and 100 mg capsules and 50 mg chewable tablets. Oral suspension—30 and 125 mg per 5 ml. IV—50 mg/ml in 2 and 5 ml ampules and 2 ml syringes.

Implementation

Dosage and administration. Adults: PO—250 mg 4 times during the first day, 500 mg daily on days 2 and 3, and 300 to 400 mg on subsequent days. Administer with food or milk to minimize gastric irritation. If an oral suspension is used, shake well first. Encourage the use of an oral syringe for accurate measurement. IM—not recommended because of erratic absorption and pain on injection. IV—250 mg initially, at a rate no faster than 50 mg per minute until the arrhythmia is abolished, a total of 1000 mg has been given, or side effects appear. If given too rapidly, bradycardia and severe hypotension may result. The diluent propylene glycol will also potentiate the hypotensive effect of phenytoin and cause ECG changes. Cardiac and respiratory arrest may occur with excessive dosage and speed of administration. Blood pressure and ECG should be monitored carefully, especially during administration.

Note: Phenytoin should *not* be mixed with any drugs or added to any IV infusion solutions. The solubility is highly pH dependent, and use with other medications or solutions will result in a white precipitate. Each IV injection should be followed by an injection of sterile saline through the same needle or IV catheter to avoid local venous irritation.

Evaluation

Side effects to expect

NAUSEA, VOMITING, INDIGESTION. These effects are common during initiation of therapy. Gradual increases in therapy and administration with food or milk will minimize gastric irritation.

SEDATION, DROWSINESS, DIZZINESS, BLURRED VISION. These symptoms tend to disappear with continued therapy and possible readjustment of dosage. Encourage the patient not to discontinue therapy without first consulting the physician.

Provide for patient safety during episodes of dizziness. Report for further evaluation.

Caution the patient that blurred vision may occur and make appropriate suggestions for personal safety.

CONFUSION. Perform a baseline assessment of the patient's degree of alertness and orientation to name, place, and time *before* initiating therapy. Make regularly scheduled subsequent mental status evaluations and compare findings. Report development of alterations.

Side effects to report

DERMATOLOGIC REACTIONS. Report a rash or pruritis immediately and withhold additional doses pending approval by the physician.

Drug interactions

DRUGS THAT ENHANCE THERAPEUTIC AND TOXIC EFFECTS. Warfarin, disulfiram, phenylbutazone, isoniazid, carbamazepine, amiodarone, chloramphenicol, cimetidine, and the sulfonamide antimicrobial agents. Monitor patients with concurrent therapy for signs of phenytoin toxicity: nystagmus, sedation, and lethargy. Serum levels may be ordered, and a reduced dosage of phenytoin may be required.

DRUGS THAT DECREASE THERAPEUTIC EFFECTS. Barbiturates, folic acid, and antacids. Monitor patients with concurrent therapy for increased seizure activity or arrhythmias. Monitoring changes in serum levels should help warn of possible increased seizure or arrhythmic activity.

DISOPYRAMIDE, QUINIDINE, MEXILETINE. Phenytoin decreases serum levels of these agents. Monitor patients for redevelopment of arrhythmias.

PREDNISOLONE, DEXAMETHASONE. Phenytoin decreases serum levels of these agents. Monitor patients for reduced antiinflammatory activity.

ORAL CONTRACEPTIVES. Spotting or bleeding may be an indication of reduced contraceptive activity. Use of alternative forms of birth control is recommended.

THEOPHYLLINE. Phenytoin decreases serum levels of theophylline derivatives. Monitor patients for a greater frequency of respiratory difficulty. The theophylline dose may have to be increased 50% to 100% to maintain the same therapeutic response.

VALPROIC ACID. This agent may increase or decrease the activity of phenytoin. Monitor for increased frequency of seizure activity. Monitoring changes in serum levels should help warn of possible increased seizure activity. Monitor patients with concurrent therapy for signs of phenytoin toxicity: nystagmus, sedation, and lethargy. Serum levels may be ordered, and a reduced dosage of phenytoin may be required.

KETOCONAZOLE. Concurrent administration with ketoconazole may alter the metabolism of one or both drugs. Monitoring for both is recommended.

CYCLOSPORINE. Phenytoin enhances the metabolism of cyclosporine. Increased doses of cyclosporine may be necessary in patients receiving concomitant therapy.

procainamide hydrochloride (pro'kane'ah-myd)
Pronestyl (pro-nes'til), **Procan SR** (pro-kan')

Actions

Procainamide is an effective synthetic class Ia antiarrhythmic agent that has many cardiac effects similar to those of quinidine but generally with fewer side effects.

Uses

Procainamide is used to treat a wide variety of ventricular and supraventricular arrhythmias, atrial fibrillation, and flutter. It is usually not as effective in the last two disorders as quinidine.

Therapeutic Outcomes

The primary therapeutic outcome expected from procainamide therapy is conversion of arrhythmia to normal sinus rhythm.

Nursing Process

Premedication Assessment

Obtain data relating to the six cardinal signs of cardiovascular disease to be used as a baseline for subsequent evaluation of response to therapy.

Planning

Availability. PO—250, 375, and 500 mg tablets and capsules; 250, 500, 750, and 1000 mg sustained-release tablets. IV—100 mg/ml in 10 ml ampules and 500 mg/ml in 2 ml ampules.

Implementation

Dosage and administration. Note: Do not use in complete atrioventricular block, and use with extreme caution in partial atrioventricular block.

Adult: PO—loading dose: 1 to 1.25 g. Follow with 750 mg 1 hour later if the arrhythmia is still present. Maintain the dosage at 0.5 to 1 g every 4 to 6 hours. Some patients may require maintenance doses every 3 to 4 hours to maintain adequate control of arrhythmias. Administer in divided doses around the clock. If gastric irritation is a problem administer with food or milk. IM—0.5 to 1 g every 6 hours until PO therapy is possible. IV—100 mg every 5 minutes at 25 to 50 mg per minute until arrhythmias are suppressed, a maximum of 1 g has been administered, or side effects develop. Patients should have ECG and blood pressure monitoring when receiving intravenous doses of procainamide.

Once arrhythmias are suppressed, a continuous infusion may be started at 25 to 30 mg/kg per minute. If arrhythmias recur, suppress the arrhythmias with bolus therapy and increase the rate of infusion.

Serum levels of procainamide are performed to measure the amount of procainamide in the bloodstream. Blood should be drawn before the daily dose of medication or at least 6 hours after administration. It is important to be consistent in the time of drawing the blood and administering the dose if more than one serum level is to be drawn in the same patient. Therapeutic blood levels are 4 to 8 mg/L.

Evaluation

Side effects to expect

DROWSINESS, SEDATION, DIZZINESS. Tell patients they may experience these symptoms early in therapy, as the dosage is being adjusted. Instruct patients to use caution in operating power equipment or driving.

HYPOTENSION. Hypotension may be observed while therapy is being initiated, particularly by the intravenous route. Hypotension is usually transient and can be avoided by rising slowly from supine and sitting positions.

Side effects to report

FEVER, CHILLS, JOINT AND MUSCLE PAIN, SKIN ERUPTIONS. Tell patients to report the development of these symptoms. Monitor laboratory reports for leukocyte counts and the antinuclear antibody (ANA) titer.

Drug interactions

DRUGS THAT ENHANCE THERAPEUTIC AND TOXIC EFFECTS. Digitalis, cimetidine, ranitidine, quinidine, trimethoprim, and beta-adrenergic blocking agents (timolol, nadolol, propranolol, and others). Monitor for an increase in severity of side effects such as bradycardia and hypotension.

NEUROMUSCULAR BLOCKAGE, RESPIRATORY DEPRESSION. Surgical muscle relaxants (tubocurarine, succinylcholine, and gallamine triethiodide) and aminoglycoside antibiotics (gentamicin, streptomycin, amikacin, kanamycin, netilmycin, and others). Monitor the patient's respiratory rate and depth. Observe for signs of cyanosis and additional arrhythmias.

Patients who are on respirators may require additional time to be weaned off ventilatory assistance.

HYPOTENSION. Diuretics and antihypertensive agents: Instruct patients to rise slowly from a supine position. If symptoms begin to recur more frequently, report to the physician.

propafenone (pro-pah'fen-own)
Rythmol (rith'mohl)

Actions

Propafenone is classified as a class Ic antiarrhythmic agent. It also has weak beta-blocking and calcium channel–blocking effects.

Uses

Propafenone is used for the treatment of paroxysmal atrial fibrillation and life-threatening ventricular arrhythmias such as ventricular tachycardia. Because of its ability to cause additional arrhythmias, its use is reserved for those patients in whom the benefits outweigh the potential risks.

Therapeutic Outcomes

The primary therapeutic outcome expected from propafenone therapy is conversion of arrhythmia to normal sinus rhythm.

Nursing Process

Premedication Assessment

1. Obtain data relating to the six cardinal signs of cardiovascular disease to be used as a baseline for subsequent evaluation of response to therapy.
2. Record data relating to any gastrointestinal symptoms present before initiation of therapy.

Planning

Availability. PO—150 and 300 mg tablets.

Implementation

Dosage and administration. Note: Because propafenone has mild beta-adrenergic blocking properties, it should not be used in patients with asthma.

PO—initially 150 mg every 8 hours. At 3- to 4-day intervals the dosage may be increased to 225 mg every 8 hours, then 300 mg every 8 hours (900 mg per day).

Administer in divided dosages around the clock. If a patient misses a dose of propafenone, the next dose should not be doubled because of an increased risk of adverse reactions.

Evaluation

Side effects to expect

DIZZINESS. This may occur, particularly during initiation of therapy. It usually subsides within a few days. Instruct the patient to rise slowly from a supine position. Monitor the patient's blood pressure.

NAUSEA, VOMITING, CONSTIPATION. Gastrointestinal complaints occur in approximately 11% of patients, but discontinuation of therapy is rarely required. Administer with food or milk to alleviate nausea. Encourage the patient not to discontinue therapy without first consulting a physician.

Side effects to report

ARRHYTHMIAS. Propafenone may induce or aggravate arrhythmias. Patients with more serious arrhythmias, such as sustained ventricular tachycardia, are more susceptible to myocardial toxicity. The patient should be instructed to contact the physician for further evaluation if sensations of a jumping or racing heart develop.

Drug interactions

DRUGS THAT ENHANCE THERAPEUTIC AND TOXIC EFFECTS. Quinidine and cimetidine. Monitor for an increase in severity of side effects from propafenone such as hypotension, somnolence, bradycardia, and arrhythmias.

DRUGS THAT DECREASE THERAPEUTIC EFFECTS. Rifampin. Monitor patients with concurrent therapy for increased frequency of arrhythmias.

DIGOXIN. Propafenone produces dose-related increases in serum digoxin levels. Measure plasma digoxin levels and reduce digoxin dosage when propafenone is started.

PROPRANOLOL, METOPROLOL. Propafenone appears to inhibit the metabolism of these beta-blocking agents. A reduction in beta-blocker dosage may be necessary during concurrent therapy with propafenone.

WARFARIN. Propafenone increases plasma warfarin concentrations by inhibiting warfarin metabolism, thus prolonging prothrombin time. Observe for the development of petechiae, ecchymoses, nosebleeds, bleeding gums, dark tarry stools, and bright red or coffee-ground emesis. Monitor the prothrombin time and reduce the dosage of warfarin if necessary.

quinidine (kwin'i-din)

Actions

Quinidine, originally obtained from cinchona bark, has been used as an antiarrhythmic agent for several decades. It is classified as a class Ia antiarrhythmic agent, working on the muscle of the heart and stabilizing the rate of conduction of impulses. It slows the heart and changes a rapid, irregular pulse to a slow, regular pulse.

Uses

Quinidine is used most frequently to suppress atrial fibrillation, atrial flutter, paroxysmal supraventricular and ventricular tachycardia, and premature ventricular contractions. Use with extreme caution in patients with digitalis intoxication or heart block.

Therapeutic Outcomes

The primary therapeutic outcome expected from quinidine therapy is conversion of arrhythmia to normal sinus rhythm.

Nursing Process

Premedication Assessment
1. Obtain data relating to the six cardinal signs of cardiovascular disease to be used as a baseline for subsequent evaluation of response to therapy.
2. Assess and record data relating to the patient's usual pattern of bowel elimination.

Planning
Availability. Quinidine sulfate: PO—100, 200, and 300 mg tablets; 200 and 300 mg capsules; 300 mg sustained-release tablets. IM, IV—200 mg/ml in 1 ml ampules.

Quinidine gluconate: PO—324 mg and 330 mg sustained-release tablets. IM, IV—80 mg/ml in 10 ml vials.

Implementation
Dosage and administration. Adult: PO—quinidine sulfate: 200 to 400 mg 3 to 5 times daily. Higher doses may be used, but the maximum single dose should not exceed 600 to 800 mg. Administer with food or milk if gastric irritation develops. IM—quinidine gluconate: 600 mg initially, then 400 mg every 2 hours as needed. IV—quinidine gluconate: 800 mg diluted to 40 ml with dextrose 5% and infused at a rate of 1 ml per minute.

Note: IV administration is extremely hazardous. Blood pressure and ECG readings should be monitored continuously because hypotension and arrhythmias may occur. Therapeutic blood levels are 1.5 to 3 mg/L.

Pediatric: PO—quinidine sulfate: 30 mg/kg per 24 hours divided into 4 to 6 doses. IM—quinidine gluconate: as for PO administration.

Serum levels of quinidine are performed to measure the amount of quinidine in the bloodstream. Blood should be drawn before the daily dose of medication or at least 6 hours after administration. It is important to be consistent in the time of drawing the blood and administering the dose if more than one serum level is to be drawn in the same patient.

Evaluation
Side effects to expect
DIARRHEA. Diarrhea is common during initiation of therapy. It usually subsides, but occasionally a different medication may need to be administered because of adverse effect. Chart the frequency and consistency of the diarrhea, and monitor the patient for dehydration and electrolyte imbalance.

DIZZINESS, FAINTNESS. These may occur, particularly during initiation of therapy. They usually subside within a few days. Instruct the patient to rise slowly from a supine position. Monitor the patient's blood pressure.

Side effects to report
CINCHONISM. Monitor patients for signs of **cinchonism** and report the development of rash, chills, fever, ringing in the ears (**tinnitus**), and increasing mental confusion.

Drug interactions
DRUGS THAT ENHANCE THERAPEUTIC AND TOXIC EFFECTS. Cimetidine, phenothiazines, procainamide, digitalis, and beta-adrenergic blocking agents (propranolol, atenolol, timolol, and others). Monitor for increases in severity of drug effects such as bradycardia, tachycardia, and hypotension.

DRUGS THAT REDUCE THERAPEUTIC EFFECTS. Rifampin. Monitor for an increase in arrhythmias.

NEUROMUSCULAR BLOCKADE, RESPIRATORY DEPRESSION. Surgical muscle relaxants (tubocurarine, succinylcholine, and gallamine triethiodide) and aminoglycoside antibiotics (gentamicin, streptomycin, kanamycin, netilmycin, and others). Monitor the patient's respiratory rate and depth. Observe for signs of cyanosis and additional arrhythmias.

Patients who are on respirators may require additional time to be weaned from ventilatory assistance.

DIGITALIS. Quinidine may increase the effects of digitalis. Monitor the patient for symptoms of anorexia, nausea, vomiting, headaches, blurred or colored vision, and bradycardia. A digitalis serum level and quinidine serum level may be ordered by the physician.

WARFARIN. Quinidine may increase the anticoagulant effects of warfarin. Monitor for signs of increased bleeding: bleeding gums, increased menstrual flow, petechiae, and bruises.

Monitor the laboratory report and notify the physician immediately if the prothrombin time or the internationalized ratio (INR) is abnormally high.

HYPOTENSION. Diuretics and antihypertensive agents: Instruct the patient to rise slowly from a supine position. If symptoms become excessive, report to the physician.

tocainide (toe-kayn'ayd)
Tonocard (toe-no'kard)

Actions

Tocainide hydrochloride is the first available derivative of lidocaine with antiarrhythmic activity when administered orally. Like lidocaine, it is a class Ib antiarrhythmic agent.

Uses

Tocainide is indicated for the suppression of ventricular arrhythmias, including frequent premature ventricular contractions, unifocal or multifocal couplets, and ventricular tachycardia. Most patients who respond to lidocaine will also respond to tocainide. It is useful in patients whose arrhythmias have been initially controlled with intravenously administered lidocaine.

Therapeutic Outcomes

The primary therapeutic outcome expected from tocainide therapy is conversion of arrhythmia to normal sinus rhythm.

Nursing Process

Premedication Assessment

1. Obtain data relating to the six cardinal signs of cardiovascular disease to be used as a baseline for subsequent evaluation of response to therapy.
2. Record data relating to any gastrointestinal symptoms present before initiation of therapy.
3. Initiate request for laboratory tests to evaluate hematologic status of patient before initiation of therapy (for example, complete blood cell count [CBC] with differential).

Planning

Availability. PO—400 and 600 mg tablets.

Implementation

Dosage and administration. Note: Tocainide should not be used in patients with second- or third-degree atrioventricular block in the absence of an artificial ventricular pacemaker and must be used with caution in patients with known heart failure. Monitor the ECG readings before and during therapy.

PO—initially 400 mg every 8 hours. The usual maintenance dose is 1200 to 1800 mg daily given in equally divided doses every 8 hours. Maximum daily doses are usually less than 2400 mg.

Conversion from lidocaine—A 600 mg oral dose of tocainide is given 6 hours before cessation of lidocaine therapy and repeated 6 hours later, at the time of lidocaine discontinuation. Maintenance doses may be started 6 to 8 hours later. Patients should be monitored closely during this transition.

Evaluation

Side effects to expect

NAUSEA, VOMITING, ANOREXIA, ABDOMINAL PAIN. These side effects are usually mild and tend to resolve with continued therapy. Encourage the patient not to discontinue therapy without first consulting a physician.

Side effects to report

DIZZINESS, CONFUSION, NUMBNESS, TINGLING. Perform a baseline assessment of the patient's degree of alertness and orientation to name, place, and time before initiating therapy. Make regularly scheduled subsequent mental status evaluations and compare findings. Report development of alterations. Provide for patient safety during episodes of dizziness.

DYSPNEA, WHEEZING, COUGH. Adverse pulmonary effects associated with tocainide therapy are usually characterized by pulmonary radiographic changes, including bilateral infiltrates, and are clinically manifested by dyspnea, wheezing, and cough. Symptoms usually occur within 3 to 18 weeks after initiation of therapy. If these adverse effects develop, tocainide therapy should be discontinued.

THROMBOCYTOPENIA, LEUKOPENIA, ANEMIA. Hematologic effects such as anemia, leukopenia, agranulocytosis, and thrombocytopenia have occurred in less than 1% of patients. These effects usually occur 2 to 12 weeks after initiation of therapy. Blood cell counts usually return to normal within 1 month after discontinuation of therapy.

Routine laboratory studies (red blood cell count, platelets, white blood cell count, and differential counts) should be scheduled. Stress the importance of returning for this laboratory work.

Monitor patients for the development of sore throat, fever, purpura, jaundice, or excessive, progressive weakness.

Drug interactions

DRUGS THAT ENHANCE THERAPEUTIC AND TOXIC EFFECTS. Procainamide, disopyramide, quinidine, phenytoin, and beta-adrenergic blocking agents. Monitor for an increase in severity of side effects such as bradycardia and hypotension.

DRUGS THAT REDUCE THERAPEUTIC EFFECTS. Cimetidine and rifampin. Monitor for an increased frequency in arrhythmias.

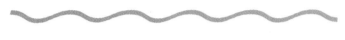

CHAPTER REVIEW

Arrhythmias are complex in origin, severity, and treatment for control. Many of the agents used to treat arrhythmias have serious adverse effects and must be monitored closely. Nurses can play a significant role in public education efforts, monitor patient response to therapy, monitor for noncompliance, and encourage patients to participate in their own therapy.

MATH REVIEW

1. Ordered: Quinidine 0.8 g, PO TID.
   On hand: Quinidine 200 mg tablets.
   Give: _____ tablets per dose.
   Give: _____ total g in 24 hours.

2. Ordered: Procainamide hydrochloride (Pronestyl) 1 g PO q6h.
   On hand: Procainamide hydrochloride (Pronestyl) 250 mg capsules.
   Give: _____ capsules per dose.

CRITICAL THINKING QUESTIONS

Situation:

Adenosine (Adenocard) 6 mg IV bolus was given stat to a patient in the emergency room today being treated for paroxysmal supraventricular tachycardia. At postconference the instructor discusses this case with the student nurses. Using any reference books, answer the following questions:

1. What is paroxysmal supraventricular tachycardia, and why is this dangerous to the patient?

2. What is the normal conduction of impulses through the heart?

3. The instructor requests the students to look up the following information for the drug adenosine:

Drug action
Dosage
Preparation of drug for IV use
    Dilution: Yes   No
    Solutions that can be used to dilute the IV
    medication
    Rate of administration
    Incompatability
    Side effects to expect
Situation:
Physician order is quinidine sulfate 200 mg PO QID.
1. What time schedule would be used to fulfill this order?
   When a quinidine serum level is ordered, based on the time schedule established, when would the laboratory draw the blood sample?
2. What nursing assessments should be made during the administration of quinidine sulfate? What health teaching should be done?
Situation:
The physician orders disopyramide (Norpace) 150 mg PO q6h.
1. What time schedule would be used to administer the drug?
2. After a week of therapy the therapeutic blood level report from the laboratory is 8 mg/L. What nursing actions would be initiated?

23

Drugs Used to Treat Angina Pectoris

CHAPTER CONTENT

Objectives

1. Describe the actions of nitrates, beta-adrenergic blockers, and calcium channel blockers on the myocardial tissue of the heart.
2. Identify assessment data needed to evaluate an anginal attack.
3. Implement medication therapy health teaching to an anginal patient in the clinical setting.

Key Words

angina pectoris
ischemic heart disease
chronic stable angina

unstable angina
variant angina

ANGINA PECTORIS

Coronary heart disease is the leading cause of disability, socioeconomic loss, and death in the United States, and angina pectoris is the first clinical indication of underlying disease in many patients. **Angina pectoris** is the name given to a feeling of chest discomfort arising from the heart because of lack of oxygen to heart cells. It is a symptom of coronary artery disease, also called ischemic heart disease. **Ischemic heart disease** develops when the supply of oxygen needed by heart cells is inadequate. The lack of oxygen is caused by reduced blood flow through the coronary arteries caused by atherosclerosis or spasm of the arteries. Atherosclerosis can develop as localized plaques or as a generalized narrowing of the coronary arteries. Patients are usually asymptomatic until there is at least 50% narrowing of the artery. Coronary artery disease caused by atherosclerosis is a progressive disease; however, progression can be slowed by diet control and possibly by use of cholesterol-lowering agents. (See Chapter 19.)

The presentation of angina pectoris is highly variable. The sensation of discomfort is often described variously as squeezing, tightness, choking, pressure, burning, or heaviness. This discomfort may radiate to the neck, lower jaw, shoulder, and arms. The usual anginal attack begins gradually, reaches a peak intensity over the next several minutes, and then gradually subsides after the person stops activity and rests. Attacks can last from 30 seconds to 30 minutes. Anginal episodes are usually precipitated by factors that require an increased oxygen supply (for example, physical activity such as climbing a flight of stairs or lifting). Other precipitating factors include exposure to cold temperatures, emotional stress, sexual intercourse, and eating a large meal.

Angina pectoris is classified as chronic stable, unstable, or variant angina. **Chronic stable angina** is precipitated by physical exertion or stress, lasts only a few minutes, and is relieved by rest or nitroglycerin. It is usually caused by fixed atherosclerotic obstruction in the coronary arteries. **Unstable angina** is unpredictable; it changes in ease of onset, frequency, duration, and intensity. It is probably caused by a combination of atherosclerotic narrowing, vasospasm, and thrombus formation. **Variant angina** occurs while the patient is at rest, is characterized by specific electrocardiographic changes, and is caused by vasospasm of a coronary artery reducing blood flow. The type of angina pectoris is diagnosed by a combination of history, electrocardiographic changes during an anginal attack, and exercise tolerance testing with or without thallium-201 scintigraphy.

Treatment

The goals in treatment of angina pectoris are to relieve anginal pain symptoms; improve the quality of life by preventing additional anginal attacks; prevent complications such as sudden death, myocardial infarction, and arrhythmias; and prolong life expectancy. All patients should receive extensive patient education to help them reduce the risks of coronary heart disease. Avoidance of activities that can precipitate attacks (for example, strenuous exercise, exposure to cold weather, use of caffeine-containing beverages, cigarette smoking, eating heavy meals, and emotional stress) should be attempted. Risk factors such as diabetes mellitus, hypertension, and hypercholesterolemia must also be treated. A structured exercise program designed for each specific patient can also be successful in fostering weight reduction in overweight patients and improving cardiovascular health. Healthy muscle tissue requires less oxygen. Medications are effective in preventing the onset of anginal attacks.

Drug Therapy

Actions

The underlying pathophysiology of ischemic heart disease is an imbalance between the oxygen demands of the heart and the ability of coronary arteries to deliver the oxygen, spasticity of coronary arteries, platelet aggregation, and thrombus formation. The oxygen demand of the heart is determined by the heart rate, contractility, and ventricular volume. Therefore the pharmacologic treatment of angina is aimed at decreasing oxygen demand by decreasing heart rate, myocardial contractility, and

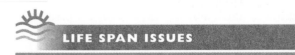

LIFE SPAN ISSUES

ANGINAL ATTACKS

The goal of treatment of an anginal attack, which most often occur in the elderly, is relief of pain, not simply a reduction of pain. If pain relief is not achieved with the use of nitroglycerin, the patient should immediately contact the physician or be seen in the emergency room. Do not administer analgesics in an attempt to eliminate the pain.

ventricular volume. Because platelet aggregation, blood flow turbulence, and blood viscosity also play a role, especially in unstable angina, platelet-active agents are also prescribed to prevent anginal attacks. (See Chapter 26.)

Uses

At present, four groups of drugs are used to treat angina pectoris: nitrates, beta-adrenergic blocking agents, calcium ion antagonists, and platelet-active agents. Combination therapy is beneficial in many patients.

Drug therapy for patients with angina must be individualized. Most patients will be given prescriptions (for example, nitroglycerin sublingual tablets or lingual spray) for treating acute attacks and a prescription for prophylactic therapy to prevent recurrent attacks. Prophylactic therapy consists of a long-acting nitrate, a beta blocker, or a calcium ion antagonist. The decision of which to use is dependent on other diseases the patient may have and the expected adverse effects of therapy. Aspirin, a platelet-active agent, may also be considered to slow platelet aggregation.

Nursing Process for Anginal Therapy

Assessment

History of anginal attacks. Ask specific questions to identify the onset, duration, and intensity of the pain. Ask the patient to describe the chest sensation and the pattern of occurrence (for example, under the sternum; in the jaw, neck, and shoulder; or radiation down the left arm, right arm, or both into the hand and fingers). What activities precipitate an attack? Does the pain occur with or without exertion? Is the pain relieved by rest? Does the chest pain occur shortly after eating?

Medication history. What medications are being used for the treatment of the angina? What effect does taking nitroglycerin have on the anginal pain? How many nitroglycerin tablets are required to obtain pain relief during an attack? How many nitroglycerin tablets are being taken per day? How old is the nitroglycerin being used sublingually? Is it stored properly? Have the prescribed medications been taken regularly? If not, determine reasons for noncompliance.

Central nervous system. • Mental status: Identify the individual's level of consciousness and clarity of thought. Check for orientation to date, time, and place and level of confusion, restlessness, or irritability. These factors are indicators of cerebral perfusion. • Syncope: Ask the patient to describe the conditions surrounding any episodes of syncope. Record the degree of presenting symptoms such as general mental weakness, inability to stand upright, feeling faint, or loss of consciousness. Record what activities, if any, bring on these episodes. • Anxiety: What degree of apprehension is present? Were there stressful events that precipitated the attack?

Cardiovascular system. • Palpitations: Record the patient's description of palpitations, such as "my heart skips some beats" or "it began to feel like it was racing." Ask if these conditions are preceded by mild or strenuous exercise and how long the palpitations last. • Heart rate: Count and record the rate, rhythm, and quality of the pulse. • Blood pressure: Record the blood pressure. It may be increased or decreased during an attack. Compare to previous baseline readings. • Respirations: The patient may be dyspneic. Ask whether the attack occurred while at rest or during exertion. • Cardiovascular history: What concurrent cardiovascular diseases does the patient have (for example, hypertension or hypercholesterolemia)? • Peripheral perfusion: Check for peripheral perfusion by taking pedal pulses and checking skin color and temperature. Check hair pattern on feet and lower legs. • Smoking: Does the patient smoke? How much? What understanding of the effects of smoking on the cardiovascular system does the patient have? *Nutritional history.* Diet: Is the patient on a special diet (for example, low sodium, low fat)? Is the patient being treated for high cholesterol?

Nursing Diagnosis
- Pain, acute (indication)
- Tissue perfusion, altered (indication)
- Activity intolerance (indication)
- Injury, risk for (side effects)

Planning
History of anginal attacks. Review the history of anginal attacks to identify precipitating factors. Work with the patient to plan interventions that will minimize factors that trigger attacks.

Medication history. Review medications being taken and establish whether they are being taken correctly. Analyze noncompliance issues and plan interventions with the patient. Plan to review drug administration as needed.

Central nervous system. Plan for stress reduction education and discussion of effective means of coping with stressful events.

Cardiovascular system. Identify the degree of cardiovascular symptoms produced by the anginal attack. Develop a plan to intervene to improve tissue oxygenation and provide for patient safety.

Nutritional history. Examine the dietary history to establish whether a referral to a nutritionist would benefit the individual's understanding of the diet regimen. Plan interventions needed to deal with dietary noncompliance.

Implementation
- Adequate tissue perfusion is essential. Instruct the patient to take measures to avoid fatigue and cold weather, which can cause vasoconstriction, and provide for personal safety when symptoms of hypoxia are present (for example, light-headedness, dyspnea, and chest pain).
- When pain is present, comfort measures must be implemented to allow the individual to decrease the pain. Fatigue may increase pain perception; spacing activities so that fatigue does not occur is recommended.
- Medication administration—see individual monographs.

Patient Education and Health Promotion
Medications
- Teach the signs and symptoms of hypotension, which is known to occur when nitrates are taken. Weakness, dizziness, or faintness can usually be relieved by increasing muscular activity (alternately flexing and relaxing muscles

in legs) or by sitting or lying down. Resting for 10 to 15 minutes after taking medication may also assist in management of hypotension. Because light-headedness or fainting is a possibility when taking nitroglycerin, safety measures to prevent injury from the transient orthostatic hypotension must be stressed.
- Explain that a headache may occur with the use of nitroglycerin, but it should subside within 20 to 30 minutes.
- Teach specific administration techniques to the patient for the type of medication prescribed, for example, sublingual, transmucosal tablets, translingual spray, topical ointment, and transdermal disks.

Lifestyle modifications
- Lifestyle modifications are essential for many individuals with angina. Teach appropriate behavioral changes, such as stress management (relaxation techniques, meditation, three-part breathing, etc.).
- The patient must resume activities of daily living within the boundaries set by the physician. (Such activities as regular, moderate exercise, meal preparation, resumption of usual sexual activities, and social interactions all need to be encouraged.)
- Individuals unable to attain the degree of activity hoped for through drug therapy may become frustrated. Allow for verbalization of feelings, and then implement actions appropriate to the circumstances.
- Participation in regular exercise is essential. Follow guidelines of the American Heart Association regarding an exercise program. Increase exercise demands gradually, and monitor effects on the cardiovascular system. Changes in the level of exercise may require participation in a supervised program, that is, cardiac rehabilitation. Tell the patient to avoid overexertion. Anginal pain may occur with exercise, and taking nitroglycerin before exercise or performing certain activities may be recommended. Instruct the patient to always *stop exercising* or performing any activity *when chest pain is present.*
- Discuss the need for smoking cessation and make referrals to available self-help programs in the area. Smoking causes vasoconstriction; encourage drastic reduction and preferably elimination of smoking.
- Dietary modification aimed at decreasing the cholesterol level and a reducing program to maintain ideal weight are usually prescribed by the physician. Depending on coexisting conditions, other dietary modifications such as low sodium may be suggested. Discourage the use of caffeine-containing products because they may precipitate an anginal attack when taken in excess.
- If hypertension accompanies the angina, stress the importance of following prescribed emotional, dietary, and medicinal regimens to control the disease.
- Instruct the patient not to ingest alcohol while receiving nitroglycerin therapy. Alcohol causes vasodilation, potentially resulting in postural hypotension.
- Teach proper storage of medication in a dark, airtight container, especially sublingual nitroglycerin.
- Always report poor pain control to the physician.

Fostering health maintenance
- Throughout the course of treatment, discuss medication information and how it will benefit the patient.

• Drug therapy is essential to maintain adequate oxygenation of the myocardial cells and body tissues. Although medications can control the anginal attacks, lifestyle changes to deal with the management of precipitating factors must also occur.
• Provide the patient and significant others with the important information contained in the specific drug monograph for the drugs prescribed. Additional health teaching and nursing interventions for side effects to expect and report will be described in the drug monographs that follow.
• Seek cooperation and understanding of the following points so that medication compliance is increased: name of medication, dosage, route and times of administration, side effects to expect, and side effects to report.
• Enlist the patient's aid in developing and maintaining a written record of monitoring parameters, such as blood pressure, pulse, degree of pain relief, exercise tolerance, and side effects experienced (see the Patient Education and Monitoring Form in Chapter 21, p. 282). Instruct the patient to bring the written record to follow-up visits.

Drug Class: Nitrates

Actions

The nitrates are the oldest effective therapy for angina pectoris. Although they have been termed *coronary vasodilators,* these agents do not increase total coronary blood flow. First, nitrates relieve angina pectoris by inducing relaxation of peripheral vascular smooth muscles, resulting in dilatation of arteries and veins. This reduces venous blood return (reduced preload) to the heart, which in turn leads to decreased oxygen demands on the heart. Second, nitrates increase myocardial oxygen supply by dilating large coronary arteries and redistributing blood flow, enhancing oxygen supply to ischemic areas.

Uses

Nitroglycerin is currently the drug of choice for treatment of angina pectoris. It is available in different dosages for adjustment to the patient's needs. Sublingual tablets dissolve rapidly and are used primarily for acute attacks of angina. The sustained-release tablets and capsules, ointment, transmucosal tablets, and transdermal patches are used prophylactically to prevent anginal attacks. The translingual spray may be used for both acute treatment and prophylaxis of anginal attacks.

Amyl nitrite is a volatile liquid, available in small glass ampules. The ampules are encased in a loosely woven material so that the ampule can be crushed easily under the patient's nostrils for inhalation. The onset of action is less than 1 minute, but the duration is only about 10 minutes.

With continued use of transdermal nitroglycerin patches and frequent doses of oral nitrates and sustained-release nitrates, tolerance and loss of antianginal response develop. The best way to avoid tolerance is to have periodic nitrate-free periods. An 8- to 12-hour nitrate-free period will eliminate the development of tolerance. Depending on the type of angina, patients will be told when not to use nitrates (for example, bedtime) unless they have an acute attack. Other agents such as beta blockers or calcium ion antagonists may also be prescribed to help provide prophylaxis against attacks during nitrate-free periods.

Therapeutic Outcomes

The primary therapeutic outcomes from nitrate therapy are as follows:
• Relief of anginal pain during an attack
• Reduced frequency and severity of anginal attacks
• Increased tolerance of activities

Nursing Process

Premedication Assessment
1. Assess pain level, location, duration, intensity, and pattern.
2. Ask when the last dose of nitrates was taken and what degree of relief was obtained.

Planning
Availability.   See Table 23-1.

Implementation
Dosage and administration.   See Table 23-1.
Sublingual administration
1. Instruct the patient to sit or lie down at the first sign of an oncoming anginal attack.
2. Place a tablet under the tongue and allow it to dissolve; encourage the patient not to swallow the saliva immediately.
3. If more than 3 tablets within 15 minutes are required to control pain, the patient should seek medical attention.
4. One or two tablets may be taken prophylactically a few minutes before engaging in activities that may trigger an anginal attack.
5. Chart the patient's ability to place the sublingual medication under the tongue correctly.
   Medication deterioration.   Every 3 months, the nitroglycerin prescription should be refilled and the old tablets safely discarded. (Be sure the patient knows how to have the prescription refilled).)
   Medication storage.   Store nitroglycerin in the original, dark-colored glass container with a tight lid.
   Medication accessibility.   Nonhospitalized patients should carry nitroglycerin at all times, but not in a pocket directly next to the body because heat hastens the deterioration of the medication. When taken, the drug should produce a slight stinging or burning sensation, which usually indicates that the drug is still potent.
   Allow the hospitalized patient to keep the nitroglycerin at bedside or on person if ambulatory. Check hospital policy to see if a fresh supply of medicine should be issued rather than using the agents brought from home. (Remember, the nurse is still responsible for gathering and charting relevant data regarding all medication taken by the patient when the medication is left at bedside.)
Sustained-release tablet administration. This type of nitroglycerin is usually taken on an empty stomach every 8 to 12 hours. If gastritis develops, it may be necessary to take the sustained-release tablet with food.
Transmucosal tablet administration.   When placed under the upper lip or buccal pouch, it releases nitroglycerin for absorption by the oral mucosa over the next 3 to 5 hours. Patients may eat, drink, and talk while the tablet is in place. The usual initial dose is one tablet 3 times daily: one on

Table 23-1

Nitrates

GENERIC NAME	BRAND NAME	AVAILABILITY	ONSET	DURATION	DOSAGE
Amyl nitrite		Inhalation: 0.3 ml ampules in a woven sack for crushing	0.5 min	3-5 min	Inhalation: I ampule crushed in sack and placed under patient's nostrils for inhalation at time of acute attack
Isosorbide dinitrate	Isordil	Sublingual tablets: 2.5, 5, 10 mg	2-3 min	I-3 hr	Sublingual: 2.5-10 mg for acute attack
		Oral tablets: 5, 10, 20, 30, 40 mg	0.5-I hr	4-6 hr	PO: 2.5-30 mg 3-4 times daily on empty stomach
		Chewable tablets: 5, 10 mg	3 min	0.5-2 hr	PO: initially, chew 5 mg; if needed, chew 5-10 mg
		Sustained-release tablets and capsules: 40 mg	0.5-I hr	6-8 hr	PO: 20-40 mg every 6-8 hr or 80 mg every 8-12 hr
Isosorbide mononitrate	Monoket ISMO Imdur	Oral tablets: 10 mg Oral tablets: 20 mg Sustained-release tablets: 60 mg	30-60 min 3-4 hr	NA 8-12 hr	PO: 20 mg twice daily, 7 hr apart PO: 30-240 mg once daily; do not crush or chew tablets
Nitroglycerin	Nitrostat	Sublingual tablets: 0.3, 0.4, and 0.6 mg	I-2 min	>30 min	Sublingual: 0.3-0.6 mg for prophylactic use before activity that may induce angina pectoris or at time of acute attack
	Nitrong	Oral sustained-release tablets and capsules: 2.5, 6.5, 9 mg	30-45 min	3-8 hr	PO: 2.5-9 mg 3-4 times daily for prophylaxis
	Nitro-Bid	Ointment: 2%	30 min	3 hr	Topical: 0.5-4 inch of ointment using special applicator every 4-6 hr
	Nitrogard	Transmucosal: 1, 2, and 3 mg tablets	2-3 min	3-5 hr	Buccal: place 1-3 mg between cheek and gum every 3-5 hr
	Nitro-Dur	Transdermal: 0.1, 0.2, 0.3, 0.4, 0.6, and 0.8 mg/hr patches	30-60 min	<24 hr	Topical: I patch applied for 24 hrs; patient should wait 12-24 hr after removing old patch before applying new patch
	Nitrolingual	Translingual: 0.4 mg metered spray	2 min	30-60 min	Spray: 1-2 sprays for acute attack; repeat if needed in 3-5 min; may be used prophylactically 5-10 min before exercise
	Nitro-Bid IV	Intravenous: 0.5, 0.8, 5, and 10 mg/ml in 1, 5, 10, and 20 ml vials and ampules	I-2 min	3-5 min	IV: initially, 5 μg/min through an infusion pump; adjust dosage as needed

arising, one after lunch, and one after the evening meal. Do not administer more than one tablet every 2 hours.

Translingual spray administration. Patients should be instructed to familiarize themselves with the position of the spray orifice, which can be identified by the finger rest on top of the valve. This can be particularly helpful for administration at night.

The spray is highly flammable. Instruct the patient not to use it where it might be ignited.

1. At the time of administration, the patient should preferably be in a sitting position.
2. The canister should be held vertically with the valve head uppermost and the spray orifice as close to the mouth as possible. Do not shake the container because bubbles formed may slow the release of nitroglycerin.
3. The dose should be sprayed onto or under the tongue by pressing the button firmly.
4. The mouth should be closed immediately after each dose. THE SPRAY SHOULD NOT BE SWALLOWED OR INHALED.

If more than three doses are required within 15 minutes, medical attention should be sought.

Topical ointment administration

1. Position the dose-measuring applicator paper with the printed side down.
2. Squeeze the proper amount (usually 1 to 2 inches) of ointment onto the applicator paper.
3. Place the measuring applicator on the skin, ointment down, spreading in a thin, uniform layer. Do not massage or rub in. Any area without hair may be used; however, many people prefer the chest, flank, or upper arm. The lower extremities are not used, especially if there is reduced peripheral perfusion. (Because of the potential for skin irritation, do not shave an area to apply the medication.)
4. Help the patient develop a site rotation schedule to prevent skin irritation. Tell the patient not to apply the ointment to an area that shows signs of irritation. Use of the applicator allows measuring of the proper dose and also prevents absorption through the fingertips.
5. Cover the area where the patch is placed with a clear plastic wrap and tape in place. (Caution the patient that the medication may discolor clothing.)
6. Close the tube tightly and store in a cool place.
7. When terminating the use of the topical ointment, gradually reduce the dose and frequency of application over 4 to 6 weeks.

Transdermal disk administration. This dosage form provides a controlled release of nitroglycerin through a semipermeable membrane for 24 hours when applied to intact skin. The dosage released depends on the surface area of the disk. Therapeutic effect can be observed in about 30 minutes after attachment and continues for about 30 minutes after removal.

1. The disk should be applied to a clean, dry, hairless area of skin. Do not apply to shaved areas. Skin irritation may alter drug absorption. If hair is likely to interfere with patch adhesion or removal, trim the hair but do not shave. Optimal locations for patch placement are on the upper chest or side; pelvis; and inner, upper arm. Avoid scars, skin folds, and wounds. Rotate skin sites daily. (Help the patient develop a rotation chart.)
2. Wash hands before applying and after removing the product.
3. See individual product information to determine whether a patch can be worn while swimming, bathing, or showering.

4. If a disk becomes partially dislodged, discard it and replace with a new disk.
5. Sublingual nitroglycerin may be necessary for anginal attacks, especially while the dosage is being adjusted.
6. Dispose of used patches out of reach of children. Discarded patches still contain enough active ingredient to be dangerous to children.

Intravenous nitroglycerin administration. This drug is used in an intensive care setting and requires continuous monitoring of vital signs: blood pressure, pulse, respirations, and central venous pressure.

An infusion pump must be used to monitor the precise delivery of the infusion. Dose is titrated to achieve the desired clinical response. Gradual weaning is needed under controlled conditions to prevent a rebound action.

This medication is never mixed with other medications and is administered only with administration sets made specifically for nitroglycerin because most plastic administration sets absorb the drug. See the manufacturer's literature for exact directions recommended for preparation and administration.

Evaluation
Side effects to report

EXCESSIVE HYPOTENSION. This side effect of the nitrates is an extension of its pharmacologic activity. Other possible side effects include dizziness, nausea, flushing, and rarely syncope or hypotension. Report these adverse effects so that more appropriate dosage adjustment may be made.

PROLONGED HEADACHE. The most common side effect of the nitrate therapy is headache. This can range from a mild sensation of fullness in the head to an intense and severe generalized headache. Most patients develop a tolerance within a few weeks of starting therapy. Analgesics such as acetaminophen may be used if needed. Report these adverse effects so that more appropriate dosage adjustment may be made.

TOLERANCE (INCREASING DOSES TO ATTAIN RELIEF). Tolerance to the nitrate dosages can develop rapidly, particularly if large doses are administered frequently. Tolerance can appear within a few days and may be well established within a few weeks. The smallest dose to give satisfactory results should be used to minimize the development of tolerance. Tolerance is broken by withdrawing the drug for a short period.

Drug interactions

ALCOHOL. Alcohol accentuates the vasodilation and postural hypotension of the nitrates. Patients should be warned that drinking alcohol while on therapy may cause hypotension.

CALCIUM ION ANTAGONISTS, BETA-ADRENERGIC BLOCKING AGENTS. Calcium ion antagonists and nitrates may significantly lower blood pressure. Dosage adjustments may be necessary.

Drug Class: Beta-Adrenergic Blocking Agents
Actions

The beta-adrenergic blocking agents (beta blockers) (see Table 11-3) reduce myocardial oxygen demand by blocking the beta-adrenergic receptors in the heart, preventing stimulation from norepinephrine and epinephrine that would normally cause an increased heart rate. The beta blockers also reduce blood pressure. (See Chapter 20.)

Uses

The goal of beta-blocker therapy is to reduce the number of anginal attacks, reduce nitroglycerin use, and improve exercise tolerance while minimizing side effects. All beta blockers are effective in treating angina pectoris, so product selection should be based on other conditions the patient may have (for example, diabetes, chronic obstructive airway disease, peripheral vascular disease) and compliance issues. The cardioselective agents (see Chapter 11) will have less effect on the beta-2 receptors of the lungs and peripheral vasculature, minimizing side effects from these body systems. Acebutolol, atenolol, betaxolol, and metoprolol are examples of beta blockers that can be administered once daily to minimize anginal attacks if compliance is a problem. Dosages of beta blockers needed to control angina are extremely patient specific; therefore therapy should be started at low doses and worked upward, depending on the patient's need. Optimally, exercise stressing should be used to determine the most appropriate dosage.

Therapeutic Outcomes

The primary therapeutic outcomes expected from beta-blocker therapy are as follows:
- Decreased frequency and severity of anginal attacks
- Increased tolerance of activities
- Reduced use of nitroglycerin for acute anginal attacks

Nursing Process

Premedication Assessment

1. Take blood pressure in supine and standing positions.
2. Check history for respiratory disorders, for example, bronchospasm, chronic bronchitis, emphysema, and asthma.
3. Check for history of diabetes. If present, determine baseline serum glucose before initiation of therapy.

See Chapter 11 for further discussion of patient education and nursing process associated with beta-adrenergic inhibition.

Drug Class: Calcium Ion Antagonists

Actions

These agents are known variously as calcium antagonists, calcium channel blockers, slow channel blockers, and calcium ion influx inhibitors. Regardless of their names, they all share the ability to inhibit the movement of calcium ions across a cell membrane.

Calcium ion antagonists (Table 23-2) may be used to treat angina pectoris by decreasing myocardial oxygen demand (decreasing workload) and increasing myocardial blood supply by coronary artery dilatation. By inhibiting smooth muscle contraction, the calcium ion antagonists dilate blood vessels and decrease resistance to blood flow.

Table 23-2

Calcium Ion Antagonists Used to Treat Angina Pectoris

GENERIC NAME	BRAND NAME	AVAILABILITY	DOSAGE RANGE
Amlodipine	Norvasc	Tablets: 2.5, 5, 10 mg	PO: initial—5 mg once daily; adjust over 7-14 days to a maximum of 10 mg/day
Diltiazem	Cardizem	Tablets: 30, 60, 90, 120 mg Sustained-release capsules: 60, 90, 120, 180, 240, 300 mg	PO: initial—30 mg 4 times daily, gradually increasing dosage to 180-360 mg in 3-4 divided doses PO: initial—120-180 mg sustained-release capsule once daily; adjust as needed after 14 days Maintenance—240-480 mg daily
Bepridil	Vascor	Tablets: 200, 300, 400 mg	PO: initial—200 mg daily; adjust after 10 days depending on response Maintenance—300 mg daily Maximum—400 mg daily
Nicardipine	Cardene	Capsules: 20, 30 mg	PO: initial—20 mg 3 times daily Maximal response may require 2 wk of therapy Allow at least 3 days between dosage adjustments Maintenance—20 to 40 mg 3 times daily
Nifedipine	Procardia	Capsules: 10, 20 mg Sustained-release tablets: 30, 60, 90 mg	PO: initial—10 mg 3 times daily Adjust over 7-14 days to balance antianginal and hypotensive activity Maintenance—10-20 mg 3 times daily Sustained-release tablets are administered once daily Maximum—capsules: 180 mg daily; sustained-release tablets: 120 mg daily
Verapamil	Calan, Isoptin	Tablets: 40, 80, 120 mg	PO: initial—40-120 mg 3 times daily Maintenance—120-480 mg daily Administer with food

Dilatation of peripheral vessels reduces the workload of the heart. Coronary artery dilatation improves coronary blood flow.

Uses

Although each of these agents act by calcium ion inhibition, there are significant differences in clinical use. Their clinical effects also depend on the type and severity of the patient's disease. The primary calcium ion antagonists used to treat angina are verapamil, diltiazem, nifedipine, nicardipine, and bepridil. The overall effect of calcium ion antagonists will be the combined effects of vasodilator and myocardial actions with reflex-mediated adrenergic activity. Nifedipine, a potent peripheral arterial vasodilator, reduces peripheral vascular resistance, which may cause a reflex tachycardia. Verapamil and diltiazem also have myocardial depressant effects that prevent tachycardia. They must, however, be used with extreme caution in patients who may be developing heart failure.

Therapeutic Outcomes

The primary therapeutic outcomes expected from calcium ion antagonists are as follows:
• Decreased frequency and severity of anginal attacks
• Increased tolerance of activities

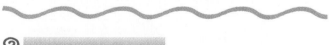

Nursing Process

Premedication Assessment

1. Take blood pressure in supine and standing positions.
2. Check for history of heart failure; withhold drug and consult physician if present.
3. Check laboratory values for hepatotoxicity.

Planning

Availability. See Table 23-2.

Implementation

Dosage and administration. See Table 23-2. See Chapter 20 for further discussion of patient education and nursing process associated with calcium ion antagonist therapy.

CHAPTER REVIEW

Coronary heart disease is the leading cause of disability, socioeconomic loss, and death in the United States. Angina pectoris is the first clinical indication of underlying disease in many patients. The frequency of anginal attacks can be reduced by controlling risk factors and avoiding precipitating causes such as stress. Medicines such as the nitrates, beta blockers, and calcium ion antagonists can help control symptomatology. Nurses can play a significant role in public education efforts, monitor for noncompliance, monitor

patient response to therapy, and encourage patients to make changes in lifestyle to reduce the severity of angina pectoris.

MATH REVIEW

1. Ordered: nitroglycerin 0.3 mg, sublingual, prn chest pain.
   On hand: nitroglycerin 0.15 mg sublingual tablets.
   Give:_____ tablets.

2. Ordered: nifedipine (Procardia XL) 30 mg PO q6h.
   On hand: nifedipine 10 mg capsules.
   Give:_____ capsules per dose.
   Give:_____ mg nifedipine in 24 hours.

3. Ordered: nifedipine (Procardia) 10 mg, sublingual for acute pain.
   On hand: nifedipine (Procardia) 10 mg capsules.
   Give:_____ capsules.
   Explain the procedure for sublingual administration of the nifedipine.

4. Ordered: propranolol hydrochloride (Inderal) 160 mg PO once daily.
   On hand: propranolol hydrochloride (Inderal) concentrated oral solution 80 mg/ml.
   Give:_____ ml.

CRITICAL THINKING QUESTIONS

Situation:
Pablo Sanchez, a 64-year-old man, comes to the emergency room with acute chest pain. He is holding his chest with his fist directly over the sternum. He appears diaphoretic. He is in work clothes and has been mowing the lawn. It is 98° F outside.

1. What nursing actions would be appropriate immediately?

2. What drugs would likely be ordered if this is acute angina pectoris?

3. Describe the correct procedure for administering sublingual nitroglycerin.

4. If a stat dose of nitroglycerin sublingual spray is ordered, explain how you would instruct the patient to give it.

Situation:
When giving morning medications in the nursing home, the nurse comes to an order to apply Nitro-Dur patch 2.5 mg to Mrs. Ignazeous. The medication administration record (MAR) indicates that the previous patch was applied to the right scapula area. The patch is not there. How would you proceed to execute the order?

Drugs Used to Treat Peripheral Vascular Disease

Objectives

1. List the baseline assessments needed to evaluate a patient with peripheral vascular disease.

2. Identify specific measures the patient can use to improve peripheral circulation and prevent complications from peripheral vascular disease.

3. Identify the systemic effects to expect when peripheral vasodilating agents are administered.

4. Explain why hypotension and tachycardia occur frequently with the use of peripheral vasodilators.

5. Develop measurable objectives for patient education for patients with peripheral vascular disease.

6. State both pharmacologic and nonpharmacologic goals of treatment for peripheral vascular disease.

Key Words

arteriosclerosis obliterans   vasospasm

intermittent claudication   Raynaud's disease

paresthesias

PERIPHERAL VASCULAR DISEASE

The classification "peripheral vascular disease" can be applied to a wide variety of illnesses associated with blood vessels outside the heart, but it generally refers to diseases of the blood vessels of the arms and legs (the extremities). These illnesses can be subdivided into two types based on arterial or venous origin: peripheral arterial disease and venous disorders such as acute deep vein thrombosis. (See Chapter 26.) The arterial disorders are subdivided into those that result from arterial narrowing and occlusion (obstructive) and those caused by arterial spasm (vasospastic).

The most common form of obstructive arterial disease is **arteriosclerosis obliterans**, also called atherosclerosis obliterans. It results from atherosclerotic plaque formation with narrowing of the lower aorta and the major arteries that provide circulation to the legs. As with atherosclerosis of the coronary arteries, the risk factors that play an important role in the development of this disease are high levels of low-density lipoprotein cholesterol (LDL-C), hypertension, cigarette smoking, low levels of LDL-C, and diabetes mellitus.

Patients tend to remain symptom free until there is significant narrowing (75% to 90%) in key locations of the major arteries and arterioles of the legs. The typical pain pattern described is one of aching, cramping, tightness, or weakness that occurs during exercise. The primary pathophysiology is obstruction of blood flow through the arteries resulting in ischemia to the tissues supplied by those arteries. A term commonly applied to this condition is **intermittent claudication**, the symptom of which is pain secondary to lack of oxygen to muscles during exercise. In the earlier stages of symptomatology, the patient finds relief by stopping the exercise for a few minutes. As the disease progresses over time without treatment, the arteries become obstructed, resulting in thrombosis and the potential for gangrene. Additional symptoms that develop are pain at rest, numbness, and **paresthesias** (numbness with a tingling sensation). The disease is often accompanied by increased blood viscosity. Physical findings are reduced arterial pulsations on palpation, systolic bruits over the involved arteries, waxy, pale, dry coloration, lower temperature of the skin of the extremity, edema, and numbness to sensation.

Peripheral vascular disease caused by arterial **vasospasm** is known as **Raynaud's disease**, named after the man who first described the illness in 1862. Unfortunately, more than a century later, the pathophysiology and treatment are still not well defined. Raynaud's disease is classified as primary, in which the cause is unknown, or secondary, in which other conditions contribute to the symptomatology. Secondary causes are frequent exposure to cold weather, obstructive arterial disease, occupational trauma (for example, pneumatic hammer users, typists, pianists) and certain drugs (for example, beta blockers, imipramine, nicotine, bromocriptine, vinblastine, clonidine). Heredity may also play a role in this disease. The onset of the disease is usually during the teen years to the forties and it occurs four times more frequently in women.

Raynaud's disease is thought to be caused by vasospasm (vasoconstriction of blood vessels) and subsequent ischemia of the arteries of the skin of the hands, fingers, and sometimes toes. The physiologic mechanisms that trigger the vasospasm are unknown. Sudden coldness applied to the extremity, such as cold water, will induce an attack. The signs and symptoms associated with Raynaud's disease are numbness, tingling and sense of skin tightness in the affected area, and blanching of the skin because of sudden vasoconstriction followed by cyanosis. As the attack subsides, vasodilation causes a redness, or *rubor,* to the pale skin. The skin appears normal except during spasm. In the early years of the illness, only the tips of fingers of both hands are involved, but as the disease progresses the skin of the hands is also affected by the arteriospasm.

Treatment

The goals of treatment of arteriosclerosis obliterans are reversal of the progression of the atherosclerosis, improved blood flow, pain relief, and prevention of skin ulceration and gangrene. An important concept that must be stressed to most patients is that other diseases they may have, such as diabetes, hypertension, angina, and hyperlipidemia, are all interrelated. Control of diet, high blood pressure, smoking, weight, and diabetes will significantly help all of these diseases. Implementation of a step 1 American Heart Association diet can arrest the progression of atherosclerosis. Lipid-lowering agents can be started if diet is not successful in treating the hypercholesterolemia. A daily exercise program (usually walking) can significantly improve collateral blood circulation around areas of obstruction and reduce the frequency of intermittent claudication. Proper foot care (keeping them warm and dry, with properly fitting shoes), especially if the patient is a diabetic, is also extremely important in preventing the ulcerative complications. Other nonpharmacologic treatments that may improve blood flow to the extremities are avoidance of cold, elevation of the head of the bed 12 to 16 inches, and arterial angioplasty and surgery.

Most vasospastic attacks of Rayaud's disease can by stopped by avoidance of cold temperatures, emotional stress, tobacco, and drugs known to induce attacks. Keeping the hands and feet warm with gloves and socks and using foam "wraparounds" when handling iced beverages can reduce exposure to cold.

Drug Therapy

Actions

As the causes of peripheral vascular disease have become better understood, clinical studies have defined which pharmacologic therapies are truly successful. It has been shown that the nonpharmacologic treatment of arteriosclerosis obliterans is substantially more successful in treating the underlying pathology. Pentoxifylline has had modest success. Pentoxifylline is classified as a hemorheologic agent. It acts by enhancing red blood cell flexibility, which reduces blood viscosity, thus providing better oxygenation to muscle tissue to stop intermittent claudication. Vasodilator therapy, the mainstay of treatment until the 1980s, has little long-term benefit in most cases. When drug therapy for Raynaud's disease is required, such as when the disease interferes with the ability to work, medicines with a vasodilating effect are used.

Uses

Pentoxifylline is the first, and so far only, available agent approved by the Food and Drug Administration (FDA) that is specifically indicated for the treatment of intermittent claudication caused by chronic occlusive arterial disease of the limbs.

Classes of drugs that have been somewhat successful in treating Raynaud's disease are the calcium ion antagonists, adrenergic antagonists, angiotensin-converting enzyme (ACE) inhibitors, and direct vasodilators.

The three calcium ion antagonists studied for the treatment of Raynaud's disease are diltiazem, verapamil, and nifedipine. Of the three, nifedipine has had the greatest success in reducing the frequency of vasospastic attack in about two thirds of patients.

Adrenergic antagonists (for example prazosin, reserpine, guanethidine, and methyldopa) have been used for many years in the treatment of Raynaud's disease. Unfortunately, treatment has been only moderately successful, and many side effects are associated with these drugs.

The ACE inhibitors cause an increase in bradykinin, a potent vasodilator. Captopril has been most extensively tested and causes a reduction in both frequency and severity of attacks.

For more than 50 years nitroglycerin, a direct vasodilator, has been applied as an ointment base to the hands of patients suffering from Raynaud's disease. The treatment reduces the frequency and severity of attacks, but the side effects of dizziness, headache, and postural hypotension limit its use. Other vasodilators, such as papaverine, isoxsuprine, and cyclandelate, have been used extensively over the years but have not been tested in controlled studies. They are, however, still occasionally used as adjunctive therapy to treat peripheral vascular diseases.

Nursing Process for Peripheral Vascular Disease Therapy

Assessment

A baseline assessment of the individual patient should be completed. It should include the following data to evaluate the history and degree of oxygenation that exists in the extremities. Subsequent regular assessments should be performed for comparison and analysis of therapeutic effectiveness or lack of response to all treatments initiated.

History of risk factors. Ask age, note gender and race, and take family history of incidence of symptoms of peripheral vascular disease.

Hypertension. Take blood pressure in supine and lying positions daily. Ask about medications that have been prescribed. Are the medications being taken regularly? If not, why not?

Smoking. Obtain a history of the number of cigarettes or cigars smoked daily. How long has the person smoked? Has the person ever tried to stop smoking? Ask if the patient understands what effect smoking has on the vascular system. How does the individual feel about modifying the smoking habit?

Dietary habits. • Obtain a dietary history. Ask specific questions to obtain data relating to foods eaten that are high in fat, cholesterol, refined carbohydrates, and sodium. Using a calorie counter, ask the person to estimate the number of calories eaten per day. How much meat, fish, and poultry is eaten daily (size and number of servings)? Estimate the percent

of total daily calories provided by fat. • Discuss food preparation—for example, baked, broiled, fried foods. How many servings of fruits and vegetables are eaten daily? What types of oils and fats are used in food preparation? See a nutrition text for further dietary history questions. • What are the frequency and volume of alcoholic beverages consumed?
Glucose intolerance. Ask specific questions regarding whether the individual has now or has ever had elevated serum glucose (blood sugar). If yes, what dietary modifications have been made? How successful are they? What medications are being taken for the elevated serum glucose (for example, oral hypoglycemic agents or insulin)?
Elevated serum lipids. Find out whether the patient is aware of having elevated lipids, triglycerides, or cholesterol. If elevated, what measures has the patient tried for reduction and how much impact have the interventions had on the blood levels at subsequent examinations? Review laboratory data available (for example, LDL and very low density lipoprotien [VLDL]).
Obesity. Weigh the patient. Ask about any recent weight gains or losses and whether intentional or unintentional.
Psychomotor functions. • *Type of lifestyle.* Ask the patient to describe the exercise level in terms of amount (for example, walking 3 blocks), intensity (for example, how long does it take to walk 3 blocks), and frequency (for example, walking every other day). Is the patient's job physically demanding or of a sedentary nature? • *Psychologic stress.* How much stress does the individual estimate having in life? How does the individual cope with stressful situations at home and in the work setting?
Assessment of tissue. • *Oxygenation.* Observe the color of each hand, finger, leg, and foot; report cyanosis or reddish-blue locations. Examine the skin of the extremities for any signs of ulceration. • *Temperature.* Feel the temperature in each hand, finger, leg, and foot. Report paleness and coldness. (Note that these symptoms will be increased if the limb is elevated above the level of the heart.) • *Edema.* Assess, record, and report edema and its extent, and determine whether it is relieved or unchanged when the limb is in a dependent position. • *Peripheral pulses.* Record the pedal and radial pulses at least every 4 hours if circulatory impairment is found in that limb. Compare findings between each of the extremities; report diminished or absent pulses immediately. When pulses are difficult to palpate or are absent, use of a Doppler ultrasound device may aid in determining peripheral blood flow. • *Limb pain.* Assess pain in the patient carefully. Pain during exercise that is relieved by rest may be from claudication. Conversely, pain when the patient is at rest may be from sudden obstruction by a thrombus or embolus. Check the apprehension level of the patient, pedal and radial pulses, details of onset and location of pain, and vital signs, and determine whether pain is increased by dorsiflexion of the foot. Until status of patient's limb pain is established, have the patient remain on bed rest and administer analgesic if ordered. Notify physician of findings.

Nursing Diagnosis
• Tissue perfusion, alteration in (indication)
• Pain, acute and chronic (indication)
• Activity intolerance (indication)
• Injury, risk for (indication)

Planning
History of risk factors. • Review the modifiable risk factors and plan interventions and health teaching needed for appropriate alterations in lifestyle. • Review ordered medications to be used concurrently with lifestyle modifications for health teaching needed regarding their use. • Order baseline laboratory studies requested by the physician (for example, lipid profile studies, liver function tests, and clotting time).
Assessment of tissue. Schedule assessment of pertinent data on the care plan and Kardex at regular intervals that correlate with the patient's status.
Psychomotor function and lifestyle pattern. Examine assessment data to decide on an appropriate teaching plan that will incorporate changes in lifestyle issues (for example, control of hypertension, smoking cessation, dietary alterations, stress-related factors, and the disease process itself) and drug therapy prescribed.
Medication administration. Plan drug administration in accordance with recommendations in individual drug monographs to avoid possible interference with the absorption of other drugs ordered.

Implementation
• Prepare the patient for diagnostic tests (for example, ultrasonography, pulse volume recordings, segmental limb pressure, and exercise testing) and possible invasive procedures such as arteriography.
• Do not place pillows in the popliteal space or flex the knee rest on the bed. Use a cradle or footboard to prevent bedsheets from constricting the circulation.
• Always check with the physician before initiating elevation of the extremities. It is *contraindicated* in patients with *arterial* insufficiency.
• Perform baseline assessments of tissue perfusion (for example, skin temperature, peripheral pulses) at intervals appropriate to the patient's status (at least every 4 hours).
• Implement pain management measures.

Patient Education and Health Promotion
Promoting tissue perfusion
• Teach self-care measures that promote peripheral circulation.
• Smoking causes vasoconstriction of the blood vessels. Therefore encourage drastic reduction and preferably total abstinence from smoking.
• Encourage patients to wear nothing that constricts peripheral blood flow, such as tight-fitting anklets, socks, or garters. Tell the patient *not* to elevate the extremities above the level of the heart without specific orders to do so from the physician. The physician *may* order the patient's bed elevated at night.
• Meticulous foot and hand care is essential. Teach proper self-care of the limbs, including visual inspection techniques, and explain how to take femoral, popliteal, and pedal pulses.
• The need to inspect the extremities for possible skin breakdown or signs of infection must be stressed. Notify the physician immediately of sudden changes in color, such as mottling or a more purplish color. Cold temperatures will increase pain or decrease sensations in the extremities.

- Areas of discoloration in nails, cracking of skin, calluses, or blisters on the extremities require complete follow-up. Listen to the patient's description of changes noted. Tell the patient that going barefoot can be dangerous because of potential injuries to the feet.
- Because of the possible decrease in sensation in the extremities, encourage the patient to test the water temperature before immersing the hands or feet. After bathing, gently pat, do not vigorously rub the feet and hands to dry them.
- To avoid skin breakdown, the patient should alternate pairs of shoes to allow for thorough drying between wearings, change socks or hose daily, and avoid rubber-soled shoes.
- Standing or sitting for prolonged periods should be avoided. Persons who must sit for extended periods of time must have a properly fitting chair. The seat must be of the correct depth so that no pressure is exerted on the popliteal space. Encourage individuals not to sit with knees or ankles crossed and to take frequent short breaks for walks. Furthermore, persons who must stand for long periods of time should seek aspects of the job that can be performed sitting down in a properly fitting chair or other alternatives.

Psychomotor functions. • Maximum mobility should be maintained. Devise a daily activity plan that includes walks and usual activities of daily living, such as shopping and housework. • Pain management and the psychologic aspects of dealing with a prolonged illness with persistent symptoms are a major challenge to the patient and the nurse. (See Chapter 18 for pain management information.)

Environment. During periods of exposure to cold temperature, the patient should wear several layers of lightweight clothing. Caution should be exercised during exposure to the cold to avoid frostbite. Because of decreased sensations in the extremities, frostbite can occur without the patient's awareness.

Nutritional aspects. • Dietary education is strongly indicated in the treatment of peripheral vascular disease. It is particularly important to control obesity and cholesterol and triglyceride levels. • When ulcerations are present, encourage a high-protein diet with adequate intake of vitamins to promote the healing process. • Unless other medical conditions contraindicate, instruct the patient to drink eight 8-ounce glasses of water daily to promote adequate hydration of body tissues. Maintaining blood volume will help reduce peripheral vasoconstriction. Check with the physician regarding recommendations for fluid or caffeine restriction.

Medication regimen. • Certain medications for the treatment of peripheral vascular disease cause vasodilation of blood vessels. As a result, orthostatic hypotension may occur. Teach patients to rise slowly from a sitting or lying position, steady themselves, flex the leg muscles, and then proceed with movement. • Teach the individual to take and record own blood pressure. • Administer prescribed medicines.

Fostering health maintenance. • Throughout the course of treatment, discuss medication information and explain how the medication will benefit the patient. • Drug therapy is not a total solution for atherosclerosis. The patient may not be committed to the lifestyle changes needed to control the modifiable aspects of the disease. Often, setting short-term goals to control the pain and finding other interventions that will allow the patient to view efforts positively will help encourage permanent adoption of the needed changes. • Patients who are unresponsive to lifestyle modifications and drug therapy may require surgical interventions to reestablish blood flow to the affected area. Such procedures as a bypass graft, endarterectomy, or angioplasty may be appropriate. Failure to reestablish blood flow to an extremity may result in an amputation. • Provide the patient and significant others with important information contained in the specific drug monograph for the drugs prescribed. Additional health teaching and nursing interventions for side effects to expect and report are described in each drug monograph. • Seek cooperation and understanding of the following points so that medication compliance is increased: name of medication, dosage, route and times of administration, side effects to expect, and side effects to report. • Enlist the patient's aid in developing and maintaining a written record of monitoring parameters (for example, color of limb, pain in limb, temperature and pulses in limb, and amount of edema present). Instruct the patient to bring the written record to follow-up visits.

Drug Class: Hemorheologic Agents

 pentoxifylline (pen-tox-ē′fi′-leen)
Trental (tren′tahl)

Actions

Pentoxifylline is not an anticoagulant, but it is thought to increase erythrocyte flexibility, decrease the concentration of fibrinogen in blood, and prevent aggregation of red blood cells and platelets. These actions decrease the viscosity of blood and improve its flow properties, resulting in increased blood flow to the affected microcirculation to enhance tissue oxygenation.

Uses

Pentoxifylline is the agent approved for the treatment of intermittent claudication. Pentoxifylline therapy should be considered an adjunct to, not a replacement for, smoking cessation, weight loss, exercise therapy, surgical bypass, or removal of arterial obstructions in the treatment of peripheral vascular disease.

Therapeutic Outcomes

The primary therapeutic outcome expected from pentoxifylline is improved tissue perfusion with a reduced frequency of pain, improved tolerance to exercise, and improved peripheral pulses.

Nursing Process

Premedication Assessment

1. Perform baseline gastrointestinal assessments to determine if nausea, vomiting, dyspepsia, or intolerance to caffeine products exists.
2. Assess for the presence of dizziness or headache.
3. Ask specifically about any cardiac symptoms. Report to physician if present.
4. Obtain baseline data on degree of pain present in the extremities.

Planning
Availability. PO—400 mg tablets.

Implementation
Dosage and administration. PO—400 mg 3 times daily. If adverse gastrointestinal (GI) or central nervous system (CNS) effects develop, dosage should be reduced to 400 mg twice daily. If adverse effects persist, therapy should be discontinued. Symptomatic relief may start within 2 to 4 weeks, but treatment should be continued for at least 8 weeks to determine maximal efficacy.

Evaluation
Side effects to expect
NAUSEA, VOMITING, DYSPEPSIA. Dyspepsia, nausea, and vomiting occur in about 1% to 3% of patients. Belching and flatus occur in less than 1% of patients. These side effects are usually mild and tend to resolve with continued therapy. Administration with food or milk may help minimize discomfort. Encourage the patient not to discontinue therapy without first consulting a physician.
DIZZINESS, HEADACHE. Central nervous system disturbances characterized by dizziness occur in about 2% of patients, and headache and tremor occur less frequently. These side effects are usually mild and tend to resolve with continued therapy. Provide for patient safety during episodes of dizziness. Encourage the patient to sit down if feeling faint. Encourage the patient not to discontinue therapy without first consulting a physician.
Side effects to report
CHEST PAIN, ARRHYTHMIAS, SHORTNESS OF BREATH. Without causing undue alarm, strongly encourage the patient to seek a physician's attention for further evaluation.
INTOLERANCE TO CAFFEINE, THEOPHYLLINE, THEOBROMINE. Pentoxifylline is a xanthine derivative. Patients should be asked specifically about intolerance to xanthine derivatives before initiating therapy.
Drug interactions
ANTIHYPERTENSIVE AGENTS. Although pentoxifylline is not an antihypertensive agent, patients receiving pentoxifylline therapy frequently display a small reduction in systemic blood pressure. Blood pressure should be monitored to observe for hypotension. The dosage of antihypertensive therapy may have to be reduced to minimize adverse effects.

Drug Class: Vasodilators

🔹 **cyclandelate** (sī-klan′de-layt)
Cyclospasmol (sī-klo-spaz′mol)

Actions
Cyclandelate has a direct relaxation effect on the smooth muscles of peripheral arterial blood vessels, increasing circulation to the extremities.

Uses
Cyclandelate is considered possibly effective in treating patients with intermittent claudication, arteriosclerosis obliterans, vasospasm associated with thrombophlebitis, nocturnal leg cramps, and Raynaud's disease.

Therapeutic Outcomes
The primary therapeutic outcome expected from Cyclospasmol is improved tissue perfusion with a reduced frequency of pain, improved tolerance to exercise, and improved peripheral pulses.

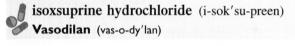

Nursing Process

Premedication Assessment
Obtain baseline assessment of degree of pain present and symptoms of peripheral vascular constriction.

Planning
Availability. PO—200 and 400 mg capsules.

Implementation
Dosage and administration. PO—It is often advantageous to initiate therapy at higher dosages: 1200 to 1600 mg daily in divided doses before meals and at bedtime. When a clinical response is noted, the dosage can be decreased in 200 mg increments until the maintenance dosage is reached. The usual maintenance dose is between 400 and 800 mg per day in 2 to 4 divided doses. Administer at meals or with milk to decrease gastric irritation.

Evaluation
Side effects to expect
FLUSHING, TINGLING, SWEATING. Explain to the patient that these side effects may occur during the initial phase of therapy; however, these symptoms resolve with continued therapy.
Drug interactions. None specifically associated with cyclandelate have been reported.

🔹 **isoxsuprine hydrochloride** (i-sok′su-preen)
Vasodilan (vas-o-dy′lan)

Actions
Isoxsuprine hydrochloride is a beta-adrenergic stimulant that causes vasodilation of the smooth muscles of the blood vessels.

Uses
Isoxsuprine is used to treat the symptoms of peripheral vascular spasm, cerebral vascular insufficiency, Raynaud's and Buerger's diseases, and arteriosclerosis obliterans.

Therapeutic Outcomes
The primary therapeutic outcome expected from isoxsuprine therapy is improved tissue perfusion with a reduced frequency of pain, improved tolerance to exercise, and improved peripheral pulses.

Nursing Process

Premedication Assessment
1. Obtain baseline assessment of degree of pain present and symptoms of peripheral vascular constriction.
2. Take baseline vital signs.

Planning
Availability. PO—10 and 20 mg tablets.

Implementation
Dosage and administration. PO—10 to 20 mg 3 or 4 times daily. IM—5 to 10 mg 2 or 3 times daily. Intramuscular administration may be used initially in acute conditions.

Evaluation
Side effects to expect
FLUSHING, TINGLING, SWEATING, NAUSEA, VOMITING. Explain to the patient that these side effects may occur during the initial phase of therapy; however, these symptoms resolve with continued therapy.
Side effects to report
HYPOTENSION, TACHYCARDIA. Monitor blood pressure and pulse throughout the course of therapy. Prevent hypotensive episodes by having the patient rise slowly from a supine or sitting position and perform exercises to prevent blood pooling when standing or sitting in one position for prolonged periods. Have the patient sit or lie down if feeling faint.
SEVERE RASH. Discontinue medication if a severe rash develops. Notify the physician so that appropriate alternative agents may be prescribed.
NERVOUSNESS AND WEAKNESS. As therapy progresses, these symptoms may develop. Tell the patient to discuss them with the physician if they become a problem.
Drug interactions
DRUGS THAT ENHANCE THERAPEUTIC AND TOXIC EFFECTS. Antihypertensive agents: The vasodilating action of isoxsuprine and antihypertensive agents may result in excessive hypotensive effects. Assess the blood pressure at regular intervals to monitor the combined effects. Monitor the patient for hypotension, light-headedness, dizziness, and tachycardia. Provide for patient safety; prevent falls.
DRUGS THAT REDUCE THERAPEUTIC EFFECTS. Warn the patient against taking over-the-counter cough and cold preparations without first consulting the physician or pharmacist. Many of these products will counteract the effects of isoxsuprine.

papaverine hydrochloride (pah-pav'er-in)
Pavabid (pah-vah'bid)

Actions
Papaverine relaxes smooth muscle, vasodilates cerebral and coronary blood vessels, and inhibits atrial and ventricular premature contractions and ventricular arrhythmias.

Uses
Papaverine is a drug that has been tried for many illnesses for many years. Even so, there is little objective evidence to indicate that it has any therapeutic value. Papaverine is used orally as a smooth muscle relaxant to treat cerebral and peripheral ischemia associated with arterial spasm and myocardial ischemia complicated by arrhythmias.

Therapeutic Outcomes
The primary therapeutic outcome expected from papaverine is improved tissue perfusion with a reduced frequency of pain, improved tolerance to exercise, and improved peripheral pulses.

Nursing Process
Premedication Assessment
1. Obtain baseline assessment of degree of pain present and symptoms of peripheral vascular constriction.
2. Take baseline vital signs.

Planning
Availability. PO—150 mg timed-release capsules. IV—30 mg/ml in 2 ml ampules and 10 ml vials.

Implementation
Dosage and administration. PO—60 to 300 mg 1 to 5 times daily. Timed-release products: 150 mg every 12 hours. In difficult cases, increase to 150 mg every 8 hours or 300 mg every 12 hours.

Evaluation
Side effects to expect and report
FLUSHING, SWEATING, NAUSEA, ABDOMINAL DISTRESS, TACHYCARDIA, VERTIGO, DROWSINESS, HEADACHE. These side effects are usually mild and are dose related. Monitor vital signs (blood pressure, pulse, and respirations) and report deviations from baseline data for the physician's evaluation.
Drug interactions
DRUGS THAT ENHANCE THERAPEUTIC AND TOXIC EFFECTS. Antihypertensive agents: The vasodilating action of papaverine and antihypertensive agents may result in excessive hypotensive effects. Assess blood pressure at regular intervals to monitor the combined effects. Monitor the patient for hypotension, light-headedness, dizziness, and tachycardia. Provide for patient safety; prevent falls.
DRUGS THAT REDUCE THERAPEUTIC EFFECTS. Warn the patient against taking over-the-counter cough and cold preparations without first consulting the physician or pharmacist. Many of these products will counteract the effects of papaverine.

phenoxybenzamine hydrochloride
(fe-nok-se-ben'zah-meen)
Dibenzyline (di-ben'zi-leen)

Actions
Phenoxybenzamine is an alpha-adrenergic blocking agent that relaxes the smooth muscle of blood vessels, resulting in vasodilation and improved blood flow to peripheral tissues.

Uses
Phenoxybenzamine is used in blood vessel disorders, such as Raynaud's disease, leg ulceration, and the complications of frostbite.

Therapeutic Outcomes
The primary therapeutic outcome expected from phenoxybenzamine is improved tissue perfusion with a reduced frequency of pain, improved tolerance to exercise, and improved peripheral pulses.

Nursing Process

Premedication Assessment

1. Obtain baseline assessment of degree of pain present and symptoms of peripheral vascular constriction.
2. Take baseline vital signs.

Planning

Availability. PO—10 mg capsules.

Implementation

Dosage and administration. PO—initially 10 mg per day. After determining response for 4 or more days, increase the dose by 10 mg increments every few days to a maximum of 60 mg per day. Several weeks of therapy are usually required to observe full therapeutic benefits.

Evaluation

Side effects to expect and report

NASAL STUFFINESS, MIOSIS, HYPOTENSION, AND TACHYCARDIA. Monitor blood pressure and pulse. Prevent hypotensive episodes by instructing the patient to rise slowly from a supine or sitting position and perform exercises to prevent blood pooling when standing or sitting in one position for prolonged periods. Have the patient sit or lie down if feeling faint. Report increasing episodes so that dosage is adjusted accordingly.

Drug interactions

DRUGS THAT ENHANCE THERAPEUTIC AND TOXIC EFFECTS. Antihypertensive agents and alcohol: The vasodilating action of phenoxybenzamine and antihypertensive agents may result in excessive hypotensive effects. Assess the blood pressure at regular intervals to monitor the combined effects. Monitor the patient for hypotension, light-headedness, dizziness, and tachycardia. Provide for patient safety; prevent falls.

DRUGS THAT REDUCE THERAPEUTIC EFFECTS. Warn the patient against taking over-the-counter cough and cold preparations without first consulting the physician or pharmacist. Many of these products will counteract the effects of phenoxybenzamine.

tolazoline (tol-az′o-leen)
Priscoline (pris′ko-leen)

Actions

Tolazoline acts directly on the smooth muscle of the blood vessels to produce vasodilation and increase blood flow.

Uses

Tolazoline is approved by the FDA for treating persistent pulmonary hypertension in the neonatal infant. It is also occasionally used to improve the circulation of patients with diabetes, Raynaud's disease, chronic ulcers, gangrene, frostbite, and other spastic peripheral vascular diseases. It should be used cautiously in patients with peptic ulcers because it causes stimulation of gastric secretions that might aggravate peptic ulcers.

Therapeutic Outcomes

The primary therapeutic outcome expected from tolazoline is improved tissue perfusion with a reduced frequency of pain, improved tolerance to exercise, and improved peripheral pulses.

Nursing Process

Premedication Assessment

1. Obtain baseline assessment of degree of pain present and symptoms of peripheral vascular constriction.
2. Report preexisting cardiovascular conditions to the physician before initiating drug therapy.

Planning

Availability. Parenteral—25 mg/ml in 4 ml ampules.

Implementation

Dosage and administration. IV, SC, IM—Dosage must be individualized. General dosage requirements are 10 to 50 mg 4 times daily. Start with lower dosages, increasing gradually until therapeutic response (localized flushing) is observed. Keeping the patient warm will often increase effectiveness of the medication.

Evaluation

Side effects to expect

FLUSHING OF THE FACE, NECK, CHEST, AND BACK. Tell the patient to expect that these areas will become increasingly red; this is a desirable effect. Keeping the patient warm enhances the effectiveness of the drug.

TINGLING, SWEATING, NAUSEA, VOMITING. Explain to the patient that these side effects may occur during the initial phase of therapy; however, these symptoms are self-limiting.

Side effects to report

ARRHYTHMIAS, TACHYCARDIA, ANGINAL PAIN. Monitor the pulse rate and report changes in rhythm. Anginal pain should be reported and the time of onset, frequency, duration, and intensity documented in the nurse's notes for hospitalized patients.

CONFUSION, HALLUCINATIONS. These adverse effects are rare, but monitor patients carefully for progressive symptoms of restlessness, agitation, anxiety, hallucinations, and euphoria. Act calmly with the excited, anxious, or euphoric patient. Provide safety and fulfillment of the patient's needs. Report this alteration in the patient's response to the physician as soon as possible.

Drug interactions

DRUGS THAT ENHANCE THERAPEUTIC AND TOXIC EFFECTS. Antihypertensive agents and alcohol: The vasodilating action of tolazoline and antihypertensive agents may result in excessive hypotensive effects.

Assess the blood pressure at regular intervals to monitor the combined effects.

Monitor the patient for hypotension, light-headedness, dizziness, and tachycardia.

Provide for patient safety; prevent falls.

DRUGS THAT REDUCE THERAPEUTIC EFFECTS. Warn the patient against taking over-the-counter cough and cold preparations without first consulting the physician or pharmacist. Many of these products will counteract the effects of tolazoline.

CHAPTER REVIEW

Peripheral vascular disease is a cause of significant morbidity in the United States. Major treatable causes of peripheral vascular disease are hypertension, cigarette smoking, and atherosclerosis.

The most cost-effective and successful forms of treatment are smoking cessation, weight reduction, exercise, and dietary modification. Patients should be fully informed of the significance of peripheral vascular disease, the potential complications of not modifying lifestyles, and the use of drug therapy.

MATH REVIEW

1. Ordered: cyclandelate (Cyclospasmol) 200 mg PO QID for 4 days, then 400 mg per day BID.
   On hand: cyclandelate (Cyclospasmol) 200 mg and 400 mg tablets.
   How many 200 mg tablets would be needed to administer the first 4 days of dosages?
   How many 400 mg tablets would be needed to administer the next 5 days of dosages?

2. Ordered: papaverine hydrochloride (Pavabid) 300 mg PO every 12 hours.
   On hand: papaverine hydrochloride (Pavabid) 150 mg time-released capsules.
   Give: _____ capsules per dose.

CRITICAL THINKING QUESTIONS

Situation:

Mrs. Dunbar tells you that when she and her husband go for their daily walks he can go only two blocks and then must sit down because of pain in the calves of his legs. They rest a while, walk another two blocks, and the pain is back. She asks your advice. What would you tell her?

Two days later, Mr. Dunbar is assigned to you for nursing care. His primary nursing diagnosis is altered tissue perfusion related to insufficient oxygenation of the lower limbs manifested by pain on walking two blocks and diminished popliteal pulses bilaterally.

What nursing assessments would you plan to make? What health teaching would be needed in relation to his drug therapy? He is prescribed a 10 mg capsule daily of phenoxybenzamine hydrochloride (Dibenzyline). Review the drug monograph and discuss the drug's action and side effects to anticipate.

Situation:

Mr. Canterbury, age 76, has been suffering from arteriosclerosis obliterans with intermittent claudication. He refuses to give up smoking. At his last office visit, a prescription for Trental 400 mg 4 times daily PO with meals was written. After leaving the examination room he tells you, the office nurse, that the physician did not explain how this would work to improve his "leg pain."

Give him a simple explanation of what is thought to be the mechanism of action, and draw a diagram that depicts "erythrocyte flexibility." Use the visual aid to help him understand how the drug could improve his leg pain.

A week later, Mr. Canterbury calls the office and says, "That new medication you gave me for my leg pain isn't working." How should you respond?

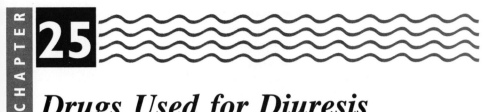

Drugs Used for Diuresis

CHAPTER CONTENT

Objectives

1. Cite nursing assessments used to evaluate a patient's state of hydration.
2. Review possible underlying pathology that may contribute to the development of excess fluid volume in the body.
3. State which electrolytes may be altered by diuretic therapy.
4. Cite nursing assessments used to evaluate renal function.
5. Identify the effects of diuretics on blood pressure, electrolytes, and diabetic or prediabetic patients.
6. Review the signs and symptoms of electrolyte imbalance and normal laboratory values of potassium, sodium, and chloride.
7. Identify the action of diuretics.
8. Explain the rationale for administering diuretics cautiously to elderly patients and persons with impaired renal function, cirrhosis of the liver, or diabetes mellitus.
9. Describe the goal of administering diuretics to treat hypertension, heart failure, or increased intraocular pressure or before vascular surgery in the brain.
10. List side effects that can be anticipated whenever a diuretic is administered.
11. Cite alterations in diet that may be prescribed concurrently with loop, thiazide, or potassium-sparing diuretic therapy.
12. State the nursing assessments needed to monitor the therapeutic response or the development of side effects to expect or report from diuretic therapy.
13. Develop objectives for patient education for patients taking loop, thiazide, and potassium-sparing diuretics.

Key Words

aldosterone	orthostatic hypotension
tubule	electrolyte imbalance
loop of Henle	hyperuricemia

DIURETICS

Drug Therapy

Actions

Diuretics are drugs that act to increase the flow of urine. The purpose of diuretics is to increase the net loss of water. To achieve this, they act on the kidneys in different locations to enhance the excretion of sodium. The methylxanthines increase glomerular filtration, spironolactone inhibits tubular reabsorption of sodium by inhibiting **aldosterone,** and the thiazides and loop diuretics act directly on the kidney tubules to inhibit the reabsorption of sodium and chloride from the lumen of the **tubule.** Sodium and chloride that are not reabsorbed are excreted into the collecting ducts and then into the ureters to the bladder, taking large volumes of water to be excreted from the body through urination (Figure 25-1).

Uses

Diuretics are mainstays of treatment in two major diseases affecting the cardiovascular system: heart failure and hypertension. They are routinely used in heart failure to remove excessive sodium and water to relieve symptoms associated with pulmonary congestion and edema. The Fifth Report of the Joint National Committee on Detection, Evaluation, and Treatment of High Blood Pressure (JNC V) recommends that after lifestyle modifications diuretics be used as primary agents to treat hypertension because they have been shown to reduce cardiovascular morbidity and mortality associated with hypertension.

Diuretics have a variety of other medical uses as well. Mannitol reduces cerebral edema, acetazolamide is used to reduce intraocular pressure associated with glaucoma, spironolactone can be effective in reducing ascites associated with liver disease, and furosemide may be used to treat hypercalcemia.

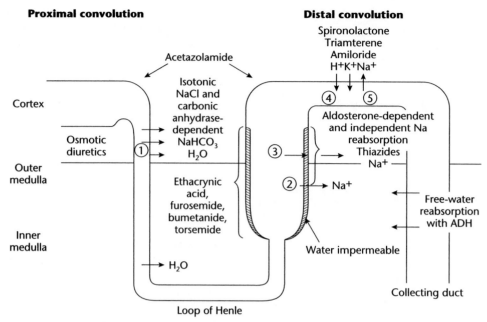

Figure 25-1 *Sites of actions of diuretics within the nephron.*

Nursing Process for Diuretic Therapy

The information the nurse obtains about the patient's general clinical symptoms is important to the physician when analyzing data for diagnosis and success of therapy. In addition to assessing overall clinical symptoms, the nurse should include the following data for subsequent evaluation of the patient's response to prescribed therapeutic modalities that act on the urinary system.

Assessment

History of related causative disorders/factors. Ask questions relating to any history of disorders that contribute to fluid volume excess: heart disorders (for example, myocardial infarction, heart failure, valvular disease, and arrhythmias); liver disease (for example, ascites, cirrhosis, and cancer); renal disease (for example, renal failure); and factors such as immobility, hypertension, pregnancy, and use of corticosteroid agents.

History of current symptoms. Ask questions to ascertain information relating to the onset, duration, and progression of specific symptoms relating to edema, weakness, fatigue, dyspnea, productive cough, and weight gain.

Pattern of urination. Ask the patient to describe current urination pattern and to cite changes. Such details as frequency, dysuria, incontinence, changes in the stream, hesitancy in starting to void, hematuria, nocturia, and urgency are all of significance.

Medication history. Obtain information on all prescribed and over-the-counter medications being taken. Tactfully ask questions regarding compliance.

Hydration status. Obtain baseline vital signs; note pulse that is bounding and full or irregular (indicating possible arrhythmias); check respiratory rate and quality; listen to lung sounds to detect presence of rales or rhonchi; ask for a history of recent weight gain or loss; and assess for neck vein distention. Blood pressure may be elevated.

Dehydration. Assess, report, and record significant signs of dehydration in the patient. Observe for poor skin turgor, sticky oral mucous membranes, a shrunken or deeply furrowed tongue, crusted lips, weight loss, deteriorating vital signs, soft or sunken eyeballs, weak pedal pulses, delayed capillary filling, excessive thirst, high urine specific gravity (or no urine output), and possible mental confusion.

Skin turgor. Check skin turgor by *gently* pinching the skin together over the sternum, on the forehead, or on the forearm. Elasticity is present and the skin rapidly returns to a flat position in the well-hydrated patient. In dehydrated patients the skin will remain in a "peaked" or "pinched" position and return slowly to the flat, normal position.

Oral mucous membranes. With adequate hydration, the membranes of the mouth feel smooth and glisten. With dehydration, they appear dull and are sticky.

Assess skin turgor, oral mucosa, and firmness of eyeballs.

Laboratory changes. The values of the hematocrit, hemoglobin, blood urea nitrogen (BUN), and electrolytes will appear to fluctuate, based on the state of hydration. When a patient is overhydrated, the values appear to drop as a result of hemodilution. A dehydrated patient will show higher values because of hemoconcentration.

Overhydration. Increases in abdominal girth, weight gain, neck vein engorgement, and circumference of the medial malleolus are indications of overhydration. Measure the abdominal girth daily at the umbilical level. Measure the extremities bilaterally daily at a level approximately 5 cm above the medial malleolus. Weigh the patient daily using the same scale, at the same time, in similar clothing.

Edema. *Edema* is a term used to describe excess fluid accumulation in the extracellular spaces. Edema is considered "pitting" when an indentation remains in the tissue after pressure is exerted against a bony part such as the shin, ankle, or sacrum. The degree is usually recorded as 1+ (slight) to 4+ (deep).

Pale, cool, tight, shiny skin is another sign of edema. Also listen to lung sounds to detect the presence of excess fluid.

Assess for the presence of edema (record degree of pitting), obtain baseline measurement of abdominal girth when edema is present, and check for the presence of fluid waves in the abdomen.

Electrolyte imbalance. Because the symptoms of most electrolyte imbalances are similar, the nurse should gather data relative to changes in the patient's mental status (alertness, orientation, and confusion), muscle strength, muscle cramps, tremors, nausea, and general appearance.

Susceptible persons. Those who are particularly susceptible to the development of electrolyte disturbances frequently have a history of renal or cardiac disease, hormonal disorders, or massive trauma or burns or are on diuretic or steroid therapy.

Review available electrolyte studies.

Hypokalemia. Serum potassium (K$^+$) levels below 3.5 mEq/L. Hypokalemia is especially likely to occur when a patient exhibits vomiting, diarrhea, or heavy diuresis. All diuretics, except the potassium-sparing type, are likely to cause hypokalemia.

Hyperkalemia. Serum potassium (K$^+$) levels above 5.5 mEq/L. Hyperkalemia occurs most commonly when a patient is given excessive amounts of potassium supplementation, either intravenously or orally. It may also occur as an adverse effect of potassium-sparing diuretics.

Hyponatremia. Serum sodium (Na$^+$) below 135 mEq/L. Remember the phrase, "Where sodium goes, water goes." Because diuretics act by excreting sodium, monitor the patient for hyponatremia during and after diuresis.

Hypernatremia. Serum sodium (Na$^+$) above 145 mEq/L. Hypernatremia occurs most frequently when a patient is given intravenous (IV) fluids in excess of fluid excreted.

Nursing Diagnosis
- Fluid volume, excess (indication)
- Cardiac output, decreased (indication)
- Fluid volume, deficit (side effect)
- Injury, potential for (side effect)

Planning

History of causative disorder/factors. Review the patient's history to identify the underlying diagnosis for which the diuretic therapy is prescribed.

History of current symptoms. Plan to perform a focused assessment at least every shift to identify any changes in the patient's status.

Pattern of urination. Schedule appropriate nursing interventions for identified problems relating to the pattern of urinary elimination. Be sure to provide assistance with voiding for persons with impaired mobility, fatigue, or other impairment.

Medications. Schedule prescribed medications on the medication administration record (MAR). Remember to administer diuretics in the morning whenever possible to prevent nocturia.

Hydration. Schedule intake and output (I&O) every shift or more frequently depending on patient status. Place information to be assessed for status of hydration on the Kardex (for example, measure abdominal girth every shift, record degree of edema present in legs every shift).

Renal diagnostics. Many laboratory tests are ordered throughout the treatment of renal dysfunction (BUN, serum creatinine, creatinine clearance, serum osmolalities, and urine osmolalities). Plan schedules for appropriate timing of collections of blood and urine samples.

Nutrition. Patients with edema are routinely placed on a restricted sodium diet to help control edema associated with heart failure.

Diet therapy for renal disease is directed at keeping a normal equilibrium of the body while decreasing the excretory load on the kidneys. See a nutrition text for modifications specific to acute and chronic renal failure.

Implementation

Intake and output. Intake and output should be recorded accurately every shift and totaled every 24 hours for all patients having renal evaluations or receiving diuretics.

Intake. Measure and record *accurately* all fluids taken (oral, parenteral, rectal, and via tubes). Ice chips and foods such as gelatin that turn to a liquid state must be included. Irrigation solutions should be carefully measured so that the difference between that instilled and that returned can be recorded as intake.

Remember to enlist the help of the patient, family, and other visitors in this process. Ask them to keep a record of how many glasses of water or juice or cups of coffee were consumed. Then convert the household measurements to milliliters.

Output. Record all output from the mouth, urethra, rectum, wounds, and tubes (surgical drains, nasogastric tubes, and indwelling catheters). Liquid stools should be recorded according to consistency, color, and quantity. Urine output should include information on quantity, color, pH, odor, and specific gravity.

All other secretions should be characterized by color, consistency, volume, and changes from previous collections, if possible.

Daily output is usually 1200 to 1500 cc, or 30 to 50 cc per hour. Always report urine output below this hourly rate. Low hourly output may indicate dehydration, renal failure, or cardiac disease.

Keep the urinal or bedpan readily available.

Tell patients and their visitors the importance of not "helping" by dumping the bedpan or urinal. Instruct them to use the call light and allow hospital personnel to empty and record all output.

Serum electrolytes. Monitor serum electrolyte reports; notify physicians of deviations from normal values.

Nutrition. Order prescribed special diet depending on underlying pathology. If fluid restrictions are prescribed, state the

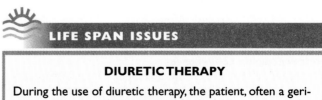

LIFE SPAN ISSUES

DIURETIC THERAPY

During the use of diuretic therapy, the patient, often a geriatric patient, must be monitored for hydration status and electrolyte balance as well as for the response of the presenting symptoms to the therapy. Patients taking digoxin or digitoxin are particularly susceptible to digitalis toxicity as a result of electrolyte imbalance.

amount of fluid to be taken on each tray and the amount that may be taken orally each shift on the Kardex and have this information posted on the head of the patient's bed.

Laboratory diagnostics. Order requested laboratory studies relating to the disease process.

Patient Education and Health Promotion

Purposes of diuresis

- If the disease process is hypertension, stress the importance of following the prescribed ways to deal with emotions and the dietary and medicinal regimens that can control the disease. (See under Nursing Process for Hypertensive Therapy, Chapter 20.)
- Teach the patient and significant others the functional changes that hypertension and heart failure cause. Emphasize the need for lifelong treatment and adherence to drug therapy, diet, and exercise regimens to obtain maximum control of the disease process.
- Diuretics are used in the treatment of several disease processes, for example, glaucoma, asthma, ascites, hypercalcemia, and renal disease. Be certain the patient understands the medication administration schedule and desired therapeutic outcome for the prescribed therapy.

Medication considerations

- Diuretics should be taken in the morning to avoid nocturia.
- When the diuretic is prescribed on a scheduled pattern other than daily, assist the patient with the development of ways to remember when to take the medication (for example, using a calendar on which to mark dosages or using a medication holder that is marked with the days of the week and is loaded weekly with the medications to be taken).
- Instruct the patient to perform daily weights using the same scale, in similar clothing, at the same time daily—usually before breakfast. Record and report significant weight changes because weight gains and losses are the best indicators of fluid loss or gain. Usually a gain of 2 pounds in 2 days should be reported.
- Potassium supplements may be prescribed concurrently with diuretics other than potassium-sparing diuretics.
- Diuretic therapy may produce postural hypotension. Teach the patient to rise slowly from a supine or sitting position, and encourage the patient to sit or lie down if feeling faint.

Nutrition

- The physician usually prescribes dietary modifications appropriate to the underlying pathology, for example, weight reduction and sodium restriction.
- Patients receiving potassium-sparing diuretics should be taught which foods are high in potassium content. These foods should be moderately restricted but not withheld from the diet. Salt substitutes should be avoided because they are high in potassium content.
- When taking diuretics other than the potassium-sparing type, the patient is required to eat potassium-rich foods.

Fostering health maintenance

- Throughout the course of treatment, discuss medication information and how it will benefit the patient. Stress the importance of the nonpharmacologic interventions and the long-term effects that compliance with the treatment regimen can provide.
- Provide the patient and significant others with important information contained in the specific drug monograph for the medicines prescribed. Additional health teaching and

nursing interventions for the side effects to expect and report are described in the drug monographs that follow.

- Seek cooperation and understanding of the following points so that medication compliance is increased: name of medication, dosage, route and times of administration, side effects to expect, and side effects to report.
- Enlist the patient's aid in developing and maintaining a written record of monitoring parameters (see box on p. 323). Instruct the patient to bring the written record to follow-up visits.

Drug Class: Carbonic Anhydrase Inhibitor

acetazolamide (ah-see-tah-zol'a-myd)
Diamox (dy'ah-moks)

Actions

Acetazolamide is a weak diuretic that acts by inhibiting the enzyme carbonic anhydrase within the kidney, brain, and eye. As a diuretic, it promotes the excretion of sodium, potassium, water, and bicarbonate.

Uses

Currently this agent is not used frequently as a diuretic because of the availability of more effective medications. However, it is used to reduce intraocular pressure in patients with glaucoma and to reduce seizure activity in patients with certain types of epilepsy. (See Chapters 17 and 40.)

Drug Class: Methylxanthine

aminophylline (ah-mi-noff'ih-lin)

Actions

Aminophylline is a methylxanthine derivative used for its diuretic effects in cardiorenal disease and as a bronchodilator in patients with pulmonary disease. The methylxanthine derivatives include theophylline, caffeine, and theobromine, all of which display weak diuretic properties. All act by improving blood flow to the kidneys.

Uses

Aminophylline is now rarely used as a diuretic because of the availability of more effective diuretic agents. However, a diuresis is occasionally noted when aminophylline is used in the treatment of asthma. For discussion of aminophylline as a bronchodilator, see Chapter 28.

Drug Class: Loop Diuretics

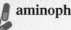

bumetanide (bu-met'an-eyd)
Bumex (bu'mex)

Actions

Bumetanide is a potent diuretic that acts primarily by inhibiting sodium and chloride reabsorption from the ascending limb of the **loop of Henle** in the kidneys. It also acts by increasing renal

PATIENT EDUCATION & MONITORING FORM | Diuretics or Urinary Antibiotics

MEDICATIONS	COLOR	TO BE TAKEN

Name _____

Physician _____

Physician's phone _____

Next appt.* _____

PARAMETERS		DAY OF DISCHARGE								COMMENTS
Weight										
Blood Pressure										
Pulse										
Faintness, dizziness	At rest									
	On exertion									
	No. of occurrences									
Muscle weakness	With exertion									
	When at rest									
Pain pattern and severity										
Severe — Moderate — Low; 10, 5, 1. Description: On urination, Without urination, Flank area, Suprapubic area										
Voiding and frequency	___ times voiding per day									
	___ times voiding per hr									
Fluid intake	___ glasses per day									
	___ cups per day									
Urine	Color (check one): Straw / Dark / Red									
	Odor: usual or unusual									

*Please bring this record with you to your next appointment.
Use the back of this sheet for additional information.

blood flow into the glomeruli and inhibits electrolyte absorption in the proximal tubule, enhancing sodium, chloride, phosphate, and bicarbonate excretion into the urine. Its diuretic activity starts within 30 to 60 minutes after administration; peak activity is within 1 to 2 hours and lasts for 4 to 6 hours.

Uses

Bumetanide is used to treat edema resulting from heart failure, cirrhosis of the liver, and renal disease, including nephrotic syndrome.

Therapeutic Outcomes

The primary therapeutic outcome associated with bumetanide therapy is diuresis with reduction of edema and improvement in symptoms related to excessive fluid accumulation.

Nursing Process

Premedication Assessment

1. Obtain baseline data before initiation of therapy, such as vital signs, lung sounds, weight, degree of edema present, laboratory studies (for example, serum electrolytes and liver and renal function tests).
2. Obtain data relating to the patient's mental status (orientation, alertness, and confusion), muscle strength, muscle cramps, tremors, nausea, and general appearance.
3. Patients with diabetes require baseline measurement of blood glucose levels.

Planning

Availability. PO—0.5, 1, and 2 mg tablets. IV—0.25 mg/ml in 2, 4, and 10 ml ampules.

Implementation

Dosage and administration. Adult: PO—initially 0.5 to 2 mg is administered as a single, daily dose. If additional diuresis is required, additional doses may be administered at 4- to 5-hour intervals. Do not exceed a maximum daily dose of 10 mg. Administer with food or milk to reduce gastric irritation. DO NOT administer after midafternoon to prevent nocturia. IM or IV—initially 0.5 to 1 ml administered over 1 to 2 minutes. Additional doses may be administered at 2- to 3-hour intervals, as necessary. Do not exceed 10 mg per 24 hours.

Evaluation

Side effects to expect

ORAL IRRITATION, DRY MOUTH. Start regular oral hygiene measures when the therapy is initiated. Suggest the use of 1 teaspoon of hydrogen peroxide in 6 to 8 ounces of water as a mouthwash. Commercial mouthwashes contain alcohol, which may cause further drying and oral irritation.

Other methods to alleviate dryness include sucking on ice chips or hard candy.

ORTHOSTATIC HYPOTENSION (DIZZINESS, WEAKNESS, FAINTNESS). Although this effect is infrequent and generally mild, all diuretics may cause some degree of orthostatic hypotension manifested by dizziness and weakness, particularly when therapy is being initiated.

Monitor the blood pressure daily in both the supine and erect positions.

Anticipate the development of postural hypotension and take measures to prevent an occurrence. Teach the patient to rise slowly from a supine or sitting position, and encourage the patient to sit or lie down if feeling faint.

Side effects to report

GASTRIC IRRITATION, ABDOMINAL PAIN. If gastric irritation occurs, administer with food or milk. If symptoms persist or increase in severity, report for physician evaluation.

ELECTROLYTE IMBALANCE, DEHYDRATION. The electrolytes most commonly altered are potassium (K^+), sodium (Na^+), and chloride (Cl^-). Hypokalemia is most likely to occur.

Many symptoms associated with altered fluid and electrolyte balance are subtle and interspersed with general symptoms of drug toxicity or the disease process itself.

Gather data about changes in the patient's mental status (alertness, orientation, and confusion), muscle strength, muscle cramps, tremors, nausea, and general appearance.

Always check the electrolyte reports for early indications of electrolyte imbalance.

Keep accurate records of I & O, daily weights, and vital signs.

HIVES, PRURITUS, RASH. Report symptoms for further evaluation by the physician. Pruritus may be relieved by adding baking soda to the bath water.

Drug interactions

ALCOHOL, BARBITURATES, NARCOTICS. Orthostatic hypotension associated with bumetanide therapy may be aggravated by these agents.

DIGITALIS GLYCOSIDES. Bumetanide may cause excessive potassium excretion, leading to hypokalemia. If the patient is also receiving a digitalis glycoside, monitor closely for digitalis toxicity (anorexia, nausea, fatigue, blurred or colored vision, bradycardia, and arrhythmias).

AMINOGLYCOSIDES (GENTAMICIN, AMIKACIN, NETILMICIN, OTHERS). The potential for ototoxicity from the aminoglycosides is increased. Assess the patient for gradual, often subtle, changes in hearing. Note if the patient seems to speak more loudly, asks for statements to be repeated, or turns the television or radio progressively louder.

CISPLATIN. The potential for ototoxicity from combination of cisplatin and bumetanide is increased. Assess the patient for gradual, often subtle, changes in hearing. Note if the patient seems to speak more loudly, asks for statements to be repeated, or turns the television or radio progressively louder.

NONSTEROIDAL ANTIINFLAMMATORY DRUGS (INDOMETHACIN, IBUPROFEN, NAPROXEN, OTHERS). Nonsteroidal antiinflammatory drugs (NSAIDs) inhibit the diuretic activity of this agent. The dose of bumetanide may have to be increased or the NSAID discontinued. Maintain accurate I&O records and monitor for a decrease in diuretic activity.

CORTICOSTEROIDS (PREDNISONE, OTHERS). Corticosteroids may enhance the loss of potassium. Check potassium levels and monitor more closely for hypokalemia when these two agents are used concurrently.

PROBENECID. Probenecid inhibits the diuretic activity of bumetanide. In general, do not use concurrently.

ethacrynic acid (eth-ah-krin'ik)
Edecrin (eh'deh-krin)

Actions

Ethacrynic acid is another diuretic that acts primarily on the ascending limb of the loop of Henle to prevent sodium and chloride reabsorption. Ethacrynic acid does not appear to affect renal blood flow or glomerular filtration rate. Its diuretic activity begins within 30 minutes, peaks in approximately 2 hours, and lasts 6 to 8 hours.

Uses

Ethacrynic acid is used to treat edema resulting from heart failure, cirrhosis of the liver, renal disease, and malignancy, and for hospitalized pediatric patients with congenital heart disease. It is thought that because ethacrynic acid inhibits the reabsorption of sodium to a much greater extent than other diuretics, it may be more effective in patients with significant renal failure. It is also used in conjunction with 0.9% sodium chloride infusions to enhance excretion of calcium in patients with hypercalcemia.

Therapeutic Outcomes

The primary therapeutic outcome associated with ethacrynic acid therapy is diuresis with reduction of edema and improvement in symptoms related to excessive fluid accumulation.

Nursing Process

Premedication Assessment

1. Obtain baseline data before initiation of therapy, such as vital signs, lung sounds, weight, degree of edema present, and laboratory studies (for example, serum electrolytes and liver and renal function tests).
2. Obtain data relating to the patient's mental status (orientation, alertness, and confusion), muscle strength, muscle cramps, tremors, nausea, and general appearance.
3. Patients with diabetes require baseline measurement of blood glucose levels.

Planning

Availability. PO—25 and 50 mg tablets. IV—50 mg per vial.

Implementation

Dosage and administration. Adult: PO—50 to 100 mg initially followed by 50 to 200 mg daily. Do not exceed 400 mg per day. Administer with food or milk to reduce gastric irritation. DO NOT administer after midafternoon to prevent nocturia. IV—50 mg or 0.5 to 1 mg/kg. Add 50 ml of dextrose 5% or saline solution to 50 mg of ethacrynic acid. This solution is stable for 24 hours. Administer over several minutes through the tubing of a running infusion or by direct IV.

Occasionally the addition of a diluent may result in an opalescent solution. These solutions should not be used. Do not mix with blood derivatives.

Pediatric: PO—initially 25 mg daily. Increase the dosage in increments of 25 mg to the desired effects. IV—1 mg/kg. Dilute with dextrose 5% and administer over 5 minutes through a running infusion. DO NOT use IV solution if it turns opalescent when the diluent is added.

Always monitor vital signs and I&O at regular intervals when administering this agent intravenously. Report blood pressure that decreases steadily or a narrowing pulse pressure, which may indicate hypovolemia.

Evaluation

Side effects to expect

ORTHOSTATIC HYPOTENSION (DIZZINESS, WEAKNESS, FAINTNESS). Although this effect is infrequent and generally mild, all diuretics may cause some degree of orthostatic hypotension manifested by dizziness and weakness, particularly when therapy is being initiated.

Monitor the blood pressure daily in both the supine and erect positions.

Anticipate the development of postural hypotension and take measures to prevent its occurrence. Teach the patient to rise slowly from a supine or sitting position, and encourage the patient to sit or lie down if feeling faint.

Side effects to report

ELECTROLYTE IMBALANCE, DEHYDRATION. The electrolytes most commonly altered are potassium (K^+), sodium (Na^+), and chloride (Cl^-). Hypokalemia is most likely to occur.

Many symptoms associated with electrolyte imbalance are subtle and interspersed with general symptoms of drug toxicity or the disease process itself.

Gather data about changes in the patient's mental status (alertness, orientation, and confusion), muscle strength, muscle cramps, tremors, nausea, and general appearance.

Always check the electrolyte reports for early indications of electrolyte imbalance.

Keep accurate records of I&O, daily weights, and vital signs.

GASTROINTESTINAL BLEEDING. Observe for "coffee-ground" vomitus or dark tarry stools, particularly in patients receiving IV therapy.

DIZZINESS, DEAFNESS, TINNITUS. Persons with impaired renal function may experience these symptoms. Assess the patient for gradual, often subtle, changes in balance and hearing. Note if the patient seems more unsteady when standing, speaks loudly, asks for statements to be repeated, or turns the television or radio progressively louder.

DIARRHEA. Diarrhea may become severe. Report to the physician and monitor the patient for dehydration and fluid and electrolyte imbalance.

HYPERGLYCEMIA. Diabetic or prediabetic patients must be monitored for the development of hyperglycemia, particularly during the early weeks of therapy.

Assess regularly for glycosuria and report if it occurs with any frequency.

Patients receiving oral hypoglycemic agents or insulin may require an adjustment in dosage.

Drug interactions

AMINOGLYCOSIDES (GENTAMICIN, AMIKACIN, NETILMICIN, TOBRAMYCIN, OTHERS). The potential for ototoxicity from the aminoglycosides is increased. Assess the patient for gradual, often subtle, changes in hearing.

Note if the patient seems to speak loudly, asks for statements to be repeated, or turns the television or radio progressively louder.

CISPLATIN. The potential for ototoxicity from combination of cisplatin and ethacrynic acid is increased. Assess the patient for gradual, often subtle, changes in hearing. Note if the patient seems to speak more loudly, asks for statements to be repeated, or turns the television or radio progressively louder.

NSAIDS (INDOMETHACIN, IBUPROFEN, NAPROXEN, OTHERS). NSAIDs inhibit the diuretic activity of this agent. The dose of ethacrynic acid may have to be increased or the NSAID discontinued. Maintain accurate I&O records and monitor for a decrease in diuretic activity.

DIGITALIS GLYCOSIDES. This diuretic may cause excess potassium excretion, leading to hypokalemia. If the patient is also receiving a digitalis glycoside, monitor closely for digitalis toxicity (anorexia, nausea, fatigue, blurred or colored vision, bradycardia, and arrhythmias).

CORTICOSTEROIDS (PREDNISONE, OTHERS). Corticosteroids may enhance the loss of potassium. Check potassium levels and monitor more closely for hypokalemia when these two agents are used concurrently.

furosemide (fuhr-oh'sah-myd)
Lasix (lay'siks)

Actions

Furosemide acts primarily on the ascending limb of the loop of Henle but also on the proximal and distal portions of the tubule to prevent sodium and chloride reabsorption. Furosemide diuresis results in enhanced excretion of sodium, chloride, potassium, hydrogen, calcium, magnesium, ammonium, bicarbonate, and possibly phosphate. Maximum diuretic effect occurs in 1 to 2 hours after oral administration and lasts 4 to 6 hours. Diuresis occurs within 5 to 10 minutes after IV administration, peaks within 30 minutes, and lasts approximately 2 hours.

Uses

Furosemide is one of the most potent and effective diuretics currently available. In addition to treating edema caused by heart failure, renal disease, and cirrhosis of the liver, furosemide may also be used for the treatment of hypertension, alone or in combination with other antihypertensive therapy. It is also used in conjunction with 0.9% sodium chloride infusions to enhance excretion of calcium in patients with hypercalcemia.

Therapeutic Outcomes

The primary therapeutic outcome associated with furosemide therapy is diuresis with reduction of edema and improvement in symptoms related to excessive fluid accumulation.

Nursing Process

Premedication Assessment

1. Obtain baseline data before initiation of therapy, such as vital signs, lung sounds, weight, degree of edema present, and laboratory studies (for example, serum electrolytes and liver and renal function tests).
2. Obtain data relating to the patient's mental status (orientation, alertness, and confusion), muscle strength, muscle cramps, tremors, nausea, and general appearance.
3. Patients with diabetes require baseline measurement of blood glucose levels.
4. Note any reduction in hearing.

Planning

Availability. PO—20, 40, and 80 mg tablets; 10 mg/ml and 40 mg per 5 ml oral solution. IV—10 mg/ml in 2, 4, 5, 6, 8, 10, and 12 ml ampules, vials, and prefilled syringes.

Implementation

Note: Patients who are allergic to sulfonamides may also be allergic to furosemide.

Dosage and administration. Adult: PO—20 to 80 mg as a single dose given preferably in the morning. If a second dose is necessary, administer 6 to 8 hours later. Increase in increments of 20 to 40 mg per day. Administer with food or milk to reduce gastric irritation. DO NOT administer after midafternoon to prevent nocturia. IV—20 to 40 mg given over 1 to 2 minutes. Much larger doses are frequently administered IV. The rate of administration should not exceed 4 mg per minute. Do not exceed 1000 mg per day. Always monitor vital signs and I&O at regular intervals with IV administration of this agent. Report blood pressure that decreases steadily or a narrowing pulse pressure, which may indicate hypovolemia.

Pediatric: PO—initially 1 to 2 mg/kg. If the response is not satisfactory, increase by 1 to 2 mg/kg every 6 hours. IV—initially 1 mg/kg. If diuresis is not satisfactory, increase by 1 mg/kg every 2 hours to a maximum of 6 mg/kg.

Evaluation

Side effects to expect

ORAL IRRITATION, DRY MOUTH. Start regular oral hygiene measures when therapy is initiated. Suggest the use of 1 teaspoon of hydrogen peroxide in 6 to 8 ounces of water as a mouthwash. Commercial mouthwashes contain alcohol and may cause further drying and oral irritation.

Other measures to alleviate dryness include sucking on ice chips or hard candy.

ORTHOSTATIC HYPOTENSION (DIZZINESS, WEAKNESS, FAINTNESS). Although this effect is infrequent and generally mild, all diuretics may cause some degree of orthostatic hypotension manifested by dizziness and weakness, particularly when therapy is being initiated.

Monitor the blood pressure daily in both the supine and erect positions.

Anticipate the development of postural hypotension and take measures to prevent an occurrence. Teach the patient to rise slowly from a supine or sitting position, and encourage the patient to sit or lie down if feeling faint.

Side effects to report

ELECTROLYTE IMBALANCE, DEHYDRATION. The electrolytes most commonly altered are potassium (K^+), sodium (Na^+), and chloride (Cl^-). Hypokalemia is most likely to occur.

Many symptoms associated with altered fluid and electrolyte balance are subtle and interspersed with general symptoms of drug toxicity or the disease process itself.

Gather data about changes in the patient's mental status (alertness, orientation, and confusion), muscle strength, muscle cramps, tremors, nausea, and general appearance.

Always check the electrolyte reports for early indications of electrolyte imbalance.

Keep accurate records of I&O, daily weights, and vital signs.

HYPERURICEMIA. This diuretic may inhibit the excretion of uric acid, resulting in hyperuricemia. Patients who have had previous attacks of gouty arthritis are particularly susceptible to additional attacks as a result of hyperuricemia.

Monitor the laboratory reports for early indications of hyperuricemia. Report to the physician, who may then add a uricosuric agent or allopurinol to the patient's medication regimen.

HYPERGLYCEMIA. Diabetic or prediabetic patients must be monitored for the development of hyperglycemia, particularly during the early weeks of therapy.

Assess regularly for glycosuria and report if it occurs with any frequency.

Patients receiving oral hypoglycemic agents or insulin may require an adjustment in dosage.

HIVES, PRURITUS, RASH. Report symptoms for further evaluation by the physician. Pruritus may be relieved by adding baking soda to the bath water.

Drug interactions

DIGITALIS GLYCOSIDES. This diuretic may cause excessive excretion of potassium, resulting in hypokalemia. If the patient is also receiving a digitalis glycoside, monitor closely for digitalis toxicity (anorexia, nausea, fatigue, blurred or colored vision, bradycardia, and arrhythmias).

PROPRANOLOL. The action of propranolol may be increased. Monitor for hypotension and bradycardia. Dosage adjustment may be necessary.

THEOPHYLLINE DERIVATIVES. The action of theophylline derivatives may be increased. Assess patients for signs of theophylline toxicity (restlessness, irritability, insomnia, nausea, vomiting, tachycardia, and arrhythmias). Serum levels of theophylline may be beneficial in dosage adjustment.

AMINOGLYCOSIDES (GENTAMICIN, AMIKACIN, NETILMICIN, TOBRAMYCIN, OTHERS). The potential for ototoxicity from the aminoglycosides is increased. Assess the patient for gradual, often subtle, changes in balance and hearing. Note if the patient seems more unsteady when standing, speaks loudly, asks for statements to be repeated, or turns the television or radio progressively louder.

CISPLATIN. The potential for ototoxicity from combination of cisplatin and furosemide is increased. Assess the patient for gradual, often subtle, changes in hearing. Note if the patient seems to speak more loudly, asks for statements to be repeated, or turns the television or radio progressively louder.

NSAIDS (INDOMETHACIN, IBUPROFEN, NAPROXEN, OTHERS). NSAIDs inhibit the diuretic activity of this agent. The dose of furosemide may have to be increased or the NSAID discontinued. Maintain accurate I&O records and monitor for a decrease in diuretic activity.

SALICYLATES. The potential for salicylate toxicity may be increased if taken concurrently for several days. Monitor patients for nausea, tinnitus, fever, sweating, dizziness, mental confusion, lethargy, and impaired hearing. Serum levels of salicylates may be beneficial in determining the amounts of salicylate dosage reduction.

METOLAZONE. When used concurrently, there is a considerably greater diuresis than that when either agent is used alone. Monitor closely for dehydration and electrolyte imbalance.

PHENYTOIN. Phenytoin may inhibit the absorption of orally administered furosemide. The dosage of furosemide may have to be increased based on the clinical response of the patient to normal doses.

torsemide (tohr-sah'myd)
Demadex (dehm'ah-dex)

Actions

Torsemide is a new sulfonamide type of loop diuretic similar to furosemide. It acts on the ascending limb of the loop of Henle to prevent sodium and chloride reabsorption. Torsemide does not appear to affect glomerular filtration rate or renal blood flow. Maximum diuretic effect occurs within 1 to 2 hours after oral administration and lasts 6 to 8 hours. Diuresis occurs within 5 to 10 minutes after IV administration, peaks within 60 minutes, and lasts up to 6 hours.

Uses

Torsemide is used to treat edema caused by heart failure, renal disease, and cirrhosis of the liver. Torsemide may also be used for the treatment of hypertension, alone or in combination with other antihypertensive therapy.

Therapeutic Outcomes

The primary therapeutic outcome associated with torsemide therapy is diuresis with reduction of edema and improvement in symptoms related to excessive fluid accumulation.

Nursing Process

Premedication Assessment

1. Obtain baseline data before initiation of therapy, such as vital signs, lung sounds, weight, degree of edema present, and laboratory studies (for example, serum electrolytes and liver and renal function tests).
2. Obtain data relating to the patient's mental status (orientation, alertness, and confusion), muscle strength, muscle cramps, tremors, nausea, and general appearance.
3. Patients with diabetes require baseline measurement of blood glucose levels.
4. Note any reduction in hearing.

Planning

Availability. PO—5, 10, 20, and 100 mg tablets. IV—10 mg/ml in 2 and 5 ml ampules.

Implementation

NOTE: Patients who are allergic to sulfonamides may also be allergic to furosemide.

Dosage and administration. PO—initially 5 to 20 mg once daily. If the dose is inadequate, increase the dose upward by doubling it until the desired diuretic response is achieved. IV—same as for PO dosages. Administer slowly over 2 or more minutes.

Evaluation

Side effects to expect

ORAL IRRITATION, DRY MOUTH. Start regular oral hygiene measures when therapy is initiated. Suggest the use of 1 teaspoon of hydrogen peroxide in 6 to 8 ounces of water as a mouthwash. Commercial mouthwashes contain alcohol and may cause further drying and oral irritation.

Other measures to alleviate dryness include sucking on ice chips or hard candy.

ORTHOSTATIC HYPOTENSION (DIZZINESS, WEAKNESS, FAINTNESS). Although this effect is infrequent and generally mild, all diuretics may cause some degree of orthostatic hypotension manifested by dizziness and weakness, particularly when therapy is being initiated.

Monitor the blood pressure daily in both the supine and erect positions.

Anticipate the development of postural hypotension and take measures to prevent an occurrence. Teach the patient to rise slowly from a supine or sitting position, and encourage the patient to sit or lie down if feeling faint.

Side effects to report

ELECTROLYTE IMBALANCE, DEHYDRATION. The electrolytes most commonly altered are potassium (K^+), sodium (Na^+), and chloride (Cl^-). Hypokalemia is most likely to occur.

Many symptoms associated with altered fluid and electrolyte balance are subtle and interspersed with general symptoms of drug toxicity or the disease process itself.

Gather data about changes in the patient's mental status (alertness, orientation, and confusion), muscle strength, muscle cramps, tremors, nausea, and general appearance.

Always check the electrolyte reports for early indications of electrolyte imbalance.

Keep accurate records of I&O, daily weights, and vital signs.

HYPERURICEMIA. Torsemide may inhibit the excretion of uric acid, resulting in hyperuricemia. Patients who have had previous attacks of gouty arthritis are particularly susceptible to additional attacks as a result of hyperuricemia.

Monitor the laboratory reports for early indications of hyperuricemia. Report to the physician, who may then add a uricosuric agent or allopurinol to the patient's medication regimen.

HYPERGLYCEMIA. Diabetic or prediabetic patients must be monitored for the development of hyperglycemia, particularly during the early weeks of therapy.

Assess regularly for glycosuria and report if it occurs with any frequency.

Patients receiving oral hypoglycemic agents or insulin may require an adjustment in dosage.

HIVES, PRURITUS, RASH. Report symptoms for further evaluation by the physician. Pruritus may be relieved by adding baking soda to the bath water.

Drug interactions

DIGITALIS GLYCOSIDES. This diuretic may cause excessive excretion of potassium, resulting in hypokalemia. If the patient is also receiving a digitalis glycoside, monitor closely for digitalis toxicity (anorexia, nausea, fatigue, blurred or colored vision, bradycardia, and arrhythmias).

THEOPHYLLINE DERIVATIVES. The action of theophylline derivatives may be increased. Assess patients for signs of theophylline toxicity (restlessness, irritability, insomnia, nausea, vomiting, tachycardia, and arrhythmias). Serum levels of theophylline may be beneficial in dosage adjustment.

AMINOGLYCOSIDES (GENTAMICIN, AMIKACIN, NETILMICIN, TOBRAMYCIN, OTHERS). The potential for ototoxicity from the aminoglycosides is increased. Assess the patient for gradual, often subtle, changes in balance and hearing. Note if the patient seems more unsteady when standing or speaks loudly, asks for statements to be repeated, or turns the television or radio progressively louder.

CISPLATIN. The potential for ototoxicity from combination of cisplatin and torsemide is increased. Assess the patient for gradual, often subtle, changes in hearing. Note if the patient seems to speak more loudly, asks for statements to be repeated, or turns the television or radio progressively louder.

NSAIDS (INDOMETHACIN, IBUPROFEN, NAPROXEN, OTHERS). NSAIDs inhibit the diuretic activity of this agent. The dose of torsemide may have to be increased or the NSAID discontinued. Maintain accurate I&O records and monitor for a decrease in diuretic activity.

SALICYLATES. The potential for salicylate toxicity may be increased if taken concurrently for several days. Monitor patients for nausea, tinnitus, fever, sweating, dizziness, mental confusion, lethargy, and impaired hearing. Serum levels of salicylates may be beneficial in determining the amounts of salicylate dosage reduction.

METOLAZONE. When used concurrently, there is a considerably greater diuresis than that when either agent is used alone. Monitor closely for dehydration and electrolyte imbalance.

Drug Class: Thiazide Diuretics

Actions

The benzothiadiazides, more commonly called the thiazides, have been an important and useful class of diuretic and antihypertensive agents for the past two decades. As diuretics, thiazides act primarily on the distal tubules of the kidney to block the reabsorption of sodium and chloride ions from the tubule. The unreabsorbed sodium and chloride ions are passed into the collecting ducts, taking molecules of water with them, thus resulting in a diuresis.

Uses

The thiazides are used as diuretics in the treatment of edema associated with heart failure, renal disease, hepatic disease, pregnancy, obesity, premenstrual syndrome, and administration of adrenocortical steroids. The antihypertensive properties of the thiazides result from a direct vasodilatory action on the peripheral arterioles. (See Chapter 20.)

Therapeutic Outcomes

The primary therapeutic outcomes associated with thiazide therapy are as follows:
- Diuresis with reduction of edema and improvement in symptoms related to excessive fluid accumulation
- Reduction in elevated blood pressure

Nursing Process

Premedication Assessment

1. Obtain baseline data before initiation of therapy, such as vital signs, lung sounds, weight, degree of edema present, and laboratory studies (for example, serum electrolytes and liver and renal function tests).

Table 25-1

Thiazide Diuretic Products

THIAZIDE	BRAND NAME	DOSAGE RANGE (MG)	DOSAGE FORMS AVAILABLE
Bendroflumethiazide	Naturetin	2.5-15	Tablets: 5 and 10 mg
Benzthiazide	Exna, Hydrex, Proaqua	50-150	Tablets: 50 mg
Chlorothiazide	Diuril	1000-2000	Tablets: 250 and 500 mg Oral suspension: 250 mg/5 ml Injection: 500 mg/20 ml
Hydrochlorothiazide	Esidrix, HydroDiuril, Oretic	25-100	Tablets: 25, 50, and 100 mg
Hydroflumethiazide	Saluron, Diucardin	25-100	Tablets: 50 mg
Methyclothiazide	Enduron, Aquatensen	2.5-5	Tablets: 2.5 and 5 mg
Polythiazide	Renese	1-4	Tablets: 1, 2, and 4 mg
Trichlormethiazide	Naqua, Metahydrin, Aquazide, Diurese	1-4	Tablets: 2 and 4 mg

Table 25-2

Thiazide-Related Products

DIURETIC	BRAND NAME	DOSAGE RANGE (MG)	DOSAGE FORMS AVAILABLE
Chlorthalidone	Hygroton	50-200	Tablets: 25, 50, and 100 mg
Indapamide	Lozol	2.5-5	Tablets: 2.5 mg
Metolazone	Zaroxolyn, Mykrox	2.5-10	Tablets: 0.5, 2.5, 5, and 10 mg

2. Obtain data relating to the patient's mental status (orientation, alertness, and confusion), muscle strength, muscle cramps, tremors, nausea, and general appearance.
3. Patients with diabetes require baseline measurement of blood glucose levels.
4. Note any reduction in hearing.
5. Check for any symptoms of acute gout. If present, notify the physician.

Planning
Availability. Tables 25-1 and 25-2 provide a list of thiazide diuretics and those diuretics chemically related to the thiazides. Most of the diuretics listed are administered in divided daily doses for the treatment of hypertension. However, single daily dosages may be most effective for mobilization of edema fluid.

Implementation
DO NOT administer after midafternoon to prevent nocturia.
Dosage and administration. See Tables 25-1 and 25-2. Administer with food or milk to reduce gastric irritation.

Evaluation
Side effects to expect
ORTHOSTATIC HYPOTENSION (DIZZINESS, WEAKNESS, FAINTNESS). Although this effect is infrequent and generally mild, all diuretics may cause some degree of orthostatic hypotension manifested by dizziness and weakness, particularly when therapy is being initiated.

Monitor the blood pressure daily in both the supine and erect positions.

Anticipate the development of postural hypotension and take measures to prevent an occurrence. Teach the patient to rise slowly from a supine or sitting position, and encourage the patient to sit or lie down if feeling faint.
Side effects to report
GASTRIC IRRITATION, NAUSEA, VOMITING, CONSTIPATION. If gastric irritation occurs, administer with food or milk. If symptoms persist or increase in severity, report to the physician for evaluation.

ELECTROLYTE IMBALANCE, DEHYDRATION. Use of thiazides may cause or aggravate electrolyte imbalance; therefore patients should be observed regularly for signs such as dry mouth, drowsiness, confusion, muscular weakness, and nausea. The electrolytes most commonly altered are potassium (K^+), sodium (Na^+), and chloride (Cl^-). Hypokalemia is most likely to occur, and supplementary potassium is often prescribed to prevent or treat hypokalemia.

Many symptoms associated with altered fluid and electrolyte balance are subtle and interspersed with general symptoms of drug toxicity or the disease process itself.

Gather data about changes in the patient's mental status (alertness, orientation, and confusion), muscle strength, muscle cramps, tremors, nausea, and general appearance.

Always check the electrolyte reports for early indications of electrolyte imbalance.

Keep accurate records of I&O, daily weights, and vital signs.

HYPERURICEMIA. Plasma uric acid is frequently elevated by the thiazides, which inhibit the excretion of uric acid. Patients who have had previous episodes of hyperuricemia or attacks of gouty arthritis are particularly susceptible to additional attacks when receiving thiazide therapy.

Monitor the laboratory reports for early indications of hyperuricemia. Report to the physician, who then may add a uricosuric agent or allopurinol to the patient's medication regimen.

HYPERGLYCEMIA. The thiazides may induce hyperglycemia and aggravate cases of preexisting diabetes mellitus. Diabetic or prediabetic patients must be monitored for the development of hyperglycemia, particularly during the early weeks of therapy.

Assess regularly for glycosuria and report if it occurs with any frequency.

Dosages of oral hypoglycemic agents and insulin may have adjustment in patients with diabetes mellitus who also require diuretic therapy.

HIVES, PRURITUS, RASH. Report symptoms for further evaluation by the physician. Pruritus may be relieved by adding baking soda to the bath water.

Drug interactions

DIGITALIS GLYCOSIDES. This diuretic may cause excessive potassium excretion, resulting in hypokalemia. If the patient is also receiving a digitalis glycoside, monitor closely for digitalis toxicity (anorexia, nausea, fatigue, blurred or colored vision, bradycardia, and arrhythmias).

CORTICOSTEROIDS (PREDNISONE, OTHERS). Corticosteroids may enhance the loss of potassium. Check potassium levels and monitor more closely for hypokalemia when these two agents are used concurrently.

LITHIUM: Thiazide diuretics may induce lithium toxicity. Monitor patients for lithium toxicity manifested by nausea, anorexia, fine tremors, persistent vomiting, profuse diarrhea, hyperreflexia, lethargy, and weakness.

NSAIDS (INDOMETHACIN, IBUPROFEN, NAPROXEN, OTHERS). NSAIDs inhibit the diuretic activity of this agent. The dose of thiazide may have to be increased or the NSAID discontinued. Maintain accurate I&O records and monitor for a decrease in diuretic activity.

ORAL HYPOGLYCEMIC AGENTS, INSULIN. Because of the hyperglycemic effects of the thiazide diuretics, dosages of insulin and oral hypoglycemic agents are frequently required.

Drug Class: Potassium-Sparing Diuretics

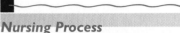

amiloride (am-ihl-or'eyd)
Midamor (my-da'mor)

Actions

Amiloride is a potassium-sparing diuretic that has weak antihypertensive activity. Its mechanism of action is unknown, but it acts at the distal renal tubule to retain potassium and excrete sodium, resulting in a mild diuresis.

Uses

Amiloride is usually used in combination with other diuretics in patients with hypertension or heart failure to help prevent hypokalemia that may result from other diuretic therapy.

Therapeutic Outcomes

The primary therapeutic outcome associated with amiloride therapy is diuresis with reduction of edema and improvement in symptoms related to excessive fluid accumulation.

Nursing Process

Premedication Assessment

1. Obtain baseline data before initiation of therapy, such as vital signs, lung sounds, weight, degree of edema present, and laboratory studies (for example, serum electrolytes and liver and renal function tests).
2. Obtain data relating to the patient's mental status (orientation, alertness, and confusion), muscle strength, muscle cramps, tremors, nausea, and general appearance.

Planning

Availability. PO—5 mg tablets.

Implementation

Dosage and administration. Adult: PO—initially 5 mg daily. Dosages may be increased in 5 mg increments up to 20 mg daily with close monitoring of electrolytes. Administer with food or milk to reduce gastric irritation. DO NOT administer after midafternoon to prevent nocturia.

Evaluation

Side effects to expect

ANOREXIA, NAUSEA, VOMITING, FLATULENCE. These side effects should be mild, particularly if the dose is administered with food. Persistent nausea and vomiting should be evaluated for other causes, as well as for the development of electrolyte imbalance.

HEADACHE. Monitor the blood pressure at regularly scheduled intervals because this agent is used for hypertension. Additional readings should be taken during headaches to determine if headaches are caused by the agents or by the hypertension. Report persistence of headaches.

Side effects to report

ELECTROLYTE IMBALANCE, DEHYDRATION. The electrolytes most commonly altered are potassium (K^+), sodium (Na^+), and chloride (Cl^-). Hyperkalemia is most likely to occur. Report potassium levels above 5 mEq/L.

Many symptoms associated with altered fluid and electrolyte balance are subtle and interspersed with general symptoms of drug toxicity or the disease process itself.

Gather data about changes in the patient's mental status (alertness, orientation, and confusion), muscle strength, muscle cramps, tremors, nausea, and general appearance.

Always check the electrolyte reports for early indications of electrolyte imbalance.

Keep accurate records of I&O, daily weights, and vital signs.

Drug interactions

LITHIUM. Amiloride may induce lithium toxicity. Monitor patients for lithium toxicity as manifested by nausea, anorexia, fine tremors, persistent vomiting, profuse diarrhea, hyperreflexia, lethargy, and weakness.

POTASSIUM SUPPLEMENTS, SALT SUBSTITUTES. Amiloride inhibits potassium excretion. Do NOT administer with potassium supplements or use salt substitutes high in potassium because of the potentially dangerous effects of hyperkalemia.

 spironolactone (spy-ro-no-lak'tone)
Aldactone (al-dak'tone)

Actions

Spironolactone blocks the sodium-retaining and potassium-excreting properties of aldosterone, resulting in a loss of water with the increased sodium excretion.

Uses

Spironolactone is a diuretic that is particularly useful in relieving edema and ascites that do not respond to the usual diuretics. This drug may be given with thiazide diuretics to increase its effect and reduce the hypokalemia often induced by the thiazides.

Therapeutic Outcomes

The primary therapeutic outcome associated with spironolactone therapy is diuresis with reduction of edema and improvement in symptoms related to excessive fluid accumulation.

Nursing Process

Premedication Assessment

1. Obtain baseline data before initiation of therapy, such as vital signs, lung sounds, weight, degree of edema present, and laboratory studies (for example, serum electrolytes and liver and renal function tests).
2. Obtain data relating to the patient's mental status (orientation, alertness, and confusion), muscle strength, muscle cramps, tremors, nausea, and general appearance.
3. Tactfully ask about any preexisting problems with libido.

Planning

Availability. PO—25, 50, and 100 mg tablets.

Implementation

Dosage and administration. Adult: PO—initially 50 to 100 mg daily. Maintenance dosage is usually 100 to 200 mg daily, but doses up to 400 mg may be prescribed. Administer with food or milk to reduce gastric irritation. Do NOT administer after midafternoon to prevent nocturia.

Pediatric: PO—1.5 to 3.5 mg/kg per day in divided doses every 6 to 24 hours. Readjust the dosage every 3 to 5 days.

Evaluation

Side effects to expect and report

MENTAL CONFUSION. Perform a baseline assessment of the patient's alertness, drowsiness, lethargy, and orientation to time, date, and place before initiating drug therapy. Compare subsequent mental status and analyze on a regular basis.

HEADACHE. Monitor blood pressure at regularly scheduled intervals because this agent is used for hypertension. Additional readings should be taken during headaches to determine if headaches are caused by the agent or the hypertension. Report persistence of headaches.

DIARRHEA. The onset of new symptoms occurring after initiation of the drug therapy requires evaluation if persistent.

ELECTROLYTE IMBALANCE, DEHYDRATION. The electrolytes most commonly altered are potassium (K$^+$), sodium (Na$^+$), and chloride (Cl$^-$). Hyperkalemia is most likely to occur. Report potassium levels above 5 mEq/L.

Many symptoms associated with altered fluid and electrolyte balance are subtle and interspersed with general symptoms of drug toxicity or the disease process itself.

Gather data about changes in the patient's mental status (alertness, orientation, and confusion), muscle strength, muscle cramps, tremors, nausea, and general appearance.

Always check the electrolyte reports for early indications of electrolyte imbalance.

Keep accurate records of I&O, daily weights, and vital signs.

GYNECOMASTIA, REDUCED LIBIDO, BREAST TENDERNESS. Because the chemical structure of spironolactone is similar to that of estrogenic hormones, an occasional male patient will report gynecomastia, reduced libido, and diminished erection. Women may complain of breast soreness and menstrual irregularities. These effects are reversible after discontinuation of therapy.

Drug interactions

POTASSIUM SUPPLEMENTS, SALT SUBSTITUTES. Spironolactone inhibits potassium excretion. Do NOT administer with potassium supplements or use salt substitutes high in potassium because of potentially dangerous effects from hyperkalemia.

triamterene (try-am'ter-een)
Dyrenium (dy-reen'ee-um)

Actions

Triamterene is a mild diuretic that acts by blocking the exchange of potassium for sodium in the distal tubule of the kidney, resulting in retention of potassium with excretion of sodium and water.

Uses

Triamterene is an effective agent to use in conjunction with the potassium-excreting diuretics such as the thiazides and the loop diuretics.

Therapeutic Outcomes

The primary therapeutic outcome associated with triamterene therapy is diuresis with reduction of edema and improvement in symptoms related to excessive fluid accumulation.

Nursing Process

Premedication Assessment

1. Obtain baseline data before initiation of therapy, such as vital signs, lung sounds, weight, degree of edema present, and laboratory studies (for example, serum electrolytes and liver and renal function tests).
2. Obtain data relating to the patient's mental status (orientation, alertness, and confusion), muscle strength, muscle cramps, tremors, nausea, and general appearance.

Planning

Availability. PO—50 and 100 mg capsules.

Table 25-3
Combination Diuretic Products

DIURETICS	BRAND NAME	DOSAGE RANGE
Spironolactone 25 mg, hydrochlorothiazide 25 mg	Aldactazide	1 to 8 tablets daily
Spironolactone 50 mg, hydrochlorothiazide 50 mg	Aldactazide	1 to 4 tables daily
Triamterene 37.5 mg, hydrochlorothiazide 25 mg	Dyazide	1 to 2 capsules twice daily after meals
Triamterene 37.5 mg, hydrochlorothiazide 25 mg	Maxzide, 25 mg	1 to 2 tablets daily after meals
Triamterene 75 mg, hydrochlorothiazide 50 mg	Maxzide	1 tablet daily
Amiloride 5 mg, hydrochlorothiazide 50 mg	Moduretic	1 to 2 tablets daily with meals

Implementation

Dosage and administration. Adult: PO—50 to 150 mg 2 times daily.

Evaluation

Side effects to expect and report

ELECTROLYTE IMBALANCE, DEHYDRATION, LEG CRAMPS, NAUSEA, VOMITING, WEAKNESS: The electrolytes most commonly altered are potassium (K^+), sodium (Na^+), and chloride (Cl^-). Hyperkalemia is most likely to occur. Report potassium levels above 5 mEq/L.

Many symptoms associated with altered fluid and electrolyte balance are subtle and interspersed with general symptoms of drug toxicity or the disease process itself.

Gather data about changes in the patient's mental status (alertness, orientation, and confusion), muscle strength, muscle cramps, tremors, nausea, and general appearance (drowsy, anxious, or lethargic).

Always check the electrolyte reports for early indications of electrolyte imbalance.

Keep accurate records of I&O, daily weights, and vital signs.

HIVES, PRURITUS, RASH. Report symptoms for further evaluation by the physician. Pruritus may be relieved by adding baking soda to the bath water.

Drug interactions. Triamterene inhibits potassium excretion. Do NOT administer with potassium supplements or use salt substitutes high in potassium because of the potentially dangerous effects from hyperkalemia.

Drug Class: Combination Diuretic Products

A common problem associated with thiazide diuretic therapy is hypokalemia. In an attempt to minimize this adverse effect, several products have been manufactured that contain a potassium-sparing diuretic with a thiazide diuretic (Table 25-3). The goal of the combination products is to promote diuresis and antihypertensive effect through different mechanisms of action while maintaining normal serum potassium levels. Patients receiving a combination product are at risk for side effects resulting from any of the component drugs. Many cases of hyperkalemia and hyponatremia have been reported after use of the combination products.

Combination products should not be used as initial therapy for edema or hypertension. Therapy with individual products should be adjusted for each patient. If the fixed combination represents the appropriate dosage for each component, the use of a combination product may be more convenient for patient compliance. Patients must be reevaluated periodically for appropriateness of therapy and to prevent electrolyte imbalance.

CHAPTER REVIEW

Diuretics are drugs that act to increase the flow of urine. The purpose of diuretics is to increase the net loss of water. Diuretics are mainstays in the symptomatic treatment of heart failure, hypertension, and renal disease. Diuretics also have a variety of other medical uses, such as reducing cerebral edema, intraocular pressure, ascites, and hypercalcemia. The information the nurse obtains about the patient's general clinical symptoms is important to the physician when analyzing data for diagnosis and success of therapy.

MATH REVIEW

1. Ordered: ethacrynic acid 50 mg IV in 50 ml 5% dextrose and water. The patient has an IV pump running that is calibrated in milliliters per hour. Infuse the medication over 30 minutes.
   Set the pump at _____ ml per hour.

2. Ordered: furosemide 40 mg PO, stat.
   On Hand: furosemide 20 mg, tablets.
   Give: _____ tablet(s).

CRITICAL THINKING QUESTIONS

1. The physician orders furosemide 60 mg stat IV push. The drug resource book states, "The rate of administration should not exceed 4 mg per minute." Based on this information, how long would it take to administer the furosemide? What other facts should be checked before initiating IV push of the drug?

2. Ms. Jess is being treated for hypertension with diuretic therapy. She calls the physician's office to report that she is feeling weak, light-headed, and fatigued. What additional information would be useful before discussing her symptoms with the physician?

Drugs Used to Treat Thromboembolic Disorders

Objectives

1. State the primary purposes of anticoagulant therapy.

2. Analyze Figure 26-1 to identify the site of action of warfarin, heparin, and fibrinolytic medicine.

3. Identify the effects of anticoagulant therapy on existing blood clots.

4. Describe conditions that place an individual at risk for developing blood clots.

5. Identify specific nursing interventions that can prevent clot formation.

6. Explain laboratory data used to establish dosing of anticoagulant medications.

7. Describe specific monitoring procedures to detect hemorrhage in the anticoagulated patient.

8. Describe procedures used to ensure that the correct dose of an anticoagulant is prepared and administered.

9. Explain the specific procedures and techniques used to administer heparin subcutaneously, via intermittent administration through a heparin lock, and via intravenous infusion.

10. Identify the purpose, dosing determination, and scheduling factors associated with the use of protamine sulfate.

11. State the nursing assessments needed to monitor therapeutic response and the development of side effects to expect or report from anticoagulant therapy.

12. Develop objectives for patient education for patients receiving anticoagulant therapy.

Key Words

thromboembolic diseases
thrombosis
thrombus
embolus
intrinsic clotting pathway
extrinsic clotting pathway
platelet inhibitors
anticoagulants
thrombolytic agents

THROMBOEMBOLIC DISEASE

Diseases associated with abnormal clotting within blood vessels are known as **thromboembolic diseases** and are major causes of morbidity and mortality. **Thrombosis** is the process of formation of a fibrin blood clot (**thrombus**). An **embolus** is a small fragment of a thrombus that breaks off and circulates until it becomes trapped in a capillary, causing either ischemia or infarction to the area distal to the obstruction (for example, cerebral embolism, pulmonary embolism).

Major causes of thrombus formation are immobilization with venous stasis; surgery and the postoperative period; trauma to lower limbs; certain illnesses (for example, heart failure, vasospasm, or ulcerative colitis); cancers of the lung, prostate, stomach, and pancreas; pregnancy and oral contraceptives; and heredity.

Normally, blood clot formation and dissolution is a fine balance within the cardiovascular system. The clotting proteins normally circulate in an inactive state and must be activated to form a fibrin clot. When there is a trigger, such as increased blood viscosity from bed rest and stasis or damage to a blood vessel wall, the *clotting cascade* is activated. For example, if a blood vessel is injured and collagen in the vessel wall is exposed, platelets first adhere to the site of injury and release adenosine diphosphate (ADP), leading to additional platelet aggregation that forms a "platelet plug." At the same time platelets are forming a plug, the **intrinsic clotting pathway** is triggered by the presence of collagen activating factor XII. Activated factor XIIa activates factor XI to XIa, which activates factor IX to IXa. Factor IXa, in the presence of calcium, platelet factor 3 (PF3), and factor VIII, activates factor X. Activated factor Xa, in the presence of calcium, platelet factor 3, and factor V, stimulates the conversion of prothrombin to thrombin (Figure 26-1).

Sources outside the blood vessels, such as tissue extract or thromboplastin (tissue factor), can trigger the **extrinsic clotting pathway** by activating factor VII to VIIa. Factor

VIIa can also activate factor X, which results in the formation of thrombin. After stimulation from either the intrinsic or extrinsic pathway, thrombin, in the presence of calcium, activates fibrinogen to soluble fibrin. With time and the presence of factor XIII, the loose fibrin mesh is converted to a tight, insoluble fibrin mesh clot. Thrombin also stimulates platelet aggregation and stimulates further activity of factors V, VIIa, VII, and Xa. As the fibrin clot is being formed, it also triggers the release of fibrinolysin, an enzyme that dissolves fibrin, preventing the clot from spreading.

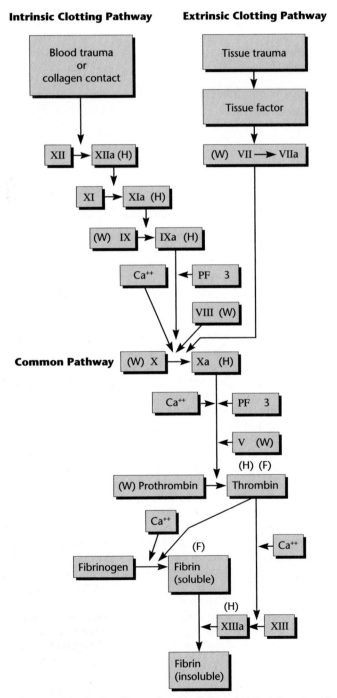

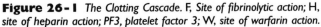

Figure 26-1 *The Clotting Cascade. F, Site of fibrinolytic action; H, site of heparin action; PF3, platelet factor 3; W, site of warfarin action.*

Historically, thrombi have been classified into red and white blood clots. A red thrombus is actually a venous thrombus and is composed almost entirely of fibrin and erythrocytes (red blood cells) with a few platelets. Venous thrombi generally form in response to venous stasis after immobility or surgery. The poor circulation prevents dilution of activated coagulation factors by rapidly circulating blood. The most common cause of red thrombus formation is deep venous thrombosis of the lower extremities. These thrombi may extend upward into the veins of the thigh and have the potential of fragmenting to cause life-threatening pulmonary emboli. White thrombi develop in arteries and are composed of platelets and fibrin. This type of thrombus forms in areas of high blood flow in response to injured vessel walls. Coronary artery occlusion leading to myocardial infarction is an example of a white thrombus.

Treatment

Diseases caused by intravascular clotting (for example, deep vein thrombosis, myocardial infarction, arrhythmias with clot formation, and coronary vasospasm leading to thrombus formation) are major causes of death. When thrombosis is suspected, patients are admitted to the hospital and often placed in an intensive care unit, where they can be closely observed for further signs and symptoms of thrombosis formation and progression and anticoagulant and thrombolytic therapy can be started. A combination of physical examination, patient history, Doppler ultrasound, phlebography, radiolabeled fibrinogen studies, and angiograms is used to diagnose the presence and etiology of a thrombus or embolism. Routine laboratory tests to assess the clotting process and ensure that occult bleeding is not in progress are: platelet count, hematocrit, prothrombin time (PT), activated partial thromboplastin time (APTT), urinalysis, and stool guiaic test.

Nonpharmacologic prevention and treatment of thromboembolic disease includes patient education on how to prevent venous stasis (for example, leg exercises and leg elevation), the use of properly fitted support stockings, and appropriate use of medications. The major pharmacologic treatments are platelet inhibitors, anticoagulants, and thrombolytic agents.

Drug Therapy

Actions

The pharmacologic agents used to treat thromboembolic disease act either to prevent platelet aggregation or inhibit a variety of steps in the fibrin clot formation cascade (Figure 26-1). See individual monographs for more detailed discussion of mechanisms of action.

Uses

Agents used in the prevention and treatment of thromboembolic disease can be divided into **platelet inhibitors**, **anticoagulants**, and **thrombolytic agents**. Antiplatelet agents (for example, aspirin) are used preventatively to reduce arterial clot formation (white thrombi) by inhibiting platelet aggregation. The anticoagulants, heparin, heparin derivatives (enoxaparin, dalteparin), and warfarin, are also used prophylactically to prevent formation of arterial and venous thrombi in predisposed patients. The primary purpose of anticoagulants is to prevent new clot formation or the extension of existing clots. They cannot dissolve an existing clot. The thrombolytic agents (for example, streptokinase and alteplase) are used to dissolve thromboemboli once formed.

Nursing Process for Anticoagulant Therapy

Assessment

History. Ask specific questions to determine whether the patient or family members have a history of any type of vascular difficulty. Patients at greater risk for clot formation are those with a history of clot formation, those with recent abdominal, thoracic, or orthopedic surgery, and those at prolonged bed rest.

Current symptoms. • Ask the patient to describe the symptoms. Is the patient now taking or has the patient recently taken anticoagulants? Individualize further questioning to obtain data that would support or rule out thrombosis formation or progression of thrombosis. • Collect data about reduced tissue perfusion—symptoms relating to cerebral, cardiopulmonary, or peripheral vascular disease, depending on underlying pathophysiology.

Medications. • Obtain a thorough medication history of both prescribed and over-the-counter medications being taken. • Ask specific questions relating to medicines being taken that affect clotting. Ask whether the patient has been complying with medication regimens and if any dosage adjustment has taken place. If anticoagulants are being taken, has the patient reported for scheduled laboratory studies?

Basic assessment. • Obtain vital signs and auscultation of breath sounds. Observe for dyspnea at rest or with exertion. • Check the mental status (for example, orientation to date, time, and place, alertness, and confusion). Use as a baseline for future comparison. • Assess for specific signs of reduced tissue perfusion. Perform a focused assessment depending on the underlying pathology (for example, cardiopulmonary, cerebral, or peripheral vascular disease). • Collect data about any pain being experienced. • Ask specific questions about the patient's state of hydration. Review intake and output.

Diagnostic studies. Review completed diagnostic studies and laboratory data (for example, PT, APTT, hematocrit, platelet count, Doppler studies, exercise testing, serum triglycerides, arteriogram, and cardiac enzyme studies).

Nursing Diagnosis
• Altered tissue perfusion (indication)
• Impaired gas exchange (indication)

Planning

History of causative disorder/factors. Review the patient's history to identify the diagnosis for which the anticoagulant or thrombolytic therapy was prescribed.

History of current symptoms. Plan to perform a focused assessment at appropriate intervals consistent with the patient's status to detect further signs and symptoms of thrombosis formation or progression.

Medications. Schedule prescribed anticoagulant medications on the medication administration record (MAR). Remember to *mark the one-time dosages clearly* because some medicines prescribed are based on the results of laboratory data completed daily or more frequently.

Hydration. Schedule intake and output (I&O) every shift or more frequently depending on the patient's status. Place information to be assessed for status of hydration on the Kardex.

Laboratory/diagnostic studies. • Order requested laboratory and diagnostic studies relating to the disease process (for example, platelet count, hematocrit, PT, APTT, arteriogram, and Doppler studies). • Mark the Kardex when additional laboratory studies are ordered, (for example, collection of stools for guiaic testing).

Prevent clot formation or extension. • Record activity level permitted on the Kardex. Place the patient on a turning schedule if on complete bed rest, or schedule activities for mobility. • Mark the Kardex with orders for use of support hose. Schedule times for removal and inspection of the legs every shift.

Implementation

Techniques for preventing clot formation. • Provide early, regular ambulation after surgery. Use active or passive leg exercises for patients on bed rest or restricted activity. • Develop and follow a specific turning schedule for persons on complete bed rest to prevent tissue breakdown and blood stasis. Implement good back care and deep breathing and coughing exercises as part of general nursing care. • Do not flex the knees or place pressure against the popliteal space with pillows. • Do not allow the patient to stand or sit motionless for prolonged periods of time. • Use elastic hose, such as thromboembolic deterent (TED) stockings. Remove stockings and inspect the skin on every shift. Make sure they are being worn properly and not becoming bunched around the knees or ankles.

Patient Assessment. Monitor vital signs and mental status every 4 to 8 hours or more frequently, depending on the patient's status.

Nutritional status. • The dietary regimen will depend on the patient's diagnosis and current clinical status. • Adequate hydration to promote fluidity of the blood is important. Unless coexisting diagnoses prohibit, give at least 6 to 8 8-ounce glasses of liquid daily.

Laboratory/diagnostic data. Monitoring and reporting laboratory results to the physician are essential during anticoagulant therapy. Coagulation tests that might be ordered include the following: whole blood clotting time (WBCT), PT, PTT, APTT, and activated coagulation time (ACT). The PT is routinely used to monitor warfarin therapy, and APTT is most commonly used to monitor heparin therapy.

Medication Administration. Never administer an anticoagulant without first checking the chart for the most recent laboratory results. Be certain that the anticoagulant to be administered has been ordered after the most recent results have been reported to the physician. Follow policy statements regarding checking of anticoagulant doses with other qualified professionals.

Patient Education and Health Promotion

Nutritional Status. • While receiving anticoagulant therapy, patients must limit intake of green leafy vegetables which contain vitamin K. (Vitamin K inhibits the action of warfarin.) • Instruct the patient to drink 6 to 8 8-ounce glasses of liquid daily, unless the physician has prescribed fluid restrictions.

Exercise and activity. • For peripheral vascular disease, Buerger Allen exercises may be recommended. Teach procedure and frequency. • Discuss the level of exercise prescribed by the physician. Walking may be prescribed to promote venous blood flow. Elevation of the legs when seated may be encouraged to promote venous blood flow. • Stress the need to prevent bodily injury. Tell the patient to avoid use of power equipment, use care in stepping up or down from curbs, not participate in contact sports, use only an electric razor, and brush teeth gently with a soft-bristled toothbrush.

Medication regimen
- Instruct the patient to take the dosage of the medication exactly as prescribed. Explain the importance of returning for laboratory blood tests to determine effectiveness and the need to adjust medicine dosages. Tell the patient to resume a regular schedule if one dose of warfarin is missed. If two or more doses are missed, the patient should consult the physician.
- Tell the patient to wear a medication alert bracelet.
- Explain symptoms the patient should report, for example, nosebleeds, tarry stools, "coffee-ground" or blood-tinged vomitus, petechiae (tiny purple or red spots occurring in various sites on the skin), ecchymoses (bruises), hematuria (blood in the urine), bleeding from the gums or any other body opening, or cuts or injuries from which the bleeding is difficult to control. If a dressing is on, check periodically for bleeding. Report excessive menstrual flow.
- In some cases the physician may want the patient to perform guaiac testing to detect blood in the stool. If ordered, specific patient education should be done to teach the patient or support person how to perform the test.
- Tell patients that because not all bleeding is clearly visible, they should report immediately a rapid, weak pulse; deep, rapid respirations; moist, clammy skin; and a general feeling of weakness or faintness.
- Tell the patient *not* to take any medication, including over-the-counter medications, without first consulting the physician or pharmacist because many drugs interact with warfarin to either increase or decrease its effectiveness.
- Patients should always inform any health care provider (for example, physician, home health care provider, dentist) that anticoagulant therapy is being taken whenever seeking care.

Fostering health maintenance
- Throughout the course of treatment, discuss medication information and how it will benefit the patient.
- Provide the patient and significant others with important information contained in the specific drug monograph for the medicines prescribed. Additional health teaching and nursing interventions for the side effects to expect and report are described in the drug monographs that follow.
- Seek cooperation and understanding of the following points so that medication compliance is increased: name of medication, dosage, route and times of administration, side effects to expect, and side effects to report.

- Enlist the patient's aid in developing and maintaining a written record of monitoring parameters (see box on page 337). Instruct the patient to bring the written record to follow-up visits.

Drug Class: Platelet Inhibitors

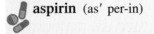 aspirin (as' per-in)

Actions

Aspirin is well known as a salicylate and nonsteroidal antiinflammatory agent. A unique property of aspirin, when compared with other salicylates, is inhibition of platelet aggregation with prolongation of bleeding time. The platelet loses its ability to aggregate and form clots for the duration of its lifetime (7 to 10 days). The mechanism of action is acetylation of the cyclooxygenase enzyme, which inhibits the synthesis of thromboxane A_2, a potent vasoconstrictor and inducer of platelet aggregation.

Uses

Aspirin is used to reduce the risk of recurrent transient ischemic attacks (TIAs) and stroke in men. There is a controversy in the literature as to whether aspirin is equally effective in women. Aspirin is also used to reduce the risk of myocardial infarction in patients with previous myocardial infarction or unstable angina pectoris.

Therapeutic Outcomes

The primary therapeutic outcomes expected from aspirin therapy when used for antiplatelet therapy are as follows:
- Reduced frequency of TIAs and stroke in men
- Reduced frequency of myocardial infarction

Nursing Process

Premedication Assessment

1. Perform baseline neurologic assessment, for example, orientation to date, time and place, mental alertness, bilateral hang grip, motor functioning (balance and hearing).
2. Monitor for gastrointestinal (GI) symptoms before and during therapy. Stool guaiac testing may be ordered if GI tract bleeding is suspected.
3. Check on concurrent use of anticoagulant agents.
4. If the patient is receiving oral hypoglycemic agents, review baseline serum glucose levels.

Planning

Availability. See Tables 18-3 and 18-4.

Implementation

Dosage and administration. Prevention of blood clots: PO—80 to 1300 mg daily. The dosage depends on whether the patient has a previous history of clot formation and other medications the patient may be receiving. The larger doses are usually subdivided into 325 mg doses 2 to 4 times daily. Administer with meals to minimize gastric irritation.

PATIENT EDUCATION & MONITORING FORM   Anticoagulants

MEDICATIONS	COLOR	TO BE TAKEN

Name _____

Physician _____

Physician's phone _____

Next appt.* _____

PARAMETERS		DAY OF DISCHARGE							COMMENTS
Weight									
Blood Pressure									
Pulse									
Color of urine	Normal								
	Red								
	Orange								
Mouth	Gums bleed with brushing								
Shaving	Bleeding—difficulty stopping blood								
Bruising	Nosebleeds— (___) of times?								
	Bruising to light touch								
Pain relief	Name limb (e.g., left leg, right leg)								
	Color of limb								
	Temperature								
Activities of daily living	Able to do								
	Done with difficulty								
	Too difficult to do								
Bowel movements	Normal								
	Diarrhea								
	Color—normal or black, tarry								
	Smell—normal or foul								
Report immediately									
	Chest pain								
	Faintness								
	Dizziness								
	Red vomitus								
	Black stools								

*Please bring this record with you to your next appointment.
Use the back of this sheet for additional information.

Evaluation

See Chapter 18.

dipyridamole (dye-per-id′ a-mole)
Persantine (per-sahn′ teen)

Actions

Dipyridamole is a platelet-adhesiveness inhibitor that is thought to work by inhibiting thromboxane A_2, increasing cyclic adenosine monophosphate (cAMP) in platelets, potentiating prostacyclin-mediated inhibition, and possibly reducing red blood cell uptake of adenosine, which also inhibits platelets.

Uses

Dipyridamole has been used extensively in combination with warfarin to prevent the formation of thromboembolism after cardiac valve replacement. It has also been prescribed in combination with aspirin for prevention of myocardial infarction, TIAs, and stroke. Recent studies, however, indicate that the combination is no more effective than aspirin alone.

Therapeutic Outcomes

The primary therapeutic outcome from dipyridamole therapy is prevention of blood clots secondary to artificial valve placement.

Nursing Process

Premedication Assessment

Obtain baseline vital signs.

Planning

Availability. PO—25, 50 and 75 mg tablets.

Implementation

Dosage and Administration. Adult: PO—75 to 100 mg 4 times daily with warfarin to prevent thromboembolism secondary to valve replacement.

Evaluation

Side effects to expect and report

DIZZINESS, ABDOMINAL DISTRESS. These symptoms are transient and disappear with continued therapy. Encourage the patient not to discontinue therapy.

Monitor the blood pressure daily in both the supine and erect positions.

Anticipate the development of postural hypotension and take measures to prevent an occurrence. Teach the patient to rise slowly from a supine or sitting position, and encourage the patient to sit or lie down if feeling faint.

Drug interactions

No clinically significant drug interactions have been reported with dipyridamole.

ticlopidine (ty-cloh′ ped-een)
Ticlid (ty′ clid)

Actions

Ticlopidine is thought to act by inhibiting the adenosine diphosphate (ADP) pathway required for platelet aggregation. The antiplatelet activity is seen after 3 to 5 days of continuous therapy. The antiaggregatory effect persists for up to 10 days after discontinuation of therapy. Ticlopidine also prolongs bleeding time. The maximal effect is seen after 5 to 6 days of continuous therapy.

Uses

Ticlopidine is used to reduce the risk of additional strokes in patients who have had a stroke and those who are at risk for a stroke. The medical histories of those patients at greatest risk include TIAs, atrial fibrillation, and carotid artery stenosis. Studies indicate that it is equally effective in men and women.

Early studies indicate that ticlopidine is more effective in reducing the risk of strokes than aspirin, but the potential for side effects (that is, neutropenia/agranulocytosis) limits its use to patients who cannot tolerate aspirin therapy (GI bleeding or hypersensitivity) or who should not take aspirin.

Therapeutic Outcomes

The primary therapeutic outcome expected from ticlopidine therapy is reduced frequency of TIA and stroke.

Nursing Process

Premedication Assessment

1. Obtain baseline vital signs.
2. Order baseline laboratory studies requested by the physician (for example, complete blood cell count [CBC]).
3. Assess and record the presence of any GI symptoms.

Planning

Availability. PO—250 mg tablets.

Implementation

Dosage and administration. Adult: PO—250 mg 2 times daily with meals.

Evaluation

Side effects to expect

NAUSEA, VOMITING, ANOREXIA, DIARRHEA. These effects tend to occur most frequently with early dosages and tend to resolve with continued therapy over 2 weeks. They can be minimized by taking the medicine with food. Encourage the patient not to discontinue therapy without first consulting a physician.

Side effects to report

NEUTROPENIA, AGRANULOCYTOSIS. Neutropenia (absolute neutrophil count less than 1200 neutrophils per mm^3) was discovered in 2.4% of patients in clinical trials. While neutropenic, patients are susceptible to infection. The neutropenic effects occur within 3 weeks to 3 months after start of therapy. The manufacturer recommends that blood counts be taken every 2 weeks for the first 3 months of therapy. Stress the importance of returning for this laboratory work.

Encourage the patient to report symptoms of infection (sore throat, fever, or excessive fatigue) to the physician as soon as possible.

BLEEDING. A normal physiologic effect of ticlopidine is prolongation of bleeding time. Patients should report any incidents of bleeding as soon as possible. Incidents to be reported include nose bleeds, easy bruising, bright red or "coffee-ground" emesis, hematuria, and dark tarry stools.

Patients should inform other health care practitioners (for example, another physician, dentist) that they are receiving platelet inhibitor therapy.

Drug interactions

CIMETIDINE. Cimetidine significantly reduces the metabolism of ticlopidine. Monitor patients closely for signs of toxicity from the ticlopidine.

Drug Class: Anticoagulants

dalteparin (dalt-eh′ pair-in)
Fragmin (frag′ min)

Actions

Dalteparin is the second (after enoxaparin) of the low molecular weight heparins (LMWHs) that are essentially the active components of the heparin protein molecule. The LMWHs have the advantage of specific action at certain steps of the coagulation pathway, resulting in less potential for hemorrhage and longer duration of action. Dalteparin enhances antithrombin activity against factors Xa and thrombin, which prevents completion of the coagulation cascade. Dalteparin has no antiplatelet activity and has only minimal effect on PT and APTT.

Uses

Dalteparin is used to prevent deep vein thrombosis after hip replacement surgery and abdominal surgery.

Therapeutic Outcomes

The primary therapeutic outcome from dalteparin therapy is prevention of deep vein thrombosis after hip replacement surgery or abdominal surgery.

Nursing Process

Premedication Assessment
1. Perform scheduled laboratory tests, including complete blood counts, platelet count, and stool occult blood tests before start of dalteparin therapy.
2. Obtain baseline vital signs.

Planning
Availability. SC—2500 IU of antifactor Xa (16 mg dalteparin) in 0.2 ml prefilled syringe with 27 gauge, ½-inch needle.

Implementation
Dosage and administration. *Note:* DO NOT INJECT INTRAMUSCULARLY! To prevent loss of drug, do not expel air bubble from syringe before injection.

Adult: SC—16 mg is injected 1 to 2 hours before surgery, and continued daily for 5 to 10 days after surgery. Administer by deep SC injection into a U-shaped area around the navel, the upper outer side of the thigh, or the upper outer quadrangle of the buttock. When the area around the navel or the thigh is used, lift up a fold of skin with the thumb and forefinger while giving the injection. Insert the entire length of the needle at a 45- to 90-degree angle. The skin fold should be held throughout the injection. Inject the drug slowly, leaving the needle in place for 10 seconds after injection. To minimize bruising, do not rub the injection site after completion of the injection. Alternate sites every 24 hours. Use the right side in the morning and the left side in the evening. Periodic complete blood counts, including platelet count, and stool occult blood tests are recommended during the course of treatment with dalteparin. No special monitoring of clotting times (that is, APTT) is required.

Evaluation

Side effects to expect
HEMATOMA FORMATION, BLEEDING AT INJECTION SITE. Inappropriate administration techniques lead to hematoma formation at the site of injection. USE PROPER TECHNIQUE!

Side effects to report
BLEEDING. Inspect the skin and mucous membranes for petechiae, ecchymoses, or hematomas. Also monitor for hematuria, bleeding gums, and melena.

Assess and record vital signs at regular intervals. Report signs and symptoms of internal bleeding (decreasing blood pressure; increasing pulse; cold, clammy skin; feeling faint; or disoriented sensorium).

Check urine and stools for blood. Urine may appear red, smoke colored, or brownish. Stools may appear to be dark and tarry. Perform a Hemoccult test on the stool, if necessary.

Vomitus may contain bright red blood or may be coffee ground in appearance.

Postoperative patients require assessment of dressings or drainage tubes for any signs of bleeding.

THROMBOCYTOPENIA. Dalteparin may induce type I and type II heparin-induced thrombocytopenia (HIT) (see the section on Heparin later in this chapter). Monitor platelet counts on a daily basis.

Drug interactions
No clinically significant drug interactions have been reported, but dalteparin should be used cautiously in patients receiving antiplatelet or warfarin therapy.

enoxaparin (en-ox′ a- pair-in)
Lovenox (lo-vehn′ ox)

Actions

Enoxaparin is the first of the LMWHs that are essentially the active components of the heparin protein molecule. The LMWHs have the advantage of specific action at certain steps of the coagulation pathway, resulting in less potential for hemorrhage and longer duration of action. Enoxaparin is specifically active against factor Xa and thrombin; it prevents completion of the coagulation cascade. Enoxaparin has no antiplatelet activity and does not affect the PT or APPT.

Uses

Enoxaparin is used to prevent deep vein thrombosis after hip replacement surgery.

Therapeutic Outcomes

The primary therapeutic outcome from enoxaparin therapy is prevention of deep vein thrombosis after hip replacement surgery.

Nursing Process

Premedication Assessment
1. Perform scheduled laboratory tests, including complete blood counts, platelet count, and stool occult blood tests before starting enoxaparin therapy.
2. Obtain baseline vital signs.

Planning
Availability. SC—30 mg (3000 IU antifactor Xa) in 0.3 ml of water for injection in a prefilled syringe with 26-gauge, ½-inch needle.

Implementation
Dosage and administration. Note: DO NOT INJECT INTRAMUSCULARLY! To prevent loss of drug, do not expel air bubble from syringe before injection.

Adults: SC—administer by deep SC injection into the anterolateral or posterolateral abdominal wall. The entire length of the needle should be introduced into a skin fold held between the thumb and forefinger; the skin fold should be held throughout the injection. Inject the drug slowly, leaving the needle in place for 10 seconds after injection. To minimize bruising, do not rub the injection site after completion of the injection. Alternate sites every 12 hours. Use the right side in the morning and the left side in the evening.

Periodic complete blood counts, including platelet count, and stool occult blood tests are recommended during the course of treatment with enoxaparin. No special monitoring of clotting times (that is, APTT) is required.

Evaluation
Side effects to expect

HEMATOMA FORMATION, BLEEDING AT INJECTION SITE. Inappropriate administration techniques lead to hematoma formation at the site of injection. USE PROPER TECHNIQUE!

Side effects to report

BLEEDING. Inspect the skin and mucous membranes for petechiae, ecchymoses, or hematomas. Also monitor for hematuria, bleeding gums, and melena.

Assess and record vital signs at regular intervals. Report signs and symptoms of internal bleeding (decreasing blood pressure; increasing pulse; cold, clammy skin; feeling faint; or disoriented sensorium).

Check urine and stools for blood. Urine may appear red, smoke colored, or brownish. Stools may appear to be dark and tarry. Perform a Hemoccult test on the stool, if necessary.

Vomitus may contain bright red blood or may be coffee-ground in appearance.

Assessment of dressings or drainage tubes for any signs of bleeding is necessary for postoperative patients.

THROMBOCYTOPENIA. Enoxaparin may induce type I and type II HIT (see the section on Heparin later in this chapter). Monitor platelet counts on a daily basis.

Drug interactions

No clinically significant drug interactions have been reported, but enoxaparin should be used cautiously in patients receiving antiplatelet or warfarin therapy.

 heparin (hep′ ahr-in)

Actions
Heparin is a natural substance that is commercially extracted from gut and lung tissue of pigs and cattle. In full therapeutic doses, heparin acts as a catalyst to accelerate the rate of action of a naturally occuring inhibitor of thrombin, antithrombin III (sometimes called the heparin cofactor). In the presence of heparin, antithrombin III rapidly neutralizes thrombin, activated factors IXa, Xa, XI, XII, and plasmin. Heparin also inhibits activation of factor VIII, the fibrin-stabilizing factor, preventing soluble fibrin clots from becoming insoluble clots (see Figure 26-1). Heparin has no fibrinolytic activity and cannot lyse established fibrin clots.

In low doses, heparin causes the neutralization of only factor Xa, preventing the conversion of prothrombin to thrombin. This allows lower dosages to be used with fewer complications from therapy. This is the rationale routinely used in prophylaxis with subcutaneous heparin to prevent the occurence of postoperative thrombi.

Uses
Heparin is used to treat deep venous thrombosis, pulmonary embolism, cerebral embolism, and acute peripheral arterial embolism. It is also used in the treatment of patients with heart valve prostheses. It is used prophylactically before and during cardiovascular surgery, in postoperative, immobilized patients, and during hemodialysis to prevent active coagulation and clot formation.

Therapeutic Outcomes
The primary therapeutic outcomes from heparin therapy are as follows:
- When used in low doses, prophylactically, heparin prevents deep venous thrombosis.
- In full doses heparin is used to treat a thromboembolism and promote neutralization of activated clotting factors, thus preventing the extension of thrombi and the formation of emboli. If therapy is started shortly after the formation of a thrombus, heparin will also prevent it from developing into an insoluble, stable thrombus, resulting in reduced tissue damage.

Nursing Process

Premedication Assessment
1. Take baseline vital signs.
2. Always check the most recent laboratory data (APTT) to ensure that the results are within recommended range for heparin therapy.

Planning
Availability. SC, IV—1000, 5000, 10,000, 20,000, and 40,000 U/ml in various sizes of ampules and vials.

Implementation
Dosage and administration. Accuracy of dose: Always confirm the dosage calculations with two nurses before subcutaneous or intravenous administration. Be certain the strength is correct. There is a *drastic difference* in clinical response from 1 ml of 1:1000 units and 1 ml of 1:10,000 units of heparin.

Dosage adjustment: Blood samples for laboratory studies (that is APTT) are usually drawn 4 to 6 hours after each subcutaneous dose or just before each intravenous dose.

Blood may be drawn every 6 to 8 hours during a continuous intravenous infusion. Do not draw blood samples from the same arm being used for heparin infusion.

Heparin dosage is considered to be in the normal therapeutic range if the APTT is 1.5 to 2.5 times the control APTT value (for example, if control is 30 seconds, the patient receiving full-dose heparin should have an APTT of 45 to 75 seconds for optimal therapy).

SC—prophylactic: 5000 U every 8 to 12 hours. Therapeutic: initially 10,000 to 15,000 U. Maintenance: 5000 to 10,000 U every 8 to 12 hours (Figure 26-2).

Subcutaneous injection is usually made into the tissue over the abdomen (see Figure 26-2). Do not inject within 2 inches of the umbilicus. The injection site should not be massaged before or after injection, and sites should be rotated for each dose to prevent the development of a massive hematoma.

Needle length and angle must be adapted to the patient's size so that the drug will be deposited into the subcutaneous tissue. (Usually a 26- or 27-gauge, ½-inch needle is used.) The injection is usually made at a 90-degree angle to the skin.

Always use a tuberculin syringe so that the dosage can be accurately measured.

Do NOT aspirate. This will increase local tissue damage and create the possibility of hematoma formation.

Do NOT inject into a hematoma or an area with any infection present.

Follow a planned site rotation schedule.

After injection, apply gentle pressure for 1 to 2 minutes to control local bleeding, but do not massage the area.

Ice packs on the site after injection may be used; check the hospital policy. At this time, there is little documented evidence that ice packs prevent hematoma formation or affect drug absorption.

IM—Not recommended because of the development of hematomas.

IV—Intermittent: Initially 10,000 U bolus; maintenance: 5000 to 10,000 U every 4 to 6 hours. A heparin lock, consisting of a 22 to 25-gauge scalp vein needle attached to a 3½-inch tubing ending in a resealing rubber diaphragm, may be used to administer intermittent IV doses of heparin.

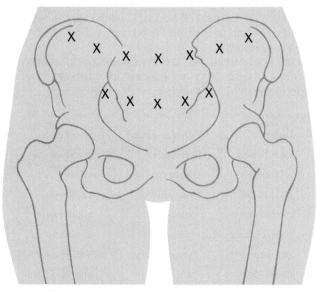

Figure 26-2 *Sites of heparin administration.*

(See Figure 9-11.) Advantages of a heparin lock are the mobility that it provides the patient and fewer venipunctures.

After injecting a bolus of heparin through the rubber diaphragm, flush the line with 1 ml of a solution containing 10 U of heparin per milliliter of saline solution. The heparin flush solution ensures that the patient will receive the entire heparin bolus, and it prevents the formation of a clot in the scalp vein needle.

IV—continuous infusion: initially 70 to 100 U/kg bolus; maintenance, 15 to 25 U/kg per hour. Continuous infusions of heparin provide the advantage of steady heparin levels in the blood. Periodic dosage adjustment is required based on the response of the patient.

When making a solution for infusion, always have two nurses confirm the calculations and the strength of the heparin to be used. As a safety measure, never make infusions that run more than 6 to 8 hours. This protects patients from receiving massive doses of heparin should the infusion "run away."

Always use an electronic control device for infusion. However, the infusion should be monitored at least every 30 to 60 minutes.

Antidote. Protamine sulfate, 1 mg, will neutralize approximately 100 U of heparin. If protamine sulfate is given more than 30 minutes after the heparin was administered, give only one half the dose of protamine sulfate. Because excessive doses of protamine may also cause excessive anticoagulation, it must be used judiciously.

Evaluation

Patients receiving full-dose heparin therapy should be monitored for hematocrit, platelet counts, APTT, and signs of bleeding.

Adverse effects of heparin therapy are most commonly caused by inappropriate administration technique or overdosage. Factors that can influence the incidence of complications include age, weight, sex, and recent trauma. The most common signs of overdosage are petechiae, hematomas, hematuria, bleeding gums, and melena.

Side effects to expect

HEMATOMA FORMATION, BLEEDING AT INJECTION SITE. Inappropriate administration techniques lead to hematoma formation at the site of injection. USE PROPER TECHNIQUE!

Side effects to report

BLEEDING. Inspect the skin and mucous membranes for petechiae, ecchymoses, or hematomas. Also monitor for hematuria, bleeding gums, and melena.

Always monitor menstrual flow to be certain that it is not excessive or prolonged.

Assess and record vital signs at regular intervals. Report signs and symptoms of internal bleeding (decreasing blood pressure; increasing pulse; cold, clammy skin; feeling faint; or disoriented sensorium).

Check urine and stools for blood. Urine may appear red, smoke colored, or brownish. Stools may appear to be dark and tarry. Perform a Hemoccult test on the stool, if necessary.

Vomitus may contain bright red blood or may be coffee ground in appearance.

Assessment of dressings and drainage tubes for any signs of bleeding is required in postoperative patients .

THROMBOCYTOPENIA. Heparin therapy may induce two types of thrombocytopenia. Type I HIT results from a direct effect of heparin on platelets causing sequestration and a fall in the platelet count to above 100,000/mm^3. The patient is asymptomatic, and heparin therapy should be continued if therapeutically indicated. Type II HIT should be suspected when the platelet count falls below 100,000/mm^3. This type of thrombocytopenia is an allergic reaction to heparin that causes aggregation of platelets. The onset of falling platelet counts is immediate after heparin therapy is started if the patient has previously received heparin or 5 to 14 days in the previously unexposed patient. Type II HIT occurs in about 3% of patients. Patients are at risk for white thrombus formation caused by sudden aggregation of platelets. Heparin therapy should be immediately discontinued if patients develop signs of clot formation, such as pain in an extremity, symptoms of a stroke, or chest pain resembling angina. Warfarin therapy may be initiated or continued, and antiplatelet therapy (aspirin) may also be started. Low molecular weight heparins are contraindicated because of the potential for cross-allergenicity. Platelet counts should be monitored daily.

Drug interactions

INCREASED THERAPEUTIC AND TOXIC EFFECTS. Concurrent use of nonsteroidal antiinflammatory drugs (NSAIDs), aspirin, dipyridamole, and ticlopidine may predispose the patient to hemorrhage.

warfarin (war' fah-rin)
Coumadin (koo' mah-din)

Actions

Warfarin is a potent anticoagulant that acts by inhibiting the activity of vitamin K, which is required for the activation of clotting factors II, VII, IX, and X in the blood. Blockade of the activation of these factors prevents clot formation (Figure 26-1).

Uses

Warfarin is used to treat or prophylactically prevent venous thrombosis, atrial fibrillation with embolism, pulmonary embolism, and coronary occlusion.

Therapeutic Outcomes

The primary therapeutic outcomes from warfarin therapy are as follows:
* Prevention and treatment of venous thrombosis and embolism
* Prevention and treatment of thromboemboli associated with atrial fibrillation
* Reduced risk of death, recurrent myocardial infarction and thromboembolic events such as stroke after myocardial infarction
* Prevention and treatment of thromboemboli associated with cardiac valve replacement

Nursing Process

Premedication Assessment
1. Obtain baseline vital signs.
2. Always check most recent PT or international normalized ratio (INR) results to determine if within the recommended range for warfarin therapy.

Planning
Availability. PO—1, 2, 2.5, 4, 5, 7.5, and 10 mg tablets.

Implementation

Dosage and administration. Dosage adjustment: Dosage during therapy is based on the prothrombin times. The PT is expressed as the INR, an internationally accepted standard for adjusting for variability in the prothrombin time assay. The optimal dosage is that which prolongs the PT and maintains the INR at 2 to 3. Certain medical conditions (for example, mechanical prosthetic valves and recurrent systemic embolism) require an INR of 2.5 to 3.5 and concurrent antiplatelet therapy.

When warfarin therapy is initiated, the patient should be monitored closely for evidence of hemorrhage because of the drug's accumulative effects.

Stress the need to comply with the prescribed regimen and the need for laboratory data to determine the correct maintenance dose.

Instruct the patient to resume a regular schedule if one dose is missed. If two or more doses are missed, the patient should consult the physician.

PO—10 mg daily for 2 to 4 days. Maintenance: 2 to 10 mg daily as determined by the PT reported as the INR.

Antidote. Vitamin K is a specific antidote for warfarin-induced hemorrhage but is rarely needed. Most cases of bleeding induced by warfarin overdose can be controlled by discontinuing warfarin therapy. An alternative in severe hemorrhage is a transfusion with plasma or whole blood.

Evaluation
Side effects to report
BLEEDING. Inspect the skin and mucous membranes for petechiae, ecchymoses, or hematomas. Also monitor for hematuria, bleeding gums, and melena.

Always monitor menstrual flow to be certain that it is not excessive or prolonged.

Assess and record vital signs at regular intervals. Report signs and symptoms of internal bleeding (decreasing blood pressure; increasing pulse; cold, clammy skin; feeling faint; or disoriented sensorium).

Check urine and stools for blood. Urine may appear red, smoke colored, or brownish. Stools may appear to be dark and tarry. Perform a Hemoccult test on the stool, if necessary. Vomitus may contain bright red blood or may be coffee ground in appearance. Assessment of dressings and drainage tubes for any signs of bleeding is required for postoperative patients.

Drug interactions

THE FOLLOWING DRUGS, WHEN USED CONCURRENTLY WITH WARFARIN, MAY ENHANCE THE THERAPEUTIC AND TOXIC EFFECTS OF WARFARIN:

acetaminophen	amiodarone	anabolic steroids
aspirin	chloral hydrate	cimetidine
ciprofloxacin	clofibrate	co-trimoxazole
disulfiram	erythromycin	ethanol
fluconazole	isoniazid	itraconazole
metronidazole	miconazole	omeprazole
phenylbutazone	phenytoin	piroxicam
propafenone	propoxyphene	propranolol
quinidine	simvastatin	salicylates
sulfinpyrazone	tamoxifen	tetracyclines

THE FOLLOWING DRUGS, WHEN USED CONCURRENTLY WITH WARFARIN, MAY DECREASE THE THERAPEUTIC ACTIVITY OF WARFARIN:

barbiturates	carbamazepine	chlordiazepoxide
cholestyramine	dicloxacillin	griseofulvin
nafcillin	rifampin	vitamin K

ALL PRESCRIPTION AND NONPRESCRIPTION MEDICATIONS. Caution the patient *not* to take *any* over-the-counter or prescription medication without first consulting the physician or pharmacist.

Drug Class: Fibrinolytic Agents

Over the past two decades there have been significant advances in the treatment of thromboemboli. Enzymes have been discovered that work within the clotting system to dissolve recently formed thrombi. The agents used are called fibrinolytic agents because of their ability to cause the dissolution of fibrin clots. The goals of fibrinolytic therapy are to lyse the thrombi during the early phase of clot formation, limit the damage to surrounding tissues by restoring circulation to the area distal to the thrombus, and reduce the morbidity and mortality after the formation of a thromboembolism.

Actions

Fibrinolytic agents activate the conversion of plasminogen to plasmin (also known as fibrinolysin), which digests fibrin, dissolving the clot. There are currently four fibrinolytic agents available: streptokinase, urokinase, anistreplase, and alteplase.

Streptokinase (Kabikinase) has the advantages of having proven clinical effectiveness, relative ease of administration, and relatively low cost. Disadvantages are potential for allergenicity if additional doses must be given in the future and potential for hemorrhage in other parts of the body.

Urokinase (Abbokinase) is effective and nonallergenic, but it is expensive and has the potential for causing hemorrhage in other parts of the body.

Anistreplase (anisoylated plasminogen streptokinase activator complex [APSAC]) (Eminase) is easy to administer and has a longer duration, but it is expensive, antigenic, and has the potential to cause hemorrhage in other parts of the body.

Alteplase (tPA–tissue plasminogen activator) (Activase) is of proven clinical effectiveness, more clot specific (a lower potential for hemorrhage elsewhere in the body), and nonantigenic. Disadvantages are a tenfold to twentyfold higher cost, a prolonged administration time, and the need for concurrent heparin therapy.

Uses

The fibrinolytic agents are used to dissolve clots secondary to coronary artery occlusion (myocardial infarction), pulmonary emboli, cerebral emboli (stroke), and deep venous thrombosis. The decision for use and selection of the agent depend on the location of the thrombus, clinical condition and age of the patient, preference of the patient care team, and the availability of alternative therapies such as angioplasty or bypass graft surgery. A key factor in the successful treatment of these conditions is the early treatment with fibrinolytic agents. Fibrinolytic agents tend to be much more successful

against the "soluble" fibrin clot, because they restore circulation to the obstructed area. Urokinase and streptokinase may also be used to reopen IV catheters, including central venous catheters, obstructed by blood clots.

Therapeutic Outcomes

The primary therapeutic outcome from fibrinolytic therapy is reperfusion of the tissues obstructed by the thrombus.

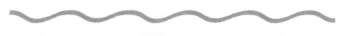

CHAPTER REVIEW

Diseases caused by intravascular clotting are major causes of death and must be treated rapidly to reduce tissue damage associated with thrombosis. The major pharmacologic treatments are platelet inhibitors, anticoagulants, and fibrinolytic agents. Nurses can play a significant role, especially in the nonpharmacologic prevention and treatment of thromboembolic disease, which includes patient education on how to prevent venous stasis, the use of properly fitted support stockings, and appropriate use of prescribed medicines.

MATH REVIEW

1. Ordered: heparin 2000 U SC stat.
   On hand: heparin 10,000 U/ml is available.
   Give: _____ ml.

2. Ordered: 100 ml D_5W with 30,000 U heparin. Infuse at a rate of 800 U per hour, IV. Set the infusion pump, calibrated in ml per hr, at _____ ml per hour.
   Three hours after the infusion is started, the physician changes the order to 1200 U per hour. How much heparin has already infused? _____ U.
   What rate would the infusion pump be adjusted to? Set infusion pump at _____ ml per hour.

3. Ordered: persantine 75 mg per day QID. With how many 75 mg tablets should the patient be dismissed in order to take the medication for the next 7 days? _____ tablets.

CRITICAL THINKING QUESTIONS

1. A patient comes from surgery after a femoral bypass with a heparin drip running through a pump. What nursing assessments should be made to monitor this patient's postoperative progress? The operative record indicates that the patient has had a total of 50,000 U of heparin during the operative procedure. The postoperative orders do not state a specific rate of flow for the heparin drip that is currently running through the pump at 8 ml per hour. What actions should be taken by the nurse?

2. Review the procedure for administration of enoxaparin subcutaneously. What monitoring of the patient should be done during therapy with this drug?

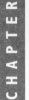

DRUGS USED TO TREAT DISORDERS OF THE RESPIRATORY SYSTEM

CHAPTER 27

Drugs Used to Treat Upper Respiratory Disease

CHAPTER CONTENT

Objectives

1. State the causes of allergic rhinitis and nasal congestion.
2. Explain the major actions (effects) of sympathomimetic, antihistaminic, and corticosteroid decongestants and cromolyn.
3. Define *rhinitis medicamentosa* and describe the patient education needed to prevent it.
4. Review the procedure for administration of medications by nose drops, sprays, and inhalation.
5. Explain why all decongestant products should be used cautiously in persons with hypertension, hyperthyroidism, diabetes mellitus, cardiac disease, increased intraocular pressure, or prostatic disease.
6. State the nursing assessments needed to monitor therapeutic response and development of side effects to expect or report from the use of decongestant drug therapy.
7. Identify essential components involved in planning patient education that will enhance compliance with the treatment regimen.

Key Words

rhinitis	histamine
rhinitis medicamentosa	rhinorrhea
sinusitis	decongestants
allergic rhinitis	antihistamines
antigen-antibody	antiinflammatory agents

UPPER RESPIRATORY TRACT ANATOMY AND PHYSIOLOGY

The respiratory system is a series of airways that start with the nose and mouth and end at the alveolar sacs within the lungs. The upper respiratory tract is composed of the nose with its turbinates, sinuses, nasopharnyx, pharynx, tonsils, eustachian tubes, and larynx (Figure 27-1). The nose and its structures serve two functions: olfactory (smell) sensation and respiratory function. The olfactory region is located in the upper part of each nostril. It is an area of specialized tissue cells (olfactory cells) that contain microscopic hairs that react to odors in the air and then stimulate the olfactory cells. The olfactory cells in turn send signals to the brain, which processes the sensation that we perceive as a particular smell.

The respiratory function of the nose is to warm, humidify, and filter the air inhaled to prepare it for the lower respiratory airways. Both nasal passages have folds of skin called turbinates that significantly increase the surface area of the passages and contain massive numbers of blood vessels. The blood circulating through the membranes lining the turbinates warms and humidifies the inhaled air. The inhaled air is also filtered of particulate matter. The hairs at the entrance to the nostrils remove large particles, and the turbinates and the narrowness of the nasal passages cause turbulence of the airflow passing through from each inhalation. All of the surfaces of the nose are coated with a thin layer of mucus secreted by goblet cells. Because of the turbulence of airflow, particles are thrown against the walls of the nasal passages and become trapped in the mucosal secretions. The epithelial cells lining the posterior two thirds of the nasal passages contain cilia that sweep the particulate matter back toward the nasopharynx and pharynx. Once in the pharynx the particulate matter is either expectorated or swallowed. The warming, humidification, and filtration processes continue as the air passes into the trachea, bronchi, and bronchioles.

The nasal structures are innervated by the autonomic nervous system. Cholinergic stimulation causes vasodilation of the blood vessels lining the nasal mucosa, and sympathetic (primarily alpha-adrenergic) stimulation causes vasoconstriction. The cholinergic fibers also innervate the secretory glands. When stimulated, they produce serous and mucus secretions within the nostrils.

The paranasal sinuses are hollow, air-filled cavities in the cranial bones on both sides and behind the nose. There are eight sinuses, four on each side. The purpose of the paranasal sinuses appears to be as resonating chambers for the voice and as a means of lightening the bones of the head. The sinuses are lined with the same mucous membranes and ciliated epithelium as those of the upper respiratory tract. The

sinuses are connected to the nasal passages by ducts and drain into the nasal cavity by activity from ciliated cells.

On either side of the oral pharynx is the pharyngeal tonsil, a collection of lymphoid tissue that is called the adenoids when enlarged. The tonsils are located in an area where mucus laden with particulate matter such as virus particles and bacteria accumulate from the ciliary action of cells in the nasopharynx above. The lymphoid tissue is rich in immunoglobulins and is thought to play a role in the immunologic defense mechanisms of the upper airway.

Sneezing is a physiologic reflex used by the body to clear the nasal passages of foreign matter. The sneeze reflex is initiated by irritation of the nasal mucosa by foreign particulate matter. It is quite similar to the cough reflex that clears the lower respiratory airways of secretions and foreign matter.

COMMON UPPER RESPIRATORY DISEASES

Rhinitis is the term used to define inflammation of the nasal mucous membranes. Signs and symptoms are sneezing, nasal discharge, and nasal congestion. Rhinitis is often subclassified into acute and chronic rhinitis based on the duration of the signs and symptoms. The most common causes of acute rhinitis are the common cold (that is, viral infection), bacterial infection, presence of a foreign body, and drug-induced congestion (**rhinitis medicamentosa**). Common causes of chronic rhinitis are allergy, nonallergic perennial rhinitis, chronic sinusitis, and a deviated septum.

The "common cold" is actually a viral infection of the upper respiratory tissues. When considering the amount of

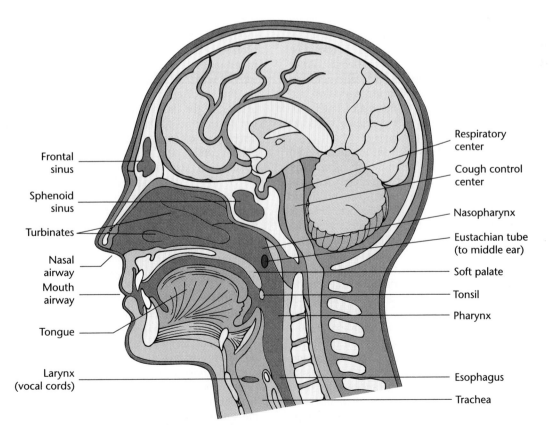

Figure 27-1 *Upper respiratory tract.*

time lost from school and work and the number of physician office visits annually, it is probably the single most expensive illness in the United States. Seasons in which viral infections reach near-epidemic proportions are midwinter, spring, and early fall, a few weeks after school starts. There are six different virus families (including 120 to 200 subtypes) that cause coldlike symptoms; the most common are the rhinoviruses and the coronaviruses. Viruses are spread from person to person by direct contact and sneezing. The earliest symptoms of a cold are a clear, watery nasal discharge and sneezing. Nasal congestion from engorgement of the nasal blood vessels and swelling of nasal turbinates quickly follows. Over the next 48 hours, the discharge becomes cloudy and much more viscous. Other symptoms include coughing, a "scratchy" or mildly sore throat (pharyngitis), and coughing and hoarseness (laryngitis). Other symptoms that occur less frequently are headache, malaise, chills and fever. A few patients may develop a fever up to 100° F. Symptoms should subside over the next 5 to 7 days.

Complications occasionally develop secondary to the challenge to the body's immune system by cold viruses. Complications also arise from thick, tenacious mucus obstructing sinus ducts or the eustachian tubes to the middle ears. Bacteria are easily trapped behind these obstructions in the sinuses and the ears, resulting in bacterial **sinusitis** or otitis media (infection of the middle ear). Viral infections are also a common cause of obstructive lung disease and of acute asthmatic attacks in susceptible individuals. If symptoms of the cold do not start to resolve over several days or if symptoms become worse or additional symptoms appear (for example, temperature over 100° F, earache), a physician should be consulted.

Allergic rhinitis is defined as inflammation of the nasal mucosa secondary to an allergic reaction. Patients with allergic rhinitis have had previous exposure to one or more allergens (for example, pollens, grasses, and house dust mites) and have developed antibodies to the allergen. After this exposure, when a person inhales the allergen, an **antigen-antibody** reaction occurs, causing inflammation and swelling of the nasal passages. One of the major causes of symptoms associated with an allergy is the release of histamine during the antigen-antibody reaction.

Histamine is a compound derived from an amino acid called histidine. It is stored in small granules in most body tissues. Its physiologic functions are not completely known, but it is released in response to allergic reactions and tissue damage from trauma or infection. When histamine is released in the area of tissue damage or at the site of an antigen-antibody reaction (such as a pollen being inhaled into the nose of a patient allergic to that specific pollen), it reacts with the H_1-receptors in the area and the following reactions take place: arterioles and capillaries in the region dilate, allowing an increased blood flow to the area that results in redness; capillaries become more permeable, resulting in the outward passage of fluid into the extracellular spaces, causing edema (manifested by congestion in the mucous membranes and turbinates of the patient's nose); and nasal, lacrimal, and bronchial secretions are released, resulting in the running nose (**rhinorrhea**) and watery eyes (conjunctivitis) noted in patients with allergies. Patients with allergic rhinitis also complain of itching of the palate, ears, and eyes. Most patients with asthma have an allergic

component to the disease that triggers acute attacks of asthma.

When large amounts of histamine are released, such as in a severe allergic reaction, there is extensive arteriolar dilatation. The blood pressure drops (hypotension), the skin becomes flushed and edematous, and severe itching (urticaria) develops. Constriction and spasm of the bronchial tubes make respiratory effort more difficult (dyspnea), and copious amounts of pulmonary and gastric secretions are released.

Allergies may be seasonal or perennial. Seasonal allergies occur at certain times of the year when the allergen is abundant. Tree pollen is prevalent from late March to early June. Ragweed is abundant from early August until the first hard freeze in October. Grasses pollinate from mid-May to mid-July. Weather conditions such as rainfall, humidity, and temperature affect the amount of pollen produced in a particular year but not the actual onset or termination of the specific allergen's season. It is common for a person to be allergic to more than one allergen simultaneously, so seasons may overlap or may occur more than once per year. Persons who have allergies to multiple antigens such as smoke, molds, animal dander, feathers, house dust mites, and pollens have varying degrees of symptomatology year round and are said to have perennial allergies. It is important that the symptoms of allergy be treated, not only for symptomatic relief but also to prevent irreversible changes within the nose. These changes include thickening of the mucosal epithelium, loss of cilia, loss of smell, recurrent sinusitis and otitis media, growth of connective tissue, and the development of nasal or sinus polyps that aggravate rhinitis and secondary infections.

Overuse of topical **decongestants** may lead to a rebound of nasal secretions known as rhinitis medicamentosa. This secondary congestion (rhinitis medicamentosa) is thought to be caused by excessive vasoconstriction of the blood vessels and by direct irritation of the nasal membranes by the solution. When the vasoconstrictor effects wear off, the irritation causes excessive blood flow to the passages, causing swelling and engorgement to reappear; the nose feels more stuffy and congested than before treatment. Over the next few weeks, a vicious cycle develops, causing more frequent use of the topical decongestant to relieve nasal passage swelling and obstruction. Rhinitis medicamentosa may develop as early as 3 to 5 days after use of the long-acting topical decongestants (for example, oxymetazoline and zylometazoline) but usually does not develop until after 2 to 3 weeks of regular use of the short-acting topical decongestants (for example phenylephrine).

Treatment
Common Cold

Treatment of the common cold is limited to relieving the symptoms associated with the rhinitis and, if present, pharyngitis and laryngitis; reducing the risk of complications; and preventing spread of viral infection to others. Decongestants are the most effective in relieving nasal congestion and rhinorrhea.

The use of **antihistamines** (H_1 receptor antagonists) in the symptomatic relief of cold symptoms has been controversial. Studies indicate that pre–school-aged children do not

DECONGESTANTS

Antihistamines and sympathomimetic amines, more commonly called decongestants, are frequently used in combination with analgesics in cold and flu products. Persons are often not fully aware of the ingredients of over-the-counter combination products.

Patients with diabetes mellitus, hypertension, or ischemic heart disease should use products containing decongestants only on the advice of a physician or pharmacist.

A paradoxic effect from antihistamines often seen in children and elderly persons is central nervous system stimulation rather than sedation, which may cause insomnia, nervousness, and irritability. Antihistamines may also cause urinary retention and should be used with caution in older men with an enlarged prostate gland.

benefit from their use but that older children, adolescents, and adults receive some benefit from antihistamines.

Depending on whether a fever, pharyngitis, or a cough is present, patients may also benefit from the use of analgesics, antipyretics (see Chapter 18), and expectorants and antitussive agents (see Chapter 28). Laryngitis should be treated by resting the vocal cords as much as possible. Inhaling cool mist vapor several times daily may be beneficial to humidify the larynx, but putting medication in the inhaled vapor is of no value. Lozenges and gargles do nothing to relieve hoarseness because they do not reach the larynx.

Allergic Rhinitis

The first step in the treatment of allergic rhinitis is to identify the allergens, usually through skin testing, to avoid future exposure, if possible. Unfortunately, it is often not possible to eliminate exposure to many allergens without severely restricting lifestyle. Medicines must then be used to block the allergic reaction or treat the symptoms. The pharmacologic agents used include antihistamines, decongestants, and intranasal **antiinflammatory agents.** Saline nasal spray can be effective in reducing nasal irritation between doses of other pharmacologic agents. If the patient is physically able, vigorous exercise for 15 to 30 minutes one or two times daily increases sympathetic output and induces vascular vasoconstriction.

Rhinitis Medicamentosa

The best treatment of rhinitis medicamentosa is prevention. Unfortunately, most patients are not aware of the condition until it becomes a problem. Following the directions for daily dosage and limiting the duration of therapy to that which is described on the topical decongestant product is the best way to avoid the condition.

Several treatment strategies have been successful in treating rhinitis medicamentosa. Regardless of the approach used, the patient must understand what caused the rebound congestion and why it is important to eliminate the problem. One strategy is to completely withdraw the topical decongestant at once. The patient is likely to be congested and

uncomfortable for the next week, but use of saline nasal spray can help moisturize irritated nasal tissues. Nasal steroid solutions can also be used, but it will take several days to reduce inflammation and congestion. Probably the most successful approach, although the longest to complete, is to have the patient work to clear one nostril at a time. Start by reducing the strength and frequency of the decongestant used in the left nostril while continuing with the "normal" dosage in the right nostril. Saline or corticosteroid nasal spray can be used every other dose in the left nostril. Eventually, the saline will be used more frequently and the decongestant can be discontinued in the left nostril. Once the patient can breathe normally through the left nostril, the same approach of reduced strength and frequency of decongestant can be started in the right nostril. Frequent follow-up with the patient and reinforcement of progress made are important to the success of this treatment.

Drug Therapy

Actions and Uses

Antihistamines or H_1-receptor antagonists, are the drugs of choice in treating allergic rhinitis. Because they are administered orally and thus distributed systemically, they also reduce the symptoms of nasal itching, sneezing, rhinorrhea, lacrimation and conjunctival itching. The antihistamines do not, however, reduce nasal congestion.

Decongestants are alpha-adrenergic stimulants that cause vasoconstriction to the nasal mucosa, which significantly reduces nasal congestion. When treating allergic rhinitis, decongestants are often administered in conjunction with antihistamines to reduce nasal congestion and counteract the sedation caused by many antihistamines.

Antiinflammatory agents administered intranasally are used to treat nasal symptoms resulting from mild to moderate allergic rhinitis. In general, antiinflammatory agents are not used to treat symptoms associated with a cold, because the symptoms start to resolve before the antiinflammatory agents can become effective. The antiinflammatory agents used to treat allergic rhinitis are corticosteroids and cromolyn sodium.

Nursing Process for Upper Respiratory Disease

Nasal congestion, allergic rhinitis, and sinusitis are treated by prescription or over-the-counter medicine. The nurse's role in the physician's office is to perform the initial assessment of symptoms and then focus on teaching the proper techniques of self-administering and monitoring the medication therapy.

Assessment

Description of symptoms. • What symptoms are present, for example, frequency of sneezing or coughing, hoarseness, nasal congestion, nasal secretions, and type (watery, viscous, color)? • When did the symptoms start? • Does the patient have a history of allergies? If yes, what are the known allergens? Are the symptoms associated with a particular time of year or the release of pollen from plants? Are the symptoms triggered by exposure to household environmental factors (for example, exposure to animal dander, dust, molds, or foods)? • Has the individual recently been exposed to someone with a common cold? • Is the individual having pain or discomfort? What is the specific area affected and the degree of pain?

History of treatment. • What prescription or over-the-counter medicines have been used? Are any effective? • When allergies are suspected, has skin testing been completed to determine what specific allergens are initiating the attacks? • If pain is present, how has pain relief been obtained? Is the degree of pain relief satisfactory?

Nursing Diagnosis
- Airway clearance, ineffective (indication)
- Knowledge deficit (side effects, treatment)

Planning
Symptoms and treatment. Establish the educational needs of the patient related to the underlying cause of the upper respiratory symptoms and the assistance needed to understand self-medication and treatments prescribed.

Implementation

Patient Education and Health Promotion
- Make sure that the patient understands the importance of adequate rest, hydration, and personal hygiene and prevention of spread of infection, when present.
- Discuss the specific medications prescribed, the therapeutic effects that can be expected, and when to contact the physician if therapy does not provide the expected benefit. Explain symptoms that should be reported to the physician

that would indicate poor response to the therapy (for example, escalation of symptoms, pain, or temperature with sinusitis).
- Make sure that the patient understands when to take the medicine; for example, if treating symptoms of allergy, antihistamines should be taken 45 to 60 minutes before exposure to the allergen.
- Proper technique is important to the success of therapy. Explain the procedures for proper installation of nose drops or nasal sprays associated with the prescribed treatment regimen. Document and verify that the patient can self-administer the medication as recommended.
- Teach the patient to monitor temperature, pulse, respirations, and blood pressure as appropriate to underlying diagnosis and the medicines used to treat the diagnosis.

Fostering health maintenance. • Throughout the course of treatment discuss medication information and how it will benefit the patient. Recognize that noncompliance may occur, especially when treatment response is not immediate. • Seek cooperation and understanding of the following points so that medication compliance is increased: name of medication, dosage, route and times of administration, side effects to expect, and side effects to report.

Drug Class: Sympathomimetic Decongestants

Actions
Sympathomimetic nasal decongestants (Table 27-1) stimulate the alpha-adrenergic receptors of the nasal mucous membranes, causing vasoconstriction. This constriction reduces blood flow in the engorged nasal area, resulting in shrinkage

Table 27-1

Nasal Decongestants

GENERIC NAME	BRAND NAME	AVAILABILITY	ADULT DOSAGE RANGE
Ephedrine	Ephedrine	Solution: 0.25%	Nasal: 2-3 drops 2-3 times daily
Epinephrine	Adrenalin	Solution: 0.1%	Nasal: 1-2 drops in each nostril every 4-6 hours
Naphazoline	Privine	Solution: 0.05%	Nasal: 2-3 drops or sprays no more than every 3 hours (drops) or 4-6 hours (spray).
Oxymetazoline	Afrin, Duration	Solution: 0.25%-0.05%	Nasal: 2-3 drops or sprays of 0.05% solution twice daily
Phenylephrine	Neo-Synephrine, Sinex	Solution: 0.125, 0.25, 0.5, 1% Jelly: 0.5%	Nasal: 0.25% every 3-4 hours
Phenylpropanolamine	Rhindecon, Propagest	Tablets: 25, 37.5, 50 mg Capsules: 75 mg	PO: 25 mg very 3-4 hours or 50 mg every 6-8 hours; do no exceed 150 mg daily
Pseudoephedrine	Sudafed, Seudotabs, Novafed	Tablets: 30, 60, 120 mg Liquid: 15, 30 mg/5 ml Drops: 7.5 mg/0.8 ml	PO: 60 mg every 6 hours; do not exceed 240 mg/24 hours
Tetrahydrozoline	Tyzine	Solution: 0.05%-0.1%	Nasal: 2-4 drops of 0.1% solution every 4-6 hours
Xylometazoline	Otrivin	Solution: 0.05%, 0.1%	Nasal: 2-3 sprays every 8-10 hours

of the engorged turbinates and mucous membranes. This promotes sinus drainage, improves nasal air passage, and relieves the feeling of stuffiness and obstruction.

Uses

Decongestants are the drugs of choice in relieving congestion associated with rhinitis caused by the common cold. They are also often used in conjunction with antihistamines when treating allergic rhinitis to reduce nasal congestion and to counteract the sedation caused by many antihistamines.

Decongestants used to treat rhinitis can be administered orally or applied directly to the nose (topically) in the form of nasal spray or drops. An advantage of topical administration is that essentially no systemic effects result. Disadvantages to the nasal sprays and drops are lack of effect on conjunctival symptoms, inconvenience, and the potential to cause rhinitis medicamentosa.

The use of nasal decongestants provides temporary relief of symptoms, but it is important for the patient to follow directions on the label carefully. Initially, the stuffiness or blocked sensation is relieved. However, misuse by patients, including excessive use or frequency of administration, may cause a rebound swelling (rhinitis medicamentosa) of the nasal passages.

Alpha-adrenergic agents used as nasal decongestants have the ability to stimulate alpha receptors at other sites in the body as well. Therefore they should be used with caution when taken orally in patients with hypertension, hyperthyroidism, diabetes mellitus, cardiac disease, increased intraocular pressure, or prostatic hypertrophy.

Therapeutic Outcomes

The primary therapeutic outcome associated with sympathomimetic decongestant therapy is reduced nasal congestion with easier breathing.

Nursing Process

Premedication Assessment
1. Check the patient's history for evidence of hypertension, hyperthyroidism, diabetes mellitus, cardiac arrhythmias, glaucoma, or prostatic hypertrophy. If present, consult with the physician before starting therapy.
2. Take baseline vital signs.

Planning
Availability. See Table 27-1.

Implementation
Dosage and administration. See Table 27-1. See also Chapter 10 for techniques to administer nose drops and nasal spray.

Evaluation
Side effects to expect

MILD NASAL IRRITATION. A burning or stinging sensation may be experienced when administered to the nasal membranes. This may be avoided by using a weaker strength of solution.

Side effects to report

HYPERTENSION. Excessive use of decongestants may result in significant hypertension. Patients already receiving antihypertensive therapy should avoid the use of decongestants. When used, blood pressure monitoring should be initiated and the physician contacted if blood pressure becomes elevated.

Drug interactions

DRUGS THAT ENHANCE TOXIC EFFECTS. Beta-adrenergic blocking agents (such as propranolol, timolol, atenolol, nadolol, and others) and monoamine oxidase inhibitors (tranylcypromine and pargyline). Excessive use may result in significant hypertension. Patients already receiving antihypertensive therapy should avoid the use of decongestants.

METHYLDOPA, RESERPINE. Frequent use of decongestants inhibits the antihypertensive activity of these agents. Concurrent therapy is not recommended.

Drug Class: Antihistamines

Actions

Antihistamines, or H_1-receptor antagonists, are chemical agents that act by competing with the allergy-liberated histamine for H_1-receptor sites in the patient's arterioles, capillaries, and secretory glands in mucous membranes. Antihistamines do not prevent histamine release but reduce the symptoms of an allergic reaction if the concentration of the antihistamine exceeds the concentration of histamine at the receptor site. Antihistamines are therefore more effective if taken before histamine is released or when the symptoms are first appearing.

Uses

Antihistamines are the drugs of choice for the systemic treatment of allergic rhinitis and conjunctivitis. These agents reduce rhinorrhea, lacrimation, nasal and conjunctival pruritis, and sneezing. The antihistamines do not, however, stop nasal congestion. The antihistamines shown in Table 27-2 have similar histamine-blocking effects when taken in recommended dosages but vary in duration of action, sedative effects, and anticholinergic effects. Occasionally a patient may develop a tolerance to the antihistaminic effects. Changing to another antihistamine is usually effective.

Antihistamines are best taken on a scheduled rather than as needed (prn) basis during the allergy season. These agents are much more effective if taken before exposure to the allergen, such as 45 to 60 minutes before going outdoors during the pollen season.

The most common side effect of many of the antihistaminic agents is sedation. Most patients acquire a tolerance to this adverse effect with continued therapy. However, reduction in dosage or a change to another antihistamine may occasionally be necessary.

All antihistamines cause anticholinergic side effects, particularly when higher dosages are used. Symptoms include dry mouth, stuffy nose, blurred vision, constipation, and urinary retention. Patients with asthma, prostatic enlargement, or glaucoma should take antihistamines only under a physician's supervision. The drying effects may also make respiratory mucus more viscous and tenacious. Antihistamines should be used cautiously in patients with a productive cough. If the cough continues but becomes nonproductive, consider additional hydration of the patient and discontinuation of the antihistamine.

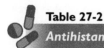

Table 27-2

Antihistamines*

GENERIC NAME	BRAND NAME	AVAILABILITY	SEDATION[†]	ADULT DOSAGE RANGE	MAXIMUM DAILY DOSE (MG)
Astemizole	Hismanal	Tablets	±	10 mg daily	30
Azatadine maleate	Optimine	Tablets	+ +	1-2 mg twice daily	4
Brompheniramine maleate	Veltane, Dimetane, Bromphen	Injection, tablets, elixir	+	4 mg 4-6 times daily	24
Chlorpheniramine maleate	Chlorate, Chlor-Trimeton, Teldrin	Tablets, capsules, syrup	+	4 mg 3-6 times daily	24
Clemastine fumarate	Tavist	Tablets, syrup		1.34-2.68 mg 3 times daily	8
Cyproheptadine hydrochloride	Periactin	Tablets, syrup	+	4 mg 3 times daily	32
Diphenhydramine hydrochloride	Benadryl, AllerMax	Injection, capsules, tablets, syrup, elixir	+ + +	25-50 mg 3-4 times daily	300
Loratidine	Claritin	Tablets	±	10 mg daily	10
Promethazine hydrochloride[‡]	Phenergan, Prorex	Injection, tablets, syrup, suppository	+ + +	12.5-25 mg 3-4 times daily	100
Terfenadine	Seldane	Tablets	±	60 mg twice daily	120
Tripelennamine	PBZ, Pelamine	Tablets, elixir	+ +	25-50 mg every 4-6 hours	300

*Many of these antihistamines are also available in combination with decongestants.
[†]Sedation index: + + +, high; + +, moderate; +, low; ±, low to none.
[‡]Promethazine is a phenothiazine with antihistaminic properties.

Therapeutic Outcomes

The primary therapeutic outcome associated with antihistamine therapy is reduced symptoms of allergic rhinitis (for example, rhinorrhea, lacrimation, itching, and conjunctivitis).

Nursing Process

Premedication Assessment

1. Review the patient's history for evidence of glaucoma, prostatic hypertrophy, or asthma. If present, consult with the physician before initiating therapy.
2. Assess the patient's work environment and consider whether drowsiness will affect safety and work performance.
3. Because antihistamines are prescribed for a variety of symptoms, such as hay fever, dermatologic reactions, drug hypersensitivity, rhinitis, and transfusion reactions, it is necessary for the nurse to individualize the patient assessments with the underlying pathology.

Planning
Availability. See Table 27-2.

Implementation
Dosage and administration. See Table 27-2.

Evaluation
Side effects to expect

SEDATIVE EFFECTS. Different antihistamines produce different degrees of sedation. Tolerance may be produced over a period of time, thus diminishing the effect.

Operating power equipment or driving may be hazardous. Caution patients to provide for personal safety in these situations.

DRYING EFFECTS. Monitor the patient's cough and degree of sputum production when antihistamines are administered. Because of their drying effects, antihistamines may impair expectoration.

FLUID INTAKE. Give adequate fluids concurrently with the use of antihistamines. Maintain fluid intake at 8 to 12 8-ounce glasses of water daily.

BLURRED VISION, CONSTIPATION, URINARY RETENTION, DRYNESS OF MUCOSA OF THE MOUTH, THROAT, AND NOSE. These symptoms are the anticholinergic effects produced by antihistamines. Patients taking these medications should be monitored for the development of these side effects.

Dryness of the mucosa may be alleviated by sucking hard candy or ice chips or chewing gum.

Caution the patient that blurred vision may occur, and make appropriate suggestions for personal safety of the individual.
Drug interactions

CENTRAL NERVOUS SYSTEM DEPRESSANTS. Central nervous system depressants, including sleep aids, analgesics,

Table 27-3

Intranasal Corticosteroids

GENERIC NAME	BRAND NAME	AVAILABILITY	ADULT DOSAGE RANGE
Beclomethasone dipropionate	Beconase, Vancerase	Nasal aerosol: 200 doses/canister	1 inhalation (42 μg) in each nostril 2 to 4 times daily
Beclomethasone dipropionate, monohydrate	Beconase AQ Vancerase AQ	Nasal spray: 200 doses/canister	1-2 sprays (42-84μg) in each nostril 2 times daily
Budesonide	Rhinocort	Nasal aerosol: 200 doses/canister	2 inhalations in each nostril morning and evening
Dexamethasone sodium phosphate	Decadron Turbinaire	Nasal aerosol: 170 doses/cartridge	2 sprays (168 μg) in each nostril 2 to 3 times daily; maximum daily dose is 12 sprays (1008 μg) in 24 hours
Flunisolide	Nasalide, ✽Rhinalar	Nasal spray: 200 doses/bottle	2 sprays (50 μg) in each nostril 2 times daily; maximum daily dose is 8 sprays (400 μg) in 24 hours
Fluticasone	Flonase	Nasal spray: 60 and 120 actuations/bottle	2 sprays in each nostril once daily
Triamcinolone	Nasacort	Nasal spray: 100 doses/bottle	2 sprays (110 μg) in each nostril once daily; maximum daily dose is 4 sprays in 24 hours

✽ Available in Canada only.

tranquilizers, and alcohol, potentiate the sedative effects of antihistamines. People who work around machinery, drive a car, pour and give medicines, or perform other duties in which they must remain mentally alert should not take these medications while working.

Drug Class: Respiratory Antiinflammatory Agents

intranasal corticosteroids

Actions
The exact mechanism by which corticosteroids reduce inflammation is not known.

Uses
Patients with allergic seasonal rhinitis who do not respond to antihistamines and sympathomimetic agents may be placed on corticosteroids to provide relief of allergic symptoms. Corticosteroids, whether applied topically or administered systemically, have been shown to be highly effective in the treatment of allergic rhinitis. Intranasal corticosteroids are successful in controlling nasal symptoms associated with mild to moderate allergic rhinitis, but systemic steroids are required for severe cases.

The newer topically active aerosol steroids, such as beclomethasone, budesonide, fluticasone and flunisolide, are highly effective and causes minimal side effects. The therapeutic effect (reduction of sneezing, nasal itching, stuffiness, and rhinorrhea) is usually observed by the third day, although the maximal effects may not be evident for 2 weeks. If symp-

toms are not improved within 3 weeks, therapy is discontinued. Dexamethasone intranasal aerosol causes a higher incidence of systemic side effects and is generally not used unless therapy with the other intranasal corticosteroids is not effective. To minimize the development of adrenal suppression, these corticosteroids should be used only for short courses of therapy for acute seasonal allergies.

Therapeutic Outcomes
The primary therapeutic outcome associated with intranasal corticosteroid therapy is reduced rhinorrhea, rhinitis, itching, and sneezing.

Nursing Process

Premedication Assessment
1. Blocked nasal passages should be treated with a topical decongestant just before initiation of intranasal corticosteroids.
2. Instruct the patient to blow the nose thoroughly before administering nasal therapy.

Planning
Availability. See Table 27-3.

Implementation
Dosage and administration. See Table 27-3. See also Chapter 10 for techniques to administer nasal spray.
Counseling. The therapeutic effects, unlike those of sympathomimetic decongestants, are not immediate. This should be explained to the patient in advance to ensure cooperation and continuation of treatment with the

prescribed dosage regimen. Full therapeutic benefit requires regular use and is usually evident within a few days, although a few patients may require up to 3 weeks of therapy for maximum benefit.

Preparation before administration. Patients with blocked nasal passages should be encouraged to use a decongestant just before intranasal corticosteroid administration to ensure adequate penetration. Patients should also be advised to clear the nasal passages of secretions before use.

Maintenance therapy. After the desired clinical effect is obtained, the maintenance dose should be reduced to the smallest amount necessary to control the symptoms.

Evaluation

Side effects to expect

NASAL BURNING. This side effect is usually mild and tends to resolve with continued therapy. Encourage the patient not to discontinue therapy without first consulting the physician.

cromolyn sodium (kro'mo-lin)
Nasalcrom

Actions

Cromolyn sodium is an antiinflammatory agent, but its mechanism of action is unknown. It inhibits the release of histamine and other mediators of inflammation. It must be administered before the body receives a stimulus to release histamine, such as an antigen that initiates an antigen-antibody allergic reaction.

Uses

Cromolyn is recommended for use in conjunction with other medications in the treatment of patients with severe allergic rhinitis to prevent the release of histamine that results in symptoms of allergic rhinitis.

Cromolyn has no direct bronchodilatory, antihistaminic, or anticholinergic activity and does not relieve nasal congestion. The concomitant use of antihistamines or nasal decongestants may be necessary during initial treatment with cromolyn. A 2- to 4-week course of therapy is usually required to determine clinical response. Therapy should be continued only if there is a decrease in the severity of allergic symptoms during treatment.

Therapeutic Outcomes

The primary therapeutic outcome associated with cromolyn therapy is reduced frequency of rhinorrhea, itching, and sneezing.

Nursing Process

Premedication Assessment

1. This medication must be taken before exposure to the stimulus that initiates an attack or allergic rhinitis.
2. Check to see if the concurrent use of antihistamines or nasal decongestants has been ordered by the physician, especially during start of cromolyn therapy.
3. Have the patient blow the nose before nasal instillation.

Planning

Availability. Nasal spray—40 mg/ml in 13 and 26 ml metered spray devices.

Implementation

Dosage and administration. See Chapter 10 for techniques to administer nasal spray.

Counseling. The therapeutic effects, unlike those of sympathomimetic amines, are not immediate. This should be explained to the patient in advance to ensure cooperation and continuation of treatment with the prescribed dosage regimen. Full therapeutic benefit requires regular use and is usually evident within 2 to 4 weeks. Therapy must be continued even if the patient is symptom free.

Nasal spray. Patients with blocked nasal passages should be encouraged to use a decongestant just before intranasal cromolyn administration to ensure adequate penetration. Patients should also be advised to clear the nasal passages of secretions and then inhale through the nose during administration. One spray in each nostril 3 to 4 times daily at regular intervals. Maximum is 6 sprays in each nostril daily.

Evaluation

Side effects to expect

NASAL IRRITATION. The most common side effect is irritation manifested by sneezing, nasal itching, burning, and stuffiness. Patients usually develop tolerance to the irritation. Rarely is this a cause for discontinuation of intranasal therapy.

Side effects to report

BRONCHOSPASM, COUGHING. Notify the physician if inhalation causes these symptoms.

Drug interactions. No significant drug interactions have been reported.

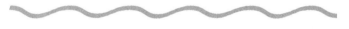

CHAPTER REVIEW

Rhinitis is defined as inflammation of the nasal mucous membranes. Signs and symptoms are sneezing, nasal discharge, and nasal congestion. The most common causes of acute rhinitis are the common cold, allergies, bacterial infection, presence of a foreign body, and drug-induced congestion (rhinitis medicamentosa). The nurse's role in working with patients with rhinitis is to perform the initial assessment of symptoms and then focus on teaching the proper techniques of self-administering and monitoring of the medication therapy. Frequent follow-up with the patient and reinforcement of progress made are important to the success of these treatments.

CRITICAL THINKING QUESTIONS

1. Mr. Longmeadow has been using phenylephrine nasal drops 2 to 3 times per day for the past 3 weeks. He comes to the physician's office complaining that his symptoms are worse than when he initiated treatment. What assessments should the nurse make?

2. Mrs. Canterville has been using chlorpheniramine maleate tablets 3 times per day and is now having considerable sedation. Her once productive cough has become nonproductive. What nursing actions should be considered?

3. One of the physician's patients calls the office and asks the nurse how she can tell if her inhaler is almost empty. What would your response be?

ADMINISTRATION QUESTIONS

1. Explain how to properly administer a medication by inhalation such as fluticasone, two sprays in each nostril once daily.

2. Perform health teaching for the proper administration of nose drops.

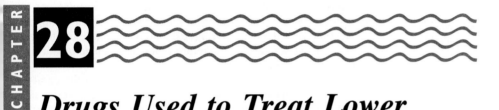

CHAPTER 28

Drugs Used to Treat Lower Respiratory Disease

CHAPTER CONTENT

Objectives

1. Compare the physiologic responses of the respiratory system to emphysema, chronic bronchitis, and asthma.

2. Describe the physiology of respirations.

3. Identify components of blood gases.

4. Cite nursing assessments used to evaluate the respiratory status of a patient.

5. Implement patient education for patients receiving drug therapy for lower respiratory disease.

6. Distinguish the mechanisms of action of expectorants, antitussives, and mucolytic agents.

7. Review the procedures for administration of medication by inhalation.

8. State the nursing assessments needed to monitor therapeutic response and the development of side effects to expect or report from expectorant, antitussive, and mucolytic therapy.

9. State the nursing assessments needed to monitor therapeutic response and the development of side effects to expect or report from sympathomimetic bronchodilator therapy.

10. State the nursing assessments needed to monitor therapeutic response and the development of side effects to expect or report from anticholinergic bronchodilator therapy.

11. List side effects known to occur with the use of xanthine derivatives, and correlate these with the needed nursing assessments and interventions.

12. State the nursing assessments needed to monitor therapeutic response and the development of side effects to expect or report from corticosteroid inhalant therapy.

ventilation

perfusion

diffusion

goblet cells

obstructive airway disease

bronchospasm

chronic obstructive
  pulmonary disease

restrictive airway disease

arterial blood gases

oxygen saturation

spirometry

cough

asthma

bronchitis

emphysema

expectorant

antitussive

mucolytic

LOWER RESPIRATORY TRACT ANATOMY AND PHYSIOLOGY

The respiratory system is a series of airways that start with the nose and mouth and end at the alveolar sacs. The nose and mouth airways connect at the pharynx. Passing out of the pharynx the airways divide into the esophagus of the gastrointestinal tract and the larynx (voicebox) and trachea of the respiratory tract. The trachea divides into the right and left mainstem bronchi, which enter the lungs. The bronchi subdivide in each lung into many smaller bronchioles. The bronchioles further subdivide into many smaller airways called alveolar ducts, which terminate in alveolar sacs. The alveolar sacs are surrounded by capillaries of the blood circulatory system. Human lungs contain between 300 and 500 million sacs for gaseous exchange and have a surface area approximately equal to that of a tennis court. The anatomic parts of the body associated with the lower respiratory system are the larynx, trachea, bronchi, bronchioles and the alveolar sacs (Figure 28-1).

The primary function of the lower respiratory tract is the ventilatory cycle. **Ventilation** is the movement of the air in and out of the lungs. It is the process of transport (inhalation) of air containing oxygen to the alveolar sacs, exchange of oxygen for carbon dioxide across the alveolar membranes containing blood capillaries, and exhalation of "stale air," including carbon dioxide. Ventilation of the lungs is accomplished by contraction and relaxation of the diaphragmatic and intercostal muscles (muscles between the ribs). During inspiration, the diaphragmatic and intercostal muscles contract, creating a vacuum in the lungs, pulling air in through the mouth and nose. During exhalation, relaxation of the muscles allows the chest to return to its unexpanded position, forcing air out of the lungs.

Blood flow through the pulmonary arteries to the capillaries surrounding the alveoli to the pulmonary veins is called **perfusion. Diffusion** is the process by which oxygen (O_2) passes across the alveolar membrane to the blood in the capillaries and carbon dioxide (CO_2) passes from the blood to the alveolar sacs. Oxygen is transported by combining with hemoglobin in red blood cells or by dissolving in the blood plasma. Blood circulation provides distribution of

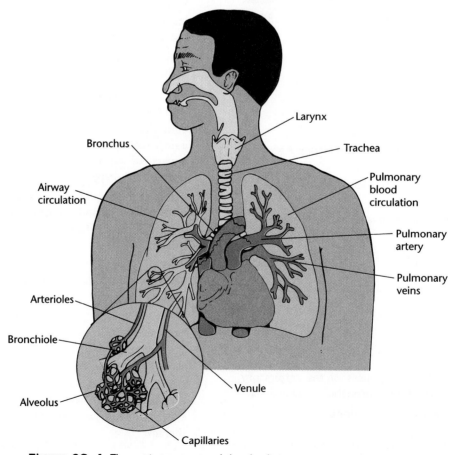

Figure 28-1 *The respiratory tract and the alveoli.* DesignPointe Communications/Atlanta

oxygen to the body's cells for the sustenance of life. Ventilation and perfusion must be equal to maintain homeostasis.

The fluids of the respiratory tract originate from specialized mucous glands (**goblet cells**) and serous glands that line the respiratory tract. The goblet cells produce a gelatinous mucus that forms a thin layer over the interior surfaces of the trachea, bronchi, and bronchioles. Secretion of mucus is increased by exposure to irritants such as smoke, airborne particulate matter, and bacteria. The serous glands are controlled by the cholinergic nervous system. When stimulated, the serous glands secrete a watery fluid to the interior surface of the bronchial tree. There, the mucus secretions of the goblet cells and the watery secretions of the serous glands combine to form respiratory tract fluid.

Normally, respiratory tract fluid forms a protective layer over the trachea, bronchi, and bronchioles. Foreign bodies such as smoke particles and bacteria are caught in the respiratory tract fluid and are swept upward by ciliary hairs that line the bronchi and trachea to the larynx, where they are removed by the cough reflex. The expectorated (coughed up) material contains pulmonary mucus secretions, foreign particulate matter such as smoke and bacteria, and epithelial cells sloughed from the lining of the airways. Common names given to the expectorated mass are sputum or phlegm. If too much mucus is secreted as a result of chronic irritation, cilia are destroyed by chronic inhalation of smoke, dehydration dries the mucus, or anticholinergic agents inhibit watery

secretions from the serous glands, the mucus becomes viscous, forming thick plugs in the bronchiolar airways (Figure 28-2). These thick plugs are difficult to eliminate. Colonization of pathogenic microorganisms in the lower respiratory tract results, which causes additional mucus secretions and the possible development of pneumonia from trapped bacteria.

The smooth muscle of the tracheobronchial tree is innervated by the parasympathetic and sympathetic branches of the autonomic nervous system. Stimulation of the cholinergic nerves causes bronchial constriction and increased mucus secretion. Sympathetic stimulation of adrenergic nerves causes dilation of bronchial and bronchiolar airways and inhibition of respiratory tract fluids. Both β_1- and β_2-adrenergic receptors are present, but the β_2-receptors predominate.

COMMON RESPIRATORY DISEASES

Respiratory diseases are often divided into two types: obstructive and restrictive. **Obstructive airway diseases** are those that narrow air passages, create turbulence, and increase resistance to airflow. Diseases cause narrowing of the airways through smooth muscle constriction (**bronchospasm**), edema, inflammation of the bronchial walls, or excessive mucus secretion. Examples of obstructive lung disease are asthma and acute bronchitis. Chronic obstructive

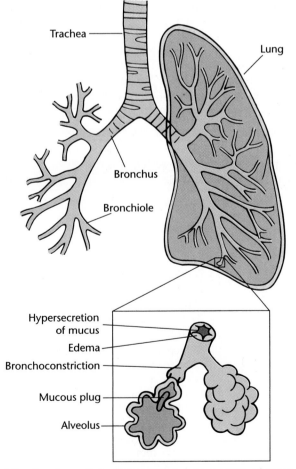

Figure 28-2 *Factors restricting the airway. Major factors include hypersecretion of mucus, mucosal edema, and bronchoconstriction. Mucous plugs may form in the alveoli.*

illnesses are also referred to as chronic obstructive lung disease (COLD), **chronic obstructive pulmonary disease** (COPD), and chronic obstructive airway disease (COAD). **Restrictive airway diseases** are those in which lung expansion is limited from loss of elasticity (for example, pulmonary fibrosis) or physical deformity of the chest (for example, kyphoscoliosis). Chronic bronchitis and emphysema are examples of both a restrictive and obstructive lung disease.

Pulmonary function tests have been developed to assess both the ventilation and diffusion capacity of the lungs to assist in diagnosis and to give an objective assessment of improvement or deterioration of the patient's clinical condition. The best indicator of overall pulmonary function (ventilation and diffusion) are the **arterial blood gases** (ABGs) (that is, PaO_2, $PaCO_2$, and pH) (Table 28-1). To determine ABGs, a sample of arterial blood must be drawn and immediately analyzed to measure the pH and partial pressures of oxygen and carbon dioxide in the blood. Another measure that is more readily available and noninvasive is the oxygen saturation of hemoglobin. **Oxygen saturation** (SaO_2) is the ratio, expressed as a percent, of the oxygen bound to hemoglobin compared with the maximum amount of oxygen that could be bound to hemoglobin (Table 28-1). Oxygen saturation is routinely used because a transcutaneous monitor (oximeter) is easily attached to the skin to continuously measure and report oxygen saturation.

Spirometry studies are routinely used to assess the capabilities of the patient's lungs, thorax, and respiratory muscles in moving volumes of air during inhalation and exhalation. A spirometer measures volumes of air. Terms used with spirometry are listed in Table 28-2. Patients with obstructive disease have difficulty with expiration and usually have a normal total lung capacity (TLC), a decreased vital capacity (VC), and an increased residual capacity (RC). Patients with restrictive disease have a decrease in all measured lung volumes. The forced expiratory volume in one second (FEV_1) and the forced vital capacity (FVC) are the most commonly used of the pulmonary function tests. The FEV_1 is used to determine the reversibility of airway disease and the effectiveness of bronchodilator therapy. The peak expiratory flow rate (PEFR) meter is not as accurate but is much less costly and more readily available than other pulmonary function tests. This meter is routinely used both by patients at home and by physicians to assess the benefits of therapy in treating acute and chronic asthmatic symptoms. A patient is considered to have significant reversibility of airway obstruction if there is a 15% to 20% improvement in the FEV_1 or PEFR after bronchodilator therapy.

One of the first symptoms of a respiratory disease is the presence of a **cough.** A cough is a reflex initiated by irritation of the airway. It is a protective, beneficial mechanism for clearing excess secretions from the tracheobronchial tree. The same irritants responsible for asthma or allergy may stimulate the cough receptors, or congestion of the nasal mucosa from a cold may cause a postnasal drip into the back of the throat that stimulates the cough.

A cough is productive if it helps remove accumulated secretions and phlegm from the tracheobronchial tree. A nonproductive cough results when irritants repeatedly stimulate the cough receptors but are not removed by the coughing reflex. Excessive coughing, particularly if it is dry and nonproductive, is not only discomforting but also tends to be self-perpetuating because the rapid air expulsion further irritates the tracheobronchial mucosa.

Asthma is a common chronic airway disease that affects 10 to 12 million people of all ages in the United States. It is the most common chronic illness of children and accounts for about 50% of emergency room visits by children under the age of 18. Asthma is a highly variable disease in terms of onset and frequency of attacks, length of remission, and stimuli that cause attacks. For unknown reasons, the prevalence of cases of asthma is increasing in the United States.

Table 28-1

Laboratory Tests Used to Assess Respiratory Function

TEST	NORMAL VALUE	RESULTS
pH	7.35-7.45 (arterial)	>7.45 = Alkalosis <7.35 = Acidosis
P_aCO_2	35-45 mm Hg	Abnormalities indicate respiratory acid-base imbalance. ↑ = Hypercapnea = respiratory acidosis ↓ = Hypocapnea = respiratory alkalosis
HCO_3	21-28 mEq/L	Abnormalities indicate metabolic acid-base imbalance. ↑ = Metabolic alkalosis ↓ = Metabolic acidosis
P_aO_2	80-100 mm HG	Measures the amount of oxygen moving through pulmonary alveoli into blood for transport to other tissues; depends on the amount of inspired oxygen. ↓ = Hypoxemia, hypoventilation ↑ = Hyperventilation
SaO_2	95%	Measures the ratio of oxygen content of hemoglobin compared with the hemoglobin's oxygen-carrying capacity. When decreased, either there is an impairment of oxygen binding to hemoglobin (for example, metabolic acidosis) or inadequate amounts of oxygen are being inspired.

Asthma is a disease of bronchi and bronchioles that are inflamed, reversibly obstructed (bronchoconstricted), and overresponsive to a variety of stimuli. Examples of stimuli that trigger bronchospasm and inflammation are respiratory viral infections, inhaled allergens, cold air, dry air, emotional stress and smoke. Symptoms of asthma include cough, wheezing, shortness of breath, tightness of the chest, and increased mucus production. The exact causes of asthma are unknown. Asthmatic patients are often subdivided into categories based on severity of disease: patients with mild asthma need less than one inhaled bronchodilator treatment daily; those with moderate asthma need daily antiinflammatory maintenance therapy, plus intermittent or routine bronchodilators; and those with severe asthma require higher doses of inhaled steroids, plus routine bronchodilators and frequent bursts of prednisone.

Chronic **bronchitis** is a condition in which chronic irritation causes inflammation and edema with excessive mucus secretion leading to airflow obstruction. Common causes of chronic irritation are cigarette smoke, grain and coal dust exposure, and air pollution. A persistent, productive cough present on most days is one of the earliest signs of the disease. The classic patient with chronic bronchitis has a chronic productive cough and moderate dyspnea, is often obese, and suffers from significant hypoxia with cyanosis. The ABGs will confirm hypoxia and respiratory acidosis. This type of patient is often called a "blue-bloater." Because of mucus overproduction and formation of mucus plugs, these patients are prone to recurrent respiratory infections. As this disease progresses, patients often develop polycythemia (increased red blood cell production) to transport oxygen and right-sided heart failure (cor pulmonale) secondary to the lung disease and pulmonary hypertension.

Emphysema is a disease of alveolar tissue destruction without fibrosis. Alveolar sacs lose elasticity and collapse during exhalation, trapping air within the lung. The classic patient with emphysema is short of breath with minimal exertion (dyspneic), breathes through pursed lips, is thin because of weight loss, is barrel-chested from increased use of accessory muscles, and has only scanty sputum production with a minimal cough. These patients are often called "pink-puffers" because they maintain normal oxygenation by increased breathing rate.

Treatment

Cough

Treatment of the cough is of secondary importance; primary treatment is aimed at the underlying disorder. If the air is dry, a vaporizer or humidifier may be used to liquefy the secretions so that they do not become irritating. A dehydrated state thickens respiratory secretions; therefore drinking large amounts of fluids will help reduce the viscosity (thickness) of the secretions. Patients can also suck on hard candies to increase the flow of saliva to coat the throat, thereby reducing irritation. If these simple measures do not reduce the frequency of the cough, an expectorant or a cough suppressant (antitussive) may be used. The therapeutic objective is to decrease the intensity and frequency of the cough yet permit adequate elimination of tracheobronchial phlegm. In severe cases of pulmonary congestion, a mucolytic agent may be required.

Asthma

The National Institutes of Health (NIH) recommends the following goals of therapy for asthma: maintain normal activity levels; maintain near-normal pulmonary function rates; prevent chronic and troublesome symptoms (for example, coughing or breathlessness in the night, in the early morning, or after exertion); prevent recurrent exacerbations of asthma; and avoid adverse effects from asthma medications. The NIH describes four components to asthma therapy: patient education, environmental control, comprehensive pharmacologic therapy, and objective monitoring measures (regular use of a peak flow meter). The NIH also recommends a stepwise approach to asthma therapy (Figure 28-3). Medicines used to treat asthma can be divided into two groups: bronchodilators and antiinflammatory agents. Three classes of bronchodilators are available: beta-adrenergic agonists, xanthine derivatives, and anticholinergic agents. Corticosteroids, cromolyn, and nedocromil are the antiinflammatory agents used to treat asthma.

Table 28-2

Terminology Used with Spirometry	
TERM	**DEFINITION**
Tidal volume (TV)	Volume of air inspired or expired during normal breathing
Vital capacity (VC)	Volume of air exhaled after maximal inspiration to full expiration
Residual volume (RV)	Volume of air left in lungs after maximal exhalation
Functional residual capacity (FRC)	Volume of air left in lungs after normal exhalation
Total lung capacity (TLC)	Vital capacity plus residual volume; $VC + RV = TLC$
Forced expiratory volume (FEV)	Volume of air forced out of the lungs by maximal exhalation
Forced expiratory volume in I second (FEV_1)	Volume of air forced out in I second to give the rate of flow
Forced vital capacity (FVC)	Maximum volume of air exhaled with maximum forced effort after maximum inhalation
Peak expiratory flow rate (PEFR)	Maximal rate of airflow produced during forced expiration

Management of Asthma in Adults

Clinical Characteristics	Therapy (Must include patient education)	Outcome

Clinical Characteristics

Step 1

Mild asthma
- Intermittent brief symptoms <1-2 times/week
- <1-2 nocturnal symptoms/month
- Asymptomatic between episodes
- PEFR or FEV_1
  - >80% predicted
  - <20% variability

Step 2 and 3

Moderate asthma
- Symptoms >1-2 times/week
- Nocturnal episodes >2/month
- Exacerbations may last several days
- Occasional emergency care
- PEFR or FEV_1
  - <80% predicted
  - >20-30% variability when symptomatic

Therapy (Must include patient education)

- Inhaled short-acting β agonist (no more than 3 times/week)
- Inhaled cromolyn or nedocromil
  or
  Inhaled short-acting β agonist before allergen exposure or before exercise

- Inhaled short-acting β agonist (prn,up to 3-4 times/day)

+

- Antiinflammatory agents
  - Inhaled corticosteroids (2-4 puffs daily)
  or
  - Cromolyn or nedocromil (2 puffs 4 times daily)

Outcome

- Symptoms controlled
- PEFR or FEV_1 values optimal for patient
- Reduced PEFR variability
- Normal activity level
- Rarely awakened at night
- Infrequent exacerbations
- Reduced frequency of prn inhaled β agonist

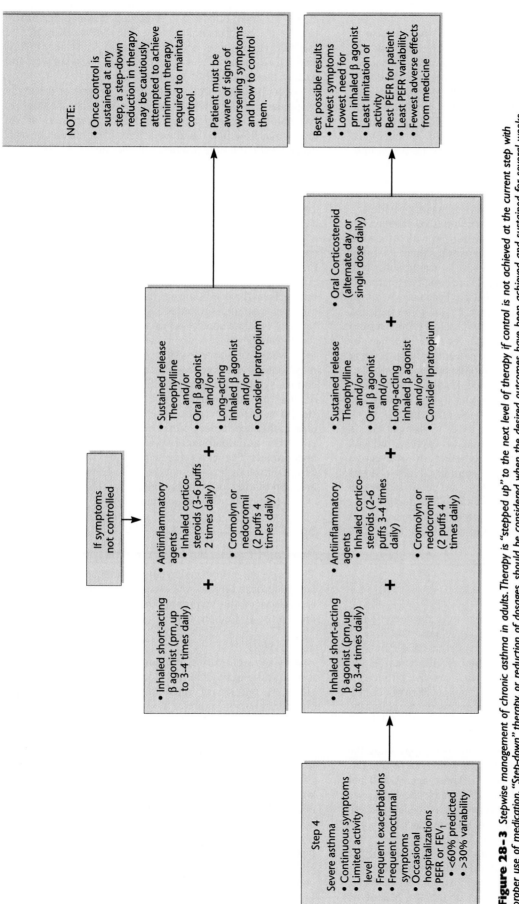

Figure 28–3 *Stepwise management of chronic asthma in adults. Therapy is "stepped up" to the next level of therapy if control is not achieved at the current step with proper use of medication. "Step-down" therapy, or reduction of dosages, should be considered when the desired outcomes have been achieved and sustained for several weeks at the current step. Step-down therapy is desired to identify the minimum dosages of therapy required to maintain the desired outcomes. FEV, Forced expiratory volume; PEFR, peak expiratory flow rate; prn, as required.* (Modified from Management of asthma, *J Allergy Clin Immunol* 88(part 2):477, 1991.)

Bronchitis and Emphysema

It is common for patients with obstructive lung disease to have symptoms of more than one of these diseases, but one disease is usually predominant. Overall treatment of obstructive disease is similar. Management principles include ensuring that the patient understands the disease process, the rationale for various procedures used to treat the disease, and the goals of therapy. Spirometry tests should be completed periodically to assess the success of treatment. Patients must also be taught appropriate nutrition, exercise, proper coughing techniques, chest percussion, postural drainage to mobilize mucus secretions and plugs, and elimination of risk factors such as smoking. All of these efforts must be balanced with the patient's perceptions of quality of life.

The bronchodilators are the cornerstones of chronic obstructive pulmonary disease, but the extent to which they are effective depends on how much reversibility there is to the patient's airway narrowing. Ipratropium, an anticholinergic agent, and the beta-adrenergic agonists are equally effective to start therapy. An oral, long-acting theophylline may be added if additional bronchodilation is necessary. In some patients, such as those with both asthma and COPD, a corticosteroid (such as prednisone) may be added for short courses of therapy during an acute exacerbation of asthma. Each of these agents should be used sequentially and the patient reevaluated at each step before a new drug is added. If spirometry tests do not show improvement with a particular agent, it should be discontinued to avoid side effects of the medicine.

Oxygen therapy may also be used if the patient is chronically hypoxemic, has nocturnal or exercise-induced hypoxemia, or has an acute exacerbation of obstructive disease and the PO_2 drops below 55 mm Hg. Normal doses are 2 to 3 L per minute. Patients must be cautioned not to increase the dose because patients with COPD depend on a certain CO_2 level in the blood to stimulate respirations. A significantly increased PO_2 level will reduce the CO_2 level and cause hypoventilation.

Drug Therapy

Actions and Uses

Expectorants liquefy mucus by stimulating the secretion of natural lubricant fluids from the serous glands. The flow of serous fluids helps liquefy thick mucus masses that may plug the narrow bronchioles. A combination of ciliary action and coughing will then expel the phlegm from the pulmonary system. Expectorants are used to treat nonproductive coughs, bronchitis, and pneumonia, in which mucus plugs inhibit the expulsion of irritants and bacteria that cause the bronchitis or pneumonia.

Cough suppressants (**antitussives**) act by suppressing the cough center in the brain. They are used when the patient has a dry, hacking, nonproductive cough. These agents will not stop the cough completely but should decrease the frequency of the cough and suppress the severe spasms, which prevent adequate rest at night. Under normal circumstances, it is not appropriate to suppress a productive cough.

Mucolytic agents reduce the stickiness and viscosity of pulmonary secretions by acting directly on the mucus plugs to cause dissolution. This eases the removal of the secretions by suction, postural drainage, and coughing. Mucolytic

agents are most effective in removing mucus plugs obstructing the tracheobronchial airway. They are used in the treatment of patients with acute and chronic pulmonary disorders and before and after bronchoscopy, after chest surgery, and as part of the treatment of tracheostomy care.

Bronchodilators relax the smooth muscle of the tracheobronchial tree. This allows an increase in the opening of the bronchioles and alveolar ducts, which decreases the resistance to airflow into the alveolar sacs. Asthma and bronchitis cause reversible obstruction of the airways. The airway constriction associated with emphysema is somewhat reversible depending on the severity and duration of the disease. The primary bronchodilators used in the treatment of airway-obstructive diseases include beta-adrenergic agents, anticholinergic aerosols, and the xanthine derivatives.

Antiinflammatory agents play an important role in the treatment of asthma to reduce inflammation. Corticosteroid therapy is the most effective antiinflammatory agent. Most commonly used are those administered by inhalation because this places the medicine at the site of inflammation with minimal systemic side effects. Depending on frequency and severity of acute attacks, some asthmatic patients will require short "bursts" of systemic steroids, usually prednisone, for 1 to 2 weeks of therapy. An occasional patient with asthma may require alternate-day or daily steroid administration to control symptomatology. All effort must be made to optimize other forms of treatment before resorting to regular systemic steroid administration because of the potential serious side effects that accompany steroid administration.

Other antiinflammatory agents used are cromolyn and nedocromil. The exact mechanism by which these agents help control asthma is not known. These agents have no bronchodilating properties and are useless in patients with chronic obstructive pulmonary disease.

Nursing Process for Lower Respiratory Disease

The nurse must first understand normal respiratory function before proceeding to the assessment of pathophysiologic conditions of the respiratory tract such as asthma, chronic bronchitis, and emphysema.

Assessment

History of respiratory symptoms. • What pulmonary symptoms has the individual had (for example, childhood or adult allergies, pulmonary infections, pneumonia, tuberculosis, chest trauma, or surgeries)? • What is the work environment of the individual? Ask about exposure to allergens, dust, and chemicals. • Ask specifically for details of smoking or exposure to secondhand smoke. History of smoking is usually recorded in pack-years. (Multiply the number of packs of cigarettes smoked per day times the number of years of smoking. Example: if a person smoked 1½ packs of cigarettes per day for 20 years, the patient is said to have a [1.5 × 20 = 30] 30 pack-year history of smoking.) • Is there a family history of respiratory disease or disorders? If so, obtain details (for example, diagnosis of disease, persons affected).

History of respiratory medication. • What prescribed medications or over-the-counter medications have been used now or in the past for the treatment of the same or similar respiratory problems? • How effective have the medications been in the treatment of prior or current symptoms?

Description of current symptoms. • What is the patient's chief complaint? • When did the symptoms start? Does the patient have any idea what triggered them? • Ask the patient to describe the symptoms being experienced. What effect do the symptoms have on the patient's ability to carry on activities of daily living?

Respiratory assessment. *Note:* The extent of the pulmonary examination (inspection, palpation, percussion, and auscultation) must be adapted to the nurse's education level and assessment skills (for example beginning student, practical nurse, or registered nurse).

- Observe the patient's general appearance and degree of respiratory impairment. Adapt the assessment and prioritizing of the examination to the degree of respiratory impairment present.
- Take and record baseline vital signs.
- *Respiratory pattern.* Assess the rate, depth, and regularity of the patient's breathing. The normal respiratory rate is approximately 14 to 22 breaths per minute in adults and up to 44 breaths per minute in infants.

Rapid, shallow breathing may be caused by an elevated diaphragm, restrictive lung disease, or pleuritic chest pain.
  - Rapid, deep breathing may be caused by exercise, anxiety, and metabolic acidosis. *Kussmaul's respiration* is deep breathing associated with metabolic acidosis. It may be fast, normal, or slow in rate. It is most often associated with patients with diabetic ketoacidosis.
  - Breathing associated with obstructive lung disease has a prolonged expiratory phase because of increased airway resistance. If the respiratory rate increases, the patient lacks time for full expiration. The chest overexpands with trapped air and breathing becomes more shallow.
  - *Cheyne-Stokes* respiration is a cyclic breathing pattern in which periods of deep breathing alternate with periods of apnea. Children and the elderly normally show this pattern while asleep. Other causes include heart failure, drug-induced respiratory depression, uremia, and stroke.
- *Cough.* Note whether a cough is productive or nonproductive. Record sputum color, consistency, amount, and any appearance of frothiness or blood (hemoptysis).
- *Mental status.* As the oxygen level in the body diminishes and carbon dioxide accumulates, the mental status will deteriorate from alertness to progressively lower levels of functioning (alert→restless→drowsy→unconscious→dead).

Inspection
- *Skin color.* Does the patient have normal skin color or is the patient cyanotic? Where is the cyanosis visible? Peripheral cyanosis is defined as a bluish coloring of an isolated area of the body (such as the earlobes, toes, feet, or fingers). Central cyanosis indicates a general lack of oxygen in the hemoglobin. The entire body has a slight bluish-white tinge. It is most readily observed on the lips and mucous membranes of the mouth.
- *Dyspnea.* Note whether dyspnea occurs at rest or with exertion. Observe the breathing pattern (for example, purse-lipped, exertion required to exhale).
- *Muscle involvement.* Elevation of the shoulders, retraction of the spaces between ribs, and use of the abdominal muscles is associated with advanced respiratory disease.

- *Posture.* Dyspneic patients usually sit upright or lean forward from the waist, resting the elbows on the knees. This helps give the chest maximal expansion.
- *Chest contour.* Note changes in contour of the chest, such as barrel chest (increased anteroposterior diameter), kyphosis, or scoliosis.
- *Clubbing of fingernails.* Assess for flattening or an increase in the angle between the fingernail and the nail base of the fingers. Clubbing has many causes, including hypoxia and lung cancer.

Palpation. Perform palpation of the chest noting any tender or painful areas, masses, and increased or decreased tactile fremitus. Note diminished expansion of the chest wall on inspiration.

Percussion. Note the presence of dullness, hyperresonance, and diaphragmatic excursion.

Auscultation. Perform auscultation of the chest; note the intensity, pitch, and relative duration of inspiratory and expiratory phases. Identify additional sounds present (for example, crackles, rhonchi, or wheezes). Are they inspiratory, expiratory, or both? Where are they located? Do they clear with deep breathing or coughing? Is bronchophony or egophony present?

Cardiovascular assessment. As appropriate to the symptoms and the diagnosis, perform a cardiovascular assessment. See under Nursing Process for Heart Failure, Chapter 21.

Psychosocial assessment. Ask specifically about the presence and degree of depression, anxiety, social isolation being experienced as a result of the disease process, and adaptive or maladaptive responses. Identify support systems in place to assist in providing for the individual's care.

Laboratory and diagnostic data. Review pulmonary function tests, ABGs, hematology, sputum tests, and x-ray reports as available and appropriate to the diagnosis.

Nursing Diagnosis
- Airway clearance, ineffective (indication)
- Activity intolerance (indication)
- Gas exchange, impaired (indication)
- Breathing pattern, ineffective (indication)

Planning
Description of current symptoms. Individualize the care plan to address the patient's degree of dyspnea, cough, pain, fatigue, sleep pattern disturbance, nutritional needs, and other relevant factors.

Medications. • Order medications prescribed, and schedule these on the medication administration record (MAR). Perform focused assessments at regularly scheduled intervals consistent with the patient's status to determine effectiveness and side effects to expect or report. • Ensure that as-needed (prn) medications are ordered and readily available for use. • Plan appropriate teaching for medication administration techniques and drug therapy.

Hydration. Mark the Kardex with fluid recommendations to maintain patient hydration consistent with any coexisting diagnoses (for example, heart failure). Order a vaporizer or humidifier, as prescribed.

Respiratory and cardiovascular assessment. Schedule assessments of respiratory and cardiovascular status at least once per shift and more frequently as indicated by the patient's status. ***Laboratory/diagnostics studies.*** Order stat and subsequent laboratory studies (for example, sputum collection, ABGs, pulmonary function tests, hematology, and x-rays).

Implementation

- Perform physical assessments of the patient in accordance with clinical setting policies (for example, every 4 or 8 hours depending on the patient's status).
- Assist the patient, as needed, to perform self-care and activities. Make note of the degree of impairment or dyspnea seen with and without oxygen.
- Administer oxygen as ordered and prn.
- Administer prescribed medications and treatments that can best alleviate the patient's symptoms and provide maximum level of comfort.
- Encourage physical activity as prescribed. Do not allow the patient to overexert or become fatigued.
- Institute measures to reduce anxiety. Support the patient in a calm manner.

Patient Education and Health Promotion

Avoiding irritants. Smoking, pollen, and environmental pollutants frequently aggravate respiratory disorders.

Activity and exercise. Fatigue and resulting dyspnea may require adjustments in physical activity and employment. Support the patient's concerns. Plan for rest periods to alternate with activity. Provide for oxygenation before or during activities as appropriate to the patient's needs.

Nutritional status. A well-balanced diet that prevents excessive weight loss or gain is important. Encourage patients with dyspnea to eat several small meals throughout the day and to take small bites.

Preventing infections. Encourage patients to avoid exposure to persons with infection; practice good hygiene, such as hand washing; get adequate rest; and dispose of secretions properly. Patients should seek medical attention at the earliest sign of suspected infection (for example, increased cough, increased fatigue, dyspnea, temperature elevation, or change in characteristics of secretions).

Increased fluid intake. Unless contraindicated, encourage patients to increase fluid intake. This will aid in decreasing the viscosity of secretions.

Environmental elements. People experiencing difficulty in breathing can benefit from proper temperature, humidification of the air, or ventilation of the immediate surroundings. Moist air from a humidifier or vaporizer can readily relieve dryness of the nose or throat.

Breathing techniques. If ordered by the physician, teach postural drainage and pursed-lip breathing or abdominal breathing and coughing.

Sleep patterns. Discuss adaptations the individual can make in daily routines to ensure adequate rest. As the disease progresses, sleeping in a recliner or in an upright position may be necessary.

Psychosocial

- Encourage open discussion of the person's fears and expectations regarding therapy. Discuss the expectations of therapy (such as level of exercise; degree of pain relief, if present; tolerance; frequency of use of therapy; relief of dyspnea; ability to maintain activities of daily living and

work; and other issues as indicated by the underlying pathology).
- Identify support persons who can assist the individual during periods of breathlessness and make them, as well as the patient, aware of community resources available such as the Visiting Nurse's Association and home health care agencies.

Medications

- Explain the purpose and method of administration of each prescribed medication. Be certain the individual understands the delivery method for administration of the medication (for example, aerosol therapy, metered-dose inhalers, nebulizer, peak expiratory flow meter). The care and cleansing of equipment used for delivery of drugs to the respiratory tract should be explained to prevent bacterial growth.
- When administering medicines by aerosol therapy to a child or to an elderly patient, make sure that the patient has the strength and dexterity to operate the equipment before discharge. When muscle coordination is not fully developed, as in a younger child, or when dexterity has diminished in a geriatric patient, it may be beneficial to use a spacer device for medicines administered by inhalation (Figure 28-4).
- Oxygen therapy must be explained in detail. The patient who is in a continuous hypoxic state must understand that it is not beneficial and may be harmful to increase the oxygen flow above the prescribed rate.
- Persons receiving theophylline therapy must understand the importance of reporting for laboratory studies to determine the plasma level of the drug. Because cigarette smoking can alter the blood level of this medicine, the individual must understand the ramifications of starting, stopping, or altering level of smoking.
- Be certain the individual understands the proper use of bronchodilators and antiinflammatory agents prescribed. Drugs prescribed for prn use or use during an acute attack of asthma must be thoroughly explained.

Fostering health maintenance

- Throughout the course of treatment discuss medication information, the importance of adequate airway clearance, dietary and hydration needs, breathing exercises, physical exercise, pulmonary hygiene, environmental control, the need to balance activities with abilities, and stress reduc-

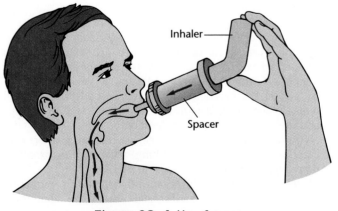

Figure 28-4 *Use of spacer.*

tion and how each of these measures can benefit the patient.
- Seek cooperation and understanding of the following points so that medication compliance is increased: name of medication, dosage, route and times of administration, side effects to expect, and side effects to report.
- Enlist the patient's aid in developing and maintaining a written record (see box on p. 364) of monitoring parameters (such as respirations, pulse, daily weights, degree of dyspnea relief, exercise tolerance, and secretions being expectorated) and response to prescribed therapies for discussion with the physician. Patients should be encouraged to take this record with them on follow-up visits.

Drug Class: Expectorants

guaifenesin (gwi-feh-neh′sin)
Robitussin (row-bih-tus′sin)

Actions

Guaifenesin is an expectorant that acts by enhancing the output of respiratory tract fluid. The increased flow of secretions decreases mucus viscosity and promotes ciliary action. A combination of ciliary action and coughing then expels the phlegm from the pulmonary system.

Uses

Guaifenesin is used for the symptomatic relief of conditions characterized by a dry, nonproductive cough and as well as to remove mucus plugs from the respiratory tract. Such conditions include the common cold, bronchitis, laryngitis, pharyngitis, and sinusitis. Guaifenesin is often combined with bronchodilators, decongestants, antihistamines, or antitussive agents to aid in making a nonproductive cough more productive. Guaifenesin is more effective if the patient is well hydrated at the time of therapy.

Guaifenesin should not be given to a patient with a dry, persistent cough that lasts more than 1 week; if there is a chronic, persistent cough such as that which accompanies asthma, bronchitis, and emphysema; or if the cough is accompanied by excessive production of phlegm. These may be indications of more serious conditions for which the patient should seek medical attention.

Therapeutic Outcomes

The primary therapeutic outcome expected from guaifenesin therapy is reduced frequency of nonproductive cough.

Nursing Process

Premedication Assessment
Record characteristics of the cough before initiation of therapy.

Planning
Availability. PO—100, 200, and 600 mg tablets, 200 and 300 mg capsules, 100 and 200 mg per 5 ml liquid. It is also available in individual products in combination with pseudoephedrine, dextromethorphan, codeine phosphate, and phenylpropanolamine.

Implementation
Dosage and administration. Adult: PO—100 to 400 mg every 4 to 6 hours. Do not exceed 2400 mg per day. Pediatric: PO—ages 6 to 12, 100 to 200 mg every 4 hours. Do not exceed 1200 mg per day. Ages 2 to 6, 50 to 100 mg every 4 hours. Do not exceed 600 mg per day.
Fluid intake. Maintain fluid intake at 8 to 12 8-ounce glasses of water daily.
Humidification. Suggest the concurrent use of a humidifier.

Evaluation
Side effects to expect
GASTROINTESTINAL UPSET, NAUSEA, VOMITING. Development of these side effects is rare.
Drug interactions
No significant drug interactions have been reported.

potassium iodide
SSKI

Actions

Potassium iodide acts as an expectorant by stimulating increased secretions from the bronchial glands to decrease the viscosity of mucus plugs, making it easier for patients to cough up the dry, hardened plugs blocking the bronchial tubes.

Uses

Potassium iodide is used in the symptomatic treatment of chronic pulmonary diseases such as bronchial asthma, bronchitis, and pulmonary emphysema in which tenacious mucus is present. It is often used in combination with bronchodilators, sympathomimetic amines, and antitussives for more effective removal of mucus.

Therapeutic Outcomes

The primary therapeutic outcome expected from potassium iodide therapy is reduction of mucus viscosity allowing a more productive cough to remove accumulated phlegm.

Nursing Process

Premedication Assessment
1. Record characteristics of cough before initiation of therapy.
2. Ask if the patient is pregnant before administration. Excessive use of iodine-containing products may result in goiter in the newborn.

Planning
Availability. PO—1 g/ml solution in 30 mg and 237 ml containers.

Implementation
Dosage and administration. Adult: PO—0.3 ml (300 mg) to 0.6 ml (600 mg) diluted in one glassful of water, fruit juice, or milk 3 to 4 times daily. Take with food to minimize gastric irritation.
Fluid intake. Maintain fluid intake of 8 to 12 8-ounce glasses of water daily.
Humidification. Suggest the concurrent use of a humidifier.

PATIENT EDUCATION & MONITORING FORM   Respiratory Agents

MEDICATIONS	COLOR	TO BE TAKEN

Name _____

Physician _____

Physician's phone _____

Next appt.* _____

PARAMETERS		DAY OF DISCHARGE							COMMENTS
Peak Flow Meter	AM L/min								
	Noon								
	PM								
Postural drainage	Times of day performed (e.g. 8 AM, 2 PM)								
	Response: productive cough, nonproductive								
Describe cough	Frequent, intermittent								
	Secretions: Color:								
	Thickness of secretions: thick, thin								
How do you feel today? (Record 2 times per day.) Awful—Improving—Good 10 5 1		AM / PM	AM / PM	AM / PM	AM / PM	AM / PM	AM / PM	AM / PM	
Exercise level: degree of tiredness with exercise Extremely—Moderate—Normal 10 5 1									
Activities of daily living	Walk (___) of stairs								
	Walk (___) of blocks								
	Can or cannot perform daily activities Yes/No								
Pain pattern	Pain is on L (left) or R (right) side								
	Pain on inspiration = I								
	Pain on expiration = E								
Difficulty breathing	Sleep with (___) pillows								
	Difficulty on exertion								
	Difficulty during stress								
	Difficulty when resting								
Appetite Poor—Decreased—Normal 10 5 1									

*Please bring this record with you to your next appointment.
Use the back of this sheet for additional information.

Thyroid function tests. Long-term use may induce goiter, particularly in children with cystic fibrosis. Always inform the physician of the use of this product if thyroid function tests are to be scheduled.

Evaluation
Side effects to expect
NAUSEA, VOMITING, DIARRHEA. Symptoms are usually mild. Take with food or milk to minimize gastric irritation. If symptoms become bothersome, report them to physician.
Drug interactions
POTASSIUM SUPPLEMENTS, SALT SUBSTITUTES, POTASSIUM-SPARING DIURETICS. Do NOT administer with potassium-sparing diuretics (amiloride, triamterene, or spironolactone). Do not use potassium supplements or salt substitutes high in potassium because of potentially dangerous effects from hyperkalemia.

LITHIUM, ANTITHYROID AGENTS. Concurrent use with lithium and antithyroid medications (methimazole and propylthiouracil) may result in hypothyroidism.

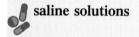 **saline solutions**

Actions
Saline solutions act by hydrating mucus, reducing its viscosity.

Uses
Saline solutions of varying concentrations can be effective expectorants when administered by nebulization. When administered by inhalation, hypotonic solutions (0.45% sodium chloride) are thought to provide deeper penetration into the more distant airways: a hypertonic solution (1.8% sodium chloride) hydrates and stimulates a productive cough by irritating the respiratory passages. Isotonic saline solutions (0.9% sodium chloride) administered by nebulization are used to hydrate respiratory secretions.

Saline nose drops are sometimes ordered for patients experiencing nasal congestion secondary to low humidity to clear the nasal passage and aid in breathing.

Therapeutic Outcomes
The primary therapeutic outcomes expected from nasal and respiratory saline therapy are as follows:
- Moisturized mucous membranes for less irritation from dryness
- More productive coughing because of less viscous mucus

Nursing Process
Premedication Assessment
Record characteristics of cough before initiation of therapy.

Drug Class: Antitussive Agents
Actions
Antitussive agents (cough suppressants) act by suppressing the cough center in the brain.

Uses
Antitussive agents are used when the patient has a bothersome dry, hacking, nonproductive cough. These agents will not stop the cough completely but should decrease the frequency of the cough and suppress the severe spasms, which prevent adequate rest at night. Under normal circumstances, it is not appropriate to suppress a productive cough.

Codeine is an effective cough suppressant and the standard against which other antitussive agents are compared. In the relatively low doses and short duration used to suppress cough, addiction is not a problem; dependence may develop, however, after long-term, continuous use. Codeine should not be used in patients with chronic pulmonary disease who may have respiratory depression or in patients who have a documented allergy to codeine (rash, pruritus).

Dextromethorphan is almost as effective a cough suppressant as codeine. It does not cause respiratory depression or addiction and is usually the drug of choice for cough suppression in children. Allergy is rare.

Diphenhydramine is an anticholinergic agent with both antihistaminic and antitussive properties. As with most other antihistamines, diphenhydramine has significant sedative properties. This is often detrimental during the day, especially if the person must be mentally alert, but it is an excellent agent to suppress cough during sleep. Like other anticholinergic agents, diphenhydramine should not be taken by patients with angle-closure glaucoma or prostatic hypertrophy. It also may cause drying of mucus secretions, making mucus more viscous, especially if the patient is not well hydrated. It should also be used cautiously with other central nervous system (CNS) depressants such as sedatives, hypnotics, alcohol, or antidepressants.

Therapeutic Outcomes
The primary therapeutic outcome expected from antitussive therapy is reduced frequency of nonproductive cough.

Nursing Process
Premedication Assessment
Record characteristics of cough before initiation of therapy.

Planning
Availability. See Table 28-3.

Implementation
Dosage and administration. See Table 28-3.

Evaluation
Side effects to expect
DROWSINESS, CONSTIPATION. All of the antitussive agents cause some sedation, but diphenhydramine has the most sedative effect. Caution patients about being alert and operating machinery.

Codeine is the most constipating of the antitussive agents. This effect can be minimized by keeping the patient well hydrated and by the use of bulk stool softeners if the patient requires more than 1 to 2 days of codeine therapy.

Table 28-3

Antitussive Agents

GENERIC NAME	BRAND NAME	AVAILABILITY	ADULT ORAL DOSAGE RANGE
Benzonatate	Tessalon Perles	Capsules: 100 mg	100 mg 3 times daily
Codeine*		Tablets: 15, 30, 60 mg	10-20 mg every 4-6 hr
Dextromethorphan	Sucrets, Delsym, Benylin DM	Lozenges: 2.5, 5, 15 mg Syrup: 3.5, 5, 7.5, 10, 15 mg/5 ml Liquid: 3.5, 5, 7.5, 30 mg/5 ml	10-30 mg every 4-8 hr; do not exceed 60-120 mg/24 hr
Diphenhydramine	Benylin, Diphen, Tusstat	Syrup: 12.5 mg/5 ml	25 mg every 4 hr; do not exceed 150 mg/24 hr
Hydrocodone*			5 mg every 4-6 hr

*Often an ingredient in combination antitussive products.

Drug interactions

CENTRAL NERVOUS SYSTEM DEPRESSANTS. The following drugs may enhance the depressant effects of antitussive agents: phenothiazines, antidepressants, sedative-hypnotics, antihistamines, and alcohol.

Drug Class: Mucolytic Agents

acetylcysteine (a-see'-til-cist-een)
Mucomyst (mu'-co-mist)

Actions

Acetylcysteine acts by dissolving chemical bonds within the mucus itself, causing it to separate and liquefy, thereby reducing viscosity.

Uses

Acetylcysteine is used to dissolve abnormally viscous mucus secretions that may occur in chronic emphysema, emphysema with bronchitis, asthmatic bronchitis, and pneumonia. The reduced viscosity allows easier removal of secretions by coughing, percussion, and postural drainage.

Therapeutic Outcomes

The primary therapeutic outcome expected from acetylcysteine therapy is improved airway flow with more comfortable breathing.

Nursing Process

Premedication Assessment

1. Record the characteristics of cough and bronchial secretions before staring therapy.
2. Obtain and record baseline vital signs.
3. Observe for and record any gastrointestinal symptoms present before starting therapy.
4. Perform a baseline assessment of the patient's mental status (for example, degree of anxiety, nervousness, and alertness).

Planning

Availability. Inhalation—10% and 20% solutions in 4, 10, 30, and 100 ml vials.

Implementation

Dosage and administration. Adult: inhalation—the recommended dosage for most patients is 3 to 5 ml of the 20% solution 3 to 4 times daily. It may be administered by nebulization, direct application, or intratracheal instillation.

After administration, the volume of bronchial secretions may increase. Some patients with inadequate cough reflex may require mechanical suctioning to maintain an open airway.

Nebulizer. This solution tends to concentrate as the solution is used. When three fourths of the original amount in the nebulizer is used, dilute the remaining solution with sterile water.

After therapy, wash the patient's face and hands because the drug is sticky and irritating. Thoroughly cleanse equipment used.

Storage. Store the opened solution of the drug in a refrigerator for up to 96 hours. Discard the unused portion after that time.

Discoloration. Use medication stored only in plastic or glass containers. Contact with metals other than stainless steel can cause discoloration of the solution.

Evaluation

Side effects to expect

NAUSEA, VOMITING. This drug has a pungent odor (similar to rotten eggs) that may cause nausea and vomiting. Have an emesis basin available in case vomiting should occur. (Do not, however, suggest it by having the basin in clear view.)

Side effects to report

BRONCHOSPASM. This agent may occasionally cause bronchoconstriction and bronchospasm. Concurrent use of a bronchodilator may be necessary.

Drug interactions

ANTIBIOTICS. Acetylcysteine inactivates most antibiotics. Do not mix together for aerosol administration. Schedule administration of inhalation antibiotics 1 hour after administration of acetylcysteine.

Drug Class: Beta-Adrenergic Bronchodilating Agents

Actions

The beta-adrenergic agonists stimulate the beta-receptors within the smooth muscle of the tracheobronchial tree to relax, thereby opening the airway passages to greater volumes of air.

Uses

Beta-adrenergic bronchodilators are now the mainstay of all asthma therapy. They are used to reverse airway constriction caused by acute and chronic bronchial asthma, bronchitis, and emphysema. Those agents with more selective beta-2 receptor activity (such as albuterol and terbutaline) have more direct bronchodilating activity with fewer other systemic side effects. (See Chapter 11 on selective beta-receptor activity.)

Unfortunately, the receptors stimulated by sympathomimetic agents, causing relaxation of the smooth muscle in the tracheobronchial tree, are found in other tissues as well as the pulmonary system. The receptors are also found in the muscles of the heart, blood vessels, uterus, and gastrointestinal, urinary, and central nervous systems. They also help regulate fat and carbohydrate metabolism. For this reason, there are many side effects from these agents, particularly if used too frequently or in higher than recommended doses. Those administered by inhalation generally have fewer systemic effects because inhalation places the drug at the site of action so that smaller dosages may be used.

The short-acting beta agonists (albuterol, bitolterol, metaproterenol, pirbuterol, and terbutaline) have a rapid onset (a few minutes) and are used to treat acute bronchospasm. During acute exacerbations, these agents can be used up to every 3 to 4 hours. If a patient is using an increased amount of these inhaled bronchodilators on a daily basis, it is an indication of worsening asthma. Patients then must be reassessed for compliance and inhalation technique and improved environmental control.

Salmeterol is a long-acting form of inhaled bronchodilator. It is not to be used for acute episodes but for patients with nocturnal asthma and for those who wheeze with exercise. The onset of action is 15 to 30 minutes, but the duration of action is up to 12 hours. Therefore it is used to prevent acute exacerbations of asthma.

Patients known to have hypertension, hyperthyroidism, diabetes mellitus, or cardiac disease with arrhythmias may be particularly sensitive to adverse reactions and must be observed closely.

Therapeutic Outcomes

The primary therapeutic outcome associated with beta-adrenergic bronchodilator therapy is easier breathing with reduced wheezing.

Nursing Process

Premedication Assessment
1. Obtain and record baseline vital signs.
2. Assess for the presence of palpitations and arrhythmias before administration of beta-adrenergic agents. If suspected, notify the physician and ask whether therapy should be started.
3. Perform an assessment of the patient's baseline mental status (for example, degree of anxiety, nervousness, and alertness).

Planning
Availability. See Table 28-4.

Implementation
Dosage and administration. See Table 28-4. Patients using inhaled bronchodilators should wait approximately 10 minutes between inhalations. This allows the medicine to dilate the bronchioles so that the second dose can be inhaled more deeply into the lungs for more therapeutic effect.

Ensure that patients understand how to use the inhaler as described in the manufacturer's leaflet for the patient.

Evaluation
Side effects to report
TACHYCARDIA, PALPITATIONS. Because most symptoms are dose related, alterations should be reported to the physician. Monitor the patient's heart rate and rhythm at regular intervals throughout therapy with bronchodilators. An increase of 20 beats or more per minute after treatment should be reported to the physician. Always report palpitations and suspected arrhythmias.

TREMORS. Tell the patient to notify the physician if tremors develop after starting any of these medications. A dosage adjustment may be necessary.

NERVOUSNESS, ANXIETY, RESTLESSNESS, HEADACHE. Perform a baseline assessment of the patient's mental status (degree of anxiety, nervousness, and alertness); compare subsequent, regular assessments to the findings obtained. Report escalation of tension.

NAUSEA, VOMITING. Monitor all aspects of the development of these symptoms. Question the patient concerning other medications being taken and any other symptoms that have also developed. Administer the medication with food and a full glass of water or milk. Report if the symptoms are not relieved.

DIZZINESS. Provide for patient safety during episodes of dizziness. Report for further evaluation.

Drug interactions
DRUGS THAT ENHANCE TOXIC EFFECTS. Ticlopidine, tricyclic antidepressants (imipramine, amitriptyline, nortriptyline, doxepin, and others), monoamine oxidase inhibitors (tranylcypromine and pargyline), and other sympathomimetic agents (metaproterenol, isoproterenol, and others). Monitor for increases in severity of drug effects such as nervousness, tachycardia, tremors, and arrhythmias.

DRUGS THAT REDUCE THERAPEUTIC EFFECTS. Beta-adrenergic blocking agents (propanolol, timolol, nadolol, pindolol, and others). Higher doses or use of another class of bronchodilator may be required.

ANTIHYPERTENSIVE AGENTS. Sympathomimetic agents may reduce the therapeutic effects of antihypertensive agents. Monitor blood pressure for an indication of loss of antihypertensive control.

Drug Class: Anticholinergic Bronchodilating Agents

Anticholinergic agents have been used as bronchodilators in the treatment of obstructive pulmonary disease for more than 200 years, but the potent anticholinergic adverse effects (throat irritation, dry mouth, reduced mucus secretions, increased viscosity of secretions, mydriasis, cycloplegia, urinary retention, and tachycardia) and the availability of selective sympathomimetic agents have limited their use in pulmonary disorders.

Table 28-4

Bronchodilators

GENERIC NAME	BRAND NAME	AVAILABILITY	ADULT DOSAGE RANGE
Beta-adrenergic agonists			
Albuterol	Proventil, Ventolin, Volmax	Tablets: 2, 4 mg Aerosol: 90 µg Capsule, inhalation 0.5% (20 ml) Syrup: 2 mg/5 ml Tablets, extended release: 4, 8 mg	PO: 2-4 mg 3-4 times daily Inhale: 2 inhalations every 4-6 hr
Bitolterol	Tornalate	Aerosol: 0.37 mg/puff	Inhale: 2-3 inhalations every 8 hr Wait 2-3 min between each inhalation
Ephedrine	Efedron	Capsules: 25, 50 mg Injection: 50 mg/ml Spray: 0.25%	PO: 25-50 mg every 3-4 hr SC, IM, IV: 25-50 mg
Epinephrine	Primatene, Bronitin, Bronkaid Mist	Nebulization: 1:100 Aerosol: 0.3 mg Injection: 0.1, 1 mg/ml	See manufacturer's recommendations
Ethylnorepinephrine	Bronkephrine	Injection: 2 mg/ml in 1 ml amps	SC or IM: 0.5-1 ml
Isoetharine	Bronkosol, Bronkometer	Nebulization: 0.125, 0.167, 0.2, 0.25, 0.5, 1% Aerosol: 0.34 mg/puff	See manufacturer's recommendations
Isoproterenol	Isuprel	Nebulization: 0.25, 0.5, 1% Aerosol: 0.2, 0.25% Injection: 0.02, 0.2 mg/ml SL: 10, 15 mg tabs	See manufacturer's recommendations
Metaproterenol	Alupent, Metaprel	Tablets: 10, 20 mg Syrup: 10 mg/5 ml Aerosol: 0.65 mg/puff Nebulization: 0.6, 5%	See manufacturer's recommendations
Pirbuterol	Maxair	Aerosol: 0.2 mg/puff	Inhale: 1-2 inhalations every 4-6 hr
Salmeterol	Serevent	Aerosol: 6.5, 13 mg	Inhale: 2 inhalations every 12 hr
Terbutaline	Brethine, Bricanyl, Brethaire	Tablets: 2.5, 5 mg Injection: 1 mg/ml Aerosol: 0.2 mg/puff	PO: 5 mg every 6 hr SC: 0.25 mg; repeat, if needed, in 30 min Aerosol: 2 inhalations every 4-6 hr

continued

ipratropium bromide (ihp-rah'trop-eum)
Atrovent (at'roh-vent)

Actions

In 1987 a new anticholinergic agent with significantly fewer side effects became available. Ipratropium bromide is administered by aerosol inhalation and produces bronchodilation by competitive inhibition of cholinergic receptors on bronchial smooth muscle. It has minimal effect on ciliary activity, mucus secretion, sputum volume, and viscosity.

Uses

Ipratropium is used as a bronchodilator for long-term treatment of reversible bronchospasm associated with

chronic obstructive pulmonary disease. It may also be used in combination with beta-adrenergic bronchodilators in patients with asthma. Initial bronchodilation is evident within the first few minutes after inhalation, but maximal effects are seen in 1 to 2 hours. The duration of significant bronchodilation is 4 to 6 hours with usual doses. Because its maximal effects are not seen immediately, the drug is more appropriately used for prophylaxis and maintenance treatment of bronchospasm associated with chronic obstructive lungdisease than for acute episodes of bronchospasm associated with asthma.

Ipratropium nasal spray is used for the symptomatic relief of rhinorrhea associated with allergic and nonallergic perennial rhinitis and the common cold. It does not relieve

Table 28-4

Bronchodilators—cont'd

GENERIC NAME	BRAND NAME	AVAILABILITY	ADULT DOSAGE RANGE
Xanthine derivatives			
Aminophylline		Tablets: 100, 200 mg Elixir: 250 mg/15 ml Liquid: 105 mg/5 ml Suppositories: 250, 500 mg Injection: 250, 500 ml Others	See manufacturer's recommendations
Dyphylline	Dilor, Lufyllin, ♣ Protophylline	Tablets: 200, 400 mg Elixir: 100, 160 mg/15 ml Injection: 250 mg/ml	PO: 15 mg/kg, 5 times daily IM: 250-500 mg slowly
Oxtriphylline	Choledyl, Choledyl SA	Tablets: 200, 400, 600 mg	200 mg 4 times daily
Theophylline	Bronkodyl, Elixophyllin, Theolair, others	Tablets: 100, 125, 200, 225, 250, 300 mg Capsules: 65, 100, 200, 250 mg Elixir: 26.7 mg/5 ml Liquid: 26.7 mg/5 ml Syrup: 26.7 mg/5 ml Others	9-20 mg/kg/24 hr in 4 divided doses

♣ Available in Canada only.

nasal congestion, sneezing, or postnasal drip associated with these conditions.

Therapeutic Outcomes

The primary therapeutic outcomes associated with ipratropium therapy are as follows:
- Easier breathing with less effort when the inhaler is used
- Reduced rhinorrhea when the nasal solution is used

Nursing Process

Premedication Assessment
1. Record baseline vital signs.
2. Check the medical record to determine whether the patient has a history of angle-closure glaucoma. If so, reconfirm the administration order with the physician before administration of ipratropium.

Planning
Availability. Inhalation—aerosol canister containing approximately 200 inhalations (18 µg per metered dose) with metered-dose inhaler mouthpiece. Nasal spray—0.03% (30 ml) and 0.06% (15 ml) nasal spray pumps.

Implementation
Note: Ipratropium bromide should not be used in the initial treatment of acute episodes of bronchospasm in which rapid response is required. Use with caution in patients with the potential for angle-closure glaucoma.
Dosage and administration. Inhalation—the usual dose is two inhalations (36 µg) 4 times a day. Patients may take additional inhalations as required but should not exceed 12 inhalations in 24 hours.

ENSURE THAT PATIENT UNDERSTANDS HOW TO INHALE MEDICATION:
1. Clear throat and mouth of sputum.
2. Insert the metal canister into the clear end of the mouthpiece.
3. Remove the protective cap, invert the canister, and shake thoroughly.
4. Enclose the mouthpiece with the lips. The base of the canister should be held vertically. (Keep the eyes closed because temporary blurring of vision may result if the aerosol is sprayed into the eyes.)
5. Exhale deeply through the mouth or nose, then inhale slowly through the mouthpiece and at the same time firmly press once on the upended canister base; continue to inhale deeply.
6. Hold breath for a few seconds, then remove the mouthpiece from the mouth and exhale slowly. Wait approximately 15 seconds and repeat the second inhalation as outlined in steps 4 and 5.
7. Replace the protective cap after use.
8. Keep the mouthpiece clean. Wash with hot water. If soap is used, rinse thoroughly with plain water.

Nasal spray—Rhinorrhea secondary to allergic and non-allergic perennial rhinitis: 2 sprays (42 µg) of 0.3% solution in each nostril 2 or 3 times daily. Rhinorrhea secondary to the common cold: 2 sprays (84 µg) of 0.6% solution in each nostril 3 or 4 times daily.

ENSURE THAT PATIENT UNDERSTANDS HOW TO PRIME AND USE THE PUMP AS DESCRIBED IN THE MANUFACTURER'S LEAFLET FOR THE PATIENT.

Evaluation
Side effects to expect
DRYNESS OF MOUTH, THROAT IRRITATION. These side effects are usually mild and tend to resolve with continued

therapy. Encourage the patient not to discontinue therapy without first consulting the physician.

Ensure that regular oral hygiene measures are continued. Suggest the use of 1 teaspoon of hydrogen peroxide in 6 to 8 ounces of water as a mouthwash. Commercial mouthwashes contain alcohol, which may cause further drying and oral irritation.

Other measures to alleviate dryness include sucking on ice chips or hard candy.

Side effects to report

TACHYCARDIA, URINARY RETENTION, EXACERBATION OF PULMONARY SYMPTOMS. Instruct the patient to consult a physician before continuing with further therapy.

Drug interactions

No significant interactions have been reported.

Drug Class: Xanthine-Derivative Bronchodilating Agents

Actions

Methylxanthines, more commonly known as xanthine derivatives, act directly on the smooth muscle of the tracheobronchial tree to dilate the bronchi, thus increasing airflow in and out of the alveolar sacs.

Uses

Xanthine-derivative bronchodilators are used in combination with sympathomimetic bronchodilators to reverse airway constriction caused by acute and chronic bronchial asthma, bronchitis, and emphysema.

Therapeutic Outcomes

The primary therapeutic outcome associated with xanthine-derivative bronchodilator therapy is easier breathing with less effort.

Nursing Process

Premedication Assessment

1. Check the patient's history for diagnoses of angina pectoris, peptic ulcer disease, hyperthyroidism, glaucoma, or diabetes mellitus.
2. Obtain and record baseline vital signs.
3. Perform baseline assessment of the patient's mental status (for example, degree of anxiety present, nervousness, and alertness).

Planning

Availability. See Table 28-4.

Implementation

Dosage and administration. See Table 28-4.
Plasma levels. To maintain consistent plasma levels, administer the medication around the clock.

Evaluation

Side effects to expect

NAUSEA, VOMITING, EPIGASTRIC PAIN, ABDOMINAL CRAMPS. These symptoms may occur from gastric irritation caused by increased gastric acid secretions stimulated by these agents.

If gastric irritation occurs, administer with food or milk. If symptoms persist or increase in severity, report for physician evaluation.

Side effects to report

TACHYCARDIA, PALPITATIONS. Because most symptoms are dose related, alterations should be reported to the physician. Monitor the patient's heart rate and rhythm at regular intervals throughout therapy with bronchodilators.

Report heart rates significantly higher than baseline values.

Always report palpitations and suspected arrhythmias.

TREMORS. Tell the patient to notify the physician if tremors develop after starting any of these medications. A dosage adjustment may be necessary.

NERVOUSNESS, ANXIETY, RESTLESSNESS, HEADACHE. Perform a baseline assessment of the patient's mental status (degree of anxiety, nervousness, and alertness); compare subsequent, regular assessments to the findings obtained. Report escalation of tension.

Drug interactions

DRUGS THAT ENHANCE TOXIC EFFECTS. Cimetidine, erythromycin, troleandomycin, diltiazem, nifedipine, verapamil, moricizine, thiabendazole, influenza vaccine, propranolol, and allopurinol. Monitor for increases in severity of drug effects such as nervousness, agitation, nausea, tachycardia, and arrhythmias.

DRUGS THAT REDUCE THERAPEUTIC EFFECTS. Tobacco or marijuana smoking. Higher doses of the bronchodilator may be required.

LITHIUM. Xanthine derivatives may increase the renal excretion of lithium carbonate. Higher doses of lithium are required to maintain therapeutic effects. Monitor for the return of manic or depressive activity. Enlist the aid of family and friends to help identify early symptoms.

BETA-ADRENERGIC BLOCKING AGENTS. Xanthine derivatives and beta-adrenergic blocking agents (propranolol, timolol, nadolol, atenolol, and others) may have mutually antagonistic actions. Patients must be observed for inhibition of either drug.

Drug Class: Respiratory Antiinflammatory Agents

corticosteroids used for obstructive airway disease

Actions

Corticosteroids (see Chapter 35), whether applied by aerosol or administered systemically, have been shown to be highly effective for the treatment of obstructive lung disease. The mechanisms of action are not completely known, but corticosteroids have a direct effect on smooth muscle relaxation; they enhance the effect of beta-adrenergic bronchodilators and inhibit inflammatory responses that may result in bronchoconstriction.

Uses

Patients with severe asthma or chronic obstructive lung disease who are becoming unresponse to sympathomimetic agents or xanthine derivatives may have corticosteroids added to the medication regimen to provide enhanced bronchodilation.

The first course of therapy is often a short course (5 to 7 days) of systemic corticosteroids (such as prednisone), with intervals of several weeks or months without steroid treatment. Alternate-day therapy (that is, a single dose every other morning) is the next preferable program. Aerosolized corticosteroids may be used daily for certain patients instead of alternate-day therapy. If the patient has not previously been receiving corticosteroid therapy, several weeks may pass before the full benefits from the aerosolized medication are achieved, but a single aerosol "burst" does produce noticeable benefits in reduction of bronchoconstriction. It is important to remember that the corticosteroid aerosols should not be regarded as true bronchodilators and should not be used for rapid relief of bronchospasm. (See Chapter 27 for the use of intranasal corticosteroids.)

Therapeutic Outcomes

The primary therapeutic outcome associated with corticosteroid therapy is easier breathing with less effort.

Nursing Process

Premedication Assessment

Inspect the oral cavity for the presence of any type of infection.

Planning

Availability. See Table 28-5.

Implementation

Dosage and administration. Counseling, compliance: The therapeutic effects, unlike those of sympathomimetic bronchodilators, are not immediate. This should be explained to the patient in advance to ensure cooperation and continuation of treatment with the prescribed dosage regimen, even when asymptomatic. Full therapeutic benefit requires regular use and may require up to 4 weeks of therapy for maximum benefit.

Preparation before administration. Patients receiving bronchodilators by inhalation should be advised to use the bronchodilator before the corticosteroid inhalant to enhance penetration of the corticosteroid into the bronchial tree. Wait several minutes before the corticosteroid is inhaled to allow time for the bronchodilator to relax the smooth muscle.

Maintenance therapy. After the desired clinical effect is obtained, the maintenance dose should be reduced to the smallest amount necessary to control the symptoms.

Severe stress or asthma attack. During periods of stress or a severe asthma attack, patients may require treatment with systemic steroids. Exacerbation of asthma that occurs during the course of corticosteroid inhalant therapy should be treated with a short course of systemic steroid. Instruct patients not to attempt to use the inhaler because the aerosol not only may cause irritation and exacerbate symptoms but also may not penetrate deeply into the bronchial tree for maximal effect.

Evaluation

Side effects to expect

HOARSENESS, DRY MOUTH. These side effects are usually mild and tend to resolve with continued therapy. Encourage the patient not to discontinue therapy without first consulting the physician.

Side effects to report

FUNGAL INFECTIONS (THRUSH). Increased risk factors for the development of oral thrush include concomitant antibiotic use, diabetes, improper aerosol administration, large oral doses of corticosteroids, and poor dental hygiene.

The patient should be instructed on good oral hygiene technique and told to gargle and rinse the mouth after each aerosol treatment with a mouthwash, such as 1 teaspoon of hydrogen peroxide in 6 to 8 ounces of water. Commercial mouthwashes contain alcohol, which may cause further drying and oral irritation.

If thrush should develop, it is usually not sufficiently troublesome to require discontinuation of the steroid aerosol therapy. An antifungal mouthwash such as nystatin (Mycostatin, Nilstat) will usually eradicate the oral candidiasis.

Table 28-5

Inhalant Corticosteroids

GENERIC NAME	BRAND NAME	AVAILABILITY	ADULT DOSAGE RANGE
Beclomethasone dipropionate	Beclovent, Vanceril	Aerosol: 200 doses/inhaler	2 inhalations (84 μg) 3-4 times daily; maximum of 840 μg (20 inhalations) daily
Dexamethasone sodium phosphate	Decadron Respihaler	Aerosol: 170 doses/container	3 inhalations (168 μg) 3-4 times daily; maximum of 12 inhalations daily
Flunisolide	AeroBid, ✺Bronalide	Aerosol: 100 doses/inhaler	2 inhalations (500 μg) twice daily; do not exceed 2 mg (8 inhalations) daily
Triamcinolone acetonide	Azmacort	Aerosol: 50 doses/inhaler	2 inhalations (200 μg) 3-4 times daily; do not exceed 1600 μg (16 inhalations) daily

✺ Available in Canada only.

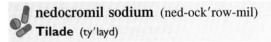

cromolyn sodium (kro'mo-lin)
Intal (in-tahl')

Actions

Cromolyn sodium is an antiinflammatory agent with unknown mechanism of action. It inhibits the release of histamine and other mediators of inflammation. It must be administered before the body receives a stimulus to release histamine, such as an antigen that initiates an antigen-antibody allergic reaction.

Uses

Cromolyn is recommended for use in conjunction with other medications in the treatment of patients with severe bronchial asthma or allergic rhinitis to prevent the release of histamine that results in asthmatic attacks or symptoms of allergic rhinitis.

Cromolyn has no direct bronchodilatory, antihistaminic, or anticholinergic activity. The concomitant use of antihistamines or nasal decongestants may be necessary during initial treatment with cromolyn. A 2- to 4-week course of therapy is usually required to determine clinical response. Therapy should be continued only if there is a decrease in the severity of asthmatic symptoms.

Therapeutic Outcomes

The primary therapeutic outcome associated with cromolyn therapy is reduced frequency of episodes of allergic rhinitis and asthmatic attacks.

Nursing Process

Premedication Assessment

1. This medication must be taken before exposure to the stimulus that initiates an attack of allergic rhinitis or severe bronchial asthma. Inhalation during an attack of bronchospasm or asthma may exacerbate symptoms.
2. Check to see if the concurrent use of antihistamines or nasal decongestants has been ordered by the physician, especially during initiation of cromolyn therapy.

Planning

Availability. Inhalation—20 mg capsules, 20 mg per 2 ml solution for nebulizer, and 112 and 200 metered-dose spray aerosols.

Implementation

Dosage and administration. Counseling: The therapeutic effects, unlike those of beta-adrenergic decongestants, are not immediate. This should be explained to the patient in advance to ensure cooperation and continuation of treatment with the prescribed dosage regimen. Full therapeutic benefit requires regular use and is usually evident within 2 to 4 weeks. Therapy must be continued even if the patient is symptom free.

Adult: PO—patients must be advised that the capsules are not absorbed when swallowed and that the drug is inactive when administered by this route. Inhalation—40 mg (2 capsule), via inhaler, 4 times daily. Inhalation during an acute asthma attack may aggravate symptoms because

the powder form of the drug can increase the irritation in the respiratory passage and result in more bronchospasm.

Proper technique is important to the success of therapy. Document and verify that the patient can do the following:
1. Load the inhaler with a capsule and pierce (only once) the capsule immediately before use.
2. Hold the inhaler away from the mouth and exhale, emptying as much air from the lungs as possible.
3. With the head tilted back and teeth apart, close lips around the mouthpiece.
4. Inhale deeply and rapidly through the inhaler with a steady, even breath.
5. Remove the inhaler and hold the breath for a few seconds, then exhale. (Instruct not to exhale through the inhaler because moisture from the breath will interfere with proper function of the inhaler.)
6. Repeat several times until the powder is inhaled. (A light dusting of powder remaining in the capsule is normal.)

Aerosol—2 metered-dose sprays inhaled 4 times daily at regular intervals.

For prevention of exercise-induced bronchospasm or bronchospasm associated with cold air or environmental substances, administer 2 metered-dose sprays at least 10 minutes before and no more than 60 minutes before exposure to the precipitating factor.

Evaluation
Side effects to expect

ORAL IRRITATION, DRY MOUTH. The most common side effect is irritation of the throat and trachea caused by inhalation of the dry powder. This irritation may be manifested by nasal itching and burning, nasal stuffiness, sneezing, coughing, and bronchospasm. Start regular oral hygiene measures when the therapy is initiated. Suggest the use of 1 teaspoon of hydrogen peroxide in 6 to 8 ounces of water as a mouthwash. Commercial mouthwashes contain alcohol, which may cause further drying and oral irritation.

Other measures to alleviate dryness include sucking on ice chips or hard candy.

Side effects to report

BRONCHOSPASM, COUGHING. Notify the physician if inhalation causes these symptoms.

Drug interactions

No significant drug interactions have been reported.

nedocromil sodium (ned-ock'row-mil)
Tilade (ty'layd)

Actions

Nedocromil sodium is an antiinflammatory agent similar to cromolyn sodium. Its mechanism of action is unknown, but it prevents the release of histamine and other mediators that cause inflammation. It must be administered before the body receives a stimulus to release histamine, such as an antigen that initiates an antigen-antibody allergic reaction.

Uses

Nedocromil is recommended for use in conjunction with other medications in the treatment of patients with mild to moderate bronchial asthma to prevent the release of histamine and other inflammatory mediators that results in asthmatic attacks.

Nedocromil has no direct bronchodilatory, antihistaminic, or anticholinergic activity. The concomitant use of antihistamines or nasal decongestants may be necessary during initial treatment with nedocromil. A 2- to 4-week course of therapy is usually required to determine clinical response. Therapy should be continued only if there is a decrease in the severity of asthmatic symptoms.

Therapeutic Outcomes

The primary therapeutic outcome associated with nedocromil therapy is fewer episodes of acute asthmatic symptoms.

Nursing Process

Premedication Assessment

1. This medication must be taken before exposure to the stimulus that initiates an attack of allergic rhinitis or severe bronchial asthma. Inhalation during an attack of bronchospasm or asthma may exacerbate symptoms.
2. Check to see if the concurrent use of antihistamines and bronchodilators has been ordered by the physician, especially during start of nedocromil therapy.

Planning

Availability. Inhalation—1.75 mg per actuation in 112-dose, dose-metered inhalation aerosol.

Implementation

Dosage and administration. Counseling: The therapeutic effects, unlike those of beta-adrenergic decongestants, are not immediate. This should be explained to the patient in advance to ensure cooperation and continuation of treatment with the prescribed dosage regimen. Full therapeutic benefit requires regular use and is usually evident within 2 to 4 weeks. Therapy must be continued even if the patient is symptom free.

Adult: inhalation—2 metered-dose sprays inhaled 4 times daily at regular intervals. Ensure that the patient understands how to use the inhaler as described in the manufacturer's leaflet for the patient. Continue other therapy for asthma as prescribed.

Evaluation

Side effects to expect

ORAL IRRITATION, DRY MOUTH. The most common side effect is irritation of the throat and trachea caused by inhalation of the medicine. This irritation may be manifested by coughing, sore throat, runny nose, and bronchospasm. Start regular oral hygiene measures when the therapy is initiated. Suggest the use of 1 teaspoon of hydrogen peroxide in 6 to 8 ounces of water as a mouthwash. Commercial mouthwashes contain alcohol, which may cause further drying and oral irritation.

Other measures to alleviate dryness include sucking on ice chips or hard candy.

Side effects to report

BRONCHOSPASM, COUGHING. Notify the physician if inhalation causes these symptoms.

Drug interactions

No significant drug interactions have been reported.

CHAPTER REVIEW

Chronic obstructive lung disease is a preventable disease. It is a long-term, progressive disease that usually causes death after a debilitating illness. It places immeasurable stress on the family both emotionally and financially and costs society billions of dollars annually. The single major cause is smoking. Nurses can play a significant role in public education efforts, monitor for noncompliance, and encourage patients to make changes in lifestyle to reduce the severity of obstructive lung disease.

MATH REVIEW

1. Ordered: diphenhydramine (Benylin) 25 mg q4h.
   On hand: diphenhydramine (Benylin) 13.3 mg per 5 ml.
   Give: _____ ml or _____ tsp.

2. Ordered: terbutaline (Brethine) 0.25 mg SC.
   On hand: terbutaline 1 mg/ml.
   Give: _____ ml.

3. Ordered: theophylline elixir 9 mg/kg per 24 hours in 4 divided doses. The patient weights 86 pounds.
   Give: _____ mg per *individual dose*.
   On hand: theophylline elixir 50 mg per 5 ml.
   Give: _____ml per *individual dose*.

CRITICAL THINKING QUESTIONS

1. Explain why the action of a beta-adrenergic blocking agent may interfere with the therapeutic effects of bronchodilating agents such as albuterol (Proventil).

2. Differentiate among the action of acetylcysteine, guaifenesin, and potassium iodide on mucus in the respiratory tract.

Unit Six
DRUGS AFFECTING THE DIGESTIVE SYSTEM

CHAPTER 29

Drugs Used to Treat Oral Disorders

CHAPTER CONTENT

Objectives

1. Cite the treatment alternatives and associated nursing assessments to monitor response to drug therapy for common mouth disorders.

2. Identify baseline data the nurse should collect on a continuous basis for comparison and evaluation of drug effectiveness.

3. Identify important nursing assessments and interventions associated with the drug therapy and treatment of diseases of the mouth.

Key Words

cold sores	tartar
fever blisters	gingivitis
canker sores	halitosis
candidiasis	xerostomia
stomatitis	dentifrice
plaque	mouthwashes
dental caries	

MOUTH DISORDERS

Common disorders affecting the mouth are cold sores on the lip; canker sores and candidal infections of soft tissues of the

tongue, cheeks, and gums; and plaque and calculus affecting the gums and teeth. Xerostomia, or lack of saliva, originates from nonoral causes. Halitosis can arise from oral or nonoral diseases. A much less common problem, but one that causes significant discomfort, is oral stomatitis.

Cold sores (**fever blisters**) are caused by the herpes simplex type 1 virus (herpes simplex labialis) and are most commonly found at the junction of the mucous membrane and the skin of the lips or nostrils, although they can occur inside the mouth, especially affecting the gums and roof of the mouth. It is estimated that at least one half of all Americans aged 20 to 40 years have had fever blisters. Most victims were infected before 5 years of age. About half of patients develop recurrent outbreaks of the lesions, often in the same location, separated by latent periods. The recurrence rate and extent of lesions are highly variable. Patients often predict when an outbreak may occur because of predisposing factors such as a systemic illness accompanied by fever, cold (hence the names fever blister and cold sore), or flu; menstruation; extreme physical stress and fatigue; or sun and wind exposure.

Patients often report that a flare-up of the sores is preceded by a prodrome of burning, itching, and numbness in the area where the lesion develops. The lesions first become visible as small, red papules that develop into fluid-filled vesicles (blisters) 1 to 3 mm in diameter. Smaller lesions often coalesce into larger lesions. Pain is intense, fever may be present, and increased salivation and mouth odor occur. Often the glands in the neck are swollen because of the body's response to infection. Over the next 10 to 14 days, a crust develops over the top of many coalesced, burst vesicles; the base is erythematous. The liquid from the vesicles contains live virus that is contagious if transferred to other persons by direct contact (for example, kissing). If pus develops in the vesicles or under the crust of a cold sore, a secondary bacterial infection may be present and should be evaluated for antibiotic therapy.

Canker sores affect 20% to 50% of Americans. The exact cause is unknown but is thought to be a hypersensitivity to antigenic components of *Streptococcus sanquis*, a bacterium found in the mouth. The lesions are not viral infections as was once thought, and they are not contagious. There appears to be a familial factor, as well as nutritional, emotional, and physiologic factors. They can develop at any age and affect both sexes in equal numbers. Canker sores can appear as an ulcer 0.5 to 3 cm in diameter on surfaces that are not attached to bone such as the tongue, gums, or inner lining of the cheeks and lips. The lesion is usually gray to whitish yellow with an erythematous halo of inflamed tissue surrounding the ulcer crater. They do not form blisters and usually do not grow together. Patients may experience a single lesion or as many as 30 or more at a time. The lesions can be painful and can inhibit normal eating, drinking, talking, and swallowing, as well as oral hygiene. There are usually no swollen lymph glands or fever unless the sores become secondarily infected. Most canker sores last for 10 to 14 days and heal without scarring.

Candidiasis is a fungal infection caused by *Candida albicans*, the most common organism associated with oral infections. It is often called "the disease of the diseased" because it appears in debilitated patients and patients taking a variety of medicines. The most common predisposing factors include physiologic factors (early infancy, pregnancy, and old age), diabetes mellitus, malnutrition, malignancies, and radiation therapy. Medicines that predispose a patient to candidiasis are those that depress defense mechanisms (immunosuppressives, corticosteroids, cytotoxics, and broad-spectrum antibiotics) and those that cause xerostomia (anticholinergics, antidepressants, antipsychotics, antihypertensives, and antihistamines).

There are several forms of candidiasis, but the most common is the acute, pseudomembranous form that is often referred to as thrush. It is characterized by white, "milk curd"–appearing plaques that are attached to the oral mucosa. These plaques usually can be easily detached, and erythematous, bleeding, sore areas appear beneath them. Thrush is most common in infants, pregnant women, and debilitated patients. Treatment of candidiasis requires local or systemic therapy with antifungal agents such as nystatin, mycostatin suspension, or clotrimazole troches. (See Chapter 43.)

Stomatitis is a general term used to describe a painful inflammation of the mucous membranes of the mouth. It is commonly associated with chemotherapy and radiation therapy. Stomatitis starts to develop 5 to 7 days after antineoplastic therapy or radiation therapy is administered. The sores are erythematous ulcerations intermixed with white patchy mucous membranes. Candidal infections are often present. A scale is often used to standardize evaluation of stomatitis (see box on lower left).

Plaque is the primary cause of most tooth, gum (gingiva), and periodontal disease. Plaque, the whitish-yellow substance that builds up on teeth and gum lines around the teeth, is thought to originate from saliva. Plaque forms a sticky "meshwork" that traps bacteria and food particles. If not removed regularly, it thickens, and bacteria proliferate. The bacteria secrete acids that eat into the enamel of teeth, causing **dental caries** (cavities). If the plaque is not removed within 24 hours, it begins to calcify, forming calculus, or **tartar**. The calculus forms a foundation for additional plaque to form, eventually eroding under the gumline causing inflammation (**gingivitis**) and periodontal disease.

Halitosis is the term used to describe a foul odor that comes from the mouth. A temporary foul odor at certain times is normal in healthy individuals, such as "morning breath" or after eating certain foods (for example, garlic or onions). Halitosis can also be a sign of underlying pathology. Halitosis comes from oral and nonoral sources. Nonoral causes of halitosis include sinusitis, tonsillitis, and rhinitis; pulmonary diseases such as tuberculosis or bronchiectasis; and elimination of chemicals from the blood such as acetone exhaled by patients with diabetic ketoacidosis. Paraldehyde and dimethyl sulfoxide (DMSO) are two medicines that are excreted primarily through the lungs and leave a characteristic foul odor to the breath. "Smoker's breath" caused by smoking is a fairly common cause of halitosis. Oral causes of halitosis include decaying food particles, plaque-coated tongue and teeth, dental caries, poor oral or denture hygiene, periodontal disease, and xerostomia.

Xerostomia is a condition in which the flow of saliva is either partially or completely stopped. About 20% of persons over the age of 65 report a change in consistency, a decrease in production, or a discontinuation of salivary flow. Xerostomia causes loss of taste, difficulty in chewing and swallowing food, and difficulty in talking, and it increases tooth decay. Xerostomia can also cause a burning sensation of the tongue, stomatitis, and a reduction in the amount of time daily that dentures can be worn. The most common causes of xerostomia are medicines (anticholinergic agents, diuretics, antidepressants, certain antihypertensive agents), diseases (diabetes mellitus, depression), and functional conditions (for example, smoking or mouth breathing).

Stomatitis Scale

0	=	Pink, moist, intact mucosa; absence of pain/burning
+1	=	Generalized erythema with or without pain or burning; scalloped/ridging on tongue or buccal mucosal surfaces
+2	=	Isolated small ulcerations and/or white plaques
+3	=	Confluent ulcerations with or without white plaques > 25% of mucosal surface
+4	=	Hemorrhagic ulcerations on > 25% of mucosal surface

From Engelking C: Managing stomatitis: a nursing process approach. In *Supportive care for the patient with cancer,* ed 1, Richmond, Va, 1988, Robins.

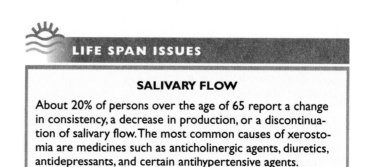

LIFE SPAN ISSUES

SALIVARY FLOW

About 20% of persons over the age of 65 report a change in consistency, a decrease in production, or a discontinuation of salivary flow. The most common causes of xerostomia are medicines such as anticholinergic agents, diuretics, antidepressants, and certain antihypertensive agents.

Drug Therapy

Cold Sores

The goals of treatment are to control discomfort, allow healing, and prevent complications. Local anesthetics (benzocaine, dibucaine) in emollient creams, petrolatum or protectants such as Orabase Lip Healer (benzocaine 5%, allantoin, menthol, and petrolatum) can temporarily relieve the pain and itching. Oral analgesics (for example, aspirin, acetaminophen, and ibuprofen) may also provide significant pain relief. The use of broad-brimmed hats and ultraviolet blockers (for example, Chapstick Sunblock, Lipkote) with a sun protection factor (SPF) of at least 15 can be used for patients who associate occurrence of cold sores with sun exposure. Secondary infections can be treated with topical antibiotic ointments such as Neosporin or Mycitracin.

Canker Sores

The goals of treatment are similar to those for cold sores: to control discomfort and promote healing. Topical anesthetics such as benzocaine (Orabase-B—benzocaine 20% in plasticized hydrocarbon gel) or butacaine are particularly effective if applied just before eating or performing oral hygiene. Oral analgesics (for example, aspirin, acetaminophen, and ibuprofen) may also provide significant pain relief. Aspirin should not be placed on the lesions because of the high risk of severe chemical burns with necrosis. Oxygen-releasing agents (carbamide peroxide, hydrogen peroxide, and perborates) can be used as debriding and cleansing agents up to 4 times daily for 7 days. Long-term safety has not been established, and tissue irritation and black, hairy tongue have been reported. Saline rinses (1 to 3 teaspoons of table salt) in 4 to 8 ounces of warm tap water may be soothing and can be used before topical application of medication. Sustained use of products containing menthol, phenol, camphor, and eugenol should be discouraged because they cause tissue irritation and damage or systemic toxicity if overused. Silver nitrate should not be used to "cauterize" lesions because it may damage healthy tissue surrounding the lesion and predispose the area to later infection.

Stomatitis

Although it takes 5 to 7 days for stomatitis to develop after chemotherapy or radiation therapy, oral hygiene regimens should be started when chemotherapy is initiated. Measures such as oral hygiene, oral irrigations and methods to relieve dry mouth and lips can be effective in providing comfort.

Pain associated with oral stomatitis can be a major complication that contributes to poor nutrition and hydration. To be effective, topical applications of medications for pain must come in contact with the tissue. Therefore, it is advisable to schedule these routines immediately after the cleansing of the oral cavity. The following are routine approaches to treating pain in the oral area:

- Lidocaine: viscous lidocaine 2% before meals to relieve pain. Care must be taken to make sure the patient is not burned by the food because the entire mouth and throat are anesthetized.
- Milk of magnesia can be used to rinse the mouth and coat the mucous membranes.
- Kaopectate stirred in water may be used as a mouthwash to coat painful oral lesions.

- Nystatin liquid can be swished in the mouth for 1 minute and then swallowed ("swish and swallow" routine), or clotrimazole lozenges may be chewed or sucked and then swallowed to reduce candidal oral infections.
- Sucralfate suspensions applied topically have been reported to provide effective pain relief.
- Oral or parenteral analgesics may be administered for severe pain.

Plaque

Plaque is controlled by tooth brushing, dental flossing between teeth, and certain mouthwashes. If plaque is removed regularly, calculus will not form. Using a dentifrice (toothpaste) with the toothbrush helps remove dental plaque and stain, resulting in less halitosis and periodontal disease and fewer dental caries. Other devices such as oral irrigators (Water Pik), sponge-tipped applicators, or electric toothbrushes can be used for patients who wear orthodontic appliances, who are physically or mentally handicapped, or who lack manual dexterity and require someone else to clean their teeth. Therapeutic mouthwashes will also help reduce plaque accumulated above the gumline.

Halitosis

Halitosis is treated most easily by eliminating causes such smoking and certain foods. Regular brushing of the teeth or dentures and the use of dental floss between teeth can remove particles of decaying food. Mouthwashes and "breath mints" can mask halitosis but usually last less than an hour. If halitosis is persistent without a readily identifiable cause such as smoking or diet, a dentist should be consulted for a thorough examination to ensure that no other pathology is the underlying cause.

Xerostomia

Xerostomia is treated by attempting to change the medicines that cause dry mouth or with artificial saliva. Artificial saliva products do not stimulate natural saliva production but mimic the viscosity, mineral content, and taste of saliva. Patients with xerostomia should be seen by a dentist regularly to help avoid additional dental caries and ensure proper denture fit to prevent irritation of the gums. Commercially available saliva substitutes include Salivart, Mouth Kote, Saliva Substitute, Oral Balance and Xero-Lube.

Nursing Process for Oral Health Therapy

Assessment

Drug history. Obtain a history of recent drug therapy. Some drugs, such as Dilantin, may cause alterations in the gums, and oral stomatitis is common after chemotherapy and radiation therapy.

Dental history. • Obtain a dental history that includes frequency of visits to the dentist and a brief summary of dental procedures that have been performed within the last 1 to 3 years. • Ask about usual hygiene practices, for example, number of times per day brushing or flossing is done, type of toothbrush used, and oral products used (toothpaste, mouthwashes). • Ask about the use of tobacco and alcohol—

frequency and amounts. Ask about any difficulty chewing, swallowing, or with speaking. • Ask about any recent changes in the taste of foods or alterations within the mouth such as burning or tingling.

Oral cavity. • Put on gloves and inspect the oral cavity with the aid of a flashlight and tongue blade. Visually inspect the mucous membranes covering the lips, hard and soft palates, gums, tongue, pharynx, and teeth. • Note the color of the mucous membranes and the moisture present. • Inspect the mucous membranes for inflamed or receding gums, ulcerations, crusts, changes in color such as white patches, and sores from poorly fitting dentures. Inquire how well the dentures fit and how long each day they are worn. Assess for the presence of teeth, dental caries, and tooth plaque. • Observe the amount and consistency of the saliva present. • Note the presence or absence of halitosis (foul-smelling breath). Presence may indicate poor dental hygiene practices or an oral infection. Some odors occur from a variety of causes (garlic, smoking, ingestion of alcohol) and some systemic diseases (acetone from diabetes, ammonia from liver disease).

Nursing Diagnosis
- Alteration in comfort (indication)
- Impaired tissue integrity (indication)
- Body-image disturbances (indication)
- Knowledge deficit related to hygiene practices, medication regimen (indication)

Planning
- Develop a schedule for oral hygiene measures to be performed consistent with type and severity of mouth disorder.
- Make necessary referrals to the dentist, especially before starting chemotherapy.
- Order prescribed oral hygiene supplies and medications; list medications used as rinses or "swish and swallows" in the medication administration record (MAR).

Implementation
Cold Sores. • Cold sores should be kept clean by gentle washing with mild soap solutions. The cold sore should be kept moist to prevent drying and cracking. Cracking may render it more susceptible to secondary bacterial infection, may delay healing, and usually increases discomfort. Therefore products that are highly astringent should be avoided (for example, tannic acid, zinc sulfate). • Apply local anesthetics and ultraviolet blockers or oral analgesics, as prescribed. • When secondary infections are present, apply topical antibiotic ointment to the cold sore.

Canker sores. • Apply topical anesthetics before the patient eats or performs oral hygiene. • Administer oral analgesics; apply oxygen-releasing agents for debridement and cleansing agents at appropriate intervals. • Saline rinses using 1 to 3 teaspoons of table salt in 4 to 8 ounces of warm tap water may be soothing and can be used prior to topical application of medications. • Changes in diet can also reduce irritation to the sores. Avoid sharp-edged foods such as potato chips and crackers, spicy foods, pineapple, citrus fruits and chocolate. Drinking acidic juices and soft drinks through a straw can minimize contact with and irritation of the canker sores.

Stomatitis
- Oral hygiene regimens should be started at the time chemotherapy or radiation therapy is started. Oral hygiene should include using a soft-bristled brush, Water Pik on low setting, or sponge-tipped applicators (in the case of severe lesions) to remove debris. With advanced lesions, pain and discomfort may be severe and other devices such as a gravity flow irrigating system or an oral syringe may be used to irrigate and cleanse the mouth.
- Commercially prepared mouthwashes containing alcohol are usually not recommended because they further dry the mouth and irritate rather than relieve symptoms of stomatitis. Alternative solutions for oral hygiene are 1 tablespoon of salt or hydrogen peroxide in 8 ounces of water or $\frac{1}{2}$ teaspoon of baking soda in 8 ounces of water as the mouthwash. Although there are disadvantages to each of these solutions, they remain the hallmark of irrigating solutions in use at this time.
- The frequency of the oral irrigations is important. Irrigations should be performed immediately before and after meals and at bedtime if symptoms are mild. With moderate lesions, increase the frequency to every 2 hours. In patients with severe symptoms, the mouth may be rinsed hourly. When fungal infections are present, the cleansing regimen should be performed immediately before administering the topical agents (nystatin liquids as a swish or clotrimazole lozenges). Performing the cleansing routine immediately before the medication is given will improve the contact of the medicine with the denuded surface. Caution the patient not to take food or drink for approximately 15 minutes after the medication.
- Dryness in the mouth can be relieved by chewing gum and sucking on ice chips or popsicles. Dry lips can be coated with cocoa butter, K-Y lubricating jelly, petroleum jelly, or lip balm. Artificial saliva is available.
- Administer pain preparations according to prescribed routines using products such as viscous lidocaine 2%, milk of magnesia or kaopectate rinses, nystatin liquid as a swish and swallow routine, or sucralfate suspension topically. Oral or parenteral analgesics may be used for severe pain.

Plaque. Perform toothbrushing and dental flossing and use mouthwashes on a scheduled basis daily to prevent plaque.

Halitosis. Regular brushing of the teeth and dentures and the use of dental floss between teeth can remove particles of decaying food. Mouthwashes and breath mints can mask halitosis but usually last less than an hour.

Xerostomia. Monitor the medication routine. Report xerostomia to the physician and apply artificial saliva if prescribed.

Dentures. Dentures should be cleaned each time oral hygiene is performed. For neutropenic patients, dentures should be worn only to eat meals. Poorly fitting dentures must be repaired to prevent further tissue breakdown.

Patient Education and Health Promotion
- Teach the patient proper cleansing techniques for oral hygiene consistent with the conditions present (for example, normal healthy tissue stomatitis, jaw wiring).
- Instruct persons who are to receive radiation or chemotherapy to start oral hygiene on a scheduled regimen immediately. Don't wait until stomatitis develops.

- Teach the patient with pain the proper use of prescribed analgesics and comfort measures.
- Discuss dietary practices that may relieve symptoms, for example, bland foods. For dry mouth, instruct the person to use gravies or sauces to moisten foods more thoroughly for eating. When the mucous membranes are irritated, suggest avoiding hot and spicy foods, alcohol, and tobacco.
- Persistent halitosis that is not relieved by brushing and flossing may have a medical basis. The individual should be told to discuss the matter with the physician or dentist to ensure appropriate therapy.
- Fluoride supplements may be recommended in areas of the country in which the water supply is not fluoridated or the fluoride level is low.

Fostering health maintenance. • Discuss hygiene practices and medications prescribed for discomfort, infections, or prevention of mucosal breakdown. • Seek cooperation and understanding of the following points so that medication compliance is increased: name of medications, dosage, route and times of administration, side effects to expect, and side effects to report. • Discuss a specific schedule for performing oral hygiene measures and include details of products to be used to relieve oral dryness or pain. • Report to the physician conditions that are not relieved by the prescribed therapies.

Drug Class: Dentifrices

Actions

Dentifrices contain one or more abrasive agents, a foaming agent, and flavoring materials. They are available in powder, paste, or gel forms and are used as an aid in the mechanical cleansing provided by a soft nylon toothbrush. Although dentifrices vary in the degree of abrasiveness, abrasiveness is an essential property for removal of plaque from teeth. Some toothpastes contain higher concentrations of abrasive agents and are advertised as "smoker's toothpastes" to remove tobacco stains. The most common therapeutic agent added to dentifrices is fluoride for its anticaries activity. Chemicals such as sanquinarine, zinc citrate, triclosan, thymol, and eucalyptol have antibacterial properties that may reduce plaque accumulation. Dentifrices advertised as "tooth whiteners" contain oxidizing ingredients such as hydrogen peroxide, carbamide peroxide, and perhydrol urea.

Uses

If possible, all persons should brush at least twice daily with a fluoride toothpaste. If the teeth and gums are normal, select a fluoride-containing dentifrice that has acceptable taste. All age groups should use toothpastes that are the least abrasive to the teeth while controlling tooth decay and gum disease. This is especially important to patients with receding gums. Colgate Regular and Peak toothpastes contain fluoride and are the least abrasive; smokers' products, such as Close-Up Paste and Mint Gel, Topol, and Aim Regular-Strength Gel, contain fluoride but are the most abrasive. Examples of products containing fluoride with moderate abrasives are Ultra-Brite Original, Crest, Close-Up Tartar Control Gel and Aquafresh Tartar Control. Baking soda is a mild abrasive

agent and can be effective and inexpensive as a dentifrice. The only disadvantages to baking soda are its slightly bitter taste and lack of fluoride. Denquel is a mildly abrasive toothpaste that also contains a desensitizing agent. This type of toothpaste is used for relieving sensitivity to hot and cold in otherwise normal teeth.

Therapeutic Outcomes

The primary therapeutic outcomes expected from dentifrices are as follows:
- Reduction in plaque formation and cavities
- A pleasant, refreshing taste in the mouth

Drug Class: Mouthwashes

Toothbrushing and flossing are optimal for good oral hygiene; however, this may not be possible for the patient who has undergone oral surgery or who has suffered facial trauma. **Mouthwashes** may be temporarily effective in removing disagreeable tastes and reducing halitosis. Therapeutic mouthwashes are also available to reduce plaque formation.

Actions

Mouthwashes are solutions of flavoring, coloring, water, surfactants, and sometimes therapeutic ingredients. Flavoring agents are used to give a pleasant taste and freshen the breath. Coloring helps imply a certain type of mouthwash; green or blue for minty, red for spicy, and brown for medicinal. Surfactants are foaming agents that aid in removal of debris. Alcohol is often present, adding a "bite," enhancing flavor, especially in the medicinal type of products, and solubilizing other ingredients. Therapeutic ingredients include fluoride for anticaries protection and antimicrobial agents (benzoic acid, thymol, eucalyptol, menthol, cetylpyridinium chloride, domiphen bromide, and chlorhexidine) to kill bacteria to reduce plaque formation and decaying food odor. Phenol is a local anesthetic, antiseptic, and antibacterial agent that penetrates and reduces plaque formation. Zinc citrate and zinc chloride are astringents that neutralize sulfur-smelling compounds from decaying debris in the mouth.

Uses

Mouthwashes can be subdivided into cosmetic and therapeutic products based on ingredients. Cosmetic mouthwashes freshen the breath and rinse out some debris, although the odor-reducing effect lasts only 10 to 30 minutes. Certain mouthwashes are recommended for specific purposes. The most common are the fluoride-containing mouthwashes used to prevent dental caries. Medicinal mouthwashes (for example, Listerine) are recommended to reducing plaque accumulation and gingivitis. Chlorhexidine (Peridex) is an antibacterial agent used to treat oral stomatitis. Products containing zinc chloride are used as astringents for temporary decrease of bleeding or irritation. A 0.9% solution of sodium chloride (normal saline) is an effective gargle. It can be used to provide temporary, soothing relief of pharyngeal irritation from nasogastric tubes, endotracheal tubes, sore throat, or oral surgery. Solutions containing hydrogen peroxide may be used to cleanse and debride minor lesions. However, use should be limited to 7 to 10 days to prevent further tissue irritation. Lidocaine, a local anesthetic, is available in both an oral spray solution (Xylocaine 10% oral spray) and an oral viscous solution (Xylocaine 2% viscous solution). The spray solution is used as a short-term, topical anesthetic for the mucous membranes in the mouth. The viscous solution has a longer-lasting local anesthetic and can be used as a gargle for patients with sore throats or mouth ulcers. This product is frequently used in immunosuppressed patients with painful candidal infections of the mouth and throat.

Unless a mouthwash is being used to treat a specific medical condition (for example, oral stomatitis), it should be remembered that mouthwashes should not become a substitute for normal oral hygiene. Primary oral hygiene is proper toothbrushing and flossing.

All mouthwashes have specific dosage recommendations. It is important not to exceed these recommendations without a physician's order because many of the therapeutic ingredients (for example, lidocaine, fluoride) can be systemically absorbed, resulting in accumulation of toxic levels. Most mouthwashes are designed to be used as a rinse (the mouthwash is held in the mouth, swished around, and expectorated). Again, prolonged swallowing of mouthwashes may lead to systemic toxicities. Patients should be advised to refrain from smoking, eating, or drinking for at least 30 minutes after use.

Therapeutic Outcomes

The primary therapeutic outcomes expected from mouthwashes are as follows:
- Temporary reduction in bleeding or irritation
- Relief of discomfort
- A refreshing taste in the mouth
- Improvement in halitosis

CHAPTER REVIEW

Common disorders affecting the mouth are cold sores on the lip; canker sores and candidal infections of soft tissues of the tongue, cheeks, and gums; and plaque and calculus affecting the gums and teeth. Xerostomia (lack of saliva) originates from nonoral causes. Halitosis can arise from oral or nonoral causes. A much less common problem, but one that causes significant discomfort, is oral stomatitis.

CRITICAL THINKING QUESTION

1. Compare oral hygiene measures appropriate in a healthy mouth with those needed in mild to severe mouth disorders.

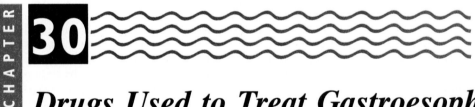

CHAPTER 30

Drugs Used to Treat Gastroesophageal Reflux and Peptic Ulcer Disease

CHAPTER CONTENT

Objectives

1. Cite common stomach disorders that require drug therapy.
2. Identify factors that prevent breakdown of the body's normal defense barriers resulting in ulcer formation.
3. State the drug classifications and actions used to treat stomach disorders.
4. Develop health teaching for an individual with stomach disorders that incorporates pharmacologic and nonpharmacologic treatment modalities.

parietal cells

hydrochloric acid

gastroesophageal reflux
 disease (GERD)

heartburn

peptic ulcer disease (PUD)

Helicobacter pylori

PHYSIOLOGY OF THE STOMACH

As a major part of the gastrointestinal (GI) tract, the stomach has three primary functions: storage of food until it can be utilized in the lower GI tract; mixing of food with gastric secretions until it is a partially digested, semisolid mixture known as chyme; and slow emptying of the stomach at a rate that allows proper digestion and absorption of nutrients and medicine from the small intestine.

Three types of secretory cells line portions of the stomach: chief cells, parietal cells, and mucous cells. The chief cells secrete pepsinogen, an inactive enzyme. The **parietal cells** are stimulated by acetylcholine from cholinergic nerve fibers, gastrin, and histamine to secrete hydrochloric acid. **Hydrochloric acid** activates pepsinogen to pepsin and provides the optimal pH for pepsin to start protein digestion. Normal pH in the stomach ranges between 2 and 5, depending on presence of food and medications. Hydrochloric acid also breaks down muscle fibers and connective tissue ingested as food and kills bacteria that enter the digestive tract through the mouth. The parietal cells also secrete intrinsic factor needed for absorption of vitamin B_{12}. The mucous cells secrete a mucus that coats the stomach wall. The 1 mm thick mucous coat is alkaline and protects the stomach wall from damage by hydrochloric acid and the digestive enzyme pepsin. It also contributes lubrication for food transport. Small amounts of other enzymes are also secreted in the stomach. Lipases start the digestion of fats, and gastric amylase digests carbohydrates. Other digestive enzymes are also carried into the stomach from swallowed saliva.

Prostaglandins also play a major role in protecting the stomach walls from injury by stomach acids and enzymes. The prostaglandins are produced by cells lining the stomach and prevent injury by inhibiting gastric acid secretion, maintaining blood flow, and stimulating mucus and bicarbonate production.

COMMON STOMACH DISORDERS

Gastroesophageal reflux disease (GERD), more commonly referred to as **heartburn,** acid indigestion, or sour stomach, is a common stomach disorder. Approximately one third of the American population suffer from heartburn once a month, and 5% to 7% suffer from heartburn daily. Common symptoms are a burning sensation, bloating, belching, and regurgitation. Other symptoms that are reported less frequently are nausea, a "lump in the throat," hiccups, and chest pain.

Gastroesophageal reflux disease is the reflux of gastric secretions, primarily pepsin and hydrochloric acid, up into the esophagus. Causes of GERD are a weakened lower esophageal sphincter, delayed gastric emptying, hiatal hernia, obesity, overeating, tight-fitting clothing, and increased acid se-

cretion. Acid secretions are increased by smoking, alcohol, carbonated beverages, coffee, and spicy foods.

Most cases of GERD pass quickly with only mild discomfort, but frequent or prolonged bouts of acid reflux cause inflammation, tissue erosion, and ulcerations in the lower esophagus. Any person who suffers from recurrent or continuous symptoms of reflux, especially if the symptoms interfere with activities, should be referred to a physician. These symptoms may also accompany more serious conditions such as ischemic heart disease, scleroderma, and gastric malignancy.

Peptic ulcer disease (PUD) is actually several stomach disorders that result from an imbalance between acidic stomach contents and the body's normal defense barriers, causing ulcerations in the GI tract. The most common illnesses are gastric and duodenal ulcers. It is estimated that approximately 10% of all Americans will develop an ulcer sometime in their lives. The incidence in men and women is approximately the same. Race, economic status, and psychologic stress do not correlate with the frequency of ulcer disease. Often the only symptom that is reported is epigastric pain, described as "burning," gnawing, or aching. Patients often report that varying degrees of pain were present for a few weeks, then gone only to recur a few weeks later. The pain is most often noticed when the stomach is empty, such as at night or between meals, and is relieved by food or antacids. Other symptoms that cause patients to seek medical attention are bloating, nausea, vomiting, and anorexia.

The formation of ulcers appears to be caused by a combination of the presence of acid and a breakdown in the body's defense mechanisms that protect the stomach wall. Proposed mechanisms are oversecretion of hydrochloric acid by excessive numbers of parietal cells, injury to the mucosal barrier such as that resulting from prostaglandin inhibitors (including aspirin), and infection of the mucosal wall by *Helicobacter pylori.* It had been thought that no bacterium could survive in the highly acidic environment of the stomach. However, *H. pylori* was first isolated from patients with gastritis in 1983. It appears that the bacteria is able to live below the mucous barrier, where it is protected from stomach acid and pepsin. The exact mechanism by which *H. pylori* contributes to ulcer formation is not known, but several hypotheses are being tested.

Several risk factors increase the likelihood of peptic ulcer disease.

1. There appears to be a genetic predisposition to PUD. Some families have a much greater history of PUD than others.
2. It is a commonly held belief that stress causes ulcers, but no well-controlled studies have supported this.
3. Cigarette smoking increases acid secretion, alters blood flow in the stomach wall, and retards prostaglandin synthesis needed for defense mechanisms.
4. Nonsteroidal antiinflammatory drugs (NSAIDs) have a twofold effect: NSAIDs inhibit prostaglandins that protect the mucosa and directly irritate the stomach wall. Once ulcerations form, NSAIDs also slow healing.
5. It is commonly thought that certain foods (for example, spicy foods) and alcohol contribute to ulcer formation. It is true that certain foods increase acid secretion and that alcohol irritates the stomach lining, but results from studies have not corroborated induction of ulcer formation by food or alcohol.

Treatment

The goals of treatment of GERD are to relieve symptoms, decrease the frequency and duration of reflux, heal tissue injury, and prevent recurrence. The most important treatment is a change in lifestyle: weight loss (if significantly over the ideal body weight), reduction or avoidance of foods and beverages that increase acid production, reduction or cessation of smoking, avoidance of alcohol, and consumption of smaller meals. Additional therapy includes remaining upright for 2 hours after meals, not eating before bedtime, and avoiding tight clothing over the abdominal area. Lozenges may be used to increase saliva production, and antacids and alginic acid therapy may be used to provide relief in patients who experience infrequent heartburn. If the patient's symptoms do not improve within 2 to 3 weeks or if the patient's condition is severe, additional pharmacologic measures should be tried to reduce irritation. About 5% to 10% of patients with GERD require surgery.

The treatment of PUD and GERD is somewhat similar: relieve symptoms, promote healing, and prevent recurrence. Lifestyle changes that eliminate risk factors such as cigarette smoking and foods (and alcohol) that increase acid secretion should be initiated. Patients rarely need to be restricted to a bland diet. If NSAIDs are being taken, consideration should be given to switching to acetaminophen, if feasible. For decades, the treatment of ulcers has focused on reducing acid secretions (anticholinergic agents, H_2 antagonists, gastric acid pump inhibitors), neutralizing acid (antacids), or coating ulcer craters to hasten healing (sucralfate). Major changes in therapy may become available, however, if the Food and Drug Administration (FDA) approves the use of antibiotics to eradicate *H. pylori*. Several large studies are currently being done to test both the healing and recurrence rate of ulcers treated with antibiotics.

Drug Therapy

Actions

- Antacids neutralize gastric acid, thereby causing the gastric contents to be less acidic.
- Coating agents provide a protective covering over the ulcer crater.
- H_2 antagonists decrease the volume of hydrochloric acid produced, increasing the gastric pH and thereby resulting in decreased irritation to the gastric mucosa.
- Gastric acid pump inhibitors block the formation of hydrochloric acid, reducing irritation of the gastric mucosa.
- Prokinetic agents increase the lower esophageal sphincter muscle pressure and peristalsis, hastening emptying of the stomach to reduce reflux.
- Antispasmodic agents reduce the secretion of saliva, hydrochloric acid, pepsin, bile, and other enzymatic fluids necessary for digestion and decrease gastrointestinal motility and secretions.

Uses

- Antacids decrease hyperacidity associated with PUD, GERD, gastritis, and hiatal hernia.
- Coating agents provide a protective barrier for the mucosal lining where hydrochloric acid may come in contact with inflamed, eroded areas. They are used to treat existing ulcer craters on the gastric mucosa.

- H_2 antagonists are used in the treatment of acute gastric and duodenal ulcers and gastroesophageal disease and also for maintenance to prevent recurrence of ulcers.
- Gastric acid pump inhibitors are used in treatment of hyperacidity conditions (for example, GERD and Zollinger-Ellison syndrome).
- Prokinetic agents are used to treat GERD.
- Antispasmodic agents decrease gastric secretions by inhibiting vagal stimulation. They are used in treatment of gastrointestinal disorders requiring decreased gastric motility or decreased gastric secretions.

Nursing Process for Agents Used for Stomach Disorders

Assessment

Nutritional assessment. Obtain patient data about current height, weight, and any recent weight gain or loss. Identify the normal pattern of eating, including snacking habits. Use the food pyramid as a guide when asking questions to identify the usual foods eaten by the individual.

Esophagus, stomach. Ask patients to describe any symptoms in their own words. Question in detail what is meant by the terms *indigestion, heartburn, upset stomach, nausea,* and *belching.*

Pain, discomfort. Ask the patient to describe the onset, duration, location, and characteristics of pain or discomfort. Determine whether there is a relationship between the ingestion of certain types of food or drinks and the onset of pain. Ask specifically about the intake of coffee, tea, colas, chocolate, and alcohol. What has the patient done in the past to relieve the pain or discomfort? Have there been any changes in taste (for example, bitterness or sourness)?

Activity, exercise. Ask specifically what type of work or activities the individual performs that may increase intraabdominal pressure (for example, lifting heavy objects or bending over frequently).

Medication history. What self-medications have been tried? What prescribed medications are being taken? What is the schedule of medication administration (for example, how frequently and when are antacids taken)?

Anxiety/stress level. Ask the patient to describe lifestyle. What does the patient think are stressors, and how often do they occur?

Smoking. What is the frequency of smoking?

Nursing Diagnosis
- Alteration in comfort (indication)
- Altered nutrition: risk for less than body requirements (indication)
- Knowledge deficit related to medications and lifestyle changes (indications)

Planning
- Planning should be based on the assessment data, and interventions should be individualized to address patient needs.
- Routine orders: most physicians order antacids 1 hour before meals, 2 to 3 hours after meals, and at bedtime. As-needed (prn) medication dosages also must be discussed.

- Each type of medication used to treat GERD or PUD may require somewhat different scheduling to avoid drug interactions. When developing the time frames for administration of medications on the medication administration record (MAR), schedule the other prescribed drugs 1 hour before or 2 hours after antacids are given.
- Changes in diet require careful planning with the patient as well as the person responsible for purchasing and cooking the meals. Schedule teaching sessions appropriately. Not only may some foods need to be altered, but the number of meals per day may need to be increased with a smaller serving at each meal.
- Plan with the patient and family for needed changes at home, for example, elevation of the head of the bed on 6- to 12-inch blocks or the use of a foam wedge for sleeping.
- Lifestyle changes must be introduced, and planning for implementation agreed to mutually (smoking cessation or reduction, work-related changes to decrease intraabdominal pressure, or measures to decrease stress).
- Schedule laboratory studies, as ordered, to detect possible gastrointestinal bleeding.

Implementation

Patient Education and Health Promotion

Nutrition. Implement prescribed dietary changes—eat small, more frequent meals to support optimal energy requirements and healing; avoid overdistention of the stomach; avoid milk and seasonings that are intolerable or that aggravate the condition; and avoid coffee, teas, colas, alcohol beverages (including beer), and citric juices, which may produce discomfort in persons with GERD. Observe for foods that aggravate the condition and eliminate these from the diet.

Pain, discomfort. Keep a written record of the onset, duration, location, and precipitating factors for any pain experienced.

Medications. • Take prescribed medications at recommended times to promote optimal healing. See individual drug monographs for suggested scheduling. • Avoid NSAIDs and aspirin-containing medicines, which are irritating to the gastric mucosa. Consult with the physician or pharmacist regarding scheduling of or discontinuation of these medications.

Lifestyle changes. Discuss stress and its effects on the person and implement needed lifestyle changes that are feasible. Encourage a significant reduction or cessation of smoking. Implement plans to gain sufficient rest.

Fostering health maintenance. • Discuss medication information and how it will benefit the course of treatment to produce an optimal response. Medications used in the treatment of hyperacidity are important measures to alleviate the irritating effects on the mucosal tissue; stress the importance of not discontinuing treatment and the need for continued medical follow-up. • Seek cooperation and understanding of the following points so that medication compliance is increased: name of medication, dosage, route and times of administration, side effects to expect, and side effects to report. • Enlist the patient's aid in developing and maintaining a written record of monitoring parameters (such as list of foods causing problems, degree of pain relief [see box on p. 384], and response to prescribed therapies) for discussion with the physician. Instruct the patient to bring the written record to follow-up visits.

Drug Class: Antacids

Actions

Antacids lower the acidity of gastric secretions by buffering the hydrochloric acid (normal pH is 1 or 2) to a lower hydrogen ion concentration. Buffering hydrochloric acid to a pH of 3 or 4 is highly desired because the proteolytic action of pepsin is reduced and the gastric juice loses its corrosive effect.

Uses

Antacid products account for one of the largest sales volumes (over $1 billion annually) of medication that may be purchased without prescription. Antacids are commonly used for treatment of heartburn, excessive eating and drinking, and PUD. However, nurses and patients must be aware that not all antacids are alike. They should be used judiciously, particularly by certain types of patients. Long-term self-treatment with antacids may also mask symptoms of serious underlying diseases, such as bleeding ulcer.

The most effective antacids available are combinations of aluminum hydroxide, magnesium oxide or hydroxide, magnesium trisilicate, and calcium carbonate. All act by neutralizing gastric acid. Combinations of these ingredients must be used because any compound used alone in therapeutic quantities may also produce severe systemic side effects. Other ingredients found in antacid combination products include simethicone, alginic acid, and bismuth. Simethicone is a defoaming agent that breaks up gas bubbles in the stomach, reducing stomach distention and heartburn. It is effective for use in patients who have overeaten or who suffer from heartburn, but it is not effective in the treatment of PUD. Alginic acid produces a highly viscous solution of sodium alginate that floats on top of the gastric contents. It may be effective only in the patient being treated for GERD or hiatal hernia and should not be used in the patient with acute gastritis or PUD. Bismuth compounds have little acid-neutralizing capacity and are therefore poor antacids.

The following principles should be considered when antacid therapy is being planned:
- For indigestion, antacids should not be administered for more than 2 weeks. If after this time the patient is still experiencing discomfort, a physician should be contacted.
- Patients with edema, congestive heart failure, hypertension, renal failure, pregnancy, or salt-restricted diets should use low-sodium antacids. These products include Riopan, Maalox, and Mylanta II. Therapy should continue only on the recommendation of a physician.
- Antacid tablets should be used only for the patient with occasional indigestion or heartburn. Tablets *do not* contain enough antacid to be effective in treating PUD.
- A common complaint of patients consuming large quantities of calcium carbonate or aluminum hydroxide is constipation. Excess magnesium results in diarrhea. If a patient experiences these symptoms and is still suffering from stomach discomfort, a physician should be consulted.
- Effective management of *acute* ulcer disease requires large volumes of antacids. The selection of an antacid and the quantity to be taken depend on the neutralizing capacity of

PATIENT EDUCATION & MONITORING FORM   Agents Affecting the Digestive System

MEDICATIONS	COLOR	TO BE TAKEN

Name _____

Physician _____

Physician's phone _____

Next appt.* _____

PARAMETERS		DAY OF DISCHARGE							COMMENTS
Bloating	Time it occurs—night, after eating, midday								
	Causes, e.g., food eaten								
Pain: Severity of pain	Time-before/after meals								
	Location								
Severe 10 Moderate 5 Dull 0									
Nausea	Vomiting—describe amount, color, time of day								
	Nausea—no vomiting								
Bowels	Color?								
	No. of stools per day?								
	Soft, watery, or hard?								
Diet: List foods that cause problems									
Degree of relief from medications? Great 10 Good 5 Poor 1									
Appetite? Excellent 10 Good 5 Poor 1									

*Please bring this record with you to your next appointment.
Use the back of this sheet for additional information.

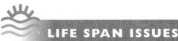

ANTACIDS

Persons over the age of 65 are the most frequent purchasers of antacids. Gastrointestinal disorders occur more often in this age group, such as peptic ulcer disease, NSAID-induced ulcers, and gastroesophageal reflux disease. Magnesium-containing antacids are often used as a laxative. Whereas the symptom of ulcer disease in a younger person is usually burning epigastric pain, the symptoms in an elderly person, if present at all, are usually vague abdominal discomfort, anorexia, and weight loss.

the antacid. Any patient with "coffee ground" hematemesis, bloody stools, or recurrent abdominal pain should seek medical attention immediately and must not attempt to self-treat the disorder.

- Calcium carbonate and sodium bicarbonate may cause rebound hyperacidity.
- Patients with renal failure should not use large quantities of antacids containing magnesium. The magnesium ions cannot be excreted and may produce hypermagnesemia and toxicity.
- Most antacids have similar ingredients. Selection of an antacid for occasional use should be determined by quantity of each ingredient, cost, taste, and frequency of side effects. Patients may need to try more than one product and weigh the advantages and disadvantages of each.

Therapeutic Outcomes

The primary therapeutic outcomes expected from antacid therapy are as follows:
- Relief of discomfort
- Reduced frequency of heartburn
- Healing of irritated tissues

Nursing Process

Premedication Assessment

1. Check renal function studies to ensure that renal function is normal. When renal failure is present, patients should not take large quantities of antacids containing magnesium. Magnesium ions cannot be excreted and may produce hypermagnesemia and toxicity.
2. Check the pattern of bowel elimination for diarrhea or constipation.
3. Record the pattern of gastric pain being experienced; report coffee ground emesis, bloody stools, or recurrent abdominal pain to the physician for prompt attention.
4. If the patient has edema, congestive heart failure, hypertension, or salt restrictions, or is pregnant, ensure that a low-sodium antacid has been prescribed.
5. Schedule other medications prescribed 1 hour before or 2 hours after antacids are to be administered.

Planning

Availability. See Table 30-1. Liquid forms of antacids should be used for treatment of PUD because tablets do not contain enough active ingredients to be effective. Antacid tablets may be used for occasional episodes of heartburn. They should be well chewed before swallowing for a more rapid onset of action.

Implementation

Dosage and administration. See Table 30-1. Follow directions on the product container.

Evaluation

Side effects to expect

CHALKY TASTE. This is a common problem with antacids. Suggest a change in brands or flavors. Suggest using a liquid dosage form instead of tablets.

Side Effects to report

DIARRHEA OR CONSTIPATION. This is a common problem when antacids are being used in therapeutic dosages to treat ulcers. Alternating between calcium- or aluminum-containing compounds and magnesium-containing compounds should help alleviate the problem.

Drug interactions

TETRACYCLINE ANTIBIOTICS, CIPROFLOXACIN, KETOCONAZOLE, DIGOXIN, DIGITOXIN, IRON COMPOUNDS. The absorption of these medicines is inhibited by antacids. These medications should be administered 1 hour before or 2 to 3 hours after the administration of antacids.

LEVODOPA. Levodopa absorption is increased by antacids. When antacid therapy is added, toxicity may result in the parkinsonian patient who is well controlled taking a certain dosage of levodopa. If the patient's parkinsonism is well controlled on levodopa *and* antacid therapy, withdrawal of antacids may result in a recurrence of parkinsonian symptomatology.

QUINIDINE, AMPHETAMINES. Frequent use of antacid therapy may result in increased urinary pH. Renal excretion of quinidine and amphetamines may be inhibited, and toxicity may occur.

Drug Class: Histamine (H₂) Antagonists

Actions

One of the primary mechanisms of hydrochloric acid secretion is stimulation of H₂ receptors on the parietal cells of the stomach by histamine. The H₂ antagonists act by blocking H₂ receptors, resulting in a decrease of the volume of acid secreted. The pH of the stomach contents rises as a result of a reduction in acid.

Uses

The H₂ antagonists—cimetidine, ranitidine, nizatidine, and famotidine—are now being used to treat duodenal ulcers and pathologic hypersecretory conditions, such as Zollinger-Ellison syndrome, and for the prevention and treatment of stress ulcers in critically ill patients. Unapproved uses include prevention of aspiration pneumonitis, GERD, acute upper GI bleeding, and hyperparathyroidism.

Famotidine is similar in action and use to cimetidine but has the apparent advantages of one dose daily, fewer drug interactions, and no antiandrogenic effect (which causes gynecomastia). Ranitidine is similar in action and use to cimetidine but has the apparent advantages of twice-daily dosing, fewer drug interactions, and no antiandrogenic effect. Nizatidine, in contrast to the other agents, is not available in a parenteral dosage form.

Table 30-1

Ingredients of Commonly Used Antacids

PRODUCT	FORM	CALCIUM CARBONATE	ALUMINUM HYDROXIDE	ALUMINUM CARBONATE	MAGNESIUM OXIDE OR HYDROXIDE	MAGNESIUM CARBONATE	SODIUM BICARBONATE	SIMETHICONE	OTHER INGREDIENTS
Aludrox	Tablet, suspension		X		X			X	
Amphojel	Tablet, suspension		X						
Basaljel	Tablet, capsule, suspension			X					
BiSoDol	Tablet, powder				X	X			
Di-Gel	Tablet, liquid		X		X			X	
Gelusil II	Tablet, suspension		X		X			X	
Maalox	Tablet, suspension		X		X				
Maalox Plus	Tablet, suspension		X		X			X	
Mylanta	Tablet, suspension		X		X			X	
Mylanta II	Tablet, suspension		X		X			X	
Phillip's Milk of Magnesia	Tablet, suspension				X				
Phosphaljel*	Suspension								Aluminum phosphate
Riopan	Tablet, suspension								Magaldrate
Riopan Plus	Tablet, suspension							X	Magaldrate
Rolaids	Tablet								Dihydroxyaluminum sodium carbonate
Titralac	Tablet, suspension	X							Glycine
Tums	Tablet	X							
WinGel	Tablet, suspension		X		X				

*No longer classified as an antacid. Used to reduce fecal excretion of phosphates.

Therapeutic Outcomes

The primary therapeutic outcomes expected from H$_2$ antagonist therapy are as follows:
- Relief of discomfort
- Reduced frequency of heartburn
- Healing of irritated tissues

Nursing Process

Premedication Assessment

Perform baseline assessment of the patient's mental status for comparison with subsequent mental status evaluations to detect central nervous system (CNS) alterations that may occur, particularly with cimetidine therapy.

Planning

Availability. See Table 30-2.

Implementation

Dosage and administration. See Table 30-2. Administer cimetidine, famotidine, and ranitidine with food. Nizatidine may be administered with or without food. Because antacid therapy is often continued during early therapy of PUD, administer 1 hour before or 2 hours after the H$_2$ antagonist dose.

Evaluation

Side effects to expect

DIZZINESS, HEADACHES, DIARRHEA, CONSTIPATION, SOMNOLENCE. Approximately 1% to 3% of patients develop these side effects. They are usually mild and resolve with continued therapy. Encourage the patient not to discontinue therapy without first consulting the physician.

Provide for patient safety during episodes of dizziness. If patients develop somnolence and lethargy, encourage them to use caution when working around machinery or driving a car.

Maintain the patient's state of hydration, and obtain an order for stool softeners or bulk-forming laxatives, if necessary. Encourage the inclusion of sufficient roughage (fresh fruits, vegetables, and whole-grain products) in the diet.

Side effects to report

CONFUSION, DISORIENTATION, HALLUCINATIONS. If high dosages are used in patients with liver or renal disease or in patients over 50 years of age, mental confusion, slurred

Table 30-2

Histamine-2 Receptor Antagonists

GENERIC NAME	BRAND NAME	AVAILABILITY	DOSAGE RANGE
Cimetidine	Tagamet, Tagamet HB	Tablets: 100, 200, 300, 400, 800 mg Suspension: 300 mg/5 ml Inj: 300 mg/2 ml	Duodenal and gastric ulcers—PO: 800-1600 mg at bedtime, 400 mg twice daily, or 300 mg four times daily; IM, IV: 300 mg every 6-8 hours GERD—PO: 800 mg twice daily or 400 mg four times daily
Famotodine	Pepcid, Pepcid AC	Tablets: 10, 20, 40 mg Suspension: 40 mg/5 ml Inj: 10 mg/1 ml	Duodenal and gastric ulcers—PO: 40 mg once daily at bedtime or 20 mg twice daily GERD—PO: 20 mg twice daily
Nizatidine	Axid	Capsules: 150, 300 mg	Duodenal and gastric ulcers—PO: 300 mg at bedtime or 150 mg twice daily GERD—PO: 150 mg twice daily
Ranitidine	Zantac, Zantac 75	Tablets: 75, 150, 300 mg Capsules: 150, 300 mg Efferdose granules: 150 mg Efferdose tablets: 150 mg Syrup: 15 mg/ml Inj: 25 mg/ml	Duodenal and gastric ulcers—PO: 300 mg at bedtime or 150 mg twice daily GERD—PO: 150 mg twice daily

speech, disorientation, and hallucinations may occur. This adverse effect dissipates over 3 to 4 days after therapy has been discontinued.

Perform a baseline assessment of the patient's degree of alertness and orientation to name, place, and time before initiating therapy. Make regularly scheduled subsequent mental status evaluations and compare findings. Report development of alterations.

GYNECOMASTIA. Mild bilateral gynecomastia and breast soreness may occur with long-term use (longer than 1 month) of cimetidine but resolve after discontinuation of therapy. Report for further observation and possible laboratory tests.

HEPATOTOXICITY. Although rare, hepatotoxicity has been reported with H$_2$ antagonists. The symptoms of hepatotoxicity are anorexia, nausea, vomiting, jaundice, hepatomegaly, splenomegaly, and abnormal liver function tests (elevated bilirubin, aspartate transaminase [AST], alanine aminotransferase [ALT], gamma glutamyltransferase [GGT], alkaline phosphatase, and prothrombin time).

Drug interactions

BENZODIAZEPINES. Cimetidine inhibits the metabolism or excretion of the following benzodiazepines: alprazolam, chlordiazepoxide, diazepam, clorazepate, flurazepam, halazepam, prazepam, and triazolam.

Patients taking cimetidine and a benzodiazepine concurrently should be observed for increased sedation; a reduction in dosage of the benzodiazepine may be required. The metabolism of temazepam and lorazepam does not appear to be affected.

THEOPHYLLINE DERIVATIVES. Cimetidine inhibits the metabolism or excretion of the following xanthine derivatives: aminophylline, oxtriphylline, dyphylline, and theophylline.

Patients at greater risk include those receiving larger doses of theophylline and those with liver disease. Observe for restlessness, vomiting, dizziness, and cardiac arrhythmias. The dosage of theophylline may need to be reduced.

BETA-ADRENERGIC BLOCKING AGENTS. Beta-adrenergic blocking agents (propranolol, labetalol, and metoprolol) may accumulate as a result of inhibited metabolism. Monitor for signs of toxicity, such as hypotension and bradycardia.

PHENYTOIN. Cimetidine inhibits the metabolism of phenytoin. Monitor patients with concurrent therapy for signs of phenytoin toxicity: nystagmus, sedation, and lethargy. Serum levels may be ordered, and a reduced dosage of phenytoin may be required.

LIDOCAINE, QUINIDINE, PROCAINAMIDE. Cimetidine may inhibit the metabolism of these agents. Monitor patients for signs of toxicity (bradycardia, additional arrhythmias, hyperactivity, and sedation) and reduce the dose if necessary.

ANTACIDS. Administer 1 hour before or 2 hours after administration of cimetidine.

WARFARIN. Cimetidine may enhance the anticoagulant effects of warfarin. Observe for the development of petechiae, ecchymoses, nosebleeds, bleeding gums, dark tarry stools, and bright red or coffee ground emesis. Monitor the prothrombin time and reduce the dosage of warfarin if necessary.

CALCIUM ANTAGONISTS. Cimetidine may inhibit the metabolism of diltiazem, nifedipine, and verapamil. Patients should be monitored for increased effects from the calcium antagonists (bradycardia, hypotension, arrhythmias, and fatigue).

TRICYCLIC ANTIDEPRESSANTS. Cimetidine may inhibit the excretion of imipramine, desipramine, and nortriptyline, usually within 3 to 5 days after the start of cimetidine therapy. If anticholinergic effects or toxicity becomes apparent, a decreased dose of the antidepressant may be required. If cimetidine is discontinued, the patient should be monitored for a decreased response to the antidepressant.

FAMOTIDINE, NIZATIDINE, RANITIDINE. In general, there appear to be only minor interactions with these H₂ antagonists. There are conflicting data, however. Studies indicate that patients receiving higher doses of ranitidine may be more susceptible to drug interactions with ranitidine and other drugs. When used concurrently, monitor for toxic effects of warfarin, theophylline, procainamide, and glipizide.

Drug Class: Gastrointestinal Prostaglandin

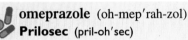

misoprostol (mis-oh′pros-tohl)
Cytotec (site-oh′tech)

Actions

Misoprostol is the first of a new synthetic prostaglandin E series to be used to treat gastrointestinal disorders. Prostaglandins are normally present in the gastrointestinal tract to inhibit gastric acid and pepsin secretion to protect the stomach and duodenal lining against ulceration. The prostaglandin E analogs may also induce uterine contractions.

Uses

Misoprostol is used to prevent and treat gastric ulcers caused by NSAIDs, including aspirin. Whereas prostaglandin inhibition is effective in reducing pain and inflammation, especially in arthritis, prostaglandin inhibition in the stomach makes the patient more predisposed to peptic ulcers.

Therapeutic Outcomes

The primary therapeutic outcomes expected from misoprostol therapy are as follows:
• Relief of discomfort
• Healing of irritated tissues

Nursing Process

Premedication Assessment

1. Determine if the patient is pregnant. This drug is a uterine stimulant and may induce miscarriage.
2. Check the pattern of bowel elimination; misoprostol may induce diarrhea.

Planning

Availability. 100 and 200 µg tablets. WARNING: Misoprostol is contraindicated during pregnancy and in women at risk of becoming pregnant. As a uterine stimulant, it may induce miscarriage.

Implementation

Dosage and administration. Adult: PO—100 to 200 µg tablets 4 times daily with food during NSAID therapy.

Evaluation

Side effects to expect

DIARRHEA. Diarrhea associated with misoprostol therapy is dose related and usually develops after approximately 2 weeks of therapy. It often resolves after about 8 days, but a few patients require discontinuation of misoprostol therapy. Diarrhea can be minimized by taking misoprostol with meals and at bedtime and avoiding magnesium-containing antacids (Maalox, Mylanta).

Encourage the patient not to discontinue therapy without first consulting the physician.

Encourage the inclusion of sufficient roughage (fresh fruits, vegetables, and whole-grain products) in the diet.

Side effects to report

PREGNANCY. Although pregnancy is obviously not a side effect of misoprostol therapy, it is crucial that misoprostol therapy be discontinued if the patient is pregnant. The patient must receive care from the physician who prescribed the misoprostol and an obstetrician. The question of alternative therapies to NSAIDs must also be considered.

Drug interactions

No significant drug interactions have been reported.

Drug Class: Gastric Acid Pump Inhibitors

omeprazole (oh-mep′rah-zol)
Prilosec (pril-oh′sec)

Actions

Omeprazole is the first of a new class of drugs that inhibit gastric secretion by inhibiting the gastric acid pump of the parietal cells of the stomach. Omeprazole has no anticholinergic or H₂-receptor antagonist actions.

Uses

Omeprazole is used to treat severe esophagitis, GERD, gastric and duodenal ulcers, and hypersecretory disorders such as Zollinger-Ellison syndrome.

Therapeutic Outcomes

The primary therapeutic outcomes expected from omeprazole therapy are as follows:
• Relief of discomfort
• Reduced frequency of heartburn
• Healing of irritated tissues

Nursing Process

Premedication Assessment

Check pattern of bowel elimination; omeprazole may induce diarrhea.

Planning

Availability. PO—20 mg sustained-release capsules.

Implementation

Dosage and administration. PO—initially, 20 mg once daily. Dosages up to 120 mg daily in divided doses may be required for certain hypersecretory conditions. Administer before a meal. The capsule should be swallowed whole; instruct the patient not to open, chew, or crush.

Evaluation
Side effects to expect
DIARRHEA, HEADACHE, MUSCLE PAIN, FATIGUE. These symptoms are relatively mild and rarely result in the discontinuation of therapy. Encourage the patient not to discontinue therapy without first consulting the physician.

Maintain the patient's state of hydration. Encourage the inclusion of sufficient roughage (fresh fruits, vegetables, and whole-grain products) in the diet.

Side effects to report
RASH. Persistent vesicular rash may be cause for discontinuation of therapy. Report for further observation and possible laboratory tests.

Drug interactions
DIAZEPAM. Omeprazole significantly increases the half-life of diazepam by inhibiting its metabolism. Observe patients for increased sedative effect of diazepam. Caution against hazardous tasks such as driving and operating machinery. The dosage of diazepam may have to be reduced.

PHENYTOIN. Omeprazole slows the metabolism of phenytoin. Observe for nystagmus, sedation, and lethargy. The dosage of phenytoin may have to be reduced.

WARFARIN. Omeprazole may reduce the rate of metabolism of warfarin. Monitor the patient closely for signs of bleeding tendencies and monitor the prothrombin time closely. Reduction of warfarin dosage may be required.

lansoprazole (lahn-sohp′rah-zol)
Prevacid (prehv-ah-sed′)

Actions
Lansoprazole inhibits gastric secretion by inhibiting the gastric acid pump of the parietal cells of the stomach. Lansoprazole has no anticholinergic or H_2-receptor antagonist actions. It is chemically related to omeprazole.

Uses
Lansoprazole is used to treat severe esophagitis, GERD, gastric and duodenal ulcers, and hypersecretory disorders such as Zollinger-Ellison syndrome.

Therapeutic Outcomes
The primary therapeutic outcomes expected from lansoprazole therapy are as follows:
• Relief of discomfort
• Reduced frequency of heartburn
• Healing of irritated tissues

Nursing Process

Premedication Assessment
Check pattern of bowel elimination; lansoprazole may induce diarrhea.

Planning
Availability. PO—15 and 30 mg sustained-release, enteric-coated capsules.

Implementation
Dosage and administration. PO—initially, 15 to 30 mg once daily. Dosages up to 180 mg daily in divided doses may be required for certain hypersecretory conditions. Larger doses may be divided into a twice-daily administration. Administer before a meal. If the patient has trouble swallowing the capsule, it may be pulled apart and the contents mixed in a tablespoon of applesauce. Instruct the patient not to chew the granules when ingesting the applesauce. Antacids may be administered concomitantly with lansoprazole.

Evaluation
Side effects to expect and report
DIARRHEA, HEADACHE, FATIGUE. These symptoms are relatively mild and rarely cause discontinuation of therapy. Encourage the patient not to discontinue therapy without first consulting the physician.

Maintain the patient's state of hydration. Encourage the inclusion of sufficient roughage (fresh fruits, vegetables, and whole-grain products) in the diet.

Drug interactions
THEOPHYLLINE. Lansoprazole increases the metabolism of theophylline by approximately 10%. A slight increase in theophylline dosage may be required to maintain therapeutic activity.

ALTERED ABSORPTION. The reduction in gastric acid secretion may alter absorption of food and drugs as follows:
• DIGOXIN. Monitor for signs of decreased activity (for example, return of edema, weight gain, and congestive heart failure.
• KETOCONAZOLE, AMPICILLIN, IRON. These medicines require an acid medium for absorption. They should be administered at least 30 to 45 minutes before lansoprazole therapy.
• INSULIN. The absorption of food may be altered, and an adjustment in timing or dosage of insulin in patients with diabetes mellitus may be required.

Drug Class: Coating Agent

sucralfate (sook-rahl′fate)
Carafate (kair-ah′fate)

Actions
Sucralfate is an agent that when swallowed forms a complex that adheres to the crater of an ulcer, protecting it from aggravators such as acid, pepsin, and bile salts. Sucralfate does not inhibit gastric secretions (as do the H_2 antagonists) or alter gastric pH (as do antacids).

Uses
Sucralfate is used to treat duodenal ulcers, particularly in those patients who do not tolerate other forms of therapy.

Therapeutic Outcomes
The primary therapeutic outcomes expected from sucralfate therapy are as follows:
• Relief of discomfort
• Healing of irritated tissues

Premediation Assessment
Check pattern of bowel elimination; sucralfate may induce constipation.

Planning
Availability. PO—1 g tablets.

Implementation
Dosage and administration. Adult: PO—1 tablet 1 hour before each meal and at bedtime, all on an empty stomach. Because antacid therapy is often continued during early therapy of ulcer disease, administer antacids at least one-half hour before or after sucralfate.

Evaluation
Side effects to expect
CONSTIPATION, DRY MOUTH, DIZZINESS. These side effects are usually mild and tend to resolve with continued therapy. Encourage the patient not to discontinue therapy without first consulting the physician.

Measures to alleviate dry mouth include sucking on ice chips or hard candy. Avoid mouthwashes that contain alcohol because they cause further drying and irritation.

Maintain the patient's state of hydration, and obtain an order for stool softeners or bulk-forming laxatives if necessary. Encourage the inclusion of sufficient roughage (fresh fruits, vegetables, and whole-grain products) in the diet.

Provide for patient safety during episodes of dizziness.
Drug interactions
TETRACYCLINES. Sucralfate may interfere with the absorption of tetracycline. Administer tetracyclines 1 hour before or 2 hours after sucralfate.

Drug Class: Prokinetic Agents

cisapride (sis-ah-pried')
Propulsid (pro-puhl-sid')

Actions
Cisapride stimulates gastrointestinal motility by stimulating cholinergic nerve fibers. It may also stimulate serotonin type 4 (5-HT$_4$) receptors to promote GI motility. Cisapride increases lower esophageal sphincter pressure and esophageal motility, accelerates gastric emptying and intestinal transit, and increases colonic emptying with increased frequency of stools. Cisapride is chemically related to metoclopramide but is a much weaker dopamine antagonist, so it is unlikely to produce extrapyramidal symptoms. Cisapride does not have antiemetic activity and does not cause CNS depression.

Uses
Cisapride is used to treat the symptoms of GERD when changes in lifestyle and diet are not sufficient to relieve the patient's symptoms.

Therapeutic Outcomes
The primary therapeutic outcomes expected from cisapride therapy are as follows:
• Relief of discomfort

• Reduced frequency of heartburn
• Healing of irritated tissues

Premediation Assessment
1. Determine if other drugs being taken may induce extrapyramidal symptoms; do not administer drug concurrently.
2. Check for a history of epilepsy. If present, check with the physician before initiating drug therapy.
3. Do not give to an individual with symptoms of gastrointestinal perforation, mechanical obstruction, or hemorrhage.
4. For diabetic patients, food absorption may be altered and more frequent monitoring for hypoglycemia may be required.

Planning
Availability. PO—10 and 20 mg tablets.

Implementation
Dosage and administration. Adult: PO—initially, 10 mg 4 times daily. Administer on an empty stomach at least 15 minutes before meals to maintain relatively consistent absorption. The dosage may be increased to 20 mg 4 times daily. *Note:* If extrapyramidal symptoms should develop, treat with diphenhydramine.

Evaluation
Side effects to expect
HEADACHE, INSOMNIA, DIARRHEA, RHINITIS, NAUSEA. These side effects are usually mild and tend to resolve with continued therapy. Encourage the patient not to discontinue therapy without first consulting the physician.
Side effects to report
EXTRAPYRAMIDAL SYMPTOMS. Provide for patient safety, then report immediately.
Drug interactions
DRUGS THAT DECREASE THERAPEUTIC EFFECTS. Anticholinergic agents (atropine, benztropine, antihistamines, and dicyclomine) and narcotic analgesics (meperidine, morphine, oxycodone, and others). Instruct the patient to try to avoid the use of these agents while using cisapride.

DRUGS THAT ENHANCE TOXIC EFFECTS. Ketoconazole, itraconazole, miconazole, and troleandomycin significantly inhibit the metabolism of cisapride, leading to cardiac arrhythmias. Administration of any of these medicines with cisapride is contraindicated.

ALTERED ABSORPTION. The gastrointestinal stimulatory effects of cisapride may alter absorption of food and drugs as follows:
• DIGOXIN. Monitor for signs of decreased activity (for example, return of edema, weight gain, and heart failure).
• LEVODOPA. Monitor for signs of increased activity (for example, restlessness, nightmares, hallucinations, additional involuntary movements such as bobbing of head and neck, facial grimacing, and active tongue movements).
• ALCOHOL. Monitor for signs of sedation and drunkenness with smaller amounts of alcohol.
• INSULIN. The absorption of food may be altered; an adjustment in timing or dosage of insulin in patients with diabetes mellitus may be required.

metoclopramide (met-oh-klo′prah-myd)
Reglan (reg′lan)

Actions

Metoclopramide is a gastric stimulant the mechanisms of action of which are not fully known. It increases lower esophageal sphincter pressure reducing reflux, increases stomach contractions, relaxes the pyloric valve, and increases peristalsis in the gastrointestinal tract, resulting in an increased rate of gastric emptying and intestinal transit. Metoclopramide is thought to work as an antiemetic by blocking dopamine in the chemoreceptor trigger zone. It has also been proposed that it inhibits serotonin (5-HT$_3$) when administered in higher dosages.

Uses

Metoclopramide is used to relieve the symptoms of gastric reflux esophagitis and diabetic gastroparesis, as an aid in small bowel intubation, and to stimulate gastric emptying and intestinal transit of barium after radiologic examination of the upper GI tract. It is also an antiemetic for vomiting associated with cancer chemotherapy.

Therapeutic Outcomes

The primary therapeutic outcomes expected from metoclopramide therapy are as follows:
* Relief of discomfort
* Reduced frequency of heartburn
* Healing of irritated tissues

Nursing Process

Premedication Assessment

1. Determine if other drugs being taken may induce extrapyramidal symptoms; do not administer drug concurrently.
2. Check for a history of epilepsy. If present, check with the physician before initiating drug therapy.
3. Do not administer to an individual with symptoms of gastrointestinal perforation, mechanical obstruction, or hemorrhage.
4. For diabetic patients, food absorption may be altered and more frequent monitoring for hypoglycemia may be required.

Planning

Availability. PO—5 and 10 mg tablets and 5 mg per 5 ml syrup. Injection—5 mg per ml in 2, 10, and 30 ml ampules.
Caution. Approximately 1 in 500 patients may develop extrapyramidal symptoms manifested by restlessness, involuntary movements, facial grimacing, and possibly oculogyric crisis, torticollis, or rhythmic protrusion of the tongue. Children and young adults are most susceptible, as are those receiving higher doses of metoclopramide as an antiemetic. Metoclopramide should not be used in patients with epilepsy or in patients receiving drugs that are likely to cause extrapyramidal reactions (such as phenothiazines) because the frequency and severity of seizures or extrapyramidal reactions may be increased. Metoclopramide must not be used in patients when increased gastric motility may be dangerous, such as in cases of gastrointestinal perforation, mechanical obstruction, or hemorrhage.

Implementation

Dosage and administration. Adult: PO—diabetic gastroparesis, 10 mg 30 minutes before each meal and at bedtime. Duration of therapy is dependent on response and continued well-being after discontinuation of therapy. IV—antiemesis, initial two doses, 2 mg/kg. If vomiting is suppressed, follow with 1 mg/kg. Dilute the dose in 50 ml of parenteral solution (D$_5$W, normal saline 0.9%, D$_5$/0.45 normal saline, Ringer's solution, or lactated Ringer's solution). Infuse over at least 15 minutes, 30 minutes before beginning chemotherapy. Repeat every 2 hours for two doses, followed by one dose every 3 hours for three doses. NOTE: Rapid IV infusion may cause sudden, intense anxiety and restlessness, followed by drowsiness. If extrapyramidal symptoms should develop, treat with diphenhydramine.

Evaluation

Side effects to expect

DROWSINESS, FATIGUE, LETHARGY, DIZZINESS, NAUSEA. These side effects are usually mild and tend to resolve with continued therapy. Encourage the patient not to discontinue therapy without first consulting the physician.

People who are working around machinery, driving a car, or performing other duties that require mental alertness should be particularly cautious.

Provide for patient safety during episodes of dizziness.

Side effects to report

EXTRAPYRAMIDAL SYMPTOMS. Provide for patient safety, then report immediately.

Drug interactions

DRUGS THAT INCREASE SEDATIVE EFFECTS. Antihistamines, alcohol, analgesics, tranquilizers, and sedative-hypnotics. Monitor the patient for excessive sedation, and reduce dosage if necessary.

DRUGS THAT DECREASE THERAPEUTIC EFFECTS. Anticholinergic agents (atropine, benztropine, antihistamines, and dicyclomine) and narcotic analgesics (meperidine, morphine, oxycodone, and others). Instruct the patient to try to avoid the use of these agents while using metoclopramide.

ALTERED ABSORPTION. The gastrointestinal stimulatory effects of metoclopramide may alter absorption of food and drugs as follows:
* DIGOXIN. Monitor for signs of decreased activity (for example, return of edema, weight gain, and congestive heart failure).
* LEVODOPA. Monitor for signs of increased activity (for example, restlessness, nightmares, hallucinations, and additional involuntary movements such as bobbing of head and neck, facial grimacing, and active tongue movements).
* ALCOHOL. Monitor for signs of sedation and drunkenness with smaller amounts of alcohol.
* INSULIN. The absorption of food may be altered; an adjustment in timing or dosage of insulin in patients with diabetes mellitus may be required.

Drug Class: Antispasmodic Agents

Actions

Drugs used as antispasmodic agents are actually anticholinergic agents. The GI tract is heavily innervated by the cholinergic branch of the autonomic nervous system. Cholinergic fibers stimulate the GI tract, causing secretion of saliva, hydrochloric acid, pepsin, bile, and other enzymatic fluids necessary for digestion; relaxation of sphincter muscles; and peristalsis to move the contents of the stomach and bowel through the GI tract. The antispasmodic agents act by preventing acetylcholine from attaching to the cholinergic receptors in the GI tract. The extent of reduction of cholinergic activity depends on the amount of anticholinergic drug blocking the receptors. Inhibition of cholinergic nerve conduction results in decreased GI motility and reduced secretions.

Because cholinergic fibers innervate the entire body and these agents are not selective in their actions in the GI tract, the effects of blocking this system are seen throughout the body. To provide adequate doses to inhibit gastrointestinal motility and secretions, the following effects will occur: reduction in perspiration and oral and bronchial secretions; mydriasis (dilation of the pupils) with blurring of vision; constipation; urinary hesitancy or retention; tachycardia, possibly with palpitations; and mild, transient postural hypotension. Psychiatric disturbances, such as mental confusion, delusions, nightmares, euphoria, paranoia, and hallucinations, may be indications of overdosage.

Uses

Antispasmodic agents are used to treat irritable bowel syndrome, biliary spasm, mild ulcerative colitis, diverticulitis, pancreatitis, infant colic, and, in conjunction with diet and antacids, PUD. Since the advent of the histamine H_2 antagonists, antispasmodic agents are used much less frequently in the treatment of ulcers.

Therapeutic Outcomes

The primary therapeutic outcomes expected from antispasmodic therapy are as follows:
• Relief of discomfort
• Reduced frequency of heartburn
• Healing of irritated tissues

Nursing Process

Premedication Assessment
1. Check the patient's history to screen for presence of closed-angle glaucoma; use of antispasmodic therapy in a

Table 30-3
Antispasmodic Agents

Generic Name	Brand Name	Availability	Clinical Uses	Initial Dosage
Anisotropine	Valpin 50	Tablets: 50 mg	Peptic ulcer disease	PO: 50 mg 3 times daily
Atropine	Atropine Sulfate	Inj: 0.05, 0.1, 0.3, 0.4, 0.5, 0.8, 1 mg/ml Tablets: 0.4 mg	Treatment of pylorospasm and spastic conditions of the GI tract	PO: 0.4-0.6 mg
Belladonna	Belladonna Tincture	Tincture: 30 mg/100 ml	Indigestion, peptic ulcer Nocturnal enuresis Parkinsonism	Tincture—PO: 0.6-1 mg 3-4 times daily
Clidinium bromide	Quarzan	Capsules: 2.5, 5 mg	Peptic ulcer disease	PO: 2.5-5 mg 3-4 times daily
Dicyclomine	Bentyl, Antispas, ✿ Bentylol	Tablets: 20 mg Capsules: 10, 20 mg Syrup: 10 mg/5 ml Inj: 10 mg/ml	Irritable bowel syndrome Infant colic	Adults—PO: 20-40 mg 3-4 times daily Infants—PO: 5 mg 3-4 times daily
Glycopyrrolate	Robinul	Tablets: 1, 2 mg Inj: 0.2 mg/ml	Peptic ulcer disease	PO: 1 mg 2-3 times daily
Isopropamide	Darbid	Tablets: 5 mg	Peptic ulcer disease	PO: 5 mg every 12 hours
Mepenzolate	Cantil	Tablets: 25 mg	Peptic ulcer disease	PO: 25-50 mg 4 times daily
Methantheline	Banthine	Tablets: 50 mg	Peptic ulcer disease	PO: 50-100 mg every 6 hours
Methscopolamine	Pamine	Tablets: 2.5 mg	Peptic ulcer disease	PO: 2.5 mg 30 min before meals and 2.5-5 mg at bedtime
Propantheline	Pro-Banthine	Tablets: 7.5, 15 mg	Peptic ulcer disease	PO: 15 mg before meals and 30 mg at bedtime
Scopolamine	Scopolamine, ✿ Buscopan	Inj: 0.3, 0.4, 1 mg/ml	GI hypermotility, pylorospasm, irritable colon syndrome	SC or IM: 0.32-0.65 mg
Tridihexethyl chloride	Pathilon	Tablets: 25 mg	Peptic ulcer disease	PO: 25-50 mg 3-4 times daily before meals and at bedtime

✿ Available in Canada only.

patient with this condition could initiate an acute attack of closed-angle glaucoma.

2. Perform a baseline mental status examination for future comparison of subsequent findings; these medicines may cause confusion, depression, nightmares, or hallucinations. These symptoms should be reported if they occur.

3. Obtain a baseline blood pressure and plan to monitor blood pressure for orthostatic hypotension, a common drug side effect.

4. Use these drugs with caution in the elderly and in patients with any condition in which gastrointestinal transit time is compromised because anticholinergic agents slow peristalsis.

Planning

Availability. See Table 30-3.

Glaucoma. All patients should be screened for the presence of closed-angle glaucoma before the initiation of therapy. Patients with open-angle glaucoma can safely use anticholinergic agents. Intraocular pressure should be monitored on a regular basis.

Implementation

Dosage and administration. See Table 30-3. Administer with food or milk to minimize gastric irritation.

Evaluation

Side effects to expect

BLURRED VISION, CONSTIPATION, URINARY RETENTION, DRYNESS OF THE MOUTH, NOSE, AND THROAT. These symptoms are the anticholinergic effects produced by these agents. Patients taking these medications should be monitored for the development of these side effects.

Dryness of the mucosa may be alleviated by sucking hard candy or ice chips or by chewing gum.

If patients develop urinary hesitancy, assess for bladder distention. Report to the physician for further evaluation.

Give stool softeners as prescribed. Encourage adequate fluid intake and foods that provide sufficient bulk.

Caution the patient that blurred vision may occur, and make appropriate suggestions for personal safety of the individual.

Side effects to report

CONFUSION, DEPRESSION, NIGHTMARES, HALLUCINATIONS. Perform a baseline assessment of the patient's degree of alertness and orientation to name, place, and time *before* initiating therapy. Make regularly scheduled subsequent mental status evaluations and compare findings. Report development of alterations.

Provide for patient safety during these episodes.

Reduction in the daily dosage may control these adverse effects.

ORTHOSTATIC HYPOTENSION. All antispasmodic agents may cause some degree of orthostatic hypotension, although it is infrequent and generally mild. It is manifested by dizziness and weakness, particularly when therapy is being initiated.

Monitor the blood pressure daily in both the supine and standing positions.

Anticipate the development of postural hypotension and take measures to prevent an occurrence. Teach the patient to rise slowly from a supine or sitting position. Encourage the patient to sit or lie down if feeling faint.

PALPITATIONS, ARRHYTHMIAS. Report for further evaluation.

Drug interactions

AMANTADINE, TRICYCLIC ANTIDEPRESSANTS, PHENOTHIAZINES. These agents may potentiate the anticholinergic side effects. Development of confusion and hallucinations is characteristic of excessive anticholinergic activity.

CHAPTER REVIEW

Gastroesophageal reflux disease and peptic ulcer disease continue to be common illnesses that are initially self-treated. The nurse should solicit information about whether symptoms have decreased and whether the patient is suffering adverse effects from therapy. The nurse is also an ideal health professional to assess and make recommendations regarding lifestyle changes that are necessary to prevent recurrence of symptoms. If symptoms have not begun to diminish over 2 weeks, the nurse should encourage the person to seek medical attention.

MATH REVIEW

1. Ordered: ranitidine (Zantac) 50 mg in 100 ml D_5W IV over 20 minutes.
   Using an infusion pump, calibrated in milliliters per hour, at what rate would the infusion pump be set?
   Give at a rate of:_____ml/hr (infusion pump).

2. Ordered: Pepcid 35 mg PO stat.
   On hand, Pepcid 40 mg/ml oral suspension.
   Give_____ml.

CRITICAL THINKING QUESTIONS

1. Miss Cantell, age 45, has PUD and seems unaware that lifestyle changes are needed to treat the disorder. She has an H_2 antagonist ordered. What teaching approaches would be appropriate for her?

2. Martha Waters is complaining of intermittent diarrhea. No physical basis for the diarrhea has been identified. She also complains of heartburn. Explore self-treatments available with over-the-counter medicines that could cause the diarrhea.

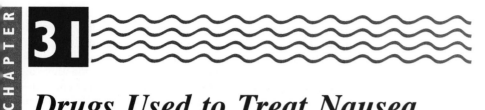

Drugs Used to Treat Nausea and Vomiting

Objectives

1. Compare the purposes of using antiemetic products.
2. State the therapeutic classes of antiemetics.
3. Discuss scheduling of antiemetics for maximum benefit.

Key Words

postoperative nausea and vomiting (PONV)

hyperemesis gravidarum

chemotherapy-induced emesis (CIE)

anticipatory nausea and vomiting

delayed emesis

NAUSEA AND VOMITING

Nausea is the sensation of abdominal discomfort that is intermittently accompanied by a desire to vomit. Vomiting is the forceful expulsion of gastric contents up the esophagus and out the mouth. Nausea may occur without vomiting, and sudden vomiting may occur without prior nausea, but the two symptoms often occur together.

Nausea and vomiting are common symptoms experienced by virtually everyone at one time or another. They are symptoms that accompany almost any illness. Nausea and vomiting may be due to a wide variety of causes (see box on right).

There are several physiologic mechanisms of nausea and vomiting, and none is well understood. It is known that the vomiting center in the brain transmits impulses after receiving certain stimuli and that the stomach and duodenum respond to these impulses in the form of nausea and vomiting.

Common Causes

Postoperative Nausea and Vomiting

Postoperative nausea and vomiting (PONV) is a relatively common complication after surgery. The incidence of nausea and vomiting varies with the surgical procedure, gender, age, anesthetic procedure, and analgesia used. A previous history of motion sickness and PONV are also indicators of the likelihood of developing this postoperative complication. Pain not treated with appropriate analgesia also induces nausea and vomiting. Surgical procedures that have a higher incidence of PONV are extraocular muscle and middle ear manipulations, testicular traction, and abdominal surgery. Women have a higher incidence of PONV, possibly because of hormonal differences, and children ages 11 to 14 have the highest incidence based on age groups. General anesthesia has a higher incidence of PONV than regional anesthesia; however, analgesics (for example, morphine, meperidine, fentanyl, alfentanil) used as premedications or with regional anesthetics frequently induce nausea and vomiting. Nitrous oxide anesthesia has a higher incidence of nausea and vomiting than halothane, enflurane, or isoflurane. Swallowed

Causes of Nausea and Vomiting

Infection
Gastrointestinal disorders such as gastritis, liver, gallbladder, or pancreatic disease
Overeating or irritation of the stomach by certain foods or liquids
Motion sickness
Drug therapy (nausea and vomiting are the most common side effects of drug therapy)
Emotional disturbances and mental illness
Pregnancy
Pain and unpleasant sights and odors
Chemotherapy and radiation therapy

blood and gas accumulation in the stomach also induce nausea and vomiting.

Motion Sickness

Nausea and vomiting associated with motion are thought to result from stimulation of the labyrinth system of the ear, with subsequent transmission of this stimulus to the vestibular network located near the vomiting center. When there is strong or frequent stimulation, such as from a rocking ship or airplane, the vestibular network is bombarded with an abnormally high number of impulses that radiate by cholinergic nerve impulses to the adjacent vomiting center. Thus drugs that inhibit the cholinergic nerve impulses from the vestibular network to the vomiting center should be effective in the treatment of motion sickness.

Nausea and Vomiting in Pregnancy

The frequency of women reporting vomiting after the first 16 weeks of gestation is relatively constant at about 40%, decreasing to 20% during the 17- to 20-week interval, with only 9% of women complaining of vomiting after 20 weeks of pregnancy. Vomiting is significantly more common among primigravidas, younger women, women with less education, nonsmokers, blacks, and obese women. Contrary to commonly held beliefs, vomiting is not more common among women who have experienced prior fetal losses or among women with hypertension, proteinuria, diabetes, or those who used diethylstilbestrol. There is also no association with vomiting and cohabitation, unplanned pregnancy, or gallbladder, liver, or thyroid disease.

Although traditionally described as "morning sickness," the majority of women report that symptoms of nausea and vomiting tend to persist to varying degrees throughout the day. The cause of morning sickness is unknown, but its occurrence and severity appear to be related to the levels of free and bound estradiol and sex hormone–binding globulin binding capacity.

A woman with severe persistent vomiting that interferes with nutrition, fluid, and electrolyte balance may be suffering from **hyperemesis gravidarum,** a condition in which starvation, dehydration, and acidosis are superimposed on the vomiting syndrome. Hospitalization for fluid, electrolyte, and nutritional therapy may be required.

Psychogenic Vomiting

Psychogenic vomiting can be self-induced, or it can occur involuntarily in response to situations that the person considers threatening or distasteful (for example, eating food whose origin is considered repulsive).

Chemotherapy-Induced Emesis

Chemotherapy-induced emesis (CIE) is the most unpleasant adverse effect associated with the use of cancer chemotherapy. Many patients regard it as the most stressful aspect of their disease, more so even than the prospect of dying. Because the object of therapy is to prolong life for a relatively short period, the effect of CIE on the quality of life must be considered.

Three types of emesis have been identified in patients receiving antineoplastic therapy: anticipatory nausea and vomiting, acute CIE, and delayed emesis.

Anticipatory nausea and vomiting is a conditioned response triggered by the sight or smell of the clinic or hospital or by the knowledge that treatment is imminent. The onset of anticipatory nausea and vomiting is usually 2 to 4 hours before treatment and is most severe at the time of chemotherapy administration. Patients who experience anticipatory nausea and vomiting are more likely be younger and to have received about twice as many courses of chemotherapy with more drugs for about three times as long as patients who do not experience this complication.

Acute CIE may be stimulated directly by chemotherapeutic agents. This type of emesis may begin within 1 to 6 hours after chemotherapy is administered and last for up to 24 hours. The emetogenic potential of antineoplastic drugs is highly variable, ranging from an incidence of almost 100% with high-dose cisplatin to less than 10% with chlorambucil. Table 31-1 summarizes chemotherapeutic agents in terms of emetogenicity. Emetogenicity is also influenced by dose, duration, and frequency of administration.

Patient factors also affect acute CIE. The incidence and severity of CIE are generally greater among older people, those in poor general health, and those with metabolic disorders (for example, uremia, dehydration, infection, or

Table 31-1

Potential of Emesis with Chemotherapeutic Agents	
AGENT	**FREQUENCY OF EMESIS**

Very high emetical potential
  Cisplatin
  Dacarbazine
  Mustine
  Streptozocin
	>90%

High emetic potential
  BCNU (carmustine)
  Cyclophosphamide
  (dose dependent)
  Mithramycin
  Procarbazine
  (dose dependent)
	60%-90%

Moderate emetic potential
  Adriamycin
  Daunorubicin
  5-Fluorouracil
	30%-60%

Low emetic potential
  Bleomycin
  Cytarabine
  Etoposide
  Methotrexate
  6-Mercaptopurine
  Tamoxifen
  Vinblastine
  (dose dependent)
	10%-30%

Very low emetic potential
  Chlorambucil
  Corticosteroids
	<10%

Modified from Borson HL, McCarthy LE: Neuropharmacology of chemotherapy-induced emesis, *Drugs* 25(suppl 1):8, 1983.

gastrointestinal obstruction). Patients with a history of motion sickness seem to be more sensitive to the emetic effects of cytotoxic agents. The patient's outlook and attitude about cancer and therapy can significantly influence the frequency and severity of emesis.

Delayed emesis occurs 24 to 120 hours after the administration of chemotherapy. The mechanism is not known, but it may be induced by metabolic by-products of the chemotherapeutic agent or by destruction of malignant cells. The emesis experienced is usually less severe than that which occurs acutely, but it can still be of significance in reducing activity, nutrition, and hydration. Events that often trigger delayed nausea and vomiting are brushing teeth, using mouthwash, manipulation of dentures, seeing food, and quickly standing up after getting out of bed in the morning.

Drug Therapy

Control of vomiting is important, not only to relieve the obvious distress associated with vomiting, but also to prevent aspiration of gastric contents into the lungs, dehydration, and electrolyte imbalance. Primary treatment of nausea and vomiting should be directed at the underlying cause. Because this is not always possible, treatment with both nondrug and drug measures is appropriate. Most medicines (antiemetics) used to treat nausea and vomiting act either by suppressing the action of the vomiting center or inhibiting the impulses going to or coming from the center. These agents are generally more effective if administered before the onset of nausea, rather than after the vomiting has already started. The six classes of agents used as antiemetics are dopamine antagonists, serotonin antagonists, anticholinergic agents, corticosteroids, benzodiazepines, and cannabinoids.

Postoperative Nausea and Vomiting

As seen from the preceding description, there is no single cause of PONV, and therefore treatment with a single pharmacologic agent for all cases is unlikely. Measures such as limiting patient movement and preventing gastric distention can reduce PONV. Adequate analgesia can also forestall this complication. Nonsteroidal antiinflammatory drugs are not emetogenic (opioids are emetogenic) and should be given consideration if appropriate to the type of surgical procedure. Antiemetics used include dopamine antagonists, anticholinergic agents, and serotonin antagonists. The H_2 antagonists (for example, cimetidine, ranitidine) are also occasionally used to reduce gastric secretions to minimize nausea and vomiting.

Postoperative nausea and vomiting is usually handled with a prn order. The first step in treating the nausea and vomiting is to identify the cause. If a nasogastric tube is in place, check its patency and placement in preventing abdominal distention. Do not move a nasogastric tube that was inserted during surgery (for example, gastric resection); in such cases there is a danger of penetrating the suture line. Irrigations of a blocked nasogastric tube may alleviate the nausea and vomiting. (A physician's order to irrigate the nasogastric tube is required.) Administration of prn antiemetics when the patient first complains of nausea often prevents vomiting.

Motion Sickness

Most agents used to reduce nausea and vomiting from motion sickness are chemically related to antihistamines. The effectiveness of antihistamines in motion sickness probably results from their anticholinergic properties, not from their ability to block histamine.

Nausea and Vomiting in Pregnancy

In most cases, morning sickness can be controlled by dietary measures alone. The woman should be advised to eat small, frequent, dry meals and to avoid fatty foods and other foods found to cause problems. Sometimes it may be difficult or impossible to work in the kitchen, and assistance in this area may be required.

In approximately 15% of cases, dietary measures alone will be insufficient and drug therapy should be considered. Drugs that have been extensively used for the treatment of morning sickness are the phenothiazines, such as promethazine and prochlorperazine, and the antihistamines, such as diphenhydramine, dimenhydrinate, meclizine, and cyclizine. From a safety standpoint, meclizine, cyclizine, or dimenhydrinate is generally recommended first. If persistent vomiting threatens maternal nutrition, promethazine may be considered. If antidopaminergic antiemetic therapy is required, prochlorperazine is the most time-tested from a safety standpoint. Metoclopramide has been shown to be an effective antiemetic in treating hyperemesis gravidarum, and no teratogenic effects have been reported to date.

Psychogenic Vomiting

When a person has chronic or recurrent vomiting, a diagnosis of psychogenic vomiting is made after elimination of all other possible causes. The person with psychogenic vomiting usually does not lose weight and is able to control vomiting in certain situations (for example, in public). The identification of the causes of psychogenic vomiting and the successful resolution of the problem may not be possible. After an extensive workup eliminates other potential causes, a short course of an antiemetic drug such as metoclopramide or an antianxiety drug may be prescribed, along with counseling.

Anticipatory Nausea and Vomiting

Persons with a negative attitude toward therapy, such as the belief that it will be of no benefit, are more likely to develop anticipatory nausea and vomiting. It tends to become more severe as treatments progress unless behavior therapy modifies the conditioned response. Such treatments include progressive muscle relaxation, mind diversion, hypnosis, self-hypnosis, and systematic desensitization. Nurses can play a significant role by maintaining a positive, supportive attitude with the patient and making sure the patient receives antiemetic therapy before each course of chemotherapy.

Chemotherapy-Induced Emesis

Antiemetic therapy to minimize acute CIE is based on the emetogenic potential of the antineoplastic agents being used. Combinations of antiemetics are often used, based on the assumption that antineoplastic agents produce emesis by more than one mechanism. In general, all patients being treated with chemotherapeutic agents of moderate to very high emetogenic potential should receive prophylactic antiemetic therapy before chemotherapy is started. Combinations of ondansetron or granisetron, high-dose metoclopramide, dexamethasone, lorazepam, and diphenhydramine are often used. Haloperidol may be substituted for metoclopramide if the latter is not tolerated by the patient. Antiemetic therapy should be continued for 4 to 7 days to prevent delayed vomiting. Emesis induced by moderately emetogenic agents may be treated prophylactically with metoclopramide and dexamethasone, and therapy should be continued for 24 hours. A phenothiazine (prochlorperazine) or dexamethasone alone is recommended if the chemotherapy is of low emetic potential. All antiemetics should be administered an adequate time before chemotherapy is initiated and should be continued an appropriate time after the antineoplastic agent has been discontinued.

Delayed Emesis

A combination of prochlorperazine, lorazepam, and diphenhydramine given orally 1 hour before meals has been successful in controlling delayed emesis.

Nursing Process for Nausea and Vomiting

Nausea and vomiting is associated with illnesses of the gastrointestinal tract and other body systems and with side effects of medications and food intolerance. Nursing care must be individualized to the patient's diagnosis and needs at all times.

Premedication Assessment

History. • Obtain a history of the patient's symptoms— onset, duration, frequency, volume, and description of the vomitus (for example, color: "coffee ground," greenish yellow, or red tinged; and consistency: undigested food particles). • Ask the patient's perception of the precipitating factors (for example, foods, odors, medications, stress, treatment [chemotherapy, radiation therapy, surgery]).

Medications. Ask the patient to give a listing of all current medications being taken that are over-the-counter or prescribed by a physician. Are any used to treat nausea and vomiting?

Basic assessment. Individualize the assessment procedure to the underlying etiology of the symptoms, if known.

Vital signs. Obtain baseline vital signs, height, and weight.

Abdomen. Assess bowel sounds in all four quadrants of the abdomen. Observe the size and shape of the abdomen. Note any signs of distention, ascites, or masses.

Hydration. Assess and record signs of hydration. Examine for poor skin turgor, sticky oral mucous membranes, excessive thirst, shrunken and deeply furrowed tongue, crusted lips, weight loss, deteriorating vital signs, soft or sunken eyeballs, delayed capillary filling, high urine specific gravity or no urine output, and possible mental confusion.

Laboratory studies. Review laboratory reports for indications of malabsorption, protein depletion, dehydration, fluid, electrolyte and acid-base imbalances, and so on (for example, K^+, Cl^-, pH, pCO_2, bicarbonate, Hgb, Hct, urinalysis [specific gravity], serum albumin, and total protein). The scope of laboratory data gathered will depend on the underlying etiology of the nausea and vomiting and severity of the symptoms.

Nursing Diagnosis
- Fluid volume, deficit (indication)
- Nutrition, altered: less than body requirements (indication)

Planning
History. Plan to perform a focused assessment consistent with the symptoms and underlying pathology.

Medications. • Schedule prescribed medications on the medication administration record (MAR) and requisition the medicines from the pharmacy. • Ensure that prechemotherapy and preradiation therapy antiemetics are marked precisely as ordered on the MAR along with around-the-clock or prn orders.

Nursing interventions. • Mark the Kardex with specific parameters to be recorded: intake and output, vital signs every shift or more frequently depending on patient's status, and daily weights. • Mark the Kardex with any requested testing of the vomitus (for example, presence of blood, pH). • Schedule oral hygiene measures.

Nutrition. • Obtain specific orders relating to nutrition. Diet orders will depend on the underlying etiology and severity of the nausea and vomiting. • Mark the Kardex regarding nutrition status (for example, nothing by mouth [NPO], nasogastric suction, intravenous [IV] fluids, enteral or parenteral nutrition). • As the patient's condition improves, obtain diet orders for a gradual progression of diet.

Laboratory studies. Order baseline laboratory studies requested by the physician, such as electrolytes, white blood cell count with differential, hemoglobin, hematocrit, and albumin. The extent of laboratory studies will depend on the underlying etiology and the patient's clinical condition.

Implementation
Maintain hydration via oral or parenteral forms as prescribed by the physician.

Adults. The usual treatment includes discontinuation of solid foods and the ingestion of oral rehydration solutions or clear juices. Depending on the severity of the condition or underlying etiology, the patient may be NPO with a nasogastric tube in place to provide a route for hydration.

As the patient's condition improves, the diet is advanced from clear liquids to small, frequent, low-fat feedings to bland diet or normal diet. Generally, high-fat foods, milk products, whole grains, and raw fruits and vegetables are initially avoided.

Infants. Generally, formula, milk products, and solid foods are discontinued. Fluids are offered every 30 to 60 minutes in small amounts (30 to 60 ml). The volume is gradually increased as tolerance improves. Oral rehydration solutions (for example, Pedialyte, dilute Jell-O water, decarbonated colas, ginger ale) may be offered.

- Monitor for intolerance to lactose when formula is reintroduced. Formula is generally given in a diluted form when reinitiated and gradually increased to full strength.
- Monitor hydration status using vital signs, skin turgor, daily weights, and moisture of mucous membranes.
- Perform a physical assessment every shift and a focused assessment at intervals consistent with the patient's status and underlying pathology.

- Initiate hygiene measures to provide for patient comfort during and after emesis. Oral hygiene should be scheduled at intervals whenever a nasogastric tube is in place, the patient has stomatitis, or the condition warrants it.
- Institute aspiration precautions, as appropriate.
- Initiate measures to eliminate factors that contribute to nausea and vomiting (for example, irritating foods, odors, or medications).
- Give antiemetics as prescribed or recommended. With post-surgical patients, administer when symptoms of nausea first occur. Administer before chemotherapy and radiation therapy; depending on treatment, schedule on an around-the-clock basis after chemotherapy and radiation therapy. Administer 30 to 60 minutes before undertaking an activity known to precipitate motion sickness. If the transdermal patch is to be worn during travel, it can be applied behind the ear 4 hours in advance of the planned activity.
- Provide diversional activities.
- Monitor nutritional needs and status on a continuum.

Patient Education and Health Promotion

Nutritional status
- Ensure that the patient, individual, parent, or significant other understands all aspects of the diet, fluid, and nutritional regimen both during hospitalization and at discharge for home management.
- Stress the importance of maintaining hydration and following the parameters that must be reported to the physician (for example, weight loss of 2 pounds in a specified time period, reoccurrence of nausea and vomiting).
- For patients receiving cancer treatments, the American Cancer Society has pamphlets available with suggestions for supplementing the dietary needs of the patient. These include, but are not limited to, giving small, frequent, low-fat meals; discussion of food temperature; and suggestions for increasing protein content of meals with the use of powdered milk added to puddings, shakes made with nutritional supplements, and frozen yogurt.
- Discuss ways to decrease environmental stimuli to vomit such as removing the emesis basin.

Medications. Verify the patient's and significant other's understanding of all prescribed medications to be given on a scheduled or prn basis.

Fostering health maintenance. • Provide the patient and significant others with important information described in the monograph for drugs prescribed. Additional health teaching and nursing interventions for side effects to expect and report are described in each monograph. • Seek cooperation and understanding of the following points so that medication compliance is increased: name of medication, dosage, route and time of administration, side effects to expect, and side effects to report. • Enlist the patient's aid in developing and maintaining a written record of monitoring parameters such as weight, details of when nausea occurs and amount and appearance of vomitus, food diary of what is being eaten, and which foods aggravate or initiate the symptoms.

Drug Class: Dopamine Antagonists
Actions

The dopamine antagonists are the phenothiazines, the butyrophenones, and metoclopramide. These medicines inhibit dopamine receptors that are part of the pathway to the vomiting center. Unfortunately, dopamine receptors in other parts of the brain are also blocked, potentially producing extrapyramidal symptoms of dystonia, parkinsonism, and tardive dyskinesia (see Chapters 16 and 30) in some patients, especially when higher doses are required.

Uses

The phenothiazines are primarily used as antiemetics for the treatment of mild to moderate nausea and vomiting associated with anesthesia and surgery, radiation therapy, and cancer chemotherapy. Prochlorperazine is the phenothiazine most widely used as an antiemetic.

The butyrophenones are also used as antiemetics in surgery and cancer chemotherapy. These agents tend to cause less hypotension than the phenothiazines, but they produce more sedation. The most widely used butyrophenone is haloperidol. Droperidol must be administered parenterally.

Metoclopramide is an antagonist of both dopamine and serotonin receptors. In addition to acting on receptors in the brain, it also acts on similar receptors in the gastrointestinal (GI) tract, thus making it particularly useful in treating nausea and vomiting associated with GI cancers, gastritis, peptic ulcer, radiation sickness, and migraine. High-dose metoclopramide is now routinely used to treat nausea and vomiting associated with certain cancer chemotherapies. In higher doses, extrapyramidal symptoms are more common; therefore many cancer chemotherapy protocols now include both high-dose metoclopramide and routine doses of diphenhydramine when highly emetogenic anticancer agents are used. Metoclopramide appears to be of little value in treating motion sickness.

Therapeutic Outcomes

The primary therapeutic outcome expected from the dopamine antagonist antiemetics is relief of nausea and vomiting.

Nursing Process

Premedication Assessment
1. Collect data regarding emesis (type, amount, and frequency, on a continuum).
2. Assess data relative to the underlying cause of nausea and vomiting (for example, pregnancy, postsurgical, chemotherapy, radiation, bowel obstruction).
3. Obtain baseline data about the patient's degree of alertness before initiation of therapy because these medications tend to produce some degree of sedation.

Planning
Availability. See Table 31-2.

Implementation
Dosage administration. See Table 31-2.

Evaluation
Phenothiazines. See Chapter 16, p. 210.
Haloperidol. See Chapter 16, p. 210.
Metoclopramide. See Chapter 30, p. 390.

Table 31-2

Antiemetic Agents

			ANTIEMETIC DOSAGE		
GENERIC NAME	BRAND NAME	AVAILABILITY	ADULTS	CHILDREN	COMMENTS
Dopamine antagonists					*Comments for all phenothiazines*
Phenothiazines Chlorpromazine	Thorazine, ♣Largactil	Tablets: 10, 25, 50, 100, 200 mg Capsules: 30, 75, 150, 200 mg Syrup: 10 mg/5 ml Concentrate: 30, 100 mg/ml Suppositories: 25, 100 mg Injection: 25 mg/ml	PO: 10-25 mg every 4-6 hr Rectal: 50-100 mg every 6-8 hr IM: 25 mg	PO: 0.25 mg/lb every 4-6 hr Rectal: 0.5 mg/lb every 6-8 hr IM: 0.25 mg/lb every 6-8 hr (Maximum IM dose: up to age 5: 40 mg/day; ages 5-12: 75 mg/day)	Phenothiazines may suppress the cough reflex. Ensure that the patient does not aspirate vomitus. Use with caution in patients, especially children, with undiagnosed vomiting. The phenothiazines can mask signs of toxicity of other drugs or mask symptoms of other diseases, such as brain tumor, Reye's syndrome, or intestinal obstruction. Use with extreme caution in patients with seizure disorders. Discontinue if rashes develop. May cause orthostatic hypotension. See Chapter 16 for a complete list of adverse effects, drug interactions, and nursing interventions.
Perphenazine	Trilafon, ♣Phenazine	Tablets: 2, 4, 8, 16 mg Concentrate: 16 mg/5 ml Injection: 5 mg/ml	PO: 4 mg every 4-6 hr IM: 5 mg	Not recommended	
Prochlorperazine	Compazine, ♣Stemetil	Tablets: 5, 10 mg Capsules: 10, 15 mg Syrup: 5 mg/5 ml Suppositories: 2.5, 5, 25 mg Inj: 5 mg/ml	PO: 5-10 mg every 6-8 hr Rectal: 25 mg 2 times daily IM: 5-10 mg	PO or rectal: 20-29 lb—2.5 mg 1-2 times daily 30-39 lb—2.5 mg 2-3 times daily 40-85 lb—2.5 mg 3 times daily IM: 0.06 mg/lb	
Thiethylperazine	Torecan	Tablets: 10 mg Suppositories: 10 mg Injection: 5 mg/ml	PO, Rectal, IM: 10-30 mg daily in divided doses	Not recommended	
Triflupromazine	Vesprin	Injection: 10-20 mg/ml	IM: 5-15 mg every 4 hr	IM:0.2-0.25 mg/kg up to 10 mg/day	

continued

Table 31-2

Antiemetic Agents—Cont'd

GENERIC NAME	BRAND NAME	AVAILABILITY	ANTIEMETIC DOSAGE		COMMENTS
			ADULTS	CHILDREN	
Dopamine antagonists—cont'd					*Comments for all phenothiazines*
Butyrophenones					
Haloperidol (see Chapter 16, p. 210)					
Metoclopramide (see Chapter 30, p. 390)					
Benzquinamide	Emete-Con	Injection: 50 mg/vial	IM: 0.5-1 mg/kg; repeat in 1 hr, then every 3-4 hr IV: 25 mg at a rate of 1 ml/min	Not recommended	Recommended for nausea and vomiting associated with anesthesia and surgery. Reconstitute with sterile water. IM route preferred.
Trimethobenzamide	Tigan	Capsules: 100, 250 mg Suppositories: 100, 200 mg Injection: 100 mg/ml	PO: 250 mg 3-4 times daily Rectal: 200 mg 3-4 times daily IM: 200 mg 3-4 times daily	PO: 30-90 lb; 100-200 mg 3-4 times daily Rectal: <30 lb: 100 mg 3-4 times daily 30-90 lb: 100-200 mg 3-4 times daily	Injectable form contains benzocaine. Do not use in patients allergic to benzocaine or local anesthetics. Inject in upper, outer quadrant of gluteal region. Avoid escape of solution along the route. May cause burning, stinging, pain on injection.
Serotonin antagonists					
Granisetron	Kytril	Tablets: 1 mg Injection: 1 mg/ml	PO: 1 mg up to 1 hr before chemotherapy, followed by a second dose 12 hr later. IV: 10 μg/kg infused over 5 min beginning 30 min before chemotherapy.	As for adults	Recommended for prevention of nausea and vomiting associated with cancer chemotherapy and postoperative nausea and vomiting.
Ondansetron	Zofran	Tablets: 4, 8 mg Injection: 2 mg/ml	PO: 8 mg 30 min before chemotherapy, followed by 8 mg 8 hr later IV: 3-0.15 mg/kg doses; (1) 30 min before chemotherapy, (2) 4 hours later, (3) 4 more hours later	As for adults	Recommended for prevention of nausea and vomiting associated with cancer chemotherapy and postoperative nausea and vomiting.

continued

Table 31-2

Antiemetic Agents—Cont'd

GENERIC NAME	BRAND NAME	AVAILABILITY	ANTIEMETIC DOSAGE ADULTS	CHILDREN	COMMENTS
Anticholinergic agents used for motion sickness					*Comments for anticholinegeric agents used for motion sickness*
Cyclizine	Marezine, ✽ Marzine	Tablets: 50 mg Inj: 50 mg/1 ml	PO: 50 mg, repeated in 4-6 hr; do not exceed 200 mg daily IM: 50 mg every 4-6 hr	PO: 6-12 yr: 25 mg up to 3 times daily	May suppress cough reflex. Ensure that patient does not aspirate vomitus. Must be administered 30-45 min before travel.
Dimenhydrinate	Dramamine, ✽ Travamine	Capsules: 50 mg Tablets: 50 mg Inj: 50 mg/ml Liquid: 12.5 mg/4 ml, 15.6 mg/5 ml	PO: 50-100 mg every 4-6 hr; do not exceed 400 mg in 24 hr IM: 50 mg, as needed	PO: 6-12 yr: 25-50 mg every 6-8 hr; do not exceed 150 mg in 24 hr 2-6 yr: up to 25 mg every 6-8 hr; do not exceed 75 mg in 24 hr	Will cause sedation. Beware of operating machinery.
Diphenhydramine	Benadryl, Dibenil, ✽ Insomnal	Tablets: 25, 50 mg Capsules: 25, 50 mg Elixir: 12.5 mg/5 ml Inj: 10, 50 mg/ml	PO: 25-50 mg 3 or 4 times daily IM: 10-50 mg; do not exceed 400 mg/24 hr	PO: over 20 lb: 12.5-25 mg 3 or 4 times daily (5 mg/kg/24 hr; do not exceed 300 mg/24 hr IM: 5 mg/kg/24 hr, in 4 divided doses; do not exceed 300 mg in 24 hr	
Hydroxyzine	Atarax, Durrax, Vistaril, ✽ Multipax	Tablets: 10, 25, 50, 100 mg Syrup: 10 mg/5 ml Inj: 25, 50 mg/ml	PO: 25-100 mg 3-4 times daily IM: as for PO	PO: Over 6 yr: 10-25 mg every 4-6 hr; under 6 yr: 10 mg every 4-6 hr IM: as for PO	
Meclizine	Antivert, ✽ Bonamine	Tablets: 12.5, 25, 50 mg	PO: 25-50 mg; may be repeated every 24 hr	PO: Not approved for use by children	
Scopolamine, Transdermal	Transderm-Scōp	Transdermal patch: delivers 0.5 mg over three days	Patch: apply to skin behind the ear at least 4 hr before antiemetic effect is required. Replace in 3 days if continued therapy is required. Do not cut patches!	Not approved for use by children	

continued

Drug Class: Serotonin Antagonists

Actions

A new group of compounds known as the serotonin (5-HT$_3$) receptor antagonists have made major inroads in the treatment of emesis associated with cancer chemotherapy, radia-

tion therapy, and postoperative nausea and vomiting over the past few years. Serotonin receptors of the 5-HT$_3$ type are located centrally in the chemoreceptor trigger zone of the medulla and in specialized cells of the GI tract and play a significant role in inducing nausea and vomiting. The sero-

Table 31-2

Antiemetic Agents—Cont'd

GENERIC NAME	BRAND NAME	AVAILABILITY	ANTIEMETIC DOSAGE		COMMENTS
			ADULTS	CHILDREN	
Corticosteroids Dexamethasone	Decadron	Tablets: 0.25, 0.5, 0.75, 1, 1.5, 2, 4, 6 mg Elixir: 0.5 mg/5 ml Injection: 4, 10, 20, 24 mg/ml	PO: 4-25 mg every 4-6 hr for 1-2 days IV: as for PO	As for adults	Recommended for prevention of nausea and vomiting associated with chemotherapy.
Benzodiazepines Lorazepam	Ativan	Tablets: 0.5, 1, 2 mg Injection: 2, 4 mg/ml	PO: 1-4 mg q 4-6 hr IV: As for PO	Not recommended	Recommended for prevention of nausea and vomiting associated with chemotherapy.
Midazolam	Versed	Inj: 1, 5 mg/ml in 1, 2, 5, 10 ml ampules	IM: 0.07 mg/kg up to 1 hr before chemotherapy	Not recommended	
Cannabinoids Dronabinol (THC)	Marinol	Capsules: 2.5, 5, 10 mg	PO: initial 5-10 mg/m^2 1-3 hr before chemotherapy, then every 2-4 hr for a total of 4-6 doses/day Maximum—15 mg/m^2/dose	Not recommended	Used for patients who have not responded to other antiemetics. Schedule II controlled substance. Common adverse effects include drowsiness, dizziness, muddled thinking, and possible impairment of coordination, sensory, and perceptual functions. Use with caution in hypertension or heart disease.

✦ Available in Canada only.

---

tonin antagonists block these receptors and have been shown to actively control nausea and vomiting associated with cisplatin and several other emetogenic chemotherapeutic agents. Two serotonin (5-HT$_3$) receptor antagonists, ondansetron and granisetron, were made available in 1991 and 1994, respectively.

Uses

Studies of ondansetron and metoclopramide demonstrate that ondansetron is more effective than metoclopramide in the control of high-dose cisplatin-induced nausea and vomiting. Two studies comparing the efficacy and safety of ondansetron and granisetron in the control of cisplatin-induced acute emesis concluded that there were no significant differences between the treatment groups with respect to emetic control, nausea, or adverse reactions. A particular advantage to this group of compounds is that there is no dopaminergic blockade, and thus no extrapyramidal adverse effects have been reported.

Therapeutic Outcomes

The primary therapeutic outcome expected from the serotonin antagonist antiemetics is relief of nausea and vomiting.

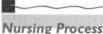

Nursing Process

Premedication Assessment

1. Collect data regarding emesis (type, amount, and frequency, on a continuum).
2. Assess data relative to the underlying cause of nausea and vomiting (for example, pregnancy, postsurgical, chemotherapy, radiation, bowel obstruction).
3. Obtain baseline data about the patient's degree of alertness before initiation of therapy because these medications tend to produce some degree of sedation.

Planning

Availability. See Table 31-2.

Implementation
Dosage administration. See Table 31-2.

Evaluation
Side effects to expect
   HEADACHE, DIARRHEA, CONSTIPATION, SEDATION. These side effects are fairly mild, especially in relation to the prevention of nausea and vomiting. Because only a few doses are administered, frequency and duration of adverse effects are minimal.
Drug interactions
No clinically significant drug interactions have been reported.

Drug Class: Anticholinergic Agents

Actions

Motion sickness is thought to be caused by an excess of acetylcholine at the chemoreceptor trigger zone and the vomiting center by cholinergic nerves receiving impulses from the vestibular network of the inner ear. Anticholinergic agents are used to counterbalance the excessive amounts of acetylcholine present.

Uses

Anticholinergic agents such as scopolamine and the antihistamines (diphenhydramine, cyclizine, meclizine, and promethazine) are used in the treatment of motion sickness and, in the case of the antihistamines, nausea and vomiting associated with pregnancy. The choice of drug depends on the period for which antinausea protection is required and the side effects. Scopolamine is the drug of choice for short periods of motion, and an antihistamine for longer periods. Of the antihistamines, promethazine is the drug of choice. Higher doses act longer, but sedation is usually a problem. Cyclizine and meclizine have fewer side effects than promethazine but have a shorter duration of action and are less effective for severe conditions. Diphenhydramine has a long duration, but excessive sedation is often a problem. For very severe conditions, sympathomimetic drugs such as ephedrine are used in combination with scopolamine or antihistamines. Anticholinergic agents are usually not effective in chemotherapy-induced nausea and vomiting.

Therapeutic Outcomes

The primary therapeutic outcome expected from the anticholinergic antiemetics is relief of nausea and vomiting.

Nursing Process

Premedication Assessment
1. Collect data regarding emesis (type, amount, and frequency, on a continuum).
2. Assess data relative to the underlying cause of nausea and vomiting (for example, pregnancy, postsurgical, chemotherapy, radiation, bowel obstruction).
3. Obtain baseline data about the patient's degree of alertness before initiation of therapy because these medications tend to produce some degree of sedation.

Planning
Availability. See Table 31-2.

Implementation
Dosage and administration. See Table 31-2.

Evaluation
Side effects to expect
   SEDATIVE EFFECTS. Tolerance may develop over a period of time, thus diminishing the effect.
   The operation of power equipment or a motor vehicle may prove hazardous. Caution patients to provide for their personal safety in these situations.
   FLUID INTAKE. Maintain fluid intake at 8 to 12 8-ounce glasses daily.
   BLURRED VISION, CONSTIPATION, URINARY RETENTION, DRYNESS OF MUCOSA OF THE MOUTH, THROAT, AND NOSE. These symptoms are the anticholinergic effects produced by these agents. Patients taking these medications should be monitored for the development of these side effects.
   Dryness of the mucosa may be relieved by sucking hard candy or ice chips or by chewing gum.
   The use of stool softeners such as docusate or the occasional use of a potent laxative such as bisacodyl may be required for constipation.
   Caution the patient that blurred vision may occur, and make appropriate suggestions for personal safety of the individual.
   Patients who develop urinary hesitancy should discontinue the medication and contact their physician for further evaluation.
Drug interactions
   ENHANCED SEDATION. Central nervous system depressants, including sleeping aids, analgesics, tranquilizers, and alcohol, will enhance the sedative effects of the antihistamines. Persons who are working around machinery, driving a car, or performing other duties in which they must remain mentally alert should not take these medications while working.

Drug Class: Corticosteroids

Actions

Several studies have shown that dexamethasone and methylprednisolone can be effective antiemetics either as single agents or in combination with other antiemetics. The mechanism of action is unknown. Other actions of the corticosteroids such as mood elevation, increased appetite, and a sense of well-being may also help in patient acceptance and control of emesis.

Uses

A particular advantage of the steroids, apart from their efficacy, is their relative lack of side effects. Because only a few doses are administered, the usual complications associated with long-term therapy do not arise.

Therapeutic Outcomes

The primary therapeutic outcome expected from the use of corticosteroids as antiemetics is relief of nausea and vomiting.

Nursing Process

Premedication Assessment
1. Collect data regarding emesis (type, amount, and frequency, on a continuum).

2. Assess data relative to the underlying cause of nausea and vomiting (for example, pregnancy, postsurgical, chemotherapy, radiation, bowel obstruction).
3. Obtain baseline data about the patient's degree of alertness before initiation of therapy because these medications tend to produce some degree of sedation.

Planning
Availability. See Table 31-2.

Implementation
Dosage and administration. See Table 31-2.

Evaluation
Side effects to expect and report
Side effects are infrequent because few doses are administered for nausea and vomiting.
 See Chapter 35, p. 443.
Drug interactions. See Chapter 35, p. 443.

Drug Class: Benzodiazepines

Actions

The benzodiazepines act as antiemetics through a combination of effects, including sedation, reduction in anxiety, possible depression of the vomiting center, and an amnesic effect. Of these actions, the amnesic effect appears to be most important as far as treating cancer patients is concerned, and in this respect lorazepam and midazolam are superior to diazepam.

Uses

The benzodiazepines (diazepam, lorazepam, and midazolam) are effective in reducing not only the frequency of nausea and vomiting but the anxiety often associated with chemotherapy. Clinically, the benzodiazepines are most useful in combination with other antiemetics such as metoclopramide, dexamethasone, and ondansetron or granisetron.

Therapeutic Outcomes

The primary therapeutic outcome expected from benzodiazepine antiemetics is relief of nausea and vomiting.

Nursing Process

Premedication Assessment
1. Collect data regarding emesis (type, amount, and frequency, on a continuum).
2. Assess data relative to the underlying cause of nausea and vomiting (for example, pregnancy, postsurgical, chemotherapy, radiation, bowel obstruction).
3. Obtain baseline data about the patient's degree of alertness before initiation of therapy because these medications tend to produce some degree of sedation.

Planning
Availability. See Table 31-2.

Implementation
Dosage and administration. See Table 31-2.

Evaluation
Side effects to expect and report. See Chapter 14, p. 188.
Drug interactions. See Chapter 14, p. 188.

Drug Class: Cannabinoids

Actions

After numerous reports that smoking marijuana reduced the frequency of nausea, the antiemetic properties of the active ingredient, tetrahydrocannabinol (THC), and synthetic analogs such as dronabinol, nabilone, and levonantradol have been studied. The cannabinoids act through several mechanisms to inhibit pathways to the vomiting center. There is no dopaminergic activity.

Uses

The cannabinoids have been shown to be more effective than placebo and equally as effective as prochlorperazine in patients receiving moderately emetogenic chemotherapy. They are less effective than metoclopramide. Because of the mind-altering effects and the potential for abuse, the cannabinoids serve as antiemetics only in patients receiving chemotherapy. The cannabinoids are of more use in those younger patients who are refractory to other antiemetic regimens and in whom combination therapy may be more effective.

Therapeutic Outcomes

The primary therapeutic outcome expected from the cannabinoids is relief of nausea and vomiting.

Nursing Process

Premedication Assessment
1. Collect data regarding emesis (type, amount, and frequency, on a continuum).
2. Assess data relative to the underlying cause of nausea and vomiting (for example, pregnancy, postsurgical, chemotherapy, radiation, bowel obstruction).
3. Obtain baseline data about the patient's degree of alertness before initiation of therapy because these medications tend to produce some degree of sedation.

Planning
Availability. See Table 31-2.

Implementation
Dosage and administration. See Table 31-2.

Evaluation
Side effects to expect and report
DYSPHORIC EFFECTS. Depressed mood, hallucinations, dreaming or fantasizing, distortion of perception, paranoid reactions, and elation are more frequent with moderate to high doses. Younger patients appear to tolerate these side effects better than older patients or patients who have not used marijuana.
 Patients should be specifically warned not to drive, operate machinery, or engage in any hazardous activity until it is determined that they are able to tolerate the drug and to perform such tasks safely.

Persons should remain under the supervision of a responsible adult during initial use of dronabinol and after dosage adjustments.

Drug interactions

DRUGS THAT INCREASE TOXIC EFFECTS. Antihistamines, alcohol, analgesics, benzodiazepines, barbiturates, antidepressants, muscle relaxants, sedative-hypnotics. Monitor the patient for excessive sedation and reduce the dosage of the other sedative agents, if necessary.

CHAPTER REVIEW

Nausea and vomiting vary from a minor inconvenience to severe debilitation. Nonpharmacologic treatments such as elimination of noxious substances, avoidance of fatty or spicy foods, and restriction of activity to bed and chair rest to avoid vestibular irritation are equally important in reducing the frequency of nausea and vomiting. The causes of nausea and vomiting should be assessed before treatment is begun, and specific therapy should be selected for each of the causes.

MATH REVIEW

1. Ordered: ondansetron (Zofran) 3 mg/kg IV in 50 ml D₅W at least 20 minutes before chemotherapy. The client weight today is 135 pounds.
   Weight is: _____ kg
   The total amount of ondansetron to administer is

   _____ .

   When administering this order, using an infusion pump calibrated in ml/hr, set the pump at _____ ml/hr.

2. Ordered: dexamethasone 6 mg by IM injection stat. On hand: dexamethasone 4 mg/ml.
   Give: _____ ml

CRITICAL THINKING QUESTIONS

1. Mr. Tanganese, age 65, has been vomiting intermittently for 3 days "with the flu." He is a resident on your unit in the nursing home. What data should be collected and reported to the physician for further evaluation and actions?

2. Tanya has been vomiting repeatedly after administration of chemotherapy and has already received metoclopramide an hour ago. What is the action of this drug, and what further actions by the nurse are appropriate?

CHAPTER

32

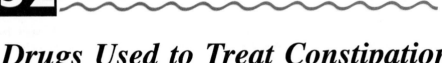

Drugs Used to Treat Constipation and Diarrhea

CHAPTER CONTENT

Objectives

1. State the underlying causes of constipation.
2. Explain the meaning of "normal" bowel habits.

3. Identify the indications for use, method of action, and onset of action for contact or stimulant laxatives, saline laxatives, lubricant or emollient laxatives, bulk-forming laxatives, and fecal softeners.

4. Describe medical conditions in which laxatives should *not* be used.

5. Cite nine causes of diarrhea.

6. State the differences between locally acting and systemically acting antidiarrheal agents.

7. Identify electrolytes that should be monitored whenever prolonged or severe diarrhea is present.

8. Describe nursing assessments needed to evaluate the patient's state of hydration when suffering from either constipation or dehydration.

9. Cite conditions that generally respond favorably to antidiarrheal agents.

10. Review medications studied to date and prepare a list of those that may cause diarrhea.

Key Words

constipation   laxatives

diarrhea

CONSTIPATION

Constipation is the infrequent, incomplete, or painful elimination of feces. It may result from decreased motility of the colon or from retention of feces in the lower colon or rectum. In either case, the longer the feces remain in the colon, the greater the reabsorption of water and the drier the stool becomes. The stool is then more difficult to expel from the anus. Causes of constipation are improper diet—too little residue or too little fluid (for example, lacking fruits and vegetables or high in constipating food such as cheese and yogurt); too little fluid intake, especially considering the climate; lack of exercise and sedentary habits; failure to respond to the normal defecation impulses; muscular weakness of the colon; diseases such as anemia and hypothyroidism; frequent use of constipating medicines (for example, morphine, codeine, anticholinergic agents); tumors of the bowel or pressure on the bowel from tumors; diseases of the rectum.

Occasional constipation is not detrimental to a person's health, although it can cause a feeling of general discomfort or abdominal fullness, anorexia, and anxiety in some persons. Habitual constipation leads to decreased intestinal muscle tone, increased straining at the stool as the person bears down in the attempt to pass the hardened stool, and an increased incidence of hemorrhoids. The daily use of laxatives or enemas should be avoided because they decrease the muscular tone and mucus production of the rectum and may result in water and electrolyte imbalance. They also become habit forming: the weakened muscle tone adds to the inability to expel the fecal contents, which leads to the continued use of enemas or laxatives.

Today, many people believe that even occasional failure of the bowel to move daily is abnormal and should be treated. Daily bowel movements are frequently not necessary. Many people have "normal" bowel habits even though they have only two or three bowel movements per week. As long as the patient's health is good and the stool is not hardened or impacted, this schedule is acceptable.

DIARRHEA

Diarrhea is an increase in the frequency or fluid content of bowel movements. Because normal patterns of defecation and the patient's perception of bowel function vary, a careful history must be obtained to determine the change in a particular patient's bowel elimination pattern. An important fact to remember about diarrhea is that diarrhea is a symptom, rather than a disease. It may be caused by any of the following:

- Intestinal infections
- Spicy or fatty foods
- Enzyme deficiencies
- Excessive use of laxatives
- Drug therapy
- Emotional stress
- Hyperthyroidism
- Inflammatory bowel disease
- Surgical bypass of the intestine

Intestinal infections are most frequently associated with ingestion of food contaminated with bacteria or protozoa (food poisoning) or eating or drinking water that contains bacteria that is foreign to the patient's gastrointestinal tract. People traveling, often to other countries, develop what is known as traveler's diarrhea from ingestion of microorganisms that are pathogenic to their gastrointestinal tracts but not to those of the local residents.

Spicy or fatty foods: Spicy or fatty foods may produce diarrhea by irritating the lining of the gastrointestinal tract. Diarrhea occurs particularly when the patient does not routinely eat these types of foods. This type of diarrhea is not uncommon on vacation (for example, eating fresh oysters daily while visiting coastal regions).

Enzyme deficiencies: Patients with deficiencies of digestive enzymes such as lactase or amylase have difficulty digesting certain foods. Diarrhea usually develops because of irritation from undigested food.

Excessive use of laxatives: Persons who use laxatives on a routine, chronic basis who are not under the care of a physician for a specific gastrointestinal problem are laxative abusers. Some persons do it for weight control, and others use laxatives under the misconception that a person is not "normal" if the bowels do not move daily.

Drug therapy: Diarrhea is a common side effect caused by the irritation of the gastrointestinal lining by ingested medication. Diarrhea may also result from the use of antibiotics that kill certain bacteria that live in the gastrointestinal tract and help digest food.

Emotional stress: Diarrhea is a common symptom of emotional stress and anxiety.

Hyperthyroidism: Hyperthyroidism induces increased gastrointestinal motility, resulting in diarrhea.

Inflammatory bowel disease: Inflammatory bowel diseases such as diverticulitis, ulcerative colitis, gastroenteritis, and Crohn's disease cause inflammation of the gastrointestinal lining, resulting in diarrhea.

Surgical bypass: Surgical bypass procedures of the intestine often result in chronic diarrhea because of the decreased absorptive area remaining after surgery. Incompletely digested food and water rapidly pass through the gastrointestinal tract.

Treatment

Constipation

Constipation that does not have a specific cause can often be treated without the use of laxatives. A high-fiber diet (fruits, grains, nuts, vegetables), adequate hydration (four to six 8-ounce glasses of water daily), and daily exercise (for physical activity and stress relief) can eliminate the vast majority of cases of constipation. Laxatives, other than treating acute constipation from a specific cause (for example, a change in routine, such as traveling for long hours in a car or plane), should be avoided. The ingredients of laxative products frequently cause side effects and may be contraindicated in certain patients. The following patients should not take laxatives and should be referred to a physician: patients with severe pain or discomfort; patients who have nausea, vomiting, or fever; patients with a preexisting condition (for example, diabetes mellitus, abdominal surgery); patients taking medicines that cause constipation (for example, iron, aluminum antacids, antispasmodics, muscle relaxants); patients who have used other laxatives without success; and patients who are laxative abusers.

Diarrhea

Diarrhea may be acute or chronic, mild or severe. Because diarrhea may be a defense mechanism to rid the body of infecting organisms or irritants, it is usually self-limiting. Chronic diarrheas may indicate a disease of the stomach or small or large intestine, may be psychogenic in origin, or may be one of the first symptoms of cancer of the colon or rectum. If diarrhea is severe or prolonged, it may cause dehydration, electrolyte depletion, and physical exhaustion. Specific antidiarrheal therapy depends on the cause of the diarrhea.

Nursing Process for Altered Elimination: Diarrhea and Constipation

Assessment

History. • Obtain a history of the patient's usual bowel pattern and changes that have taken place in the frequency, consistency, color, and number of stools per day. Ask whether the patient has a usual time of defecation daily. Does the individual respond immediately to the urge to defecate or delay toileting until a more convenient time? • Ask whether the onset of diarrhea or constipation is recent and if it can be associated with travel or stress. Has there been a change in water source or foods lately? Ask what measures the patient has already initiated, whether physician prescribed or by self-treatment, to correct the problem and the degree of success achieved. • Obtain a detailed history of the individual's health. Are any acute or chronic conditions being treated, such as cancer, gastrointestinal disorders, neurologic conditions, or intestinal obstruction?

Medications. Ask the patient to give a listing of all current medications being taken that are over-the-counter or prescribed by a physician. Are any used to treat diarrhea or constipation? Are any of these medications known to slow intestinal transit time (for example, narcotic analgesics, aluminum-containing antacids, or anticholinergic agents)? Are any known to cause diarrhea (for example, magnesium-containing antacids)?

Activity and exercise. Ask the patient about daily activity level and exercise. Does the patient play vigorous sports, take walks, and jog? Or does the patient have a sedentary job and hobby?

Nutritional history. • Ask questions to determine the patient's usual dietary practices: how much coffee, tea, soda pop (caffeinated or decaffeinated), water, fruit juice, and

alcoholic beverages are consumed daily? • Ask for a description of what the patient has eaten over the past 24 hours. Evaluate the data to identify whether foods from all levels of the food pyramid are being eaten. Are there good sources of dietary fiber? Has the patient introduced new foods not usually eaten into the diet?

Basic assessment. • Obtain baseline vital signs, height, and weight. • Assess bowel sounds in all four quadrants of the abdomen. Observe the size and shape of the abdomen. Note any signs of distention, ascites, or masses. • Assess and record signs of hydration. Examine for poor skin turgor, sticky oral mucous membranes, excessive thirst, a shrunken and deeply furrowed tongue, crusted lips, weight loss, deteriorating vital signs, soft or sunken eyeballs, delayed capillary filling, high urine specific gravity or no urine output, and possible mental confusion.

Laboratory studies. Review laboratory reports for indications of malabsorption, dehydration, fluid, electrolyte and acid-base imbalances, and so on (for example, K^+, Cl^-, pH, pCO_2, bicarbonate, Hgb, Hct, urinalysis [specific gravity], serum albumin, and total protein).

Nursing Diagnosis

Constipation. • Bowel elimination, altered: constipation (indication). • Fluid volume, deficit (indication).

Diarrhea. • Bowel elimination, altered: diarrhea (indication). • Fluid volume, deficit (indication). • Nutrition, altered: less than body requirements (indication).

Planning

History. Plan to perform a focused assessment consistent with the symptoms and underlying pathology.

Medications, treatments, and diagnostics. • Order baseline laboratory studies requested by the physician. Schedule prescribed treatments (for example, enema administration) and diagnostic procedures (for example, abdominal x-rays, colonoscopy). • Schedule prescribed medications on the medication administration record (MAR), and requisition medicines from the pharmacy.

Assessment. • Mark the Kardex with specific parameters to be recorded, such as intake and output, frequency and consistency of stools, and presence of blood. • Mark the Kardex if stool specimens are to be obtained.

Nutrition. Obtain specific orders relating to nutrition. Diet orders depend on the cause of constipation or diarrhea. A dietary consult may be indicated. Schedule intake of fluid so that fluid intake is at least 3000 ml per day, unless contraindicated by coexisting conditions (for example, heart failure or renal disease). Rehydration solutions may be required with severe diarrhea.

Activity and exercise. Mark the Kardex and care plan with specific orders regarding ambulation. Whenever possible, and not contraindicated by coexisting conditions, encourage frequent ambulation.

Implementation

• Maintain hydration with oral or parenteral solutions as prescribed by the physician. Monitor the hydration status with volume of intake by patient, urine output, skin turgor, moisturization of mucous membranes, and daily weights.

- Assess for bowel sounds in all four quadrants of the abdomen. Report absence of bowel sounds immediately to the physician.
- Give enemas prescribed according to hospital procedures. (These are not used for long-term treatment of constipation.) Oil retention enemas may be required to soften the fecal material.
- Initiate nutritional interventions, such as high-fiber foods and adequate fluid intake.
- Give prescribed laxatives or stool softeners. Monitor for effectiveness and side effects.
- Initiate hygiene measures to prevent perianal skin breakdown. Cleanse the perianal area thoroughly after each stool. Apply protective ointment (for example, zinc oxide ointment) as prescribed; with severe diarrhea, a fecal collection apparatus may be helpful.
- Monitor vital signs and daily weights, and perform a focused assessment appropriate to the underlying etiology of the constipation or diarrhea.

Patient Education and Health Promotion

Nutritional status. • Be certain the individual, parent, or significant other understands all aspects of the diet and fluid orders prescribed. • Stress the inclusion of high-fiber foods and adequate fluids to maintain hydration and alleviate constipation. • Depending on the underlying cause of the symptoms, health teaching is appropriate regarding proper food preparation, storage, and prevention of contamination. • During travel, use bottled water, when appropriate, to avoid the possibility of contaminated water.

Activity and exercise. Encourage regular exercise.

Medications. • Explain the consequences of regular use of laxatives and the benefits of handling constipation with diet, exercise, and adequate fluid intake first. • With some situations, such as the regular use of codeine or morphine for pain control in cancer patients, it is imperative that the individual know that stool softeners should be initiated and continued as long as constipating medicines are being taken. • When laxatives or enemas are prescribed to cleanse the intestines before diagnostic examination, be certain the individual has written instructions regarding the enema or drugs prescribed, the time and amount to be administered, and where the laxative or enema can be purchased. Review the correct procedure for self-administering an enema with the patient, or instruct a family member on the administration procedure. • Emphasize the need to be in close proximity to a bathroom once laxatives such as GOLYTELY are taken.

Fostering health maintenance. • Fecal-oral contamination may cause diarrhea. Teaching proper hand washing and cleansing or disinfection of the toilet, bedpan, or commode being used is important. • For diarrhea associated with chronic gastrointestinal diseases, it is imperative to reinforce all aspects of health teaching relating to the specific disease underlying the symptomatology. • Provide the patient and significant others with important information contained in individual drug monographs to identify drugs that cause constipation or diarrhea. Additional health teaching and nursing interventions for side effects to expect and report are described in each drug monograph. • Seek cooperation and understanding of the following points for judicious use of laxatives or antidiarrheals: name of medication, dosage, route and time of administration, side effects to expect, and side effects to report.

Drug Class: Laxatives

Actions

Laxatives are chemicals that act to promote the evacuation of the bowel. They are usually subclassified based on mechanism of action.

Stimulant Laxatives

Stimulant laxatives act directly on the intestine, causing an irritation that promotes peristalsis and evacuation. If given orally, these agents act within 6 to 10 hours. If administered rectally, they act within 60 to 90 minutes.

Saline Laxatives

Saline laxatives are hypertonic compounds that draw water into the intestine from surrounding tissues. The accumulated water affects stool consistency and distends the bowel, causing peristalsis. These agents usually act within 1 to 3 hours. Continued use of these products significantly alters electrolyte balance and may cause dehydration.

Polyethylene glycol–electrolyte solution is a relatively new approach to saline laxative therapy. It is a mixture of a nonabsorbable ion-exchange solution and electrolytes that acts as an osmotic agent. When taken orally, it pulls electrolytes and water into the solution in the lumen of the bowel and exchanges sodium ions to replace those removed from the body. The net result is a diarrhea that cleanses the bowel for colonoscopy and barium enema x-ray examination with no significant dehydration or loss of electrolytes.

Lubricant Laxatives

Lubricant laxatives lubricate the intestinal wall and soften the stool, allowing a smooth passage of fecal contents. Onset of action is often 6 to 8 hours but may be up to 48 hours because the action is highly dependent on the individual patient's normal gastrointestinal transit time. Peristaltic activity does not appear to be increased. If used frequently, these oils may inhibit the absorption of fat-soluble vitamins.

Bulk-Producing Laxatives

Bulk-producing laxatives must be administered with a full glass of water. The laxative causes water to be retained within the stool. This increases bulk, which stimulates peristalsis. Onset of action is usually 12 to 24 hours but may be as long as 72 hours depending on the patient's gastrointestinal transit time. Bulk-forming agents are usually considered to be the safest laxative, even when taken routinely. Fresh fruits, vegetables, and cereals such as bran are natural bulk-forming products.

Fecal Softeners

Fecal softeners, known as wetting agents, draw water into the stool, causing it to soften. They do not stimulate peristalsis and may require up to 72 hours to aid in a soft bowel movement. Action from these agents depends on the patient's state of hydration and the gastrointestinal transit time.

Uses

When using laxatives for special populations, lubricant and bulk-forming laxatives may be used in the geriatric and pregnant patient because there is little cramping accompanying their use. Pediatric patients should also be treated with a change in diet to include cereals, fruits, and grains. Constipation in infants can be treated with malt soup extract, a bulk-forming laxative, or dark corn syrup added to a feeding bottle.

Do not administer laxatives to patients with undiagnosed abdominal pain or patients with inflammation of the gastrointestinal tract such as gastritis, appendicitis, or colitis.

Bulk-Forming Laxatives

Bulk-forming laxatives are generally considered to be the drug of choice for a person who is incapacitated and needs a laxative regularly. These agents may also be used in patients with irritable bowel syndrome to provide a softer consistency to the stools if a high-fiber diet is not adequate. Bulk-forming laxatives are also used to control certain types of diarrhea by absorbance of the irritating substance, thus allowing its removal from the bowel during defecation.

It is important that bulk-forming laxatives be dispersed in a glass of water or juice before administration. If adequate volumes of water are not taken, obstruction within the gastrointestinal tract may result from a bulk laxative that forms a sticky mass.

Stimulant and Saline Laxatives

Stimulant and saline laxatives may be used to relieve acute constipation. They are also routinely used as bowel preparations to remove gas and feces before radiologic examination of the kidneys, colon, intestine, or gall bladder. These products should be used only intermittently because chronic use may cause loss of normal bowel function and dependency on the agent for bowel evacuation.

Stool Softeners

Stool softeners are routinely used for prophylactic purposes to prevent constipation or straining at stool (for example, in patients recovering from myocardial infarction or abdominal surgery).

Lubricant Laxatives

Lubricant laxatives are helpful in producing a soft stool without causing significant bowel spasm. Lubricants are also used prophylactically in patients who should not strain during defecation. Lubricants should not be administered to debilitated patients who are constantly in a recumbent position. The oil has been reported to be aspirated into the lungs, causing a lipid pneumonia.

Therapeutic Outcomes

The primary therapeutic outcomes expected from laxative therapy are as follows:

• Relief from abdominal discomfort
• Passage of bowel contents within a few hours of administration

Nursing Process

Premedication Assessment

1. Determine usual pattern of elimination.
2. Ask specifically about symptoms that may indicate undiagnosed abdominal pain such as those associated with intestinal obstruction or appendicitis.

Planning

Availability. See Table 32-1.

Implementation

Dosage and administration. PO—follow directions on the container. Be sure to give adequate water with bulk-forming agents to prevent esophageal, gastric, intestinal, or rectal obstruction.

Evaluation

Side effects to expect

GRIPPING, MINOR ABDOMINAL DISCOMFORT. The most common adverse effects are excessive bowel stimulation resulting in gripping and diarrhea. Patients who are severely constipated may develop abdominal cramps. The patient should first experience the urge to defecate, then defecate and feel a sense of relief.

Side effects to report

ABDOMINAL TENDERNESS, PAIN, BLEEDING, VOMITING, DIARRHEA, INCREASING ABDOMINAL GIRTH. Failure to defecate or defecation of only a small amount may be an indication of an impaction. These symptoms may also indicate an acute abdomen.

Drug interactions

BISACODYL. Do not administer with milk, antacids, cimetidine, famotidine, nizatidine, or ranitidine. These products may allow the enteric coating to dissolve prematurely, causing nausea, vomiting, and cramping.

PSYLLIUM. Do not administer products containing psyllium (Metamucil, Siblin, others) at the same time as salicylates, nitrofurantoin, or digitalis glycosides. The psyllium may inhibit absorption. Administer these tablets at least 1 hour before or 2 hours after the psyllium.

MINERAL OIL. Daily administration of mineral oil for more than 1 to 2 weeks may cause a deficiency of the fat-soluble vitamins.

DOCUSATE. Docusate enhances the absorption of mineral oil. Concurrent use is not recommended to prevent granuloma formation in the liver, lymph nodes, and intestinal lining.

Drug Class: Antidiarrheal Agents

Actions

Antidiarrheal agents include a wide variety of drugs, but they can be divided into two broad categories: locally acting agents and systemic agents. Locally acting agents such as activated charcoal, pectin, psyllium, and activated attapulgite adsorb excess water to cause a formed stool and to adsorb irritants or bacteria that are causing the diarrhea.

The systemic agents act through the autonomic nervous system to reduce peristalsis and motility of the gastrointesti-

Table 32-1

Laxatives

PRODUCT	CONTACT	SALINE	BULK-FORMING	LUBRICANT	FECAL SOFTENER	OTHER
Agoral	Phenolphthalein		Agar, Tragacanth, Acacia, Egg albumin	Mineral oil		
Citrate of Magnesia		Magnesium citrate				
Colace					Docusate sodium	
Colyte						Polyethylene glycol, electrolyte solution
Dialose					Docusate potassium	
Dialose Plus	Casanthranol				Docusate potassium	
Doxidan	Phenolphthalein				Docusate calcium	
Dulcolax	Bisacodyl					
Ex-lax	Phenolphthalein					
GOLYTELY						Polyethylene glycol, electrolyte solution
Haley's M-O		Magnesium hydroxide		Mineral oil		
Metamucil			Psyllium hydrophilic mucilloid			
Modane	Phenolphthalein					
Peri-Colace	Casanthranol				Docusate sodium	
Phillip's Milk of Magnesia		Magnesium hydroxide				
Phospho-Soda		Sodium phosphates				
Surfak					Docusate calcium	
X-Prep	Senna concentrate					

nal tract, allowing the mucosal lining to absorb nutrients, water, and electrolytes, leaving a formed stool from the residue remaining in the colon. Representatives of the systemically acting agents are diphenoxylate, loperamide, and certain anticholinergic agents (Table 32-2). The systemically acting agents are associated with more adverse effects (see Table 32-2). These agents should not be used to treat diarrhea caused by substances toxic to the gastrointestinal tract, such as bacterial contaminants or other irritants. Because these agents act by reducing gastrointestinal motility, the systemically acting antidiarrheals tend to allow the toxin to remain in the gastrointestinal tract longer, causing further irritation.

Uses

Although the ingredients of the antidiarrheal products are, in general, fairly benign and the majority of products are available for over-the-counter sale, the decision as to recommend treatment versus when the nurse should refer the patient to a physician is not to be taken lightly.

Antidiarrheal products are usually indicated under the following conditions:
- The diarrhea is of sudden onset, has lasted more than 2 or 3 days, and is causing significant fluid and water loss. Young children and elderly patients are more susceptible to rapid dehydration and electrolyte imbalance and therefore should start antidiarrheal therapy earlier.
- Patients with inflammatory bowel disease develop diarrhea. Rapid treatment shortens the course of the incapacitating diarrhea and allows the patient to live a more normal lifestyle. Other agents such as adrenocortical steroids or sulfonamides may also be used to control the underlying bowel disease.
- Post–gastrointestinal surgery patients develop diarrhea. These patients may require chronic antidiarrheal therapy to allow adequate absorption of fluids and electrolytes.
- The cause of the diarrhea has been diagnosed and the physician determines that an antidiarrheal product is appropriate for therapy. Because many cases of diarrhea are self-limiting, therapy may not be necessary.

GENERIC NAME	BRAND NAME	AVAILABILITY	ADULT DOSAGE	COMMENTS
Systemic action Diphenoxin with atropine	Motofen	Tablets: 1 mg diphenoxin with 0.025 mg atropine	PO: 2 tablets, then 1 tablet each loose stool. Do not exceed 8 tablets in 24 hr.	Inhibits peristalsis Atropine added to minimize potential overdose or abuse May cause drowsiness or dizziness; use caution in performing tasks requiring alertness Do not use in children less than 2 yr of age
Diphenoxylate with atropine	Lomotil, Diphenatol	Tablets: 2.5 mg diphenoxylate with 0.025 mg atropine Liquid: 2.5 mg diphenoxylate, with 0.025 mg atropine per 5 ml	PO: 5 mg 4 times daily	Inhibits peristalsis Atropine added to minimize potential overdose or abuse May cause drowsiness or dizziness; use caution in performing tasks requiring alertness Do not use in children less than 2 yr of age
Loperamide	Imodium, Imodium A-D, Diar-Aid	Tablets: 2 mg Capsules: 2 mg Liquid: 1 mg/5 ml	PO: 4 mg initially, followed by 2 mg after each unformed movement. Do not exceed 16 mg/day	Inhibits peristalsis Used in acute nonspecific diarrhea and to reduce the volume of discharge from ileostomy
Camphorated tincture of opium	Paregoric	Liquid	PO: 5-10 ml 4 times daily	Inhibits peristalsis and pain of diarrhea 5 ml of liquid = 2 mg morphine
Local action Attapulgite	Kaopectate	Tablets	PO: 2 tablets after each loose bowel movement	Used as adsorbent

continued

Therapeutic Outcomes

The primary therapeutic outcome expected from antidiarrheal therapy is relief from the incapacitation and discomfort of diarrhea.

Nursing Process

Premedication Assessment

1. Confer with patient regarding medications in use that may be contributing to diarrhea, including over-the-counter products such as antacids containing magnesium or laxative products.

2. Review history of onset of diarrhea and precipitating factors. Refer to physician if a question exists regarding advisability of administering antidiarrheal agents.

Planning

Availability. See Table 32-2.

Implementation

Dosage and administration. See Table 32-2. PO—follow directions on the container. Be sure to give adequate water with bulk-forming agents to prevent esophageal, gastric, intestinal, or rectal obstruction.

Table 32-2

Antidiarrheal Agents—cont'd

GENERIC NAME	BRAND NAME	AVAILABILITY	ADULT DOSAGE	COMMENTS
Local action—continued				
Attapulgite	Parepectolin	Suspension	PO: 15-30 ml after each loose bowel movement	Used as absorbent
Lactobacillus acidophilus	Lactinex	Capsules, granules, tablets	PO: 2-4 tablets or capsules, 2-4 times daily, with milk Granules: 1 packet added to cereal, fruit juice, milk 3-4 times daily	Bacteria used to re-colonize the gastrointestinal tract in an attempt to treat chronic diarrhea Do not use in acute diarrhea
Bismuth subsalicylate	Pepto-Bismol	Tablets, suspension	PO: 30 ml or 2 tablets chewed every 30-60 min up to 8 doses	Used as adsorbent

Evaluation

Side effects to expect

ABDOMINAL DISTENTION, NAUSEA, CONSTIPATION. The locally acting agents have essentially no adverse effects, but if used excessively, they may cause abdominal distention, nausea, and constipation.

Side effects to report

PROLONGED OR WORSENED DIARRHEA. This may be an indication that toxins are present in the gut and that the systemically acting antidiarrheal is causing retention of these toxins. Refer the patient for medical attention.

Drug interactions

DIPHENOXYLATE, DIFENOXIN. The chemical structure of these two antidiarrheal agents is similar to meperidine. These antidiarrheal agents should not be used in a patient receiving monoamine oxidase inhibitors (phenelzine, tranylcypromine). There is a theoretical potential for a hypertensive crisis.

SEDATIVES, ALCOHOL, TRANQUILIZERS. Sedation caused by diphenoxylate and difenoxin is potentiated by other medicines with central nervous system depressant properties.

CHAPTER REVIEW

Constipation and diarrhea are common disorders of the gastrointestinal tract that most people experience occa-sionally throughout their lives. Most cases are self-limiting and do not require pharmacologic treatment. Constipation is most frequently treated by adding bulk and water to the diet and by regular exercise. If drug treatment is required, laxatives that act by a variety of mechanisms are available: bulk-formers, stimulants, saline, lubricants, and surfactants.

Acute diarrhea is usually a symptom of an underlying problem, such as a gastrointestinal infection. A detailed history of recent events must be taken to assess whether to recommend treatment with antidiarrheal agents or refer the patient for medical attention.

CRITICAL THINKING QUESTIONS

1. The physician tells the office nurse to instruct the mother of a 6-month-old infant on the procedure to insert a glycerin suppository. What information would you give?

2. An 80-year-old resident asks for a laxative on a daily basis. What health teaching should be done? Would you give the prn laxative daily?

CHAPTER

33

Drugs Used to Treat Diabetes Mellitus

CHAPTER CONTENT

Objectives

1. State the current definition of diabetes mellitus.

2. Identify the extent of the disease within the United States.

3. Describe the three clinical classes of diabetes mellitus.

4. Differentiate between the symptoms of type I (IDDM) and type II (NIDDM) diabetes mellitus.

5. Identify the objectives of dietary control of diabetes mellitus.

6. Discuss the use of insulin as opposed to oral hypoglycemic agents to control diabetes mellitus.

7. Identify the major nursing considerations associated with the management of the patient with diabetes (such as nutritional evaluation, dietary prescription, activity and exercise, and psychologic considerations).

8. Differentiate between the signs, symptoms, and management of hypoglycemia and hyperglycemia.

9. Discuss the contributing factors, nursing assessments, and nursing interventions needed for patients exhibiting complications associated with diabetes mellitus.

10. Develop a health teaching plan for persons taking any type of insulin or oral hypoglycemic agent.

Key Words

diabetes mellitus
hyperglycemia
Type I insulin-dependent diabetes mellitus (IDDM)
Type II non–insulin-dependent diabetes mellitus (NIDDM)
neuropathies
paresthesia
gestational diabetes mellitus
impaired glucose tolerance (IGT)
hypoglycemia

DIABETES MELLITUS

Diabetes mellitus has traditionally been defined as a chronic, progressive disease manifested by abnormalities in carbohydrate, protein, and fat metabolism resulting from a lack of insulin. It has been redefined as a group of diseases that have glucose intolerance (**hyperglycemia**), as well as changes in protein and lipid metabolism, in common. The causes of these diseases are still unknown, but it is now recognized that different pathologic mechanisms are involved for different diseases.

Diabetes mellitus is appearing with increasing frequency in the United States as the number of older people in the population increases. In the United States, approximately 6.5 million people are being treated for diabetes. Another 2 million have undiagnosed diabetes, and 5 million more will develop diabetes during their lives. Undiagnosed diabetic adults, with few or no symptoms, present a major challenge to the health profession. Because early symptoms of diabetes are minimal, the patient does not seek medical advice. Indications of the disease are discovered only at the time of routine physical examination. Those with a predisposition to developing diabetes include people who have relatives with diabetes (they have 2.5 times greater incidence of developing the disease), obese people (85% of all diabetic patients are overweight), and older people (four out of five diabetics are over 45 years of age). The incidence of diabetes is higher in blacks, Hispanics, Native Americans, and women.

The National Diabetes Data Group of the National Institute of Health classifies diabetes by the various clinical presentations associated with the diseases. The classification includes three clinical classes, characterized by either fasting hyperglycemia or abnormalities of glucose tolerance, and two statistical risk classes, with normal glucose tolerance, that are thought to be stages in the natural course of diabetes (Table 33-1). It is possible for a person to show symptoms of both type I and type II disease.

Type I, **insulin-dependent diabetes mellitus** (IDDM), is present in 5% to 10% of the diabetic population. It frequently occurs in juveniles, but it is now recognized that patients can become symptomatic for the first time at any age. The onset

of this form of diabetes usually has a rapid progression of symptoms (a few days to a few weeks) characterized by polydipsia (increased thirst), polyphagia (increased appetite), polyuria (increased urination), increased frequency of infections, loss of weight and strength, irritability, and often ketoacidosis. There is no insulin secretion from the pancreas, and patients require administration of exogenous insulin. Insulin dosage adjustment is easily influenced by inconsistent patterns of physical activity and dietary irregularities. It is common for patients with type I diabetes mellitus to go into remission, requiring little or no exogenous insulin. This condition may last for a few months, and is referred to as the "honeymoon" period.

Type II, **non–insulin-dependent diabetes mellitus** (NIDDM), represents about 90% of the diabetic population. It usually has a more insidious onset. The pancreas still maintains some capability to produce and secrete insulin. Consequently, symptoms are minimal or absent for a prolonged period of time. The patient may seek medical attention several years later only after symptoms of the disease are apparent. Patients may complain of weight gain or loss. Blurred vision may indicate diabetic retinopathy. **Neuropathies** may be first observed as numbness or tingling of the

Table 33-1

National Diabetes Group Classification of Glucose Intolerance	
CLASS	**FORMER TERMINOLOGY**
Clinical classes	
Diabetes mellitus (DM)	
Type I: Insulin-dependent (IDDM)	Juvenile diabetes, juvenile-onset diabetes (JOD), ketosis-prone diabetes, brittle diabetes
Type II: Non–insulin-dependent (NIDDM)	Adult-onset diabetes, maturity-onset diabetes (MOD),
Nonobese NIDDM	ketosis-resistant diabetes, stable diabetes
Obese NIDDM	
Other types associated with certain conditions and syndromes	Secondary diabetes
Pancreatic disease	
Hormonol	
Drug or chemical induced	
Insulin receptor abnormalities	
Certain genetic syndromes	
Other types	
Gestational diabetes (GDM)	Gestational diabetes
Impaired glucose tolerance (IGT)	Asymptomatic diabetes, chemical diabetes, borderline diabetes,
Nonobese IGT	latent diabetes
Obese IGT	
IGT associated with certain conditions and syndromes	
Pancreatic disease	
Hormonal	
Drug or chemical induced	
Insulin receptor abnormalities	
Certain genetic syndromes	
Statistical risk classes	
Previous abnormality of glucose tolerance (PrevAGT)	Latent diabetes
Potential abnormality of glucose tolerance (PotAGT)	Prediabetes, potential diabetes

Modified from National Diabetes Data Group: *Diabetes,* Dec 1979, 28:1039.

extremities (**paresthesia**), loss of sensation, orthostatic hypotension, impotence, and difficulty in controlling urination (neurogenic bladder). Nonhealing ulcers of the lower extremities may indicate chronic vascular disease. Fasting hyperglycemia can be controlled by diet in some patients, but other patients require the use of supplemental insulin or oral hypoglycemic agents, such as tolbutamide or acetohexamide. Although the onset is usually after the fourth decade of life, NIDDM can occur in younger patients who do not require insulin for control.

The third subclass of diabetes mellitus includes additional types of diabetes that are a part of other diseases having features not generally associated with the diabetic state. Diseases that may have a diabetic component include pheochromocytoma, acromegaly, and Cushing's syndrome. Other disorders included in this category are malnutrition, drugs and chemicals that induce hyperglycemia, defects in insulin receptors, and certain genetic syndromes.

The second clinical class, known as **gestational diabetes mellitus** (GDM), is reserved for women who show abnormal glucose tolerance during pregnancy. It does not include diabetic women who become pregnant. The majority of gestational diabetics have a normal glucose tolerance postpartum. Gestational diabetics must be reclassified after delivery into the category of diabetes mellitus, impaired glucose tolerance, or previous abnormality of glucose tolerance. Gestational diabetics have been put into a separate category because of the special clinical features of diabetes that develop during pregnancy and the complications associated with fetal involvement. These women are also at a higher risk of developing diabetes 5 to 10 years after pregnancy.

The third and last clinical class is for those patients found to have an **impaired glucose tolerance** (IGT). It is now thought that patients with IGT are at a higher risk for developing NIDDM or IDDM in the future. In many of these patients, however, the glucose tolerance returns to normal or persists in the intermediate range for years. Studies indicate that these patients have an increased susceptibility to atherosclerotic disease.

There are two groups of patients at risk for diabetes or impaired glucose tolerance—those with a previous abnormality and those with a potential abnormality of glucose tolerance. Therefore the National Diabetes Data Group included two statistical risk classes in the new classification. The first risk class is for patients with a previous abnormality of glucose tolerance (PrevAGT). This class includes patients who now have normal glucose tolerance but who have a history of previous diabetes mellitus or impaired glucose tolerance. Representative of this class is the gestational diabetic who has a normal glucose tolerance after delivery or an obese patient whose glucose tolerance has returned to normal because of diet control and weight loss. It is important to realize that PrevAGT patients are not diabetics and should not be labeled as such, but they should be tested periodically for the development of diabetes.

The second statistical risk class is potential abnormality of glucose tolerance (PotAGT). This class is for patients who have never exhibited abnormal glucose tolerance but who are at an increased risk for developing abnormalities. Risk factors for the development of non–insulin-dependent diabetes include being the monozygotic twin of this type of diabetic, having a close relative (such as sibling, parent, or child) who is a non–insulin-dependent diabetic, and being obese. A person with islet cell antibodies, one who is a monozygotic twin of an insulin-dependent diabetic, or one who is a sibling of an insulin-dependent diabetic has an increased probability of becoming an insulin-dependent diabetic.

Treatment

Although the classification system of the National Diabetes Data Group was developed to facilitate clinical and epidemiologic investigation, the categorization of patients can also be helpful in determining general principles for therapy. Because a cure for diabetes mellitus is unknown at present, the minimal purpose of treatment is to prevent ketoacidosis and symptoms resulting from hyperglycemia. The long-term objective of control of the disease must involve mechanisms to stop the progression of the complications of the disease. Major determinants to success are a balanced diet, insulin or oral hypoglycemic therapy, routine exercise, and good hygiene.

Patients with diabetes can lead full and satisfying lives. However, unrestricted diets and activities are not possible. Dietary treatment of diabetes constitutes the basis for management of most patients, especially those with the type II (NIDDM) form of the disease. With adequate weight reduction and dietary control, patients may not require the use of exogenous insulin or oral hypoglycemic drug therapy. Type I (IDDM) diabetics will always require exogenous insulin as well as dietary control because the pancreas has lost the capacity to produce and secrete insulin. The aims of dietary control are the prevention of excessive postprandial hyperglycemia, the prevention of **hypoglycemia** in those patients being treated with hypoglycemic agents or insulin, the achievement and maintenance of an ideal body weight, and a reduction of lipids and cholesterol. A return to normal weight is often accompanied by a reduction in hyperglycemia. The diet should also be adjusted to reduce elevated cholesterol and triglyceride levels in an attempt to retard the progression of atherosclerosis.

To help maintain adherence to dietary restrictions, the diet should be planned using the American Diabetes Association recommendations in relation to the patient's food preferences, economic status, occupation, and physical activity. Emphasis should be placed on what food the patient may have and what exchanges are acceptable. Food should be measured for balanced portions, and the patient should be cautioned not to omit meals or between-meal and bedtime snacks.

Patient education and reinforcement are extremely important to successful therapy. The intelligence and motivation of the diabetic patient and his or her awareness of the potential complications contribute significantly to the ultimate outcome of the disease and the quality of life the patient may lead.

All diabetic patients must receive adequate instruction on personal hygiene, especially regarding care of the feet, skin, and teeth. Infection is a common precipitating cause of ketosis and acidosis and must be treated promptly.

Drug Therapy

Insulin is required to control type I diabetes and for those patients whose diabetes cannot be controlled by diet, weight reduction, or oral hypoglycemic agents. Patients normally controlled with oral hypoglycemic agents require insulin during situations of increased physiologic and psychologic stress, such as pregnancy, surgery, and infections. The dosage of insulin is usually adjusted according to the blood glucose levels and the degree of glucosuria. The patient should test blood or urine glucose before each meal and at bedtime while the insulin is being regulated.

Another adjunct in the therapy of type II diabetes is the use of oral hypoglycemic agents. They are recommended only in those patients who cannot be controlled by diet alone and who are not prone to develop ketosis, acidosis, or infections. Patients most likely to benefit from treatment are those who have developed diabetes after 40 years of age and who require less than 40 units of insulin per day.

Nursing Process for Patients with Diabetes Mellitus

A major challenge in nursing is to teach the recently diagnosed diabetic patient all the necessary information to manage self-care and the disease process and to prevent complications. The patient must be taught the entire therapeutic regimen—diet, activity level, urine or blood testing, medication, self-injection techniques, prevention of complications, and effective management of hypoglycemia or hyperglycemia. Many diabetics have difficulty understanding the critical balance among the dietary prescription, the prescribed medication, and the maintenance of general health. All are important to the control and effective management of the disease process.

Assessment
The order of performing the assessment depends on the setting and the severity of the patient's symptoms.

Description of current symptoms. • Ask the reasons for seeking the current appointment or admission. • Review symptoms and procedures used to diagnose diabetes mellitus in a general medical-surgical textbook.

Patient's understanding of diabetes mellitus. • Assess the individual's current knowledge of the treatment of diabetes mellitus. Gather additional data about the person's current educational needs with regard to self-management of the disease process. • Will other family members or significant others be providing part of the care or be participating in the health education portion of the individual's care? • Patients who are readmitted must be assessed for the understanding of the treatment regimen and for compliance with the prescribed diet, medications, and exercise.

Psychosocial assessment

Mental status. Ask specific information to evaluate the patient's current level of consciousness, alertness, comprehension, and appropriateness of responses. Evaluate the person's judgment capabilities and ability to solve problems about the management of the diabetes.

Adaptation to disease. Ask specifically about the person's adjustment to the diagnosis of diabetes mellitus; or, in a recently diagnosed individual, identify prior coping mechanisms used successfully to deal with life events.

Feelings. Assess for fears and the person's perspective of the impact of the disease on his or her life.

Support system. Obtain information regarding who can provide support for the patient. Does the individual live alone? What impact does the disease have on other members of the family structure (for example, children who are diabetics, persons with complications such as renal or visual complications)? Does the patient participate in a diabetic support group?

Nutrition. • The recently diagnosed diabetic requires a thorough nutritional assessment. Information collected by the nurse or dietitian should include identification of the patient's average daily diet, the ability and willingness to prepare foods, food budget, and level of daily activity and exercise. • Ask about diet prescription—total daily calories and distribution pattern of carbohydrates, fats, and proteins. • Have there been any problems encountered in purchasing or preparing the foods? Has it been difficult to comply with the diet? If so, what are the problems being encountered? • How much alcohol is consumed, and how often? • Has the individual experienced any weight loss or gain recently?

Activity and exercise. • Does the individual feel any weakness or fatigue with daily activities? Does the patient get regular excercise? What type, intensity, and duration is it? Has there been any major variation in the degree of exercise undertaken in the recent past? • Has the patient made any adjustments in the insulin, oral hypoglycemic agent, or diet to offset an increase or decrease in exercise? • Has there been a change in occupation that has affected the level of exercise?

Medications. What medications have been prescribed, and what is the degree of compliance with the regimen? What over-the-counter medicines does the patient take, and how often? Ask specifically about the type and amount of insulin being taken and the times of administration.

Monitoring. Ask the patient to bring a record of self-monitoring of insulin or hypoglycemic agent taken, as well as any blood glucose testing or glycosylated hemoglobin testing that were done. Has the patient done any testing for ketones? If so, what were the results? Any lipid or cholesterol monitoring? Results?

Physical assessment. Generally, data are collected about all body systems to serve as a baseline for subsequent evaluations throughout the course of treatment. Periodic focused assessments are completed to detect signs and symptoms of complications commonly associated with diabetes mellitus.

Hyperglycemia and hypoglycemia. Have there been any episodes of hypoglycemia or hyperglycemia? If so, obtain details of the occurrences (for example, has the patient eaten the prescribed diet, taken the prescribed medications, or altered the exercise level?).

Illnesses/stress. Have there been any recent illnesses, infections, or stressful events? If so, what treatments have been initiated?

Vascular changes. Obtain baseline vital signs. Does the patient have any symptoms of, or is the patient being treated for, cerebrovascular, peripheral vascular, or cardiovascular disease (including hypertension) or diabetic retinopathy or nephropathy?

Neuropathy. Ask about specific symptoms of paresthesias (numbness or tingling sensations), foot injuries and ulcerations, diarrhea, postural hypotension, impotence, or neurogenic bladder.

Nursing Diagnosis
- Knowledge deficit: (indication, side effects)
- Infection: risk for (indication)
- Fluid volume deficit: risk for (side effects)
- Nutrition, altered: less or more than body requirements (indication)

Planning

Description of current symptoms. Individualize the care plan to address the patient's symptoms (for example, hypoglycemia, hyperglycemia, diabetic ketoacidosis coma, or renal failure).

Medications. • Order medications prescribed, and schedule these on the medication administration record (MAR). • Perform focused assessments at regularly scheduled intervals consistent with the patient's status to determine the effectiveness and the side effects to expect or report. • Initiate a diabetic flow sheet.

Diet. • Order the prescribed diabetic diet, and mark the kardex or care plan clearly regarding fluid intake parameters between meals. • Schedule a consultation with a dietitian or nutritional educator appropriate to the patient's needs.

Weight. Mark the kardex or care plan with specific intervals for measurement of weight (for example, daily weights, weight every other day on even days).

Laboratory and blood studies. • Schedule the laboratory blood draws for fasting blood glucose, glucose tolerance testing, glycosylated hemoglobin, serum lipid studies, and so on as ordered by the physician. • Mark the kardex or care plan with specific intervals for the performance of finger-stick blood glucose monitoring. • Indicate clearly if the person is receiving insulin by sliding scale and where orders are written for the amount of insulin to be administered based on the sliding scale (for example, see MAR for sliding scale parameters).

Health teaching. Individualize and initiate health teaching forms used by the clinical site to educate the patient and significant others.

Implementation

- Answer questions the patient has regarding any aspect of the care being provided, including the rationale.
- Encourage expression of feelings and concerns the patient has, and address the patient's concerns first. Involve support persons, as appropriate, in the delivery of care or planning for home management of the diabetes.
- Encourage adequate nutrition by implementing the dietary regimen prescribed. Promote adequate fluid intake to maintain the hydration. Support dietary teaching by the health team, and continuously be alert for misperceptions or misunderstanding of the diet.
- Encourage activity and exercise at the prescribed level. Discuss the benefits while providing care.
- Administer prescribed medications (for example, insulin, oral hypoglycemic agent). Monitor for side effects to expect and report, and document associated monitoring parameters on the records (for example, blood glucose, ketone testing).
- If a hypoglycemic reaction occurs, notify the team leader, who will then contact the physician. The underlying cause of the hypoglycemia must be identified to prevent further occurrences. If in doubt about whether the patient is hypoglycemic or hyperglycemic, the nurse should always proceed to treat the individual for hypoglycemia to prevent neurologic damage from prolonged reduction in glucose to the nerve cells (for example, brain cells).
- With any hyperglycemic reaction, notify the team leader, who will then contact the physician. The goals of treatment include maintaining normal fluid and electrolyte balance and restoration of a normal serum glucose level.
- Perform routine physical assessments every shift as required by the clinical site. Perform focused assessments of areas where complications are anticipated, based on the admission data and subsequent data collected.

Patient Education and Health Promotion

Knowledge. Teach the individual specifics regarding the type of diabetes that has been diagnosed:
- Type I, insulin-dependent diabetes, results from damage to the beta cells of the pancreas, where insulin is normally produced. Insulin is needed to transport the glucose required by the body cells from the bloodstream to the individual cells to be used as an energy source. Without beta cells, no insulin is produced and the glucose accumulates in the blood (hyperglycemia).
- Type I, insulin-dependent diabetes, requires the administration of insulin injections to replace the insulin the body is no longer able to make. The patient must follow a prescribed diet and exercise, perform glucose testing, and, during times when hyperglycemia is present, test for ketones in the urine.
- Type II, non–insulin-dependent diabetes, requires a prescribed diet and exercise, weight loss to a near-ideal body level, glucose testing, and an oral hypoglycemic agent if unable to manage the diabetes with diet alone. During times of illness, or if the oral treatment stops being effective, insulin may be required.

Psychologic adjustment
- When first diagnosed, the patient may experience varying degrees of grief, anger, denial, or acceptance. Let the patient express these concerns, and address those items that are considered to be of greatest importance first.
- Encourage the idea that the patient can control most aspects of diabetes by careful management of diet, medications, and activities. Having a sense of control is impor-

LIFE SPAN ISSUES

INSULIN

Virtually all patients receiving insulin will experience a hypoglycemic reaction at one time or another. Symptoms of hypoglycemic reaction vary from patient to patient. Be aware that confusion and lethargy are signs of hypoglycemia but are sometimes overlooked in elderly patients with the thought that slowness and confusion are just symptoms of "age."

tant to all people. Stress that learning to manage the disease process is the best long-term approach.

- Discuss the individual's lifestyle, travel, work, school schedules, and activities, and individualize the care needs.
- Discuss the need for continued, regular monitoring of the diabetes to minimize the impact the disease may have on the patient and family.

Nutrition

- Diet is used alone or in combination with insulin or oral hypoglycemic agents to control diabetes mellitus. The diabetic patient, whether non–insulin dependent or insulin dependent, must follow a prescribed diet to achieve optimal control of the disease.
- The dietary prescription is based on providing the patient with the nutritional and energy requirements necessary to maintain an appropriate weight and lifestyle. Diabetics are encouraged to maintain a body weight slightly below an ideal weight based on height, gender, and frame size.
- The American Diabetes Association (ADA) recommends that the diet be composed of 55% to 60% carbohydrates, 30% fats (primarily unsaturated; cholesterol intake of 300 mg per day or less), and 12% to 20% proteins (0.8 g of protein per kilogram of body weight). Including high-fiber foods (for example, legumes, oats, and barley) assists in lowering both blood glucose levels and blood cholesterol. Low sodium, alcohol, and caffeine consumption is also advisable. (See a medical-surgical nursing text or a nutrition text for details on dietary calculations using the exchange list, point, constant carbohydrate, or total available glucose [TAG] systems.)
- Inclusion of sucrose is now permitted in limited amounts in the diabetic diet; however, the amount eaten must be calculated as part of the carbohydrate intake for the day.
- The American Diabetes Association approves the use of three artificial sweeteners as sugar substitutes: saccharin, aspartame (NutraSweet), and acesulfame potassium (Sweet One).
- Alcohol may be ingested in moderation by persons with good control of the diabetes. However, drinking on an empty stomach can cause hypoglycemia. Many alcoholic beverages are high in sugar and should be used with caution; light beer or dry wines are alternatives. Because alcohol does affect the blood sugar, it may be wise to test the blood glucose level before and after drinking to identify how the alcohol reacts in a particular patient.
- The American Diabetes Association has several cookbooks and a number of pamphlets available on nutrition for the diabetic.

Activity and exercise

- Maintenance of a normal lifestyle is to be encouraged. This includes exercise and activities enjoyed by the individual. The normal daily energy level is used in determining the dietary and medication requirements for the patient.
- Just as it is important for the patient to maintain a certain diet, it is equally important to maintain a certain activity level. Patients who suddenly increase or decrease activity levels are susceptible to developing episodes of hyperglycemia or hypoglycemia. Both dietary and medication prescriptions may require adjustment if the patient does not plan to resume the previous exercise level. The patient should consult with the physician before initiation of an exercise program.

- Additional self-monitoring of the blood glucose level may be advisable before, during, and approximately 30 minutes after exercise to provide the physician with data to analyze regarding the effects of exercise on the individual's blood glucose level. The ADA recommends that you not exercise if your glucose level is above 250 mg/dl. Conversely, exercising with hypoglycemia is not advisable. A snack high in carbohydrate (10 to 20 g) should be taken before exercising if the blood sugar is less than 100 mg/dl.
- Exercise helps the cells use glucose; therefore exercise lowers the glucose level.
- Drink sufficient fluids without caffeine when exercising to prevent dehydration.
- Stop exercising if feeling weak, sick, dizzy, or if experiencing any type of pain.

Medication

- Insulin or oral hypoglycemic agent therapy may be required to control diabetes mellitus. No changes in therapy should be made without medical supervision.
- A variety of combinations of insulin or insulin and oral hypoglycemic agents may be used to provide control of the blood glucose level. The goal of therapy is to consistently maintain the blood glucose level within the normal range. A variety of administration schedules have evolved over the years to accomplish this goal. The schedules most commonly used are as follows:
  1. Divided doses of intermediate-acting insulin (two thirds in the morning, one third in the evening before dinner)
  2. A combination of short-acting and intermediate-acting insulin in the morning, followed by short-acting insulin at dinner and intermediate-acting insulin before bedtime
  3. Short-acting insulin before each meal and intermediate-acting insulin at bedtime
  4. Short-acting and long-acting insulin before breakfast, short-acting insulin before lunch, and short-acting and long-acting insulin again before dinner
  5. Continuous infusion of regular insulin using a small, portable insulin infusion pump
- The regimen chosen depends on each person's response to medications, schedule of daily activities, and compliance with blood glucose monitoring, insulin injections, and diet.
- Medication preparation, dosage, frequency, storage, and refilling should be discussed and taught in detail. See p. 113 for administration of subcutaneous injections and p. 109 for mixing of insulins. Also discuss proper disposal of used syringes and needles in the home setting.
- Ensure that the patient understands how to refill prescriptions for insulin or oral hypoglycemic agents. When purchasing insulin, ask the patient to double-check the type and concentration (usually U-100) of insulin and the expiration date. The insulin should be stored in the refrigerator (not the freezer) before use. Once it is opened and being used, it can be stored at room temperature.
- If pregnancy is suspected, consult an obstetrician as soon as possible about continuation of medication therapy and necessary adjustment during pregnancy.

Hypoglycemia. Hypoglycemia, or low blood sugar, can occur from too much insulin, insufficient food intake to cover the insulin given, imbalances caused by vomiting and diarrhea, and excessive exercise without additional carbohydrate intake.

Symptoms. Recognize and assess early symptoms of hypoglycemia: nervousness, tremors, headache, apprehension, sweating, cold, clammy skin, and hunger. If uncorrected, hypoglycemia progresses to blurring of vision, lack of coordination, incoherence, coma, and death.

Treatment. If the patient is conscious and *able to swallow*, give 2 to 4 ounces of fruit juice with two teaspoons of sugar or honey in it, *or* 1 cup of skim milk, *or* 4 ounces of a non-diet soft drink, *or* give a piece of candy such as Life Savers or gum drops. An alternative is to carry a tube of cake frosting to squeeze in the mouth. (Chocolate contains fat, which is digested more slowly.) Repeat in 15 to 20 minutes if relief of symptoms is not evident. Do not use hard candy if there is a danger of aspiration. If the patient is unconscious, having a seizure, or *unable to swallow*, administer 20 to 50 ml of glucose 50% IV (only by a qualified individual). See the drug monograph on glucagon.

Hyperglycemia. Hyperglycemia (elevated blood sugar) occurs when the glucose available in the body cannot be transported into the cells for use because of a lack of insulin necessary for the transport mechanism.

Symptoms. Symptoms of hyperglycemia are headache, nausea and vomiting, abdominal pain, dizziness, rapid pulse, rapid shallow respirations, and a fruity odor to the breath from acetone. If untreated, hyperglycemia may also cause coma and death. Glucose level is over 240 mg/dl, and ketones present in the urine.

Treatment. Treatment of hyperglycemia requires hospitalization, insulin, and close monitoring of the blood glucose and urine glucose and ketones. Hyperglycemia usually occurs because of another cause; therefore the problem, often an infection, must also be identified and treated to control the hyperglycemia.

Prevention. The risk of hyperglycemia can be minimized by taking the prescribed dose of insulin or oral hypoglycemic agent; adhering to the prescribed diet and exercise; reporting fevers, infection, or prolonged vomiting or diarrhea to the physician; and maintaining an accurate written record for the physician to analyze to determine the individual patient's needs. Self-monitoring of blood glucose results and evaluation of urine ketones can provide the physician with valuable data to effectively manage the treatment of the individual.

Self-monitoring of blood glucose
- Home blood glucose monitoring (self-monitoring) is an accepted practice for the management of diabetes mellitus. It is used to evaluate the degree of control of the blood glucose being obtained. It can also be used to evaluate when additional insulin must be taken or to determine the effect of exercise on insulin needs.
- Educate the individual using the equipment for self-monitoring that will be used at home. Teach the individual all details of the operation, including calibration, care, handling, and cleansing of the glucose monitor.
- The best time to check the glucose level of the blood is just before meals, 1 to 2 hours after meals, before bed, and between 2 or 3 AM. The physician will give specific instructions regarding how often and when glucose testing

should be done. When ill, it is important to increase the frequency of glucose monitoring.
- A small sample of capillary blood is obtained, generally using an automatic finger-sticking lancet. The blood sample is applied to a reagent strip, which is then placed in an electronic device that "reads" the amount of color change and converts this into a numeric value representing the blood glucose level present. There also are meters and sensors (that do not use reagent strips) for delivering the glucose results. "Talking" glucometers are on the market for persons who are visually impaired. Written records of the blood glucose results should be maintained and taken to all follow-up visits with the physician for analysis.

Urine testing for ketones
- Teach the patient to perform urine testing for ketones. The patient should test the urine for ketones at least four times daily during times of stress, infection, or when signs or symptoms of hyperglycemia are suspected or present. (Ketone testing should be done when the blood glucose level is 240 mg/dl or above.) The physician may suggest additional times when ketones should be monitored depending on the type of regimen prescribed for control of the blood glucose. An accurate written record of the results should be maintained. Guidelines for reporting abnormal results to the physician should be discussed at the time of discharge.
- Suggest that ketone testing be initiated when an illness occurs and the serum glucose is elevated above the usual range the individual has on a daily basis. Explain when to call the physician. Suggest increasing fluid intake whenever the ketones are positive.

Other laboratory glucose testing. • Glycosylated hemoglobin (hemoglobin A_{1c}, or glycohemoglobin) test measures the percent of hemoglobin that has been irreversibly glycosylated because of high blood sugar levels. This provides a reflection of the average blood sugar level attained over the past 8 to 10 weeks. • The fructosamine test measures the amount of glucose bonded to a protein, fructosamine. This reflects the average blood level attained over the past 1 to 3 weeks.

Complications associated with diabetes mellitus
Peripheral vascular disease. The person with diabetes mellitus is more likely to suffer from peripheral vascular disease than is the general population. Reduced blood supply to the extremities may result in intermittent claudication, numbness and tingling, and a greater likelihood of foot infection. Symptoms the patient should look for and care of the extremities:
- Color. Observe the color of each hand, finger, leg, and foot; report cyanosis or reddish-blue discolorations. Inspect the skin of the extremities for any signs of ulceration.
- Temperature. Feel the temperature in each hand, finger, leg, and foot. Report paleness and coldness. Note that these symptoms will be increased if the limbs are elevated above the level of the heart.
- Edema. Report edema, its extent, and whether relieved or unchanged when in a dependent position.
- Limb pain. Pain with exercise that is relieved by rest may be from claudication and should be reported to the physician.

• Care. Prevent ulcers, injury, and infection in the lower extremities with meticulous, regular care. Inspect the feet daily for any signs of breakdown; report to physician and do not attempt to self-treat. Always cut toenails straight across and seek foot care from a podiatrist if problems exist.

Visual alterations. Visual changes are common in the patient with diabetes mellitus. These individuals frequently suffer from blurred vision associated with an elevated blood sugar. Any diabetic person with intermittently blurred vision should contact the physician for a check of the blood sugar level. Once the hyperglycemia is controlled, the blurred vision usually resolves.

Blindness. In advanced stages of diabetes mellitus, the patient may suffer from changes (microangiopathies) in the small blood vessels of the eyes. Retinal hemorrhages, degeneration of retinal vascular tissue, cataracts, and eventual blindness may occur. The diabetic patient should have regular eye exams to allow early treatment of any apparent alterations.

Renal disease. Persons with diabetes mellitus are more susceptible to urinary tract infections; therefore symptoms such as burning on urination or low back pain should be evaluated promptly.

Infection. Any type of infection can cause a significant loss of control of diabetes mellitus. Patients should observe themselves carefully for any signs of redness, tenderness, swelling, or drainage that may occur when there is any break in the skin. Patients should be taught to report immediately early signs of infection, such as fever or sore throat. During an infection, the dosage of insulin may require an adjustment to compensate for a change in metabolic rate, diet, and exercise. Contact the physician for specific directions.

Neuropathies. Explain to appropriate individuals the complication of degeneration of nerves when it exists. Ask the patient to describe any sensations (for example, numbness or tingling) being experienced in the extremities. Inspect the feet for blisters, ulcerations, ingrown toenails, or sores. Occasionally the patient will not be aware of these lesions because of the degeneration of nerves in the area. When numbness and lack of sensation are present, always test the water temperature before immersing a limb. Because of impaired sensation, it is easy to be burned and be unaware of it until later.

Patient reporting. Have patients with diabetes mellitus report nausea, diarrhea, constipation, or visual disturbances that develop.

Impotence. Impotence may occur from a number of causes and should be discussed on an individual basis with the physician should it occur.

Fostering health maintenance. • Throughout the course of treatment, discuss medication, diet, exercise, and the need to achieve and maintain good glucose control to prevent the complications associated with diabetes mellitus. The patient must achieve a high degree of understanding of diabetes mellitus and its management. The patient and family members must be included in the total educational program. • With the advent of shorter hospitalizations, it may be necessary to incorporate follow-up care by a visiting nurse association or a home health agency in the discharge planning. • Seek cooperation and understanding of the following points so that medication compliance is increased: name of medication, dosage, route and time of administration, side effects to expect, and side effects to report.

At discharge. Develop a list of specific equipment and supplies the patient will need when discharged. Keep in mind the cost of these supplies. Consider the following:
1. Syringes. Disposable syringes are convenient and presterilized but are more expensive. Be sure to tell the patient that disposable syringes are designed to be used once and then discarded. However, recent literature refers to the repeated use of the same syringe by an individual patient as long as the needle remains sharp and is kept clean and covered. CHECK with the individual physician BEFORE instituting this practice. Diabetics are prone to infection, and healing may be a problem.
2. Needles. Disposable needles are more convenient but also more expensive. Patients usually use a 27-, 28-, or 29-gauge, $\frac{1}{2}$- or $\frac{5}{8}$-inch needle, but needles should be adjusted to the individual. An obese patient may require a 1- to $1\frac{1}{2}$-inch needle length to properly inject the insulin.
3. Specialized equipment. Magni-Guides are available for the visually impaired patient. This aid holds the vial of insulin, acts as a guide in withdrawing insulin, and has a magnifying glass to make reading the syringe scale easier. Special automatic insulin syringes are available for blind patients. A talking glucose measuring device is also available for the visually impaired individual to perform self-monitoring of the capillary blood glucose levels.
4. Self-monitoring equipment for blood glucose. Be certain the individual has or understands where to purchase the supplies used with the specific brand of self-monitoring glucose machine to be used at home.

Written record. Enlist the patient's aid in developing and maintaining a written record of monitoring parameters (such as blood glucose or urine ketones, insulin dosage, pertinent stress factors, exercise level, illnesses, or major changes in diet or other routine) for discussion with the physician (see box on p. 420). Patients should be encouraged to take this record on follow-up visits.

Education. In 1991 The American Diabetes Association developed 15 areas of diabetic education. All aspects of the care outlined in these recommendations are not presented in the sample teaching plan for diabetics located in Chapter 5, p. 44. The recommendations must be adapted to the individual's needs, and it may not be possible to teach the entire program during the hospitalization period.

Drug Class: Insulins

Actions

Insulin is a hormone produced in the beta cells of the pancreas and is a key regulator of metabolism. Insulin is required for the entry of glucose into skeletal and heart muscle and fat. It also plays a significant role in protein and lipid metabolism. It is not required for glucose transport into the brain or liver tissue.

The pancreas secretes insulin at a steady rate of 0.5 to 1 unit per hour. It is released in greater quantities when the blood glucose rises above 100 mg/dl, such as after a meal.

PATIENT EDUCATION & MONITORING FORM — Antidiabetic Agents

MEDICATIONS	COLOR	TO BE TAKEN

Name _____

Physician _____

Physician's phone _____

Next appt.* _____

PARAMETERS		DAY OF DISCHARGE								COMMENTS
Insulin/Oral agent Types: AM PM	Temperature / Weight									
	Site AM / Site PM									
	Units AM / Units PM									
Urine: (use 2nd voided specimen) Sugar / Ketones	Before breakfast									
	Before lunch									
	Before supper									
	Bedtime									
Blood Glucose levels: Insert time (e.g., 1 PM)	Before breakfast: After breakfast:									
	Before lunch: After lunch:									
	Before supper: After supper:									
	Bedtime:									
	Other:									
Diet	Eat all foods allowed									
	Unable to eat									
	Overate or indulged									
Lifestyle	Usual daily activities/exercise									
	Increased amount of exercise									
	Increased stress									
	Normal day-to-day stress									
Injuries or skin integrity	No visible changes in skin of feet									
	Cuts, bruises, open sores									
Hypoglycemia	Sx: Sweating, weak, shaky, hungry									
	Blood Glucose Level: Time:									
Hyperglycemia	Sx: Urinating frequency, poor appetite, ↑thirst, weak, dizzy									
	Blood Glucose Level: Time:									

*Please bring this record with you to your next appointment.
Use the back of this sheet for additional information.

420

The average rate of insulin secretion in an adult is 30 to 50 units per day.

Insulin deficiency reduces the rate of transport of glucose into cells, producing hyperglycemia. Other metabolic reactions are also inhibited by the lack of insulin, resulting in the conversion of protein to glucose, hyperlipidemia, ketosis, and acidosis.

Insulins from the pancreases of different animals have similar activity and thus may be used in human beings. Beef and pork pancreases have been the primary sources of insulin since its discovery in 1922. Over the past decade, significant progress has been made in improving the purity of insulin to reduce allergenicity. Biosynthetic human insulin is now available for selected patients, especially newly diagnosed diabetics. It has fewer allergic reactions associated with it than beef and pork insulins.

Uses

Three factors—onset, peak, and duration—are important in the use of insulin therapy. *Onset* is the time required for the medication to have an initial effect or action; *peak* is when the agent will have the maximum effect; and *duration* is the length of time that the agent remains active in the body. When monitoring insulin therapy, it is important to understand these terms and to associate them with the type of insulin being administered to ascertain when a patient is most susceptible to hyperglycemia or hypoglycemia (Table 33-2).

Three types of insulin, based on onset, peak, and duration, are in use today: rapid-acting, intermediate-acting, and long-acting insulins.

Regular insulin is used for its immediate onset of activity and short duration of action. It is the only form of insulin that is a clear solution (not a cloudy suspension). It is the only dosage form of insulin that may be injected by both intravenous and subcutaneous routes of administration. See Table 33-2 for the activity of the regular insulins.

Neutral protamine hagedorn (NPH) insulin is an intermediate-acting insulin containing specific amounts of regular insulin and protamine. The protamine binds to the insulin. When administered subcutaneously, the insulin is slowly released from the protamine and becomes active, giving it the intermediate-acting classification.

Lente insulins are derived from a manufacturing process that produces two physical forms, one crystalline and the other noncrystalline. The long-acting, crystalline form is marketed as Ultralente; the noncrystalline, fast-acting compound is known as Semilente and is not available on the U.S. market. The intermediate-acting Lente insulin is a mixture containing approximately 30% noncrystalline Semilente and 70% crystalline Ultralente insulins.

Storage of Insulin

It is recommended that, whenever possible, insulin be stored in a refrigerator. A general rule of thumb is that the bottle of insulin should be stored in the refrigerator until opened. Because patients find it uncomfortable to inject cold insulin, the bottle may then be kept at room temperature (68 to 75° F) until gone. At sustained temperatures above room temperature, insulins lose potency rapidly.

Therapeutic Outcomes

The primary therapeutic outcomes expected from insulin therapy are as follows:

- A decrease in both fasting blood glucose levels and glycosylated hemoglobin concentrations in the range defined as acceptable for the individual patient
- Fewer long-term complications associated with poorly controlled diabetes mellitus

Nursing Process

Premedication Assessment

1. Confirm that a blood glucose level was recently measured and was acceptable for the individual patient.
2. Confirm that the patient has had a level of activity reasonable for the individual patient, and the anticipated level of activity planned for the next several hours is balanced with the insulin dose.
3. Confirm that the prescribed diet is being consumed as planned and that no changes in diet are anticipated in relation to insulin dosage over the next several hours.

Planning
Availability. See Table 33-2.

Implementation
Administration techniques. See Chapter 9.

Dosage and administration. Maintenance therapy for newly diagnosed diabetic patients: it is important to understand that effective control of diabetes mellitus requires a balanced food intake, exercise, blood glucose levels measured several times daily, and insulin dosage adjustments based on the blood glucose levels.

Several methods have been developed to initiate insulin therapy. The method chosen depends on such issues as fluctuation of the patient's blood glucose; ability of the patient to measure, mix, and administer the insulin; and compliance with planned exercise and diet.

Before starting a standardized regimen, the diet and physical exercise level must be stabilized. A standard approach is to calculate the initial total daily dose of insulin based on 0.5 to 0.8 U/kg of whole body (not lean body) weight. Neutral potamine hagedorn (human) insulin is often used to initiate therapy. This total daily dose is then split into two doses: two thirds is administered in the morning before breakfast, and one third is administered 30 minutes before supper in the evening. The insulin dose is then adjusted over the next several weeks based on blood glucose measurements taken (usually) four times daily and glycosylated hemoglobin levels. Diet and exercise may also require adjustment.

Mixing insulins. Many patients with diabetes mix rapid-acting insulin with either intermediate-acting or long-acting insulins to prevent "peaks and valleys" in blood glucose levels. See Table 33-3 and Chapter 9, p. 109, for technique in mixing insulins.

Evaluation
Side effects to expect and report

HYPERGLYCEMIA. Insulin overdose or decreased carbohydrate intake may result in hypoglycemia. If untreated, irreversible brain damage may occur. Hypoglycemia occurs most frequently when the administered insulin reaches its peak action (see Table 33-2). Hypoglycemia must be treated immediately. The following conditions may predispose a

Table 33-2

Commercially Available Forms of Insulin

TYPE OF INSULIN	MANUFACTURER	STRENGTH (UNITS/ML)	SOURCE	ONSET (HR)	PEAK (HR)	DURATION* (HR)	GLYCOSURIA†	HYPOGLYCEMIA†
Fast-acting insulin *Insulin injection*								
Humulin R (human)	Lilly	100	Semisynthetic	0.5-4	2.5-5	5-16	Early AM(1)	Before lunch(3)
Novolin R (human)	Novo Nordisk	100	Semisynthetic	0.5-4	2.5-5	5-16	Early AM	Before lunch
Regular (purified pork) insulin	Novo Nordisk	100	Pork	0.5	2.5-5	8	Early AM	Before lunch
Regular insulin	Novo Nordisk	100	Pork	0.5-1	3-6	6-8	Early AM	Before lunch
Regular Iletin I	Lilly	100	Beef and pork	0.5-1	3-6	6-8	Early AM	Before lunch
Regular Iletin II (Pork)	Lilly	100, 500	Pork	05.-1	3-6	6-8	Early AM	Before lunch
Velosulin (human)	Novo Nordisk	100	Semisynthetic	0.5	1-3	8	Early AM	Before lunch
Intermediate-acting insulin *Isophane insulin suspension (NPH)*								
Humulin N (human)	Lilly	100	Semisynthetic	1-4	4-12	16-28	Before lunch(2)	3 PM to supper(3)
Novolin N (human)	Novo Nordisk	100	Semisynthetic	1-4	4-12	16-28	Before lunch	3 PM to supper
NPH Iletin I	Lilly	100	Beef and pork	1-1.5	8-12	24	Before lunch	3 PM to supper
NPH Iletin II (Pork)	Lilly	100	Pork	1-1.5	8-12	24	Before lunch	3 PM to supper
NPH-N insulin	Novo Nordisk	100	Pork	1.5	4-12	24	Before lunch	3 PM to supper
Isophane insulin suspension and insulin injection								
Humulin 50/50 (human)	Lilly	100	Semisynthetic	0.5	4-8	24	Before lunch	3 PM to supper
Humulin 70/30 (human)	Lilly	100	Semisynthetic	0.5	4-12	24	Before lunch	3 PM to supper
Novolin 70/30 (human)	Novo Nordisk	100	Semisynthetic	0.5	4-12	24	Before lunch	3 PM to supper
Insulin zinc suspension								
Humulin L	Lilly	100	Semisynthetic	1-4	7-15	16-28	Before lunch	3 PM to supper
Lente Iletin I	Lilly	100	Beef and pork	1-1.5	8-12	24	Before lunch	3 PM to supper
Lente Iletin II	Lilly	100	Beef or pork	1-1.5	8-12	24	Before lunch	3 PM to supper
Lente (L) insulin	Novo Nordisk	100	Pork	2.5	7-15	22	Before lunch	3 PM to supper
Novolin L (human)	Novo Nordisk	100	Semisynthetic	1-4	7-15	16-28	Before lunch	3 PM to supper
Long-acting insulin *Extended insulin zinc suspension*								
Humulin U Ultralente	Lilly	100	Semisynthetic	4-8	12-18	24-28	Supper to bedtime	2 AM to breakfast

*The times listed are averages based on a newly diagnosed diabetic patient. Factors modifying these times include patient variation, site and route of administration, and dosage.
†Most frequently occurs when insulin is administered (1) at bedtime the previous night; (2) before breakfast the previous day; (3) before breakfast the same day.

Table 33-3

Compatibility of Insulin Combinations

COMBINATION	RATIO	MIX BEFORE ADMINISTRATION
Regular + NPH	Any combination	2 to 3 months
Regular + Lente	Any combination	Immediately*
Lentes	Any combination	Stable indefinitely

*Must be used immediately to retain properties of regular insulin.

diabetic patient to a hypoglycemic (insulin) reaction: improper measurement of insulin dosage, excessive exercise, insufficient food intake, concurrent ingestion of hypoglycemic drugs and discontinuation of drugs (see Drug Interactions), or conditions (such as infection or stress) causing hyperglycemia.

Diabetic or prediabetic patients must be monitored for the development of hyperglycemia, particularly during the early weeks of therapy.

Assess regularly for abnormal blood glucose and in certain patients, as requested by the physician, for glycosuria and ketones. If symptoms occur frequently, the physician should be notified, and the written records maintained by the patient that reflect the results of self-testing should be supplied to the physician for analysis.

Patients receiving insulin may require an adjustment in dosage.

HYPOGLYCEMIA. Monitor for the following signs of hypoglycemia: headache, nausea, weakness, hunger, lethargy, decreased coordination, general apprehension, sweating, and blurred or double vision.

Hypoglycemia must be treated immediately. Mild symptoms may be controlled by the oral administration of a glucose source—for example, lump of sugar, orange juice, carbonated cola beverage (not diet), candy (not chocolate)—or ingestion of a commercially prepared substance such as Glutose. Severe symptoms may be relieved by the administration of intravenous glucose, and parenteral glucagon may be prescribed in some instances. If in doubt about whether the patient is hypoglycemic or hyperglycemic, always treat the individual for hypoglycemia to prevent the possible neurologic complications that can occur from untreated hypoglycemia.

ALLERGIC REACTIONS. Allergic reactions, manifested by itching, redness, and swelling at the site of injection, have been common occurrences in patients receiving insulin therapy. These reactions may be caused by modifying proteins in NPH insulin, the insulin itself, the alcohol used to cleanse the injection site or sterilize the syringe, the patient's injection technique, or the intermittent use of insulin.

Spontaneous desensitization frequently occurs within a few weeks. Local irritation may be reduced by changing to insulin without protein modifiers (for example, go to the Lente series) or to insulins derived from biosynthetic sources (for example, "human" insulin), using unscented alcohol swabs or disposable syringes and needles, and checking the patient's injection technique. Acute rashes covering the

whole body and anaphylactic symptoms are rare but must be treated with antihistamines, epinephrine, and steroids.

LIPODYSTROPHIES. Rotation of injection sites is important to avoid atrophy or hypertrophy of subcutaneous fat tissue. This dermatologic condition may occur at the site of frequent insulin injections. The hypertrophic areas tend to be used more frequently by diabetic patients because the fat pad becomes anesthetized. In addition to the adverse cosmetic effects, the absorption rate of insulin from these sites becomes significantly prolonged and erratic. Loss of diabetic control may result, particularly in unstable type I patients.

Drug interactions

HYPERGLYCEMIA. The following drugs may cause hyperglycemia, especially in prediabetic and diabetic patients (insulin dosages may require adjustment): acetazolamide, ethanol, corticosteroids, glucagon, dextrothyroxine, lithium, diuretics (thiazides, furosemide, bumetanide), oral contraceptives, diazoxide, phenothiazines, dobutamine, phenytoin, epinephrine, salicylates, and diltiazem.

Diabetic or prediabetic patients must be monitored for the development of hyperglycemia, particularly during the early weeks of therapy.

Assess regularly for glycosuria and report if it occurs with any frequency.

HYPOGLYCEMIA. The following drugs may cause hypoglycemia, thereby decreasing insulin requirements, in diabetic patients: acetaminophen, anabolic steroids (Dianabol, Durabolin), ethanol, guanethidine, monoamine oxidase inhibitors, clofibrate, propranolol, and salicylates.

Monitor for the following signs of hypoglycemia: headache, nausea, weakness, hunger, lethargy, decreased coordination, general apprehension, sweating, and blurred or double vision.

Notify the physician if any of the aforementioned symptoms appear.

BETA-ADRENERGIC BLOCKING AGENTS. Beta-adrenergic blocking agents (propranolol, timolol, nadolol, pindolol, others) may induce hypoglycemia but may also mask many of the symptoms of hypoglycemia. Notify the physician if you suspect that any of the aforementioned symptoms appear intermittently.

Drug Class: Biguanide Oral Hypoglycemic Agent

metformin (met'for-mihn)
Glucophage (glue-ko'fahg)

Actions

Metformin represents a new class of oral hypoglycemic agent. The mechanism of action of metformin is unknown. It does not stimulate the release of insulin from the pancreas as do the sulfonylureas.

Uses

Metformin is used as an adjunct to diet to lower blood glucose in patients with type II, non–insulin-dependent diabetes mellitus whose hyperglycemia cannot be controlled by diet and exercise alone. It has the particular advantage that it will not cause hypoglycemia, as can occur with insulin and the sulfonylureas. It may also be used in combination with the sulfonylureas to lower blood glucose because the two agents act by different mechanisms.

Metformin has two other beneficial effects: it does not cause weight gain, and indeed may cause weight loss, contrary to the actions of the sulfonylureas; and metformin also has a favorable effect on triglycerides. It produces a modest decrease in concentrations of serum triglycerides and total and low-density lipoprotein (LDL) cholesterol, with modest increases in concentrations of high-density lipoprotein (HDL) cholesterol.

Therapeutic Outcomes

The primary therapeutic outcomes expected from biguanide oral hypoglycemic agent therapy are as follows:
- A decrease in both fasting blood glucose levels and the glycosylated hemoglobin concentrations in the range defined as acceptable for the individual patient
- Fewer long-term complications associated with poorly controlled type II diabetes mellitus

Nursing Process

Premedication Assessment
1. Confirm that a blood glucose level was recently measured and was acceptable for the individual patient.
2. Confirm that the patient has had a level of activity reasonable for the individual patient, and the anticipated level of activity planned for the next several hours is balanced with the oral hypoglycemic agent dose.
3. Confirm that the prescribed diet is being consumed as planned and that no changes in diet are anticipated in relation to oral hypoglycemic agent dosage over the next several hours.

Planning
Availability. 500 and 850 mg tablets.

Implementation
Dosage and administration. Adult: PO—initially, 500 mg twice daily with the morning and evening meals. Dosage is increased by adding 500 mg to the daily dose each week up to 2500 mg daily. In general, most patients require at least 1500 mg daily for therapeutic effect. At this dosage, it should be administered three times daily (1000 mg with breakfast, 500 mg with lunch, and 1000 mg with dinner). If a patient's blood glucose is not controlled with the maximum dosage, a sulfonylurea oral hypoglycemic agent may be added to the regimen.

Evaluation
Side effects to expect
NAUSEA, VOMITING, ANOREXIA, ABDOMINAL CRAMPS, FLATULENCE. These side effects are usually mild and tend to resolve with continued therapy. Taking the medicine with meals will help reduce these adverse effects. Encourage the patient not to discontinue therapy without first consulting the physician.
Side effects to report
MALAISE, MYALGIAS, RESPIRATORY DISTRESS, HYPOTENSION. A rare adverse effect of metformin is lactic acidosis. Gradual onset of these symptoms may be an early indication

of lactic acidosis developing. Patients with reduced renal function and excessive alcohol intake are most susceptible to developing lactic acidosis.

Drug interactions
DRUGS THAT MAY ENHANCE TOXIC EFFECTS. Amiloride, digoxin, morphine, procainamide, quinidine, quinine, ranitidine, cimetidine, triamterene, trimethoprim, vancomycin. These medicines are excreted by the same route through the kidneys that metformin depends on for excretion. There is a possibility that these drugs block the excretion of metformin, potentially causing lactic acidosis. Monitor for signs of lactic acidosis as discussed previously.
HYPERGLYCEMIA. The following drugs when used concurrently with metformin may decrease the therapeutic effects of metformin: corticosteroids, phenothiazines, diuretics, oral contraceptives, thyroid replacement hormones, phenytoin, diazoxide, and lithium carbonate.

Diabetic or prediabetic patients must be monitored for the development of hyperglycemia, particularly during the early weeks of therapy.

Assess regularly for glycosuria and report if it occurs with any frequency.
NIFEDIPINE. Nifedipine appears to increase the absorption of metformin. Adverse effects may be minimized by reducing the dosage of metformin.

Drug Class: Sulfonylurea Oral Hypoglycemic Agents
Actions
The sulfonylureas lower blood glucose by stimulating the release of insulin from the beta cells of the pancreas.

Uses
The sulfonylureas are effective in type II diabetic patients, in whom the pancreas still has the capacity to secrete insulin, but are of no value in the type I diabetic, who has no beta-cell function. Sulfonylureas may be effective in the treatment of type II diabetes mellitus that cannot be controlled by diet and exercise if the patient is not susceptible to developing ketosis, acidosis, or infections. Patients most likely to benefit from oral hypoglycemic treatment are those who develop signs of diabetes after age 40 and who require less than 40 units of insulin per day (indicating that some insulin is still being secreted by the beta cells).

Therapeutic Outcomes
The primary therapeutic outcomes expected from sulfonylurea oral hypoglycemic therapy are as follows:
- A decrease in both fasting blood glucose levels and the glycosylated hemoglobin concentrations in the range defined as acceptable for the individual patient
- Fewer long-term complications associated with poorly controlled diabetes mellitus

Nursing Process

Premedication Assessment
1. Confirm that a blood glucose level was recently measured and was acceptable for the individual patient.

2. Confirm that the patient has had a level of activity reasonable for the individual patient, and the anticipated level of activity planned for the next several hours is balanced with the oral hypoglycemic agent dose.
3. Confirm that the prescribed diet is being consumed as planned and that no changes in diet are anticipated in relation to the oral hypoglycemic agent dosage over the next several hours.

Planning
Availability. See Table 33-4.

Implementation
Note: Sulfonylureas generally should not be administered to patients allergic to sulfonamides. Patients may also be allergic to sulfonylureas.
Dosage and administration. See Table 33-4. Individual dosage adjustment is essential for the successful use of oral hypoglycemic agents. A patient should be given a 1-month trial on maximum doses of the sulfonylurea being used before the patient can be considered a primary failure. If a patient represents a secondary failure (a patient initially controlled on oral agents), changing to an alternative sulfonylurea is occasionally successful in controlling blood sugar.

Evaluation
Side effects to expect
NAUSEA, VOMITING, ANOREXIA, ABDOMINAL CRAMPS. These side effects are usually mild and tend to resolve with continued therapy. Encourage the patient not to discontinue therapy without first consulting the physician.
Side effects to report
HYPOGLYCEMIA. Patients receiving oral hypoglycemic therapy are as susceptible to hypoglycemia as diabetic patients on insulin therapy. Consequently, blood glucose levels must be monitored closely, especially in the early stages of therapy.

Monitor for the following signs of hypoglycemia: headache, nausea, weakness, hunger, lethargy, decreased coordination, general apprehension, sweating, blurred or double vision.

Hypoglycemia must be treated immediately. Mild symptoms may be controlled by the oral administration of a glucose source—for example, lump of sugar, orange juice, carbonated cola beverage (not diet), candy (not chocolate)—or ingestion of a commercially prepared substance such as Glutose. Severe symptoms may be relieved by the administration of intravenous glucose, and parenteral glucagon may be prescribed in some instances. If in doubt about whether the patient is hypoglycemic or hyperglycemic, always treat the individual for hypoglycemia to prevent the possible neurologic complications that can occur from untreated hypoglycemia.

Notify the physician immediately if any of the above symptoms appear. The dosage of oral hypoglycemic agents may also have to be reduced.

HEPATOTOXICITY. The symptoms of hepatotoxicity are: anorexia, nausea, vomiting, jaundice, hepatomegaly, splenomegaly, and abnormal liver function tests (elevated bilirubin, AST, ALT, GGT, alkaline phosphatase, prothrombin time).

BLOOD DYSCRASIAS. Routine laboratory studies (red blood cell count [RBC], white blood cell count [WBC], and differential counts) should be scheduled. Stress the need to return for this laboratory work.

Monitor for the development of a sore throat, fever, purpura, jaundice, or excessive and progressively increasing weakness.

DERMATOLOGIC REACTIONS. Report a rash or pruritus immediately. Withhold additional doses pending approval by the physician.
Drug interactions
HYPOGLYCEMIA. The following drugs may enhance the hypoglycemic effects of the sulfonylureas: ethanol, methandrostenolone, chloramphenicol, warfarin, propranolol,

Table 33-4
Oral Hypoglycemic Agents

Generic Name	Brand Name	Availability	Initial Dosage	Dosage Range	Duration* (Hr)
First generation					
Acetohexamide	Dymelor, ✽Dimelor	Tablets: 250, 500 mg	0.5 g daily	0.25-1.5 g daily	12-18
Chlorpropamide	Diabinese	Tablets: 100, 250 mg	100 mg daily	100-750 mg daily	24-72
Tolazamide	Tolinase	Tablets: 100, 250, 500 mg	100 mg daily	0.1-1 g daily	12-16
Tolbutamide	Orinase	Tablets: 250, 500 mg	1 g 2 times daily	0.25-3 g daily	6-12
Second generation					
Glipizide	Glucotrol	Tablets: 5, 10 mg;	2.5-5 mg daily	15-40 mg daily	10-24
Glipizide XL	Glucotrol XL	Extended release 5, 10 mg			
Glyburide	Glynase	Prestabs: 1.5, 3, 6 mg	1.5-3 mg daily	0.75-12 mg daily	24
	DiaBeta, Micronase	Tablets: 1.5, 2.5, 5 mg	2.5-5 mg daily	1.25-20 mg daily	24

*The times listed are averages based on a newly diagnosed diabetic patient. Factors modifying these times include patient variation and dosage.
✽ Available in Canada only.

salicylates, sulfisoxazole, guanethidine, oxytetracycline, monoamine oxidase inhibitors, and phenylbutazone.

Monitor for the following signs of hypoglycemia: headache, nausea, weakness, hunger, lethargy, decreased coordination, general apprehension, sweating, blurred or double vision.

Notify the physician if any of these symptoms appear.

HYPERGLYCEMIA. The following drugs when used concurrently with the sulfonylureas may decrease the therapeutic effects of the sulfonylureas: corticosteroids, phenothiazines, diuretics, oral contraceptives, thyroid replacement hormones, phenytoin, diazoxide, and lithium carbonate.

Diabetic or prediabetic patients must be monitored for the development of hyperglycemia, particularly during the early weeks of therapy.

Assess regularly for glycosuria and report if it occurs with any frequency.

Patients receiving insulin may require an adjustment in dosage.

BETA-ADRENERGIC BLOCKING AGENTS. Beta-adrenergic blocking agents (propranolol, timolol, nadolol, pindolol, others) may induce hypoglycemia but may also mask many of the symptoms of hypoglycemia. Notify the physician if any of these symptoms appear intermittently.

ALCOHOL. Ingestion of alcoholic beverages during sulfonylurea therapy may infrequently result in an Antabuse-like reaction, manifested by facial flushing, pounding headache, feeling of breathlessness, and nausea.

In patients who develop an Antabuse-like reaction to alcohol, the use of alcohol and preparations containing alcohol (such as over-the-counter cough medications and mouthwashes) should be avoided during therapy and up to 5 days after discontinuation of sulfonylurea therapy.

Drug Class: Antihyperglycemic Agent

acarbose (A'kar-bohs)
Precose (pre'kohs)

Actions

Acarbose is the first of a new type of agent called antihyperglycemic agents. It is an enzyme inhibitor that inhibits pancreatic alpha amylase and gastrointestinal alpha glycoside hydrolase enzymes used in the digestion of sugars. In patients with diabetes, this enzyme inhibition results in delayed glucose absorption and a lowering of postprandial hyperglycemia.

Uses

Acarbose is used as an adjunct to diet to lower blood glucose in patients with type II, non–insulin-dependent diabetes mellitus whose hyperglycemia cannot be controlled by diet and exercise alone. It has the particular advantage that it will not cause hypoglycemia, as can occur with insulin and the sulfonylureas. It may also be used in combination with the sulfonylureas or metformin to lower blood glucose because the agents act by different mechanisms.

Therapeutic Outcomes

The primary therapeutic outcomes expected from acarbose therapy are as follows:

- A decrease in both postprandial blood glucose levels and the glycosylated hemoglobin concentrations in the range defined as acceptable for the individual patient
- Fewer long-term complications associated with poorly controlled type II diabetes mellitus

Nursing Process

Premedication Assessment

1. If the patient is also receiving oral hypoglycemic agent or insulin therapy, ensure that the dosages of these medicines are well adjusted before starting acarbose therapy.
2. Review the patient's history to ensure that there is no gastrointestinal malabsorption syndrome or obstruction present.
3. Review the patient's medical history to ensure that no liver abnormalities are present.

Planning

Availability. 50 and 100 mg tablets.

Implementation

Dosage and administration. Adult: PO—initially, 25 mg 3 times daily at the start of each main meal. The dose is adjusted at 4- to 8-week intervals based on 1-hour postprandial blood glucose concentrations and on the severity of adverse effects. The maintenance dose is 50 to 100 mg 3 times daily. The maximum recommended dose for patients weighing less than 60 kg (132 lb) is 50 mg 3 times daily. The maximum dose for patients weighing more than 60 kg is 100 mg 3 times daily.

Evaluation

Side effects to expect

ABDOMINAL CRAMPS, DIARRHEA, FLATULENCE. These adverse effects are caused by the metabolism of carbohydrates in the large intestine that were blocked from metabolism in the small intestine by acarbose. These side effects are usually mild and tend to resolve with continued therapy. Encourage the patient not to discontinue therapy without first consulting the physician.

Side effects to report

HYPOGLYCEMIA. Although acarbose does not cause hypoglycemia by itself, it can enhance the hypoglycemia caused by a sulfonylurea or insulin. Consequently, blood glucose levels must be monitored closely, especially in the early stages of therapy.

Monitor for the following signs of hypoglycemia: headache, nausea, weakness, hunger, lethargy, decreased coordination, general apprehension, sweating, blurred or double vision.

Hypoglycemia must be treated immediately. Treatment should be initiated with oral dextrose (Glutose) because its metabolism is not blocked by acarbose. Do not use sucrose (table sugar) because its metabolism is blocked by acarbose. Severe symptoms may be relieved by the administration of intravenous glucose, and parenteral glucagon may be prescribed in some instances.

If in doubt about whether the patient is hypoglycemic or hyperglycemic, always treat the individual for hypoglycemia to prevent the possible neurologic complications that can occur from untreated hypoglycemia.

Notify the physician immediately if any of these symptoms appear. The dosage of oral hypoglycemic agents may also have to be reduced.

HEPATOTOXICITY. Acarbose has been reported to cause elevations of serum transaminases (AST and ALT). In rare cases, it has caused hyperbilirubinemia. It is recommended that serum transaminase concentrations be checked every 3 months during the first year of treatment and periodically thereafter.

Drug interactions

HYPERGLYCEMIA. The following drugs, when used concurrently with acarbose, may decrease the therapeutic effects of acarbose: corticosteroids, phenothiazines, diuretics, oral contraceptives, thyroid replacement hormones, phenytoin, diazoxide, and lithium carbonate.

Drug Class: Antihypoglycemic Agent

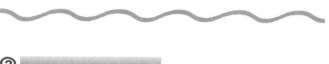

glucagon (glue′kah-gohn)

Actions

Glucagon is a hormone secreted by the alpha cells of the pancreas that breaks down stored glycogen to glucose, resulting in elevated blood glucose levels. Glucagon also aids in the conversion of amino acids to glucose (gluconeogenesis). Glucagon is dependent on the presence of glycogen for its action. It has essentially no action in cases of starvation, adrenal insufficiency, or chronic hypoglycemia.

Uses

Glucagon is used to treat hypoglycemic reactions in patients with diabetes mellitus.

Therapeutic Outcomes

The primary therapeutic outcome expected from glucagon therapy is elimination of symptoms associated with hypoglycemia.

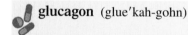

Nursing Process

Premedication Assessment

1. Confirm patient unresponsiveness before administration. If conscious, oral antihypoglycemic therapy is usually more appropriate.
2. Hypoglycemia is a medical emergency. If suspected, it should be treated by authorized personnel as soon as possible.

Planning

Availability. SC, IM, IV: 1 and 10 mg vials.

Implementation

Dosage and administration. Adult: SC, IM, IV—administer 1 mg. Response should be observed within 5 to 20 minutes. If response is minimal, 1 or 2 additional doses may be administered. If the patient is slow to arouse, consider glucose to be administered intravenously.

Evaluation

Side effects to expect and report

NAUSEA, VOMITING. These side effects may also occur with hypoglycemia. Take precautions to prevent aspiration of vomitus.

Drug interactions

WARFARIN. Glucagon may potentiate the anticoagulant effects of warfarin if used for several days. Monitor the patient's INR and reduce the dose of warfarin accordingly.

CHAPTER REVIEW

Diabetes mellitus is a complex, chronic disease with both short- and long-term complications associated with it. The long-term objective of control of the disease must involve mechanisms to stop the progression of the complications of the disease. Patient education and reinforcment are extremely important to successful therapy. Major determinants to success are the patient taking responsibility for a balanced diet, insulin or oral hypoglycemic therapy, routine exercise, and good hygiene. The nurse plays a critical role as a health educator in discussion of treatment options, planning for lifestyle changes, counseling before discharge, and reinforcement of key points during office visits. Best results are attained when the patient, family, and nurse work together in developing the care plan.

MATH REVIEW

1. Ordered: 22 U NPH (human) insulin to be administered 30 minutes before breakfast.
   Available: U-100 NPH (human) insulin.
   What volume of insulin is to be administered? _____ ml

2. Ordered: 27 U NPH (human) insulin + 7 U regular (human) insulin to be administered before breakfast.
   Available: U-100 NPH (human) insulin.
   U-100 regular (human) insulin.
   What volume of NPH insulin is to be drawn up?
   _____ ml
   What volume of regular insulin is to be drawn up?
   _____ ml
   What total volume is to be injected? _____ ml?

CRITICAL THINKING QUESTIONS

Situation:
Robbie Vanderstahl, age 18, was recently diagnosed with type I diabetes mellitus. After several days of treatment with adjustment of diet, exercise, and regular insulin, Robbie was placed on U-100 NPH (human) insulin, 20 U 30 minutes before breakfast and 10 U before the evening meal.

1. What are the nursing interventions to be considered when administering the NPH insulin?

2. Robbie is having trouble injecting himself. In a moment of frustration, he asks, "Why can't I take insulin pills like my grandfather?" What is your response?

Continuing situation: Five days later, the physician adds 5 U of regular (human) insulin to the morning dose to be administered with the NPH insulin.

3. Describe how you would teach Robbie to mix the morning insulin dose for a single administration.

4. While continuing with Robbie's education, he asks again for the difference between the symptoms of hypoglycemia and hyperglycemia. What is your response?

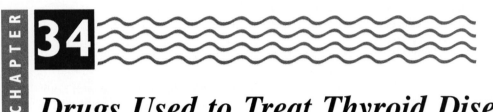

CHAPTER 34

Drugs Used to Treat Thyroid Disease

CHAPTER CONTENT

Key Words

thyroid-stimulating hormone
triiodothyronine (T_3)
thyroxine (T_4)
hypothyroidism

myxedema
cretinism
hyperthyroidism
thyrotoxicosis

Objectives

1. Describe the signs, symptoms, treatment, and nursing interventions associated with hypothyroidism and hyperthyroidism.

2. Identify the two classes of drugs used to treat thyroid disease.

3. State the drug of choice for hypothyroidism.

4. Explain the effects of hyperthyroidism on dosages of warfarin and digitalis glycosides and on persons taking oral hypoglycemic agents.

5. Cite the actions of antithyroid medications on the formation and release of the hormones produced by the thyroid gland.

6. State the three types of treatment for hyperthyroidism.

7. Explain the nutritional requirements and activity restrictions needed for an individual with hyperthyroidism.

8. Identify the types of conditions that respond favorably to the use of radioactive iodine-131.

9. Cite the action of propylthiouracil on the synthesis of T_3 and T_4.

THYROID GLAND

The thyroid gland is a large, reddish, ductless gland in front of and on either side of the trachea. It consists of two lateral lobes and a connecting isthmus and is roughly butterfly shaped. It is enclosed in a covering of areolar tissue. The thyroid is made up of numerous closed follicles containing colloid matter and is surrounded by a vascular network. This gland is one of the most richly vascularized tissues in the body.

As with other endocrine glands, thyroid gland function is regulated by the hypothalamus and the anterior pituitary gland. The hypothalamus secretes thyrotropin-releasing hormone (TRH), which stimulates the anterior pituitary gland to release **thyroid-stimulating hormone** (TSH). Thyroid-stimulating hormone stimulates the thyroid gland to release its hormones **triiodothyronine** (T_3) and **thyroxine** (T_4).

The thyroid hormones regulate general body metabolism. Imbalance in thyroid hormone production may also interfere with the following body functions: growth and maturation; carbohydrate, protein, and lipid metabolism; thermal regulation; cardiovascular function; lactation; and reproduction.

THYROID DISEASES

Hypothyroidism is the result of inadequate thyroid hormone production.

Myxedema is hypothyroidism that occurs during adult life. The onset of symptoms is usually mild and vague. Patients develop a sense of slowness in motion, speech, and mental processes. They often develop more lethargic, sedentary habits; have decreased appetites; gain weight; are constipated; cannot tolerate cold; become weak; and fatigue easily. The body temperature may be subnormal; the skin becomes dry, coarse, and thickened; and the face appears puffy. Patients often have decreased blood pressure and heart rate and develop anemia and high cholesterol levels. These patients have an increased susceptibility to infection and are sensitive to small doses of sedative-hypnotics, anesthetics, and narcotics. Myxedema may be caused by excessive use of antithyroid drugs used to treat hyperthyroidism, radiation exposure, thyroid surgery, acute viral thyroiditis, or chronic thyroiditis.

Congenital hypothyroidism occurs when a child is born without a thyroid gland or one that is hypoactive. The historical name of this disease is **cretinism**. Fortunately, this disorder is becoming rare because most states require diagnostic testing of the newborn for hypothyroidism.

Although the symptoms of hypothyroidism in both infants and adults are for the most part classical, the final diagnosis is usually not made until diagnostic tests have been completed. These tests include drawing serum levels of circulating T_3 and T_4 hormones. If the levels are low, the patient is considered to be hypothyroid. Further diagnostic testing is required to determine the cause of thyroid hypofunction.

Hyperthyroidism is caused by excess production of thyroid hormones. Disorders that may cause hyperactivity of the thyroid gland are Graves' disease, nodular goiter, thyroiditis, thyroid carcinoma, overdoses of thyroid hormones, and tumors of the pituitary gland.

The clinical manifestations of hyperthyroidism are rapid, bounding pulse (even during sleep); cardiac enlargement; palpitations; and arrhythmias. Patients are nervous and easily agitated. They develop tremors, a low-grade fever, and weight loss, despite an increased appetite. Hyperactive reflexes and insomnia are also usually present. Patients are intolerant of heat; the skin is warm, flushed, and moist, with increased sweating; edema of the tissues around the eyeballs produces characteristic eye changes, including exophthalmos. Patients develop amenorrhea; dyspnea with minor exertion; hoarse, rapid speech; and an increased susceptibility to infection. Elevated circulating thyroid hormone tests easily diagnose hyperthyroidism. Further diagnostic studies are required to determine the cause of hyperthyroidism.

Excessive formation of thyroid hormones and their secretion into the circulatory system causes hyperthyroidism, also known as **thyrotoxicosis**. Symptoms include increased metabolic rate, increased pulse rate (to perhaps 140 beats per minute), increased body temperature, restlessness, nervousness, anxiety, sweating, muscle weakness and tremors, and a sensation of feeling too warm. This condition is treated with antithyroid drugs or surgical removal of the thyroid gland.

Treatment

The primary goal of therapy for both hyperthyroidism and hypothyroidism is to return the patient to a normal thyroid (euthyroid) state. Hypothyroidism can be treated successfully by replacement of thyroid hormones (see individual agents). After therapy is initiated, the dosage of thyroid hormone is adjusted until serum levels of the thyroid hormones are within the normal range.

Three types of treatment can be used to reduce the hyperthyroid state: subtotal thyroidectomy, radioactive iodine, and antithyroid medications. Until treatment is under way, the patient requires nutritional and psychologic support.

Drug Therapy

Two general classes of drugs used to treat thyroid disorders are (1) those used to replace thyroid hormones in patients whose thyroid glandular function is inadequate to meet metabolic requirements (hypothyroidism) and (2) antithyroid agents used to suppress synthesis of thyroid hormones (hyperthyroidism). Thyroid hormone replacements available are levothyroxine (T_4), liothyronine (T_3), liotrix, thyroglobulin, and thyroid USP. Antithyroid drugs interfere with the formation or release of the hormones produced by the thyroid gland. Antithyroid agents to be discussed include iodides, propylthiouracil, and methimazole.

Nursing Process for Thyroid Disorders

Hypothyroidism and hyperthyroidism are primarily treated on an outpatient basis unless surgery is indicated or complications occur. Nurses must be able to offer guidance to the patients requiring treatment on an inpatient or ambulatory basis.

In general, body processes are slowed with hypothyroidism and accelerated with hyperthyroidism.

Assessment

History. Take a history of treatment prescribed for hypothyroidism or hyperthyroidism (for example, surgery, ^{131}I, or hormone replacement).

Medications. Request a listing of all prescribed and over-the-counter medications being taken. Ask if any of the prescribed medications are taken on a regular basis. If not taken regularly, what factors have caused the patient to decrease administration?

Description of current symptoms. Ask the patient to explain symptoms being experienced and what changes in the pattern of functioning have occurred over the past 2 to 3 months.

Focused assessment. Perform a focused assessment of the body systems generally affected by hypothyroid or hyperthyroid states.

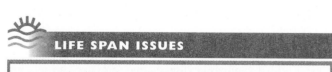

LIFE SPAN ISSUES

TREATMENT OF HYPOTHYROID STATE

During initial treatment of the hypothyroid state in the geriatric patient, be alert for and report increased frequency of angina or symptoms of heart failure.

Cardiovascular. Take current vital signs. Note bradycardia or tachycardia and any alterations in rhythm, subnormal or elevated temperature, and hypertension. Ask whether the pulse rate is decreased or elevated on awakening, before any stimulus. Does the patient experience any palpitations or a feeling that the pulse is rapid and bounding? Record heart sounds and any abnormal characteristics heard (or have a qualified nurse perform this).

Respiratory. Does the patient experience dyspnea? Is it made worse by mild exertion?

Gastrointestinal. Measure the person's height and weight. Ask for a history of any increase or decrease in weight over the past 3 months. Has there been a change in appetite? Does the individual experience any nausea and vomiting? What have the characteristics of the stools been over the past several months—constipation or diarrhea? Check and record bowel sounds.

Integumentary. Note the temperature, texture, and condition of the skin and the characteristics of the hair and nails. Does the patient complain of intolerance to heat or cold?

Musculoskeletal. What activity level is maintained? Does the person feel or act sluggish or hyperactive? Is the pattern of activity a change from the recent past? If so, when did this become apparent? Is there any muscle weakness, wasting, or discomfort? Is dependent edema present?

Neurologic. What is the patient's mental status—oriented to time, date, and place? What is the degree of alertness and pace of responsiveness (for example, sluggish and slow in contrast with quickness or fast paced). Is the individual depressed, stuporous, or hyperactive? Has the individual or family and significant others noticed any change in personality in the recent past? Has the individual had any tremors of hands, eyelids, or tongue? Has the individual experienced any insomnia?

Sensory. What is the condition of the eyes? Do the eyelids retract or is exophthalmos present?

Reproductive. Obtain a history of changes in the pattern of menses and libido that have occurred.

Immunologic. Has the individual had any recent infections?

Laboratory/diagnostic studies. Review laboratory and diagnostic studies available on the chart associated with thyroid disorders such as T_3, T_4, TSH levels, TRH stimulation test, electrocardiogram (ECG), and thyroid scan.

Nursing Diagnosis

Hyperthyroidism
- Nutrition: less than body requirements (indication)
- Alteration in elimination: diarrhea (indication)
- Sleep pattern disturbance: (indication)
- Activity intolerance, fatigue (indication)

Hypothyroidism
- Nutrition: more than body requirements (indication)
- Alteration in elimination: constipation (indication)

Note that an excess dose of thyroid medication for a person with hypothyroid disease may produce the nursing diagnoses for hyperthyroidism, which would be appropriate nursing diagnoses associated with adverse drug effects.

Planning

Environment. • For the hyperthyroid individual, plan to provide a cool, quiet, structured environment because the patient lacks the ability to respond to change and anxiety-producing situations and has an intolerance to heat. • For the hypothyroid individual, plan to provide a warm, quiet, structured environment that supports the patient's needs.

Nutrition

Hyperthyroid. Order the prescribed diet, usually a high-calorie diet of 4000 to 5000 calories per day with balanced nutrients. Mark the Kardex/care plan for no caffeine products (for example, coffee, tea, colas) or tobacco. If diarrhea is present, mark the Kardex/care plan to check trays for any foods with a laxative or stimulating effect such as bran products, fresh fruits, and fresh vegetables.

Hypothyroid. Order the prescribed diet, usually a low-calorie diet with increased bulk to alleviate constipation. Encourage adequate fluid intake, unless coexisting conditions prohibit.

Psychosocial. • Mark the Kardex/care plan to monitor the mental status at least every shift. • Plan to incorporate family into the health teaching plan because the patient may be unable to understand or implement all facets of the therapeutic regimen.

Activity and exercise. Mark the Kardex/care plan with the prescribed level of activity ordered by the physician. Institute safety precautions for individuals with muscle weakness, wasting, or pain that would place them at risk for injury.

Medications. Order the prescribed medications and transcribe orders to the medication administration record (MAR).

Assessment. • Schedule regular assessment of intake and output, vital signs, mental status, and daily weights on the Kardex/care plan. • If surgery is scheduled for hyperthyroidism, schedule routine postop vital signs, and order a tracheostomy set for bedside and a vaporizer in the room. Mark the Kardex/care plan to check dressings for bleeding, perform respiratory assessments, perform voice checks for hoarseness, and monitor for development of tetany for first 24 to 48 hours, as ordered by the physician. Have calcium gluconate and supplies needed for intravenous (IV) administration ready in the immediate environment.

Implementation

- Implement monitoring parameters for vital signs, intake and output, daily weights, and mental status checks.
- Encourage the patient to comply with dietary orders.
- Give prescribed medications and monitor for response to therapy.
- Provide support and give directions slowly and with patience because the individual may have difficulty processing the information. Incorporate the family into the provision of care, as appropriate.
- Monitor the pattern of bowel elimination and give prn medications prescribed for diarrhea or constipation.

Patient Education and Health Promotion

Medications. • Stress the need for lifelong administration of medications for the treatment of hypothyroidism and the need for periodic laboratory studies and evaluation by the physician. • Persons scheduled for outpatient diagnostics must receive detailed, written instructions regarding the prescribed medications to be taken in preparation for testing. • The patient and, as appropriate, family or significant others must understand the anticipated therapeutic response sought from prescribed medications. Teach specific indications of a satisfactory response to pharmacologic therapy. Stress the need to contact the physician if signs of an excess or deficit in dosage occur. Ensure that the individual can monitor the resting pulse.

Environment. • Explain the need for cool environment for a patient with hyperthyroidism; for a warm environment for the person with hypothyroidism. • Involve the family and significant others in identifying an appropriate home environment that will support the individual's needs until a preillness status is reached.

Nutrition. • In patients with diarrhea secondary to hyperthyroidism, explain the need for a high-calorie diet with reduced roughage. • Explain the need for a low-calorie diet with increased roughage to the individual with hypothyroidism. Encourage patients with constipation to drink 8 to 10 8-ounce glasses of water each day. • As the patient returns to a more normal thyroid function through medication, the caloric requirements of the diet will also change.

Psychosocial. The patient may have had a major personality change, may be depressed, or (at the other end of the spectrum) may be hyperactive. Explain these symptoms to the family and involve them in examining potential interventions that can be used in the home environment until the individual returns to the preillness level of functioning.

Activity and exercise. • Provide for patient safety during ambulation if muscle weakness, wasting, or discomfort is present. Discuss measures needed to provide for patient safety with family and significant others. • As the patient returns to a more normal thyroid function through medication, the activity level should change. Encourage moderate exercise.

Fostering health maintenance

- Throughout the course of treatment, discuss medication information and how it will benefit the patient. Recognize that noncompliance with lifelong treatment, when prescribed, may occur, and stress positive outcomes that occur with regular medication adherence.
- Provide the patient and significant others with important information contained in the specific drug monograph for the medicines prescribed. Additional health teaching and nursing interventions for the side effects to expect and report are described in the drug monographs.
- Seek cooperation and understanding of the following points so that medication compliance is increased: name of medication, dosage, route time of and administration, side effects to expect, and side effects to report.
- Enlist the patient's aid in developing and maintaining a written record (see boxes on pp. 432 and 433) of monitoring parameters appropriate for hypothyroid or hyperthyroid symptoms.

Drug Class: Thyroid Replacement Hormones

Actions

Hypothyroidism is treated by replacing the deficient T_3 and T_4 hormones.

Uses

The primary goal of therapy is to return the patient to a normal thyroid (euthyroid) state. Several forms of thyroid hormone replacement are available from natural and synthetic sources.

Levothyroxine (T_4) is one of the two primary hormones secreted by the thyroid gland. It is partially metabolized to liothyronine (T_3), so therapy with levothyroxine provides physiologic replacement of both hormones. It is now considered to be the drug of choice for hormone replacement in hypothyroidism.

Liothyronine is a synthetic form of the natural thyroid hormone, triiodothyronine, T_3. Its onset of action is more rapid than levothyroxine's, and it is occasionally used as a thyroid hormone replacement when prompt action is necessary. It is not recommended for patients with cardiovascular disease unless a rapid onset of activity is deemed essential.

Liotrix is a synthetic mixture of levothyroxine and liothyronine in a ratio of 4 to 1, respectively. A few endocrinologists prefer this combination because of the standardized content of the two hormones that results in consistent laboratory test results, more in agreement with the patient's clinical response. The two available commercial preparations of liotrix contain different amounts of each ingredient, so patients should not be changed from one preparation to the other unless differences in potency are considered.

Thyroglobulin is a protein obtained from a purified extract of hog thyroid. It contains thyroxine and triiodothyronine. It is effective in the treatment of inadequate thyroid hormone production. The potency of thyroglobulin is equal to that of thyroid USP but is substantially more costly.

Thyroid USP (desiccated thyroid) is derived from pig, beef, and sheep thyroid glands. Thyroid is the oldest thyroid hormone replacement available and the least expensive. Because of its lack of purity, uniformity, and stability, however, it is generally not the drug of choice for the initiation of thyroid replacement therapy.

Therapeutic Outcomes

The primary therapeutic outcome expected from thyroid hormone replacement therapy is return of the patient to a euthyroid metabolic state.

Nursing Process

Premedication Assessment

1. Record baseline vital signs, weight, and bowel elimination patterns before initiating therapy. Establish a once-daily schedule in which these assessments are retaken. Assess for patterns that may indicate early signs of hyperthyroidism.
2. Ensure that laboratory studies (for example, thyroid hormone levels) have been completed before administration of the medicine.

Planning

Availability. See Table 34-1, p. 434.

Implementation

Note: The age of the patient, severity of hypothyroidism, and other concurrent medical conditions determine the initial dosage and the interval of time necessary before increasing the dosage. Hypothyroid patients are sensitive to replacement of thyroid hormones. Monitor patients closely for adverse effects.

PATIENT EDUCATION & MONITORING FORM Thyroid Medications

MEDICATIONS	COLOR	TO BE TAKEN

Name _____

Physician _____

Physician's phone _____

Next appt.* _____

PARAMETERS	DAY OF DISCHARGE							COMMENTS
Pulse								
Temperature								
Weight								
Desire to eat: Eat all the time (10) — Normal (5) — None (1)								
Use this scale to rate tolerance of: Heat / Cold Cannot tolerate (10) — Moderate toleration (5) — Normal (1)								
Fatigue level: Tired all the time (10) — Normal (5) — Not tired; cannot stop (1)								
Skin condition: Dry, leathery Oily Normal								
How I feel about life: Feel awful (10) — Getting better (5) — Feel good (1)								
Tolerance for exercise: Difficulty breathing with exercise (10) — Normal (5) — Endless energy, no problem (1)								

*Please bring this record with you to your next appointment.
Use the back of this sheet for additional information.

PATIENT EDUCATION & MONITORING FORM   Antithyroid Medications

MEDICATIONS	COLOR	TO BE TAKEN

Name _____

Physician _____

Physician's phone _____

Next appt.* _____

PARAMETERS	DAY OF DISCHARGE						COMMENTS
Pulse							
Temperature							
Weight							
Desire to eat: Eat all the time — Normal — None 10 5 1							
Use this scale to rate tolerance of: Heat / Cold Cannot tolerate — Moderate toleration — Normal 10 5 1							
Fatigue level: Tired all the time — Normal — Not tired; cannot stop 10 5 1							
Skin condition: Dry, leathery Oily Normal							
How I feel about life: Feel awful — Getting better — Feel good 10 5 1							
Tolerance for exercise: Difficulty breathing with exercise — Normal — Endless energy, no problem 10 5 1							

*Please bring this record with you to your next appointment.
Use the back of this sheet for additional information.

Table 34-1

Thyroid Hormones

GENERIC NAME	BRAND NAME	AVAILABILITY	COMPOSITION	DOSAGE RANGE
Levothyroxine	Synthroid, Levoxyl	Tablets: 0.025, 0.05, 0.075, 0.088, 0.1, 0.112, 0.125, 0.137, 0.15, 0.175, 0.2 mg Injection: 200 and 500 μg per vial in 6 and 10 ml vials	Thyroxine (T_4)	PO: initial—0.025 mg daily; maintenance—0.1-0.2 mg daily
Liothyronine	Cytomel	Tablets: 5, 25, 50 μg Injection: 10 μg/ml in 1 ml vials	Liothyronine (T_3)	PO: initial—25 μg daily; maintenance—25-75 μg daily

Liotrix	Euthroid, Thyrolar	Euthroid
		    Tablets: 30, 60, 120, 180 mg thyroid equivalents
		Thyrolar
		    Tablets: 15, 30, 60, 180 mg thyroid equivalents
			T_4:T_3 = 4:1	PO: maintenance—60-180 mg thyroid equivalents daily

Thyroglobulin	Proloid	Tablets: 30, 60, 90, 120, 180 mg	T_4:T_3 = 2.5:1	PO: maintenance—30-180 mg daily
Thyroid USP	—	Tablets: 15, 30, 60, 90, 120, 180, 240, 300 mg Capsules: 60, 120, 180, 300 mg	Unpredictable T_4:T_3 ratio	PO: maintenance—60-180 mg daily

Dosage and administration. Adult: PO—therapy may be initiated in low doses of levothyroxine 0.025 mg daily. Dosages are gradually increased over the next few weeks to an average daily maintenance dose of 0.1 to 0.2 mg.

Evaluation

Side effects to expect and report

SIGNS OF HYPERTHYROIDISM. Adverse effects of thyroid replacement preparations are dose related and may occur 1 to 3 weeks after changes in therapy have been initiated. Symptoms of adverse effects are tachycardia, anxiety, weight loss, abdominal cramping and diarrhea, cardiac palpitations, arrhythmias, angina pectoris, fever, and intolerance to heat.

Symptoms may require a reduction or discontinuation of therapy. Patients may require up to a month without medication for toxic effects to fully dissipate.

Therapy must be restarted at lower dosages after symptoms have stopped.

Drug interactions

WARFARIN. Patients with hypothyroidism require larger doses of anticoagulants. If thyroid replacement therapy is initiated while the patient is receiving warfarin therapy, the patient should have frequent prothrombin time determinations and should be counseled to observe closely for development of petechiae, ecchymoses, nosebleeds, bleeding gums, dark tarry stools, and bright red or "coffee ground" emesis.

The dosage of warfarin may have to be reduced by one third to one half over the next 1 to 4 weeks.

DIGITALIS GLYCOSIDES. Patients with hypothyroidism require smaller doses of digitalis preparations. If thyroid replacement therapy is started while receiving digitalis glycosides, a gradual increase in the glycoside will be necessary to maintain adequate therapeutic activity.

CHOLESTYRAMINE. To prevent binding of thyroid hormones by cholestyramine, administer at least 4 hours apart.

HYPERGLYCEMIA. Diabetic or prediabetic patients must be monitored for the development of hyperglycemia, particularly during the early weeks of therapy.

Assess regularly for glycosuria and report if it occurs with any frequency.

Patients receiving oral hypoglycemic agents or insulin may require an adjustment in dosage.

Drug Class: Antithyroid Medicines

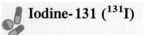 **Iodine-131 (^{131}I)**

Actions

The synthesis of thyroid hormones and their maintenance in the bloodstream in adequate amounts depend on sufficient iodine intake through food and water. Iodine is converted to iodide and stored in the thyroid gland before reaching the circulation.

Iodine-131(^{131}I) is a radioactive isotope of iodine. When administered, it is absorbed into the thyroid gland in high concentrations. The liberated radioactivity destroys the hyperactive thyroid tissue, with essentially no damage to other tissues in the body.

Uses

Radioactive iodine is most commonly used for treating hyperthyroidism in the following individuals: older patients who are beyond the childbearing years, those with severe complicating diseases (for example, heart disease), those with recurrent hyperthyroidism after previous thyroid surgery, those who are poor surgical risks, and those who have unusually small thyroid glands.

It often takes 3 to 6 months after a dose of radioactive iodine to fully assess benefits gained. Normal thyroid function occurs in about 60% of patients after one dose; the remaining patients require two or more doses. If more than one dose is required, an interval of at least 3 months between doses is required.

Therapeutic Outcomes

The primary therapeutic outcome expected from radioactive iodine is return to a normal thyroid state.

Nursing Process

Premedication Assessment
1. Review policy for both hospital personnel and the patient regarding precautions, storage, handling, administration, and disposal of radioactive substances.
2. Have all supplies immediately available in case of a spill.
3. Have all supplies needed according to hospital procedure to dispose of patient's excreta.

Planning
Availability. Each dose is prepared for an individual patient from a nuclear pharmacy.

Implementation
Administration of radioactive iodine. Administration of radioactive iodine preparations seems simple: it is added to water and swallowed. It has no color or taste. The radiation, however, is extremely dangerous.
- Minimize exposure as much as possible. Wear rubber gloves whenever administering radioactive iodine or disposing of the patient's excreta.
- If the radioactive iodine or the patient's excreta should spill, follow hospital policy. In general, collect the clothing, bedding, bedpan, urinal, and any other contaminated materials and place them in special containers for radioactive waste disposal.
- AVOID SPILLS! REPORT ANY ACCIDENTAL CONTAMINATION AT ONCE TO YOUR SUPERVISOR, AND FOLLOW DIRECTIONS FOR HOSPITAL CONTAMINATION CLEANUP TECHNIQUE.
- Complete an incident report.

Evaluation
Side effects to expect and report
TENDERNESS IN THE THYROID GLAND. Side effects include radioactive thyroiditis, which causes tenderness over the thyroid area and occurs during the first few days or few weeks after radioactive iodine therapy.

HYPERTHYROIDISM. A return of symptoms of hyperthyroidism occurs in about 40% of patients who received one dose of radioactive iodine. Additional doses may be required.

HYPOTHYROIDISM. Some patients who receive radioactive iodine develop hypothyroidism, which requires thyroid hormone replacement therapy.
Drug interactions
LITHIUM CARBONATE. Lithium and iodine may cause synergistic hypothyroid activity. Concurrent use may result

in hypothyroidism. Monitor patients for both hypothyroidism and bipolar disorder.

propylthiouracil (pro-pil-thy-o-you'rah-sil)
PTU, Propacil

methimazole (meth-im'ah-zohl)
Tapazole (tap'ah-zoal)

Actions

Propylthiouracil and methimazole are antithyroid agents that act by blocking synthesis of T_3 and T_4 in the thyroid gland. They do not destroy any T_3 or T_4 already produced, so there is usually a latent period of a few days to 3 weeks before symptoms improve once therapy is started.

Uses

Propylthiouracil and methimazole may be used for long-term treatment of hyperthyroidism or for short-term treatment before subtotal thyroidectomy. Therapy for long-term use is often continued for 1 to 2 years to control symptoms. After discontinuation, some patients gradually return to the hyperthyroid state, and antithyroid therapy must be reinitiated.

Therapeutic Outcomes

The primary therapeutic outcome expected from propylthiouracil or methimazole is gradual return to normal thyroid metabolic function.

Nursing Process

Premedication Assessment
1. Record baseline vital signs, weight, and bowel elimination patterns before initiating therapy. Establish an every-other-day schedule in which these assessments are retaken. Assess for patterns that may indicate early signs of hypothyroidism.
2. Ensure that laboratory studies (for example, thyroid hormone levels, TSH, complete blood count with differential, blood urea nitrogen (BUN), serum creatinine, liver enzymes) have been completed before administration of the medicine.

Planning
Availability. PO—propylthiouracil: 50 mg tablets; methimazole: 5 and 10 mg tablets.

Implementation
Dosage and administration. Adult: propylthiouracil, PO—initially 100 to 150 mg every 6 to 8 hours. Dosage ranges up to 900 mg daily. The maintenance dose is 50 mg 2 or 3 times daily. Methimazole, PO—initially 5 to 20 mg every 8 hours. Daily maintenance dosage is 5 to 15 mg.

Evaluation
Side effects to expect and report
PURPURIC, MACULOPAPULAR RASH. The most common reaction (in 5% of all patients) that occurs with propylthiouracil is a purpuric, maculopapular skin eruption. This skin

eruption often occurs during the first 2 weeks of therapy and usually resolves spontaneously, without treatment. If pruritus becomes severe, a change to methimazole may be necessary. Cross-sensitivity is uncommon.

HEADACHES, SALIVARY AND LYMPH NODE ENLARGEMENT, LOSS OF TASTE. These side effects are usually mild and tend to resolve with continued therapy. Encourage the patient not to discontinue therapy without first consulting the physician.

BONE MARROW SUPPRESSION. Routine laboratory studies (RBC, WBC, and differential counts) should be scheduled. Stress the importance of returning for this laboratory work.

Monitor the patient for the development of a sore throat, fever, purpura, jaundice, or excessive, progressive weakness.

HEPATOTOXICITY. The symptoms of hepatotoxicity are anorexia, nausea, vomiting, jaundice, hepatomegaly, splenomegaly, and abnormal liver function tests (elevated bilirubin, AST, ALT, GGT, alkaline phosphatase, prothrombin time).

NEPHROTOXICITY. Monitor urinalyses and kidney function tests for abnormal results. Report increased BUN and creatinine, decreased urine output or decreased urine specific gravity (despite amount of fluid intake), casts or protein in the urine, frank blood or smoky-colored urine, or RBCs in excess of 0 to 3 on the urinalysis report.

Drug interactions

WARFARIN. Patients with hyperthyroidism require smaller doses of anticoagulants. If antithyroid therapy is initiated while the patient is receiving warfarin therapy, the patient should have frequent prothrombin time determinations and should be counseled to observe closely for development of petechiae, ecchymoses, nosebleeds, bleeding gums, dark tarry stools, and bright red or coffee ground emesis.

The dosage of warfarin may have to be increased over the next 1 to 4 weeks.

DIGITALIS GLYCOSIDES. Patients with hyperthyroidism require larger doses of digitalis preparations. If antithyroid replacement therapy is started while receiving digitalis glycosides, a gradual reduction in the glycoside will be necessary to prevent signs of toxicity. Monitor for the development of arrhythmias, bradycardia, increased fatigue, or nausea, and vomiting.

CHAPTER REVIEW

Thyroid disease is a relatively common disorder that is easily treated. Most therapies require long-term treatment to maintain normal thyroid function. Nurses can play a significant role in education and reinforcement of the treatment plan. Best results are attained when the patient, family, and nurse work together in reinforcing the care plan.

MATH REVIEW

1. Ordered: Levothyroxine (Synthroid) 0.1 mg, PO, daily
   On Hand: Levothyroxine (Synthroid) 0.05 mg tablets
   Give: _____ tablets

2. Ordered: Levothyroxine (Synthroid) 200 mcg
   Convert 200 mcg to mg
   _____ mg

CRITICAL THINKING QUESTIONS

Situation:

Mr. Tanders' baseline vital signs are the following:
BP 140/60, pulse 104, respirations 24
He has been receiving levothyroxine (Synthroid) 0.1 mg PO daily for the past 6 weeks for treatment of hypothyroidism. He reports that his resting pulse, on awakening, has been between 90 and 112 during the past week. Should these findings be reported to the physician, and if so, what additional data should be assembled before initiating physician contact?

Situation:

Mrs. Travers is taking propylthiouracil 50 mg, PO, tid. What patient education should be provided to her regarding side effects to expect and side effects to report?

Corticosteroids

Objectives

1. Review the functions of the adrenal gland.
2. State the normal actions of mineralocorticoids and gluco-corticoids in the body.
3. Cite the disease states caused by hypersecretion or hyposecretion of the adrenal gland.
4. Identify the baseline assessments needed for a patient receiving corticosteroids.
5. Prepare a list of the clinical uses of mineralocorticoids and glucocorticoids.
6. Discuss the potential side effects associated with the use of corticosteroids, and give examples of specific patient education needed for the patient who will be taking these agents.
7. Develop measurable objectives for patient education for persons taking corticosteroids.

Key Words

corticosteroids
mineralocorticoids

glucocorticoids
cortisol

CORTICOSTEROIDS

Corticosteroids are hormones secreted by the adrenal cortex of the adrenal gland. Corticosteroids are divided into two categories based on structure and biologic activity. The **mineralocorticoids** (fludrocortisone and aldosterone) are used to maintain fluid and electrolyte balance and to treat adrenal insufficiency caused by hypopituitarism or Addison's disease. The **glucocorticoids** (cortisone, hydrocortisone, prednisone, and others) are used to regulate carbohydrate, protein, and fat metabolism. Glucocorticoids have antiinflammatory and antiallergic activity and are prescribed for the relief of symptoms of rheumatoid

arthritis, adrenal insufficiency, severe psoriasis, urticaria, chronic eczema, multiple myeloma, Hodgkin's disease, leukemias, and collagen diseases.

Nursing Process for Corticosteroid Therapy

Assessment

Minimum assessment data for patients receiving corticosteroids include baseline weights, blood pressure, and electrolyte studies. Monitoring of all aspects of intake, output, diet, electrolyte balance, and state of hydration is important to the long-term success of corticosteroid therapy.

Although many of the parameters used for assessment may initially be normal, it is important that a baseline for these parameters be established so that they may be used to monitor steroid therapy.

History. Ask the patient to describe the current problems that initiated this visit or admission. How long have the symptoms been present? Is this a recurrent problem? If so, how was it treated in the past?

History of pain experience. See the nursing process for pain management, Chapter 18, p. 231.

Medication history. Obtain a detailed history of all prescribed and over-the-counter medications. Ask if the patient understands why each is being taken. Tactfully determine if the prescribed medications are being taken regularly and if not, why not?

Central nervous system

Mental status. Patients receiving higher doses of corticosteroids are susceptible to psychotic behavioral changes. The most susceptible patients are those with previous histories of mental dysfunction. Perform a baseline assessment of the patient's ability to respond rationally to the environment and the diagnosis of the underlying disease. Check for orientation to date, time, and place, and assess for level of confusion, restlessness, or irritability. Make regularly scheduled mental status evaluations, and compare the findings.

Anxiety. What degree of apprehension is present? Are there stressful events that precipitated the anxiety?

History of ulcers. Patients receiving corticosteroid therapy have higher incidences of peptic ulcer disease. Ask the patient about any previous treatment for an ulcer, heartburn, or stomach pain. Periodic testing of stools for occult blood may be ordered.

Physical assessment

Blood pressure. Take a baseline blood pressure reading in both the supine and sitting positions. Because patients receiving corticosteroids accumulate fluid and gain weight, hypertension may develop.

Temperature. Record daily, and monitor more frequently if elevated. Patients receiving corticosteroids are more susceptible to infection, and fever is often an early indicator of infection. Glucocorticoids, however, sometimes suppress a febrile response to infection.

Weight. Obtain the patient's weight on admission and use as a baseline in assessing therapy. Because patients receiving corticosteroids have a tendency to accumulate fluid and gain weight, the daily weights are important tools in assessing ongoing therapy.

Pulse. Record the rate, quality, and rhythm of the pulse.

Heart and lung sounds. Nurses with advanced skills can perform auscultation and percussion to note changes in heart size and heart and lung sounds. (Consult a medical-surgical nursing textbook for details of performing these assessments.) Lung fields are assessed in a sitting position to detect abnormal lung sounds (for example, wheezes, rales, and accumulation of fluid).

Skin color. Note the color of the skin, mucous membranes, tongue, earlobes, and nailbeds. Note in particular the development of a rash or the development of ecchymoses (bruises).

Neck veins. Record any jugular vein distention. This may be an indication of fluid overload.

Status of hydration

Dehydration. Assess and record significant signs of dehydration in the patient. Observe for the following signs: poor skin turgor, sticky oral mucous membranes, a shrunken or deeply furrowed tongue, crusted lips, weight loss, deteriorating vital signs, soft or sunken eyeballs, weak pedal pulses, delayed capillary filling, excessive thirst, high urine specific gravity (or no urine output), and possible mental confusion.

Skin turgor. Check skin turgor by gently pinching the skin together over the sternum, forehead, or on the forearm. In the well-hydrated patient elasticity is present and the skin rapidly returns to a flat position. In dehydrated patients, the skin remains pinched or peaked and returns very slowly to the flat, normal position.

Oral mucous membranes. When adequately hydrated, the membranes of the mouth feel smooth and glisten. In dehydrated patients, they are sticky and appear dull.

Laboratory changes. The values of the hematocrit, hemoglobin, blood urine nitrogen (BUN), and electrolytes will appear to fluctuate, based on the state of hydration. A dehydrated patient will show higher values as a result of hemoconcentration. When a patient is overhydrated, the values appear to drop because of hemodilution.

Overhydration. Increased abdominal girth and circumference of the medial malleolus, weight gain, and neck vein engorgement are indications of overhydration. Measure the abdominal girth daily at the umbilical level. Measure the extremities bilaterally every day, approximately 5 cm above the medial malleolus.

Edema. Is edema present? It may be an indicator of fluid and electrolyte imbalance.

Laboratory tests

- Patients taking corticosteroids are particularly susceptible to the development of electrolyte imbalance. Physiologically, corticosteroids cause sodium retention (hypernatremia) and potassium excretion (hypokalemia).
- Patients most likely to develop electrolyte disturbances are those who, in addition to receiving corticosteroids, have

histories of renal or cardiac disease, hormonal disorders, massive trauma or burns, or are on diuretic therapy.

- Review laboratory tests and report abnormal results to the physician promptly. Tests include serum electrolytes, especially sodium, potassium, calcium, and magnesium; arterial blood gases; electrocardiogram (ECG); chest x-ray; urinalysis and kidney function; and hemodynamic assessments.
- Because the symptoms of most electrolyte imbalances are similar, the nurse should assess changes in the patient's mental status (alertness, orientation, and confusion), muscle strength, muscle cramps, tremors, nausea, and general appearance.

Nutrition. Obtain a history of the patient's diet. Ask questions regarding appetite and the presence of nausea and vomiting. Anorexia and nausea and vomiting are early indications of corticosteroid insufficiency.

Hyperglycemia. Corticosteroid therapy may induce hyperglycemia, particularly in prediabetic or diabetic patients. All patients must be monitored for the development of hyperglycemia, particularly during the early weeks of therapy. Assess regularly for glycosuria and blood glucose, and report any frequent occurrences.

Activity and exercise. Ask questions to obtain information about the effect of exercise on the patient's functioning. Is the person normally sedentary, moderately active, or very active? Has there been a reduction in activity level to cope with associated fatigue or dyspnea? Are the activities of daily living being performed by the person?

Nursing Diagnosis

- Activity intolerance (indication)
- Fluid volume excess (indication)
- Pain, acute or chronic (indication)
- Tissue perfusion, altered (indication)
- Injury, risk for (side effects)

Planning

Medication history. Review medications being taken, and establish whether they are being taken correctly. Analyze noncompliance issues and plan interventions with the patient. Plan to review drug administration as needed.

Medication administration. • Glucocorticoids may cause hyperglycemia, necessitating the monitoring of blood glucose levels at appropriate intervals. If elevated, insulin therapy may be required. Initiate a diabetic flow sheet, and mark the medication administration record (MAR) clearly to identify the insulin orders. • During steroid replacement therapy, the administration schedule for the replacement drugs should mimic the body's normal circadian rhythm. Therefore glucocorticoids ordered twice daily are usually scheduled with two thirds of the dose administered before 9 AM and one third of the dose in the late afternoon. Mineralocorticoids are usually given once daily in the evening. Alternate-day therapy is also used in some instances to maintain a more normal body rhythm. • Steroid replacement therapy is gradually discontinued in small increments to ensure that the patient's adrenal glands are able to start secreting steroids appropriately as the drug dosage is reduced.

Central nervous system. Plan for stress reduction education and discussion of effective means of coping with stressful events. Mark the care plan or Kardex to monitor the mental status every shift.

Fluid volume status. Plan to monitor intake and output at intervals appropriate to the patient's condition. Report intake that exceeds output.

Nutritional history. Examine the dietary history to establish whether a referral to a nutritionist would benefit the individual's understanding of the diet regimen. Plan interventions needed to deal with dietary noncompliance.

Laboratory tests. Order stat and subsequent laboratory studies.

Implementation

Medications. Order medications prescribed, and schedule these on the MAR. Perform focused assessments to determine effectiveness and side effects of pharmacologic interventions. Monitor for hyperglycemia.

Pain management. When pain is present, comfort measures must be implemented to allow the patient to decrease the pain. Fatigue may increase pain perception; spacing activities so that fatigue does not occur is recommended.

Central nervous system. • Perform neurologic assessment to determine changes in mental status. • Deal calmly with an anxious patient; offer explanations of procedures being performed; listen to concerns and intervene appropriately.

Vital signs and status of hydration. • Monitor vital signs and perform focused assessment of heart, respiratory, and hydration status at specified intervals. • Perform daily weights using the same scale, in clothing of approximately the same weight, at the same time—usually before breakfast. Record and report significant weight changes. (Weight gains and losses are the best indicators of fluid gain or loss.) As appropriate to patient's condition, obtain and record abdominal girth measurements. • When fluid restrictions are prescribed, one half of fluids is usually given with meals. The other half is given on a per shift basis. • Monitor the rate of intravenous (IV) infusions carefully; contact the physician regarding concentration of admixtures of drugs to IV infusion solution when limited fluids are indicated.

Nutrition. Schedule meetings with the nutritionist to learn how to manage specific dietary modifications prescribed (for example, a low-sodium, high-potassium diet with weight reduction parameters for obese patients). If possible, instruct the patient to practice food selections from the daily menus while still in the hospital. The nurse can then offer guidance. Teach the patient which foods are low in sodium and high in potassium. Potassium restrictions may be indicated if the patient is taking a potassium-sparing diuretic. Salt substitutes are high in potassium, therefore use must be limited.

Laboratory studies. Check for and report abnormal laboratory values (for example, hypokalemia, hyperkalemia, hypoglycemia, hyperglycemia, hyponatremia, hypernatremia) depending on the underlying disease pathology.

Patient Education and Health Promotion

Contact with physician's office. • Assess the patient's understanding of symptoms that indicate consultation with the doctor: dyspnea; productive cough; worsening fatigue; edema in the feet, ankles, or legs; weight gain; or development of angina (chest pain), palpitations, or confusion. • Instruct the patient to perform daily weights using the same scale, in clothing of approximately the same weight, at the same time—usually before breakfast. Record and report significant weight changes; weight gains and losses are the best indicators of fluid gain or loss. Usually a gain of 2 pounds in 2 days should be reported.

Skin care. Teach appropriate skin care and the need to change positions at least every 2 hours, especially when edema is present. Have the patient inspect the ankles, feet, and abdomen for edema daily. If the patient is using a recliner or bed, the sacral area should also be checked regularly for edema.

Coping with stress. • Patients receiving high doses of corticosteroids do not tolerate stress well. Patients should be instructed to notify the physician before exposure to additional stress, such as dental procedures. If a patient sustains an accidental injury or sudden emotional stress, the attending physician should be notified that the patient is receiving steroid therapy. An additional steroid dose may be needed to support the patient through a stressful situation. • Explore coping mechanisms the person uses in response to stress. Discuss how the patient is adapting to the needed changes in lifestyle to manage the disease process. Address depression issues, if present.

Avoid infections. Advise the patient to avoid crowds or people known to have infections. Report even minor signs of an infection (such as general malaise, sore throat, or low-grade fever) to the physician.

Nutritional status. • Assist the patient in developing a specific schedule for spacing daily fluid intake and planning sodium restrictions, as prescribed by the physician. • If weight gain is a specific problem (not related to fluid accumulation), plan for calorie restrictions and spacing of daily intake. • If a high-potassium diet is prescribed, help the patient become familiar with foods that should be consumed. Teach the signs and symptoms of potassium deficiency or excess, depending on medications prescribed. • Further dietary needs may include increases in vitamin D and calcium. • Fluid restrictions may be imposed; discuss specific ways to manage these limitations.

Activity and exercise. • Participation in regular exercise is essential. The patient must resume activities of daily living within the boundaries set by the physician. (Such activities as regular, moderate exercise, meal preparation, resumption of usual sexual activities, and social interactions all must be encouraged.) Help the patient plan for appropriate alterations depending on the disease process and degree of impairment. • Encourage weight-bearing measures to prevent calcium loss. Active and passive range-of-motion exercises maintain mobility and joint and muscle integrity. • Individuals unable to attain the degree of activity anticipated as a result of drug therapy may become frustrated. Allow for verbalization of feelings, and then implement actions appropriate to the circumstances.

Fostering health maintenance

• Throughout the course of treatment, discuss medication information and how the medication will benefit the patient.

• Drug therapy is one component of the treatment of illnesses for which steroids are prescribed; it is critical that the medications be taken as prescribed. Provide the patient and significant others with the important information contained in the specific drug monograph for the drugs prescribed. Additional health teaching and nursing interventions for drug side effects to expect and report are in each drug monograph.

- Seek cooperation and understanding of the following points so that medication compliance is increased: name of medication, dosage, route and times of administration, side effects to expect, and side effects to report.
- Enlist the patient's aid in developing and maintaining a written record of monitoring parameters (pulse rate, blood pressure, body weight, edema, exercise tolerance, pain relief, etc.). (See box on p. 441.) Instruct the patient to bring the written record to follow-up visits.

DRUG THERAPY

Drug Class: Mineralocorticoids

fludrocortisone (flu-droh′kort-ih-sown)
Florinef (flohr-in′ehf)

Actions

Fludrocortisone is an adrenal corticosteroid with potent mineralocorticoid and glucocorticoid effects. It affects fluid and electrolyte balance by acting on the distal renal tubules, causing sodium and water retention and potassium and hydrogen excretion.

Uses

Fludrocortisone is used in combination with glucocorticoids to replace mineralocorticoid activity in patients who suffer from adrenocortical insufficiency (Addison's disease) and for the treatment of salt-losing adrenogenital syndrome.

Therapeutic Outcomes

The primary therapeutic outcomes expected from fludrocortisone therapy are as follows:
- Control of blood pressure
- Restoration of fluid and electrolyte balance

Nursing Process

Premedication Assessment

1. Check the electrolyte reports for early indications of electrolyte imbalance.
2. Keep accurate records of intake and output, daily weights, and vital signs.
3. Question the patient about any signs and symptoms that would indicate the presence of an infection (for example, sore throat, fever, malaise, nausea, or vomiting). Corticosteroid therapy often masks symptoms of infection.
4. Perform a baseline assessment of the patient's degree of alertness; orientation to name, place, and time; and rationality of responses.
5. Ask the patient about previous treatment for an ulcer, heartburn, or stomach pain. Testing of stools for occult blood should be done periodically.

Planning
Availability. PO—0.1 mg tablets.

Implementation
Dosage and administration. Adult: PO—0.1 mg daily. Dosage may be adjusted as needed. Cortisone or hydrocortisone

is usually also administered to provide additional glucocorticoid effect.

Evaluation
Because fludrocortisone is a natural hormone, side effects are an extension of excessive use of fludrocortisone. Most side effects are associated with sodium accumulation and potassium depletion.

Side effects to expect and report
    SEE GLUCOCORTICOIDS.

Drug interactions
    SEE GLUCOCORTICOIDS.

Drug Class: Glucocorticoids

Actions

The major glucocorticoid of the adrenal cortex is **cortisol**. The hypothalamic-pituitary axis regulates the secretion of cortisol by increasing or decreasing the output of corticotropin-releasing factor (CRF) from the hypothalamus. Corticotropin-releasing factor stimulates the release of adrenocorticotropic hormone (ACTH) from the pituitary gland; ACTH then stimulates the adrenal cortex to secrete cortisol. As serum levels of cortisol increase, the amount of CRF secreted by the hypothalamus is decreased, resulting in diminished secretion of cortisol from the adrenal cortex.

Uses

Glucocorticoids are most frequently prescribed because of their antiinflammatory and antiallergic properties. They do not cure any disease but rather relieve the symptoms of tissue inflammation. When used for the control of rheumatoid arthritis, relief of symptoms is noted within a few days. Joint and muscle stiffness, muscle tenderness and weakness, joint swelling, and soreness are significantly reduced. When used for this purpose, it is important to assess the patient's predrug activity level. Relief of pain may lead to overuse of the diseased joints. Appetite, weight, and energy are increased, fever is reduced, and sedimentation rates are reduced or return to normal. Anatomic changes and joint deformities that are already present remain unchanged. Symptoms usually return a short time after withdrawal of the glucocorticoids.

Glucocorticoids are also effective for relief of allergic manifestations, such as serum sickness, severe hay fever, status asthmaticus, and exfoliative dermatitis. In addition, they may be used for the treatment of shock and collagen diseases, such as lupus erythematosus, dermatomyositis, and acute rheumatic fever.

Therapeutic Outcomes

The primary therapeutic outcomes expected from glucocorticoid therapy are as follows:
- Reduced pain and inflammation
- Minimized shock syndrome and more rapid recovery

Nursing Process

Premedication Assessment

1. Check the electrolyte reports for early indications of electrolyte imbalance.

PATIENT EDUCATION & MONITORING FORM — Corticosteroids

MEDICATIONS	COLOR	TO BE TAKEN

Name _____
Physician _____
Physician's phone _____
Next appt.* _____

PARAMETERS		DAY OF DISCHARGE						COMMENTS
Weight								
Blood Pressure								
Pulse rate								
Notify doctor of sudden stress in life	Surgery, injury, trauma, death in family or of friend, events such as fights in family							
Pain relief? No relief 10 / Improved 5 / No pain 1								
Assessment of how I feel? Good 10 / Improved 5 / Bad 1								
Breast tenderness	None							
	Occasionally uncomfortable							
	Increasing							
Hair distribution	No changes seen							
	Hair growth increased: site ____							
Edema	Swelling noted (where)? ____							
	Time of day swelling occurs?							

*Please bring this record with you to your next appointment.
Use the back of this sheet for additional information.

2. Keep accurate records of intake and output, daily weights, and vital signs.
3. Question the patient about any signs and symptoms that would indicate the presence of an infection (for example, sore throat, fever, malaise, nausea, and vomiting). Corticosteroid therapy often masks symptoms of infection.
4. Perform a baseline assessment of the patient's degree of alertness; orientation to name, place, and time; and rationality of responses.
5. Ask the patient about previous treatment for an ulcer, heartburn, or stomach pain. Testing of stools for occult blood should be done periodically.

Planning
Availability. See Table 35-1.

Implementation
Note: Glucocorticoids are potent agents that produce many undesirable side effects as well as therapeutic benefits. Unless immediate, life-threatening conditions exist, other therapeutic methods should be exhausted before corticosteroid therapy is initiated. Many of the side effects of the steroids are related to dosage and duration of therapy.

These drugs must be used with caution in patients with diabetes mellitus, heart failure, hypertension, peptic ulcer, mental disturbance, and suspected infections.

Dosage and administration. When therapeutic dosages are administered for 1 week or longer, it must be assumed that the internal production of corticosteroids is suppressed. Abrupt discontinuation of glucocorticoids may result in adrenal insufficiency. Therapy should be withdrawn gradually. The time required to decrease glucocorticoids depends on the duration of treatment, the dosage amount, the mode of administration, and the glucocorticoid being used.

Abrupt discontinuation. Patients who have received corticosteroids for at least 1 week must not abruptly discontinue therapy. Symptoms of abrupt discontinuation include fever, malaise, fatigue, weakness, anorexia, nausea, orthostatic dizziness, hypotension, fainting, dyspnea, hypoglycemia, muscle and joint pain, and possible exacerbation of the disease process.

Table 35-1
Corticosteroid Preparations*

GENERIC NAME	BRAND NAME	DOSAGE FORMS
Alclometasone	Aclovate	Cream, ointment
Amcinonide	Cyclocort	Cream, ointment, lotion
Betamethasone	Celestone, Valisone, Diprosone, Betatrex, others	Tablets, syrup, injection, cream, ointment, lotion, aerosol, gel
Clobetasol	Temovate	Cream, ointment, scalp application
Clocortolone	Cloderm	Cream
Cortisone	Cortisone	Tablets
Desonide	Tridesilon, DesOwen	Cream, ointment, lotion
Desoximetasone	Topicort	Cream, ointment, gel
Dexamethasone	Decadron, Dexone, Hexadrol, Decaspray	Cream, aerosol, gel, injection, tablets, inhalant, elixir
Diflorasone	Florone, Maxiflor	Cream, ointment
Fludrocortisone	Florinef	Tablets
Fluocinolone	Fluonid, Synalar	Cream, ointment, solution
Fluocinonide	Lidex	Cream, ointment, gel, solution
Flurandrenolide	Cordran, ✽ Drenison	Cream, ointment, tape, lotion
Fluticasone	Cutivate, Flonase	Cream, ointment, spray
Hydrocortisone	Cortef, Solu-Cortef, Hydrocortone	Cream, ointment, tablets, enema, gel, lotion, suppositories, injection
Halcinonide	Halog, Halog E	Cream, ointment, solution
Halobetasol	Ultravate	Cream, ointment
Methylprednisolone	Solu-Medrol, Depo-Medrol, Medrol	Tablets, injection, powder
Mometasone	Elocon	Cream, ointment
Prednisolone	Delta-Cortef, ✽ Novoprednisolone, Prelone	Injection, tablets, aerosol, syrup, suspension
Prednisone	Deltasone, Orasone, ✽ Apo-Prednisone	Tablets, solution
Triamcinolone	Aristocort, Kenalog, ✽ Triamcort	Cream, ointment, lotion, injection, tablets, syrup, aerosol, paste

*Ophthalmic products, Chapter 40; nasal inhalation products, Chapter 27.
✽ Available in Canada only .

Application. Topical corticosteroids are applied as directed by the manufacturer. Specific instructions regarding use of an occlusive dressing should be clarified before application.

Alternate-day therapy. Alternate-day therapy may be used to treat chronic conditions. Corticosteroids are usually administered between 6 AM and 9 AM to minimize suppression of normal adrenal function. Administer with meals to minimize gastric irritation.

Pediatric patients. The correct dosage for a child is usually based on the disease being treated rather than the weight of the patient. Monitoring of skeletal growth may be required in children if prolonged therapy is required.

Evaluation
Side effects to expect and report
ELECTROLYTE IMBALANCE, FLUID ACCUMULATION. The electrolytes most commonly altered are potassium (K^+), sodium (Na^+), and chloride (Cl^-). Hypokalemia is most likely to occur.

Many symptoms associated with altered fluid and electrolyte balance are subtle and interspersed with general symptoms of drug toxicity or the disease process itself.

Obtain data about changes in the patient's mental status (alertness, orientation, and confusion), muscle strength, muscle cramps, tremors, nausea, and general appearance (drowsy, anxious, or lethargic).

Always check the electrolyte reports for early indications of electrolyte imbalance.

Keep accurate records of intake and output, daily weights, and vital signs.

SUSCEPTIBILITY TO INFECTION. Always question the patient before initiation of therapy about any signs and symptoms that would indicate the presence of an infection. Corticosteroid therapy often masks symptoms of infection.

Monitor the patient closely for signs of infection such as sore throat, fever, malaise, nausea, and vomiting.

Encourage the patient to avoid exposure to infections.

BEHAVIORAL CHANGES. Psychotic behaviors are more likely to occur in patients with previous histories of mental instability.

Perform a baseline assessment of the patient's degree of alertness; orientation to name, place, and time; and rationality of responses before initiating therapy. Make regularly scheduled mental status evaluations, and compare the findings. Report the development of alterations.

HYPERGLYCEMIA. Diabetic or prediabetic patients must be monitored for the development of hyperglycemia, particularly during the early weeks of therapy.

Assess regularly for glycosuria and blood glucose and report any frequent occurrences.

Patients receiving oral hypoglycemic agents or insulin may require an adjustment in dosage.

PEPTIC ULCER FORMATION. Before initiating therapy, ask the patient about any previous treatment for an ulcer, heartburn, or stomach pain.

Periodic testing of stools for occult blood may be ordered. Antacids may also be recommended by the physician to minimize gastric symptoms.

DELAYED WOUND HEALING. Surgical sites of patients who have recently had surgery must be monitored closely for signs of dehiscence.

Teach surgical patients to splint wounds while coughing and breathing deeply.

Inspect surgical sites and report statements such as, "When I coughed, I felt something pop."

VISUAL DISTURBANCES. Visual disturbances noted by patients receiving long-term therapy must be reported. Glucocorticoid therapy may produce cataracts.

Drug interactions
DIURETICS (FUROSEMIDE, THIAZIDES, BUMETANIDE, OTHERS). Corticosteroids may enhance the loss of potassium. Check potassium levels and monitor the patient more closely for hypokalemia when these two agents are used concurrently.

Many symptoms associated with altered fluid and electrolyte balance are subtle and interspersed with general symptoms of drug toxicity or the disease process itself.

Obtain data about changes in the patient's mental status (alertness, orientation, and confusion), muscle strength, muscle cramps, tremors, nausea, and general appearance (drowsy, anxious, and lethargic).

Always check the electrolyte reports for early indications of electrolyte imbalance.

Keep accurate records of intake and output, daily weights, and vital signs.

WARFARIN. This medication may enhance or decrease the anticoagulant effects of warfarin. Observe for the development of petechiae, ecchymoses, nosebleeds, bleeding gums, dark tarry stools, and bright red or coffee ground emesis. Monitor the prothrombin time, and adjust the dosage of warfarin if necessary.

Because of the ulcerogenic potential of steroids, close observation of patients taking anticoagulants is necessary to reduce the possibility of hemorrhage.

HYPERGLYCEMIA. Diabetic or prediabetic patients must be monitored for the development of hyperglycemia, particularly during the early weeks of therapy.

Assess regularly for glycosuria and blood glucose, and report any frequent occurrences.

Patients receiving oral hypoglycemic agents or insulin may require an adjustment in dosage.

CHAPTER REVIEW

Corticosteroids are potent agents that produce many therapeutic benefits as well as undesirable side effects. Many of the side effects of the steroids are related to dosage and duration of therapy. These drugs must be used with caution in patients with diabetes mellitus, heart failure, hypertension, peptic ulcer, mental disturbance, and suspected infections. Nurses can play a significant role in helping patients monitor therapy and can assist them in seeking medical attention at the earliest signs of impending trouble.

MATH REVIEW

The package insert accompanying prednisone states that the physiologic replacement dose (pediatric) is 0.1 to 0.15 mg/kg per day PO in equal divided doses q12h.

Situation:

The child's weight is 22 lb.

1. 22 lb = _____ kg.

Using the dosage parameters described, calculate the minimum and maximum dose per day for this child's weight.

2. _____ mg minimum.

3. _____ mg maximum.

CRITICAL THINKING QUESTIONS

Situation:

Mr. Little is receiving prednisone for treatment of hypercalcemia associated with cancer. He tells you, with great excitement, that his young grandchildren are coming to stay at his home for the next several months. What precautions should be taught to him and immediate family members regarding exposure to the grandchildren, especially during times when pediatric immunizations may be being received?

Situation:

What data would indicate a positive clinical response after administration of adrenal cortical hormones prescribed for the treatment of Addison's disease?

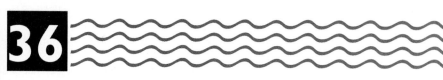

36

Gonadal Hormones

CHAPTER CONTENT

Key Words

gonads

testes

ovaries

testosterone

androgens

estrogen

progesterone

Objectives

1. Describe the body changes that can be anticipated with the administration of androgens, estrogens, or progesterone.

2. State the uses of estrogens and progestins.

3. Compare the side effects seen with the use of estrogen hormones with those seen with a combination of estrogen and progesterone.

4. Differentiate between the side effects to expect and those requiring consultation with the physician with the administration of estrogen or progesterone.

5. Identify the rationale for administering androgens to women who have certain types of breast cancer.

THE GONADS AND GONADAL HORMONES

The **gonads** are the reproductive glands: the **testes** of the male and the **ovaries** of the female. In addition to producing sperm, the testes produce **testosterone,** the male sex hormone. Testosterone controls the development of the male sex organs and influences characteristics such as voice, hair distribution, and male body form. **Androgens** are other steroid hormones that produce masculinizing effects.

The ovaries produce estrogen and progesterone. These are hormones that stimulate maturation of the female sex organs. They influence breast development, voice quality, and the broader pelvis of the female body form. Menstruation is established because of the hormone production of the ovaries. **Estrogen** is responsible for most of these changes. **Progesterone** is thought to be connected mainly with body changes that favor the implantation of the fertilized ovum, continuation of pregnancy, and preparation of the breasts for lactation.

Nursing Process for Gonadal Hormones

Assessment

History. Ask the patient to describe the current problems that initiated this visit. How long have the symptoms been present? Is this a recurrent problem? If so, how was it treated in the past?

Reproductive history. Ask the patient to describe the following, as appropriate: age of menarche; usual pattern of menses—duration, number of pads used, and last menstrual period; number of pregnancies, live births, miscarriages, and abortions; vaginal discharges, itching, infections, and how treated; and breast self-examination routine (if not being performed regularly, explain the correct procedure). Male patients should be asked whether testicular examinations are performed (if not being performed regularly, explain the correct procedure).

History of prior illnesses. Any indication of hypertension, heart or liver disease, thromboembolic disorders, or cancers of the reproductive organs is of particular concern.

Medication history. Obtain a detailed history of all prescribed and over-the-counter medications, including oral contraceptives. Ask patients if they understand why each is being taken. Tactfully determine if the prescribed medications are being taken regularly and if not, why not?

Smoking history. Does the person currently smoke?

Physical examination
- A complete physical examination is usually done as part of the preliminary workup before treatment of any disorders using gonadal hormones.
- Record basic patient data: height, weight, and vital signs. Blood pressure readings are of particular concern so that recordings on future visits can be evaluated for any change.
- Collect urine for urinalysis and blood samples for hemoglobin, hematocrit, and other laboratory studies deemed appropriate by the physician. Usually, patients with family histories of diabetes mellitus should be tested for hyperglycemia before starting gonadal hormone therapy.
- The physical examination should include a breast examination and a pelvic examination, including a Papanicolaou test. Observe the distribution of body hair and the presence of scars. Stress the need for periodic physical examinations while receiving gonadal hormones.

Nursing Diagnosis
- Fluid volume excess (side effect)
- Body image, alteration in (side effect)

Diabetes Mellitus

Patients with diabetes mellitus receiving gonadal hormones may experience alterations in the blood glucose levels. Parameters should be established and a written record for glucose monitoring maintained for reporting to the physician.

Planning
- Most gonadal hormones are prescribed to patients for prolonged self-administration. Therefore planning should stress patient education specific to the type of gonadal hormone prescribed and its intended actions, including monitoring of side effects to expect and side effects to report. Ensure that the individual understands the dosage and specific time schedule for administration of the prescribed medication.
- Schedule follow-up physician visits and laboratory studies.
- Plan to teach the individual to monitor vital signs and to perform daily weights.

Implementation
- Obtain baseline data for subsequent evaluation of therapeutic response to therapy (for example, weight, vital signs, and blood pressure in sitting, lying, and standing positions).
- Assist with the physical examination.

Patient Education and Health Promotion

Expectations of therapy. Discuss the expectations of therapy with the patient (such as degree of pain relief, frequency of use of therapy, relief of menopausal symptoms, sexual maturation, regulation of menstrual cycle, sexual activity, maintenance of mobility, and activities of daily living and work).

Smoking. Explain the risks of continuing to smoke, especially when the patient is receiving estrogen or progestin therapy. (The incidence of fatal heart attacks is increased for women over 35 years of age.)

Physical examination. Stress the need for regular periodic medical examinations and laboratory studies.

Fostering health maintenance
- Discuss medication information and how it will benefit the course of treatment to produce an optimal response.
- Seek cooperation and understanding of the following points so that medication compliance is increased: name of medication, dosage, route and times of administration, side effects to expect, and side effects to report.
- Enlist the patient's aid in developing and maintaining a written record of monitoring parameters (for example, blood pressure, pulse, daily weight, degree of pain relief, menstrual cycle information, breakthrough bleeding, nausea, vomiting, cramps, breast tenderness, hirsutism, gynecomastia, masculinization, hoarseness, headaches, sexual stimulation) and responses to prescribed therapies for discussion with the physician. Patients should be encouraged to take this record on follow-up visits.

DRUG THERAPY

Drug Class: Estrogens

Actions

The natural estrogenic hormone released from the ovaries comprises several closely related chemical compounds: estradiol, estrone, and estriol. The most potent is estradiol. It is metabolized to estrone, which is half as potent. Estrone is further metabolized to estriol, which is considerably less potent. Estrogens are responsible for the development of the sex organs during growth in the uterus and for maturation at puberty. They are also responsible for characteristics such as growth of hair, texture of skin, and distribution of body fat.

Table 36-1

Estrogens

GENERIC NAME	BRAND NAME	AVAILABILITY	USES	DOSES
Chlorotrianisene	Tace	Capsules: 12 mg	Prostatic carcinoma	PO: 12-25 mg daily
			Menopause	PO: 12-25 mg daily cyclically*
			Atrophic vaginitis	PO: 12-25 mg daily cyclically*
			Female hypogonadism	PO: 12-25 mg daily for 21 days, followed by 5 days of progestin
Conjugated estrogens	Premarin, Estrocon	Tablets: 0.3, 0.625, 0.9, 1.25, 2.5 mg	Menopause	PO: 1.25 mg daily cyclically*
		IV: 25 mg/5 ml vial	Atrophic vaginitis	PO: 0.3-1.25 mg daily cyclically*
	✽ C.E.S.	Cream: 0.625 mg/g	Female hypogonadism	PO: 2.5-7 mg daily for 20 days, followed by 10 days off
			Ovarian failure or postoophorectomy	PO: 1.25 mg daily cyclically*
			Osteoporosis	PO: 1.25 mg daily cyclically*
			Breast carcinoma	PO: 10 mg 3 times daily
			Prostatic carcinoma	PO: 1.25-2.5 mg 3 times daily
Diethylstilbestrol (DES)	Diethylstilbestrol, ✽ Honvol	Tablets: 1, 5 mg	Menopause, atrophic vaginitis	PO: 0.2-0.5 mg daily cyclically*
			Female hypogonadism, postoophorectomy, ovarian failure	Dosage range: up to 2 mg daily PO: 0.2-0.5 mg daily cyclically
			Prostatic carcinoma	PO: 1-3 mg daily
			Breast carcinoma	PO: 15 mg daily
Esterified estrogens	Estratab, Menest	Tablets: 0.3, 0.625, 1.25, 2.5 mg	Menopause, atrophic vaginitis	PO: 0.3-1.25 mg daily cyclically*
			Female hypogonadism, postoophorectomy, ovarian failure	PO: 2.5-7.5 mg daily cyclically
			Breast carcinoma	PO: 10 mg 3 times daily
			Prostatic carcinoma	PO: 1.25-2.5 mg 3 times daily

continued

Estrogens also affect the release of pituitary gonadotropins; cause capillary dilatation, fluid retention, and protein metabolism; and inhibit ovulation and postpartum breast engorgement.

Uses

Estrogen products are used for relieving the hot flash symptoms of menopause; for contraception; for hormone replacement therapy after an oophorectomy; for postpartum breast engorgement; in the treatment of osteoporosis; in conjunction with appropriate diet, calcium, and physical therapy; and to slow the disease progress (and minimize discomfort) in patients with advanced prostatic cancer and certain types of breast cancer.

Therapeutic Outcomes

The primary therapeutic outcomes expected from estrogen therapy are as follows:
- Contraception
- Hormonal balance
- Prevention of osteoporosis
- Palliative treatment of prostate and breast cancer

Nursing Process

Premedication Assessment

1. Determine whether the patient is pregnant before starting estrogen therapy; withhold the medicine and consult the physician if there is a question of pregnancy.
2. Obtain baseline weight and vital signs, especially accurate blood pressure readings.
3. Ask whether the individual has a history of thromboembolic disorders or cancer of the reproductive organs; if so, hold medication and contact physician.

Planning

Availability. See Table 36-1.

Implementation

Note: The use of estrogens during early pregnancy is contraindicated. Serious birth defects have been reported, and it has been found that female offspring have an increased risk of developing vaginal or cervical cancer later in life.

Table 36-1

Estrogens—cont'd

GENERIC NAME	BRAND NAME	AVAILABILITY	USES	DOSES
Estradiol	Estrace	Tablets: 1, 2 mg Injections: Cypionate in oil: 1, 5 mg/ml Valerate in oil: 10, 20, 40 mg/ml	Menopause, atrophic vaginitis, hypogonadism, postoophorectomy, ovarian failure Prostatic carcinoma Breast carcinoma	PO: 1-2 mg daily cyclically* IM: Cypionate: 1-5 mg every 3-4 weeks Valerate: 10-20 mg every 4 weeks PO: 1-2 mg 3 times daily IM: Valerate: 30 mg every 1-2 weeks PO: 10 mg 3 times daily
	Vivelle	Transdermal patch: 0.0375, 0.05, 0.075, 0.1 mg	Menopause Female hypogonadism Primary ovarian failure Atrophic vaginitis Postoophorectomy Prevention of osteoporosis	Transdermal system: a 0.05 mg patch should be placed on a clean, dry area of the skin on the trunk (usually abdomen or buttock) twice weekly on a cyclic schedule (3 weeks of therapy followed by 1 week without). Rotate application site; interval of 1 week between uses of same site.
Estropipate	Ogen	Tablets: 0.625, 1.25, 2.5, 5 mg Cream: Vaginal	Menopause, atrophic vaginitis Female hypogonadism, postoophorectomy, ovarian failure Osteoporosis prevention	PO: 0.625-5 mg daily cyclically* PO: 1.25-7.5 mg daily cyclically* PO: 0.625 mg daily cyclically*
Ethinyl estradiol	Estinyl, Feminone	Tablets: 0.02, 0.05, 0.5 mg	Menopause Female hypogonadism Breast carcinoma Prostatic carcinoma	PO: 0.02-0.05 mg daily cyclically* PO: 0.05 1-3 times daily for 2 weeks followed by 2 weeks of progesterone PO: 1 mg 3 times daily PO: 0.15-2 mg daily
Quinestrol	Estrovis	Tablets: 100 μg	Menopause, hypogonadism, atrophic vaginitis, postoophorectomy, ovarian failure	PO: initially, 100 μg daily for 7 days followed by 100 μg weekly starting 2 weeks after treatment starts

*Cyclically = 3 weeks of daily estrogen followed by 1 week off.
♣ Available in Canada only.

Dosage and administration. See Table 36-1.

Evaluation

Side effects to expect

WEIGHT GAIN, EDEMA, BREAST TENDERNESS, NAUSEA. These symptoms tend to be mild and resolve with continued therapy. If they do not resolve or become particularly bothersome, the patient should consult a physician.

Side effects to report

HYPERTENSION, HYPERGLYCEMIA, THROMBOPHLEBITIS, BREAKTHROUGH BLEEDING, ANY OTHER SYMPTOMS THE PATIENT RECOGNIZES AS BEING OF CONCERN. These are all complications associated with estrogen therapy. It is extremely important that the patient is evaluated by the physician to consider alternative therapy.

Drug interactions

WARFARIN. This medication may diminish the anticoagulant effects of warfarin. Monitor the prothrombin time, and increase the dosage of warfarin if necessary.

PHENYTOIN. Estrogens may inhibit the metabolism of phenytoin, resulting in phenytoin toxicity.

Monitor patients with concurrent therapy for signs of phenytoin toxicity (nystagmus, sedation, and lethargy). Serum levels may be ordered, and a reduced dosage of phenytoin may be required.

THYROID HORMONES. Patients who have no thyroid function and who begin estrogen therapy may require an increase in thyroid hormone because estrogens reduce the level of circulating thyroid hormones. Do not adjust the thyroid dosage until the patient shows clinical signs of hypothyroidism.

Drug Class: Progestins

Actions

Progesterone and its derivatives (the progestins) inhibit the secretion of pituitary gonadotropins, preventing maturation of ovarian follicles and thus inhibiting ovulation.

Uses

Progestins are used primarily to treat secondary amenorrhea, breakthrough uterine bleeding, and endometriosis, but they may also be used in combination with estrogens as contraceptives. (See the section on oral contraceptives in Chapter 38.)

Therapeutic Outcomes

The primary therapeutic outcomes expected from progestin therapy are as follows:
- Contraception
- Relief of symptoms of endometriosis
- Hormonal balance to relieve amenorrhea or abnormal uterine bleeding

Nursing Process

Premedication Assessment

1. Determine whether the patient is pregnant before starting estrogen therapy; withhold the medicine and consult the physician if there is a question of pregnancy.
2. Obtain baseline weight and vital signs, especially accurate blood pressure readings.

3. Ask whether the individual has a history of thromboembolic disorders or cancer of the reproductive organs; if so, withhold medication and contact physician.

Planning

Availability. See Table 36-2.

Implementation

Note: The use of progestins in early pregnancy has been associated with birth defects. If pregnancy is suspected, the physician should be consulted immediately.

Dosage and administration. See Table 36-2.

Evaluation

Side effects to expect

WEIGHT GAIN, EDEMA, NAUSEA, VOMITING, DIARRHEA, TIREDNESS, OILY SCALP, ACNE. These symptoms tend to be mild and resolve with continued therapy. If they do not resolve or become particularly bothersome, instruct the patient to consult the physician.

Table 36-2

Progestins

GENERIC NAME	BRAND NAME	AVAILABILITY	USES	DOSES
Hydroxyprogesterone	Duralutin Prodrox	Injection: 250 mg/ml	Amenorrhea; abnormal uterine bleeding Uterine carcinoma	IM: 375 mg IM: 1-7 g weekly
Levonorgestrel	Norplant system	Capsule implant: 36 mg	Contraception	Subdermal implant: 6 capsules implanted in first 7 days of onset of menses; insertion is subdermal in midportion of upper arm
Medroxyprogesterone	Provera, Amen, Curretab	Tablets: 2.5, 5, 10 mg	Secondary amenorrhea	PO: 5-10 mg daily for 5-10 days
			Abnormal uterine bleeding	PO: 5-10 mg daily for 5-10 days, beginning on the 16th or 21st day of the menstrual cycle
Norethindrone	Norlutin	Tablets: 5 mg	Amenorrhea, abnormal uterine bleeding	PO: 5-20 mg starting with the 5th and ending on the 25th day of the menstrual cycle
			Endometriosis	PO: 10 mg for 2 weeks; increase in increments of 5 mg/day every 2 weeks until 30 mg/day is reached
Norethindrone acetate	Aygestin	Tablets: 5 mg	Amenorrhea, abnormal uterine bleeding	PO: 2.5-10 mg starting with the 5th and ending on the 25th day of the menstrual cycle
			Endometriosis	PO: 5 mg for 2 weeks; increase in increments of 2.5 mg/day every 2 weeks until 15 mg/day is reached
Norgestrel	Ovrette	Tablets: 0.075 mg	Oral contraceptive	PO: 1 tablet daily
Progesterone	Progesterone, ✤ Gesterol	Injection: 50 mg/ml	Amenorrhea, functional uterine bleeding	IM: 5-10 mg for 6-8 consecutive days

✤ Available in Canada only.

Side effects to report

BREAKTHROUGH BLEEDING, AMENORRHEA, CONTINUING HEADACHE, CHOLESTATIC JAUNDICE, MENTAL DEPRESSION. These are all complications associated with progestin therapy. It is extremely important that the patient is evaluated by the physician to consider alternatives in therapy.

PREGNANCY. Because of the possibility of birth defects, a physician should be consulted immediately.

Drug interactions

RIFAMPIN. Rifampin may enhance the metabolism of progestins. The dosage of progestins may need to be increased to provide therapeutic benefit.

Drug Class: Androgens

Actions

The dominant male sex hormone is testosterone. It is the primary natural androgen produced by the testicles. Androgens are responsible for the normal growth and development of male sex organs and for maintenance of secondary sex characteristics. These effects include the growth and maturation of the prostate, seminal vesicles, penis, and scrotum; the development of male hair distribution; laryngeal enlargement (Adam's apple); vocal chord thickening; alterations in body musculature; and fat distribution.

Uses

Androgens are used to treat hypogonadism, eunuchism, androgen deficiency, and palliation of breast cancer in postmenopausal women with certain cell types of cancer. When androgens are used for palliation of cancer in women, they suppress cancer cell growth.

Therapeutic Outcomes

The primary therapeutic outcomes expected from androgen therapy are as follows:
- Restoration of hormonal balance in androgen deficiency
- Reduced discomfort associated with breast cancer

Nursing Process

Premedication Assessment

1. Obtain baseline vital signs and weight, and assess mental status.
2. Check baseline electrolyte values; report abnormal findings. Be especially alert for hypercalcemia.

Planning

Availability. See Table 36-3.

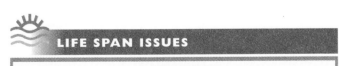

LIFE SPAN ISSUES

ANDROGENS

Male children receiving androgens must have the effects of the drug on long bones monitored by periodic x-ray of long bones. Usually, x-rays of long bones are performed every 3 to 6 months to check the status of the epiphyseal line.

Implementation

Dosage and administration. See Table 36-3.

Evaluation

Side effects to expect

GASTRIC IRRITATION. If gastric irritation occurs, administer with food or milk. If symptoms persist or increase in severity, report for physician evaluation.

Side effects to report

ELECTROLYTE IMBALANCE, EDEMA. The most commonly altered electrolytes are potassium (K^+), sodium (Na^+), and chloride (Cl^-). Hyperkalemia is most likely to occur.

Many symptoms associated with altered fluid and electrolyte balance are subtle and interspersed with general symptoms of drug toxicity or the disease process itself.

Gather data about changes in the patient's mental status (alertness, orientation, and confusion), muscle strength, muscle cramps, tremors, nausea, and general appearance (drowsy, anxious, and lethargic).

Always check the electrolyte reports for early indications of electrolyte imbalance.

Keep accurate records of intake and output, daily weights, and vital signs.

Patients should report weight gains of more than 2 pounds per week. Diuretic therapy, with or without dietary reduction of salt, may be prescribed if edema is significant.

MASCULINIZATION. Women receiving high doses of androgens may develop signs of masculinization. Women should be monitored for signs of masculinization (deepening of the voice, hoarseness, growth of facial hair, clitoral enlargement, and menstrual irregularities) during androgen therapy. The drug should usually be discontinued when mild masculinization is evident because some adverse androgenic effects (such as voice changes) may not reverse with discontinuation of therapy. In consultation with the physician, the woman may decide that some masculinization is acceptable during treatment for carcinoma of the breast. Help patients adjust to a possible change in self-image or self-esteem caused by the effects of masculinization.

Males should be carefully monitored for the development of gynecomastia, priapism, or excessive sexual stimulation. These are indications of androgen overdose.

HYPERCALCEMIA. In immobilized patients and patients with breast cancer, androgen therapy may cause hypercalcemia. Monitor patients for nausea, vomiting, constipation, poor muscle tone, and lethargy. These are indications of hypercalcemia and are indications for discontinuation of androgen therapy.

Force fluids to minimize the possibility of renal calculi. Encourage the patient to drink 8 to 12 8-ounce glasses of water daily.

Perform weight-bearing and active and passive exercises to the degree tolerated by the patient to minimize loss of calcium from bones.

HEPATOTOXICITY. The symptoms of hepatotoxicity are anorexia, nausea, vomiting, jaundice, hepatomegaly, splenomegaly, and abnormal liver function tests (elevated bilirubin, aspartate transaminase [AST], alanine aminotransferase [ALT], gamma glutamyltransferase [GGT], alkaline phosphatase, and prothrombin time).

Drug interactions

WARFARIN. Androgens may enhance the anticoagulant effects of warfarin. Observe for the development of petechiae,

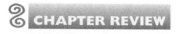

Table 36-3

Androgens

GENERIC NAME	BRAND NAME	AVAILABILITY	USES	DOSES
Short-acting				
Testosterone in water	Testosterone Aqueous, Testamone	IM: 25, 50, 100 mg/ml	Eunuchism, postpubertal cryptorchidism, impotence caused by androgen deficiency	IM: Deep gluteal muscle—25-50 mg 2-3 times daily
			Breast carcinoma	IM: Deep gluteal muscle—50-100 mg 3 times weekly
Testosterone in oil	Testosterone propionate	IM: 100 mg/ml	As above	As above
Testosterone USP in gel base	Androderm Transdermal System	Transdermal patch: 12.5 mg	Androgen deficiency	Transdermal System: 1-3 patches applied to skin, on hips, abdomen, thighs, or buttocks nightly for 24 hours; replace every 24 hours; do not apply to scrotum
Long-acting				
Testosterone enanthate	Everone, Delatestryl	IM: 100, 200 mg/ml	Eunuchism, androgen deficiency	IM: 200-400 mg every 4 weeks
			Oligospermia	IM: 100-200 mg every 4-6 weeks
Testosterone cypionate	Vigorex, Depotest, ✽ Depo-Testosterone	IM: 100, 200 mg/ml	As for testosterone enanthate	As for testosterone enanthate
Oral products				
Methyltestosterone	Oreton Methyl, Testred, Virilon, ✽ Metandren	Tablets: 10, 25 mg Capsules: 10 mg Sublingual tablets: 10 mg	Eunuchism Cryptorchidism Breast carcinoma	PO: 10-40 mg daily PO: 30 mg daily PO: 200 mg daily
Fluoxymesterone	Halotestin, Hysterone	Tablets: 2, 5, 10 mg	Male hypogonadism Female breast carcinoma	PO: 2-10 mg daily PO: 10-40 mg daily

✽ Available in Canada only.

ecchymoses, nosebleeds, bleeding gums, dark tarry stools, and bright red or coffee ground emesis. Monitor the prothrombin time, and reduce the dosage of warfarin if necessary.

ORAL HYPOGLYCEMIC AGENTS, INSULIN. Monitor for hypoglycemia: headache, weakness, decreased coordination, general apprehension, diaphoresis, hunger, and blurred or double vision.

The dosage of the hypoglycemic agent or insulin may need to be reduced. Notify the physician if any of the aforementioned symptoms appear.

CORTICOSTEROIDS. Concurrent use may increase the possibility of electrolyte imbalance and fluid retention. See earlier in this chapter for monitoring parameters.

CHAPTER REVIEW

The gonadal hormones are necessary for the body to grow and mature into the adult form and for reproduction. Male and female gonads secrete hormones. The male testes secrete predominantly androgens, and the female ovaries secrete primarily estrogens and progesterone. These hormones are responsible for the shape and secondary sex characteristics associated with the male and female body form.

MATH REVIEW

1. Ordered: hydroxyprogesterone 375 mg IM.
   On hand: hydroxyprogesterone 250 mg/ml.
   Give: _____ ml.

2. Ordered: progesterone 10 mg IM daily for 6 days.
   On hand: progesterone 50 mg/ml.
   Give: _____ ml.

CRITICAL THINKING QUESTION

Mrs. Arborbottum, age 62, is receiving methyltestosterone 200 mg PO daily for palliation of breast cancer. She asks you why she is taking this particular medication and expresses concern that this medication, like other medications she has taken for treatment of the cancer, will make her feel ill. What should you tell her?

DRUGS AFFECTING THE REPRODUCTIVE SYSTEM

37

Drugs Used in Obstetrics

Objectives

1. Describe nursing assessments and nursing interventions needed for the pregnant patient during the first, second, and third trimesters of pregnancy.

2. Identify appropriate nursing assessments, nursing interventions, and treatment options used for the following obstetric complications: infection, hyperemesis gravidarum, miscarriage, abortion, preterm labor, premature rupture of membranes, gestational diabetes and pregnancy-induced hypertension (PIH).

3. State the methods and time parameters of each approach to the termination of a pregnancy.

4. Summarize the care needs of the pregnant woman during labor and delivery and the immediate postpartal period including the patient education needed before discharge to promote safe self-care and care of the newborn.

5. State the purpose of administering glucocorticoids to certain women in preterm labor.

6. State the actions, primary uses, nursing assessment, and monitoring parameters for uterine stimulants, uterine relaxants, clomiphene citrate, magnesium sulfate, and RH_0 (D) immune globulin.

7. Compare the effects of uterine stimulants and uterine relaxants on the pregnant woman's uterus.

8. Describe specific nursing concerns and appropriate nursing actions when uterine stimulants are administered for induction of labor, augmentation of labor, and postpartum atony and hemorrhage.

9. Cite the effects of adrenergic agents on beta-1 and beta-2 receptors, then identify the relationship of these actions with the side effects to report when adrenergic agents are used to inhibit preterm labor.

10. Describe specific assessments needed before and during the use of ritodrine, terbutaline, or magnesium sulfate.

11. Identify emergency supplies that should be available in the immediate vicinity during magnesium sulfate therapy.

12. Identify the action, specific dosage, administration precautions, and proper timing of the administration of RH_0 (D) immune globulin and rubella vaccine in relation to pregnancy.

13. Summarize the immediate nursing care needs of the newborn infant after delivery.

Key Words

pregnancy-induced hypertension

lochia

precipitous labor and delivery

augmentation

dysfunctional labor

OBSTETRICS

Nursing Process for Obstetrics

Assessment

Assessment of the pregnant woman

Prenatal visit. Obtain basic historic information about the woman and family concerning diseases, surgeries, and deaths. Has the patient been treated for kidney or bladder problems; high blood pressure; heart disease; rheumatic fever; hypothyroidism or hyperthyroidism; diabetes mellitus; allergies to any foods, drugs, or environmental substances; or sexually transmitted diseases? Has the patient been exposed to any communicable diseases since becoming pregnant? Has the patient received blood or blood products? If the woman answers "yes" to any of these questions, gather more information about what physician made the diagnosis, when the disorder occurred, and how the disorder was treated.

Gather data about menstrual pattern (age of initial onset, duration and frequency of monthly periods, date of last full menstrual cycle, any bleeding since the last full menstrual period).

Gather data about contraceptive use (condoms, foam, diaphragm, sponge, oral contraceptives, or intrauterine contraceptive devices).

Take an obstetric history. Ask the woman the number of previous live births, stillbirths, miscarriages, and induced abortions. If any of the deliveries were premature, obtain additional information about the infant's age of gestation, survival of the child, any suspected causes, and infections.

Ask if $Rh_0(D)$ immune globulin (RhoGAM) has been received for Rh factor incompatibility.

Nutritional history. What is the patient's usual weight? How much weight has she gained or lost in the past 3 months?

What are the woman's favorite foods? How often does she eat? What has she eaten in the last 3 days?

Elimination pattern. What is the patient's elimination pattern? How often does she have bowel movements? What is the stool consistency and color? Is there ever any bleeding? Are laxatives ever needed? If so, how often?

Psychosocial history. Determine how the woman feels about this pregnancy (that is, excited, nervous, or is the baby unwanted).

Who makes up her support group: husband, boyfriend, friends, family?

Ask the woman about her employment status and what type of work she performs.

Determine the woman's level of education, economic status, and general interest in learning more about effective management of the pregnancy. Will referral to social services agencies be necessary?

Medication history. Ask the woman if she takes any prescribed or over-the-counter medications regularly. If she is not currently taking any medications, ask whether any have been taken over the past 6 months. Determine which have been prescribed and for what purpose.

Determine the use of alcohol or street drugs of any kind, including what, how much, and how frequently.

Physical examination. Assist the woman to undress and prepare for examination, including a pelvic examination and Papanicolaou smear.
* Height and weight: record height and weight.
* Hypertension: take the blood pressure. Ask again if any previous treatment has been given for high blood pressure. If so, inquire about the onset, treatment, and degree of control achieved.
* Heart rate: count the pulse for 1 full minute. Report irregularities in rate, rhythm, or volume. On subsequent visits, anticipate an increase in rate of approximately 10 beats per minute during the course of the pregnancy.
* Respirations: record the rate of respirations. As the pregnancy progresses, observe for hyperventilation and thoracic breathing.
* Temperature: if the temperature is elevated, ask about any signs of infection or exposure to persons with known communicable diseases.

Laboratory studies and diagnostics. Obtain a urine specimen using a clean catch method of collection.

Blood samples for complete blood count (CBC), hemoglobin, hematocrit, rubella titer, Rh factor, and sexually transmitted diseases (STDs) (for example, syphilis, gonorrhea, or *Chlamydia*) may be ordered at this initial visit. Blood tests may include an antibody, sickle cell, and thalassemia screen; folic acid level; and, as appropriate, purified protein derivative (PPD), human immunodeficiency virus (HIV), and toxicology screen.

Assessment during first, second, and third trimesters. Assessment done at routine visits during the pregnancy consists of the following: weight; measurement of blood pressure, pulse, and respirations; and examination of the abdomen with measurement of fundal height and fetal heart sounds. Any problems or concerns should be discussed. Hemoglobin and hematocrit may be periodically rechecked.

The pregnant woman who does not experience complications is usually examined once monthly for the first 6 months, every 2 weeks in the seventh and eighth months, and weekly during the last month of pregnancy. Vaginal examinations are usually performed on the initial visit and are not repeated until 2 to 3 weeks before the estimated date of confinement (EDC), or due date, at which time the cervical status, degree of engagement, and fetal presentation are evaluated.

Assessment of pregnant patients at risk. Assess for signs and symptoms of potential obstetric complications (see an obstetrics text for further details of each complication): infection, hyperemesis gravidarum, miscarriage, abortion, preterm labor, premature rupture of membranes, gestational diabetes, and **pregnancy-induced hypertension** (PIH).

Infection. Record the temperature. Report any elevations to the physician immediately for further evaluation. As appropriate obtain urine for urinalysis.

Hyperemesis gravidarum. Obtain details of any persistent, severe vomiting.

Miscarriage, placental separation, abortion. Assess for signs of bleeding. Gather specific information about the onset, duration, volume (number of pads used), and color, and report any clots or tissue seen.

Ask the patient to describe any pain being experienced. Has she had any backache or pelvic cramping, sharp abdominal pain, faintness, or pain in the shoulder area?

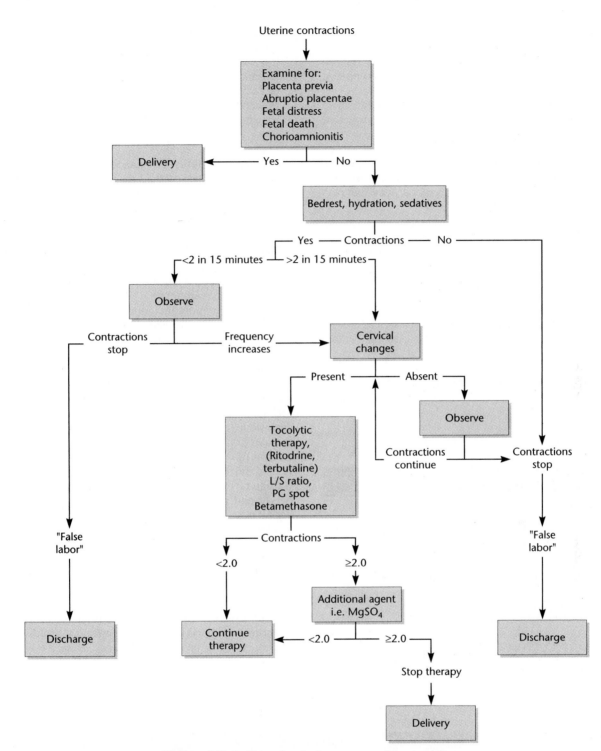

Figure 37-1 *Alternatives in the treatment of preterm labor.*

Vital signs should be taken and compared with baseline data whenever bleeding is suspected. Assess for development of shock: restlessness, perspiration, pallor, clammy skin, dyspnea, tachycardia, and blood pressure changes. Record fetal heart tones at regular intervals.

Preterm labor. Assess the status of the fetus by fetal movement counts, contraction stress testing, biophysical profile, and ultrasonography for placental placement and measurement of maturity indicators. Amniocentesis may be performed to assess fetal lung maturity (Figure 37-1).

Premature rupture of membranes. Assess for and obtain specifics of any signs of leakage of amniotic fluid from the vagina.

Gestational diabetes. Review urinalysis reports for glycosuria. Review past history of symptoms, especially during previous pregnancies.

Pregnancy-induced hypertension. Assess for and report sudden development of hypertension (an elevation of systolic pressure 30 mm Hg or more above prior readings, systolic blood pressure of 140 mm Hg or more, or diastolic pressure of 90 mm Hg or more).

Assess for edema of any body parts (fingers, hands, face, legs, ankles). Assess hydration status, and, in particular, obtain daily weights.

The status of the fetus may be assessed by fetal movement counts, contraction stress testing, biophysical profile, and ultrasonography for placental placement and measurement of maturity indicators. Amniocentesis may be performed to assess fetal lung maturity.

Review laboratory reports for abnormal electrolytes, elevated uric acid or hematocrit levels, thrombocytopenia, and the presence of red blood cells (RBCs) and protein in the urine.

Assess for signs and symptoms of seizure activity.

Monitor fetal heart rate and movements.

Assess for start of labor or signs of other complications such as pulmonary edema, disseminated intravascular coagulation, heart failure, abruptio placentae, or cerebral hemorrhage.

Assessment during normal labor and delivery

History of pregnancy. On admission to the hospital, obtain the following information:
- Name and age

- Obstetric history: gravida, para, abortions, fetal deaths, birth weight of previous children, and complications during previous deliveries
- Estimated due date, estimated gestational age, and first day of last menstrual period (LMP)
- Prenatal care: type and amount, any significant problems
- Prenatal education: type and extent of childbirth preparation
- Plan for infant feeding
- Status of membranes: intact, ruptured, time ruptured, amount and color of fluid that escaped
- Status of labor: time of onset of contractions, frequency, duration and intensity, how patient is coping with contractions
- Time of last meal

Physical examination. The physical examination should include the following:
- Height, weight, vital signs (temperature, blood pressure, pulse, and respirations)
- State of hydration, including presence of edema
- Size and contour of abdomen and fundus
- Frequency of contractions
- Fetal heart rate
- Vaginal examination: cervical dilatation and effacement, status of membranes, and presentation and position of fetus

Assessment after delivery and during postpartum care. • The vital signs should be checked every 15 minutes during the first hour or until the woman is stable, then every 30 minutes for the next 2 hours. • Inspect the perineum and note any abnormal swelling or bruising. • Assess fundal height and firmness every 15 minutes for 1 hour, then every 30 minutes for the next 4 hours. Continue to assess fundal height and position until the woman is discharged. • Describe the amount of **lochia** and the color and the presence of clots every 15 minutes for 1 hour, every 30 minutes for 4 hours, and hourly for the next 12 hours. • Assess breasts for colostrum and breast milk approximately 3 to 4 hours after delivery. Check for breast engorgement and discomfort.

Assessment of the neonate. • Ensure airway patency. • Umbilical cord is observed until pulsations cease and then clamped or ligated. • Assess neonate's health status at 1 minute and 5 minutes after delivery using the Apgar rating system (Table 37-1). • Rapid estimation of gestation age is also performed (Table 37-2).

Table 37-1

The Apgar Scoring System

SIGN	0	1	2
Heart rate	Absent	Slow (below 100)	Over 100
Respiratory effort	Absent	Slow, irregular	Good, crying
Muscle tone	Flaccid	Some flexion of extremities	Active motion
Reflex irritability	No response	Grimace	Cry
Color	Blue, pale	Body pink, extremities blue	Completely pink

Table 37-2

Gestational Age

SITES	36 WEEKS OR LESS	37-38 WEEKS	39 WEEKS OR MORE
Sole creases	Anterior transverse creases only	Occasional creases anterior two thirds	Sole covered with creases
Breast nodule diameter	2 mm	4 mm	7 mm
Scalp hair	Fine, fuzzy	Fine, fuzzy	Coarse and silky
Earlobes	Pliable, no cartilage	Some cartilage	Stiffened by thick cartilage
Testes and scrotum	Testes in lower canal, scrotum small, few rugae	Intermediate	Testes pendulous, scrotum full, extensive rugae

From Cunningham FG, MacDonald PC, Grant NF: *Williams' obstetrics,* ed 18, Norwalk, Conn, 1989, Appleton & Lange.

Nursing Diagnosis

- Altered nutrition: less than body requirements (indication)
- Altered sexuality patterns (indication)
- Body-image disturbance (indication)
- Injury, risk for (indication, side effects)
- Anxiety (indication, side effects)
- Sleep pattern disturbance (indication)

Planning

A large part of maternity care is delivered and directed from the clinic setting. Therefore the planning of care must be individualized to the patient's needs and available resources. The care plan must incorporate cultural aspects of care, education level and capabilities, family structure, economic resources, and access to health care and community resources. Health teaching is essential for maintenance of optimal health for the mother to support fetal development. An integral part of the planning must include planning for self-care to meet the following needs: nutrition, activity and exercise, elimination needs, sleep requirements, cessation of smoking and alcohol consumption, and management of the usual discomforts of pregnancy. Provide information in a timely manner regarding self-monitoring for complications and for signs of true or false labor.

Initiate discussion of infant feeding options available during the first trimester of the pregnancy. Schedule follow-up appointments, laboratory studies, and diagnostics appropriate to care needs.

Cooperatively plan with the mother (and father) for attendance at childbirth and parenting classes.

Implementation

Prenatal.　• Collect information relating to the person's health status and the pregnancy. Observe for signs of potential complications of pregnancy.　• Assist with routine prenatal examinations and diagnostic procedures.　• Review laboratory and diagnostic studies performed; report abnormal findings to the physician.　• During the first trimester of the pregnancy, initiate discussion of infant feeding options available; provide information needed for parents to make a decision.

Complications of pregnancy

Infection. Monitor for infections, and intervene according to the physician's orders when an infection is confirmed.

Hyperemesis gravidarum. (See Chapter 31.) Monitor hydration status, daily weight, and vital signs. Provide for dietary needs through intravenous therapy, nutritional supplements, and gradual progression of diet as tolerated.

Bleeding, miscarriage, abortion. Ensure that the patient adheres to bed rest, and give sedatives as prescribed. Monitor maternal vital signs, fetal heart rate and activity, and the volume (frequency of change and number of pads used) of bleeding present. When bleeding is present, blood studies for hemoglobin, hematocrit, white blood cells (WBCs), human chorionic gonadotropin (HCG) titer, and blood type and crossmatch may be ordered. Other diagnostic procedures such as culdoscopy, sonography, laparoscopy, fetoscopy, and pregnancy tests may be performed.

Preterm labor

- Monitor uterine contractions, and continue external fetal and uterine monitoring.
- Position the mother on her side, increase fluid intake, and start an intravenous (IV) line as ordered. Monitor hydration, maintain accurate intake and output records, and take daily weights.
- Assist with obtaining cervical and vaginal cultures, as ordered.
- Perform cervical examination to determine dilation and effacement.
- Take maternal vital signs. Record fetal heart rate and frequency and intensity of uterine contractions.
- Administer prescribed medications—uterine relaxants, for example, ritodrine, terbutaline, and magnesium sulfate. (See individual drug monographs for administration information and monitoring parameters.) Glucocorticoids, usually betamethasone, may be administered intramuscularly (IM) to the mother to accelerate lung maturation to minimize fetal respiratory distress syndrome. It may be used in cases in which it is anticipated that premature labor should be stopped for only 36 to 48 hours, such as with premature rupture of the membranes.
- Provide appropriate psychologic support. Involve pastoral care appropriately.

Premature rupture of membranes.　• Check fetal heart tones and fetal activity.　• Describe the color, characteristics, and amount of amniotic fluid leakage.　• Check maternal vital signs; report elevated temperature, chills, or malaise immediately.

Gestational diabetes

- Assist with the performance of glucose tolerance testing.
- Perform blood glucose testing 4 times per day, and assist the patient in administering prescribed insulin.
- Encourage adherence to diet and exercise prescribed to achieve tight glucose control to maintain desired weight gain during the pregnancy and to prevent complications (for example, neonatal hypoglycemia or stillbirth).
- Monitor for development of hypoglycemia and hyperglycemia.
- During labor, monitor glucose level every 2 hours; maintain adequate hydration.
- During the postpartum period, continue to monitor glucose levels. (Usually with gestational diabetes, the mother's glucose reverts to normal during the postpartum period. Therefore careful monitoring of glucose and adjustment of insulin dosages must occur.)

Pregnancy-induced hypertension

- Monitor maternal vital signs, fetal heart tones, and fetal movement at appropriate intervals consistent with symptoms.
- Maintain hydration by oral or intravenous routes (usually 1000 ml plus the amount of urine output over the past 24 hours). Maintain accurate intake and output, and obtain daily weights. Salt intake is generally maintained at a normal level, although heavy use should be discouraged.
- Test the urine for protein and specific gravity every hour. Report a steady decrease in hourly output or output of less than 30 ml per hour.
- Review available laboratory studies and report findings to the physician (for example, electrolyte studies, CBC with differential, thrombocytopenia, uric acid level, hematocrit, serum estriol, and L/S ratio).

- Monitor for signs of seizure activity (increased drowsiness, hyperflexia, visual disturbances, and development of severe pain). If symptoms are present, report immediately.
- If seizures occur, give supportive care, provide a nonstimulating environment, and have oxygen, suction, and padded tongue blade available. Institute seizure precautions.
- Be alert for complications (for example, start of labor, pulmonary edema, disseminated intravascular coagulation, heart failure, abruptio placentae, or cerebral edema).
- Administer prescribed drugs (for example, diazepam or phenobarbital, antihypertensive). The vasodilator hydralazine is usually administered to control blood pressure. It may be administered orally or intravenously, depending on the severity of the condition. If given IV, monitor the maternal and fetal heart rates and the mother's blood pressure every 2 to 3 minutes after the initial dose and every 10 to 15 minutes thereafter. The diastolic pressure is usually maintained at 90 to 100 mm Hg. Anticonvulsants such as magnesium sulfate may be given for treatment of seizure activity. (See drug monograph regarding administration and monitoring of the patient during drug therapy.)

Termination of pregnancy

- If bleeding occurs near the EDC, the infant may be delivered by cesarean section. If it appears that a miscarriage is occurring, the woman may be hospitalized for observation and bed rest, diagnosis for possible causes (for example, infection), and fluid replacement.
- If a pregnancy is to be terminated (aborted), the following methods may be used:
  - Before 12 weeks of gestation: suction curettage or dilatation and evacuation (D&E).
  - 12 to 20 weeks of gestation: Intraamniotic instillation of hypertonic saline (20% solution) or prostaglandin administered intraamniotically, intramuscularly, or by vaginal suppository.
  - Intrauterine fetal death after 20 weeks of gestation: prostaglandin suppositories with or without oxytocin augmentation. (See the section on uterine stimulants on p. 459.)
- Encourage the persons involved in the loss of an infant to talk about their feelings of loss, grief, sadness, or anger. Have pastoral care involved in supportive processes as appropriate. Listen and allow them to vent feelings. Give answers (if known) regarding future pregnancies. Refer for other counseling as appropriate. Anticipate that depression may develop over the next few weeks and may need treatment.
- Administer $Rh_0(D)$ immune globulin within 72 hours of the termination of pregnancy (see p. 467) to an Rh-negative mother. Also check the patient's rubella titer; if low, obtain an order for innoculation immediately after pregnancy.

Normal labor and delivery

- Perform routine admission procedures (for example, vital signs, perineal prep, and enema).
- Follow institutional guidelines regarding activity level of the mother; some permit ambulation during the early stage of labor.
- During labor, provide pain relief, alternate side-to-side positioning of mother (avoid lying flat on back), intervene with comfort measures (for example, back rubs, pelvic rocking, and effleurage). Encourage leg extension and dorsiflexion of the foot to relieve spasms and cramping.
- Provide for privacy, and support the woman and coach when necessary.
- Check for bladder distention. Have patient void every 2 hours.
- Maintain adequate hydration by giving ice chips or clear liquids. Check hydration status throughout labor—observe mucous membranes, dryness of lips, and skin turgor. Give oral hygiene frequently. Do not give solid foods unless specifically approved by the physician.
- As labor progresses, continue to monitor the maternal and fetal vital signs and the frequency, duration, and intensity of uterine contractions.
- Report contractions with a duration of 90 seconds or more and those not followed by complete uterine relaxation. Report abnormal patterns on the fetal monitor, such as decreased variability, late decelerations, and variable decelerations.
- Continue to assist the coach when necessary.
- As vaginal discharge increases, wash the perineum with warm water and dry the area. Change the bedsheets, pad, and gown when necessary.
- Monitor patient's temperature every 4 hours while membranes are intact and temperature remains within normal range. Monitor every 2 hours if the patient's temperature is elevated or if the membranes have ruptured.
- After delivery record the time of delivery and position of the infant; the type of episiotomy and type of suture used in repair, if appropriate; any anesthetic or analgesic used during repair; the time of placental delivery; and any complications (for example, additional bleeding or neonatal distress).
- Administer and record oxytocic agent, as ordered.

Immediate neonatal care. Before delivery, the maternal history through the current stage of labor should be reviewed to identify potential complications that may arise for the neonate. Although a complete physical examination of the neonate will be performed later, a preliminary assessment and recording of data must be completed at the time of birth.

The following procedures must be completed by the physician or nurse immediately after delivery.

Airway. Ensure that the airway is open and remains so. As soon as the head is delivered, the oropharynx and nasal passages are suctioned with a small bulb syringe. Immediately after delivery, the newborn baby is held with the head lowered at a 10- to 15-degree angle to help drainage of amniotic fluid, mucus, and blood. Resuction with the bulb syringe as necessary.

Clamping of the umbilical cord. When the airway is opened and the respirations have stabilized, the neonate should be held at the same level as the uterus until pulsations of the cord cease. The cord is then clamped or ligated.

Health status. The health status of the neonate is estimated at 1 minute and 5 minutes after delivery using the Apgar rating system (see Table 37-1). Rapid estimation of gestational age is also performed (see Table 37-2).

Temperature maintenance. The neonate should be dried immediately and body temperature maintained with the use of prewarmed blankets, a heated bassinet, or an infrared heat lamp. If the neonate is term and in stable condition as assessed by the Apgar score, temperature may be maintained by skin-to-skin contact with the mother.

Eye prophylaxis. It is a legal requirement that every newborn baby's eyes be treated prophylactically for *Neisseria gonorrhoea.* Another rapidly emerging neonatal conjunctival infection is chlamydial ophthalmia neonatorum, which is caused by *Chlamydia trachomatis.* The neonate may have become infected during birth if the mother is infected. Opthalmic erythromycin or tetracycline is used for prophylactic treatment of neonatal conjunctivitis caused by *Neisseria gonorrhoea* or *Chlamydia trachomatis.* Instillation of the ophthalmic agent may be delayed up to 2 hours to facilitate parent-child bonding.

Other procedures. While the parents are bonding with the newborn infant, the nurse should prepare an infant identification bracelet and place it on the baby, examine the placenta and cord for anomalies, and verify the presence of one vein and two arteries. Samples of cord blood may be collected for analysis of the Rh factor, blood grouping, and the hematocrit. The baby is then taken to the newborn nursery where it is weighed, measured, and given a complete physical examination. Some physicians also order an intramuscular injection of vitamin K to be administered to the baby as prophylaxis against hemorrhage. Evaluation of the infant's vital signs and color are performed on a continuum. Alterations from baseline are evaluated and reported.

Postpartum care. *Postpartum* is defined as the time between delivery and return of the reproductive organs to prepregnancy status.

- An Rh-negative mother may receive $Rh_0(D)$ immune globulin within 72 hours of the completion of the pregnancy.
- If the mother's rubella titer is low, an appropriate time for inoculation is immediately after pregnancy.
- Continue to assess the fundal height, position, and lochia until the woman is discharged. The lochia normally progresses from blood red (bright) to darker red with some small clots (1 to 3 days postpartum), to pinkish thin, watery consistency (4 to 10 days), to a yellowish or creamy color (11 to 21 days). The odor should be similar to that of a normal menstrual flow; a foul-smelling odor should be reported. Pads should be changed at frequent regular intervals rather than waiting for them to become heavily laden.
- On delivery, the breasts secrete a thin yellow fluid called colostrum. Within 3 to 4 days, breast milk becomes available. This may produce some discomfort for the mother as the breasts become congested. She may need to use a breast pump to prevent engorgement. Ice packs for 15 minutes alternating with breast pumping may be ordered. A warm shower or application of warm, moist heat may provide relief of breast engorgement.
- Instruct the mother to wash her breasts daily and air-dry the nipples. Express a small amount of breast milk and massage into area around nipple. In general, do not apply ointments or creams.
- The quantity of breast milk varies among mothers. Diet, fluid intake, and level of anxiety all affect lactation. Oxytocin nasal spray may be necessary to help encourage milk letdown.

- Increase the frequency of breast-feeding to stimulate flow of milk; monitor the number of infant voidings, usually 6 to 8 in 24 hours, and record stools, usually one in 24 hours.
- Weigh the infant daily. A weight gain of ¾ to 1 ounce per day indicates that the infant is receiving adequate nutritional intake.
- Help the mother to hold the baby correctly, and provide instruction and guidance on the correct technique of breast-feeding, bottle-feeding, and "bubbling" the baby.
- Non–breast-feeding mothers should wear a bra that will provide firm support; ice packs may be applied as ordered.
- Encourage the mother using formula feeding to eat a well-balanced diet with adequate protein, vitamins, and fluids to help restore the body to the optimal level.
- Continue to provide emotional support to the new mother and support persons.
- Afterpains often require a mild analgesic. For the breast-feeding mother who is experiencing afterpains, administration of a mild analgesic approximately 40 minutes before nursing may relieve the discomfort.
- Check on voiding and return of normal bowel elimination during postpartum period.
- Check vital signs every shift or more frequently when indicated.
- Monitor laboratory reports during postpartum period. The hematocrit may rise during the initial period after childbirth; WBCs, mainly neutrophils, may be elevated during this initial time span as well, making it difficult to diagnose an infection.
- Monitor for thromboembolisms during the postpartum period. Clotting factors and fibrinogen are increased during pregnancy and during the immediate postpartum period.

Patient Education and Health Promotion
- Encourage open communication with the expectant family. They must be guided to understand the need for prenatal care. Keep emphasizing those things the family can do to optimize the chances for a healthy baby, including maintenance of general health, nutritional needs, adequate rest and appropriate exercise, and continuation of prescribed medication therapy.
- The amount of information provided to the expectant mother or parents is individualized to the persons. The following health teaching is an overview of information that may be given; see a maternity textbook to cover the areas not addressed.

Adequate rest and relaxation. Assist the individual to plan for adequate rest periods throughout the day to prevent fatigue, irritability, and overexhaustion. Talk with the individual about planning rest periods during lunch breaks at work, when preschoolers are napping, or when the father is home to care for children. A short period of relaxation in a reclining chair or elevation of the feet may be beneficial when there is no time during the day for sleep. Advise the patient to avoid long periods of standing in one place and to perform some daily activities while sitting.

Activity and exercise. Usually, the woman can continue to perform common activities of daily living. New attempts at strenuous exercise (such as jogging or aerobics) should not be started during pregnancy. Daily walks in fresh air are encouraged.

Any changes in activity level should be discussed with the physician *before* starting.

Encourage good posture and participation in prenatal classes in which exercises are taught to strengthen the abdominal muscles and to relax the pelvic floor muscles.

The woman should avoid lifting heavy objects and should avoid situations that might cause physical harm, especially as the pregnancy progresses, because balance may be affected.

Employment. Advice about continued employment should be based on the type of job; working conditions; amount of lifting, standing, or exposure to toxic substances; and the individual's state of health.

General personal hygiene. Encourage maintenance of general hygiene through daily tub baths or showers. Tub baths near the end of pregnancy may be discouraged because of the danger of slipping and falling while getting in and out of the tub. Tub baths should not be taken once the membranes have ruptured.

Encourage the use of plain soap and water to cleanse the genital area and prevent odors. The woman should *not* use deodorant sprays because of possible irritation. Tell the pregnant woman that an increase in vaginal discharge is common. Discharge that is yellowish or greenish, is foul smelling, or causes irritation and itching should be reported for further evaluation.

Clothing. Encourage the mother to dress in nonconstricting clothing. As the pregnancy progresses, the mother may be more comfortable with a maternity girdle to support the abdomen. Encourage the mother to wear a well-fitting brassiere to provide proper support for the breasts. The pregnant woman should avoid restrictive circular garters, which may impede lower limb circulation. Encourage low-heeled, well-fitting shoes that provide good support. Properly fitting shoes can prevent lower back fatigue as well as tired feet.

Oral hygiene. Encourage the pregnant patient to have a thorough dental examination at the beginning of the pregnancy. She should tell the dentist she is pregnant at the time of the examination. Encourage thorough daily brushing and flossing of the teeth.

Sexual activity. Refer to an obstetrics text for discussion of alterations in sexuality during pregnancy. The wide range of feelings, needs, and intervention deserve more consideration than can be presented in this text.

Smoking and alcohol. The pregnant woman should be encouraged to abstain from smoking or drinking during pregnancy. A vast amount of data indicate that smoking and drinking are dangerous to the fetus. An increased incidence of neonatal mortality, low birth weight, and prematurity has been widely reported.

Nutritional needs. Balanced nutrition is always to be encouraged, but it is especially important throughout the course of the pregnancy. Recommended daily allowances vary based on the individual's age, weight at the time of pregnancy, and daily activity level. At all times allowances must be made to maintain the nutritional needs of the mother and fetus. Refer to a nutrition text for specific recommendations.

Encourage limiting the caffeine content of the diet during pregnancy. Limit the consumption of coffee, tea, cola beverages, and cocoa. Tell the pregnant woman to check labels for specific caffeine content because many soft drinks contain a significant quantity of caffeine. Tell the woman to avoid highly spiced foods and any foods that she knows have caused heartburn in the past.

A weight gain of 2 to 4 pounds during the first trimester, 11 pounds during the second trimester, and 11 pounds during the third trimester is usual. Stress the need to report a weight gain of 2 or more pounds in any 1 week for further evaluation.

Bowel habits. Assess the individual's usual pattern of elimination, and anticipate its continuance until later in pregnancy. Pressure on the lower bowel from the presenting part of the fetus may cause constipation and hemorrhoids. Stool softeners or a mild laxative may be prescribed if problems persist.

Encourage the consumption of fresh fruits and vegetables, whole grain, and bran products, along with an adequate intake of six to eight 8-ounce glasses of fluid daily.

Douching. Discourage any type of douching unless specifically prescribed by the physician. Be certain when douching is prescribed that the patient is given simple, explicit instructions.

Discomforts of pregnancy. Use assessment data as pregnancy progresses to determine individualized teaching needed to deal with discomforts such as development of backache, leg cramps, hemorrhoids, and edema.

Complications of pregnancy. Individualize health teaching to deal with complications as they arise. The woman should always immediately report loss of fluid vaginally; dizziness; double or blurred vision; severe headache, abdominal pain or persistent vomiting; fever; edema of the face, fingers, legs, or feet; and weight gain in excess of 2 pounds per week.

Teach signs of true and false labor and when to contact the physician.

At discharge

- Review instructions on self-care (for example, breast care, fundal height, lochia, incisional or perineal care, bowel and bladder expectations, nutritional and fluid intake, and activity). Stress signs of problems that should be reported to the physician.
- Contraceptives: discuss appropriate sexual activity and limitations. Remind the woman that breast feeding is not a form of contraception. Alternative methods of contraception should be used if the patient does not wish to become pregnant immediately.
- Review infant care needs, bathing, vital signs, fontanel assessment, care of the umbilical cord and circumcision, normal sleep pattern, and feeding.
- Stress the need for follow-up care of the mother and infant. Provide the specific date and time of physician appointments. The mother usually returns for a follow-up examination at the physician's office 6 to 8 weeks after delivery.

Fostering health maintenance

- Discuss any medications prescribed for the mother or infant and how they will benefit the course of treatment to produce optimal response.
- Seek cooperation and understanding of the following points so that medication compliance is increased; name of medication, dosage, route and times of administration, side effects to expect, and side effects to report.
- Enlist the mother's aid in developing and maintaining a written record of monitoring parameters (blood pressure, pulse, daily weights, presence and relief of discomfort, exercise tolerance, and fetal movement) and response to prescribed therapies for discussion with the physician (See boxes on p. 459 and p. 460). The woman should be encouraged to take this record to follow-up visits.

PATIENT EDUCATION & MONITORING FORM   Prenatal Care

MEDICATIONS	COLOR	TO BE TAKEN

Name _____

Physician _____

Physician's phone _____

Next appt.* _____

PARAMETERS		DAY OF EXAM						COMMENTS
Weight								
Blood Pressure								
Pulse								
Pain	Cramps?							
	Backache?							
	Abdominal pain?							
Bleeding	With cramps?							
	# pads used per day							
	Describe color (bright or dark red)							
Edema	Morning							
	Evening							
	Other							
	Location: Hands, feet, ankles?							
Fatigue								
Exercise								
Fetal movement	Normal?							
	None?							
Bowel movements								

Fatigue
```
All          After
day          exercise        Normal
|            |               |
10           5               1
```

Exercise
```
Poor         Moderate
toleration   toleration      Normal
|            |               |
10           5               1
```

Bowel movements
```
Constipated  Normal          Diarrhea
|            |               |
10           5               1
```

*Please bring this record with you to your next appointment.
Use the back of this sheet for additional information.

DRUG THERAPY WITH PREGNANCY

Drug Class: Uterine Stimulants

Uses

There are four primary clinical indications for the use of uterine stimulants: (1) induction or augmentation of labor, (2) control of postpartum atony and hemorrhage, (3) control of postsurgical hemorrhage (as in cesarean birth), and (4) induction of therapeutic abortion.

Induction of labor: Uterine stimulants, primarily oxytocin, may be prescribed in cases in which, in the physician's judgment, continuation of the pregnancy is considered to be a greater risk to the mother or fetus than the risk associated with drug-induced induction of labor. Such maternal conditions as a

PATIENT EDUCATION & MONITORING FORM — Postpartum Care

MEDICATIONS	COLOR	TO BE TAKEN

Name _____

Physician _____

Physician's phone _____

Next appt.* _____

PARAMETERS		DAY OF DISCHARGE							COMMENTS
Weight									
Blood Pressure	AM / PM								
Pulse	AM / PM									
Lochia	# pads / day								
	Color of vaginal discharge								
Cramps — Frequent 10 / Moderate 5 / None 1									
Breast tenderness	↑ discomfort								
	↓ discomfort								
	No problem								
Nipple condition	Sore								
	Cracking								
	No problem								
Sexual activity	Persistently painful								
	Uncomfortable								
	Normal								
Bowel movements	Constipation								
	Normal								

*Please bring this record with you to your next appointment.
Use the back of this sheet for additional information.

history of **precipitous labor and delivery**, postterm pregnancy, prolonged pregnancy with placental insufficiency, prolonged rupture of the membranes, or pregnancy-induced hypertension may be indications for induction of labor. Vaginal inserts and gels of prostaglandins are currently being tested as adjunctive therapy to help ripen the cervix.

Augmentation of labor: In general, oxytocin should not be used to hasten labor. The type and force of contraction induced by the oxytocin may be harmful to the mother and fetus. In occasional cases of **dysfunctional labor**, there is a prolonged latent phase of cervical dilatation or arrest of descent through the birth canal. Oxytocin infusions starting with low dosages and continuous fetal monitoring may be beneficial in these cases.

Postpartum atony and hemorrhage: After delivery of the fetus and the placenta, the uterus sometimes remains flaccid and "boggy." Continued intravenous infusions of low-dose oxytocin or intramuscular injections of ergonovine or methylergonovine may be used to stimulate firm uterine contractions to reduce the risk of postpartum hemorrhage from an atonic uterus. Occasionally, oral dosages of ergonovine or methylergonovine are administered for a few days after delivery to assist in uterine involution.

Therapeutic abortion: Pharmacologic agents are usually not effective in evacuating uterine contents until several weeks into the second trimester of pregnancy. Various dosage forms of prostaglandins and hypertonic (20%) sodium chloride may be effective. Uterine smooth muscle is not very responsive to oxytocin stimulation until late in the third trimester, so even large doses of oxytocin are not indicated in therapeutic abortion. Regardless of the stage of pregnancy, stimulants such as ergonovine or methylergonovine may be prescribed after the uterus is emptied to control bleeding and maintain uterine muscle tone.

dinoprostone (die'no-prahs-tone)
Prostin E₂, Prepidil, Cervidil

Actions

Dinoprostone (prostaglandin E₂) is a natural chemical in the body that causes uterine and gastrointestinal smooth muscle stimulation. It also plays an active role in cervical softening and dilatation (cervical "ripening") unrelated to uterine muscle stimulation. When used during pregnancy, it produces cervical softening and dilatation and, in higher doses, increases the frequency and strength of uterine contractions.

Uses

Dinoprostone is used to start and continue cervical ripening at term. In larger doses it is also used to expel uterine contents in cases of intrauterine fetal death, benign hydatiform mole, missed spontaneous miscarriage, and second trimester abortion. Occasionally, oxytocin and dinoprostone are used together to shorten the duration of time required to expel uterine contents.

Therapeutic Outcomes

The primary therapeutic outcomes associated with dinoprostone therapy are as follows:
• Cervical softening and dilatation before labor
• Evacuation of uterine contents

Nursing Process

Premedication Assessment
1. Obtain baseline vital signs. Temperature and vital signs should be monitored every half hour after initiation of therapy.
2. Assess the state of hydration.
3. Assess uterine activity, including amount and characteristics of any vaginal discharge.
4. Check for antiemetic and antidiarrheal medications ordered at prescribed times or prn.

Planning
Availability. Vaginal suppository—20 mg (Prostin E₂); vaginal insert—10 mg (Cervidil); cervical gel—0.5 mg in 2.5 ml prefilled syringe (Prepidil).

Implementation
Dosage and administration. Adult: for cervical ripening, intravaginal administration—the slab (Cervidil) is placed transversely in the posterior fornix of the vagina after removal from tinfoil wrap. Patients should remain supine for 2 hours after insertion but may be ambulatory thereafter. Cervidil is removed at onset of labor or 12 hours after insertion. The product does not need to be warmed before insertion. Intracervical gel—allow the prefilled syringe of gel (0.5 mg) to warm to room temperature. Do not force the warming process with a water bath or other external source of heat. A catheter is attached to the syringe (20 mm if the cervix is less than 50% effaced; 10 mm if more than 50% effaced). The patient is placed in a dorsal position with the cervix visualized using a speculum. Using sterile technique, the gel is introduced through the catheter into the cervical canal just below the level of the internal os. The catheter is removed after placement of the gel. After administration, the patient should remain in the supine position for at least 15 to 30 minutes to minimize leakage from the cervical canal. Doses may be repeated in 6 hours. The maximum recommended cumulative dose for a 24-hour period is 1.5 mg (7.5 ml).

For evacuation of uterine contents, intravaginal suppository—before removing the tinfoil, allow the suppository (Prostin E₂) to warm to room temperature. Insert one suppository high into the posterior vaginal fornix. Patients should remain supine for at least 10 minutes after each insertion. Suppositories should be inserted every 2 to 5 hours, depending on uterine activity and tolerance to side effects.

Evaluation
Side effects to expect
NAUSEA, VOMITING, DIARRHEA. The most frequently observed gastrointestinal side effects are nausea, vomiting, and diarrhea. Premedication with an antiemetic such as prochlorperazine and an antidiarrheal agent (loperamide or diphenoxylate) will reduce, but usually not completely eliminate, these adverse effects.

FEVER. Chills and shivering may occur in patients receiving dinoprostone. Temperature elevations to approximately 38° C (100.6° F) occur within 15 to 45 minutes and continue for up to 6 hours. Sponge baths with water and maintaining fluid intake may provide symptomatic relief.

Aspirin does not inhibit dinoprostone-induced fever.

Patients should be observed for clinical indications of intrauterine infection. Monitor temperature and vital signs every half hour.

Side effects to report
ORTHOSTATIC HYPOTENSION. Transient hypotension with a drop in diastolic pressure of 20 mm Hg, dizziness, flushing, and arrhythmias have all been reported. Although these effects are infrequent and generally mild, dinoprostone may cause some degree of orthostatic hypotension manifested by dizziness, flushing, and weakness, particularly when therapy is initiated.

Monitor blood pressure in both the supine and standing positions.

Anticipate the development of postural hypotension, and take measures to prevent its occurrence. For ambulatory patients, teach the patient to rise slowly from a supine or sitting position, and encourage her to sit or lie down if feeling faint. Report rapidly falling blood pressure, bradycardia, paleness, and other alterations in vital signs.

Drug interactions

No clinically significant interactions have been reported.

ergonovine maleate (er-go-no'veen mal-ee-ate)
Ergotrate Maleate (er'go-trayt)
methylergonovine maleate (meth-il-er-go-no'veen mal-ee-ate)
Methergine (meth'er-jin)

Actions

Ergonovine and methylergonovine are structurally similar ergot derivatives that share similar actions. Both drugs directly stimulate contractions of the uterus. Small doses produce uterine contractions with normal resting muscle tone; intermediate doses cause more forceful and prolonged contractions with an elevated resting muscle tone; and large doses cause severe, prolonged contractions. Because of this sudden, intense uterine activity, which is dangerous to the fetus, these agents cannot be used for induction of labor.

Uses

Ergonovine and methylergonovine produce more sustained contractions than oxytocin and are used in small doses in postpartum patients to control bleeding and maintain uterine firmness.

Therapeutic Outcome

The primary therapeutic outcome associated with ergonovine and methylergonovine therapy is reduced postpartum blood loss.

Nursing Process

Premedication Assessment

1. Obtain baseline vital signs, especially blood pressure and pulse.
2. Assess amount and characteristics of vaginal discharge and fundal height and contractility.

Planning

Availability. PO—0.2 mg tablets. Injection—0.2 mg/ml in 1 ml ampules.

Implementation

Note: Use with extreme caution in patients with hypertension, preeclampsia, heart disease, venoatrial shunts, mitral valve stenosis, sepsis, or hepatic or renal impairment.
Dosage and administration. Adult: PO—0.2 mg every 6 to 8 hours after delivery for a maximum of 1 week. IM—0.2 mg every 2 to 4 hours to a maximum of 5 doses.

Evaluation

Side effects to expect

NAUSEA, VOMITING. These side effects are usually mild and tend to resolve with continued therapy. Encourage the patient not to discontinue therapy without first consulting the physician.

ABDOMINAL CRAMPING. This is normally an indication of therapeutic activity, but, if severe, reduction or discontinuation of dosage may be necessary.

Side effects to report

HYPERTENSION. Certain patients, especially those who are eclamptic or previously hypertensive, may be particularly sensitive to the hypertensive effects of these agents. These patients have a higher incidence of developing generalized headaches, severe arrhythmias, and strokes. Monitor the patient's blood pressure and pulse rate and rhythm. Report immediately if the patient complains of headache or palpitations.

Drug interactions

INHIBITION OF PROLACTIN. Do not use ergonovine in patients who wish to breast-feed. Methylergonovine may be used as an alternative because it will not inhibit stimulation of milk production by prolactin.

CAUDAL OR SPINAL ANESTHESIA. Hypertension and headaches may develop in patients who have received caudal or spinal anesthesia followed by a dose of either methylergonovine or ergonovine. Monitor the patient's blood pressure and heart rate and rhythm.

oxytocin (ok-se-to'sin)
Pitocin (pih-to'sin)

Actions

Oxytocin is a hormone produced in the hypothalamus and stored in the pituitary gland. When released, it stimulates the smooth muscle of the uterus, blood vessels, and the mammary glands. When administered during the third trimester of pregnancy, active labor may be initiated.

Uses

Oxytocin is the current drug of choice for inducing labor at term and for augmenting uterine contractions during the first and second stages of labor. Oxytocin is routinely administered immediately postpartum to control uterine atony and postpartum hemorrhage. Oxytocin also has been administered intranasally to promote milk letdown and to treat breast engorgement during lactation.

Therapeutic Outcomes

The primary therapeutic outcomes associated with oxytocin therapy are as follows:
* Initiation of labor
* Support of uterine contractions during the first and second stages of labor
* Control of postpartum bleeding
* Milk letdown for nursing mothers

Nursing Process

Premedication Assessment

Never leave a patient receiving an oxytocin infusion unattended. Ensure that the IV site is functional before adding oxytocin; use an infusion pump.

1. Monitor maternal vital signs, especially blood pressure and pulse rate.
2. Obtain baseline assessment data of the mother's hydration status. Continue to monitor urine output and intake and output throughout drug therapy.
3. Monitor characteristics of uterine contractions, for example, frequency, rate, duration, and intensity.

4. Monitor fetal heart rate and rhythm. Be alert for signs of fetal distress.
5. Perform reflex testing.
6. Check amount and characteristics of vaginal discharge.

Planning

Availability. IV—10 U/ml in 1 and 10 ml vials and 1 ml disposable syringes. Nasal spray—40 U/ml in 2 and 5 ml squeeze bottles.

Implementation

Note: Overdosage of oxytocin may cause hyperstimulation of the uterus, resulting in severe contractions with possible abruptio placentae, cervical lacerations, impaired uterine blood flow, and fetal trauma.

Dosage and administration

Starting the infusion. Establish records of baseline vital signs and intake and output. Oxytocin administered IV should be added to the solution after the IV is shown to be patent and running.

Rate. Careful monitoring of the prescribed rate of infusion is imperative. Should the IV line suddenly open, the resulting severe contractions could be extremely dangerous to the mother.

Infusion pump. A constant infusion pump is recommended for control of the rate of administration. Keep in mind that a pump can still fail. Continue to monitor the number of drops per minute from the drip chamber.

Induction of labor. IV—initial rate: 1 to 2 mU per minute. It is strongly recommended that an infusion pump be used to help control the rate of oxytocin infusion. Most pregnancies close to term will respond well to 2 to 10 mU per minute. Rarely will a patient require more than 20 mU per minute. Those patients at 32 to 36 weeks of gestation often require 20 to 30 mU per minute or more to develop a laborlike contraction pattern. Rates of infusion should not be altered more frequently than every 20 to 30 minutes. It is frequently necessary to reduce or discontinue the infusion as spontaneous uterine activity develops and labor progresses.

Augmentation of labor. IV—occasionally a labor that started spontaneously may not progress satisfactorily. Labor may be augmented by oxytocin infusions at rates of 0.5 to 2 mU per minute.

Postpartum hemorrhage. IM—10 U given after delivery of the placenta. IV—10 to 40 U may be added to 100 ml of fluid and electrolyte solution and run at a rate necessary to control uterine atony.

Milk letdown. Intranasal spray—1 spray or 3 drops may be instilled into one or both nostrils 2 to 3 minutes before nursing or pumping of the breasts.

Evaluation

Side effects to expect

UTERINE CONTRACTIONS. Oxytocin infusions should be monitored by both a tocometer (an instrument that measures uterine contractions) and a fetal heart monitor.

Maintain an ongoing record of the frequency, duration, and intensity of uterine contractions. Duration of contractions over 90 seconds requires the flow rate of the oxytocin to be slowed or discontinued.

NAUSEA, VOMITING. Although infrequent, these side effects may occur. Reduction in dosage may control symptoms.

Side effects to report

FETAL DISTRESS. Fetal heart rate should be monitored continuously, but especially closely during uterine contractions. (Normal fetal heart rate is greater than 120 to 160 beats per minute.) Indications of fetal distress may be manifested by tachycardia (greater than 160 beats per minute) followed by bradycardia (less than 120 beats per minute). As the degree of distress progresses, bradycardia occurs more frequently and lasts longer than 15 seconds after contractions.

If the infant develops sudden distress, reduce the oxytocin infusion to the slowest possible rate according to hospital policy, turn the mother to the left lateral position, administer oxygen by nasal cannula or face mask, and call the physician immediately.

HYPERTENSION, HYPOTENSION. Check the mother's blood pressure and pulse rate at least every 30 minutes during oxytocin infusion. Report trends upward or downward because oxytocin may cause hypertension or hypotension.

WATER INTOXICATION. Oxytocin can alter fluid balance by stimulating antidiuretic hormone, causing the body to accumulate water. This is particularly likely to occur if oxytocin is administered with electrolyte solutions.

Symptoms of water intoxication include drowsiness, listlessness, headache, confusion, anuria, edema, and in extreme cases seizures.

DEHYDRATION. Because mothers are routinely placed on nothing by mouth (NPO) status during labor, an occasional patient may develop dehydration even though an IV is running. Monitor urine output, dry crusted lips, and requests for water. Report to the physician, and request ice chips and additional IV fluids if appropriate.

POSTPARTUM HEMORRHAGE. Early postpartum hemorrhage occurs within the first 24 hours after delivery and is usually defined as a blood loss of 500 ml or greater during this time span.

The hemorrhage may be caused by uterine atony, retained fragments of placenta, or lacerations of the vaginal tract. Less frequent causes include defective blood clotting mechanisms, uterine eversion, and uterine infections.

Oxytocin is routinely administered after delivery of the placenta to cause the uterus to contract and to decrease blood loss. Always check the height of the fundus of the uterus (usually at umbilical level) every 5 minutes after delivery. Report if the uterus is not firm or the height is rising. (This may be an indication of urinary retention or a uterus filling with blood.) When the uterus becomes boggy, uterine massage is necessary until it becomes firm.

Check the vaginal flow rate on each perineal pad at least every half hour. With uterine atony or retained placental fragments, the uterus becomes boggy and dark vaginal bleeding is present; with a laceration of the cervix or vagina, the bleeding is bright red and the uterus is firm. Regardless of the cause, the woman must be observed carefully for signs of hypovolemic shock.

Monitor vital signs as ordered by the physician, or every 15 minutes until stable, every 30 minutes for 2 hours, then every hour until definitely stable. Report an increasing respiratory rate; pulse rate that increases and becomes thready; a pulse deficit; blood pressure that indicates hypotension; skin that is pale, cold, and clammy; or nail beds, lips, and mucous membranes that are pale or cyanotic. Monitor hourly urine output and report an output of 30 ml per hour or less. Observe for restlessness and complaints of thirst and for any decrease in level of consciousness.

Drug interactions

ANESTHETICS. Monitor the blood pressure and heart rate and rhythm closely. Report significant changes in the blood pressure or pulse.

For those patients receiving a local anesthetic containing epinephrine, immediately report any complaints of diaphoresis, fever, chest pain, palpitations, or severe "throbbing" headache.

Drug Class: Uterine Relaxants

Uterine relaxants are used primarily to delay or prevent preterm labor and delivery in selected patients (p. 453).

> **ritodrine hydrochloride** (rih'toh-dreen)
> **Yutopar** (u'toh-par)
> **terbutaline sulfate** (ter-bew'tal-een)
> **Bricanyl** (brih-can'il)

Actions

Ritodrine and terbutaline are beta-adrenergic receptor stimulants, acting predominantly on the beta-2 receptors, but, especially in higher dosages, on the beta-1 receptors as well. Stimulation of the beta-2 receptors produces relaxation of the uterine, bronchial, and vascular smooth muscle. Beta-1 receptor stimulation causes an increased heart rate.

Unfortunately, the receptors that are stimulated by beta receptor agents to cause relaxation of the smooth muscle of the uterus are found in other tissues as well as the reproductive system. They are found in the muscles of the heart, blood vessels, bronchopulmonary tree, and gastrointestinal, urinary, and central nervous systems. They also help regulate fat and carbohydrate metabolism. For this reason, many side effects can be expected from these agents, particularly if used too frequently or in higher than recommended doses.

Uses

Because of selective relaxant properties on the uterus causing a reduction in the intensity and frequency of uterine contractions, ritodrine and terbutaline are used to arrest premature labor in situations in which it has been determined that there is no underlying pathology that would indicate that pregnancy should not be allowed to progress to completion.

Therapeutic Outcome

The primary therapeutic outcome associated with ritodrine and terbutaline therapy is arrest of preterm labor.

Nursing Process

Assessment

1. Obtain baseline vital signs and weight.
2. Monitor maternal and fetal heart rates.
3. Perform baseline mental status examination (for example, alertness, orientation, anxiety level, muscle strength, and tremors).

Table 37-3

Guidelines for Use of Ritodrine in Premature Labor

1. Initiate a control IV of dextrose 5%, Ringer's lactate, or saline solution and administer 400 to 500 ml 15 to 20 minutes before the initiation of the medication. Then decrease to 100 to 125 ml/hr.
2. Make a ritodrine infusion solution. The usual concentration is 3 ampules in 500 ml of parenteral solution, but weaker or stronger concentrations may be used depending on the patient's fluid requirements.
3. Have the patient recline in the left lateral position to minimize hypotension.
4. The usual initial dosage is 50 to 100 μg/min. Increase by 50 μg/min every 10 minutes until labor is inhibited or side effects prevent further increases in dosage. The effective dose is usually 150 to 350 μg/min. Frequent monitoring of maternal uterine contractions, heart rate, and blood pressure and fetal heart rate is mandatory, with dosage individually titrated according to response.
5. Fluid input and output, breath sounds, and blood glucose and serum electrolyte levels must be monitored periodically to prevent fluid overload, hyperglycemia, or hypokalemia.
6. The IV infusion is maintained for 8 to 12 hours after cessation of uterine contractions.
7. Recurrence of premature labor may be treated starting the guidelines over again. Labor may be arrested on lower IV dosages, depending on the patient's compliance with the oral medication regimen.

4. Obtain baseline laboratory studies ordered (for example, electrolytes, glucose, hematocrit, and carbon dioxide).
5. In patients who have diabetes, obtain baseline glucose and plan to monitor closely for subsequent hyperglycemia and possible changes in insulin dosage.

Planning

Availability. Ritodrine: injection—10 mg/ml in 5 ml ampules; 15 mg/ml in 10 ml vials. Terbutaline: PO—2.5 and 5 mg tablets. Injection—1 mg/ml in 1 ml ampules.

Implementation

Dosage and administration. See Tables 37-3 and 37-4. IV rate: use of an infusion pump is absolutely essential for the safe delivery of these agents. PO: administer with food or milk to reduce gastric irritation.

Evaluation

Side effects to report

TACHYCARDIA, PALPITATIONS, HYPERTENSION, AND HYPOTENSION. Because most symptoms are dose related, alterations should be reported to the physician. Monitor the maternal and fetal heart rates and rhythms at regular intervals throughout therapy. Report heart rates significantly higher than baseline values. These include maternal and fetal tachycardia averaging 130 and 164 beats per minute, respectively. Maternal systolic blood pressure increases to a range of 96 to 162 mm Hg, and diastolic pressures drop to a range of 0 to 76 mm Hg.

Always report palpitations and suspected arrhythmias.

Table 37-4

Guidelines for Use of Terbutaline with Premature Labor*

1. Initiate a control IV of dextrose 5%, Ringer's lactate, or saline solution and administer 400 to 500 ml 15 to 20 minutes before the initiation of the medication. Then decrease to 100 to 125 ml/hr.

2. Add 20 mg of terbutaline to 1000 ml of dextrose 5%.

3. Place the patient in a left lateral, horizontal position with a blood pressure cuff in position.

4. Administer a loading dose of 250 μg IV over 1 to 2 minutes. Monitor closely for hypotension.

5. Start the infusion at a rate of 10 μg IV (30 ml/hr).

6. Increase the infusion rate by 3.5 μg/min (10 ml/hr) every 10 minutes until labor has stopped or a maximum dose of 26 μg/min (80 ml/hr) has been attained.

7. Maintain the effective dose for 1 hr or more, then begin decreasing the rate by 2 μg/min (6 ml/hr) every 30 minutes until the lowest effective dose is reached. Maintain the total IV fluid intake at 125 ml/hr.

8. When the lowest effective IV dose is reached, begin PO terbutaline, 2.5 mg every 4 hours.

9. If labor has stopped, discontinue the IV infusion 24 hr after PO administration was initiated if the uterus is not irritable.

10. Continue the PO regimen (2.5 mg every 4 hr or 5 mg every 8 hr) until 36 weeks gestation.

11. If labor begins again, restart the IV infusion as above.

*NOTE: Terbutaline is not approved by the FDA for use in premature labor. It may be used, however, in emergency situations when the physician judges that it is in the best interests of the patient and infant.

When terbutaline is used for premature labor, sometimes a significant drop in blood pressure (due to vasodilatory effects) can be observed at the time of the loading dose and when the infusion is started. Blood pressure and pulse monitoring should be done before and every 5 minutes after the loading dose has been administered and the infusion started, until the patient is stable. Use continuous fetal monitoring. If the maternal pulse exceeds 120 beats/min and does not decrease with an increase in fluids or when the patient is rolled on her left side, or if there is any evidence of a decrease in uterine perfusion, discontinue the infusion.

TREMORS. Instruct the patient to notify the physician if tremors develop after starting any of these medications. A dosage adjustment may be necessary.

NERVOUSNESS, ANXIETY, RESTLESSNESS, HEADACHE. Perform a baseline assessment of the patient's mental status (degree of anxiety, nervousness, and alertness); compare at regular intervals with the findings obtained. Report escalation of tension.

NAUSEA, VOMITING. Monitor all aspects of the development of these symptoms.

Administer the oral medication with food and a full glass of water or milk. Report if the symptoms are not relieved.

DIZZINESS. Provide for patient safety during episodes of dizziness; report for further evaluation.

HYPERGLYCEMIA. Ritodrine and terbutaline routinely increase serum glucose and insulin levels, although these tend to return to normal within 48 to 72 hours with continued infusion. Diabetic or prediabetic patients must be monitored for the development of hyperglycemia, particularly during the early days of therapy.

Assess regularly for glycosuria, and report if it occurs with frequency.

Insulin requirements may double in these patients during ritodrine or terbutaline therapy.

ELECTROLYTE IMBALANCE. The electrolyte most commonly altered is potassium (K^+). Hypokalemia is most likely to occur. Serum potassium levels may drop during IV administration. Urinary losses generally do not increase; most of the losses are due to intracellular redistribution, which will return to the blood after discontinuation of therapy.

Many symptoms associated with altered fluid and electrolyte balance are subtle.

Gather data relative to changes in the patient's mental status (that is, alertness, orientation, and confusion), muscle strength, muscle cramps, tremors, nausea, and general appearance (drowsy, anxious, and lethargic).

Always check the electrolyte reports for early indications of electrolyte imbalance.

Keep accurate records of intake and output, daily weights, and vital signs.

THE NEONATE. Neonatal adverse effects are infrequent, but hyperglycemia followed by hypoglycemia, hypocalcemia, hypotension, and paralytic ileus have been reported. Monitor these newborns closely over the next several hours. Make sure that the infant's sleep after birth is not masking these conditions.

Drug interactions

DRUGS THAT ENHANCE TOXIC EFFECTS. Tricyclic antidepressants (imipramine, amitriptyline, nortriptyline, doxepine, and others), monoamine oxidase inhibitors (tranylcypromine and pargyline), and other sympathomimetic agents (metaproterenol, isoproterenol and others).

Monitor for increases in severity of drug effects such as nervousness, tachycardia, tremors, and arrhythmias.

DRUGS THAT REDUCE THERAPEUTIC EFFECTS. Beta-adrenergic blocking agents (propranolol, timolol, nadolol, pindolol, and others).

CORTICOSTEROIDS. Concurrent use may rarely result in pulmonary edema. There is a higher incidence in patients with multiple pregnancy, occult cardiac disease, and fluid overload. Persistent tachycardia may be a sign of impending pulmonary edema. Observe patient closely; monitor fluid intake and output, breath sounds, and heart rate, as well as the patient's anxiety level and state of well-being.

ANTIHYPERTENSIVE AGENTS. Sympathomimetic agents may reduce the therapeutic effects of antihypertensive agents. Monitor blood pressure for an indication of loss of antihypertensive control.

ANESTHETICS. Concurrent use with general anesthetics may result in additional hypotensive effects. Monitor blood pressure and heart rate and rhythm regularly.

NAUSEA. Although it is infrequent, some patients do experience nausea.

Drug Class: Other Agents

clomiphene citrate (klom′ih-feen si′trayt)
Clomid (klo′mid)

Actions

Clomiphene is a chemical compound that is structurally similar to natural estrogens. When administered, it binds to estrogen receptor sites, reducing the number of sites available for circulating estrogens. The receptors send back signals to the hypothalamus and pituitary gland, indicating a lack of circulating estrogens. The hypothalamus responds by increasing the secretion of hypothalamic-releasing factor. This stimulates the pituitary gland to release luteinizing hormone (LH) and follicle-stimulating hormone (FSH), which in turn stimulate the ovaries to release ova for potential fertilization.

Uses

Clomiphene is used to induce ovulation in women who are not ovulating because of reduced circulating estrogen levels. Studies indicate that pregnancy occurs in 25% to 30% of patients treated. Ovulation of more than one ovum per cycle with potential of fertilization of multiple ova may occur in 5% to 10% of patients treated.

Therapeutic Outcome

The primary therapeutic outcome associated with clomiphene therapy is ovulation followed by fertilization and pregnancy.

Nursing Process

Assessment

1. Check to ensure that the patient has had a complete physical examination, including pregnancy testing, before initiating therapy.
2. Obtain baseline data regarding any gastrointestinal or visual disturbances present before initiation of therapy.

Planning

Availability. PO—50 mg tablets.

Implementation

Note: It is mandatory that patients have a complete physical examination to rule out other pathologic causes for lack of ovulation before the initiation of clomiphene therapy.

Patients must be informed of the possibility of multiple fetuses and the importance of timing sexual intercourse at the time of ovulation, usually 6 to 10 days after the last day of treatment.

Clomiphene should not be administered if pregnancy is suspected. Basal temperatures should be followed for 1 month after therapy. If the body temperature follows a biphasic distribution (peaks twice within a few days) and is not followed by menses, the next course of clomiphene therapy should not be scheduled until pregnancy tests have been completed.

Possible pregnancy. Clomiphene should not be administered if pregnancy is suspected. Instruct the patient on how to take and record basal temperatures and how to report a biphasic temperature distribution.

Timing of intercourse. The timing of intercourse is important to the success of therapy. Make sure the patient understands the importance of having intercourse during the time of ovulation, usually 6 to 10 days after the last dose of medication.

Dosage and administration. Adult: PO—50 mg daily for 5 days. Start therapy at any time if there has been no recent bleeding. If spontaneous bleeding occurs before therapy, start on or about the fifth day for 5 days.

If ovulation does not occur after the first course, give a second course of 100 mg per day for 5 days. Start this course no earlier than 30 days after the previous course.

A third course may be administered at 100 mg per day for 5 days. However, most patients who respond will have done so in the first 2 courses. Reevaluation of the patient is necessary.

Evaluation

Side effects to expect

NAUSEA, VOMITING, DIARRHEA, CONSTIPATION, "HOT FLASHES," ABDOMINAL CRAMPS. These side effects are usually mild and tend to resolve with continued therapy. Encourage the patient not to discontinue therapy without first consulting the physician.

Side effects to report

SEVERE ABDOMINAL CRAMPS. Patients should be informed to report significant abdominal or pelvic pain and bloating that develop during therapy.

VISUAL DISTURBANCES. Patients developing visual blurring, spots, or double vision should report for an eye examination. The drug is usually discontinued, and visual disturbances pass within a few days to weeks after discontinuation.

Caution the patient to temporarily avoid tasks that require visual acuity, such as driving or operating power machinery.

DIZZINESS. Provide for patient safety during episodes of dizziness; report for further evaluation.

Drug interactions

No clinically significant drug interactions have been reported.

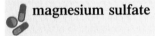 **magnesium sulfate**

Actions

Magnesium is an ion normally found in the blood in concentrations of 1.8 to 3 mEq/L. When administered parenterally in doses sufficient to produce levels above 4 mEq/L, the drug may depress the central nervous system and block peripheral nerve transmission, producing anticonvulsant effects and smooth muscle relaxation.

Uses

Magnesium sulfate is used in obstetrics primarily for the control of seizure activity associated with preeclampsia or eclampsia. It may also be used to inhibit premature labor in patients who cannot tolerate ritodrine. When used as an anticonvulsant or to inhibit labor, blood levels should be maintained at 4 to 8 mEq/L.

Patients maintained at a magnesium serum level between 3 and 5 mEq/L rarely show any side effects from hypermagnesemia. At levels approximately 5 to 8 mEq/L, patients begin to show increasing signs of toxicity that correlate fairly well with serum levels. Early signs of maternal toxicity are complaints of "feeling hot all over" and "being thirsty all the time," flushed skin color, and diaphoresis. Patients may then become hypotensive; have depressed patellar, radial, and biceps reflexes; and have flaccid muscles. Later signs of hypermagnesemia are central nervous system depression shown first by anxiety, followed by confusion, lethargy, and drowsiness. If serum levels continue to increase, cardiac depression and respiratory paralysis may result. Magnesium sulfate should be administered with extreme caution to patients with impaired renal function and patients whose urine output is less than 100 ml over the past 4 hours.

Therapeutic Outcomes

The primary therapeutic outcomes associated with magnesium sulfate therapy are as follows:
* Elimination of seizure activity
* Arrest of preterm labor

Nursing Process

Premedication Assessment

1. Obtain baseline vital signs, especially blood pressure, pulse, and respirations.
2. Perform a mental status examination: level of consciousness, orientation, and anxiety level.
3. Check deep tendon reflexes; report hyporeflexia or absence of reflexes.
4. Review intake and output record; report declining output.
5. Have calcium gluconate or calcium chloride and equipment for IV administration available if needed.
7. Obtain baseline laboratory values (for example, $MgSO_4$).
8. Monitor fetal heart rate and uterine activity; report distress.

Planning

Availability. Injection—10%, 12.5%, 25%, and 50% solutions.

Implementation

Dosage and administration. IM: intramuscular injection is extremely painful. Avoid if possible, or administer in conjunction with a local anesthetic. IV: it is absolutely essential that an infusion pump be used to help control the infusion of the loading dose and continuous drip.

Anticonvulsant. IM—loading dose: 10 g of 50% solution (20 ml) is divided into 2 doses of 5 g each (10 ml) and is injected by deep intramuscular injection into each buttock; 1% lidocaine or procaine may be added to each syringe to reduce the pain on injection. The IM loading dose is usually administered at the same time that 4 g are administered intravenously. Maintenance dose: 4 to 5 g of 50% solution (10 ml) IM every 4 hours in alternate buttocks. IV—loading dose: 4 g of magnesium sulfate are added to 250 ml of 5% dextrose in water and infused slowly at a rate of 10 ml per minute. (The IV loading dose is usually administered at the same time as a 10 g IM loading dose.) Maintenance dose: 1 to 2 g per hour by continuous infusion.

Preterm labor. IV—loading dose: 4 g of magnesium sulfate intravenously over 15 to 20 minutes. Maintenance dose: 1 to 3 g per hour by continuous infusion.

Note: Deep tendon reflexes, intake and output, vital signs, and orientation to the environment must be monitored on a regular, ongoing basis.

Evaluation

Side effects to report

DEEP TENDON REFLEXES. The presence or absence of patellar reflex (knee jerk reflex), biceps reflex, or radial reflex are primary monitoring parameters for magnesium sulfate therapy.

The patellar reflex should be monitored hourly if the patient is receiving a continuous IV infusion or before every dose if being administered intermittently IM or IV. If the reflex is absent, further dosages should be withheld until it returns. If the patellar reflex cannot be used because of epidural anesthesia, the biceps or radial reflex may be used.

INTAKE AND OUTPUT. Magnesium toxicity is more likely to occur in patients with reduced renal output. Report urine outputs of less than 30 ml per hour or less than 100 ml over a 4-hour period. Observe the color, and measure the specific gravity.

Note any other fluid and electrolyte loss such as vaginal bleeding, diarrhea, or vomiting.

VITAL SIGNS. Vital signs (blood pressure and heart rate and rhythm) should be measured every 15 to 30 minutes when a patient is receiving a continuous IV infusion. Take vital signs before and after each administration for patients receiving intermittent therapy.

The respiratory rate should be at least 16 breaths per minute before the administration of further doses of magnesium sulfate.

Do not administer additional doses if there is a reduced respiratory rate, a drop in blood pressure or fetal heart rate, or other signs of fetal distress.

CONFUSION. Perform a baseline assessment of the patient's degree of alertness and orientation to name, place, and time *before* initiating therapy. Make regularly scheduled mental status evaluations to ensure that the patient is oriented.

OVERDOSE. The antidote for magnesium intoxication (shown by respiratory depression and heart block) is calcium gluconate. A 10% solution of calcium gluconate should be kept at the patient's bedside ready for use. The dosage is 5 to 10 mEq (10 to 20 ml) IV over a 3-minute period.

Administer cardiopulmonary resuscitation until the patient responds appropriately.

NEONATES. Infants born of mothers who receive magnesium sulfate must be monitored for hypotension, hyporeflexia, and respiratory depression.

Drug interactions

CENTRAL NERVOUS SYSTEM DEPRESSANTS. Central nervous system depressants, including barbiturates, analgesics, general anesthetics, tranquilizers, and alcohol, will potentiate the central nervous system depressant effects of magnesium sulfate.

Periodically check the patient's orientation to make sure the patient is not suffering from magnesium toxicity.

NEUROMUSCULAR BLOCKADE. Concurrent use of neuromuscular blocking agents and magnesium sulfate will further depress muscular activity. Monitor the patient closely for depressed reflexes and respiration.

Rh₀(D) immune globulin (human)
RhoGAM, HypRho-D, Gamulin Rh, MICRhoGAM, Mini-Gamulin Rh

Actions

$Rh_0(D)$ immune globulin suppresses the stimulation of active immunity by Rh-positive foreign red blood cells that enter the maternal circulation either at the time of delivery, at the termination of a pregnancy, or during a transfusion of inadequately typed blood.

Rh hemolytic disease of the newborn can be prevented in subsequent pregnancies by administering $Rh_0(D)$ immune globulin (Rh$_0$[D] antibody) to the Rh-negative mother shortly after delivery of an Rh-positive child.

Uses

Rh$_0$(D) immune globulin (human) is used to prevent Rh immunization of the Rh-negative patient exposed to Rh-positive blood as the result of a transfusion accident, during termination of a pregnancy, or as the result of a delivery of an Rh-positive infant.

Therapeutic Outcome

The primary therapeutic outcome associated with Rh$_0$(D) immune globulin (human) therapy is prevention of Rh hemolytic disease.

Nursing Process

Premedication Assessment

Check Rh status of mother; she must be Rh negative. Has the mother previously been sensitized to Rh factor through blood transfusion or previous pregnancy?

Planning

Availability. Rh$_0$(D) immune globulin microdose (MI-CRhoGAM, Mini-Gamulin Rh): single-dose vial. Rh$_0$(D) immune globulin (Gamulin Rh, Hyp-Rho-D, RhoGAM): single-dose vial or prefilled syringe.

Implementation

Dosage and administration

Previous immunization. Although there is no need to administer Rh$_0$(D) immune globulin to a woman who is already sensitized to the Rh factor, the risk is no more than that when given to a woman who is not sensitized. When in doubt, administer Rh$_0$(D) immune globulin.

> *Before administration*
> 1. *Never* administer intravenously.
> 2. *Never* administer to a neonate.
> 3. *Never* administer to an Rh-negative patient who has been previously sensitized to the Rh antigen.
> 4. *Confirm* that the mother is Rh negative.

Pregnancy. Postpartum prophylaxis—1 standard dose vial IM. Additional vials may be necessary if there was unusually large fetal-maternal hemorrhage. Antepartum prophylaxis—1 standard dose vial IM at about 28 weeks of gestational age. This must be followed by another vial administered within 72 hours of delivery. After amniocentesis, miscarriage, abortion, or ectopic pregnancy—less than 13 weeks of gestation: 1 microdose vial IM within 72 hours; 13 or more weeks of gestation: 1 standard dose vial IM within 72 hours.

Transfusion accident. Rh-negative, premenopausal women who receive Rh-positive red cells by transfusion: 1 standard dose vial IM for each 15 ml of transfused packed red cells.

Evaluation

Side effects to expect

LOCALIZED TENDERNESS. Inform patients that they may experience stiffness at the site of injection for a few days.

FEVER, ARTHRALGIAS, GENERALIZED ACHES, PAINS. Monitor on a regular basis for the development of these symptoms. Follow routine orders of the physician or hospital concerning the use of analgesics (usually acetaminophen; do not use aspirin or other antiinflammatory agents) for patient discomfort.

Side effects to report

URTICARIA, TACHYCARDIA, HYPOTENSION. Allergic reactions require immediate treatment. Monitor patients for 20 to 30 minutes after administration. Have emergency supplies readily available.

Drug interactions

No significant drug interactions have been reported.

Neonatal Ophthalmic Solutions

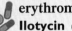
erythromycin ophthalmic ointment
Ilotycin (eye-lo′ty-sin)

Action and Use

Erythromycin (Ilotycin) is a macrolide antibiotic used prophylactically to prevent ophthalmia neonatorum, which is caused by *Neisseria gonorrhea*. It is also effective against *Chlamydia trachomatis*.

Therapeutic Outcome

The primary therapeutic outcome associated with erythromycin ophthalmic ointment therapy is prevention of postpartum gonorrhea or *Chlamydia* eye infection.

Nursing Process

Premedication Assessment

Describe any drainage present in the eye or on the lids; cleanse thoroughly.

Planning

Availability. Ophthalmic ointment— 1, 3.5, and 3.75 g tubes.

Implementation

Dosage and administration

Ointment. A new tube should be started for each infant.

Wash hands. Wash hands immediately before administration to prevent bacterial contamination. Put on gloves.

Cleansing the eyes. Using a separate sterile absorbent cotton or gauze pledget for each eye, wash the unopened lids from the nose outward until free of blood, mucus, or meconium.

Open the eyes, instill medication. Separate the eyelids and instill a narrow ribbon of erythromycin ointment along the lower conjunctival surface.

Instillation. Instill a ¼-inch narrow ribbon along the lower conjunctival surface of both eyes. Administration should be done within 2 hours of birth.

Irrigation. Do NOT irrigate the eyes after instillation.

Evaluation

Side effects to expect

MILD CONJUNCTIVITIS. A mild conjunctival inflammation occurs in the neonate and may interfere with the ability to focus. This side effect generally disappears in 1 to 2 days. Assure the family that the redness is temporary and that it will disappear within 1 to 2 days.

Drug interactions

No significant drug interactions have been reported.

phytonadione (fy-toe-nah-di′own)
Aquamephyton (ak-wah-mef′i-ton)

Actions

Vitamin K is a fat-soluble vitamin necessary for the production of the blood clotting factors prothrombin (factor II), proconvertin (factor VII), plasma thromboplastin component (factor IX), and Stuart factor (factor X) in the liver. Vitamin K is absorbed from the diet and is normally produced by the bacterial flora in the gastrointestinal tract, from which it is absorbed and transported to the liver for clotting factor production. Newborn infants have not yet colonized the colon with bacteria and are often deficient in vitamin K. They also may be deficient in these clotting factors and are therefore more susceptible to hemorrhagic disease of the newborn in the first 5 to 8 days after birth.

Uses

Phytonadione is routinely administered prophylactically to protect against hemorrhagic disease of the newborn.

Therapeutic Outcome

The primary therapeutic outcome associated with phytonadione therapy is prevention of hemorrhagic disease of the newborn.

Nursing Process

Premedication Assessment
No assessment is required.

Planning
Availability. Injection—2, 10 mg/ml in 0.5, 1, 2.5, and 5 ml containers.

Implementation
IM. Do NOT administer intravenously! Severe reactions, including hypotension, cardiac arrhythmias, and respiratory arrest, have been reported.
Choice of concentration. Although the 2 mg/ml concentration is packaged to be administered to infants (0.5 ml), the 10 mg/ml concentration is often used because the volume to be administered (0.1 ml) intramuscularly is smaller. This is particularly useful in premature or small-for-gestational-age neonates.
Dosage and administration. IM—0.5 to 2 mg in the lateral aspect of the thigh.

Evaluation
Side effects to report
BRUISING, HEMORRHAGE. Observe for bleeding (usually occurring on the second or third day). Bleeding may be seen as petechiae, generalized ecchymoses, or bleeding from the umbilical stump, circumcision site, nose, or gastrointestinal tract. Assess results of serial prothrombin times.
Drug interactions
No significant drug interactions have been reported.

CHAPTER REVIEW

Today's health care system is placing more emphasis on self-care for the mother and the newborn. Shortened hospital stays have heightened the health care professional's awareness of the need to provide more education to the mother and significant others, not only in the care needs of the mother but also for the newborn.

Every exposure to the mother is an opportunity to enhance her learning and preparation for parenting. Community resources for prenatal and parenting classes should be encouraged.

The prenatal examination provides a basis for establishing the future health care needs of the mother and infant. Psychosocial and cultural aspects of care must be incorporated into the assessments and interventions planned for self-care. At subsequent prenatal visits the persons must be provided with relevant information on all aspects of self-care to enhance the normal growth and development of the fetus and to prevent or manage potential complications of pregnancy. After delivery, the mother should attend discharge classes and should be provided with telephone follow-up, home visitations, and referrals to available community resources to meet the care needs of the mother and newborn at home.

MATH REVIEW

1. Ordered: methylergonovine maleate (Methergine) 0.2 mg, IM immediately after delivery of the placenta.
   On hand: Use the drug monograph in the textbook to determine the availability of the drug.
   Give: _____ ml.

2. Ordered: magnesium sulfate 1 g/hr by continuous infusion.
   On hand: magnesium sulfate 4 g added to 250 ml 5% dextrose in water.
   Set the infusion pump at: _____ ml/hr.

CRITICAL THINKING QUESTIONS

Situation:
1. After delivery of a newborn, an Rh-negative mother asks you why she must receive RhoGAM. Give an explanation of the rationale that a nonprofessional should be able to understand.

2. Why is it necessary to prehydrate the mother before administration of terbutaline IV?

3. During administration of terbutaline IV, the woman's pulse elevates to 150 beats per minute and the fetal heart fate is 200 beats per minute. What actions would you take?

38

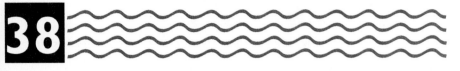

Drugs Used in Men's and Women's Health

Objectives

1. Identify common organisms known to cause leukorrhea.
2. Cite the generic and brand names of products used to treat *Candida albicans*, *Trichomonas vaginalis*, and *Gardnerella vaginalis*.
3. Review specific techniques for administering vaginal medications.
4. Develop a plan for teaching self-care to women and men with sexually transmitted diseases. Include personal hygiene measures, medication administration, methods of pain relief, and prevention of spread of infection or reinfection.
5. Discuss specific interviewing techniques that can be used to obtain a sexual history.
6. Compare the active ingredients in the two types of oral contraceptive agents.
7. Differentiate between the actions and the benefits of the combination pill and the minipill.
8. Describe the major adverse effects and contraindications to the use of oral contraceptive agents.
9. Develop specific patient education plans to be used to teach a patient to initiate oral contraceptive therapy with the combination pill and the minipill.

Key Words

leukorrhea
oligomenorrhea

amenorrhea
dysmenorrhea

VAGINITIS

Secretions from the vagina usually represent a normal physiologic process, but if the discharge becomes excessive it is known as **leukorrhea**. Leukorrhea is an abnormal, usually whitish vaginal discharge that may occur at any age. It affects almost all females at some time in their lives. Leukorrhea is not a disease but a symptom of an underlying disorder. The most common cause is an infection of the lower reproductive tract, but other physiologic and noninfectious causes of vaginal discharge are well known (Table 38-1).

The most common organisms causing the infectious type of leukorrhea are *Candida albicans*, *Trichomonas vaginalis*, and *Gardnerella vaginalis* (Table 38-2). Occasionally, *Candida albicans* infections of the mouth, gastrointestinal tract, or vagina may develop as secondary infections during the use of broad-spectrum antibiotics, such as the penicillins, tetracyclines, and cephalosporins.

Pathogens that are frequently transmitted by sexual contact are called sexually transmitted diseases (STDs) (Table 38-3). In some diseases, such as gonorrhea, syphilis, and genital herpes simplex virus infection, sexual transmission is the primary mode of transmission. In others, such as giardiasis, shigellosis, and the hepatitis viruses, other important nonsexual means of transmission also exist. Unfortunately, the true incidence of STDs is not known in the United States because of large numbers of unreported cases.

Drug Therapy for Leukorrhea and Genital Infections

See Table 38-2.

Nursing Process for Men's and Women's Health

Assessment

Past female reproductive history. Assess for the following:
- Age of menarche.
- Usual pattern of menses: duration, number of pads used, last menstrual period.
- Any pain, discomfort, spotting between periods, or extended time of menstrual flow.
- Number of pregnancies, live births, miscarriages, and abortions.
- Vaginal discharges, infections, genital lesions, or warts. Describe color, odor, and amount of discharge; describe lesions or any itching present.

Table 38-1

Causes of Vaginal Discharge

PHYSIOLOGIC	INFECTIOUS	NONINFECTIOUS
Ovulation	Vaginal	Atrophic vaginitis
Coitus	Candida	Foreign body
Oral contraceptives	Trichomonas	Vaginal adenosis
Pregnancy	Gardnerella	Allergic vulvovaginitis
Premenstruation	Toxic shock syndrome	Vulvar, vaginal carcinoma
Premenarche	Vulvar	Cervical polyps
Intrauterine device	Herpes	Cervical erosions/ulcers
	Condylomata acuminata	Uterine carcinoma
	Syphilis	Endometrial myoma
	Bartholinitis	Vesicovaginal fistula
	Lymphogranuloma venereum	Enterovaginal fistula
	Chancroid	
	Granuloma inguinale	
	Urethritis	
	Pyoderma	
	Cervical	
	Gonorrhea	
	Chlamydial or bacterial cervicitis	
	Chronic cervicitis	
	Pelvic inflammatory disease	

From Reilly BM: *Practical strategies in outpatient medicine,* Philadelphia, 1984, Saunders.

- Contraceptive methods used (for example, oral contraceptives, intrauterine device, condoms, or spermatocidal products).
- If taking oral contraceptives, what types have been taken? How long has therapy been used? What, if any, side effects to the contraceptives have been experienced? Are they taken regularly?
- Sexual orientation and number of sexual partners.
- Breast self-examination routine (if not being performed regularly, explain correct procedure).
- Age of menopause.
- Postmenopausal women: is there any vaginal bleeding?
- History of frequency of Papanicolaou smears.
- Reproductive problems (for example, endometriosis, ovarian cysts, and uterine fibroids).
- History of STDs (for example, chlamydia, syphilis, gonorrhea, yeast infections, genital herpes, human immunodeficiency virus [HIV]). If so, when, and what was the treatment?
- If the person is seeking a prescription for oral contraceptive therapy, ask about any indication of hypertension, heart or liver disease, thromboembolic disorders, or cancer of the reproductive organs. Does the individual smoke?

Past male reproductive history. Assess for the following:
- Pattern of urination. Has there been a recent change in the pattern of urination (for example, difficulty initiating urine stream, need to strain to empty the bladder, frequency of nocturia, pain on urination, frequency, urgency, hematuria, incontinence, dribbling, or urinary retention)?
- Presence of a urethral discharge or genital or perianal lesions. Is there swelling of the penis?

- Is there pain in the lower back, perineum, or pelvis?
- History of prostatitis, benign prostatic hypertrophy, or prostatic cancer.
- Testicular self-examination. How frequently?
- History of STDs. If so, when, and what was the treatment?
- History of multiple sexual partners—male, female, or both. What type of protection is used during sexual intercourse?
- History of arthralgia, fever, chills, malaise, pharyngitis, or oral lesions.
- History of prior illnesses.

History of current symptoms. Ask the patient to describe the current problem or problems that initiated this visit. How long have the symptoms existed? Is there a recurrence of symptoms that were treated previously?

Medication history
- Has the individual taken steroids or antibiotics recently? If so, what condition was being treated, and for how long? How long ago was therapy discontinued?
- Are over-the-counter, prescribed, or illegal drugs being taken? If so, what, why, and for how long?
- Are there any allergies to medications (for example, antibiotics)?
- If the patient is having a reoccurrence of an STD, what previous treatment has been taken?

Psychosocial
- Sexually transmitted diseases cause a high degree of anxiety. The intimate nature of the questioning required to obtain a sexual history may be embarrassing. Vaginal or urethral discharge may also be alarming to the patient seeking health care. When an STD diagnosis is suspected, explain the confidentiality policy of the facility before

Table 38-2

Causative Organisms and Products Used to Treat Genital Infections

CAUSATIVE ORGANISM	GENERIC NAME	BRAND NAME	DRUG MONOGRAPH, NURSING IMPLICATIONS
Vulvovaginitis			
Candida albicans (fungus)	Butoconazole vaginal cream	Femstat, Femstat 3	(p. 550)
	Clotrimazole vaginal cream, vaginal tablets	Gyne-Lotrimin, Mycelex-G	(p. 550)
	Miconazole vaginal cream, suppositories	Monistat	(p. 556)
	Terconazole vaginal cream, suppositories	Terazol 7, Terazol 3	(p. 551)
	Tioconazole vaginal ointment	Vagistat	(p. 551)
Trichomonas vaginalis (protozoa)	Metronidazole oral tablets	Flagyl	(p. 547)
	Clotrimazole (in pregnancy)	Gyne-Lotrimin, Mycelex-G	(p. 550)
Gardnerella vaginalis (bacteria)	Metronidazole oral tablets	Flagyl	(p. 547)
Gonorrhea			
Neisseria gonorrhea (bacteria)	Ceftriaxone	Rocephin	(p. 534)
	Spectinomycin	Trobicin	(p. 548)
	Cefixime	Suprax	(p. 534)
	Ciprofloxacin	Cipro	(p. 538)
Syphilis			
Treponema pallidum (spirochete)	Penicillin G, benzathine	Bicillin C-R	
	Tetracycline	Tetracycline	(p. 541)
	Erythromycin	Erythromycin	(p. 535)
Genital herpes			
Herpes simplex genitalis (virus)	Acyclovir oral capsules	Zovirax	(p. 557)
Chlamydiae			
Chlamydia trachomatis (chlamydia)	Doxycycline	Vibramycin	(p. 541)
	Erythromycin	Erythromycin	(p. 535)
	Azithromycin	Zithromax	(p. 535)

asking about sexual partners. (Many individuals do not return for follow-up appointments; this may be the only chance to obtain relevant information on contacts.)

- Ask about lifestyle orientation (for example, heterosexual, bisexual, or homosexual and number of partners). Has there been known contact with persons with STDs? Are precautions used during sexual contacts?
- Assess the level of anxiety present and adaptive responses and coping mechanisms used.

Laboratory and diagnostics

- Review reports on Gram stains and cultures from the anus, throat, and urethra for gonorrhea; Venereal Disease Research Laboratories (VDRL) and rapid plasma reagin (RPR), fluorescent treponema antibody absorption (FTA-ABS) for syphilis; tissue cultures for HSV-2, HIV testing as appropriate to test for STDs.
- Diagnostics are individualized to the suspected etiology of the signs and symptoms (for example, complete blood count, prostate specific antigen [PSA], cultures of prostatic

secretions, urine cultures, blood urea nitrogen, creatinine) for prostatic disorders.

Physical examination

- Perform routine physical examination of the woman, including pelvic examination, Papanicolaou smear, cultures, and breast examination.
- Perform routine physical examination of the man including testicular examination (rectal examination with palpation of prostate after age 40). An anorectal examination and examination of throat, tonsils, and mouth should be completed with men of homosexual or bisexual orientation.

Nursing Diagnosis

- Infection, risk for (indication)
- Health maintenance, altered (indication)
- Pain, risk for (indication)
- Knowledge deficit (indication, side effects)

Table 38-3

Sexually Transmitted Diseases

Bacteria
  Neisseria gonorrhea
  Gardnerella vaginalis
  Treponema pallidum
  Calymmatobacterium granulomatis
  Haemophilus ducreyi
  Shigella species
  Mobiluncus species
  Campylobacter species
  Group B streptococci
Chlamydiae
  Chlamydia trachomatis
Ectoparasites
  Sarcoptes scabei
  Phthirus pubis
Fungi
  Candida albicans
Mycoplasma
  Ureaplasma urealyticum
  Mycoplasma hominis
Protozoa
  Trichomonas vaginalis
  Entamoeba hystolytica
  Giardia lamblia
Viruses
  Herpes simplex virus
  Hepatitis A, B, C
  Cytomegalovirus
  Human papilloma virus
  Poxvirus
  Human immunodeficiency virus

Planning

- Most of the conditions discussed in this chapter are treated in the doctor's office and managed through self-care. Therefore planning is focused on self-care issues, prevention of transmission of infectious disorders, and seeking appropriate follow-up care.
- For patients with menstrual irregularities or needing contraceptive therapy, education regarding medications and personal health practices must be given.
- For patients with infections of the reproductive tract, education regarding personal hygiene, proper medication administration and adherence, and prevention of spread of infection and reinfection are crucial.
- Discuss sex practices, mode of transmission of STDs, prevention measures, and contact follow-up.
- Stress the need for an annual Papanicolaou smear to detect cervical cancer that originates from cervical intraepithelial neoplasia (CIN). Men need annual physical examinations after age 40 that include a rectal examination to palpate the prostate.

Implementation

- Record basic patient data (for example, height, weight, and vital signs).
- Prepare the patient for and assist with a physical examination.
- Observe distribution of body hair and presence of any scars, lesions, body rashes, pubic lice, or mites.
- Assist with specimen collection (for example, vaginal smears or cultures of discharge).
- Inspect the penis and scrotum for swelling or abnormalities, Observe for urethral discharge.
- Provide psychologic support and refer for available counseling, as appropriate.

Patient Education and Health Promotion

Instructions for women
- Refrain from the use of irritating vaginal substances such as deodorants, scented toilet paper, perfumed soaps, sprays, and douches.
- The use of warm sitz baths may help relieve vaginal or perineal irritation.
- Douching is generally avoided unless specifically prescribed by the physician. Douching alters the pH of the vagina and may actually encourage the growth of inappropriate organisms.
- Personal hygiene should include wiping from front to back after voiding and defecation, voiding before and after intercourse, thorough cleansing of genitals before and after intercourse, and changing tampons or pads frequently when having menstrual flow. Avoid wearing synthetic materials in underwear; wear cotton materials to prevent moisture accumulation.

Instructions for men
- Practice good personal hygiene measures. Keep the penis, scrotum, and perianal area thoroughly cleansed. Wash areas before and after intercourse. Urinate after intercourse. Wash hands well.
- Prostatitis is treated with antibiotics, antiinflammatory agents, and stool softener medications. The local application of heat with a sitz bath, drinking plenty of fluids, and adequate rest are also usually used for relief of the symptoms of prostatitis.

Instructions for women and men
- When infections are present, abstain from sexual intercourse. When sexual practices are resumed, use latex condoms and other protective measures such as spermicidal jellies and creams. Stress the need to prevent reinfection.
- Use sexual abstinence during the communicable phase of any disease. Avoid sexual contact with persons known to be infected. Remember that when having sex with an individual one is also having sex with all previous sexual partners when considering the infectious possibilities.
- Practice safe sex, if not abstinence. Use latex condoms. Discuss proper techniques for applying, use, removal, and discarding of condoms.
- Arrange for follow-up appointments with the physician and appropriate referrals for counseling or with social service department as needed.

Medications
  For women. Teach the patient the proper way to apply medications topically or intravaginally using ointments, tro-

ches, or suppositories. It is imperative that proper cleansing of the genital area be done regularly using soap and water; rinse and dry well. Hands should be washed before and after the application or insertion of medications and before and after toileting. Cleansing of the vaginal applicator after every use should include thoroughly washing it with soap and water and drying. After insertion of vaginal medications (creams or suppositories) the woman should remain in a recumbent position for 30 minutes to allow time for drug absorption. Wear a minipad to catch remaining drainage.

With oral contraceptive therapy, teach not only the medication schedule and dosage but also what to do if a dose is missed, frequency of follow-up care, and side effects to expect and report.

For men and women. Teach the medication regimen and who must take the medications—both partners in sexual relationship.

Fostering health maintenance

- Throughout the course of treatment, discuss medication information and how it will benefit the patient. Stress the importance of the nonpharmacologic interventions such as maintenance of general health and proper nutrition and hygiene. Stress the need for compliance with the treatment regimen.
- Provide the patient and significant others with important information contained in the specific drug monographs for the drugs prescribed. Additional health teaching and nursing interventions for drug side effects to expect and report are found in each drug monograph.
- Seek cooperation and understanding of the following points so that medication compliance is increased: name of medication, dosage, route and times of administration, side effects to expect, and side effects to report.
- Enlist the patient's aid in developing and maintaining a written record of monitoring parameters, such as blood pressure, pulse, weights, degree of relief from menstrual pain, and menstrual cycle information for persons on oral contraceptives. For persons with STDs a listing of the symptoms and degree of relief obtained may be appropriate. Instruct the patient to bring the written record to follow-up visits.

Drug Therapy for Contraception

The oral (hormonal) contraceptives (birth control pills) became available in 1960. They now represent one of the most common forms of artificial birth control in use in the United States. It is estimated that approximately one third of all women between 18 and 44 years of age use oral contraceptives.

Drug Class: Oral Contraceptives

Actions

Estrogens and progestins, to some extent, induce contraception by inhibiting ovulation. The estrogens block pituitary release of follicle-stimulating hormone (FSH), preventing the ovary from developing a follicle from which the ovum is released. Progestins inhibit pituitary release of luteinizing hormone (LH), the hormone responsible for release of the ovum from the follicle. Other mechanisms play a contribu-

tory role in preventing conception. Estrogens and progestins alter cervical mucus by making it thick and viscous, inhibiting sperm migration, mobility of uterine and oviduct muscle, reducing transport of both sperm and ovum; and the endometrium, impairing implantation of the fertilized ovum.

The minipills, or progestin-only pills, represent a relatively new direction in oral contraceptive therapy. Many of the adverse effects of combination-type contraceptives are caused by the estrogen component of the tablet. For those women particularly susceptible to adverse effects of estrogen therapy, the minipill provides an alternative. Women who might prefer the minipill are those with a history of migraine headaches, hypertension, mental depression, weight gain, and breast tenderness and those who want to breast-feed postpartum. The minipill is not without its disadvantages, however. Between 30% and 40% of women on the minipill continue to ovulate. Birth control is maintained by progestin activity on cervical mucus, uterine and fallopian transport, and implantation. There is a slightly higher incidence of both uterine and tubal pregnancy. **Dysmenorrhea,** manifested by irregular periods, infrequent periods, and spotting between periods, is common among women taking the minipill.

Uses

There are two types of oral contraceptives in general use: the combination pill, which is taken for 21 days of the menstrual cycle and contains both an estrogen and a progestin (Table 38-4); and the minipill, which is taken every day and contains only a progestin (see Table 38-4). The combination pills are subdivided into fixed-combination (monophasic), biphasic, and triphasic products. The monophasic combination pills contain a fixed ratio of estrogen and progestin given daily for 21 days beginning on day 5 of the menstrual cycle. The biphasic product contains a fixed dose of estrogen and a progestin dose on days 1 to 10 that is lower than that on days 11 to 21 of the menstrual cycle. The triphasic combination pills provide three concentrations of estrogen and progestin. The purpose of the variable concentrations of hormones is to provide contraception with the lowest necessary dose of hormones. The combination pills are also packaged in 28-tablet containers. The last 7 tablets are inert but are supplied so that there is no break in the routine of taking one tablet daily.

Therapeutic Outcome

The primary therapeutic outcome associated with oral contraceptive therapy is prevention of pregnancy.

Nursing Process

Assessment

1. Review the medical history. If there is a history of hypertension, gallbladder disease, diabetes mellitus, severe varicose veins, seizure disorders, **oligomenorrhea** or **amenorrhea,** rheumatic heart disease, thromboembolic disease, stroke, malignancy of breast or the reproductive system, renal or liver disease, severe mental depression, suspected pregnancy, or repeated contraceptive failure, consult with the physician before dispensing birth control pills.

2. Take a baseline blood pressure in the supine and sitting positions.
3. Ensure that a pregnancy test has been given and the patient is not pregnant.

Planning
Availability. See Table 38-4.

Implementation
Before initiating therapy. The patient should have a complete physical examination that includes blood pressure, pelvic and breast examination, Papanicolaou smear, urinalysis, and hemoglobin or hematocrit.

Instructions for using combination oral contraceptives. Start the first pill on the first Sunday after your period begins. Take 1 pill daily, at the same time daily, until the pack is gone. If using a 21-day pack, wait 1 week and restart on the next Sunday. If using a 28-day pack, start a new pack the day after finishing the last pack. Use another form of birth control (condoms, foam) during the first month. You may not be fully protected by the pill during the first month.

Missed pills. If you miss 1 pill, take it as soon as you remember it; take the next pill at the regularly scheduled time. If you miss 2 pills, take 2 pills as soon as you remember and 2 the next day. Spotting may occur when 2 pills are missed. Use another form of birth control (condoms, foam) until you finish this pack of pills. If you miss *3 or more*, start using another form of birth control immediately. Start a new pack of pills on the next Sunday even if you are menstruating. Discard your old packs of pills. Use other forms of birth control through the next month after missing 3 or more pills.

Missed pills and skipped periods. Return to your physician for a pregnancy test.

Skipping one period but not missing a pill. It is not uncommon for a woman to occasionally miss a period when on the pill. Start the next pack on the appropriate Sunday.

Spotting for two or more cycles. See your physician.

Periodic examinations. A yearly examination should include blood pressure tests, pelvic examination, urinalysis, breast examination, and Papanicolaou smear.

Discontinuing the pill for conception. Because of a possibility of birth defects, the pill should be discontinued 3 months before attempting pregnancy. Use other methods of contraception for these 3 months.

Duration of oral contraceptive therapy. Many physicians prefer to have patients discontinue the pill for 3 of every 28 months. This allows the body to return to a normal cycle. Be sure to use other forms of contraception during this time. Long-term use (3 or more years) must be determined on an individual basis.

Side effects to be reported as soon as possible. Severe headaches, dizziness, blurred vision, leg pain, shortness of breath, chest pain, and acute abdominal pain. Although these side effects are usually of minor consequence, absence of serious adverse effects must be confirmed.

Note: When being seen by a physician or a dentist for other reasons, be sure to mention that you are currently taking oral contraceptives.

Instructions for using the minipill. Start using the minipill on the first day of menstruation. Take 1 tablet daily, every day, regardless of when your next period is. Tablets should be taken at approximately the same time every day.

Missed pills. If you miss 1 pill, take it as soon as you remember, and take your next pill at the regularly scheduled time. Use another form of birth control until your next period.

If you miss 2 pills, take 1 of the missed pills immediately, and take your regularly scheduled pill for that day on time. The next day, take the regularly scheduled pill as well as the other missed pill. Use another method of birth control until your next period.

Missed periods. Some women note changes in the time as well as duration of their periods while using minipills. These changes are to be expected. If menses occurs every 28 to 30 days, ovulation may still be occurring. For maximal safety, use alternative forms of contraception on days 10 through 18. If irregular bleeding occurs every 25 to 45 days, ovulation is probably not occurring on a regular basis. You may feel more comfortable if you use other forms of contraception with the minipill or discuss switching to an estrogen-containing (combination) contraceptive.

If you have taken all tablets correctly but have not had a period for over 60 days, speak to your physician concerning a pregnancy test.

Note: Report sudden, severe abdominal pain, with or without nausea and vomiting, to your physician immediately. There is a higher incidence of ectopic pregnancy with the minipill because it does not inhibit ovulation in all women.

Side effects to be reported as soon as possible. Severe headaches, dizziness, blurred vision, leg pain, shortness of breath, chest pain, and acute abdominal pain. Although these side effects are usually of minor consequence, absence of serious adverse effects must be confirmed.

Duration of oral contraceptive therapy. Many physicians prefer to have patients discontinue the pill for 3 of every 18 months. This allows the body to return to a normal cycle. Be sure to use other forms of contraception during this time. Long-term use (3 or more years) must be determined on an individual basis.

Discontinuing the pill for conception. Because of a possibility of birth defects, discontinue the pill 3 months before attempting pregnancy. Use other methods of contraception for these 3 months.

Dosage and administration. The estrogenic component of the combination-type pills is responsible for most of the adverse effects associated with therapy. The Food and Drug Administration (FDA) has recommended that therapy be initiated with a product containing a low dose of estrogen. Side effects must be reviewed in relation to individual case histories, but many physicians initiate therapy with Norinyl 1 + 50 or Ortho Novum 1/50. Therapy, and therefore products, may be adjusted based on the incidence of side effects.

Evaluation
Side effects to expect
NAUSEA, WEIGHT GAIN, SPOTTING, CHANGED MENSTRUAL FLOW, MISSED PERIODS, DEPRESSION, MOOD CHANGES, CHLOASMA, HEADACHES. These are the most common side effects of hormonal contraceptive therapy. If these symptoms are not resolved after 3 months of therapy, the woman should return to the physician for reevaluation and a possible change in prescription.

Table 38-4

Oral Contraceptives

Brand Name	Progestin						Estrogen		Other Ingredients
	Norethindrone (mg)	Norethindrone Acetate (mg)	Norgestrel (mg)	Ethynodiol Diacetate (mg)	Norethynodrel (mg)	Levonorgestrel (μg)	Ethinyl Estradiol (μg)	Mestranol (μg)	
*Combination**									
Brevicon (21, 28)†	0.5						35		
Demulen 1/35 (21,28)				1			35		
Demulen 1/50 (21,28)				1			50		
Desogen (28)							30		Desogestrel 150 μg
Genora 0.5/35 (21,28)	0.5						35		
Genora 1/35 (21,28)	1						35		
Genora 1/50 (21,28)	1							50	
Levlen (21, 28)						150	30		
Levora (21,28)						150	30		
Loestrin 1/20 (21)		1					20		
Loestrin Fe 1/20 (28)		1					20		Ferrous fumarate 75 mg
Loestrin 1.5/3.0 (21)		1.5					30		
Loestrin Fe 1.5/3.0 (28)		1.5					30		Ferrous fumarate 75 mg
Lo/Ovral (21,28)			0.3				30		
Modicon (21,28)	0.5						35		
Nelova 0.5/35 E (21,28)	0.5						35		
Nelova 1/35 E (21,28)	1						35		
Nelova 1/50 M (21,28)	1							50	
Nelova 10/11 (21,28)	10 tabs 0.5 11 tabs 1.0						35		
Norcept E 1/35 (21,28)	1						35		
Nordette (21,28)						150	30		
Norethin 1/35 E (21,28)	1						35		
Norethin 1/50 M	1							50	

continued

Table 38-4
Oral Contraceptives—cont'd

BRAND NAME	PROGESTIN						ESTROGEN		OTHER INGREDIENTS
	NORETHIN-DRONE (MG)	NORETHIN-DRONE ACETATE (MG)	NORGESTREL (MG)	ETHYNODIOL DIACETATE (MG)	NORETHY-NODREL (MG)	LEVONOR-GESTREL (µG)	ETHINYL ESTRADIOL (µG)	MESTRANOL (µG)	
Norinyl 1 + 35 (21,28)	1						35		
Norinyl 1 I 50 (21,28)	1							50	
Ortho-Cept							30		Desogestrel 150 µg
Ortho-Cyclen							30		Norgestimate 250 µg
Ortho-Novum 1/35 (21,28)	1						35		
Ortho-Novum 1/50 (21,28)	1							50	
Ortho-Novum 10/11 (21,28)	10 tabs-0.5 / 11 tabs-1.0						35 / 35		
Ortho-Novum 7/7/7 (21,28)‡	7 tabs-0.5 / 7 tabs-0.75 / 7 tabs-1.0						35 / 35 / 35		
Ovcon-35 (28)	0.4						35		
Ovcon-50 (28)	1						50		
Ovral (21,28)			0.5				50		
Tri-Levlen (21,28)‡						6 tabs-50 / 5 tabs-75 / 10 tabs-125	30 / 40 / 30		
Tri-Norinyl (21,28)‡	7 tabs-0.5 / 9 tabs-1.0 / 5 tabs-0.5						35 / 35 / 35		
Triphasil-21 (21,28)‡						6 tabs-50 / 5 tabs-75 / 10 tabs-125	30 / 40 / 30	30	
Zovia 1/35 E (21,28)				1			35		
Zovia 1/50 E (21,28)				1			50		
Progestin only§									
Micronor (28)	0.35								
Nor-QD (42)	0.35								
Ovrette (28)			0.075						

*Products contain 20 or 21 hormone tablets/package.
†21 hormone tablets/package plus 7 inert tablets.
‡Triphasic oral contraceptives.
§Products contain all active hormone tablets.

477

Side effects to report

VAGINAL DISCHARGE, BREAKTHROUGH BLEEDING, YEAST INFECTION. These symptoms represent the development of secondary disorders. Examination, a change in oral contraceptive, and possible treatment with other medications may be necessary.

BLURRED VISION, SEVERE HEADACHES, DIZZINESS, LEG PAIN, CHEST PAIN, SHORTNESS OF BREATH, ACUTE ABDOMINAL PAIN. Report as soon as possible. These side effects are usually of minor consequence, but they may be early indications of serious adverse effects.

Drug interactions

WARFARIN. This medication may diminish the anticoagulant effects of warfarin. Monitor the prothrombin time, and increase the dosage of warfarin if necessary.

PHENYTOIN. Monitor patients with concurrent therapy for signs of phenytoin toxicity: nystagmus, sedation, and lethargy. Serum levels may be ordered, and a reduced dosage of phenytoin may be required.

THYROID HORMONES. Patients who have no thyroid function and who start on estrogen therapy may require an increase in thyroid hormone because the estrogens reduce the level of circulating thyroid hormones. The thyroid dosage is not adjusted until the patient shows clinical signs of hypothyroidism.

PHENOBARBITAL. Phenobarbital may enhance the metabolism of estrogens to the extent that there is inadequate contraceptive protection. Changing to an oral contraceptive with a higher estrogen content or using another form of contraception (foam, condoms) is recommended.

AMPICILLIN, ISONIAZID, RIFAMPIN. The use of another form of contraception (foam, condoms) is recommended.

BENZODIAZEPINES. Oral contraceptives appear to have a variable effect on the metabolism of benzodiazepines. Those that have reduced metabolism with an increase in therapeutic response are alprazolam, chlorazepate, chlordiazepoxide, diazepam, flurazepam, halazepam, and prazepam. Benzodiazepines that have enhanced metabolism and reduced therapeutic activity when taken with oral contraceptives are lorazepam, oxazepam, and temazepam. Adjust the dosage of benzodiazepine accordingly.

PHENYTOIN, PRIMIDONE, CARBAMAZEPINE. The efficacy of the oral contraceptive may be impaired. Breakthrough bleeding may be an indication of this interaction. Adjustment in dosage of oral contraceptive and the use of other methods of contraception (foam, condoms) should be considered.

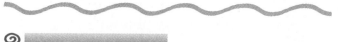

CHAPTER REVIEW

There is a great need for counseling about contraception and about modes of transmission of STDs for all persons who are sexually active. Nurses must be leaders in encouraging persons to report STDs and seek health care as soon as an STD is suspected.

MATH REVIEW

1. Ordered: acyclovir (Zovirax) 200 mg PO q4h while awake for a total of 5 capsules per day.
   The total daily dose would be _____ mg.
   A prescription that is to last for 2 weeks, until the patient is seen in the clinic again, would need to contain a total of _____ capsules.

2. Ordered: doxycycline (Doryx) 100 mg q12h PO for the first day followed by 100 mg per day PO for 10 days. When the prescription comes from the pharmacy, how many capsules should be in the bottle (the product is available in 100 mg capsules)?
   _____ capsules.

CRITICAL THINKING QUESTIONS

1. Ms. Johansen is being started on a combination oral contraceptive. You are to give her the initial health teaching regarding the prescription. What would you explain?

2. Ms. White comes to the clinic for an annual physical examination and renewal of her oral contraceptives. She tests positive for *Chlamydia* and becomes very upset when informed of this. How would you handle this situation?

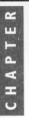

39

Drugs Used to Treat Disorders of the Urinary System

CHAPTER CONTENT

Objectives

1. Explain the major action and effects of drugs used to treat disorders of the urinary tract.

2. Identify baseline data the nurse should collect on a continuous basis for comparison and evaluation of drug effectiveness.

3. Identify important nursing assessments and interventions associated with the drug therapy and treatment of diseases of the urinary system.

4. Identify essential components involved in planning patient education that will enhance compliance with the treatment regimen.

5. Analyze Table 39-1 and identify specific portions of a urinalysis report that would indicate proteinuria, dehydration, infection, or renal disease.

6. Prepare a chart of antimicrobial agents used to treat urinary tract infections. Give the drug names, the organisms treated, and special considerations (such as the need for acidic urine, changes in urine color, and effect on urine tests).

7. Develop a health teaching plan for an individual who has repeated urinary tract infections.

Key Words

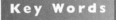

pyelonephritis
cystitis
prostatitis
urethritis

antispasmodic agent
acidification
neurogenic bladder

URINARY TRACT INFECTIONS

Urinary tract infections are some of the most common infectious diseases in humans, second only to upper respiratory tract infection as a cause of morbidity from infection. Urinary tract infections encompass several different types of infection of local tissue: **pyelonephritis** (the kidney), **cystitis** (the bladder), **prostatitis** (the prostate gland), and **urethritis** (the urethra).

The incidence of urinary tract infections in women is approximately 10 times higher than in men. The incidence increases in women with age, so that by 60 years of age, up to 20% of women will have suffered from at least one urinary tract infection in their lives.

Most urinary tract infections are caused by gram-negative aerobic bacilli from the gastrointestinal tract. *Escherichia coli* accounts for about 80% of noninstitutionally acquired uncomplicated urinary tract infections. Other common infecting organisms are *Klebsiella, Enterobacter, Proteus mirabilis,* and *Pseudomonas aeruginosa.* Nosocomial urinary tract infections and those associated with urinary tract pathologic abnormalities are considered to be complicated urinary tract infections. The pathogens tend to be the same types of bacteria, but they are frequently more resistant to the antibiotics commonly used. This requires the use of more potent antibiotics for longer courses of therapy, placing the patient at a greater risk for complications secondary to drug therapy.

The use of an indwelling urinary catheter should be avoided if possible. When used, adherence to strict aseptic technique and attachment to a closed drainage system is necessary to reduce the rate of infection.

URINARY TRACT INFECTIONS

In children and adult males, urinary tract infections may have a more serious etiology than that in a case of cystitis. Therefore all urinary tract infections must be thoroughly investigated to identify the underlying etiology.

Nursing Process for Urinary System Disease

The information the nurse gains through assessment of the patient's clinical signs and symptoms is important to the physician when analyzing data for diagnosis and for evaluation of the patient's response to prescribed treatment.

Assessment

History of urinary tract symptoms. • Does the individual have a history of a congenital disorder of the urinary tract, sexually transmitted disease, recent delivery of a baby, prostatic disease, recent catheterization, urologic instrumentation or surgical procedure, renal calculi, urinary tract infection, or bladder dysfunction of neurologic origin? Obtain details applicable to the responses the patient makes. • Is there a problem with defecation? When was the last bowel movement?

History of current symptoms. Has the individual had chills, fever, general malaise, or a change in mental status? New confusion in an elderly patient may be the only sign of a urinary tract infection. Ask questions relating to personal hygiene practices and sexual intercourse to evaluate for the possibility of bacterial contamination as an underlying cause of cystitis.

Pattern of urination. Ask the individual to describe the symptoms being experienced affecting the ability to void. What is the current urination pattern, and have there been recent changes? Such details as frequency, dysuria, incontinence, changes in the stream, hesitancy in starting to void, hematuria, nocturia, and urgency are all of significance. State the onset, course of progression of the symptoms, and any self-treatment that has been attempted and response achieved.

Pattern of pain. Record the details of any pain the patient describes: frequency, intensity, duration, and location. Pain associated with renal pathology usually occurs at the groin, back, flank, and suprapubic area and on urination (dysuria). Does the pain radiate? If so, obtain details.

Intake and output. Ask specifically about the individual's usual daily fluid intake. How frequently does the patient usually void? What is the amount of each voiding?

Medication history. Ask for a list of all prescribed and over-the-counter (OTC) medicines being taken. Many pharmacologic agents (for example, anticholinergic agents, cholinergic agents, antihistamines, antihypertensives, chemotherapeutic agents, and immunosuppressants) can induce urinary retention, an altered urinary elimination pattern, or urologic symptoms.

Nutritional history. Has the individual been fasting for any prolonged period? How much alcoholic beverage has been consumed?

Laboratory and diagnostic studies. Review diagnostic and laboratory reports (for example, urinalysis, renal function tests, voiding evaluatory procedures, cystoscopy, and complete blood count [CBC] with differential).

Urinalysis. The urinalysis is the most routine test the nurse encounters. An understanding of the significant data that this basic test can reveal is imperative in monitoring the patient. Refer to Table 39-1 for a description of the data. See a general medical-surgical text for details of collecting urine samples correctly.

Nursing Diagnosis

- Pain, acute (indication)
- Incontinence (functional, stress, reflex, total, urge) (indication)
- Infection (indication)

Planning

- Individualize the care plan to address the type of urinary tract disorder the individual has (for example, retention, incontinence, and cystitis).
- Order medications prescribed and list on the medication administration record (MAR).
- Schedule diagnostic procedures ordered; transcribe orders relating to preparation for diagnostic procedures.
- Order laboratory studies (for example, urinalysis, CBC with differential, and creatinine clearance).
- Mark dietary orders on Kardex and care plan; indicate the amount of fluid to be taken every shift to maintain an adequate intake.
- Mark the care plan and Kardex for daily weights and accurate intake and output, and, as appropriate to diagnosis, indicate if bladder training, Kegel's exercises, and so on are to be taught and encouraged.
- Indicate the level of activity or exercise permitted.

Implementation

- Perform focused assessment of symptoms (for example, retention, urinary frequency, and pain).
- Monitor the pain level, and provide appropriate supportive and pharmacologic interventions.
- Administer prescribed medications; monitor response and side effects.
- Maintain adequate fluid intake and accurate intake and output record. Instruct the patient to avoid foods known to be bladder irritants, such as spicy foods, citrus juices, alcohol, and caffeine.
- For inability to void, institute techniques to stimulate voiding (for example, proper positioning to void, running water in sink, and pouring warm water over perineum).
- For incontinence, establish a regular toileting schedule and initiate bladder training measures as appropriate and as ordered. Start measures to prevent perineal irritation. Apply external urinary diversion devices as ordered, such as external condom (Texas catheter). Use incontinent pads as needed. Keep the urinal or bedpan readily available.
- Implement measures to maintain the individual's dignity and privacy and to prevent embarrassment when incontinence is present.
- Maintain the activity and exercise level prescribed.

Table 39-1

Urinalysis

	NORMAL DATA	ABNORMAL DATA
Color	Straw, clear yellow, or amber	Dark smoky color, reddish, or brown may indicate blood. White or cloudy may indicate urinary tract infection or chyluria. Dark yellow to amber may indicate dehydration. Green, deep yellow, or brown may indicate liver or biliary disease. Some drugs may also alter urine color: phenazopyridine—orange; methylene blue—blue.
Odor	Ammonia-like on standing	Foul smell may indicate an infection. The dehydrated patient's urine is concentrated and the ammonia smell is apparent.
Protein	0	Foamy or frothy-appearing urine may indicate protein. Proteinuria is associated with kidney disease and toxemia of pregnancy; it may be present after vigorous exercise.
Glucose	0-trace	Presence is usually associated with diabetes mellitus or low renal threshold with glucose "spillage." Also seen at times of stress, such as major infection, or after a high-carbohydrate meal.
pH	4.6-8.0	Medications can be prescribed to produce an alkaline or acid urine; pH of urine increases if urine is tested after standing 4 hr or more.
Red blood cell count	0-3	Indicative of bleeding at some location in the urinary tract: infection, obstruction, calculi, renal failure, or tumors. (Be sure urine is not contaminated by menses.)
Casts	Rare	May indicate dehydration, possible infection within renal tubules, or other types of renal disease.
White blood cell count	0-4	An increase indicates infection somewhere in the urinary tract.
Specific gravity	1.003-1.030	Used as an indicator of the state of hydration (in absence of renal pathology). Above 1.018 is early sign of dehydration; below 1.010 is "dilute urine" and may indicate fluid accumulation. A fixed specific gravity at around 1.010 may indicate renal disease.
Bacteria	0	May indicate urinary tract infection.

Patient Education and Health Promotion

For incontinence

- Teach personal hygiene measures to keep the skin clean and dry and prevent perineal breakdown. Explore available appliances and incontinence products available for personal use.
- Teach Kegel's exercises and bladder training, and stress importance of responding to the urge to void.
- Teach women the proper method of wiping after defecation or urination to prevent bacterial contamination.

For urinary tract infections

- Teach women the following measures to avoid future urinary tract infections: Avoid nylon underwear (use cotton) and tight, constrictive clothing in the perineal area; avoid frequent use of bubble bath; avoid colored toilet paper because the dyes may be irritating; wash the perineal area immediately before and after sexual intercourse; and urinate immediately after intercourse.
- Explain the correct procedure for obtaining a clean-catch urine sample and the importance of having follow-up urine cultures collected as requested by the physician.
- Teach comfort measures such as the use of a sitz bath.
- Stress the importance of adequate fluid intake and its effect of diluting the urine, decreasing bladder irritability, and helping to remove organisms present in the bladder. Define

"adequate intake of fluid" to the individual in terms of the number and size of glasses of liquid to be consumed during the day.
- Explain the signs of improvement or worsening of the urinary condition appropriate to the individual's diagnosis. Emphasize symptoms that should be reported to the physician.

For urinary retention.
Teach self-examination to assess for bladder distention; Crede's maneuver to aid in emptying the bladder; and, as appropriate, self-catheterization.

Medications

- For urinary retention, explain side effects to anticipate with the prescribed medications.
- For the urinary analgesic phenazopyridine hydrochloride, explain that the urine will have a reddish-orange color. If discoloration of the skin or sclera occurs, contact the physician.
- For urinary tract infections, instruct patients to take the medicines exactly as prescribed for the entire course of medication. Discontinuing the antimicrobial agent when the symptoms improve may result in another infection after approximately 2 weeks that will be resistant to antimicrobial treatment. See individual drug monographs for specific instructions relating to **acidification** of the urine and instructions on taking medications with food or milk to avoid gastric irritation.

- See individual drug monographs regarding treatment of acute attacks and length of time before response can be anticipated. Stress the need for follow-up laboratory evaluation to evaluate response to therapy.

Fostering health maintenance

- Discuss medication information and how it will benefit the course of treatment to produce an optimal response. Stress maintenance of adequate urine volume as a part of the overall treatment of urinary tract disorders.
- Seek cooperation and understanding of the following points so that medication compliance is increased: name of medication, dosage, route and times of administration, side effects to expect, and side effects to report. See individual drug monographs for additional teaching.
- Enlist the patient's aid in developing and maintaining a written record of monitoring parameters for urinary antimicrobial agents (see below). Instruct the patient to bring the written record to the follow-up visits.

DRUG THERAPY
Urinary Antimicrobial Agents

Actions

Urinary antimicrobial agents are substances that are secreted and concentrated in the urine in sufficient amounts to have an antiseptic effect on the urine and the urinary tract.

Uses

Selection of the product to be used is based on identification of the pathogens by Gram stain or by urine culture in severe, recurrent, or chronic infections.

Cinoxacin, enoxacin, methenamine mandelate, nitrofurantoin, and nalidixic acid are used only for urinary tract infections. Other antibiotics that are also used to treat urinary infections are ampicillin, sulfisoxazole, co-trimoxazole, sulfamethizole, ciprofloxacin, lomefloxacin, norfloxacin, tetracycline, doxycycline, gentamicin, and carbenicillin. These

---

PATIENT EDUCATION & MONITORING FORM — Urinary Antibiotics

MEDICATIONS	COLOR	TO BE TAKEN

Name _____

Physician _____

Physician's phone _____

Next appt.* _____

PARAMETERS		DAY OF DISCHARGE						COMMENTS
Temperature								
Pain pattern and severity Severe — Moderate — Low 10 — 5 — 1 Description: On urination Without urination Flank area Suprapubic area								
Voiding and frequency	___ times voiding per day							
	___ times voiding per hour							
Fluid intake	___ glasses per day							
	___ cups per day							
Urine	Color (check one) Straw / Dark / Red							
	Odor: usual or unusual							

*Please bring this record with you to your next appointment.
Use the back of this sheet for additional information.

agents are effective in a variety of tissue infections against many different microorganisms. Because of their use in multiple organ systems, they are discussed in detail (with nursing process) in Chapter 43.

Fluid intake should be encouraged so that there will be at least 2000 ml of urinary output daily. Duration of treatment is dependent on whether the infection is uncomplicated or complicated, or acute, chronic, or recurrent; the pathogen being treated; the antimicrobial agent being used for treatment; and whether a follow-up culture can be collected to assess success of therapy.

Drug Class: Quinolone Antibiotics

Actions

The antibacterial actions of the quinolones (cinoxacin, enoxacin, nalidixic acid, and norfloxacin) have not been fully determined, but it is known that they act as antibacterial agents by inhibiting DNA gyrase enzymes needed for DNA replication in bacteria.

Uses

Cinoxacin and nalidixic acid are effective in treating initial and recurrent urinary tract infections caused by *E. coli, Proteus mirabilis,* and other gram-negative microorganisms. They are not effective against *Pseudomonas* species, common pathogens in chronic urinary tract infections. Clinical studies indicate that cinoxacin may have milder side effects than nalidixic acid.

Norfloxacin and enoxacin have an advantage over other quinolones because they have a much broader spectrum of activity against gram-positive and gram-negative microorganisms. Because of expense, however, they should be reserved to treat resistant, recurrent urinary tract infections caused by *E. coli, Proteus mirabilis, Pseudomonas, Staphylococcus aureus, Staphylococcus epidermidis,* and other gram-positive and gram-negative microorganisms no longer sensitive to the penicillins, cephalosporins, or sulfonamides. Because these antibiotics are administered orally, they may also be useful in treating patients on an outpatient basis who would have required hospitalization for parenteral therapy.

Therapeutic Outcome

The primary therapeutic outcome associated with quinolone therapy is resolution of the urinary tract infection.

Nursing Process

Premedication Assessment

1. Record voiding characteristics—frequency, amount, color, odor, and associated symptoms such as burning and pain to serve as a baseline for monitoring therapy.
2. When using nalidixic acid, check for history of glucose-6-phosphate dehydrogenase deficiency; if present, withhold drug and contact physician.
3. When using cinoxacin or nalidixic acid, record any associated complaints of visual disturbances present before initiation of therapy (for example, altered color perception, difficulty focusing, and double vision).
4. Assess for and record any existing gastrointestinal complaints before initiation of therapy.
5. Record baseline vital signs.

Planning

Availability See Table 39-2.

Implementation

Dosage and administration. See Table 39-2.

Evaluation

Side effects to expect

NAUSEA, VOMITING, ANOREXIA, ABDOMINAL CRAMPS, FLATULENCE. These side effects are usually mild and tend to resolve with continued therapy. Encourage the patient not to discontinue therapy without first consulting the physician.

DROWSINESS, HEADACHE, DIZZINESS. These side effects are usually mild and tend to resolve with continued therapy. Encourage the patient not to discontinue therapy without first consulting the physician.

Provide for patient safety during episodes of dizziness; report for further evaluation if recurrent.

VISUAL DISTURBANCES. During the first few days of therapy with nalidixic acid, difficulty focusing, double vision, and changes in brightness and colors may occur shortly after each dose is given. If these symptoms persist or occur later in therapy, notify the physician for further evaluation.

PHOTOSENSITIVITY. Patients should avoid exposure to direct sunlight and wear sunshades and long-sleeved garments outdoors while taking this medication. A severe sunburn requires medical attention.

Table 39-2

Quinolone Urinary Antibiotics

GENERIC NAME	BRAND NAME	AVAILABILITY	DOSAGE RANGE
Cinoxacin	Cinobac	Capsules: 250, 500 mg	PO: 1 g daily in 2-4 divided doses for 7-14 days; take with meals
Enoxacin	Penetrex	Tablets: 200, 400 mg	PO: 200-400 mg every 12 hr for 7-14 days; take 1 hr before or 2 hr after meals with a large glass of fluid
Nalidixic acid	NegGram	Tablets: 0.25, 0.5, 1 g	PO: 1 g 4 times daily for 7-14 days; take with meals
Norfloxacin	Noroxin	Tablets: 400 mg	PO: 400 mg twice daily for 7-10 days; take 1 hr before or 2 hr after meals with a large glass of fluid; do not exceed 800 mg daily

Side effects to report

HEMATURIA. Although rare, crystal formation has been reported when high doses of norfloxacin have been used or when the patient is dehydrated. The crystals may cause hematuria. Report bloody urine to the physician immediately. Encourage the patient to drink 8 to 12 8-ounce glasses of water daily.

PERINEAL BURNING, URTICARIA, PRURITUS, HIVES. Burning with urination may be produced by the infection itself. However, a small percentage of patients receiving quinolones also develop these symptoms secondary to therapy.

Notify the physician if any of these symptoms develop. Symptomatic relief may be obtained by the use of cornstarch or baking soda in the bath water. The use of antihistamines or topical steroids is rarely required.

HEADACHE, TINNITUS, DIZZINESS, TINGLING SENSATIONS, PHOTOPHOBIA. Report these symptoms for further evaluation.

Drug interactions

PROBENECID. Probenecid may reduce urinary excretion of cinoxacin and norfloxacin, thereby causing inadequate antimicrobial therapy and the possibility of developing resistant strains of microorganisms.

WARFARIN. The quinolones may enhance the anticoagulant effects of warfarin. Observe for the development of petechiae, ecchymoses, nosebleeds, bleeding gums, dark tarry stools, and bright red or coffee ground emesis. Monitor the prothrombin time, and reduce the dosage of warfarin if necessary.

ANTACIDS, SUCRALFATE, MINERAL SUPPLEMENTS CONTAINING IRON, MAGNESIUM, CALCIUM, OR ALUMINUM. These ingredients will decrease absorption of the quinolones. Administer the quinolone 1 hour before or 2 hours after therapy with these agents.

NITROFURANTOIN. Nitrofurantoin may antagonize the antibacterial effects of norfloxacin. Do not use concurrently.

CLINITEST. Nalidixic acid may produce false-positive Clinitest results. Use Clinistix or Tes-Tape to measure urine glucose.

methenamine mandelate (meth'en-a-meen man-del'ate)
Mandelamine (man-del'ah-min)

Actions

Methenamine mandelate combines the action of methenamine and mandelic acid. Methenamine yields formaldehyde in the presence of an acidic urine. The formaldehyde released helps suppress the growth and multiplication of bacteria that may cause recurrent infection. Mandelic acid is present to help maintain the acidic urine. Ascorbic acid (vitamin C) is also frequently prescribed to help maintain the acidity of the urine.

Uses

Methenamine mandelate is used only in patients susceptible to chronic, recurrent urinary tract infections. It is not potent enough to be effective in patients suffering from a preexisting infection. The infection should be treated with antibiotics until the urine is sterile; methenamine should then be given to help prevent recurrence of the infection.

Therapeutic Outcome

The primary therapeutic outcome associated with methenamine mandelate therapy is resolution of the urinary tract infection.

Nursing Process

Premedication Assessment

1. Record voiding characteristics—frequency, amount, color, odor, and associated symptoms such as burning and pain to serve as a baseline for monitoring therapy.
2. Check urine for acidification; give prescribed vitamin C; recheck urine for acidification.
3. Record baseline vital signs.

Planning

Availability. PO—0.5 and 1 g enteric-coated tablets; 0.25 and 0.5 g per 5 ml suspension; 1 g packets of granules.

Implementation

Dosage and administration. Adult: PO—1 g 4 times daily after meals and at bedtime. Gastrointestinal symptoms may be minimized by administering with meals.

DO NOT crush the tablets. This will allow the formation of formaldehyde in the stomach, resulting in nausea and belching.

pH testing. Perform urine testing for pH at regular intervals. Report values above 5.5.

Evaluation

Side effects to expect

NAUSEA, VOMITING, BELCHING. These side effects are usually mild and tend to resolve with continued therapy. Encourage the patient not to discontinue therapy without first consulting the physician.

Side effects to report

HIVES, PRURITUS, RASH. Report symptoms for further evaluation by the physician. Pruritus may be relieved by adding baking soda to the bath water.

BLADDER IRRITATION, DYSURIA, FREQUENCY. Notify the physician of these symptoms because they may indicate the presence of another urinary tract infection.

Drug interactions

ACETAZOLAMIDE, SODIUM BICARBONATE. Acetazolamide and sodium bicarbonate produce an alkaline urine, preventing the conversion of methenamine to formaldehyde, thereby inactivating the medication.

SULFAMETHIZOLE. Sulfamethizole may form an insoluble precipitate in acidic urine. Therefore concurrent treatment with sulfamethizole and methenamine should be avoided.

nitrofurantoin (ny-tro-fuhr-an'toe-in)
Furadantin (fuhr-ah-dan'tin),
Macrodantin (mak-ro-dan'tin)

Actions

Nitrofurantoin is an antibiotic that acts by interfering with several bacterial enzyme systems.

Uses

This antibiotic is not effective against microorganisms in the blood or in tissues outside the urinary tract. It is active against many gram-positive and gram-negative organisms, such as *Streptococcus faecalis, E. coli,* and *Proteus* species. It is not active against *Pseudomonas aeruginosa* or *Serratia* species.

Therapeutic Outcome

The primary therapeutic outcome associated with nitrofurantoin therapy is resolution of the urinary tract infection.

Nursing Process

Assessment

1. Record voiding characteristics—frequency, amount, color, odor, and associated symptoms such as burning and pain to serve as a baseline for monitoring therapy.
2. Assess for and record any gastrointestinal complaints present before initiation of drug therapy.
3. When using nitrofurantoin, check for history of glucose-6-phosphate dehydrogenase deficiency; if present, withhold drug and contact physician.
4. To serve as a baseline, assess for the presence of peripheral neuropathies before initiating therapy.
5. Record baseline vital signs.

Planning

Availability. PO—50 and 100 mg tablets and capsules; 25 mg per 5 ml suspension.

Implementation

Note: Nitrofurantoin must be in the bladder in sufficient concentrations to be therapeutically effective. Nitrofurantoin therapy is *not* recommended for use in patients with a creatinine clearance of less than 40 ml per minute.
Dosage and administration. Adult: PO—50 to 100 mg 4 times daily for 10 to 14 days. Administer with food or milk to reduce gastrointestinal side effects. To maintain adequate urine concentrations, space the dosage at even intervals around the clock. Pediatric: do not administer to infants under 1 month of age. PO—5 to 7 mg/kg per 24 hours in 4 divided doses.

Suspension. Store in a dark amber container away from bright light.

Evaluation

Side effects to expect

NAUSEA, VOMITING, ANOREXIA. Administer with food or milk to reduce gastric irritation.

URINE DISCOLORATION. Tell the patient that urine may be tinted rust-brown to yellow and that this should not be cause for alarm.

Side effects to report

DYSPNEA, CHILLS, FEVER, ERYTHEMATOUS RASH, PRURITUS. These symptoms are the early indications of an allergic reaction to nitrofurantoin.

Acute reactions usually occur within 8 hours in previously sensitized individuals and within 7 to 10 days in patients who develop sensitivity during the course of therapy. Discontinue the drug and notify the physician.

PERIPHERAL NEUROPATHIES. Nitrofurantoin may cause peripheral neuropathies, particularly in patients with renal impairment, anemia, diabetes, electrolyte imbalance, or vita-

min B deficiency. Nitrofurantoin should be discontinued at the first sign of numbness or tingling in the extremities.

SECOND INFECTION. Report immediately the development of dysuria, pungent-smelling urine, or fever. These symptoms may be the early indications of a second infection by an organism resistant to nitrofurantoin.

Drug interactions

CLINITEST. This drug may produce false-positive Clinitest results. Use Clinistix or Tes-Tape to measure urine glucose.

ANTACIDS. Encourage the patient *not* to take products containing magnesium trisilicate (Escot Capsules, Gaviscon, and Gelusil) concurrently with nitrofurantoin because the antacid may inhibit absorption of the nitrofurantoin.

Bladder-Active Drugs

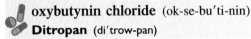

oxybutynin chloride (ok-se-bu'ti-nin)
Ditropan (di'trow-pan)

Actions

Oxybutynin chloride is an **antispasmodic** agent that acts directly on the smooth muscle of the bladder.

Uses

Oxybutynin is used to reduce the frequency of bladder contractions and delay the initial desire to void in patients with **neurogenic bladder.** It should not be used in patients with glaucoma, myasthenia gravis, bowel disease such as ulcerative colitis, or obstructive uropathy such as prostatitis.

Therapeutic Outcome

The primary therapeutic outcome expected from oxybutynin is control of incontinence associated with neurogenic bladder.

Nursing Process

Premedication Assessment

1. Record voiding characteristics—frequency, amount, color, odor, and associated symptoms such as burning and pain to serve as a baseline for monitoring therapy.
2. Obtain baseline vital signs.

Planning

Availability. PO—5 mg tablets; 5 mg per 5 ml syrup.

Implementation

Dosage and administration. Adult: PO—5 mg 2 or 3 times daily, maximum dose 20 mg daily. Pediatric (over 5 years of age): PO—5 mg twice daily, maximum dose 15 mg daily.

Evaluation

Side effects to expect

DRY MOUTH, URINARY HESITANCE, RETENTION. These side effects are usually dose related and respond to a reduction in dose.

Instruct the patient to relieve dry mouth by sucking on ice chips or hard candy or by chewing gum.

CONSTIPATION, BLOATING. Encourage balanced nutrition and inclusion of fresh fruits and vegetables for roughage and an adequate fluid intake to help alleviate this complication. If this approach is unsuccessful, suggest a stool softener or bulk-forming supplement. Avoid laxatives.

BLURRED VISION. Caution patients not to drive or operate power equipment until they have adjusted to this side effect.

Side effects to report

If any of the aforementioned side effects intensifies, it should be reported to the physician for evaluation.

Drug interactions

No clinically significant interactions have been reported.

bethanechol chloride (beth-an′ek-ol)
Urecholine (u-reh-ko′leen)

Actions

Bethanechol is a parasympathetic nerve stimulant that causes contraction of the detrusor urinae muscle in the bladder, usually resulting in urination. It may also stimulate gastric motility, increase gastric tone, and restore impaired rhythmic peristalsis.

Uses

Bethanechol is used in nonobstructive urinary retention, particularly in postoperative and postpartum patients, to restore bladder tone and urination.

Therapeutic Outcome

The primary therapeutic outcome associated with bethanechol therapy is restoration of bladder tone and urination.

Nursing Process

Premedication Assessment

1. Record voiding characteristics—frequency, amount, color, odor, and associated symptoms such as burning and pain to serve as a baseline for monitoring therapy.
2. Record any gastrointestinal symptoms present to serve as a baseline for monitoring therapy.

Planning

Availability. PO—5, 10, 25, and 50 mg tablets. SC—5 mg/ml in 1 ml vials.

Implementation

Dosage and administration. Adult: PO—10 to 50 mg 2 to 4 times daily. The maximum daily dose is 120 mg. SC—2.5 to 5 mg. Atropine sulfate must be available to counteract serious adverse effects.

Note: If overdosage occurs, the pharmacologic actions of the drug can immediately be abolished by atropine.

Evaluation

Side effects to expect

FLUSHING OF SKIN, HEADACHE. A pharmacologic property of the drug results in dilated blood vessels.

Side effects to report

NAUSEA, VOMITING, SWEATING, COLICKY PAIN, ABDOMINAL CRAMPS, DIARRHEA, BELCHING, INVOLUNTARY DEFECATION. These effects are caused by a pharmacologic property of the drug. Consult the physician; a dosage adjustment may control these adverse effects.

Support the patient who develops diarrhea or involuntary defecation.

Drug interactions

QUINIDINE, PROCAINAMIDE. Do not use concurrently with bethanechol. The pharmacologic properties of these agents counteract those of bethanechol.

neostigmine (nee-oh-stig′meen)
Prostigmin (pro-stig′mihn)

Actions

Neostigmine is an anticholinesterase agent that binds to cholinesterase, preventing the destruction of acetylcholine. Because cholinesterase is bound to neostigmine, it cannot metabolize acetylcholine. The acetylcholine accumulates at cholinergic synapses, and its effects become prolonged and exaggerated. This produces a general cholinergic response manifested by miosis; increased tone of intestinal, skeletal, and bladder muscles; bradycardia; stimulation of secretions of the salivary and sweat glands; and constriction of the bronchi and ureters.

Uses

In patients with urinary tract disorders, neostigmine is used to prevent and treat postoperative distention and urinary retention.

Therapeutic Outcome

The primary therapeutic outcome expected from neostigmine is prevention or treatment of postoperative or postpartum urinary retention.

Nursing Process

Premedication Assessment

1. Check for pregnancy, intestinal or urinary tract obstruction, and peritonitis; if present, withhold drug and contact physician.
2. Take baseline vital signs; if bradycardia is present, withhold drug and contact physician.
3. Check for a recent coronary event, hyperthyroidism, epilepsy, asthma, or peptic ulcer; if present, this drug must be used with caution. Depending on symptoms, contact the physician for approval before administering the drug.
4. Record voiding characteristics—frequency, amount, color, odor, and associated symptoms such as burning and pain to serve as a baseline for monitoring therapy.

phenazopyridine hydrochloride
(fen-ay-zoh-peer′i-deen)
Pyridium (py-rid′ee-um)

Actions

Phenazopyridine is an agent that, as it is excreted through the urinary tract, produces a local anesthetic effect on the mucosa of the ureters and bladder. It acts within about 30 minutes after oral administration.

Uses

Phenazopyridine relieves burning, pain, urgency, and frequency associated with urinary tract infections. It also reduces bladder spasm, which relieves the resulting urinary retention. Phenazopyridine is also used for preoperative and postoperative surface analgesia in urologic surgical procedures and after diagnostic tests in which instrumentation is necessary. It is occasionally used to relieve the discomfort caused by the presence of an indwelling catheter.

Therapeutic Outcome

The primary therapeutic outcome associated with phenazopyridine therapy is relief of burning, frequency, pain, and urgency associated with urinary tract infection.

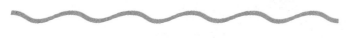

Nursing Process

Premedication Assessment

Record skin color before initiation of therapy.

Planning

Availability. PO—100 and 200 mg tablets.

Implementation

Dosage and administration. Adult: PO—200 mg 3 times daily. Pediatric (6 to 12 years of age): PO—100 mg 3 times daily.

Evaluation

Side effects to expect

REDDISH-ORANGE URINE DISCOLORATION. Be certain the patient understands that the color of the urine will become reddish-orange when this drug is used and that there is no need for alarm.

Side effects to report

YELLOW SCLERA OR SKIN. The patient should report any yellowish tinge developing in the sclera (white portion) of the eye.

Drug interactions

URINE COLORIMETRIC PROCEDURES. This medication will interfere with colorimetric diagnostic tests performed on urine. Consult the hospital laboratory for alternative measures.

CHAPTER REVIEW

Urinary tract infections are some of the most common types of infections and are found in all patient care settings. The nurse can provide significant care by understanding and reporting the early symptoms associated with acute and chronic infections. Nurses can also play a significant role in discretely assisting patients who have difficulty with urinary retention and incontinence.

MATH REVIEW

1. Ordered: bethanechol chloride (Urecholine) 2.5 mg SC stat.
   On hand: bethanechol chloride 5 mg/ml.
   Give: _____ ml.

2. Ordered: methenamine mandelate (Mandelamine) 750 mg PO.
   On hand: methenamine mandelate 0.5 g per 5 ml suspension.
   Give: _____ ml.

CRITICAL THINKING QUESTION

Situation:

Martha Contelli, age 64, a resident of Longmeadow Nursing Home, has developed her third urinary tract infection in the past 4 months. What assessments should be made? Discuss appropriate nursing actions during the treatment of the current urinary tract infection and measures to be instituted to prevent another episode.

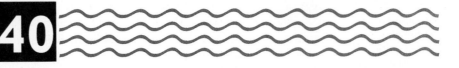

40

Drugs Used to Treat Glaucoma and Other Eye Disorders

Key Words

cornea	near point
sclera	zonular fibers
iris	cycloplegia
sphincter muscle	lacrimal canaliculi
miosis	intraocular pressure
dilator muscle	closed-angle glaucoma
mydriasis	open-angle glaucoma
lens	

ANATOMY AND PHYSIOLOGY OF THE EYE

The eyeball has three coats, or layers: the protective external, or corneoscleral, coat; the nutritive middle vascular layer, called the choroid; and the light-sensitive inner layer, or retina (Figure 40-1).

The **cornea,** the outermost sheath of the anterior eyeball, is transparent so that light can enter the eye. The cornea has no blood vessels; it receives its nutrition from the aqueous humor and its oxygen supply by diffusion from the air and surrounding vascular structures. There is a thin layer of

Objectives

1. Describe the normal flow of aqueous humor in the eye.

2. Identify the changes in normal flow of aqueous humor caused by open-angle and closed-angle glaucoma.

3. Explain baseline data that should be gathered when an eye disorder exists.

4. Review the correct procedures for instilling eye drops and eye ointments.

5. Develop teaching plans for a person with an eye infection and a person receiving glaucoma medication.

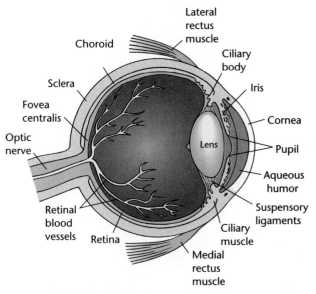

Figure 40-1 *Cross section of the eye.*

epithelial cells on the external surface of the cornea that is resistant to infection. An abraded cornea, however, is highly susceptible to infection. The cornea has sensory fibers, and any damage to the corneal epithelium will cause pain. Seriously injured corneal tissue is replaced by scar tissue that is usually not transparent. The **sclera,** the eye's white portion, is continuous with the cornea and nontransparent.

The **iris** is a diaphragm that surrounds the pupil and gives the eye its blue, green, hazel, brown, or gray color. The **sphincter muscle** within the iris encircles the pupil and is innervated by the parasympathetic nervous system. **Miosis** is contraction of the iris sphincter muscle, which causes the pupil to narrow. The **dilator muscle,** which runs radially from the pupillary margin to the iris periphery, is sympathetically innervated. **Mydriasis** is contraction of the dilator muscle and relaxation of the sphincter muscle, which causes the pupil to dilate (Figure 40-2). Constriction of the pupil normally occurs with light or when the eye is focusing on nearby objects. Dilation of the pupil normally occurs in dim light or when the eye is focusing on distant objects.

The **lens** is a transparent, gelatinous mass of fibers encased in an elastic capsule situated behind the iris. Its function is to ensure that the image on the retina is in sharp focus. It does this by changing shape (accommodation). This occurs readily in youth, but with age the lens becomes more

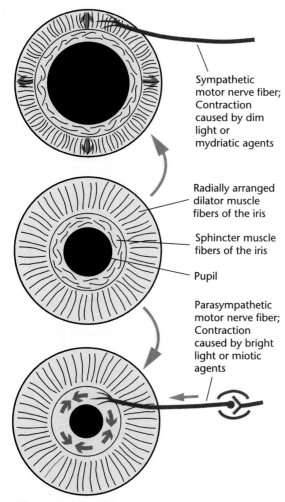

Figure 40-2 *Effect of light or ophthalmic agents on the iris of the eye.*

Sympathetic motor nerve fiber; Contraction caused by dim light or mydriatic agents

Radially arranged dilator muscle fibers of the iris

Sphincter muscle fibers of the iris

Pupil

Parasympathetic motor nerve fiber; Contraction caused by bright light or miotic agents

rigid and the ability to focus on close objects is lost. The **near point,** the closest point that can be seen clearly, recedes. With age, the lens may lose its transparency and become opaque, forming a cataract. Blindness can occur unless the cataract can be treated or surgically removed.

The lens has ligaments around its edge called **zonular fibers** that connect with the ciliary body. Tension on the zonular fibers helps change the shape of the lens. In the unaccommodated eye, the ciliary muscle is relaxed and the zonular fibers are taut. For near vision, the ciliary muscle fibers contract, relaxing the pull on the ligaments and allowing the lens to increase in thickness. Accommodation depends on two factors: the ability of the lens to assume a more biconvex shape when tension on the ligaments is relaxed and ciliary muscle contraction. Paralysis of the ciliary muscle is termed **cycloplegia.** The ciliary muscle is innervated by parasympathetic nerve fibers.

The ciliary body secretes aqueous humor, which bathes and feeds the lens, posterior surface of the cornea, and iris. After it is formed the fluid flows forward between the lens and the iris into the anterior chamber. It drains out of the eye through drainage channels located near the junction of the cornea and sclera into a meshwork that leads into Schlemm's canal and into the venous system of the eye.

Eyelids, eyelashes, tears, and blinking all protect the eye. There are about 200 eyelashes for each eye. The eyelashes cause a blink reflex whenever a foreign body touches them, closing the lids for a fraction of a second to prevent the foreign body from entering the eye. Blinking, which is bilateral, occurs every few seconds during waking hours. It keeps the corneal surface free from mucus and spreads the lacrimal fluid evenly over the cornea. Tears are secreted by lacrimal glands and contain lysozyme, a mucolytic lubrication for lid movements. They wash away foreign agents and form a thin film over the cornea, providing it with a good optical surface. Tear fluid is lost by drainage into two small ducts, the **lacrimal canaliculi,** at the inner corners of the eyelids and by evaporation.

GLAUCOMA

Glaucoma is an eye disease characterized by abnormally elevated **intraocular pressure** (IOP), which may result from excessive production of the aqueous humor or from diminished ocular fluid outflow. Increased pressure, if persistent and sufficiently elevated, may lead to permanent blindness. There are three major types of glaucoma: primary, secondary, and congenital. Primary includes **closed-angle glaucoma** and **open-angle glaucoma.** These are diagnosed by the iridocorneal angle of the anterior chamber, where aqueous humor reabsorption takes place. Secondary glaucoma may result from previous eye disease or may occur after a cataract extraction and may require drug therapy for an indefinite period. Congenital glaucoma requires surgical treatment.

Open-angle glaucoma develops insidiously over the years as pathologic changes at the iridocorneal angle prevent the outflow of aqueous humor through the trabecular network to Schlemm's canal and into the veins of the eye. (See Figure 40-3 for the normal pathway of aqueous flow.) In cases of open-angle glaucoma, there is reduced outflow of aqueous humor through the trabecular network and Schlemm's canal

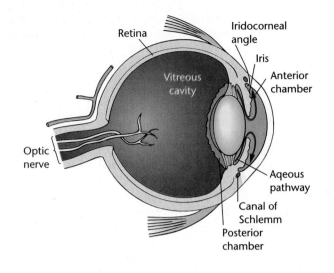

Figure 40-3 *Anterior and posterior chambers of the eye. Arrows indicate the pathway of aqueous flow.*

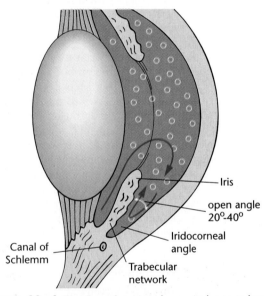

Figure 40-4 *The flow of aqueous humor is due to reduced outflow at Schlemm's canal in the trabecular network. There is no obstruction from closure of the iridocorneal angle.*

because of resistance of outflow of the aqueous humor; the iridocorneal angle is open (Figure 40-4). Intraocular pressure builds up and, if not treated, will damage the optic disk. Initially, the patient has no symptoms, but over the years there is a gradual loss of peripheral vision. If untreated, total blindness may result.

Acute closed-angle glaucoma occurs when there is a sudden increase in IOP caused by a mechanical obstruction of the trabecular network in the iridocorneal angle (Figure 40-5). This occurs in patients who have narrow anterior chamber angles. Symptoms develop gradually and appear intermittently for short periods, especially when the pupil is dilated. (Dilation of the pupil pushes the iris against the trabecular meshwork, causing the obstruction.) Symptoms often reported are blurred vision, halos around white lights,

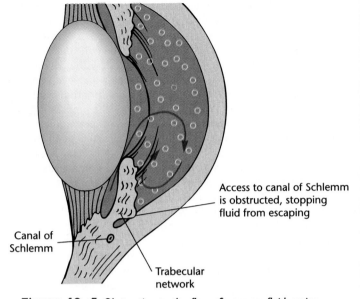

Figure 40-5 *Obstruction to the flow of aqueous fluid, casing closed-angle glaucoma.*

frontal headache, and eye pain. Patients often associate the symptoms with stress or fatigue. An attack can also be precipitated by administration of a mydriatic agent such as atropine or scopolamine for eye examination.

Drug Therapy

The principle for treatment of open-angle glaucoma is maintenance of IOP at normal levels to prevent further blindness. Historically, miotic agents (for example, pilocarpine) have been the most commonly used to increase outflow of aqueous humor. In recent years, however, the beta-adrenergic blocking agents (for example, timolol maleate) have become the initial drugs of choice. Other agents that may also be used are sympathomimetic agents (for example, epinephrine), the carbonic anhydrase inhibitors (for example, acetazolamide), and the cholinesterase inhibitors (for example, echothiophate iodide). The selection of the drug is determined to a great extent by the requirements of the individual patient.

Acute angle-closure glaucoma requires immediate treatment with the administration of miotic agents to relieve the pressure of the iris against the trabecular network and allow drainage of the aqueous humor. Mannitol, an osmotic diuretic, may be administered to draw aqueous humor from the eye, and acetazolamide may be administered to reduce formation of aqueous humor. Analgesics and antiemetics may be administered if pain and vomiting persist. Surgery is then required to correct the abnormality.

Nursing Process for Eye Disorders

The nurse has an important role in educating the public and promoting safety measures to protect the eye from potential sources of injury. Health professionals can participate in this role during their daily contacts with people in the community. The use of safety glasses in potentially hazardous situations, prevention of chemical burns from common household cleansing items or other agents at home or work, proper cleaning and wearing of contact lenses or glasses, and the selection of safe toys and play activities for children are examples of areas about which the nurse can teach the public. These safety measures can significantly reduce the number of injuries that occur annually.

Nurses also play an important role in detection and implementation of the treatment process. An example of this would be in patients with diabetes mellitus. Encourage annual or more frequent eye examinations to detect and prevent complications associated with the disease process.

The primary delivery of eye care is through self-administration of drugs. One of the greatest challenges in the care of chronic eye disorders such as glaucoma is convincing the patient of the need for long-term treatment and compliance with the therapeutic regimen.

Assessment

Eye examination. • Observe for eyelid edema. It may be an indication of a systemic disease process or tumor. Report if present. • Assess pupils for equality of size, roundness, and response to light. Report irregular contour, unequal size, or decreased response to light. • Observe for and report nystagmus. • Observe for any redness or drainage present in the eyes. • Observe for complete closure of the eyelid. This is essential for protection of the cornea. Patients who have received corneal anesthesia, who have had fifth cranial nerve surgery, who have exophthalmus, or who are unconscious must have the cornea protected to prevent damage. • Ask whether glasses or contact lenses are worn. • Inspect the eye dressings and report immediately for evaluation if any drainage is observed. Never remove the dressing to inspect the eye.

History of symptoms. • Ask the patient to describe the symptoms for which treatment is being sought. • Has the person had any noticeable pain, blurred or halo vision, or loss of vision? • Ask whether there is any difficulty in adjusting vision when going from a dark to a brightly lighted area or vice versa. • Are colors clear and crisp, or do they lack clarity? • Has there been an increase in tearing or discharge from the eye? If so, ask for details of appearance and amount of drainage. • Has there been any recent nausea and vomiting?

Diagnostics. Ask the patient to describe what eye diagnostic procedures have been completed before admission.

Medications. Ask for a list of all prescribed and over-the-counter (OTC) medications being taken. Ask for details on medicines, dosage, schedule, and degree of compliance.

Nursing Diagnosis
• Injury, risk for (indication, side effects)
• Pain, actual (indicator)
• Sensory alteration, visual (indication, side effects)
• Self-care deficit, actual (indication, side effect)

Planning
• Schedule diagnostic procedures, surgery, and laboratory studies as ordered.
• List all ordered medications on the medication administration record (MAR). If beta blockers are being taken, list the pulse on the MAR as a preassessment to administration of the ophthalmic drops.
• Mark the Kardex and care plan with parameters relating to prevention of injury, activity and exercise level permitted, and diet orders.

Implementation
• Perform assessments every shift consistent with the patient's status and diagnosis.
• Prepare the patient for eye examinations, diagnostics, or eye surgery.
• Administer cycloplegic and mydriatic medicines prescribed for dilation of the eye before an eye examination or ophthalmic surgery.
• Administer miotic medicine to produce constriction of the eye after eye examination or diagnostic procedures, as prescribed.
• Administer all ophthalmic medicines prescribed for identified disease process (for example, glaucoma) after correct clinical procedure. Maintain aseptic technique to prevent the transfer of infection from one eye to the other.
• Protect the cornea from damage during anesthesia or in an unconscious patient through the use of ophthalmic ointment or "artificial tears" to prevent corneal drying.
• Assist with diagnostic procedures (for example, visual fields, tonometry, and visual acuity).
• Take baseline vital signs.
• Institute appropriate comfort measures.
• If eye surgery is performed (for example, trabeculectomy), institute routine postoperative care measures. Position the patient as ordered, usually on the back or on the unoperated side. With the scleral buckling procedure, positioning orders may be extremely specific.
• Ensure that an eye patch and shield are applied properly to protect the eye from further injury.
• Explain and enforce activity and exercise restrictions. To prevent an increase in IOP, instruct the patient to avoid heavy lifting, straining on defecation, coughing, or bending and placing the head in a dependent position.
• A blind or disoriented patient or a patient with both eyes patched may suffer from sensory deprivation. Always speak before touching the person with impaired vision. Check on the patient at frequent intervals; hold conversations and regularly orient the patient to date, time, and place. Try to arrange for a semiprivate room with an alert roommate who can provide stimulation. If the patient is agitated, contact the physician; it may be necessary to obtain an order to remove one eye patch or sedate the patient.
• Provide emotional support.

Patient Education and Health Promotion

Disease or disorder
• Reinforce the teaching of pertinent facts regarding the diagnosis and disease process.
• If the patient is being treated for glaucoma, stress the need for lifelong treatment and use of medications. Explain that compliance with the drug regimen can help prevent blindness.
• If an infectious process is present, teach personal hygiene measures to prevent introduction of an infection.
  • Wash hands thoroughly each time the area is touched (before or after any eye treatments or instillation of medications).

- Use only sterile medications or dressings on the eye.
- Wipe one eye from the inner canthus outward; discard the tissue or cotton ball used; wash hands before proceeding to the second eye.
- When an infection is present, prevent cross-contamination; always use a separate source of medication and droppers for each eye.
- Never touch the eyeball or face with the tip of the dropper or opening of the ointment container. Demonstrate the proper way to set the lid down so that the inside is not contaminated.
- When inserting or removing contact lenses, wash hands first, and then follow the manufacturer's instructions regarding the cleansing and care of the lenses.
- Report any persistent redness or drainage from the eyes.

Visual acuity. Provide for patient safety.

- Assess whether diminished visual acuity will reduce the ability of the patient to perform his or her usual activities of daily living. Teach adaptation methods appropriate to the situation.
- Restrict the operation of tools or power equipment, as appropriate, to the degree of alteration present.

Medications. Review the details of medication administration.

- Ensure that directions are printed in large, bold print that the individual is capable of reading.
- Have the patient store all medications in an area separate from other containers so that the person cannot inadvertently put things other than medicine in the eye.
- Have the person demonstrate the ability to self-administer the eye medications to ensure manual dexterity to perform the procedures.
- Keep an extra bottle of eye medications on hand, particularly those used to reduce IOP.

Fostering health maintenance

- Discuss medication information and how it will benefit the course of treatment (for example, reduction of IOP or elimination of an infection).
- Seek cooperation and understanding of the following points so that medication compliance is increased: name of medication, dosage, route and times of administration, side effects to expect, and side effects to report. Verify ability to self-administer all medications. Additional health teaching is included in individual drug monographs.
- Encourage the patient to discuss any side effects the medications may produce to plan mutually with the health

provider for ways to minimize these effects or make adaptation rather than reduce the frequency or eliminate the use of the medications.

- Enlist the patient's aid in developing and maintaining a written record (see p. 493) of monitoring parameters (for example, blood pressure and pulse with adrenergic and beta-adrenergic blocking agents, degree of visual disturbance, and progression of impairment) and response to prescribed therapies for discussion with the physician. Encourage the patient to take this record to all follow-up visits.

DRUGS USED TO LOWER INTRAOCULAR PRESSURE

Drug Class: Osmotic Agents

Actions

Osmotic agents are administered intravenously, orally, or topically to reduce IOP. These agents elevate the osmotic pressure of the plasma, causing fluid from the extravascular spaces to be drawn into the blood. The effect on the eye is reduction of volume of intraocular fluid, which produces a decrease in IOP.

Uses

The osmotic agents are used to reduce IOP in patients with acute narrow-angle glaucoma; before iridectomy; preoperatively and postoperatively in conditions such as congenital glaucoma, retinal detachment, cataract extraction, and keratoplasty; and in some secondary glaucomas.

Therapeutic Outcome

The primary therapeutic outcome expected from osmotic agents is reduced IOP.

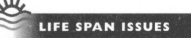

Nursing Process

Premedication Assessment

1. Initiate an intravenous (IV) line for administration of the osmotic agent. Be certain the IV site is functional and not infiltrated before hanging the osmotic agent for infusion.
2. If a Foley catheter is used, ensure that it is functional; initiate strict intake and output monitoring.
3. Assess and record baseline weight, hydration status, lung sounds, and vital signs.
4. Record predrug IOP readings and visual acuity data.

Planning

Availability. See Table 40-1.

Implementation

Dosage and administration. See Table 40-1.

    Catheter. Be certain the patient has an indwelling catheter if these drugs are used during an operative procedure; check with the physician before scrubbing for the procedure.

    Intravenous. Assess the IV site at regular intervals for any signs of infiltration. Tissue necrosis may occur from infiltration into the surrounding tissue. If it occurs, stop the IV, report, and then elevate the extremity and follow

PATIENT EDUCATION & MONITORING FORM   Eye Medications

MEDICATIONS	COLOR	TO BE TAKEN

Name _____

Physician _____

Physician's phone _____

Next appt.* _____

PARAMETERS		DAY OF EXAM							COMMENTS
Blood Pressure									
Pain in eye (Right or Left)									
No pain in eyes									
Vision (clarity)	Blurred all the time								
	Occasionally hazy								
	Clear								
Side vision	Must turn head to see								
	Can see without turning head								
Vision since starting eye medication: No improvement 10 Better 5 Much better 1									
Headache	None								
	If yes, location								
	What were you doing when it started?								
Eye color Redness	Is redness improved by medication?								
Burning	Is burning improved by medication?								
Itching, rash	None								
	Sometimes associated with medication								
	Always occurs with medication								

*Please bring this record with you to your next appointment.
Use the back of this sheet for additional information.

Table 40-1

Osmotic Agents

GENERIC NAME	BRAND NAME	AVAILABILITY	DOSAGE	COMMENTS
Glycerin	Osmoglyn	50% solutions	PO: 1-1.5 g/kg	An oral osmotic agent for reducing intraocular pressure Administer 60-90 min before surgery Use with caution in diabetic patients; monitor for hyperglycemia
Isosorbide	Ismotic	100 g in 220 ml solution (45%)	PO: 1.5 g/kg (range: 1-3 g/kg) 2-4 times daily	An oral osmotic agent for reducing intraocular pressure Onset of action is 30 min, duration is 5-6 hr With repeated doses, monitor fluids and electrolytes The solution will taste better if poured over cracked ice and sipped
Mannitol	Osmitrol	5%, 10%, 15%, 20% solutions for infusions	IV: 1.5-2 g/kg as a 25% solution over 30 min	Used intravenously when oral methods are unacceptable When used preoperatively, administer 60-90 min before surgery Use an in-line filter because mannitol has a tendency to crystallize
Urea	Ureaphil	40 g in 150 ml	IV: 1-5 g/kg	Administer as a 30% solution at an infusion rate not to exceed 4 ml/min Used when mannitol and oral methods are not available Do not exceed 120 g daily Use extreme caution against extravasation; tissue necrosis may result Do not infuse in veins of lower extremities because of the possibility of thrombus formation

hospital protocol for extravasation. *Note:* Do not use veins in lower extremities for administration of these agents. This will minimize the occurrence of phlebitis and thrombosis.

Mannitol crystals. Check the mannitol solution for crystals; do NOT administer if present. Follow directions in the literature accompanying the medication for a warm bath to dissolve the crystals, and then cool the solution before administration.

Evaluation
Side effects to report
THIRST, NAUSEA, DEHYDRATION, ELECTROLYTE IMBALANCE. The electrolytes most commonly altered are potassium (K^+), sodium (Na^+), and chloride (Cl^-).

Many symptoms associated with altered fluid and electrolyte balance are subtle and resemble general symptoms of drug toxicity or the disease process itself.

Gather data about changes in the patient's mental status (alertness, orientation, and confusion), muscle strength, muscle cramps, tremors, nausea, and general appearance (drowsy, anxious, and lethargic).

Always check the electrolyte reports for early indicators of electrolyte imbalance.

Keep accurate records of intake and output, daily weights, and vital signs.

HEADACHE. This is an indication of cerebral dehydration. It can be minimized by keeping the patient in a supine position.

CIRCULATORY OVERLOAD. These medications act on the blood volume by pulling fluid from the tissue spaces into the general circulation (blood). Assess the patient at regularly scheduled intervals for signs and symptoms of fluid overload, pulmonary edema, or heart failure. Perform lung assessments; report the development of rales and increasing dyspnea, frothy sputum, or cough.

Drug interactions
LITHIUM. Mannitol increases the excretion of lithium. Patients being treated with lithium should be monitored for low lithium levels if treated with mannitol.

Drug Class: Carbonic Anhydrase Inhibitors

Actions
These agents are inhibitors of the enzyme carbonic anhydrase. Inhibition of this enzyme results in a decrease in the production of aqueous humor, thus lowering IOP.

Uses
These agents are used in conjunction with other treatment to control IOP in cases of intraocular hypertension and closed-

angle and open-angle glaucoma. Dorzolamide has the advantage of intraocular administration with less potential for systemic side effects.

Therapeutic Outcome

The primary therapeutic outcome expected from carbonic anhydrase inhibitors is reduced IOP.

Nursing Process

Premedication Assessment

1. Establish whether the patient is pregnant; if pregnancy is suspected, withhold the medicine and contact the physician.
2. Check for allergy to sulfonamide antibiotics; withhold the medicine and contact the physician if allergy is present.
3. Ensure that contact lenses have been removed before the instillation of dorzolamide drops.
4. Ensure that baseline electrolyte laboratory studies have been drawn as ordered.
5. Assess and record baseline weight, hydration data, vital signs, and mental status.
6. Record predrug IOP readings and visual acuity data.
7. Assess for any signs of gastric symptoms before initiating drug therapy. If present, schedule medications for administration with milk or food.

Planning

Availability. See Table 40-2.

Implementation

Dosage and administration. See Table 40-2.

Sulfonamides. Do not administer to patients allergic to sulfonamide antibiotics without prior physician approval. Observe closely for the development of hypersensitivity.

Gastric irritation. If gastric irritation occurs, administer with food or milk. If symptoms persist or increase in severity, report for physician evaluation.

Evaluation

Side effects to report

ELECTROLYTE IMBALANCE, DEHYDRATION. Although infrequent, treatment with carbonic anhydrase inhibitors may lead to excessive diuresis resulting in water dehydration and electrolyte imbalance. The electrolytes most commonly altered are potassium (K^+), sodium (Na^+), and chloride (Cl^-). Hypokalemia is most likely to occur.

Many symptoms associated with altered fluid and electrolyte balance are subtle and resemble general symptoms of drug toxicity or the disease process itself.

Gather data about changes in the patient's mental status (alertness, orientation, and confusion), muscle strength, muscle cramps, tremors, nausea, and general appearance (drowsy, anxious, and lethargic).

Always check the electrolyte reports for early indications of electrolyte imbalance.

Keep accurate records of intake and output, daily weight, and vital signs.

DERMATOLOGIC, HEMATOLOGIC, NEUROLOGIC REACTIONS. Carbonic anhydrase inhibitors are sulfonamide derivatives and thus have the potential to cause adverse effects similar to those associated with sulfonamide antimicrobial therapy. These adverse effects, although rare, include dermatologic, hematologic, and neurologic reactions. (See the section on sulfonamides in Chapter 43, p. 539.)

CONFUSION. Perform a baseline assessment of the patient's degree of alertness and orientation to name, place, and time before initiating therapy. Make regularly scheduled subsequent mental status evaluations, and compare findings. Report development of alterations.

DROWSINESS. This side effect is usually mild and tends to resolve with continued therapy. Encourage the patient not to discontinue therapy without first consulting the physician.

Persons who are working around machinery, driving a car, pouring and giving medicines, or performing other duties during which they must remain mentally alert should not take these medications while working.

Drug interactions

QUINIDINE. These diuretics may inhibit the excretion of quinidine. If the patient is also receiving quinidine, monitor closely for signs of quinidine toxicity (tinnitus, vertigo, headache, confusion, bradycardia, and visual disturbances).

DIGITALIS GLYCOSIDES. Patients receiving these diuretics may excrete excess potassium, which leads to hypokalemia. If the patient is also receiving a digitalis glycoside, monitor closely for digitalis toxicity (anorexia, nausea, fatigue, blurred or colored vision, bradycardia, and arrhythmias).

Table 40-2
Carbonic Anhydrase Inhibitors

GENERIC NAME	BRAND NAME	AVAILABILITY	DOSAGE RANGE
Acetazolamide	Diamox	Tablets: 125, 250 mg; Capsules: 500 mg	PO: 250-1000 mg every 24 hr
Dichlorphenamide	Daranide	Tablets: 50 mg	PO: 25-50 mg, 1-3 times daily
Dorzolamide	Trusopt	Ophthalmic solution: 2% in 5 and 10 ml dropper bottles	Intraocular—1 drop in affected eye(s) 3 times daily; if more than one ophthalmic agent is to be administered in the same eye, separate the administration by at least 10 min
Methazolamide	Neptazine	Tablets: 25, 50 mg	PO: 50-100 mg, 2-3 times daily

CORTICOSTEROIDS (PREDNISONE, OTHERS). Corticosteroids may enhance the loss of potassium. Check potassium levels and monitor more closely for hypokalemia when these two agents are used concurrently.

Drug Class: Cholinergic Agents

Actions

Cholinergic agents produce strong contractions of the iris (miosis) and ciliary body musculature (accommodation).

Uses

Cholinergic agents lower IOP in patients with glaucoma by widening the filtration angle, which permits outflow of aqueous humor. They may also be used to counter the effects of mydriatic and cycloplegic agents after surgery or ophthalmoscopic examination.

Cholinergic agents have several advantages: they are effective in many cases of chronic glaucoma, the side effects are less severe and less frequent than those of anticholinesterase agents, and they give better control of IOP with fewer fluctuations in pressure.

Therapeutic Outcomes

The primary therapeutic outcomes expected from cholinergic agents are as follows:

• Reduced IOP in patients with glaucoma

• Reversal of mydriasis and cycloplegia secondary to ophthalmic agents used in surgery or ophthalmic examination

Nursing Process

Premedication Assessment

1. Obtain baseline vital signs.
2. Record predrug IOP readings and visual acuity data.

Planning

Availability. See Table 40-3.

Implementation

Dosage and administration. See Table 40-3.

Evaluation

Side effects to expect

REDUCED VISUAL ACUITY. A common side effect of cholinergic agents is difficulty in adjusting quickly to changes in light intensity. Reduced visual acuity may be most notable at night, particularly in areas of poor lighting, in older patients and patients developing lens opacities. Advise patients to use caution while driving at night or performing hazardous tasks in poor light.

Blurred vision occurs particularly during the first 1 to 2 hours after instilling the medication.

Table 40-3

Cholinergic Agents

GENERIC NAME	BRAND NAME	AVAILABILITY	DOSAGE	COMMENTS
Acetylcholine chloride, intraocular	Miochol Intraocular	1:100 solution	0.5-2 ml instilled into the eye during surgery	Used only during surgery to produce complete miosis within seconds; duration of action is only a few minutes, so pilocarpine may be added to maintain miosis
Carbachol, intraocular	Miostat Intraocular	0.01% solution	0.5 ml	Used only during surgery to produce complete miosis within 2-5 min
Carbachol, topical	Isopto-Carbachol	0.75%, 1.5%, 2.25% and 3% solution	1-2 drops into eye 2-4 times daily	Miotic action lasts 4-8 hr May be particularly useful in patients resistant to pilocarpine
Pilocarpine	Isopto-Carpine, Pilocar, Akarpine, Piloptic, Pilopine HS	0.25%, 0.5%, 1%, 2%, 3%, 4%, 5%, 6%, 8%, 10% solutions; 4% gel	1-2 drops up to 6 times daily; 0.5%-4% solutions used most frequently	Safest, most commonly used miotic for glaucoma Also used to reverse mydriasis after eye examination Onset is 15 minutes to 1 hr; lasts for 2-3 hr

Pilocarpine ocular therapeutic system	Ocusert Pilo-20 Ocusert Pilo-40	—	Inserted weekly, releases either 20 or 40 μg of pilocarpine per hr	A small reservoir containing pilocarpine that is placed in a corner of the eye
				Advantages:
				  Convenience, once-weekly dosing
				  Better continuous control of intraocular pressure
				  Less medication used, lower incidence of toxicity
				Disadvantages:
				  Cost
				  Weekly insertion
				  Conjunctival irritation
				  Variable duration of action
				  May fall out during sleep

Be sure to keep eye medications separate from other solutions.

The ability to read for long periods of time is decreased because of impairment of near-vision accommodation.

Provide for patient safety when visual impairment exists. In hospitals, orient to the hospital unit, furniture placement, and call light; place the bed in a low position. At home, do not move furniture or the individual's household or personal belongings.

CONJUNCTIVAL IRRITATION, ERYTHEMA, HEADACHE. These side effects are usually mild and tend to resolve with continued therapy. Encourage the patient not to discontinue therapy without first consulting the physician.

PAIN, DISCOMFORT. Because of pupillary constriction, an increase in pain or discomfort may occur, particularly in bright light. Stress the need for compliance, and assure the patient that this side effect will diminish with continued use.

Side effects to report

SYSTEMIC SIDE EFFECTS. Rarely, a patient may develop signs of systemic toxicity manifested by diaphoresis, salivation, abdominal discomfort, diarrhea, bronchospasm, muscle tremors, hypotension, arrhythmias, and bradycardia. These symptoms are indications of excessive administration.

Report to the physician for dosage adjustment. The adverse effects themselves usually do not need to be treated because they will resolve by withholding cholinergic therapy.

Prevent systemic effects by carefully blocking the inner canthus for 1 to 2 minutes after instilling the medication to prevent absorption via the nasolacrimal duct.

During drug therapy, assess blood pressure every shift, and report significant changes from the baseline data.

If accidental overdosage occurs during instillation, flush the affected eye with water or normal saline.

Drug interactions

See the following section on cholinesterase inhibitors.

Drug Class: Cholinesterase Inhibitors

Actions

Cholinesterase is an enzyme that destroys acetylcholine, the cholinergic neurotransmitter. The cholinesterase inhibitors prevent the metabolism of acetylcholine within the eye. This causes increased cholinergic activity, which results in decreased IOP and miosis.

Uses

Cholinesterase inhibitors are used in the treatment of glaucoma. Because of the higher incidence of side effects, however, they are reserved for patients who do not respond well to cholinergic agents.

Therapeutic Outcome

The primary therapeutic outcome expected from cholinesterase inhibitors is reduced IOP in patients with glaucoma.

Nursing Process

Premedication Assessment

1. Obtain baseline vital signs; withhold the medicine and contact the physician if bradycardia or any type of respiratory disorder is present.
2. Record predrug IOP readings and visual acuity data.

Planning

Availability. See Table 40-4.

Implementation

Dosage and administration. See Table 40-4.

Evaluation

Side effects to expect

REDUCED VISUAL ACUITY. A common side effect of cholinergic agents is difficulty in adjusting quickly to changes in

Table 40-4

Cholinesterase Inhibitors

GENERIC NAME	BRAND NAME	AVAILABILITY	DOSAGE	COMMENTS
Demecarium bromide	Humorsol	0.125%, 0.25% solution	1-2 drops 1-2 times daily	Onset is within 1 hr; duration may be several days Because of cumulative doses, use only the minimum dose necessary; wipe excess solution away immediately
Echothiophate iodide	Phospholine Iodide	0.03%, 0.06%, 0.125%, 0.25% solution	1 drop 1-2 times daily	Used most commonly in open-angle glaucoma Onset occurs within 10-45 min; duration may be several days After reconstitution, use within 1 mo if stored at room temperature, 6 mo if refrigerated Tolerance may develop after prolonged use; a rest period will restore response
Physostigmine	Eserine	0.25% ointment	Ointment: small quantity up to 3 times daily	May only be needed every other day Duration ranges 12-36 hr

light intensity. Reduced visual acuity may be most notable at night, particularly in areas of poor lighting, in older patients and patients developing lens opacities. Advise patients to use caution while driving at night or performing hazardous tasks in poor light.

CONJUNCTIVAL IRRITATION, ERYTHEMA, HEADACHE, LACRIMATION. These side effects are usually mild and tend to resolve with continued therapy. Encourage the patient not to discontinue therapy without first consulting the physician.

Side effects to report

SYSTEMIC SIDE EFFECTS. Rarely, a patient may develop signs of systemic toxicity manifested by diaphoresis, salivation, vomiting, abdominal cramps, urinary incontinence, diarrhea, dyspnea, bronchospasm, muscle tremors, hypotension, arrhythmias, and bradycardia. These are indications of overdosage or excessive administration. Report to the physician for treatment and dosage adjustment. If symptoms become severe, parenteral atropine should be administered. If accidental overdosage occurs during instillation, flush the affected eye with water or normal saline.

Drug interactions

CARBAMATE AND ORGANOPHOSPHATE INSECTICIDES AND PESTICIDES. Gardeners, farmers, manufacturing employees, and others who are exposed to these pesticides and insecticides and who are receiving cholinesterase inhibitors should be warned of the added risk of systemic symptoms from absorption of these chemicals through the skin and respiratory tract. Respiratory masks and frequent washing and clothing changes are advisable.

MIOTIC AGENTS (PILOCARPINE AND OTHERS). The miotic and IOP-lowering effects of the anticholinesterases is competitively inhibited by pilocarpine.

PHYSOSTIGMINE. The short-acting cholinesterase inhibitor physostigmine blocks the binding to receptors and therefore blocks the pharmacologic effect of subsequently administered long-acting cholinesterase inhibitors.

Drug Class: Adrenergic Agents

Actions

Adrenergic agents have several uses in ophthalmology. Sympathomimetic agents cause pupil dilation, increased outflow of aqueous humor, vasoconstriction, relaxation of the ciliary muscle, and a decrease in the formation of aqueous humor.

Uses

Adrenergic agents are used to lower IOP in open-angle glaucoma, relieve congestion and hyperemia, and produce mydriasis for ocular examinations. Use with caution in patients with hypertension, diabetes mellitus, hyperthyroidism, heart disease, arteriosclerosis, or long-standing bronchial asthma.

Therapeutic Outcomes

The primary therapeutic outcomes expected from adrenergic agents are as follows:
- Mydriasis for ophthalmic examination
- Reduced IOP in open-angle glaucoma
- Reduced redness of the eyes from irritation

Nursing Process

Premedication Assessment

1. Obtain baseline vital signs, including blood pressure.
2. Record predrug IOP readings and visual acuity data.

Planning

Availability. See Table 40-5.

Table 40-5
Adrenergic Agents

GENERIC NAME	BRAND NAME	AVAILABILITY	DOSAGE	COMMENTS
Apraclonidine	Iopidine	0.5%-1% solution	1 drop 1 hr before surgery	Used to control intraocular pressure after laser surgery
Dipivefrin hydrochloride	Propine	0.1% solution	1 drop every 12 hr	This drug has no activity itself but is metabolized to epinephrine; used because it can penetrate the anterior chamber more readily than epinephrine and is less irritating
Epinephrine	Epifrin, Glaucon, Epinal, Eppy/N	0.5%, 1%, 2% solutions	1-2 drops 1-2 times daily	Used to treat open-angle glaucoma, often in combination with cholinergic or beta-blocking agents Duration of action is about 12 hr
Naphazoline hydrochloride	Vasoclear, Allerest, Naphcon, Albalon Liquifilm	0.012%, 0.02%, 0.025%, 0.03%, 0.1% solutions	1-2 drops every 3-4 hr	Used as a topical vasoconstrictor
Tetrahydrozoline hydrochloride	Murine Plus, Visine, Optigene 3	0.05% solution	1-2 drops 2 or 3 times daily	Used as a topical vasoconstrictor

Implementation

Dosage and administration. See Table 40-5.

Evaluation

Side effects to expect

SENSITIVITY TO BRIGHT LIGHT. The mydriasis produced allows excessive amounts of light into the eyes, which causes the patient to squint. Use of sunglasses will help reduce the brightness. Caution the patient to temporarily avoid tasks that require visual acuity, such as driving or operating power machinery.

CONJUNCTIVAL IRRITATION, LACRIMATION. These side effects are usually mild and tend to resolve with continued therapy. Encourage the patient not to discontinue therapy without first consulting the physician.

Side effects to report

SYSTEMIC SIDE EFFECTS. Systemic effects from ophthalmic instillation are uncommon and minimal. However, systemic absorption may occur via the lacrimal drainage system into the nasal pharyngeal passages. Systemic effects are manifested by palpitations, tachycardia, arrhythmias, hypertension, faintness, trembling, and diaphoresis. These are indications of overdosage or excessive administration. Report to the physician for treatment and dosage adjustment.

Prevent systemic effects by carefully blocking the inner canthus for 1 to 2 minutes after instilling the medication to prevent absorption via the nasolacrimal duct.

Monitor pulse rate and blood pressure, and instruct the patient to continue to do this at home; report significant changes from the baseline data.

DIAPHORESIS, TREMBLING. Touch the patient and bedding to assess for diaphoresis (sweating), particularly when these agents are used in surgery in which the patient is under sterile drapes, is anesthetized, and is unable to respond to verbal questioning.

Drug interactions

TRICYCLIC ANTIDEPRESSANTS. Tricyclic antidepressants (amitriptyline, imipramine, doxepin, and others) may cause additive hypertensive effects. Monitor carefully for poor blood pressure control or a gradually increasing blood pressure.

Drug Class: Beta-Adrenergic Blocking Agents

Actions

The beta-adrenergic blocking agents are used in ophthalmology to reduce elevated IOP. The exact mechanism of action is not known, but these agents are thought to reduce the production of aqueous humor.

Uses

The beta-adrenergic blocking agents are used to reduce IOP in patients with chronic open-angle glaucoma or ocular hypertension. Unlike the anticholinergic agents, there is no blurred or dim vision or night blindness because IOP is reduced with little or no effect on pupil size or visual acuity.

Therapeutic Outcome

The primary therapeutic outcome expected from adrenergic blocking agents is reduced IOP.

Nursing Process

Premedication Assessment

1. Obtain baseline vital signs, including blood pressure; withhold medicine and contact the physician if bradycardia, hypertension, or respiratory disorders are present.
2. Record the predrug IOP readings and visual acuity data.

Planning

Availability. See Table 40-6.

Implementation

Dosage and administration. See Table 40-6.

Evaluation

Side effects to expect

CONJUNCTIVAL IRRITATION, LACRIMATION. These side effects are usually mild and tend to resolve with continued therapy. Encourage the patient not to discontinue therapy without first consulting the physician.

Side effects to report

SYSTEMIC SIDE EFFECTS. Systemic effects are uncommon but may be manifested by bradycardia, arrhythmias, hypotension, faintness, and bronchospasm. These adverse effects are more frequently observed in patients requiring higher doses of beta-adrenergic blocking agents and in patients with hypertension, diabetes mellitus, heart disease, arteriosclerosis, or long-standing bronchial asthma. Report to the physician for treatment and dosage adjustment.

Record the blood pressure and pulse rate at specific intervals.

Drug interactions

BETA-ADRENERGIC BLOCKING AGENTS. Propranolol, atenolol, acebutolol, nadolol, pindolol, labetalol, and metoprolol may enhance the systemic therapeutic and toxic effects of ophthalmic beta-adrenergic blocking agents. Monitor for an increase in severity of side effects such as fatigue, hypotension, bronchospasm, and bradycardia.

OTHER OPHTHALMIC AGENTS

Drug Class: Anticholinergic Agents

Actions

Anticholinergic agents cause the smooth muscle of the ciliary body and iris to relax, producing mydriasis (extreme dilation of the pupil) and cycloplegia (paralysis of the ciliary muscle).

Uses

Ophthalmologists use these pharmacologic effects to examine the interior of the eye, measure the proper strength of lenses for eyeglasses (refraction), and rest the eye in inflammatory conditions of the uveal tract.

Therapeutic Outcomes

The primary therapeutic outcomes expected from anticholinergic ophthalmic use are as follows:

• Visualization of intraocular structures
• Reduced uveal tract inflammation

Table 40-6

Beta-Adrenergic Blocking Agents

GENERIC NAME	BRAND NAME	AVAILABILITY	INITIAL DOSAGE	COMMENTS
Betaxolol hydrochloride	Betoptic	0.25%, 0.5% solutions in 5 and 10 ml dropper bottles	1 drop twice daily	A beta-1 selective agent; onset in 30 min, duration is 12 hr; several weeks of therapy may be required to determine optimal dosage
Carteolol	Occupress	1% solution in 5 and 10 ml bottles	1 drop twice daily	A beta-1,2 agent; duration is up to 12 hr
Levobunolol hydrochloride	Betagan	0.5% solution in 5 and 10 ml dropper bottles	1 drop once or twice daily	A beta-1,2 agent; onset within 60 min, duration is up to 24 hr
Metipranolol	OptiPranolol	0.3% solution in 5 and 10 ml dropper bottles	1 drop twice daily in affected eye(s)	A beta-1,2 agent; onset within 30 min, duration is 12-24 hr
Timolol maleate	Timoptic	0.25%, 0.5% solutions in 5, 10, and 15 ml dropper bottles	1 drop of 0.25% solution twice daily	A beta-1,2 agent; onset within 30 min, duration is up to 24 hr

Nursing Process

Premedication Assessment

1. Check for the existence of increased IOP. If present, withhold the medicine and contact the physician for approval before instillation of the anticholinergic agent.
2. Take vital signs; if the patient has hypertension, contact the physician for approval before instillation of the anticholinergic agent.

Planning

Availability. See Table 40-7.

Implementation

Note: The pharmacologic effects of anticholinergic agents cause an increase in intraocular pressure. Use these agents with extreme caution in patients with narrow anterior chamber angles; in infants, children, and the elderly; and in patients with hypertension, hyperthyroidism, and diabetes. Discontinue therapy if signs of increased IOP or systemic effects develop.

Dosage and administration. See Table 40-7.

Evaluation

Side effects to expect

SENSITIVITY TO BRIGHT LIGHT. The mydriasis produced allows excessive light into the eyes, causing the patient to squint. Use of sunglasses will help reduce the brightness. Caution the patient to temporarily avoid tasks that require visual acuity, such as driving or operating power machinery.

CONJUNCTIVAL IRRITATION, LACRIMATION. These side effects are usually mild and tend to resolve with continued therapy. Encourage the patient not to discontinue therapy without first consulting the physician.

Side effects to report

SYSTEMIC SIDE EFFECTS. Prolonged use may result in systemic effects manifested by flushing and dryness of the skin, dry mouth, blurred vision, tachycardia, arrhythmias, urinary hesitancy and retention, vasodilation, and constipation. These are indications of overdosage or excessive administration. Report to the physician for treatment and dosage adjustment. Children are particularly prone to develop systemic reactions.

Drug interactions

No clinically significant drug interactions have been reported.

Drug Class: Antifungal Agents

natamycin (na-tah-my′sin)
Natacyn (na′tah-sin)

Actions

Natamycin acts by altering the cell wall of the fungus to prevent it from serving as a selective barrier, therefore causing loss of fluids and electrolytes.

Uses

Natamycin is an antifungal agent effective against a variety of yeasts, including *Candida, Aspergillus,* and *Fusarium.* It is effective in the treatment of fungal blepharitis, conjunctivitis, and keratitis caused by susceptible organisms. If little or no improvement is noted after 7 to 10 days of treatment, resistance to the antifungal agent may have developed. Topical administration does not appear to result in systemic effects.

Therapeutic Outcome

The primary therapeutic outcome expected from natamycin is eradication of fungal infection.

Table 40-7

Anticholinergic Agents

GENERIC NAME	BRAND NAME	AVAILABILITY	DOSAGE	COMMENTS
Atropine sulfate	Isopto-Atropine, Atropisol	1% ointment, 0.5%, 1% solution	Uveitis: 1-2 drops up to 3 times daily	Onset of mydriasis and cycloplegia is 30-40 min, duration is 7-12 days Do not use in infants
Cyclopentolate hydrochloride	Cyclogyl, AK Pentolate	0.5%, 1%, 2% solutions	Refraction: 1 drop followed by another drop in 5-10 min	For mydriasis and cycloplegia necessary for diagnostic procedures 1-2 drops of 1%-2% pilocarpine allows full recovery within 3-6 hr Central nervous system (CNS) disturbances of hallucinations, loss of orientation, restlessness, and incoherent speech have been reported in children
Homatropine hydrobromide	Isopto-Homatropine	2% and 5 % solutions	Uveitis: 1-2 drops every 3-4 hr	Onset of mydriasis and cycloplegia is 40-60 min; duration is 1-3 days
Scopolamine hydrobromide	Isopto-Hyoscine	0.25% solution	Uveitis: 1-2 drops up to 3 times daily	Onset of mydriasis and cycloplegia is 20-30 min; duration is 3-7 days
Tropicamide	Mydriacyl	0.5% and 1% solutions	Refraction: 1 or 2 drops, repeated in 5 min	Onset of mydriasis and cycloplegia is 20-40 min; duration is 6 hours CNS disturbances of hallucinations, loss of orientation, restlessness, and incoherent speech have been reported in children

Nursing Process

Premedication Assessment

1. Collect ordered cultures or smears before initiating drug therapy.
2. Record baseline data relating to symptoms accompanying the fungal infection and the degree of visual impairment that exists.

Planning

Availability. Ophthalmic—5% suspension.

Implementation

Dosage and administration. Fungal keratitis: 1 drop in the conjunctival sac at 1- or 2-hour intervals for the first 3 to 4 days. The dosage may then be reduced to 1 drop every 3 to 4 hours. Continue therapy for 14 to 21 days.

Evaluation

Side effects to expect

SENSITIVITY TO BRIGHT LIGHT. The slight mydriasis produced allows an excessive amount of light into the eyes, causing the patient to squint. Use of sunglasses will help reduce the brightness. Caution the patient to temporarily avoid tasks that require visual acuity, such as driving or operating power machinery.

BLURRED VISION, LACRIMATION, REDNESS. Provide for patient safety during temporary visual impairment. Instruct the patient not to rub the eyes forcefully while tearing.

These side effects are usually mild and tend to resolve with continued therapy. Encourage the patient not to discontinue therapy without first consulting the physician.

Side effects to report

EYE PAIN. If eye pain develops, discontinue use and consult an ophthalmologist immediately.

THERAPEUTIC EFFECT. If, after several days of therapy, the symptoms do not improve or gradually worsen, consult the physician treating the patient.

Drug interactions

No significant drug interactions have been reported.

Drug Class: Antiviral Agents

Actions

The ophthalmic antiviral agents act by inhibiting viral replication.

Uses

Idoxuridine and trifluridine are chemically related compounds used to treat herpes simplex keratitis. Idoxuridine is particularly effective against initial infections but is not as effective against deep infections or chronic, recurrent infections. Trifluridine is used to treat recurrent infections in patients who are intolerant of or resistant to idoxuridine or vidarabine therapy; cross-sensitivity with these other agents has not been reported.

Vidarabine is used topically as an ophthalmic ointment to treat keratitis and keratoconjunctivitis caused by herpes simplex virus types 1 and 2. Vidarabine does not show cross-sensitivity to idoxuridine or trifluridine and may be effective in treating recurrent keratitis that is resistant to idoxuridine and trifluridine.

These antiviral agents are not effective against infections caused by bacteria, fungi, or *Chlamydia*.

Therapeutic Outcome

The primary therapeutic outcome expected from antiviral agents is eradication of the viral infection.

Nursing Process

Premedication Assessment

Record baseline data concerning the symptoms and the degree of visual impairment.

Planning

Availability. See Table 40-8.

Implementation

Dosage and administration. See Table 40-8.

Note: If significant improvement has not occurred in 7 to 14 days, other therapy should be considered. Do not exceed 21 days of continuous therapy because of potential ocular toxicity.

Storage. Trifluridine should be stored in the refrigerator.

Evaluation

Side effects to expect

VISUAL HAZE, LACRIMATION, REDNESS, BURNING. Patients may notice a mild, transient stinging, burning, and redness of the conjunctiva and sclera on instillation. Provide for patient safety during temporary visual impairment. Instruct the patient not to rub the eyes forcefully while tearing.

These side effects are usually mild and tend to resolve with continued therapy. Encourage the patient not to discontinue therapy without first consulting the physician.

SENSITIVITY TO BRIGHT LIGHT. The slight mydriasis produced allows excessive light into the eyes, causing the patient to squint. Use of sunglasses will help reduce the brightness. Caution the patient to temporarily avoid tasks that require visual acuity, such as driving or operating power machinery.

Side effects to report

ALLERGIC REACTIONS. Discontinue therapy and consult an ophthalmologist immediately.

Drug interactions

No significant drug interactions have been reported.

Drug Class: Antibacterial Agents

Uses

Antibacterial agents (Table 40-9) are used in the treatment of superficial eye infections and for prophylaxis against gonorrhea infection in the eyes of newborn infants (ophthalmia neonatorum). Prolonged or frequent intermittent use of topical antibiotics should be avoided because of the possibility of hypersensitivity reactions and the development of resistant organisms, including fungi. If hypersensitivities or new infections appear during use, consult an ophthalmologist immediately. Refer to the Index for a discussion of these antibiotics.

Drug Class: Corticosteroids

Uses

Corticosteroid therapy (Table 40-10) is used for allergic reactions of the eye and other acute, noninfectious inflammatory conditions of the conjunctiva, sclera, cornea, and ante-

Table 40-8
Antiviral Agents

GENERIC NAME	BRAND NAME	AVAILABILITY	DOSAGE RANGE
Idoxuridine	Herplex	Ophthalmic solution: 0.1% in 15 ml dropper bottle	Intraocular—initially 1 drop in each infected eye every hr during the day and every 2 hr after bedtime; after significant improvement, as shown by loss of staining with fluorescein, reduce the dose to 1 drop every 2 hr during the day and every 4 hr at night; continue therapy for 3 to 5 days after healing appears to be complete to minimize recurrences
Trifluridine	Viroptic	Ophthalmic solution: 1% in 7.5 ml	Intraocular—place 1 drop onto the cornea of the affected eye every 2 hr during waking hours; do not exceed 9 drops daily; continue for 7 more days to prevent recurrence, using 1 drop every 4 hr (5 drops daily)
Vidarabine	Vira-A	Ophthalmic ointment: 3% in 3.5 g tube	Intraocular—place a 1 cm ribbon of ointment inside the lower conjunctival sac of the infected eye 5 times daily at 3-hr intervals; continue for an additional 5 to 7 days at a dosage of 1 cm twice daily after significant improvement has occurred to prevent recurrence of the infection

Table 40-9
Ophthalmic Antibiotics

ANTIBIOTIC	BRAND NAME	AVAILABILITY
Bacitracin	Bacitracin Ophthalmic	Ointment
Chloramphenicol	Chloromycetin Ophthalmic, Chloroptic, Ocu-Chlor	Drops, ointment
Chlortetracycline	Aureomycin Ophthalmic	Ointment
Ciprofloxacin	Ciloxan	Drops
Erythromycin	Ilotycin Ophthalmic	Ointment
Gentamicin	Garamycin Ophthalmic	Drops, ointment
Norfloxacin	Chibroxin	Drops
Polymyxin B	Polymyxin B Sulfate	Drops
Sulfacetamide	Sulf-10, Isopto-Cetamide	Drops, ointment
Tetracycline	Tetracycline Ophthalmic	Ointment
Tobramycin	Tobrex Ophthalmic	Drops, ointment
Combinations		
Trimethoprim/Polymyxin B	Polytrim Ophthalmic	Drops
Neomycin/Polymyxin B/Bacitracin	Ocu-Spor-B, Ocutricin	Ointment
Neomycin/Polymyxin B/Gramicidin	Neosporin Ophthalmic	Drops

Table 40-10
Corticosteroids

GENERIC NAME	BRAND NAME	AVAILABILITY
Dexamethasone	Ocu-Trol	Ointment
	Maxitrol	Suspension
Fluorometholone	FML Liquifilm	Suspension
Medrysone	HMS Liquifilm	Suspension
Prednisolone	Econopred Plus	Solution
	Ocu-Pred-A	Suspension

rior uveal tract. Corticosteroid therapy must not be used in bacterial, fungal, or viral infections of the eye because corticosteroids decrease defense mechanisms and reduce resistance to pathologic organisms. This therapy should be used for a limited time only, and the eye should be checked frequently for an increase in IOP. Prolonged ocular steroid therapy may cause glaucoma and cataracts. Refer to the Index for further discussion of the corticosteroids.

Ophthalmic Antiinflammatory Agents

Flurbiprofen sodium, ketorolac tromethamine, suprofen, and diclofenac sodium are topical nonsteroidal antiinflammatory agents for ophthalmic use. These agents have been shown to have antiinflammatory, antipyretic, and analgesic activity by inhibiting the biosynthesis of prostaglandins that are responsible for an increase in intraocular inflammation and pressure. They also inhibit prostaglandin-mediated constriction of the iris (miosis) that is independent of cholinergic mechanisms. Flurbiprofen and suprofen are used primarily to inhibit miosis during cataract surgery. Diclofenac sodium is used to treat postoperative inflammation after cataract extraction. Flurbiprofen is available as a 0.03% solution (Ocufen) that should be used by instilling 1 drop in the appropriate eye every 30 minutes, beginning 2 hours before surgery (for a total of 4 drops). Suprofen (Profenal) is available as a 1% solution that is instilled (2 drops) into the conjunctival sac 3 hours, 2 hours, and 1 hour before surgery. Diclofenac sodium (Voltaren) is available as a 0.1% solution. One drop is applied to the affected eye 4 times daily beginning 24 hours after surgery and continued for 2 weeks. Ketorolac tromethamine is available as a 0.5% solution. One drop is applied to each eye four times daily to relieve ocular itching associated with seasonal allergic conjunctivitis.

Antiallergic Agent

Uses

Cromolyn sodium is a stabilizing agent that inhibits the release of histamine and slow-reacting substance of anaphylaxis (SRS-A) from mast cells after exposure to specific antigens. It is used to treat allergic ocular disorders such as vernal keratoconjunctivitis, vernal keratitis, and allergic keratoconjunctivitis. It is available as a 4% solution (Opticrom); 1 to 2 drops are applied in each eye 4 to 6 times daily at regular intervals.

Sodium Fluorescein

Uses

Sodium fluorescein is used in fitting hard contact lenses and as a diagnostic aid in identifying foreign bodies in the eye and abraded or ulcerated areas of the cornea. It is also useful for evaluating retinal vasculature for abnormal circulation.

When sodium fluorescein is instilled in the eye, it stains the pathologic tissues green if observed under normal light and bright yellow if viewed under cobalt blue light. Sodium fluorescein is available in 2% topical solution; 0.6, 1, and 9 mg strips for topical application; and 5%, 10%, and 25% solutions for injection into the aqueous humor. The strips have the advantage of being used once and then discarded. The solution carries the risk of bacterial contamination if used for several different patients. Product names include Fluorescite, Funduscein-25, Ful-Glo, and Fluor-I-Strip.

Artificial Tear Solutions

Uses

Artificial tear solutions are products made to mimic natural secretions of the eye. They provide lubrication for dry eyes. They may also be used as lubricants for artificial eyes. Most products contain variable concentrations of methylcellulose, polyvinyl alcohol, and polyethylene glycol. The dosage is 1 to 3 drops in each eye 3 to 4 times daily, as needed. Product names include Isopto Plain, Lacril, Tears Naturale, Moisture Drops, and Liquifilm Tears Drops.

Ophthalmic Irrigants

Uses

These products are sterile solutions used for soothing and cleansing the eye, for removing foreign bodies, in conjunction with hard contact lenses, or with fluorescein. Product names include Eye-Stream, Lavoptik Eye Wash, Lauro Eye Wash, and Trisol Eye Wash.

CHAPTER REVIEW

The nurse has an important role in educating the public and promoting safety measures to protect the eyes from potential sources of injury. Examples of areas in which the nurse can teach the public are the use of safety glasses in potentially hazardous situations, prevention of chemical burns from common household cleansing items or other agents at home or work, proper cleaning and wearing of contact lenses or glasses, and the selection of safe toys and play activities for children. These safety measures can significantly reduce the number of injuries that occur annually.

MATH REVIEW

1. Ordered: 1.5 g/kg mannitol 15% solution, IV over 30 minutes.
   The patient weight is 156 pounds.
   The total dose of mannitol to administer would be:
   _____ g.

CRITICAL THINKING QUESTIONS

1. While working in the eye clinic, the nurse observes that several of the patients being treated for glaucoma complain that the medications cause pain and headache and that reading ability is diminished. How would the nurse respond to these statements?

2. Develop a teaching plan for a patient who is to self-administer Betoptic 1 drop twice daily.

Drugs Affecting Neoplasms

Objectives

1. Cite the goals of chemotherapy.

2. Explain the normal cycle for cell replication and describe the effects of cell cycle–specific and cell cycle–nonspecific drugs within this process.

3. Cite the rationale for giving chemotherapeutic drugs on a precise time schedule.

4. State which types of chemotherapeutic agents are cell-cycle specific and those that are cell-cycle nonspecific.

5. Study the nursing assessments and interventions needed for persons experiencing adverse effects from chemotherapy.

6. Develop patient education objectives for a patient receiving chemotherapy.

Key Words

cancer
metastases
cell-cycle specific

cell cycle-nonspecific
palliation

CANCER AND THE USE OF ANTINEOPLASTIC AGENTS

Cancer is a disorder of cellular growth. It is a group of abnormal cells that generally proliferate (multiply) more rapidly than do normal cells, lose the ability to perform specialized functions, invade surrounding tissues, and develop growths in other tissues distant to the site of original growth (**metastases**).

Cancer is a leading cause of death in the United States. Unfortunately, the number of persons dying from malignant diseases increases each year. The American Cancer Society estimates new cancer cases in *Facts and Figures* annually as a means of projecting cancer incidence for the upcoming year. Early diagnosis and treatment is still one of the most important factors in providing a more optimistic prognosis for those patients stricken with the many forms of neoplastic disease.

Treatment of cancer often requires a combination of surgery, radiation, chemotherapy, and immunotherapy. Recent advancements in carcinogenesis, cellular and molecular biology, and tumor immunology have enhanced the role that antineoplastic agents may play in therapy. It is beyond the scope of this chapter to delve into the interrelationships of chemotherapy and neoplastic disease; however, a short discussion of the concepts of cancer chemotherapy will be presented. As a result of rapidly changing approaches to the treatment of specific malignancies and the changing nature of chemotherapeutic regimens, specific agents and dosages have not been discussed.

All cells, whether normal or malignant, pass through a similar series of phases during their lifetime, although duration of time spent in each phase differs with the type of cell.

Mitosis is the phase of cellular proliferation in which the cell divides into two equal daughter cells. Phase G_1 follows mitosis and is considered a resting phase before the S phase, the stage of active DNA synthesis. Phase G_2 is a postsynthetic phase in which the cell contains a double complement of DNA. After a period of apparently minimal cellular activity in phase G_2, the mitosis phase again divides the cell into two G_1 daughter cells. The G_1 cells may advance again to the S phase or pass into a nonproliferative stage known as G_0. The time required to complete one cycle is called the generation time.

Many antineoplastic agents are **cell-cycle specific;** that is, the drug is selectively toxic when the cell is in a specific phase of growth. Thus those malignancies most amenable to chemotherapy proliferate rapidly. **Cell cycle–nonspecific** drugs are active throughout the cell cycle and may be more effective against slowly proliferating neoplastic tissue. One implication of cell-cycle specificity is the importance of correlating the dosage schedule of anticancer therapy with the known cellular kinetics of that type of neoplasm. Drugs are usually administered when the cell is most susceptible to the cytotoxic effects of the agent for a greater "kill rate" of neoplastic cells. Table 41-1 (see p. 511) lists the more common commercially available drugs, their dosage range, major toxicities, and major indications.

Drug Therapy

The overall goal of cancer chemotherapy is to give a dose large enough to be lethal (cytotoxic) to the cancer cells but small enough to be tolerable for normal cells. It is hoped that a long-term survival or cure can be achieved by this means. A second goal may be control of the disease (arresting of the tumor growth). When a cancer is beyond control, the goal of treatment may be **palliation** (alleviation) of symptoms. Finally, in some types of cancer in which no tumor is detectable yet the patient is known to be at risk of developing a particular cancer or having recurrence of a cancer, prophylactic chemotherapy may be administered.

Chemotherapy is most effective when the tumor is small and the cell replication is rapid. The cancer cells are the most sensitive to chemotherapy when the cells are dividing rapidly. This is when phase-specific drugs are most effectively used. As a tumor enlarges, more of the cells are in the resting G_0 phase. These cells respond better to phase-nonspecific chemotherapeutic agents. Combination therapy, using cell cycle–specific and cell cycle–nonspecific agents, is superior in therapeutic effect than the use of single-agent chemotherapy. The use of combination drug therapy allows for cell death during different phases of the cell cycle, but the agents often have toxic effects on different organs at different time intervals after administration. The choice of chemotherapeutic agents depends on the type of tumor cells, their rate of growth, and the size of the tumor.

Chemotherapeutic agents currently used are classified as alkylating agents, antimetabolites, natural products, and hormones. The mechanisms by which these agents cause cell death have not yet been fully determined.

Nursing Process for Chemotherapy

Assessment

History of risk factors

- Ask age, gender, and race. Take a family history of the incidence of cancer.
- Ask about job-related exposure to known chemical carcinogens (for example, benzene, vinyl chloride, asbestos, soots, tars, or oils).
- Ask about exposure to tobacco smoke. Obtain a history of the number of cigarettes or cigars smoked daily. How long has the person smoked? Has the person ever tried to stop smoking? How does the person feel about modifying the smoking habit? Is there chronic exposure to "passive" smoke at home or at work?
- Obtain a drug history to acquire information on pharmacologic agents that have the potential to become carcinogens (for example, diethylstilbestrol, cyclophosphamide, melphalan, and azathioprine).
- Ask about a history of viral diseases suspected of being associated with carcinogenesis (for example, Epstein-Barr virus, hepatitis B virus, and human immunodeficiency virus [HIV]).
- Is there a history of exposure to or treatment with radiation?

Dietary habits

- Take a dietary history. Ask specific questions to obtain data relating to foods eaten that are high in fat, animal protein (especially red meats; salt-cured, smoked, or charcoaled foods; and nitrate and nitrite additives). Are whole grains included in the diet? How many servings of fruits and vegetables are eaten daily? What types of vegetables are eaten daily? Estimate the number of calories consumed per day.
- Ask the patient about normal eating patterns, food likes and dislikes, and elimination pattern.
- Ask whether certain foods cause bloating, indigestion, or diarrhea, and how much seasoning and spices are put on food.
- What is the usual fluid intake daily? How much coffee, tea, soft drinks, and fruit juices are consumed? Determine the frequency and volume of alcoholic beverages consumed.
- Is the person experiencing anorexia, nausea, and vomiting? If so, what measures are being used to control these symptoms?
- Obtain a baseline height and weight. Has there been a weight gain or loss in the past year?

Preexisting health problems. Ask about any preexisting health problems for which the patient is or has been receiving treatment.

Diagnosis. • Ask the patient to explain his or her understanding of the current diagnosis and plan of treatment. • Review the admission notes or old charts to determine the details relating to the diagnostic test data, type of cancer, the staging of the disease, laboratory values, and treatments to date.

Adaptation to the diagnosis

- Determine whether this is the initial or a subsequent cycle of chemotherapy. Gather data regarding the patient's and support person's or family's understanding of the disease and the planned course of treatment.
- Ask how the patient normally copes with stressful situations. Does the patient have an individual in whom to confide who is supportive and understanding?
- Observe both the verbal and nonverbal messages conveyed during the interview. Take note of the patient's general appearance, tone of voice, inflections, and gestures. Try to pick up on subtle clues and confirm their meanings with the patient.
- Inquire regarding psychologic issues that the patient is perceiving—loss of control, self-esteem, body parts guilt, and so on.
- Review the physician's progress notes for information being imparted to the patient and family throughout the course of treatment.

Psychomotor functions. • Type of lifestyle. Ask the patient to describe exercise level in terms of amount tolerated, the degree of fatigue present, and the ability to perform activities of daily living. • Is the patient having any difficulty performing normal roles (for example, housewife, provider, mother, father)?

Safety. Assess for weakness, confusion, orthostatic hypotension, or similar symptoms that could signal impending potential for injury problems.

Symptoms of pharmacologic side effects. Ask specific questions to determine whether the individual has been or is experiencing symptoms associated with the type of drugs being administered, such as myelosuppression, anemia, bleeding, stomatitis, altered bowel patterns (diarrhea or constipation), alopecia, neurotoxicity, anorexia, nausea, or vomiting.

Physical assessment. • Perform a baseline physical, psychosocial, and spiritual assessment of the individual to serve as the database for ongoing assessments throughout the course of care. • Throughout the course of therapy perform daily assessments of the physical, psychosocial, and spiritual needs of the individual and family. Perform a focused assessment on the body systems affected by the disease process and those likely to be affected by metastasis.

Sexual assessment. Discuss birth control and reproductive counseling issues at the time of initiation of therapy. The couple may wish to use a sperm bank or begin a contraceptive method.

Pain. Ask whether the person is having any pain and what interventions are being used to manage the pain. Obtain a rating of pain level and the degree of relief being gained from current medications and supportive practices (for example, relaxation or guided imagery).

Nursing Diagnosis
* Infection, risk for (side effect)
* Nutrition, altered: less than body requirements (side effect)
* Activity intolerance (side effect)
* Injury, risk for (side effect)
* Knowledge deficit (chemotherapy treatment, side effects)
* Body-image alterations (side effect)

Planning
History of risk factors. Review assessment data to determine needed interventions for the individual and support persons.

Dietary habits. After obtaining the dietary history, develop a plan to meet the individual's nutritional needs based on the number of calories being eaten, current weight, and calculated needs to meet the demands of the disease process. Consult with dietitian as appropriate to circumstances.

Smoking. Discuss smoking habits with the patient, and plan a mutually agreeable way to handle this habit, both while hospitalized and when at home. Does the patient wish to modify the habit?

Preexisting health problems. Plan interventions to continue treatment of any preexisting health problems (for example, angina, congestive heart failure, or asthma).

Diagnosis and adaptation to diagnosis. Analyze data to determine effectiveness of current coping strategies being used to adapt to the diagnosis. Attempt to identify adaptive coping strategies that could be tried when maladaptive ones are evident.

Psychomotor functions. • Schedule nursing care needs so the individual will have adequate rest periods between needed care delivery. • Plan a referral to social services for needed guidance for the patient or support persons to assist in the management of problems relating to inability to work, home care, and so forth.

Safety. Determine the amount of assistance needed with self-care, ambulation, and so on, and mark the Kardex clearly so that all caregivers will provide adequately for the individual's safety needs.

Symptoms of pharmacologic side effects. Research the specific drugs prescribed to identify the usual side effects to expect, and plan to institute measures to minimize or prevent their occurrence.

Physical assessment. Schedule physical, psychosocial, and spiritual assessments on a regular basis. Usually these are done once per shift while hospitalized and more frequently when specific problems exist.

Medication administration
* Plan drug administration exactly at the time intervals prescribed to promote maximum cytotoxicity of the chemotherapy agents and maximum effectiveness of drug therapy. See individual drug monographs.
* Review drug orders for any premedication or hydration prescribed, and schedule initiation at appropriate intervals in advance of the chemotherapy.
* Schedule oral hygiene measures using prescribed local anesthetic and antimicrobial solutions. Perform before and after meals and at bedtime if symptoms are mild. With moderate lesions, increase the frequency to every 2 hours. In patients with severe symptoms, the mouth is rinsed hourly while the patient is awake.

Implementation
* Implement planned interventions consistent with assessment data and identified individual needs of the patient (for example, nutritional support, blood component therapy, growth factor therapy, fatigue, alopecia, anemia, constipation, diarrhea, nausea and vomiting, neutropenia, pain, and thrombocytopenia).
* Examine laboratory data on a continuum. Monitor for the development of cancer emergencies (for example, hypercalcemia, superior vena cava syndrome, or disseminated intravascular coagulation).
* Monitor vital signs, including temperature, pulse, respirations, and blood pressure, at least every shift or more frequently depending on recommended monitoring parameters of specific drugs prescribed.
* Hydration: Monitor the patient's state of hydration. Check skin turgor, mucous membranes, and softness of the eyeballs. Electrolyte reports require vigilant observation; report abnormal findings to the physician. Fluid replacement via intravenous (IV) administration or total parenteral nutrition may be appropriate in some circumstances.
* Infection: Report even the slightest sign of infection for evaluation (for example, elevating temperature, chills, malaise, hypotension, and pallor).
* Nausea, vomiting: There are three patterns of emesis associated with antineoplastic therapy: acute, delayed, and anticipatory. (See Chapter 31 for the treatment of nausea and vomiting associated with chemotherapy.)

  Chart the degree of effectiveness achieved when antiemetics are given. Report poor control to the physician. Changing the antiemetic medication ordered or the route of administration may improve control. Patients experiencing nausea and vomiting must be weighed daily and monitored for electrolyte values and accurate intake and output.
* Positioning: Hospitalized patients may be sedated. Position the patient on one side to prevent aspiration.
* Diarrhea: Record the color, frequency, and consistency of stool. Include an estimate of the volume of watery stools in the output record. Check for occult blood. Provide for

adequate hydration, and administer any drugs ordered to relieve the symptoms.

Encourage adequate fluid intake and dietary alterations, such as eliminating spicy foods and those high in fat content. It may be necessary to switch to a clear liquid diet followed by a diet low in roughage. Diarrhea may require high-protein foods with high caloric value and vitamin and mineral supplements. Patients with diarrhea should be weighed daily and monitored for fluid intake and output and electrolyte values.

Check the anal area for irritation, provide for hygiene measures, and protect from excoriation with products such as A and D ointment or zinc oxide ointment.

- Constipation: Compare this symptom with the patient's usual pattern of elimination. Many persons do not normally defecate daily.

Perform daily assessment of bowel sounds when the patient is hospitalized. When a patient is constipated, the physician usually orders stool softeners or laxatives, fluids, and a diet that enhances normal defecation. Observe carefully for signs of an impaction (the urge to defecate with little to no stool or seepage of watery stool.)

- Stomatitis: Use meticulous oral hygiene measures. (See Chapter 29.)
- Bleeding: Observe and report signs and symptoms of bleeding, for example, epistaxis, hematuria, bruises, petechiae, dark tarry stools, "coffee ground" emesis, or blurred vision. Instruct female patients to report menstrual flow that is excessive, bright in color, or lasts for a prolonged period of time. Check laboratory reports for changes in hematologic status, electrolytes, and so on; report abnormal or changing values to the physician.
- Pain. Administer pain medications prescribed at scheduled intervals to maintain a constant blood level of the analgesic and thereby promote maximum pain control. Maintain a record of pain medications administered and the patient's rating of the degree of pain relief achieved. (See Chapter 18.)

Report insufficient pain relief. Obtain orders for the treatment of the pain, or institute prn analgesics prescribed for "breakthrough" pain episodes.

- Anxiety: Monitor the degree of anxiety being exhibited, and intervene appropriately to alleviate. Give prescribed medications; discuss issues about which the patient or significant others are concerned. Keep the patient involved in making appropriate decisions regarding self-care to give some degree of control over the situation; discuss when prescribed treatments are to be performed.

Implement relaxation techniques (use of biofeedback, visual imagery) as prescribed. Deal with stress-related issues that arise within the support or family group.

Patient Education and Health Promotion
Nutrition
- Teach the patient specific ways to implement dietary needs (for example, ways to support increased protein and caloric intake such as adding powdered milk to puddings, creamed soups, and so on). Suggest using nutritional supplements such as Ensure or Carnation Instant Breakfast. Suggest obtaining educational materials from the American Cancer Society on dietary interventions during the treatment of cancer.

- If the patient is receiving enteral tube feedings, peripheral parenteral nutrition, or total parenteral nutrition, arrange for necessary at-home support for administration and monitoring of therapy.

Preexisting health problems. Continue prescribed medications and regimens for preexisting health problems.

Diagnosis and adaptation to diagnosis
- Encourage the patient and support group to discuss concerns about the disease, prognosis, and treatment.
- Present the patient with appropriate choices that allow involvement in the decisions concerning selection of care. Encourage the patient to maintain the best health possible. Include the patient in selection of diet, planning activities, scheduling rest periods, and personal care. Stress what the patient *can* do, not what the patient cannot do.
- Limit the amount of information to the facts that are significant at this point in the care plan and to the degree of symptoms present. Emphasize the prevention of complications through maintenance of nutrition and hydration and commitment to hygiene practices.

Psychomotor. Discuss activities the patient is able to perform independently and those requiring assistance. Provide for patient safety on a continuum. Include the support group in the development of a plan to provide for self-care at home. Arrange appropriate referrals to support the self-care needs of the person in the home environment.

Nausea and vomiting. • Teach the person when and how to take prescribed antiemetics. • Make suggestions for comfort measures to minimize nausea (for example, rinsing mouth frequently, cool cloth to wash face, and relaxation and distraction techniques). • Teach the patient to take weight daily and give parameters of weight loss that must be reported to the physician.

Diarrhea or constipation
- Teach the patient the proper use of prn medications prescribed to treat either constipation or diarrhea.
- Explain measures to prevent constipation, such as drinking sufficient fluids daily, eating high-fiber foods, and avoiding foods that cause constipation. Instruct the individual to report failure to have stools in a usual pattern of elimination or seeping, loose watery stools while feeling the need to defecate (may be an indication of an impaction).
- When diarrhea is present, instruct the patient to avoid foods that irritate or stimulate peristalsis, for example, coffee, tea, and hot or cold beverages. Encourage the increased intake of potassium-containing foods. Teach personal hygiene measures to provide for skin care and to prevent skin breakdown.

Neutropenia
- Explain the measures the individual should initiate to minimize the chance of infection when neutropenia is present (for example, hand washing; avoidance of exposure to individuals known to have an infection; no fresh flowers, vegetables, or receptacles with freestanding water such as denture cups or humidifiers; and avoidance of persons receiving immunizations and pets).
- Teach signs and symptoms of infection and when to report symptoms present. Be certain the person understands how to take temperature and that even minor elevations should be reported.

- Teach self-care of central lines, when present, consistent with the patient or significant others' abilities to perform the procedure while maintaining strict aseptic technique. Arrange for referral to community or home care agency as indicated.

Pain

- Discuss beliefs about pain with the patient, family, and significant others as a baseline for health teaching needed.
- Instruct the patient to record the intensity of the pain being experienced and degree of pain relief being obtained from prescribed medications. (See Chapter 18 for a pain scale.)
- Emphasize the need to report pain that is not being controlled or new symptoms of pain being felt.
- Stress the importance of taking pain medications at prescribed intervals to obtain maximum relief.
- Determine whether the patient has access to medications for pain. (Does the patient have sufficient money to purchase or obtain prescribed medication?)
- Stress the need to start stool softeners and to take them regularly to prevent constipation when morphine or codeine therapy is used.
- Oral medications are frequently used to provide pain relief. Several analgesics are also available as rectal suppositories. (Pain control must be achieved. When oral and rectal forms of pain management no longer suffice, patients may require hospitalization for stabilization on parenteral forms of narcotic analgesics. Infusion pumps are frequently used, and spinal morphine may be delivered effectively via epidural or intrathecal catheters. Patients must understand that they can be kept comfortable.)

Anemia. Teach the patient the possible causes and related self-care needed when anemia is present (for example, management of fatigue by spacing of activities and prevention of orthostatic hypotension by rising slowly, sitting and resting, and then standing). Instruct the patient not to drive or operate power equipment for safety reasons.

Thrombocytopenia. • Teach self-monitoring for other blood-related symptoms (for example, bleeding, bruising, hematuria, epistaxis, coffee ground emesis, or excessive or prolonged menstrual flow). • Suggest safety measures when at home (for example, avoiding use of sharp knives, shaving with an electric razor, or wearing a thimble when sewing). • Stress that the patient should not take any aspirin or aspirin-containing products.

Anxiety. Assist the patient to practice stress reduction techniques, and make the patient aware of cancer support resources available (for example, Make Today Count).

Fostering health maintenance

- Throughout the course of treatment, discuss medication information and how the medication will benefit the patient.
- Drug therapy will be individualized for the patient and type of cancer being treated. The need to follow the established regimen precisely must be emphasized to obtain maximum cytotoxic effects while minimizing side effects. Side effects to the drug therapy should be expected, and the patient and significant others must be educated in the management of the side effects to expect and those that should be reported. Additional teaching must be individualized to the patient for equipment used to administer drug therapy or nutritional support.
- Seek cooperation and understanding of the following points so that medication compliance is increased: name of medication, dosage, route and times of administration, side effects to expect, and side effects to report.
- Patients should be encouraged to maintain basic good health practices throughout treatment (for example, adequate rest, exercise consistent with abilities, stress management or stress reduction techniques, and maintenance of usual spiritual beliefs).
- Enlist the patient's aid in developing and maintaining a written record of monitoring parameters (nausea, vomiting, pain relief, constipation, diarrhea, and so on). (See box on p. 510.) Instruct the patient to bring the written record to follow-up visits.

Drug Class: Alkylating Agents

Actions

The alkylating agents are highly reactive chemical compounds that bond with DNA molecules, causing cross-linking of DNA strands. The interstrand binding prevents the separation of the double-coiled DNA molecule that is necessary for cellular division. Alkylating agents are cell-cycle nonspecific—that is, they are capable of combining with cellular components at any phase of the cell cycle. Generally, the development of resistance to one alkylating agent imparts cross-resistance to other alkylators.

Uses

See Table 41-1.

Therapeutic Outcomes

The primary therapeutic outcome from alkylating agent therapy is eradication of malignant cells.

Nursing Process

Premedication Assessment

1. Check laboratory reports for baseline data reflecting hepatic and renal function.
2. Assess the patient's state of hydration, and review doctor's orders for oral and intravenous hydration instructions before drug therapy (for example, cisplatin). Initiate intake and output monitoring if not already in effect.
3. Administer prechemotherapy drugs prescribed at time intervals specified (for example, mesna).
4. Review laboratory data for baseline hematologic studies that reflect the degree of myelosuppression present before initiation of chemotherapy.
5. Discuss birth control methods and sperm storage before initiation of therapy.

Drug Class: Antimetabolites

Actions

The antimetabolites (subclassified as folic acid, purine, and pyrimidine antagonists) inhibit key enzymes in the biosynthetic pathways of DNA and RNA synthesis. Many of the antagonists are cell-cycle specific, killing cells during the S phase of cell maturation.

Text continues on p. 516.

PATIENT EDUCATION & MONITORING FORM   Antineoplastic Agents

MEDICATIONS	COLOR	TO BE TAKEN

Name _____

Physician _____

Physician's phone _____

Next appt.* _____

PARAMETERS		DAY OF DISCHARGE								COMMENTS
Temperature	AM / PM									
Pain level — Severe 10, Moderate 5, None 1	8 AM									
	Noon									
	6 PM									
	Night									
Fatigue level — Exhausted with minimal activities 10, Tired with performance of activities of daily living 5, Normal 1										
Fear and anxiety — Anxious 10, 5, Calm 1										
Nausea: Degree of relief — Good 10, Moderate 5, Poor 1	Time of day									
Appetite — Good 10, Normal 5, Poor 1										
Oral hygiene — Normal 10, Moderate pain 5, Severe pain 1										
Bleeding (Yes or No)	Nosebleeds									
	Bruising									
Bowel movements	Color: brown, tarry									
	Diarrhea: Number of stools									
	Normal									

*Please bring this record with you to your next appointment.
Use the back of this sheet for additional information.

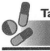

Table 41-1

Cancer Chemotherapeutic Agents

		TOXICITY		
DRUG	**USUAL DOSAGE**	**ACUTE**	**DELAYED**	**MAJOR INDICATIONS**
Alkylating agents				
Busulfan (Myleran)	2-8 mg/day for 2-3 wk PO; stop for recovery; then maintenance	None	Bone marrow depression	Chronic granulocytic leukemia
Carboplatin (Paraplatin)	360 mg/m² every 4 wk	Nausea, vomiting	Bone marrow suppression, anemia, nephrotoxicity	Ovarian carcinoma
Carmustine (BCNU; ✿ BiCNU)	As single agent: 100-200 mg/m² IV; over 1-2 hr infusion every 6-8 wk In combination: 30-60 mg/m² IV Use gloves because solution may cause skin discoloration	Nausea and vomiting; pain along vein of infusion	Granulocyte and platelet suppression Hepatic and renal toxicity	Brain, colon, breast, lung, Hodgkin's disease, lymphosarcoma, myeloma, malignant melanoma
Chlorambucil (Leukeran)	Start 0.1-0.2 mg/kg/day PO; adjust for maintenance	None	Bone marrow depression (anemia, leukopenia, thrombocytopenia) can be severe with excessive dosage	Chronic lymphocytic leukemia, Hodgkin's disease, non-Hodgkin's lymphoma, trophoblastic neoplasms
Cisplatin (Platinol)	20-100 mg/m² IV; frequency highly variable	Nausea, vomiting	Nephrotoxicity, ototoxicity, blurred vision, changes in color perception	Testicular and ovarian cancers; bladder cancer
Cyclophosphamide (Cytoxan)	40-50 mg/kg IV in single or in 2-8 daily doses or 2-4 mg/kg/day PO for 10 days; adjust for maintenance	Nausea and vomiting	Bone marrow depression, alopecia, cystitis	Hodgkin's disease and other lymphomas, multiple myeloma, lymphocytic leukemia, many solid cancers
Fludarabine (Fludara)	25 mg/m² daily IV over 30 min for 5 days	Nausea, vomiting	Fever, chills, cough, edema, rash	Chronic lymphocytic leukemia; lymphomas, Hodgkin's disease
Ifosfamide (Ifex)	1.2 g/m²/day for 5 days IV	Nausea, vomiting, diarrhea	Hematuria, alopecia	Testicular, lung, breast, ovarian, pancreatic, gastric cancer
Lomustine (CCNU) CeeNU	130 mg/m² PO once every 6 wk	Severe nausea and vomiting; anorexia	Thrombocytopenia, leukopenia, alopecia, confusion, lethargy, ataxia	Brain, colon, Hodgkin's disease, lymphosarcoma, malignant melanoma
Mechlorethamine (nitrogen mustard; Mustargen)	0.4 mg/kg IV in single or divided doses	Nausea and vomiting	Moderate depression of peripheral blood count	Hodgkin's disease and other lymphomas, bronchogenic carcinoma

✿ Available in Canada only.

continued

Table 41-1

Cancer Chemotherapeutic Agents—cont'd

DRUG	USUAL DOSAGE	TOXICITY		MAJOR INDICATIONS
		ACUTE	**DELAYED**	
Alkylating agents—cont'd				
Melphalan (Alkeran)	0.25 mg/kg/day for 4 days PO; 2-4 mg/day as maintenance or 0.1-0.15 mg/kg/day for 2-3 wk	None	Bone marrow depression	Multiple myeloma, malignant melanoma, ovarian carcinoma, testicular seminoma
Streptozocin (Zanosar)	As single agent: 1.0-1.5 mg/m^2/wk for 6 consecutive wk with 4 wk of observation In combination: 400-500 mg/m^2 for 4-5 consecutive days with 6 wk of observation	Hypoglycemia, severe nausea and vomiting	Moderate but transient renal and hepatic toxicity, hypoglycemia, mild anemia, leukopenia	Pancreatic islet cell tumors
Thiotepa	0.2 mg/kg IV for 5 days	None	Bone marrow depression	Hodgkin's disease, bronchogenic and breast carcinomas
Antimetabolites				
Cytarabine hydrochloride (Cytosar)	2-3 mg/kg/day IV until response or toxicity or 1-3 mg/kg IV over 24 hr for up to 10 days	Nausea and vomiting	Bone marrow depression megaloblastosis	Acute leukemia
Fluorouracil (5-FU, FU)	12.5 mg/kg/day IV for 3-5 days or 15 mg/kg/wk for 6 wk	Nausea	Oral and GI ulceration, stomatitis and diarrhea, bone marrow depression	Breast, large bowel, ovarian carcinoma
Mercaptopurine (6-MP, Purinethol)	2.5 mg/kg/day PO	Occasional nausea and vomiting, usually well tolerated	Bone marrow depression, occasional hepatic damage	Acute lymphocytic and granulocytic leukemia, chronic granulocytic leukemia
Methotrexate (MTX)	2.5-5.0 mg/day PO; 0.4 mg/kg rapid IV daily 4-5 days (not over 25 mg) or 0.4 mg/kg rapid IV twice/wk	Occasional diarrhea, hepatic necrosis	Oral and GI ulceration, bone marrow depression (anemia, leukopenia, thrombocytopenia), cirrhosis	Acute lymphocytic leukemia, choriocarcinoma, carcinoma of cervix and head and neck area, mycosis fungoides, solid cancers
Thioguanine ✤ (Lanvis)	2 mg/kg/day PO	Occasional nausea and vomiting, usually well tolerated	Bone marrow depression	Acute leukemia

✤ Available in Canada only.

continued

Table 41-1

Cancer Chemotherapeutic Agents—cont'd

| | | TOXICITY | | |
| | | ACUTE | DELAYED | |
DRUG	USUAL DOSAGE	ACUTE	DELAYED	MAJOR INDICATIONS
Natural products				
Etoposide (VePesid)	50-100 mg/m^2 daily for 5 days IV; cycles of therapy are given every 3-4 wk	Nausea (15%), vomiting, stomatitis, diarrhea	Leukopenia, nadir in 10-14 days, recovery in 3 wk; thrombocytopenia; alopecia	Testicular tumors, small cell carcinoma of the lung, Hodgkin's disease and non-Hodgkin's lymphoma, acute nonlymphocytic leukemia, breast carcinoma, Kaposi's sarcoma
Vinblastine sulfate (Velban; ✿ Velbe)	0.1-0.2 mg/kg/wk IV or every 2 wk	Nausea and vomiting, local irritant	Alopecia, stomatitis, bone marrow depression, loss of reflexes	Hodgkin's disease and other lymphomas, solid cancers
Vincristine sulfate (Oncovin)	0.01-0.03 mg/kg/ wk IV	Local irritant	Areflexia, peripheral neuritis, paralytic ileus, mild bone marrow depression	Acute lymphocytic leukemia, Hodgkin's disease and other lymphomas, solid cancers
Antibiotics				
Bleomycin (Blenoxane)	10-15 mg/m^2 once or twice a wk, IV or IM to total dose 300-400 mg	Nausea and vomiting, fever, very toxic	Edema of hands, pulmonary fibrosis, stomatitis, alopecia	Hodgkin's disease, non-Hodgkin's lymphoma, squamous cell carcinoma of head and neck, testicular carcinoma
Dactinomycin (actinomycin D; Cosmegen)	0.015-0.05 mg/kg/ wk (1-2.5 mg) for 3-5 wk IV; wait for marrow recovery (3-4 wk), then repeat course	Nausea and vomiting, local irritant	Stomatitis, oral ulcers, diarrhea, alopecia, mental depression, bone marrow depression	Testicular carcinoma, Wilms' tumor, rhabdomyosarcoma, Ewing's and osteogenic sarcoma, and other solid tumors
Daunorubicin (Cerubidine)	30-45 mg/m^2/day for 2 or 3 days of combination therapy; never give IM or SC	Nausea, vomiting, diarrhea, fever, chills	Bone marrow suppression, reversible alopecia	Acute nonlymphocytic leukemia in adults; acute lymphocytic leukemia in children and adults
Doxorubicin (Adriamycin)	60-90 mg/m^2 IV, single dose or over 3 days; repeat every 3 wk up to total dose 500 mg/m^2	Nausea, red urine (not hematuria)	Bone marrow depression, cardiotoxicity, alopecia, stomatitis	Soft tissue, osteogenic and miscellaneous sarcomas, Hodgkin's disease, non-Hodgkin's lymphoma, bronchogenic and breast carcinoma, thyroid cancer, leukemias

✿ Available in Canada only.

continued

Table 41-1

Cancer Chemotherapeutic Agents—cont'd

| | | TOXICITY | | |
DRUG	USUAL DOSAGE	ACUTE	DELAYED	MAJOR INDICATIONS
Antibiotics—cont'd				
Idarubicin (Idamycin)	12 mg/m²/day for 3 days by slow (10-15 min) IV; do not give IM or SC	Nausea, vomiting, diarrhea	Bone marrow suppression, cardiotoxicity, mucositis, hemorrhage	Acute myelocytic leukemia
Mitomycin C (Mutamycin)	0.05 mg/kg/day IV for 5 days	Nausea and vomiting, flulike syndrome	Bone marrow depression, skin toxicity; pulmonary, renal, CNS effects	Squamous cell carcinoma of head and neck, lungs, and cervix; adenocarcinoma of the stomach, pancreas, colon, rectum; adenocarcinoma and duct cell carcinoma of the breast
Mitoxantrone (Novantrone)	12 mg/m²/day for 2-3 days by IV infusion	Nausea, vomiting, diarrhea	Heart failure; GI bleeding; cough, dyspnea	Acute nonlymphocytic leukemia, non-Hodgkin's lymphoma, breast cancer
Plicamycin (Mithracin)	0.025-0.050 mg/kg every 2 days for up to 8 doses IV	Nausea and vomiting, hepatotoxicity	Bone marrow depression (thrombocytopenia), hypocalcemia	Testicular carcinoma, trophoblastic neoplasms
Other synthetic agents				
Altretamine (Hexalen) ✿ (Hexastat)	260 mg/m²/day for 14 or 21 days in a 28 day cycle; give daily doses as 4 divided oral doses	Nausea, vomiting	Anemia, leukopenia, thrombocytopenia, peripheral neuropathy	Ovarian cancer
Dacarbazine (DTIC-Dome; DIC)	4.5 mg/kg/day IV for 10 days; repeated every 28 days	Nausea and vomiting, flulike syndrome	Bone marrow depression (rare)	Metastatic malignant melanoma
Hydroxyurea (Hydrea)	80 mg/kg PO single dose every 3 days or 20-30 mg/kg/day PO	Mild nausea and vomiting	Bone marrow depression	Chronic granulocytic leukemia
Interferon alfa-2a (Roferon-a)	3 million units daily IM or SC	Flulike syndrome	Bone marrow depression	Hairy cell leukemia
Interferon alfa-2b (Intron a)	2 million μ/m² IM or SC 3 times/wk	Flulike syndrome	Bone marrow depression	Hairy cell leukemia
Interferon (alfa-n3)	Highly variable	Fever, muscle aches, headache, nausea	Bone marrow suppression	Condylomata acuminata; carcinoid tumor; non-Hodgkin's lymphoma
Levamisole (Ergamisol)	50 mg PO every 8 hr for 3 days every 2 wk	Nausea, diarrhea	Dermatitis, alopecia, leukopenia	Colon cancer
Leuprolide acetate (Lupron)	1 mg SC daily	Hot flashes; initial exacerbation of symptoms	Arrhythmias, edema	Prostatic carcinoma, breast carcinoma

✿ Available in Canada only.

continued

Table 41-1

Cancer Chemotherapeutic Agents—cont'd

		TOXICITY		
DRUG	**USUAL DOSAGE**	**ACUTE**	**DELAYED**	**MAJOR INDICATIONS**
Other synthetic agents—cont'd				
Mitotane (Lysodren)	6-15 mg/kg/day PO	Nausea and vomiting	Dermatitis, diarrhea, mental depression	Adrenal cortical carcinoma
Procarbazine hydrochloride (Matulane; ✿ Natulan)	Start 1-2 mg/kg/day PO; increase over 1 wk to 3 mg/kg; maintain for 3 wk, then reduce to 2 mg/kg/day until toxicity	Nausea and vomiting	Bone marrow depression, CNS depression	Hodgkin's disease, non-Hodgkin's lymphoma, bronchogenic carcinoma
Tamoxifen (Nolvadex)	20-40 mg daily in two divided doses	Nausea, vomiting, hot flashes	Increased bone and tumor pain, thrombocytopenia, leukopenia, edema, hypercalcemia	Breast cancer (estrogen sensitive)
Hormones				
Diethylstilbestrol (DES)	15 mg/day PO (1 mg in prostate cancer)	None	Fluid retention, hypercalcemia, feminization, uterine bleeding; if during pregnancy, may cause vaginal carcinoma in offspring	Breast and prostate carcinomas
Ethinyl estradiol	3 mg/day PO	None	Fluid retention, hypercalcemia, feminization, uterine bleeding	Breast and prostate carcinomas
Fluoxymesterone (Halotestin)	10-20 mg/day PO	None	Fluid retention, masculinization, cholestatic jaundice	Breast carcinoma
Flutamide (Eulexin) ✿ (Euflex)	2 capsules PO 3 times daily at 8 hr intervals	Nausea, vomiting	Hot flashes, loss of libido, impotence, gynecomastia	Metastatic prostatic carcinoma
Goserelin (Zoladex)	3.6 mg SC every 28 days in upper abdominal wall; local anesthesia may be used	Anorexia, dizziness, pain	Hot flashes, sexual dysfunction	Carcinoma of the prostate
Hydroxyprogesterone caproate	1 g IM twice a wk	None	None	Endometrial carcinoma
Medroxyprogesterone acetate	100-200 mg/day PO; 200-600 mg twice a wk	None	None	Endometrial carcinoma, renal cell, breast cancer
Prednisone	10-100 mg/day PO	None	Hyperadrenocorticism	Acute and chronic lymphocytic leukemia, Hodgkin's disease, non-Hodgkin's lymphomas
Testolactone (Teslac)	100 mg 3 times a wk IM	None	Fluid retention, masculinization	Breast carcinoma
Testosterone enanthate	600-1200 mg/wk IM	None	Fluid retention, masculinization	Breast carcinoma
Testosterone propionate	50-100 mg, IM 3 times a wk	None	Fluid retention, masculinization	Breast carcinoma

CNS, Central nervous system; *GI,* gastrointestinal.

✿ Available in Canada only.

Uses

See Table 41-1.

Therapeutic Outcome

The primary therapeutic outcome from antimetabolite therapy is eradication of malignant cells.

Nursing Process

Premedication Assessment

1. Check laboratory reports for baseline data reflecting hepatic and renal function.
2. Assess gastrointestinal symptoms before initiation of therapy to serve as baseline data, for example, status of mouth (ulcerations and stomatitis), bowel pattern (diarrhea), anorexia, nausea, and vomiting.
3. Review baseline laboratory data for degree of myelosuppression present.
4. Discuss birth control methods and sperm storage before initiation of therapy.

Drug Class: Natural Products

Actions

Vinca Alkaloids

Vincristine and vinblastine are natural derivatives of the periwinkle plant. They are cell cycle–specific agents that block the formation of the mitotic spindle during mitosis, thus inhibiting cell division. Even though there is close structural similarity, cross-resistance does not usually develop between the two agents.

Antibiotics

Through various mechanisms, the antibiotics bind with cellular DNA, preventing its replication as well as RNA synthesis, which is required for subsequent protein synthesis.

Uses

See Table 41-1.

Therapeutic Outcome

The primary therapeutic outcome from natural product therapy is eradication of malignant cells.

Nursing Process

Premedication Assessment

1. Check laboratory reports for baseline data reflecting hepatic function.
2. Assess for peripheral neuropathy, mentation, orientation, gait, and motor weakness before initiation of therapy with the natural products.
3. Assess the patient's history for cardiac disease before use of antineoplastic antibiotics. Report presence to the physician before initiation of therapy.
4. Assess respiratory function and review the chart for any tests that may indicate compromised respiratory function before treatment with bleomycin.

5. Review baseline laboratory data for degree of myelosuppression present.
6. Discuss birth control methods and sperm storage before initiation of therapy.

Drug Class: Hormones

Actions

Corticosteroids (usually prednisone) may be beneficial in treating lymphomas and acute leukemia because of their lympholytic effects and their ability to suppress mitosis in lymphocytes. Steroids are also used to help reduce edema secondary to radiation therapy and as palliative therapy in temporarily suppressing fever, diaphoresis, and pain and in restoring, to some degree, appetite, weight, strength, and a sense of well-being in critically ill patients. With symptomatic relief, it is hoped that the patient's general physical condition may be improved sufficiently to permit further definitive therapy.

Uses

Estrogens and androgens are used in malignancies of sexual organs based on the assumption that these malignancies have hormonal requirements similar to those of nonmalignant sexual organs. Estrogens (usually diethylstilbestrol) may be used in prostatic carcinoma. There are regressions in the primary tumor and in soft tissue metastases, with significant symptomatic relief from the point of view of the patient. Androgens may be used in the treatment of metastatic breast cancer in any age group, and estrogens may be used in postmenopausal women with metastatic breast cancer. (See Table 41-1.)

Therapeutic Outcomes

The primary therapeutic outcome from hormone therapy is reduction in rate of growth and proliferation of malignant cells.

Nursing Process

Premedication Assessment

1. Obtain baseline weight and vital signs, especially blood pressure.
2. Discuss birth control methods and sperm storage before initiation of therapy.
3. Check baseline electrolytes (for example, calcium with diethylstilbestrol, tamoxifen, and testosterone).

CHAPTER REVIEW

Nurses play a crucial role in the treatment of patients with cancer. No other disease seems to evoke fear and anxiety equal to the effect that the diagnosis of cancer has on the patient and family. Nurses are often the contact between the physician, patient, and family in helping with adaptation to the diagnosis and entry into the health care system for treatment. Nurses are often the first persons to identify complications of therapy, such as recognizing and reporting early symptoms of infection in an immunocompromised patient. Early recognition and prompt action often reduce the severity of the complications. Nurses are active providers of public information on wellness. They also co-ordinate screening programs for the early detection of cancer.

MATH REVIEW

1. Ordered: cefazolin 1 g IV, q8h.
   On hand: cefazolin 1 g diluted in 50 ml 5% D/W
   To administer this medication over a 30-minute period on a pump that is calibrated in milliliters per hour, at what rate would the pump be set?

2. Ordered: PCA morphine sulfate 1 mg per dose with 6-minute lockout. Maximum 30 mg q4h.
   Discuss how to initiate the PCA setup on this patient, how to set up the initial settings on the PCA pump, and when and how to record the amount of morphine sulfate used each shift.

CRITICAL THINKING QUESTIONS

Situation:
Mr. Kentworth, age 65, has small cell cancer of the lung with brain and liver metastases. He has had several grand mal seizures in the past month.

His orders read:
1. Daily weight.
2. Assist with ambulation as tolerated.
3. Routine vitals.
4. Seizure precautions.
5. Intake and output.
6. Heparin lock the IV.
7. Physical therapy consult to assist with plan for self-care at home.
8. IV site dressing change every 72 hours.

9. Medications:
   Folic acid 1 mg PO, daily.
   Multivitamin 1, PO, daily.
   Ensure 1 can TID.
   KCl 20 mEq, PO, BID.
   Normal saline flush 2.5 ml, heparin lock after meds.
   Ranitidine 300 mg PO hs.
   Ondansetron 32 mg IV 30 minutes before chemotherapy.
   Dexamethasone 4 mg IV q12h.
   Phenytoin 200 mg, PO daily.
   Lorazepam 1 mg PO q12h.

Develop a Kardex for this patient and a medication administration record (MAR) that includes the scheduling of each medication.

For each medication prescribed, state the action, side effects to expect, and side effects to report.

For IV medications prescribed, state the action, rate of administration, dilution for administration, monitoring required, and what type of IV setup would be required to initiate the IV delivery of the medications.
Situation:
Mrs. Oakley, age 68, has gastric cancer with liver metastasis. She has the following medication orders:
   5% D/0.45% NS at 100 ml per hour.
   Ondansetron 32 mg IV in 50 ml 5% D/W to run for 15 minutes.
   Cisplatin 35 mg in 250 ml NS to run for 30 minutes.
   Add mannitol 12.5 g to cisplatin.
   Leucovorin 20 mg IV push.

To carry out these orders, what type of an IV setup would be required? Because you are not "chemo certified" and could not start the chemotherapy drugs as a student nurse, what nursing responsibilities would you have during the execution of these drug orders? What is the action of each medication, side effects to expect, and side effects to report?

How would you set a pump to deliver the ondansetron in 15 minutes? (The pump is calibrated in milliliters per hour.) What rate would the same type of pump be set at to administer the cisplatin?

Drugs Used to Treat the Muscular System

Key Words

cerebral palsy
multiple sclerosis
neuromuscular blocking agents
hypercapnia

muscle spasticity
hyperreflexia
clonus
stroke syndrome

Objectives

1. Prepare a list of assessment data needed to evaluate a patient with a skeletal muscle disorder.

2. State the nursing assessments needed to monitor therapeutic response and the development of side effects to expect and report from skeletal muscle relaxant therapy.

3. Develop a health teaching plan for patients with skeletal muscle relaxant therapy.

4. Describe the effect of centrally acting skeletal muscle relaxants on the central nervous system and the safety precautions required during use.

5. Describe essential components of patient assessment used for patients receiving neuromuscular blocking agents.

6. State where information on the use of these agents is found in the patient's chart.

7. List the equipment that should be available in the immediate patient care area when neuromuscular blocking agents are to be administered.

8. Describe the physiologic effects of neuromuscular blocking agents.

9. Cite four uses of neuromuscular blocking agents.

10. Identify the effect of neuromuscular blocking agents on consciousness, memory, and the pain threshold.

11. Describe disease conditions that may affect the patient's ability to tolerate the use of neuromuscular blocking agents.

12. List steps required to treat respiratory depression.

MUSCLE RELAXANTS AND NEUROMUSCULAR BLOCKING AGENTS

Nursing Process for Skeletal Muscle Relaxants and Neuromuscular Blocking Agents

Assessment

Assessment for skeletal muscle disorders. Musculoskeletal disorders may produce varying degrees of pain and immobility impairing the individual's ability to perform the activities of daily living. The nursing assessments performed are individualized to the muscles affected and the underlying disease.

Current history. • What is the reason for seeking treatment now? Request a brief history of any symptoms present. • What is the degree of impairment present (for example, strength, gait, conservation effect, and compensatory action)? • Assess the pain level and extent, frequency of analgesic use, precipitating factors, and any measures the patient has identified that alleviate pain. • Assess the extent of muscle spasticity and the muscle groups affected.

History. • Ask the patient to describe diagnoses that cause musculoskeletal impairment (for example, scoliosis, poliomyelitis, rickets, osteoarthritis, **cerebral palsy, multiple sclerosis,** muscular dystrophy, spinal cord injury, or stroke). • Have there been any injuries to or surgeries on the musculoskeletal system (for example, dislocations, sprains, fractures, or joint replacements)? If so, obtain details.

Medication history. • Ask the patient to list all prescribed and over-the-counter medications taken within the past 6 months. Ask specifically about antiinflammatory or corticosteroid use. • What has been the response to the medications taken (for example, antiinflammatory, analgesics, or skeletal muscle relaxants)? • What are the medications most recently taken and when?

Activity and exercise. • What is the extent of usual daily exercise? • Determine which activities of daily living can

be performed independently and which require assistance.
• Ask about any assistive devices used (for example, cane or walker).

Elimination. Ask specifically about the ability to toilet independently. Does mobility interfere with this function? Is constipation, diarrhea, or incontinence a problem? If so, how is it managed?

Nutrition. • Take a diet history. Are the four food groups included? Are supplemental vitamins and minerals (for example, calcium) taken daily? • Weigh the individual and ask whether there has been a weight gain or loss over the past 6 months. If so, obtain details.

Physical examination. • Inspect the affected part for swelling, edema, bruises, redness, localized tenderness, deformities, or malalignments. (Be gentle during the inspection.) • During examination, note differences in circumference, symmetry, or length of limbs. • Record any abnormalities present (for example, scoliosis, contractures, and atrophy). • Record range of motion present in joints, gait, and degree of mobility.

Laboratory and diagnostics. • Review diagnostic studies performed (for example, x-rays, magnetic resonance imaging [MRI], computed tomography [CT], arthroscopic reports and bone scan). • Examine laboratory reports associated with the disease process present (for example, calcium, phosphorous, lupus testing, rheumatoid factor, uric acid level, and creatine kinase).

Assessment for neuromuscular blocking agents

• Assessment of the patient's vital signs, mental status, and particularly, respiratory function is mandatory for persons having received **neuromuscular blocking agents.** The side effects associated with these drugs may occur 48 hours or more after administration. Close observation of respiratory function, ability to swallow secretions, and the presence of a cough reflex is necessary. Suction, oxygen, mechanical ventilators, and resuscitation equipment should be available in the immediate area.

• Monitor blood pressure, pulse, and respirations. Review the baseline readings of the patient's vital signs before administration of anesthetic and neuromuscular blocking agents. Generally, changes from the baseline should be reported.

• Monitor the patient closely for clinical signs of hypoxia and **hypercapnia** (tachycardia, hypotension, and cyanosis). Arterial blood gases (ABGs) (see Table 28-1) may be drawn to accurately confirm the clinical observations.

Detection of respiratory depression

• Early signs of diminished ventilation are difficult to detect, particularly in the immediate postoperative period. Often the signs of restlessness, anxiety, lethargy, decreased mental alertness, and headache are early, subtle clues to distress.

• Use of the abdominal, intercostal, or neck muscles is an indication of respiratory distress. Flaring of the nostrils may be present in severe cases.

• As respiratory distress progresses, respirations become shallow and rapid. Assess for asymmetric chest movements.

• The development of cyanosis is a late sign of respiratory complications. Respiratory distress should be detected early through close observation before cyanosis develops.

• Assess muscle strength by asking the patient to lift his or her head off the pillow and hold a few seconds.

Pain assessment. Assess the degree of pain present because neuromuscular blocking agents paralyze the muscles but do NOT relieve pain.

Nursing Diagnosis
• Pain (indication)
• Activity intolerance (indication, side effect)
• Body-image disturbance (indication)
• Self-care deficit (indication)
• Injury, risk for (indication, side effect)

Planning

Planning must be done cooperatively with the patient and significant others. Adaptations in care needs must be based on the individual's ability to perform the activities of daily living and self-care.

Medications. • When on an inpatient service, the prescribed medications and schedule are listed on the medication administration record (MAR). For persons being instructed in self-care at home, obtain prescriptions and perform health teaching. • Develop a written record for the patient to maintain and take to the physician to track response to the prescribed treatment. See box on p. 521.

Activity and exercise. • Discuss the specifics of the prescribed regimen—degree of exercise allowed, bed rest, immobilization, and so forth. • Review treatments prescribed, such as hot and cold applications.

Psychosocial. • Plan with the patient for at-home management of the musculoskeletal problems and needed supportive services or referrals. • When self-care is no longer possible, involve appropriate resource persons in patient placement in a care facility.

Implementation

Nursing interventions with musculoskeletal disorders

• Assist with physical examination, drawing of blood samples, obtaining vital signs, and weighing for preparation for diagnostic procedures.

• Adapt procedures to meet the self-care abilities of the individual patient.

• Administer prescribed medications (for example, antiinflammatories, analgesics, and muscle relaxants).

• Provide specific instructions on the application of hot or cold packs. Generally, ice packs alleviate swelling immediately after muscle injury. Later in the course of treatment, application of heat provides comfort.

• Elevating the extremity immediately after injury decreases swelling and to some degree alleviates pain.

• Maintain the activity level prescribed (for example, bed rest and immobilization of muscle group or limb). During the initial phase of treatment, immobilizing the affected part will decrease muscle spasms and therefore decrease pain. Maintenance of proper alignment of the affected part will also relieve pain and swelling. Various approaches may be used for immobilization, including elastic bandages, splinting, casts, bed rest, or modified activity levels.

• Range-of-motion exercises may be prescribed to maintain joint function and to prevent muscle atrophy and contractures. The activity plan prescribed must be individualized to the diagnosis and should be carefully followed for maximum effectiveness.

* Increased anxiety produces stress on the body's muscles. Implement measures to produce relaxation and provide for the psychologic needs of the individual.

Nursing interventions with neuromuscular blockers

* Neuromuscular blockers are used during anesthesia and surgery to relax muscle groups and during the use of mechanical ventilation to improve air flow and oxygenation of the patient. See a general medical-surgical nursing text for a detailed discussion of nursing care while the patient is receiving mechanical ventilation. The patient must be intubated and receiving mechanical ventilation before administration of neuromuscular blocking agents.

* Monitor airway patency, respiratory rate, and tidal volume in accordance with hospital policy.

* The histamine release caused by these drugs may produce increased salivation. In patients who are paralyzed or who have incomplete return of control over swallowing, coughing, and deep breathing, these secretions may obstruct the airway.

* Assess for dyspnea and loud or gurgling sounds with respirations. Suction secretions according to hospital policies and procedures. If qualified, palpate for coarse chest wall vibrations and listen for rales or rhonchi.

* Deep-breathing exercises can allow the opportunity to assess the patient's cough reflex. Assist the patient by splinting any abdominal or thoracic incisions. Have the patient take 3 or 4 deep breaths and then cough. During this process, assess the patient's ability to breathe deeply. Cupping your hand and holding it a few inches from the patient's mouth while the patient breathes allows you to feel the air being exhaled.

* Patients can usually cough better in a semi-Fowler's or high Fowler's position; therefore, depending on the situation and stability of the patient's vital signs, elevating the head of the bed may assist coughing and breathing. For unconscious or semiconscious individuals, position on the side, using good body alignment. Keep the siderails up.

* Persons still paralyzed by the effects of these agents may experience pain and be unable to speak to request medication. Ensure that analgesics are scheduled on a regular basis and administered on time.

* Deal calmly with the patient experiencing respiratory dysfunction. The inability to breathe may cause the patient to panic. Give reassurance while initiating measures to assist the patient.

* Question antibiotic orders that prescribe aminoglycosides or tetracycline when neuromuscular blockers have been used. These drugs may potentiate the neuromuscular blocking activity.

Patient Education and Health Promotion

Pain relief. • The degree of musculoskeletal pain relief with and without activity must be discussed. Make modifications appropriate to the diagnosis and degree of impairment.
• Teach procedures designed to relieve pain (for example, application of cold or heat, elevation of body part, and proper body alignment).

Activities and exercise. The patient must resume activities of daily living within the boundaries set by the physician. (Such activities as regular moderate exercise, meal preparation, resumption of usual sexual activities, and social interaction all must be encouraged once specific orders are obtained.)

Psychosocial. For disorders of a chronic nature, encourage the patient to express feelings regarding chronic illness. The adjustment to this situation involves working through great personal fears, frustrations, hostilities, and resentments associated with the loss of personal control within one's life.

Medications. Many of the medications used in the treatment of musculoskeletal disorders produce sedation. Teach the patient about maintaining safety precautions such as avoiding operating power equipment or driving while taking these medications.

Fostering health maintenance

* Throughout the course of treatment discuss medication information and the individual's expectations of therapy. Ensure that the individual understands the activity level prescribed, pain relief methods, and safety precautions to ensure personal safety during mobility.

* Seek cooperation and understanding of the following points so that medication compliance is increased: name of medication, dosage, route and times of administration, side effects to expect, and side effects to report.

* Enlist the patient's aid in developing and maintaining a written record (box on p. 521) of monitoring parameters (such as level, location, and duration of pain; areas or muscles affected; degree of impairment with improvement in mobility; and exercise tolerance) and response to prescribed therapies for discussion with the physician. Episodes of nausea, vomiting, or diarrhea should also be reported for the physician's evaluation if it is a new symptom.

DRUG THERAPY

Drug Class: Centrally Acting Skeletal Muscle Relaxants

Actions

The centrally acting skeletal muscle relaxants belong to a class of compounds used to relieve acute muscle spasm. The exact mechanism of action of the centrally acting skeletal muscle relaxants is not known, except that they act by central nervous system (CNS) depression. They do not have any direct effect on muscles, nerve conduction, or myoneural junctions. All of these muscle relaxants produce some degree of sedation, and most physicians believe that the benefits of these agents come from their sedative effects rather than from actual muscle relaxation.

Uses

The centrally acting skeletal muscle relaxants are used in combination with physical therapy, rest, and analgesics to relieve muscle spasm associated with acute, painful musculoskeletal conditions. They should not be used in muscle spasticity associated with cerebral or spinal cord disease because they may reduce the strength of remaining active muscle fibers and produce further impairment and debilitation.

PATIENT EDUCATION & MONITORING FORM — Muscle Relaxants

MEDICATIONS	COLOR	TO BE TAKEN

Name _____

Physician _____

Physician's phone _____

Next appt.* _____

PARAMETERS			DAY OF DISCHARGE							COMMENTS
Muscle areas affected	List areas: 1. ____ 2. ____ 3. ____ 4. ____		AM	AM	AM	AM	AM	AM	AM	
Chart areas affected 2 times per day	Example: 1. Arm, lower 2. Lower back 3. 4.	AM 1, 2 PM 1, 2	PM	PM	PM	PM	PM	PM	PM	
Exercise and range of motion pain No improvement Moderate improvement Much improvement 10 5 1										
Pattern of pain	Location									
	Time of day pain occurs									
	Relieved by									
	Made worse by									
Impairment(s) and improvement	Example: Could not comb hair—can now. Could not turn head without pain—can now.									
Physical therapy prescribed	Example: Application of cold packs at 8 AM-4 PM and bedtime	Therapy								
		Time of day								
		Feeling, response								

*Please bring this record with you to your next appointment.
Use the back of this sheet for additional information.

Therapeutic Outcome

The primary therapeutic outcome expected from centrally acting skeletal muscle relaxant therapy is relief from muscle spasm.

Nursing Process

Premedication Assessment

1. Obtain baseline vital signs and mental status of patient.
2. Have ordered laboratory studies drawn (for example, liver function studies and complete blood count [CBC]).

Planning

Availability. See Table 42-1.

Implementation

Dosage and administration. See Table 42-1.

Evaluation

Side effects to expect

SEDATION, WEAKNESS, LETHARGY, GASTROINTESTINAL COMPLAINTS. These side effects are usually mild and tend to resolve with continued therapy. Encourage the patient not to discontinue therapy without first consulting the physician.

Provide for patient safety for the duration of these symptoms. Patients must avoid operating power equipment or driving.

DIZZINESS. Provide for patient safety during episodes of dizziness; report for further evaluation.

Side effects to report

HEPATOTOXICITY. The symptoms of hepatotoxicity are anorexia, nausea, vomiting, jaundice, hepatomegaly, splenomegaly, and abnormal liver function tests (elevated bilirubin, aspartate aminotransferase [AST], alanine aminotransferase [ALT], gamma glutamyltransferase [GGT], alkaline phosphatase, and prothrombin time).

BLOOD DYSCRASIAS. Routine laboratory studies (red blood cell [RBC], white blood cell [WBC], and differential counts) are scheduled for patients taking these agents for 30 days or longer. Stress returning for this laboratory work.

Monitor for the development of sore throat, fever, purpura, jaundice, or excessive progressive weakness.

Drug interactions

CNS DEPRESSANTS. Alcohol, narcotics, barbiturates, anticonvulsants, sedative-hypnotics, tranquilizers, phenothiazines, antidepressants. Persons who are working around machinery, driving a car, pouring and giving medicines, or performing other duties in which they must remain mentally alert should not take these medications while working.

baclofen (bak'lo-fen)
Lioresal (ly-or'e-sahl)

Actions

Baclofen is a skeletal muscle relaxant that apparently acts somewhat differently from the centrally acting musculoskeletal agents. Its complete mechanism of action is unknown, although reflex activity at the spinal cord is partially inhibited.

Uses

Baclofen is used in the management of **muscle spasticity** resulting from multiple sclerosis, spinal cord injuries, and other spinal cord diseases. It is not recommended for use in spasticity associated with Parkinson's disease, cerebral palsy, stroke, or rheumatic disorders. Use with caution in patients who must use spasticity to maintain an upright posture and balance in moving.

Table 42-1

Centrally Acting Muscle Relaxants

GENERIC NAME	BRAND NAME	ADULT DOSAGE (PO)	COMMENTS
Carisoprodol	Rela, Soma	350 mg 4 times daily	Onset of action—30 min; duration–4 to 6 hr
Chlorphenesin carbamate	Maolate	400-800 mg 3 to 4 times daily	Recommended only for short-term treatment (8 wk) of muscle spasm induced by trauma or inflammation; may cause blood dyscrasias
Chlorzoxazone	Paraflex	250-750 mg 3 to 4 times daily	Commonly causes gastrointestinal discomfort; may be hepatotoxic
Cyclobenzaprine	Flexeril	10 mg 3 times daily; do not exceed 60 mg daily	Recommended only for short-term treatment (2-3 wk) of painful musculoskeletal conditions
Metaxalone	Skelaxin	800 mg 3 to 4 times daily	Use with caution in patients with liver disease; causes false-positive Clinitest reaction
Methocarbamol	Robaxin, Delaxin	1-1.5 g 4 times daily	Parenteral forms also available
Orphenadrine citrate	Norflex, Flexon, Myolin	100 mg 2 times daily	Also has analgesic properties; do not use in patients with glaucoma or prostatic hypertrophy

Therapeutic Outcome

The primary therapeutic outcome expected from baclofen therapy is relief from muscle spasm.

Nursing Process

Premedication Assessment

1. Check history for any spastic disorders (for example, Parkinson's disease, cerebral palsy, stroke, or rheumatic disorders). If present, withhold medication and check with physician.
2. Perform a baseline mental status examination.

Planning

Availability. PO—10 and 20 mg tablets.

Implementation

Dosage and administration. Adult: PO—initially 5 mg 3 times daily. Increase the dosage by 5 mg every 3 to 7 days based on response. Optimum effects are usually noted at dosages of 40 to 80 mg daily but may take several weeks to achieve.

Note: Do not abruptly discontinue therapy. Severe exacerbation of spasticity and hallucinations may result.

Evaluation

Side effects to expect

NAUSEA, FATIGUE, HEADACHE, DROWSINESS. These side effects are usually mild and tend to resolve with continued therapy. Encourage the patient not to discontinue therapy without first consulting the physician.

DIZZINESS. Provide for patient safety during episodes of dizziness; report for further evaluation.

Drug interactions

CNS DEPRESSANTS. CNS depressants, including sleep aids, analgesics, tranquilizers, and alcohol, potentiate the sedative effects of baclofen. Persons who are working around machinery, driving a car, pouring and giving medicines, or performing other duties in which they must remain mentally alert should not take these medications while working.

Drug Class: Direct-Acting Skeletal Muscle Relaxant

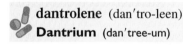

dantrolene (dan'tro-leen)
Dantrium (dan'tree-um)

Actions

Dantrolene is a muscle relaxant that acts directly on skeletal muscle. It produces generalized mild weakness of skeletal muscles and decreases the force of reflex muscle contractions, **hyperreflexia, clonus,** muscle stiffness, involuntary muscle movements, and spasticity.

Uses

Dantrolene is used to control the spasticity of chronic disorders such as cerebral palsy, multiple sclerosis, spinal cord injury, and **stroke syndrome.** It is also used to treat neuroleptic malignant syndrome associated with the use of antipsychotic agents (see p. 212).

Therapeutic Outcomes

The primary therapeutic outcome expected from dantrolene therapy is relief from muscle spasm.

Nursing Process

Premedication Assessment

1. When used for neuroleptic malignant syndrome, perform a baseline assessment of vital signs, especially temperature.
2. Establish a baseline of degree of muscle symptoms present.

Planning

Availability. PO—25, 50, and 100 mg capsules. IV—0.32 mg/ml in 70 ml vials.

Implementation

Dosage and administration. Adult: PO—initially 25 mg daily. Increase to 25 mg 2, 3, or 4 times daily at 4- to 7-day intervals, then gradually increase the dosage up to 100 mg 2, 3, or 4 times daily. A small number of patients may require 200 mg 4 times daily.

Evaluation

Side effects to expect

WEAKNESS, DIARRHEA, DROWSINESS. These side effects are usually mild and tend to resolve with continued therapy. They can often be minimized by starting therapy with low doses. Encourage the patient not to discontinue therapy without first consulting the physician.

DIZZINESS, LIGHT-HEADEDNESS. Provide for patient safety during episodes of dizziness; report for further evaluation.

RESPONSE TO THERAPY. Tell the patient that effectiveness of the drug may not be apparent for 1 week or longer. Encourage the patient not to discontinue therapy without first consulting the physician.

Side effects to report

PHOTOSENSITIVITY. The patient should be cautioned to avoid exposure to sunlight and ultraviolet light. Suggest wearing long-sleeved clothing, hat, and sunglasses while exposed to sunlight. The patient must not use artificial tanning lamps. The patient should not discontinue therapy without notifying the physician.

HEPATOTOXICITY. The symptoms of hepatotoxicity are anorexia, nausea, vomiting, jaundice, hepatomegaly, splenomegaly, and abnormal liver function tests (elevated bilirubin, AST, ALT, GGT, alkaline phosphatase, prothrombin time).

Drug interactions

CNS DEPRESSANTS. CNS depressants, including sleep aids, analgesics, tranquilizers, and alcohol, potentiate the sedative effects of dantrolene. Persons who are working around machinery, driving a car, pouring and giving medicines, or performing other duties in which they must remain mentally alert should not take these medications while working.

Drug Class: Neuromuscular Blocking Agents

Actions

Neuromuscular blocking agents act by interrupting transmission of impulses from motor nerves to muscles at the skeletal neuromuscular junction. Neuromuscular blocking agents have no effect on consciousness, memory, or the pain threshold. Reassurance by nursing personnel is essential to paralyzed patients (such as those on respirators), and analgesics must be administered on schedule. These patients may suffer extreme pain and may be unable to ask for analgesics.

Uses

Neuromuscular blocking agents are important skeletal muscle relaxants. These agents are used to produce adequate muscle relaxation during anesthesia to reduce the use (and side effects) of general anesthetics, ease endotracheal intubation and prevent laryngospasm, decrease muscular activity in electroshock therapy, and aid in the muscle spasms associated with tetanus.

Therapeutic Outcome

The primary therapeutic outcome expected from neuromuscular blocking therapy is smooth and skeletal muscle relaxation.

Nursing Process

Premedication Assessment

1. These drugs are administered by anesthetist or anesthesiologist during surgical anesthesia or when a patient is placed or being maintained on a respirator. Check hospital policy for who may administer these drugs and specific monitoring parameters.
2. Check history for hepatic, pulmonary, or renal disease or neurologic disorders such as myasthenia gravis, spinal cord injury, or multiple sclerosis. If present, tag the chart appropriately before administration of anesthesia.
3. Have oxygen, suction, and artificial respiration equipment available in the immediate area whenever these drugs are to be used. Also have antidotes (for example, neostigmine methylsulfate [Prostigmin], pyridostigmine bromide [Mestinon, Regonal], and edrophonium chloride [Tensilon]) available.

Planning

Availability. See Table 42-2.

Implementation

Administration. These agents are usually given intravenously but may also be given intramuscularly. Because they are potent drugs, they should be used only by persons thoroughly familiar with their effects, such as an anesthetist or anesthesiologist, and under conditions in which the patient can receive constant, close attention for signs of respiratory failure. Adequate equipment for artificial respiration, antidotes, and other measures for prompt treatment of toxicity must be readily available.

Patients with hepatic, pulmonary, or renal disease or neurologic disorders such as myasthenia gravis, spinal cord injury, or multiple sclerosis must be fully evaluated to assess their ability to tolerate neuromuscular blocking agents. Much smaller doses are often necessary when these diseases are present. Neonates and elderly patients also require adjustments in dosage because of the insensitivity of their neuromuscular junction.

Treatment of overdose. Treatment of overdose includes artificial respiration with oxygen and antidotes such as neostigmine methylsulfate (Prostigmin), pyridostigmine bromide (Mestinon, Regonal), and edrophonium chloride (Tensilon). Atropine sulfate is usually administered with neostigmine or pyridostigmine to block bradycardia, hypotension, and salivation induced by these agents. There is no antidote for the early blockade induced by succinylcholine. Fortunately, it is of short duration and does not require reversal.

Evaluation

Side effects to expect

SALIVATION. Neuromuscular blocking agents cause histamine release, which may cause bronchospasm, bronchial and salivary secretions, flushing, edema, and urticaria. Ensure that the airway is patent and that secretions are suctioned regularly to prevent obstruction. Report evidence of bronchospasm, edema, and urticaria immediately.

Table 42-2

Neuromuscular Blocking Agents

GENERIC NAME	BRAND NAME	AVAILABILITY
Atracurium besylate	Tracrium	10 mg/ml in 5 and 10 ml ampules
Doxacurium chloride	Nuromax	1 mg/ml in 5 ml vials
Metocurine iodide	Metubine Iodide	2 mg/ml in 20 vials
Mivacurium chloride	Mivacron	Infusion: 0.5 mg/ml in 50 ml D_5W Injection: 2 mg/ml in 5 and 10 ml vials
Pancuronium bromide	Pavulon	1 mg/ml in 10 ml vials; 2 mg/ml in 2 and 5 ml ampules
Pipecuronium bromide	Arduan	1 mg/ml in 10 ml vials
Succinylcholine	Anectine, Quelicin, Sucostrin	20 mg/ml in 10 ml vials, 50 mg/ml in 10 ml ampules, 100 mg/ml in 5, 10, 20 ml vials
Tubocurarine chloride	Tubocurarine Chloride	3 mg/ml in 5, 10 and 20 mg vials
Vecuronium bromide	Norcuron	10 mg in 5 and 10 ml vials

MILD DISCOMFORT. Mild to moderate discomfort, particularly in the neck, upper back, lower intercostal, and abdominal muscles, will be noted when the patient first ambulates after use.

Side effects to report

SIGNS OF RESPIRATORY DISTRESS. Monitor vital signs for a prolonged period after administration of neuromuscular blocking agents.

DIMINISHED COUGH REFLEX, INABILITY TO SWALLOW. Assess deep breathing and coughing at regular intervals. Have suction and oxygen equipment available, and be familiar with emergency code practices at your hospital.

Drug interactions

DRUGS THAT ENHANCE THERAPEUTIC AND TOXIC EFFECTS. General anesthetics (ether, fluroxene, methoxyflurane, enflurane, halothane, and cyclopropane), aminoglycoside antibiotics (kanamycin, gentamicin, neomycin, streptomycin, netilmicin, tobramycin, and amikacin), quinidine, quinine, beta-adrenergic blocking agents (propranolol, timolol, pindolol, nadolol, and others), and agents that deplete potassium (thiazide diuretics, furosemide, torsemide, bumetanide, ethacrynic acid, chlorthalidone, amphotericin B, and corticosteroids), inhibit neuromuscular transmission, thus prolonging neuromuscular blockage.

Label charts of patients scheduled for surgery who are taking any of these agents. These combinations may potentiate respiratory depression. Check the anesthetist's records of surgical patients; monitor postoperative patients for respiratory depression for a prolonged period. This may occur 48 hours or more after drug administration.

DRUGS THAT REDUCE THERAPEUTIC EFFECTS. Neostigmine methylsulfate, pyridostigmine bromide, and edrophonium chloride. These agents are used as antidotes in case of overdosage of the neuromuscular blocking agents.

RESPIRATORY DEPRESSANTS. Analgesics, sedatives, and tranquilizers. These agents, in combination with muscle relaxants, may potentiate respiratory depression. Check the anesthetist's records of surgical patients. Monitor postoperative patients for respiratory depression for a prolonged period. This may occur 48 hours or more after drug administration.

CHAPTER REVIEW

Nurses can play an important role in providing counseling and guidance to patients and family in understanding muscle spasticity and pain and how to maintain an appropriate balance between daily activities and timing of analgesics to optimize quality of life. Nurses also play a crucial role in providing comfort and monitoring to patients who have received neuromuscular blocking agents. It is mandatory that nurses know how to recognize and respond quickly when respiratory emergencies arise.

MATH REVIEW

1. Ordered: methocarbamol (Robaxin) 1.5 g QID. Convert 1.5 g to _____ mg.

CRITICAL THINKING QUESTIONS

Situation:
Mr. Conway was working in his garden and "pulled a muscle" in his back. The doctor prescribed cyclobenzaprine 10 mg, TID for 1 week. Before the patient leaves the physician's office, what health teaching should you provide for the medication and temporary lifestyle changes?

Situation:
After an extensive major surgical procedure, the patient is transferred to the postanesthesia recovery unit with an endotracheal tube in place. During the surgical procedure the anesthesia record notes the administration of tubocurarine chloride. What criteria should be used to determine when to remove the endotracheal tube? What monitoring of the patient should be done to check for residual effects of the neuromuscular blocking agent?

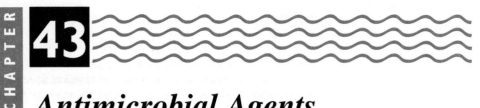

CHAPTER 43

Antimicrobial Agents

CHAPTER CONTENT

Objectives

1. Identify significant data in a patient history that could alert the medical team that a patient is likely to experience an allergic reaction.

2. Identify baseline data the nurse should collect on a continuous basis for comparison and evaluation of antimicrobial drug effectiveness.

3. Describe basic principles of patient care that can be implemented to enhance an individual's therapeutic response during an infection.

4. Identify criteria used to select an effective antimicrobial agent.

5. Differentiate between gram-negative and gram-positive microorganisms and between anaerobic and aerobic properties of microorganisms.

6. Explain the major action and effects of drugs used to treat infectious diseases.

7. Describe the nursing assessments and interventions for the common side effects associated with antimicrobial

agents: allergic reaction; direct tissue damage (nephrotoxicity, ototoxicity, or hepatotoxicity); secondary infection; and other considerations, such as photosensitivity, peripheral neuropathy, and neuromuscular blockage.

8. Review parenteral administration techniques and the procedure for vaginal insertion of drugs.

9. Develop a plan for implementing patient education for patients receiving aminoglycosides, cephalosporins, penicillins, quinolones, sulfonamides, tetracyclines, antifungal agents, and antiviral agents.

Key Words

pathogenic
antibiotics
nephrotoxicity
ototoxicity
gram-negative
  microorganisms
gram-positive
  microorganisms

hypoprothrombinemia
thrombophlebitis
bacteriostatic
bactericidal
penicillinase-resistant
  penicillins

ANTIMICROBIAL AGENTS

Antimicrobial agents are chemicals that eliminate living microorganisms that are **pathogenic** to the patient. Antimicrobial agents may be of chemical origin, such as the sulfonamides, or they may be derived from other living organisms. Those derived from other living microorganisms are called **antibiotics**; for example, penicillin was first derived from the mold *Penicillium notatum*. Most antibiotics used today are harvested from large colonies of microorganisms that are purified and chemically modified into semisynthetic antimicrobial agents. The chemical modification makes the antibiotic more effective against certain specific pathogenic organisms. Antimicrobial agents are often first classified according to the type of pathogen to be destroyed, such as bacteria (antibacterial agents), fungus (antifungal agents), or virus (antiviral agents). The antimicrobial agents are then subdivided by chemical families into drug classes such as the penicillins, tetracyclines, and aminoglycosides.

The selection of the antimicrobial agent must be based on the sensitivity of the pathogen and the possible toxicity to the patient. If at all possible, the infecting organisms should first be isolated and identified. Culture and sensitivity tests should be completed. The antimicrobial therapy is then started based on the sensitivity results and the clinical judgment of the physician.

Nursing Process for Antimicrobial Therapy

Nurses must consider the entire patient when administering and monitoring antimicrobial therapy. It is essential that the nurse be knowledgeable about the drugs themselves, including physiologic parameters for monitoring expected therapeutic activity and potential adverse effects. It is important to teach the individual with an infection basic principles of self-care that will enhance the recovery process and measures to prevent the spread of the infection. In the case of communicable diseases, exposed individuals must be contacted for follow-up testing and appropriate treatment.

Assessment

History of current infection

* What symptoms are described by the patient? Extend questioning to help the patient focus—for example, when did the symptoms begin? Have they worsened? Is there fever, night sweats, malaise, chronic fatigue, weight loss, arthralgia, cough (type of secretions), diarrhea, painful urination, nausea, vomiting, lesions or skin rash on the body, discharge, or drainage? Has the patient been treated previously for an infection similar to this?
* When treating patients with sexually transmitted diseases, ask about the number of sexual partners, sexual orientation, and use of precautions during intercourse. (See Chapter 38 for further details.)

Past history. Ask the patient about previously treated conditions. What treatments were used, and what was the response to therapy? Focus on areas that may impinge on antimicrobial therapy, such as reduced renal or hepatic function, immunocompromised conditions, blood dyscrasias, partial deafness, and gastrointestinal complaints.

Allergies. Is the patient allergic to certain medicines, dust, weeds, foods, or other environmental substances?

Medication history

* Ask the patient to list all prescribed and over-the-counter medications currently being taken or taken in the past 6 months. Ask specifically about any medicines, such as corticosteroids, chemotherapy, or transplant suppressants, that may affect the immune status of the individual.
* Does the person take any type of allergy "shots" or medications?
* Is the person immunized against childhood diseases?
* Has the person been treated for an infection in the recent past? If so, what medications were taken and were there any allergic responses? If so, ask for details of the symptoms of the "allergic reaction."
* Has the patient taken this medication before? If so, what symptoms (such as nausea, vomiting, diarrhea, rash, itching, or hives) developed when taking it that led the patient to state now that there is an allergy? Ask the patient to describe the appearance of the rash, where it started, and the course of recovery. How soon after starting the medication did the symptoms develop?
* Ask if the patient has ever developed a secondary infection (black furry tongue, white patches in mouth, or vaginal

infection) when taking an antibiotic. For example, women taking antibiotics may develop a vaginal infection because of suppression of normal flora.

Physical examination. • Perform a head-to-toe body or functional assessment, focusing on the areas pertinent to the admitting diagnosis. • Assess for risk factors that may contribute to development of infection, such as extensive surgical procedures, obesity, underlying contributory conditions (chronic obstructive pulmonary disease, diabetes), immunotherapy drugs, malnutrition, and age extremes (infant or elderly).

Psychosocial. For an individual with a serious communicable disease, assess the response and adaptive processes being used to cope with the disease and its treatments.

Laboratory tests and diagnostics. • Review laboratory reports on the chart (for example, complete blood count [CBC], urinalysis, creatinine clearance, blood urea nitrogen [BUN], aspartate aminotransferase [AST], alanine aminotransferase [ALT], culture reports, electrolytes, screening tests for sexually transmitted diseases). • Tuberculin skin testing and chest x-rays are done to screen for exposure to tuberculosis. Sputum cultures are collected to confirm the presence of *M. tuberculosis*.

Assessment during antimicrobial therapy. Read each drug monograph for specific side effects to expect and side effects to report, and individualize the assessments for the drugs prescribed. Nausea, vomiting, diarrhea, allergies, anaphylaxis, **nephrotoxicity,** hepatotoxicity, **ototoxicity,** hematologic dyscrasias, secondary infection, and photosensitivity are found with recurring frequency in the antimicrobial drug monographs.

Nausea, vomiting, and diarrhea. These conditions are the "big three" commonly occurring side effects associated with antimicrobial drug therapy. When they occur, gather further data: (1) Did the patient have a history of nausea, vomiting, or diarrhea before starting the drug therapy? (2) How soon after starting the medication did the symptoms start? (3) Since starting the medication, has the diet or water source changed in any way? (4) Was the patient taking other drugs, either prescription or over-the-counter medications, before the initiation of antibiotic therapy? (5) How much fluid is the patient consuming when taking medications? Inadequate fluid intake sometimes causes gastritis manifested by nausea. (6) For diarrhea, what was the pattern of elimination before drug therapy? Report diarrhea and the character and frequency of stools as well as any abdominal pain promptly. Nausea, vomiting, and diarrhea effects are often dose related and result from changes in normal bacterial flora in the bowel, from irritation, and from secondary infection. Symptoms resolve within a few days, and discontinuation of therapy is rarely required.

Secondary infection. Assess for symptoms of secondary infection such as oral infection. Observe for a black, furry-appearing tongue, white patches in the oral cavity, cold sores, canker sores, and glossitis. There may be lesions and itching in the vaginal and anal areas. Secondary infection of the intestine can produce severe, life-threatening diarrhea.

Allergies and anaphylaxis. The severity of allergic reaction ranges from a mild rash to fatal anaphylaxis. Allergic reactions may develop within 30 minutes of administration (anaphylaxis, laryngeal edema, shock, dyspnea, or skin reactions) or may occur several days after discontinuance of therapy (skin rashes or fever). All patients must be questioned for previous allergic reactions, and allergy-prone patients must be observed closely. It is important that a patient not be labeled "allergic" to a particular medication without adequate documentation. The medication to which a patient claims an allergy may be a life-saving drug for that patient.

Nephrotoxicity. Assess for an increasing BUN and creatinine, decreasing urine output, decreasing urine specific gravity, casts or protein in the urine, frank blood or smoky-colored urine, or red blood cells (RBCs) in excess of 0 to 3 on the urinalysis report.

Hepatotoxicity. Assess for preexisting hepatic disease such as cirrhosis or hepatitis. Review laboratory studies (for example, bilirubin, AST, ALT, gamma glutamyltransferase [GGT], alkaline phosphatase, and prothrombin time) and report abnormal findings to the physician.

Ototoxicity. Damage to the eighth cranial nerve can occur from drug therapy, particularly from aminoglycosides. This may initially be manifested by dizziness, tinnitus, and progressive hearing loss. Assess the patient for difficulty in walking unaided, and assess the level of hearing daily. Intentionally speak to patients softly; note if they are aware that you said anything. Take particular notice of the patient who repeatedly says, "What did you say?" or who starts talking more loudly or progressively increases the volume on the television or radio.

Blood dyscrasias. (1) Ask specifically about any history of blood disorders that have been diagnosed and treatments prescribed. (2) Ask specifically about any types of anemia (for example, aplastic, hemolytic, or megaloblastic) or deficiencies of folic acid, vitamin B_{12}, or glucose-6-phosphate dehydrogenase (G6PD). (3) Ask whether the individual has received chemotherapy, radiation therapy, or transplant therapy, all of which may induce an immunocompromised state and changes in the blood. (4) Has the patient received blood cell stimulator drugs such as Epogen or Neupogen? (5) Does the patient have any bleeding disorders, such as hemophilia or thrombocytopenia? (6) Observe for bleeding gums, prolonged bleeding at an injection site, petechiae, and nosebleeds. (6) Review admission laboratory studies and report abnormalities (for example, CBC with differential, hemoglobin, and hematocrit).

Photosensitivity. Assess for the development of dermatologic symptoms such as exaggerated sunburn, itching, rash, urticaria, pruritus, and scaling.

Nursing Diagnoses
- Infection: actual (indication)
- Risk for infection transmission (indication)
- Fluid volume deficit (indication, side effect)
- Injury: risk for (side effect)

Planning
Medication
- Order medications prescribed, and schedule these on the medication administration record (MAR).
- In scheduling the times of administration of antibiotic therapy, other drugs prescribed and the potential interactions (for example, antacids) should be taken into

consideration. Antibiotics are usually given at even intervals over a 24-hour period to maintain cyclic blood levels of the medication. Orders such as 4 times daily (qid) should be clarified to determine whether the physician meant 8-12-4-8 o'clock or 12-6-12-6 o'clock administration times.
- Have any cultures been ordered taken before initiation of antimicrobial therapy? Mark the Kardex and care plan when blood draws for serum level peak or trough are ordered.
- Request necessary infusion equipment for administration of prescribed antimicrobials (for example, syringe pump or infusion pump).
- If a definite drug allergy is identified, the patient's chart, unit Kardex, and an identification bracelet should be carefully marked to alert all personnel to the specific drugs the patient should not receive.

Laboratory tests.
Order any stat or subsequent laboratory studies (for example, culture and sensitivity, urinalysis, CBC, baseline electrolytes, and renal or hepatic function tests).

Nursing care.
Individualize the nursing care plan for the type and severity of the infectious process. Monitor symptoms present, vital signs, and response to therapy. Provide supportive nursing measures appropriate to the type of infection. Plan to provide health teaching to the patient and significant others regarding the patient's basic care, prevention of spread of the infection, and medication regimen.

Implementation
- Routine monitoring of all individuals receiving antimicrobial therapy should include status of hydration, temperature, pulse, respirations, and blood pressure. Monitor at least every 4 hours and more frequently as the patient's clinical status warrants.
- Use Centers for Disease Control (CDC)–recommended precautions for infection transmission: (1) category-specific precautions, (2) disease-specific precautions, (3) universal precautions, including those that call for reverse isolation for immunocompromised individuals with neutropenia, leukemia, or lymphomas.
- Monitor for the development of phlebitis when antimicrobials are administered intravenously.
- Administer antimicrobials as prescribed on the time schedule established:
  - In some instances, a second drug (for example, probenecid) may be administered concurrently to inhibit the excretion of the antibiotic (penicillin or cephalosporins). When this is done, monitor extremely closely for adverse effects.
  - Some oral antimicrobials can be administered without regard for meals; others should be given 1 hour before or 2 hours after meals.
  - Always give oral antibiotics with sufficient water, and maintain adequate hydration throughout therapy. Drugs such as sulfonamides require forcing fluids unless contraindicated by coexisting medical conditions.
  - Check the drug monograph for drug-drug or drug-food interactions and establish administration times accordingly. An example of this would be tetracyclines, which need to be administered 1 hour before or 2 hours after ingesting antacids, milk and other dairy products, or

products containing calcium, aluminum, magnesium, or iron (such as vitamins).

- Monitor for adaptive or maladaptive responses to the diagnosis and intervene appropriately by providing support and information and by making appropriate referrals.

Nausea, vomiting and diarrhea. When drug therapy causes nausea and vomiting, the physician may elect to give the antibiotic with food to decrease irritation even though absorption may be slightly decreased, or the physician may choose to switch to a parenteral dosage form. When reporting any incidence of nausea and vomiting, all significant data should be collected and reported. (See also Chapters 31 and 32.) Administer prescribed antiemetics or antidiarrheal agents.

Secondary infection. Secondary infection may occur in patients receiving broad-spectrum antibiotic therapy, particularly those who are immunosuppressed. Monitor for the development of symptoms of secondary infection, and notify the physician if this occurs. Initiate prescribed treatment consistent with the etiology of the symptoms. Obtain cultures as ordered, and administer additional antibiotics effective against the new organism. Instruct the patient to minimize exposure to people known to have an infection and practice good personal hygiene measures.

Allergies and anaphylaxis. Monitor closely all patients, particularly those with histories of allergies, asthma, or rhinitis or who are taking multiple drug preparations, for an allergic response during antimicrobial therapy. All patients should be watched carefully for possible allergic reactions for at least 20 to 30 minutes after administration of a medication. However, some drug reactions may not occur for several days.

Hold the prescribed antimicrobial medication if the person reports possible allergy; share all information obtained with the physician, who will decide whether to administer the drug. The elderly, because of physiologic changes of aging, require close observation for therapeutic response or for toxicity to drugs. Learn the location of the hospital emergency cart and the procedure for summoning it. In the event of suspected anaphylaxis, summon the physician and the emergency cart immediately.

Although a serious reaction may occur with the first administration of a drug, repeated exposures to a previously sensitized substance can be fatal. Respond immediately to any signs of reaction, including swelling, redness, or pain at the site of injection, hives, nasal congestion and discharge, wheezing progressing to dyspnea, pulmonary edema, stridor, and sternal retractions.

When symptoms of an allergic response occur, follow hospital protocol, which will usually include the following steps:

- Activate the patient emergency care system.
- Establish and maintain a patent airway; administer oxygen, elevate head of bed.
- Monitor the patient's vital signs continuously and lung sounds frequently. Report hypotension, increasing pulse, respirations that become labored and shallow, and abnormal breath sounds.
- Have emergency equipment and drugs available for administration.
- An intravenous infusion should be initiated if not already available.

Nephrotoxicity. Report abnormal laboratory results relating to kidney function. Maintain an accurate intake and output record; report declining output or output below 30 ml per hour.

Many antimicrobial agents are potentially nephrotoxic (aminoglycosides, tetracyclines, and cephalosporins). Concomitant therapy with diuretics enhances the likelihood of toxicity, particularly in the elderly or debilitated patient. When renal function is impaired, most drug dosages must be decreased or alternate drug therapy used.

Hepatotoxicity. Several drugs to be studied in this unit are potentially hepatotoxic (isoniazid, and sulfonamides). The liver is active in the metabolism of many drugs, and drug-induced hepatitis may occur. The actual liver damage may occur shortly after exposure to the pharmacologic agent or may not appear for several weeks after initial exposure. The symptoms of hepatotoxicity are anorexia, nausea, vomiting, jaundice, hepatomegaly, splenomegaly, and abnormal liver function tests (elevated bilirubin, AST, ALT, GGT, alkaline phosphatase, and prothrombin time). Patients with preexisting hepatic disease such as cirrhosis or hepatitis will require lower doses of drugs metabolized by the liver.

Ototoxicity. Report preexisting hearing impairment or the development of symptoms of developing hearing deficits to the physician, and initiate orders prescribed. Provide for patient safety if tinnitus or dizziness accompanies the symptoms of hearing impairment.

Blood dyscrasias. Individualize care to the type of blood dyscrasia present. When hypothrombinemia is present the usual treatment is administration of vitamin K. Serious and possibly fatal bone marrow suppression may occur after therapy is initiated with some antibiotics (for example, chloramphenicol). Monitor for signs and symptoms, including sore throat, fatigue, elevated temperature, small petechial hemorrhages, and bruises on the skin. If present report immediately.

Photosensitivity. This adverse effect is seldom evident during hospitalization. It is more commonly seen in ambulatory practice.

When the drug monograph mentions this as a potential side effect to report, the nurse should provide health teaching to prevent its occurrence. Instruct the patient to avoid exposure to sunlight and ultraviolet light (sunlamps, tanning beds); wear long-sleeved clothing, a hat, and sunglasses; and apply a sunscreen when going into the sun.

Medication history. Ask the patient to list all prescribed or purchased over-the-counter medications currently being taken. Ask specifically about the recent use of corticosteroids, chemotherapy, or transplant suppressants.

Does the patient have any allergies? If so, obtain details of medications and actual symptoms that occur when an allergic reaction occurs. What treatment was used for any past allergic responses? What antibiotics have been taken in the past? Were there any problems during antibiotic therapy?

Patient Education and Health Promotion

The following basic principles of patient care should not be overlooked when treating a patient with infections:

- Adequate rest with as little stress as possible; rest also decreases metabolic needs and enhances the physiologic repair process.

- Nutritional management, including attention to hydration, proteins, fats, carbohydrates, minerals, and vitamins, to support the body's needs during an inflammatory response. Adequate nutrients to meet energy needs, especially during times of fever, are essential so that the body will not break down its protein stores to meet energy requirements. The dietary teaching must be individualized to the patient's diagnosis and point of recovery.
- Extensive teaching, individualized to the circumstances and mode of transmission of the disease, should be given to individuals with communicable infections. This should include contacting exposed individuals in accordance with institutional policies for disease screening, treatment, and follow-up counseling.
- Explain personal hygiene measures, such as hand-washing techniques, management of excretions such as sputum, and wound care.
- Instruct the patient to refrain from sexual intercourse during therapy for sexually transmitted disease infections.

Medications
- Drug therapy specific for the type of microorganism causing the infection should be explained in detail so the patient will realize the need for compliance with the prescribed regimen.
- Examine each drug monograph to identify suggestions to the patient for how to handle the common side effects associated with antimicrobial therapy. The patients must also be taught the signs and symptoms that must be reported to the physician. Stress to the patient not to discontinue the medication prescribed until the side effects have been discussed with the physician.
- Develop a medication schedule with the patient for at-home medications prescribed. Ensure that the patient understands why it is important to take antimicrobials for the entire course of drug therapy and not discontinue when feeling improved. Finally, patients must know self-monitoring parameters for the prescribed drug therapy.
- Nursing mothers should remind their physicians that they are breast-feeding so that antibiotics may be selected that will have no impact on the infant.
- After an allergic reaction, the patient and family should be alerted to inform anyone treating the patient in the future of the allergy to a specific drug.

Fostering health maintenance
- Throughout the course of treatment discuss medication information and continue to emphasize those factors the patient can control to alter the progression of the disease: maintenance of general health, nutritional needs, adequate rest and appropriate exercise, and continuation of prescribed medication therapy until the entire course of prescribed medication has been completed.
- Discuss expectations of therapy so that the patient understands whether a satisfactory response to drug therapy is being achieved, such as the relief of symptoms for which treatment was sought (for example, relief of burning with urination and frequency of urination, relief of cough, and end of drainage and healing of a wound).
- Enlist the patient's aid in developing and maintaining a written record of monitoring parameters (list presenting symptoms: cough with a large amount of phlegm, wound drainage, temperature, and exercise tolerance) and re-

sponse to prescribed therapies for discussion with the physician (see box on p. 531). Patients should be encouraged to take this record to follow-up visits.

DRUG THERAPY FOR INFECTIOUS DISEASE

Drug Class: Aminoglycosides

Actions

The aminoglycosides kill bacteria primarily by inhibiting protein synthesis. Other mechanisms of action are not yet fully defined.

Uses

The aminoglycoside antibiotics are used primarily against **gram-negative microorganisms** that cause urinary tract infections, meningitis, wound infections, and life-threatening septicemias. They are the mainstays in the treatment of nosocomial gram-negative infections (for example, *Acinetobacter, Citrobacter, Enterobacter, Escherichia coli, Klebsiella, Providencia, Pseudomonas, Salmonella,* and *Shigella*). Kanamycin and neomycin may also be used before surgery to reduce the normal flora content of the intestinal tract.

Therapeutic Outcome

The primary therapeutic outcome expected from aminoglycoside therapy is elimination of bacterial infection.

Nursing Process

Premedication Assessment
1. Obtain baseline assessments of presenting symptoms.
2. Record temperature, pulse, respirations, blood pressure, and hydration status.
3. Assess for any allergies and symptoms of hearing loss or renal disease. If present, withhold drug and report findings to physician.
4. If patient has had anesthesia within the past 48 to 72 hours, check to see if skeletal muscle relaxants were administered. If used, withhold drug and notify physician.
5. Check for time scheduling of laboratory aminoglycoside serum level testing. After levels are determined, assess whether results are normal or toxic. Contact the physician, as appropriate.
6. Obtain baseline laboratory studies ordered (for example, CBC with differential).

Planning
Availability. See Table 43-1.

Implementation
Dosage and administration. See Table 43-1.
Compatibilities. Do NOT mix different drugs in the same syringe or infuse together with other drugs. See under Drug Interactions for incompatibilities.
Laboratory. Check with the hospital laboratory regarding timing of aminoglycoside blood level tests. After levels have been determined, assess whether results are normal or toxic.

PATIENT EDUCATION & MONITORING FORM Antibiotics

MEDICATIONS	COLOR	TO BE TAKEN

Name _____

Physician _____

Physician's phone _____

Next appt.* _____

PARAMETERS		DAY OF DISCHARGE								COMMENTS
Temperature	On arising / 12 noon									
	5 PM / 9 PM									
Aspirin Aceta-minophen	Time; # tabs, e.g. 8AM2									
	Time; # tabs, e.g. 12N2									
Site of infection Scale	Redness									
	Pain									
+ Small ++++ Severe	Drainage									
Cough and sputum	Color									
	Thickness									
Productive:	No cough									
Mouth and throat	Sore throat									
	No problem									
Dizziness	Walk unaided									
	Must use support									
	Walk with help									
Hearing	Had to ↑ volume of radio–TV									
	No difficulty									
Skin	Rash with itching									
	Rash–fine red									
	No itching									
	No rash									
Vaginal itching (Yes or No)										
Rectal itching (Yes or No)										

*Please bring this record with you to your next appointment.
Use the back of this sheet for additional information.

Table 43-1

The Aminoglycosides

GENERIC NAME	BRAND NAME	AVAILABILITY	ADULT DOSAGE RANGE
Amikacin	Amikin	100 mg/2 ml vial 500 mg/2 ml vial 1 g/4 ml vial	IM, IV: 15 mg/kg/24 hr
Gentamicin	Garamycin	2, 10, 40 mg/ml 60 mg/1.5 ml 80 mg/2 ml 100 mg/100 ml	IM, IV: Up to 240 mg/24 hr
Kanamycin	Kantrex	75,500 mg, 1 g vials	IM, IV: Up to 15 mg/kg/24 hr hr, not to exceed 1.5 g/24 hr
Neomycin	Mycifradin	125 mg/5 ml in 480 ml bottle	PO: 4-12 g daily in 4 divided doses
Netilmicin	Netromycin	100 mg/ml in 1.5 ml vials	IM, IV: 3-6.5 mg/kg/24 hr
Streptomycin	Streptomycin	400 mg/ml, 1 and 5 g vials	IM: 1-4 g/24 hr
Tobramycin	Nebcin	10 mg/ml in 2 ml vials 40 mg/ml in 1.5 g vials 40 mg/ml in 2 ml vials	IM, IV: Up to 5 mg/kg/24 hr

Rate of Infusion. Consult with a pharmacist or see the individual package literature.

Evaluation

Side effects to report

OTOTOXICITY. Damage to the eighth cranial nerve can occur as a result of aminoglycoside therapy. This may initially be manifested by dizziness, tinnitus, and progressive hearing loss. Continue to observe patients for ototoxicity after therapy has been discontinued. These adverse effects may appear several days later.

Assess each patient for difficulty in walking unaided and assess the level of hearing daily. Intentionally speak softly; note if the patient is aware that you said anything. Take particular notice of the patient who repeatedly says, "What did you say?" or who starts talking more loudly or progressively increases the volume on the television or radio.

NEPHROTOXICITY. Monitor urinalysis and kidney function tests for abnormal results. Report an increasing BUN and creatinine, decreasing urine output or decreasing urine specific gravity (despite amount of fluid intake), casts or protein in the urine, frank blood or smoky-colored urine, or RBCs in excess of 0 to 3 on the urinalysis report.

Drug interactions

NEPHROTOXIC POTENTIAL. Cephalosporins and diuretics, when combined with aminoglycosides, may increase the nephrotoxic potential. Monitor the urinalysis and kidney function tests for abnormal results.

OTOTOXIC POTENTIAL. Aminoglycosides, when combined with ethacrynic acid, bumetanide, and furosemide, may increase ototoxicity. Therefore nursing assessments for tinnitus, dizziness, and decreased hearing should be done regularly every shift.

NEUROMUSCULAR BLOCKADE. Aminoglycoside antibiotics in combination with skeletal muscle relaxants may produce respiratory depression.

Check the anesthesia record in postoperative patients to determine if skeletal muscle relaxants such as succinylcholine or pancuronium bromide were administered during surgery.

The nurse should monitor and assess the respiratory rate, depth of respirations, and chest movement and report apnea immediately. Because these effects may be seen for up to 48 hours after administration of skeletal muscle relaxants, continue monitoring respirations, pulse, and blood pressure beyond the usual postsurgical vital signs routine.

HEPARIN. Gentamicin and heparin are physically incompatible. Do NOT mix together before infusion.

AMPICILLIN, PIPERACILLIN, TICARCILLIN, MEZLOCILLIN. These penicillins rapidly inactivate aminoglycoside antibiotics. Do NOT mix together or administer together at the same IV site.

Drug Class: Cephalosporins

Actions

The cephalosporins are chemically related to the penicillins and have a similar mechanism of activity. The cephalosporins act by inhibiting cell wall synthesis in bacteria. The cephalosporins may be divided into groups, or "generations," based primarily on antimicrobial activity. The first-generation cephalosporins have effective activity against **gram-positive microorganisms** (*Staphylococcus aureus, S. epidermidis; Streptococcus pyogenes, Streptococcus pneumoniae*) and relatively mild activity against gram-negative microorganisms (*Escherichia coli, Klebsiella pneumoniae, Proteus mirabilis*). The second-generation cephalosporins have somewhat increased activity against gram-negative bacteria but are much less active than the third-generation agents. Third-generation cephalosporins are generally less active than first-generation agents against gram-positive cocci, although they are much more active against the penicillinase-producing bacteria.

Some of the third-generation cephalosporins are also active against *Pseudomonas aeruginosa*, a potent gram-negative microorganism. Fourth generation cephalosporins are considered "broad spectrum" with both gram-negative and gram-positive coverage.

Uses

The cephalosporins may be used with caution as alternatives when patients are allergic to the penicillins, unless they are also allergic to the cephalosporins. The cephalosporins are used for certain urinary and respiratory tract infections, abdominal infections, septicemia, meningitis, and osteomyelitis.

Therapeutic Outcome

The primary therapeutic outcome expected from cephalosporin therapy is elimination of bacterial infection.

Nursing Process

Premedication Assessment

1. Obtain baseline assessments of presenting symptoms.
2. Record temperature, pulse, respirations, blood pressure, and hydration status.
3. Assess for any allergies, symptoms of renal disease, or bleeding disorders. If present, withhold drug and report findings to the physician.
4. Obtain baseline laboratory studies ordered (for example, CBC with differential).

Planning

Availability. See Table 43-2.

Implementation

Dosage and administration. See Table 43-2.

Evaluation

Side effects to report

DIARRHEA. Cephalosporins cause diarrhea by altering the bacterial flora of the gastrointestinal tract. The diarrhea is usually not severe enough to warrant discontinuing medication. Encourage the patient not to discontinue therapy without consulting the physician. When diarrhea persists, monitor the patient for signs of dehydration.

SECONDARY INFECTIONS. Oral thrush, genital and anal pruritus, vaginitis, and vaginal discharge may occur with cephalosporin therapy. Report promptly because these infections are resistant to the original antibiotic used.

Teach the importance of meticulous oral and perineal personal hygiene.

ABNORMAL LIVER AND RENAL FUNCTION TESTS. Transient elevations of liver function tests (AST, ALT, and alkaline phosphatase) and renal function tests (BUN and serum creatinine) have been reported. Renal toxicity, as evidenced by proteinuria, hematuria, casts, decreased creatinine clearance, and decreased urine output, has also developed.

Monitor returning laboratory data and report abnormal findings to the physician.

HYPOPROTHROMBINEMIA. **Hypoprothrombinemia,** with and without bleeding, has been reported. These rare occurrences are most frequent in elderly, debilitated, or otherwise

compromised patients with borderline vitamin K deficiency. Treatment with broad-spectrum antibiotics eliminates enough gastrointestinal flora to cause a further reduction in vitamin K synthesis.

Assess the patient for ecchymosis after minimal trauma, prolonged bleeding at an infusion site or from a surgical wound, or the development of petechiae, bleeding gums, or nosebleeds. Notify the physician of any of the signs of hypoprothrombinemia. The usual treatment is administration of vitamin K.

THROMBOPHLEBITIS. Phlebitis and **thrombophlebitis** are recurrent problems associated with intravenous administration of cephalosporins. Use small IV needles, large veins, and alternating infusion sites if possible to minimize irritation.

Carefully assess patients receiving IV cephalosporins for the development of thrombophlebitis.

Inspect the IV area frequently while providing care; inspect during dressing changes and at times when the IV is changed to a new site. Always investigate pain at the IV site. Report redness, warmth, tenderness to touch, or edema in the affected part. If in lower extremities, dorsiflexion of the foot may cause pain in the calf area (Homans' sign). Compare findings in the affected limb with those in the unaffected limb.

ELECTROLYTE IMBALANCE. If a patient develops hyperkalemia or hypernatremia, consider the electrolyte content of the antibiotics. Most of the cephalosporins have a high electrolyte content.

Drug interactions

NEPHROTOXIC POTENTIAL. Patients receiving cephalosporins, aminoglycosides, polymyxin B, vancomycin, and diuretics concurrently should be assessed for signs of nephrotoxicity. Monitor urinalysis and kidney function tests for abnormal results. Report an increasing BUN and creatinine, decreasing urine output or decreasing urine specific gravity (despite amount of fluid intake), casts or protein in the urine, frank blood or smoky-colored urine, or RBCs in excess of 0 to 3 on the urinalysis report.

PROBENECID. Patients receiving probenecid in combination with cephalosporins are more susceptible to toxicity because of the inhibition of excretion of the cephalosporins by probenecid. Monitor closely for adverse effects.

ALCOHOL. Instruct the patient to avoid alcohol consumption during cefamandole, cefmetazole, cefoperazone, cefotetan, and possibly ceftizoxime therapy. Patients ingesting alcohol during and for 24 to 72 hours after administration of these cephalosporins will become flushed, tremulous, dyspneic, tachycardic, and hypotensive. Also tell the patient not to use over-the-counter preparations containing alcohol, such as mouthwash (Cepacol) or cough preparations because of the alcohol content.

Drug Class: Macrolides

Actions

The macrolide antibiotics act by inhibiting protein synthesis in susceptible bacteria. They are **bacteriostatic** and **bactericidal,** depending on the organism and the concentration of medicine present. Erythromycin is effective against gram-positive microorganisms and gram-negative cocci. Azithromycin is less active against gram-positive organisms than erythromycin but has greater activity against gram-negative

Table 43-2

The Cephalosporins

GENERIC NAME	BRAND NAME	GENERATION	AVAILABILITY	ADULT DOSAGE RANGE
Cefaclor	Ceclor	2	250, 500 mg capsules 125, 187, 250, 375 mg/5 ml suspension	PO: 250-500 every 8 hr; do not exceed 4 g/day
Cefadroxil	Duricef	1	500 mg capsules 1000 mg tablets 125, 250, 500 mg/5 ml suspension	PO: 1-2 g daily in 1-2 doses daily
Cefamandole	Mandol	2	500 mg, 1, 2, 10 g vials	IM, IV: 0.5-1 g every 4-8 hr; do not exceed 12 g/24 hr
Cefazolin	Ancef, Kefzol, Zolicef	1	250, 500 mg, 1, 10, 20 g vials	IM, IV: 250 mg to 1.5 g every 6-8 hr
Cefepime	Maxipime	4	500 mg, 1, 2 g vials	IM, IV: 0.5-2 g every 12 hr
Cefixime	Suprax	3	200, 400 mg capsules 100 mg/5 ml suspension	PO: 200 mg every 12 hr or 400 mg once daily
Cefmetazole	Zefazone	2	1, 2 g vials	IV: 2 g every 6-12 hr
Cefonicid	Monocid	2	500 mg, 1, 10 g vials	IM, IV: 0.5-1 g once daily; do not exceed 2 g daily
Cefoperazone	Cefobid	3	1, 2 g vials	IV: 1-3 g every 6-8 hr
Cefotaxime	Claforan	3	500 mg, 1, 2, 10 g vials	IV: 1-2 g every 4-8 hr; do not exceed 12 g/day
Cefotetan	Cefotan	3	1, 2, 10 g vials	IM, IV: 1-2 g every 12 hr; do not exceed 6 g/day
Cefoxitin	Mefoxin	2	1, 2, 10 g vials	IM, IV: 1-2 g every 6-8 hr; do not exceed 12 g/day
Cefpodoxime	Vantin	3	100, 200 mg tablets 50, 100 mg/5 ml suspension	PO: 200 mg every 12 hr for 7-14 days
Cefprozil	Cefzil	2	250, 500 mg tablets 125, 250 mg/5 ml suspension	PO: 250-500 mg every 12 hr for 10 days
Ceftazidime	Fortaz, Tazidime, ✽ Magnacef	3	500 mg, 1, 2, 6, 10 g vials	IM, IV: 1-2 g every 12 hr
Ceftibuten	Cedax	3	400 mg capsules 90, 180 mg/5 ml suspension	PO: 400 mg once daily 2 hr before or 1 hr after meals for 10 days
Ceftizoxime	Cefizox	3	500 mg, 1, 2, 10 g vials	IV: 1-2 g every 8-12 hr
Ceftriaxone	Rocephin	3	250, 500 mg, 1, 2, 10 g vials	IM, IV: 1-2 g once daily; do not exceed 4 g daily
Cefuroxime	Zinacef, Kefurox, Ceftin	2	125, 250, 500 mg tablets; 750 mg, 1.5 g vials	PO: 250-500 mg every 12 hr IV: 750 mg to 1.5 g every 8 hr
Cephalexin	Keflex, ✽ Ceporex	1	250, 500 mg capsules, tablets 1000 mg tablets 125, 250 mg/5 ml suspension	PO: 250-1000 mg every 6 hr
Cephalothin	Keflin, ✽ Ceporacin	1	1, 2, 20 g vials	IM, IV: 500 mg to 2 g every 4-6 hr
Cephapirin	Cefadyl	1	500 mg, 1, 2, 4, 20 g vials	IM, IV: 500 mg to 1 g every 4-6 hr
Cephradine	Velosef	1	250, 500 mg capsules 125, 250 mg/5 ml suspension 250, 500 mg, 1, 2 g vials	PO: 250-500 mg every 6 hr IM, IV: 500 mg to 1 g every 6 hr; do not exceed 8 g/day
Loracarbef	Lorabid	2	200 mg capsules 100 mg/5 ml suspension	PO: 200-400 mg every 12 hr 1 hr before or 2 hr after a meal for 7-14 days

✽ Available in Canada only.

organisms that are resistant to erythromycin. Clarithromycin has a spectrum of activity similar to that of erythromycin but has considerably greater potency. Dirithromycin is a prodrug, the active metabolite of which is erythromycylamine. Erythromycylamine has a spectrum of activity somewhat similar to that of erythromycin. Dirithromycin also has a tentative advantage over the other macrolide antibiotics in that it does not affect liver metabolism of other drugs; thus it has fewer interactions. Troleandomycin is less effective than erythromycin and offers no advantages over the other macrolide antibiotics.

Uses

The macrolides are used for respiratory, gastrointestinal tract, skin, and soft tissue infections and sexually transmitted diseases, especially when penicillins, cephalosporins, and tetracyclines cannot be used.

Therapeutic Outcome

The primary therapeutic outcome expected from macrolide therapy is elimination of bacterial infection.

Nursing Process

Premedication Assessment

1. Obtain baseline assessments of presenting symptoms.
2. Record temperature, pulse, respirations, blood pressure, and hydration status.
3. Assess for and record any gastric symptoms present before initiation of therapy.
4. Assess for any allergies.
5. Obtain baseline laboratory studies ordered (for example, CBC with differential).

Planning
Availability. See Table 43-3.

Implementation
Dosage and administration. See Table 43-3. PO—azithromycin and erythromycin should be administered at least 1 hour before or 2 hours after meals. Clarithromycin and troleandomycin may be taken without regard to meals. IM—because of pain on injection and the possibility of sterile abscess formation, intramuscular administration of erythromycin is generally not recommended for multiple-dose therapy. IV—dilute the dosage of erythromycin in 100 to 250 ml of saline solution or 5% dextrose and administer over 20 to 60 minutes. Thrombophlebitis after IV infusion is a relatively common side effect.

Evaluation
Side effects to expect
GASTRIC IRRITATION. The most common side effects of oral macrolide therapy are diarrhea, nausea and vomiting, and abnormal taste. These side effects are usually mild and tend to resolve with continued therapy. Encourage the patient not to discontinue therapy without first consulting the physician.

Side effects to report
THROMBOPHLEBITIS. Carefully assess patients receiving IV erythromycin for the development of thrombophlebitis.

Table 43-3
The Macrolides

GENERIC NAME	BRAND NAME	AVAILABILITY	ADULT DOSAGE RANGE
Azithromycin	Zithromax	PO: 250 mg capsules; 100, 200 mg/5 ml suspension	PO: 500 mg as a single dose on day 1, followed by 250 mg once daily on days 2-5 for a total dose of 1.5 g
Clarithromycin	Biaxin	PO: 250, 500 mg tablets; 125, 250 mg/5 ml suspension	PO: 250-500 mg every 12 hr for 7-14 days
Dirithromycin	Dynabac	PO: 250 mg tablets	PO: 500 mg as a single dose daily; take with food or within 1 hr of having eaten; take for 7-14 days
Erythromycin	Eryc, Ilosone, E-Mycin, many others	PO: 250, 333, 500 mg enteric-coated tablets; 200, 250, 500 mg chewable tablets; 250, 500 mg film-coated tablets; 125, 250 mg enteric-coated pellets in capsules; 125, 200, 250, 400 mg/5 mg suspension; 100 mg/ml and 100 mg/2.5 ml drops IV: 500, 1000 mg vials for reconstitution	PO: 250 mg 4 times daily for 10-14 days IM: 100 mg every 4-6 hr IV: 15-20 mg/kg/24 hr; up to 4 g/24 hr
Troleandomycin	Tao	PO: 250 mg capsules	PO: 250-500 mg 4 times daily for 10 days

Inspect the IV area frequently while providing care; inspect during dressing changes and when the IV is changed to a new site. Always investigate pain at the IV site. Report redness and edema in the affected part. If in lower extremities, dorsiflexion of the foot may cause pain in the calf area (Homans' sign). Compare the affected limb with the unaffected limb.

Drug interactions

TOXICITY CAUSED BY MACROLIDES. Macrolide antibiotics may inhibit the metabolism of several drugs, causing accumulation and potential toxicity. These drugs are alfentanil, terfenadine, astemizole, cisapride, warfarin, bromocriptine, carbamazepine, cyclosporine, digoxin, disopyramide, triazolam, tacrolimus, and theophyllines. Read individual monographs for monitoring parameters of toxicity from these agents.

Drug Class: Penicillins

Actions

The penicillins were the first true antibiotics to be grown and used against pathogenic bacteria in human beings. They currently remain one of the most widely used classes of antibiotics.

The penicillins act by interfering with the synthesis of bacterial cell walls. The resulting cell wall is weakened because of defective structure, and the bacteria are subsequently destroyed by osmotic lysis. The penicillins are most effective against bacteria that multiply rapidly. They do not hinder growth of human cells because human cells have protective membranes but no cell wall.

Many bacteria that are initially sensitive to the penicillins develop a protective mechanism and become resistant to penicillin therapy. These bacteria produce the enzyme penicillinase (beta-lactamase), which can destroy the antibacterial activity of most bacteria. Penicillinase inactivates the penicillin antibiotics by splitting open the beta-lactam ring of the penicillin molecule. Researchers have developed two mechanisms to prevent this inactivation. The first is to modify the penicillin molecule to "protect" the ring structure while retaining antimicrobial activity. This mechanism culminated in the development of the **penicillinase-resistant penicillins** (methicillin, nafcillin, oxacillin, cloxacillin, and dicloxacillin). The second method is to add another chemical with similar structure that will more readily bond to the penicillinase enzymes than the penicillin, leaving the free penicillin to inhibit cell wall synthesis. Potassium clavulanate is now added to amoxicillin (Augmentin) and ticarcillin (Timentin) to bond to penicillinases that would normally destroy these antibiotics. Sulbactam has been added to ampicillin (Unasyn) and tazobactam to piperacillin (Zosyn) for similar reasons.

Uses

The penicillins are used to treat middle ear infections (otitis media), pneumonia, meningitis, urinary tract infections, syphilis, and gonorrhea and as a prophylactic antibiotic before surgery or dental procedures for patients with histories of rheumatic fever.

Therapeutic Outcome

The primary therapeutic outcome expected from penicillin therapy is elimination of bacterial infection.

Nursing Process

Premedication Assessment

1. Obtain baseline assessments of presenting symptoms.
2. Record temperature, pulse, respirations, blood pressure, and hydration status.
3. Assess for and record any allergies, symptoms of diarrhea, and abnormal liver or renal function tests. If present, withhold drug and report findings to the physician.
4. Obtain baseline laboratory studies ordered (for example, CBC with differential).

Planning

Availability. See Table 43-4.

Implementation

Dosage and administration. See Table 43-4.
Compatibilities. Do NOT mix with other drugs in the same syringe or infuse together with other drugs. See under Drug Interactions for incompatibilities.
Rate of infusion. Consult with a pharmacist or see package literature.

Evaluation

Side effects to report

DIARRHEA. Penicillins cause diarrhea by altering the bacterial flora of the gastrointestinal tract. The diarrhea is usually not severe enough to warrant discontinuation. Encourage the patient not to discontinue therapy without first consulting the physician. If diarrhea persists, monitor the patient for signs of dehydration.

ABNORMAL LIVER AND RENAL FUNCTION TESTS. Monitor returning laboratory data and report abnormal findings to the physician.

THROMBOPHLEBITIS. Carefully assess patients receiving IV penicillins for the development of thrombophlebitis.

Inspect the IV area frequently while providing care; inspect during dressing changes and at times the IV is changed to a new site. Always investigate pain at the IV site. Report redness, warmth, tenderness to touch, and edema in the affected part. If in lower extremities, dorsiflexion of the foot may cause pain in the calf area (Homans' sign). Compare the affected limb with the unaffected limb.

ELECTROLYTE IMBALANCE. The electrolyte content of the antibiotics may cause hyperkalemia or hypernatremia. Most of the penicillins have a high electrolyte content.

Drug interactions

PROBENECID. Patients receiving probenecid in combination with penicillins are more susceptible to toxicity because probenecid inhibits excretion of the penicillins. Monitor closely for adverse effects.

This combination may be used to advantage in the treatment of gonorrhea and other infections in which high levels are indicated.

AMPICILLIN AND ALLOPURINOL. When used concurrently, these two agents are associated with a high incidence of rash. Do not label the patient as allergic to penicillins until further skin testing has verified that there is a true hypersensitivity to penicillins.

ANTACIDS. Excessive use of antacids may diminish the absorption of oral penicillins.

Table 43-4

The Penicillins

GENERIC NAME	BRAND NAME	AVAILABILITY	ADULT DOSAGE RANGE
Amoxicillin	Amoxil, Trimox, Wymox	125 and 250 mg chewable tablets 250 and 500 mg capsules 50, 125 and 250 mg/5 ml suspension	PO: 250-500 mg/8 hr
Ampicillin	Marcillin, Omnipen, Principen, ✷ Apo-Amp, Totacillin	0.125, 0.25, 0.5, 1, and 2 g vials 250 and 500 mg capsules 125, 250, 500 mg/5 ml suspension	IM, IV: 0.5 to 1 g/4-6 hr PO: 250-500 mg/6 hr
Carbenicillin	Geocillin	382 mg tablets	PO: 382-764 mg 4 times daily
Cloxacillin	Cloxapen	250 and 500 mg capsules 125 mg/5 ml suspension	PO: 250-500 mg/6 hr
Dicloxacillin	Dynapen, Dycill	250 and 500 mg capsules 62.5 mg/5 ml suspension	PO: 125-500 mg/6 hr
Methicillin	Staphcillin	1, 4, 10 g vials	IM, IV: 1 g/4-6 hr
Mezlocillin	Mezlin	1, 2, 3, 4 g vials	IM, IV: Do not exceed 24 g/24 hr
Nafcillin	Nallpen, Unipen	0.5, 1, 2 g vials 250 mg capsules 250 mg/5 ml suspension	IM, IV: 0.5-1 g/4-6 hr PO: 250-500 mg/4-6 hr
Oxacillin	Bactocill	0.25, 0.5, 1, 2, 4 g vials 250 and 500 mg capsules 250 mg/5 ml suspension	IM, IV: 0.5-1g/4-6hr PO: 250-500 mg/4-6 hr
Penicillin G, potassium or sodium	Pfizerpen, Pentids, ✷ Crystapen	Vials of 0.2, 0.5, 1, 2, 3, 5 and 10, 20 million units	IM, IV: 600,000 to 30 million units daily
Penicillin V potassium	V-Cillin K, Pen-Vee K, Veetids	250 and 500 mg tablets 125 and 250 mg/5 ml suspension	PO: 250-500 mg/6 hr
Piperacillin	Pipracil	2, 3, 4 g vials	IM, IV: 3-4 g every 4-6 hr, not to exceed 24 g/24 hr
Ticarcillin	Ticar	1, 3, and 20 g vials	IM: Do not exceed 2 g/injection site IV: Up to 18 g/24 hr
Combination products			
Amoxicillin and potassium clavulanate	Augmentin, ✷ Clavulin	125, 250, 500, and 875 mg tablets 125 and 250 mg/5 ml suspension	PO: 250-600 mg every 8 hr IV: 3.1-3.2 g every 4-6 hr
Ticarcillin and potassium clavulanate	Timentin	3 g ticarcillin/100 mg clavulanate/vial	
Ampicillin and sulbactam sodium	Unasyn	1.5, 3 g bottles and vials	IM, IV: 1.5-3 g every 6 hr
Piperacillin and tazobactam	Zosyn	2, 3, 4 g vials	IV: 3 g every 6 hr

✷ Available in Canada only.

Drug Class: Quinolones

Actions

The quinolone antibiotics are rapidly emerging as an important class of therapeutic agents. This class is not new; the original members—nalidixic acid and cinoxacin—have been available for the treatment of urinary tract infections (see Chapter 39, p. 483) for well over two decades. A new subclass known as the fluoroquinolones is showing great promise against a wide range of gram-positive and gram-negative bacteria, including some anaerobes. The fluoroquinolones act by inhibiting the activity of DNA gyrase, an enzyme that is essential for the replication of bacterial DNA.

Uses

Ciprofloxacin is the first well-tolerated, broad-spectrum oral antibiotic in the quinolone series. It demonstrates rapid bactericidal activity against the bacterial pathogens that cause nosocomial and community-acquired urinary tract infections; most of the strains that cause enteritis; gonococci, meningococci, *Legionella*, *Pasteurella*, *Haemophilus influenzae*, and methicillin-resistant staphylococci; and some gram-negative bacteria, including *Pseudomonas aeruginosa*. The activity of ciprofloxacin against gram-positive and gram-negative cocci is equal to or better than that of the penicillins, cephalosporins, and aminoglycosides, but most anaerobic organisms are resistant.

Lomefloxacin is used to treat adults with mild to moderate lower respiratory infections (*Haemophilus influenzae* and *Moraxella catarrhalis*) and urinary tract infections (*Escherichia coli*, *Klebsiella pneumoniae*, *Proteus mirabilis*, and *Enterobacter cloacae*). Lomefloxacin should not be used empirically to treat acute exacerbations of chronic bronchitis when it is probable that *Streptococcus pneumoniae* is the pathogen. This organism is resistant to lomefloxacin.

Ofloxacin has broad-spectrum activity against gram-negative, gram-positive, and anaerobic bacteria. It differs from ciprofloxacin in that it has less activity against *Pseudomonas aeruginosa* but greater activity against sexually transmitted diseases such as *Neisseria gonorrhoeae*, *Chlamydia trachomatis*, and genital ureaplasma. Ofloxacin is also less susceptible to drug interactions than other fluoroquinolones. Ofloxacin is used to treat urinary tract infections, prostatitis, skin infections (cellulitis and impetigo), lower respiratory pneumonia, and sexually transmitted diseases other than syphilis.

Cinoxacin, enoxacin, nalidixic acid, and norfloxacin are used to treat urinary tract infections. (See Chapter 39.)

Therapeutic Outcome

The primary therapeutic outcome expected from quinolone therapy is elimination of bacterial infection.

Nursing Process

Premedication Assessment
1. Obtain baseline assessments of presenting symptoms.
2. Record temperature, pulse, respirations, blood pressure, and hydration status.
3. Assess for and record any gastric symptoms present before initiation of therapy.
4. Assess for any allergies.
5. Obtain baseline laboratory studies ordered (for example, CBC with differential).
6. Ensure that the patient is not pregnant.
7. Warn patients of possible phototoxicity to lomefloxacin. (See under Side Effects to Report.)

Planning
Availability. See Table 43-5.

Implementation
Dosage and administration. See Table 43-5.
Children. Pediatric therapy is not recommended because of the potential for permanent cartilage damage.
Pregnancy. Quinolone therapy is not recommended during pregnancy unless the benefit of therapy outweighs the risk. No studies have been completed in human patients, but animal studies have demonstrated various teratogenic effects.

Evaluation
Side effects to expect
NAUSEA, VOMITING, DIARRHEA, DISCOMFORT. These side effects are usually mild and tend to resolve with continued therapy. Encourage the patient not to discontinue therapy without first consulting the physician. If the patient should become debilitated, contact the physician.

Table 43-5

The Quinolones

GENERIC NAME	BRAND NAME	AVAILABILITY	ADULT DOSAGE RANGE
Cinoxacin	Cinobac	Capsules: 250 and 500 mg	PO: 1 g daily in 2-4 divided doses for 7-14 days; take with meals
Ciprofloxacin	Cipro	Tablets: 250, 500, and 750 mg; Injection: 200 and 400 mg vials	PO: 0.5-1.5 g daily in 2 divided doses 2 hr after meals; IV: 400-800 mg daily in 2 divided doses every 12 hr
Enoxacin	Penetrex	Tablets: 200 and 400 mg	PO: 200-400 mg every 12 hr for 7-14 days; take 1 hr before or 2 hr after meals with a large glass of fluid
Lomefloxacin	Maxaquin	Tablets: 400 mg	PO: 400 mg once daily; may be taken without regard to meals
Nalidixic acid	NegGram	Tablets: 0.25, 0.5, and 1 g	PO: 1 g 4 times daily for 7-14 days; take with meals
Norfloxacin	Noroxin	Tablets: 400 mg	PO: 400 mg twice daily for 7-10 days; take 1 hr before or 2 hr after meals with a large glass of fluid; do not exceed 800 mg daily
Ofloxacin	Floxin	Tablets: 200, 300, and 400 mg; Injection: 200 and 400 mg vials	PO: 600-800 mg daily in 2 divided doses every 12 hr, 1 hr before or 2 hr after meals with a large glass of fluid; IV: 600-800 mg every 12 hr

DIZZINESS, LIGHT-HEADEDNESS. Although infrequent, ciprofloxacin may cause these disturbances. They tend to be self-limiting, and therapy should not be discontinued until the patient consults a physician.

Caution the patient against driving or performing hazardous tasks until adjustment to the effects of the medication has been achieved.

Side effects to report

PHOTOTOXICITY. Phototoxic reactions have been reported in patients treated with lomefloxacin. Exposure to direct and indirect sunlight and the use of sunlamps should be avoided. These reactions have occurred with and without the use of sunblocks and sunscreens with single doses of lomefloxacin. The patient should not take additional doses and should contact the physician if a sensation of skin burning, redness, swelling, blisters, rash, itching, or dermatitis develops. Suggest wearing long-sleeved clothing, a hat, and sunglasses when exposed to sunlight.

RASH. Report a rash or pruritus immediately and withhold additional doses pending approval by the physician.

ABNORMAL LABORATORY TESTS. Monitor returning laboratory data and report abnormal findings to the physician.

NEUROLOGIC EFFECTS. Report the development of tinnitus, headache, dizziness, mental depression, drowsiness, or confusion.

Drug interactions

IRON, ANTACIDS, AND SUCRALFATE. Iron salts, sucralfate, and antacids containing magnesium hydroxide or aluminum hydroxide decrease the absorption of the quinolones. Administer at least 4 hours before or 2 hours after ingestion of antacids, sucralfate, or iron-containing products.

PROBENECID. Patients receiving probenecid in combination with quinolones are more susceptible to toxicity because probenecid inhibits excretion of the quinolones. Monitor closely for toxic effects.

The combination may be used advantageously in the treatment of serious or resistant infections in which high serum levels of a quinolone are required.

DIDANOSINE. Do not administer quinolone antibiotics within 2 hours of administration of didanosine tablets or pediatric powder for oral solution. The antacid present in these formulations inhibits the absorption of the quinolones.

THEOPHYLLINE. Quinolones, when given with theophylline, may result in theophylline toxicity. Observe for vomiting, dizziness, restlessness, and cardiac arrhythmias. Monitor theophylline serum levels. The dosage of theophylline may need to be reduced.

Drug Class: Sulfonamides

Actions

The sulfonamides are not true antibiotics because they are not synthesized by microorganisms. However, they are highly effective antibacterial agents. Sulfonamides act by inhibiting bacterial biosynthesis of folic acid, which eventually results in bacterial cell death. Human cells do not synthesize folic acid and therefore are not affected.

Uses

Sulfonamides are used primarily to treat urinary tract infections and otitis media. They may also be used to prevent streptococcal infection or rheumatic fever in persons who are allergic to penicillin.

Because of an increasing frequency of organisms developing resistance to sulfonamide therapy and the unreliability of in vitro sulfonamide sensitivity tests, patients should be monitored closely for continued therapeutic response to treatment. This is particularly important in patients being treated for chronic and recurrent urinary tract infections.

The most routinely used sulfonamide today is actually a combination of trimethoprim and sulfamethoxazole (co-trimoxazole, TMP-SMZ). This combination blocks two steps in the pathway of folic acid production; therefore fewer resistant strains of microorganisms have developed. Co-trimoxazole is frequently used for treatment of urinary tract infections, otitis media in children, traveler's diarrhea, acute exacerbations of chronic bronchitis in adults, and prophylaxis and treatment of *Pneumocystis carinii* pneumonia (PCP) in immunocompromised patients.

Therapeutic Outcome

The primary therapeutic outcome expected from sulfonamide therapy is elimination of bacterial infection.

Nursing Process

Premedication Assessment

1. Obtain baseline assessments of presenting symptoms.
2. Record temperature, pulse, respirations, blood pressure, and hydration status.
3. Assess for and record any gastric symptoms present before initiation of therapy.
4. Assess for any allergies.
5. Obtain baseline laboratory studies ordered (for example, CBC with differential).

Planning

Availability. See Table 43-6.

Implementation

Dosage and administration. See Table 43-6. *Note:* Patients should be encouraged to drink water several times daily while receiving sulfonamide therapy. In rare situations, crystals form in the urinary tract if the patient becomes too dehydrated.

Evaluation

Side effects to report

NAUSEA, VOMITING, ANOREXIA, DIARRHEA. These side effects are usually mild and tend to resolve with continued therapy. Encourage the patient not to discontinue therapy without first consulting the physician.

If the patient becomes debilitated, contact the physician.

DERMATOLOGIC REACTIONS. Report a rash or pruritus immediately and withhold additional doses pending approval by the physician.

PHOTOSENSITIVITY. The patient should be cautioned to avoid exposure to sunlight and ultraviolet light. Suggest wearing long-sleeved clothing, a hat, and sunglasses when exposed to sunlight. Discourage the use of artificial tanning lamps.

HEMATOLOGIC REACTIONS. Routine laboratory studies (RBC, white blood cell [WBC], and differential counts) are

Table 43-6

The Sulfonamides

GENERIC NAME	BRAND NAME	AVAILABILITY	ADULT DOSAGE RANGE
Sulfadiazine	Sulfadiazine	500 mg tablets	PO: Initial dose—2-4 g, then 4-8 g/24 hr in divided doses
Sulfamethizole	Thiosulfil Forte	500 mg tablets	PO: 0.5-1 g 3-4 times daily
Sulfamethoxazole	Gantanol, Urobak	500 mg tablets	PO: Initial dose—2 g, then 1 g/12 hr
Sulfasalazine	Azulfidine	500 mg tablets	PO: Initial therapy—3-4 g daily in divided doses; maintenance dose is 2 g daily
Sulfisoxazole	Gantrisin	500 mg tablets 500 mg/5 ml syrup	PO, IM, IV: Initial dose—2-4 g; maintenance dose is 4-8 g/24 hr divided into 3-6 doses
Co-trimoxazole	Bactrim, Septra	Tablets, suspension, infusion	PO: 2-4 tablets daily, depending on strength, disease being treated IV: 15-20 mg/kg/24 hr (based on trimethoprim) in 3-4 divided doses for up to 14 days
Erythromycin-sulfisoxazole	Pediazole, Eryzole	Suspension	PO: 2.5-10 ml every 6 hr depending on weight of patient

scheduled for patients taking sulfonamides for 14 days or longer. Stress the importance of returning for this laboratory work.

Monitor for the development of a sore throat, fever, purpura, jaundice, or excessive and progressive weakness.

NEUROLOGIC EFFECTS. Report the development of tinnitus, headache, dizziness, mental depression, drowsiness, or confusion.

Drug interactions

ORAL HYPOGLYCEMIC AGENTS. Sulfonamides may displace sulfonylurea oral hypoglycemic agents (tolbutamide, acetohexamide, tolazamide, and chlorpropamide) from protein-binding sites, resulting in hypoglycemia.

Monitor for hypoglycemia, headache, weakness, decreased coordination, general apprehension, diaphoresis, hunger, and blurred or double vision.

The dosage of the hypoglycemic agent may need to be reduced. Notify the physician if any of the above-mentioned symptoms appear.

CLINITEST. A false-positive reaction for glucose in the urine may occur with Clinitest tablets but not with Tes-Tape or Diastix.

WARFARIN. This medication may enhance the anticoagulant effects of warfarin. Observe for the development of petechiae, ecchymoses, nosebleeds, bleeding gums, dark tarry stools, and bright red or coffee ground emesis. Monitor the prothrombin time and reduce the dosage of warfarin if necessary.

METHOTREXATE. Sulfonamides may produce methotrexate toxicity when given simultaneously. Monitor patients on concurrent therapy for oral stomatitis and for signs of nephrotoxicity (oliguria, hematuria, proteinuria, casts, and so on).

PHENYTOIN. Sulfisoxazole may displace phenytoin from protein-binding sites, resulting in phenytoin toxicity.

Monitor patients on concurrent therapy for signs of phenytoin toxicity: nystagmus, sedation, and lethargy (serum levels may be ordered). A reduced dosage of phenytoin may be required.

Drug Class: Tetracyclines

Actions

The tetracyclines are a class of antibiotics that are effective against both gram-negative and gram-positive bacteria. They act by inhibiting protein synthesis by bacterial cells.

Uses

The tetracyclines are often used for patients allergic to the penicillins for the treatment of certain venereal diseases, urinary tract infections, upper respiratory tract infections, pneumonia, and meningitis. They are particularly effective against skin (acne), rickettsial, and mycoplasmic infections.

Tetracyclines administered during the ages of tooth development (the last half of pregnancy through 8 years of age) may cause enamel hypoplasia and permanent staining of the teeth to a yellow, gray, or brown color. Tetracyclines are secreted in breast milk, so nursing mothers on tetracycline therapy are advised to feed their infants formula or cow's milk, as appropriate.

Therapeutic Outcome

The primary therapeutic outcome expected from tetracycline therapy is elimination of bacterial infection.

Nursing Process

Premedication Assessment

1. Obtain baseline assessments of presenting symptoms.
2. Record temperature, pulse, respirations, blood pressure and hydration status.
3. Assess for and record any gastric symptoms present before initiation of therapy.
4. Assess for any allergies.
5. Obtain baseline laboratory studies ordered (for example, CBC with differential).

Planning

Availability. See Table 43-7.

Implementation

Dosage and administration. See Table 43-7. PO—Emphasize the importance of taking medication 1 hour before or 2 hours after ingesting antacids, milk or other dairy products, or products containing calcium, aluminum, magnesium, or iron (such as vitamins). *Exception:* food or milk does not interfere with the absorption of doxycycline.

Evaluation

Side effects to report

NAUSEA, VOMITING, ANOREXIA, ABDOMINAL CRAMPS, DIARRHEA. These side effects are usually mild and tend to resolve with continued therapy. Encourage the patient not to discontinue therapy without first consulting the physician.

PHOTOSENSITIVITY. Photosensitivity resulting in an exaggerated sunburn after short exposure has been reported. The patient should be cautioned to avoid exposure to sunlight and ultraviolet light. Suggest wearing long-sleeved clothing, a hat, and sunglasses when exposed to sunlight. Discourage the use of artificial tanning lamps. Notify the physician for the advisability of continuing therapy.

Drug interactions

WARFARIN. This medication may enhance the anticoagulant effects of warfarin. Observe for the development of petechiae, ecchymoses, nosebleeds, bleeding gums, dark tarry stools, and bright red or coffee ground emesis. Monitor the prothrombin time and reduce the dosage of warfarin if necessary.

METHOXYFLURANE. If patients are receiving tetracycline and are scheduled for surgery, label the front of the chart "taking tetracycline." Fatal nephrotoxicity has been reported when methoxyflurane is administered to a person taking tetracycline.

IMPAIRED ABSORPTION. Iron; calcium-containing foods (milk and other dairy products); calcium, aluminum, or magnesium preparations (antacids); and alkaline products (sodium bicarbonate) decrease absorption of tetracycline. Administer all tetracycline products 1 hour before or 2 hours after ingestion of these foods or products.

Exception: food or milk does not interfere with the absorption of doxycycline.

PHENYTOIN, CARBAMAZEPINE. These agents reduce the half-life of doxycycline. Monitor patients for lack of clinical improvement from the infection.

TOOTH DEVELOPMENT. Do not administer tetracyclines to pregnant patients or children under 8 years of age. The infant's or child's tooth enamel may be permanently stained (yellow, gray, or brown).

LACTATION. Nursing mothers must switch their babies to formula while taking tetracyclines because tetracyclines are present in the breast milk.

DIDANOSINE. Do not administer tetracycline antibiotics within 2 hours of taking didanosine tablets or pediatric

Table 43-7

The Tetracyclines

GENERIC NAME	BRAND NAME	AVAILABILITY	ADULT DOSAGE RANGE
Demeclocycline	Declomycin	150 and 300 mg tablets	PO: 150 mg 4 times daily or 300 mg 2 times daily
Doxycycline	Vibramycin	100 and 200 mg vials 100 mg tablets 50 and 100 mg capsules 25 and 50 mg/5 ml syrup	IV: 100-200 mg 1 or 2 times daily PO: 200 mg on day 1, then 100 mg divided in 2 doses
Minocycline	Minocin	100 mg vial 50 and 100 mg capsules, tablets 50 mg/5 ml syrup	PO, IV: 200 mg, followed by 100 mg/12 hr
Oxytetracycline	Terramycin	250 mg capsules	PO: 250-500 mg 4 times daily
Tetracycline	Panmycin, Robitet, Sumycin	250 and 500 mg capsules and tablets 125 mg/5 ml syrup	PO: 250-500 mg 4 times daily

powder for oral solution. The antacid present in these formulations inhibits the absorption of the quinolones.

Drug Class: Antitubercular Agents

ethambutol (e-tham'bu-tol)
Myambutol (my-am'bu-tol)

Actions

Ethambutol inhibits tuberculosis bacterial growth by altering cellular RNA synthesis and phosphate metabolism.

Uses

Ethambutol is an antitubercular agent. It must be used in combination with other antitubercular agents to prevent the development of resistant organisms.

Therapeutic Outcome

The primary therapeutic outcome expected from ethambutol therapy is elimination of tuberculosis.

Nursing Process

Premedication Assessment

1. Obtain baseline assessments of presenting symptoms.
2. Record temperature, pulse, respirations, blood pressure, and hydration status.
3. Assess for and record any gastric symptoms present before initiation of therapy.
4. Assess for any allergies.
5. Perform baseline mental status assessment (orientation and alertness), assess for gastrointestinal symptoms, and test color vision (red-green discrimination) before initiation of therapy.
6. Review laboratory data of tuberculin testing on the patient's chart.

Planning

Availability. PO—100 and 400 mg tablets.

Implementation

Dosage and administration. Adults: PO—initial treatment: 15 mg/kg administered as a single dose every 24 hours. Retreatment: 25 mg/kg as a single daily dose. After 60 days, reduce the dose to 15 mg/kg and administer as a single dose every 24 hours. Administer once daily with food or milk to minimize gastric irritation.

Counseling. The patient should be warned that omission or interrupted intake may result in drug resistance, reversal of clinical improvement, and increased susceptibility of family members and others to tuberculosis.

Evaluation

Side effects to expect

NAUSEA, VOMITING, ANOREXIA, ABDOMINAL CRAMPS. These side effects are usually mild and tend to resolve with continued therapy. Encourage the patient not to discontinue therapy without first consulting the physician. Administer daily dose with food to minimize nausea and vomiting.

Side effects to report

CONFUSION, HALLUCINATIONS. Perform a baseline assessment of the patient's degree of alertness and orientation to name, place, and time *before* initiating therapy. Make regularly scheduled subsequent mental status evaluations, and compare findings. Report development of alterations. Provide for patient safety during episodes of altered behavior or periods of dizziness.

BLURRED VISION, RED-GREEN COLOR CHANGES. Check for any visual alterations using a color vision chart before initiating therapy. Schedule subsequent evaluations on a regular basis. Report the development of visual disturbances for the physician's evaluation. These adverse effects disappear within a few weeks after therapy is discontinued.

Drug interactions

No clinically significant interactions have been reported.

isoniazid (i-so-ny'ah-zid)
INH, Nydrazid (ny'dra-zid), **✦Rimifon** (rhim-ih-fon')

Actions

Isoniazid has been a mainstay in the prevention and treatment of tuberculosis for many years. Despite this, its mechanism of action is still not fully known. It appears to disrupt the *Mycobacterium tuberculosis* cell wall and inhibit replication.

Uses

Isoniazid is used for the prophylaxis and treatment of tuberculosis. It should be used in combination with other antitubercular agents for therapy of active disease.

Therapeutic Outcomes

The primary therapeutic outcomes expected from isoniazid therapy are as follows:
- Prevention of tuberculosis in persons with positive skin test
- Elimination of tuberculosis in persons with active disease

Nursing Process

Premedication Assessment

1. Obtain baseline assessments of presenting symptoms.
2. Record temperature, pulse, respirations, blood pressure, and hydration status.
3. Assess for and record any gastric symptoms, abnormal liver function tests, or paresthesias present before initiation of therapy.
4. Assess for any allergies.
5. Check medication orders for concurrent administration of other antituberculin drugs and for an order for pyridoxine.

Planning

Availability. PO—50, 100, and 300 mg tablets; 50 mg/ml syrup. IM—100 mg/ml in 10 ml vials.

Implementation

Dosage and administration. Adult: PO—treatment of active tuberculosis: 5 mg/kg to a maximum of 300 mg daily.

Isoniazid should be used in conjunction with other effective antitubercular agents. Prophylactic therapy: 300 mg daily in single or divided doses. Administer on an empty stomach for maximum effectiveness. It is usually given as a single daily dose but may be given in divided doses. Pyridoxine, 25 to 50 mg daily, is frequently given concurrently with isoniazid to diminish peripheral neuropathies, dizziness, and ataxia. IM—as for PO administration.

Pediatric: PO—10 to 30 mg/kg per 24 hours in single or divided doses. Infants and children tolerate larger doses than adults. Maximum dose is 500 mg daily.

Evaluation
Side effects to expect and report
TINGLING, NUMBNESS, NAUSEA, VOMITING. Tingling and numbness of the hands and feet and nausea and vomiting are relatively common side effects of isoniazid and are dose related. Concurrent use of pyridoxine, 25 to 50 mg daily, will usually prevent the development of these symptoms.

When paresthesias are present, the patient must be cautioned to inspect the extremities for any possible skin breakdown because of the diminished sensation. Caution patients not to immerse feet or hands in water without first testing the temperature.

Monitor patients with paresthesias for adequate nutrition.

DIZZINESS, ATAXIA. Provide for patient safety and assistance in ambulation until either a dose adjustment or addition of pyridoxine provides symptomatic relief.

HEPATOTOXICITY. The incidence of hepatotoxicity increases with age and the consumption of alcohol. This reaction usually occurs within the first 3 months of therapy and is thought to be an allergic reaction.

The symptoms of hepatotoxicity are anorexia, nausea, vomiting, jaundice, hepatomegaly, splenomegaly, and abnormal liver function tests (elevated bilirubin, AST, ALT, GGT, alkaline phosphatase, and prothrombin time).

Drug interactions
DISULFIRAM. Patients may experience changes in physical coordination and mental affect and behavior. Provide for patient safety, and monitor the patient's mental status before and during therapy. If possible, avoid concomitant therapy.

CARBAMAZEPINE. Isoniazid may inhibit the metabolism of carbamazepine. Monitor patients receiving concurrent therapy for signs of carbamazepine toxicity: ataxia, headache, vomiting, blurred vision, drowsiness, and confusion.

PHENYTOIN. Isoniazid may inhibit the metabolism of phenytoin. Monitor patients receiving concurrent therapy for signs of phenytoin toxicity: nystagmus, sedation, and lethargy. Serum levels may be ordered and the dosage of phenytoin reduced.

CLINITEST. This drug may produce false-positive Clinitest results. Use Clinistix or Tes-Tape to measure urine glucose.

rifampin (rif′am-pin)
Rifadin (rif′ah-din)

Actions
Rifampin prevents RNA synthesis in mycobacterium by inhibiting DNA-dependent RNA polymerase. This action blocks key metabolic pathways needed for mycobacterium cells to grow and replicate.

Uses
Rifampin is used in combination with other agents in treatment of tuberculosis. Rifampin is also used to eliminate meningococci from the nasopharynx of asymptomatic *Neisseria meningitidis* carriers and to eliminate *Haemophilus influenzae* type b (Hib) from the nasopharynx of asymptomatic carriers.

Therapeutic Outcomes
The primary therapeutic outcomes expected from rifampin therapy are as follows:
- Elimination of tuberculosis
- Eradication of meningococci or Hib from asymptomatic carriers of these diseases

Nursing Process
Premedication Assessment
1. Obtain baseline assessments of presenting symptoms.
2. Record temperature, pulse, respirations, blood pressure, and hydration status.
3. Assess for and record any gastric symptoms present before initiation of therapy.
4. Assess for any allergies.
5. Obtain baseline laboratory studies ordered (for example, CBC with differential, tuberculin tests, and chest x-ray).

Planning
Availability. PO—150 and 300 mg capsules. IV—600 mg vials.

Implementation
Dosage and administration. Adult: PO—600 mg once daily either 1 hour before or 2 hours after a meal. IV—As for PO.

Pediatric: PO—10 to 20 mg/kg per 24 hours with a maximum daily dose of 600 mg. IV—As for PO.

Note: Patients should be warned that omission or interrupted intake may result in drug resistance, reversal of clinical improvement, and increased susceptibility of family members to tuberculosis.

Evaluation
Side effects to expect
REDDISH-ORANGE SECRETIONS. Urine, feces, saliva, sputum, sweat, and tears may be tinged a reddish-orange color. The effect is harmless and will disappear after discontinuation of therapy. Rifampin may permanently discolor soft contact lenses.
Side effects to report
NAUSEA, VOMITING, ANOREXIA, ABDOMINAL CRAMPS. These side effects are usually mild and tend to resolve with continued therapy. Encourage the patient not to discontinue therapy without first consulting the physician. If these symptoms are accompanied by fever, chills, or muscle and bone pain or if unusual bruising or a yellowish discoloration of the skin or eyes appears, contact the patient's physician.
Drug interactions
WARFARIN. This medication may diminish the anticoagulant effects of warfarin. Monitor the prothrombin time and increase the dosage of warfarin if necessary.

ISONIAZID. Concurrent therapy may rarely result in hepatotoxicity. Patients on combined therapy should have liver function tests monitored periodically.

QUINIDINE, DIAZEPAM, VERAPAMIL, MEXILETINE, THEOPHYLLINE, BETA-BLOCKING AGENTS, DISOPYRAMIDE, BARBITURATES, ORAL ANTIDIABETIC AGENTS, MANY OTHER DRUGS. Rifampin stimulates the metabolism of these agents. Long-term combined therapy may require an increase in dosages for therapeutic effect.

PROBENECID. Probenecid may reduce hepatic metabolism of rifampin. Monitor closely for rifampin toxicity.

KETOCONAZOLE. Administration of rifampin and ketoconazole decreases serum levels of both drugs. Avoid concurrent use if possible.

ORAL CONTRACEPTIVES. Rifampin interferes with the contraceptive activity oral contraceptives. Counseling regarding alternative methods of birth control should be planned.

Drug Class: Miscellaneous Antibiotics

aztreonam (aze'tree-on-am)
Azactam (aze'ak-tam)

Actions

Aztreonam is the first in a new class of synthetic, bactericidal antibiotics called monobactams. The monobactams act by inhibiting cell wall synthesis.

Uses

The monobactams have a high degree of activity against beta-lactamase–producing aerobic gram-negative bacteria, including *Pseudomonas aeruginosa*. Aztreonam has essentially no activity against anaerobes or gram-positive microorganisms. Aztreonam is used to treat urinary tract, lower respiratory tract, skin, intraabdominal, gynecologic, and septicemic infections and meningitides caused by *Pseudomonas aeruginosa, Neisseria gonorrhoeae, Salmonella, Shigella*, and ampicillin-resistant *H. influenzae*. It is recommended that aztreonam be combined with a broad-spectrum antibiotic in the initial treatment of an infection of unknown cause to treat susceptible anaerobes or gram-positive organisms.

Therapeutic Outcome

The primary therapeutic outcome expected from aztreonam therapy is elimination of bacterial infection.

Nursing Process

Premedication Assessment

1. Obtain baseline assessments of presenting symptoms.
2. Record temperature, pulse, respirations, blood pressure, and hydration status.
3. Assess for and record any gastric symptoms present before initiation of therapy.
4. Assess for any allergies.
5. Obtain baseline laboratory studies ordered (for example, CBC with differential).

Planning

Availability. Injection—500 mg, 1 and 2 g powders in 15 ml and 100 ml bottles for reconstitution.

Implementation

Dosage and administration. Adult: IM or IV—urinary tract infections, 0.5 to 1 g every 8 to 12 hours; moderately severe systemic infections, 1 to 2 g every 8 to 12 hours; life-threatening infections, 2 g every 6 to 8 hours. IM—reconstitute a 15 ml vial with at least 3 ml of diluent per gram of aztreonam. After adding diluent to container, shake immediately and vigorously. Inject deeply into the large muscle mass of the gluteus maximus. Discard unused portion of vial. IV bolus—reconstitute a 15 ml vial with 6 to 10 ml of diluent. Shake immediately and vigorously. Inject directly into a vein or into the tubing of a suitable IV set over 3 to 5 minutes. Discard any unused portion of the vial. IV infusion—reconstitute the 100 ml bottle with at least 50 ml of diluent. Shake immediately and vigorously. Infuse over the next 30 to 60 minutes.

Evaluation

Side effects to expect

NAUSEA, VOMITING, DIARRHEA. These side effects are usually mild and tend to resolve with continued therapy.

Side effects to report

PHLEBITIS. Avoid IV infusion in the lower extremities or in areas with varicosities. Use proper technique in starting the intravenous solution.

Carefully assess at regularly scheduled intervals for signs of developing phlebitis. Inspect for redness, warmth, tenderness to touch, edema, or pain.

Always assess complaints of pain at the infusion site. If signs of inflammation accompany complaints, discontinue and restart elsewhere.

SECONDARY INFECTIONS. Oral thrush, genital and anal pruritus, vaginitis, and vaginal discharge may occur. Report promptly because these infections are resistant to the original antibiotic used.

Teach the importance of meticulous oral and perineal personal hygiene measures.

Drug interactions

CEFOXITIN, IMIPENEM. These antibiotics induce beta-lactamase production in some gram-negative organisms resulting in possible antagonism with a beta-lactam antibiotic such as aztreonam. It is recommended that beta-lactamase stimulating antibiotics not be used concurrently with aztreonam.

chloramphenicol (klo-ram-fen'i-kol)
Chloromycetin (klo-ro-my-se'tin)

Actions

Chloramphenicol is an antibiotic that acts by inhibiting bacterial protein synthesis of a variety of gram-positive and gram-negative organisms.

Uses

Chloramphenicol is particularly effective in treating rickettsial infections, meningitis, and typhoid fever. It must not be used in the treatment of trivial infections or when it is not indicated, such as in colds, influenza, throat infections, or as a prophylactic agent to prevent bacterial infection.

Therapeutic Outcome

The primary therapeutic outcome expected from chloramphenicol therapy is elimination of bacterial infection.

Nursing Process

Premedication Assessment

1. Obtain baseline assessments of presenting symptoms.
2. Record temperature, pulse, respirations, blood pressure, and hydration status.
3. Assess for and record any gastric symptoms present before initiation of therapy.
4. Assess for any allergies.
5. Obtain baseline laboratory studies ordered (for example, CBC with differential).

Planning

Availability. PO—250 mg capsules, 150 mg/5 ml suspension. IV—100 mg/ml in 1 g vials.

Implementation

Dosage and administration. Adult: PO—50 to 100 mg/kg every 6 hours. IM—not recommended because of poor absorption and clinical response. IV—as for PO administration. Reconstitute by adding 10 ml of sterile water for injection or dextrose 5% to 1 g of chloramphenicol to make a solution containing 100 mg/ml. Administer the calculated dose intravenously over a 1-minute period.

Pediatric: PO—neonates: 25 mg/kg per 24 hours in 4 equally divided doses. Infants over 2 weeks of age: 50 mg/kg per 24 hours in 4 equally divided doses. IM—not recommended. IV—as for PO administration. Administer over 1 minute. Use only chloramphenicol sodium succinate intravenously in children.

Evaluation

Side effects to report

HEMATOLOGIC. Serious and possibly fatal bone marrow suppression may occur after therapy is initiated with chloramphenicol. Early signs include sore throat, a feeling of fatigue, elevated temperature, and small petechial hemorrhages and bruises on the skin. If patients describe any of these symptoms, report them to the supervisor immediately. Routine laboratory studies (RBC, WBC, and differential counts) are scheduled for patients taking chloramphenicol 14 days or longer. Stress the importance of returning for this laboratory work.

Monitor for the development of sore throat, fever, purpura, jaundice, or excessive and progressive weakness.

SECONDARY INFECTIONS. Oral thrush, genital and anal pruritus, vaginitis, and vaginal discharge may occur. Report promptly because these infections are resistant to the original antibiotic used.

Teach the importance of meticulous oral and perineal personal hygiene.

Drug interactions

WARFARIN. This medication may enhance the anticoagulant effects of warfarin. Observe for the development of petechiae, ecchymoses, nosebleeds, bleeding gums, dark tarry stools, and bright red or coffee ground emesis. Monitor the prothrombin time and reduce the dosage of warfarin if necessary.

ORAL HYPOGLYCEMIC AGENTS. Monitor for hypoglycemia: headache, weakness, decreased coordination, general apprehension, diaphoresis, hunger, and blurred or double vision.

The dosage of the hypoglycemic agent may need to be reduced. Notify the physician if any of the above-mentioned symptoms appear.

CLINITEST. Chloramphenicol may cause a false-positive urinary glucose reaction when Clinitest is used. Tes-Tape or Diastix may be used instead to test for the presence of glucose.

PHENYTOIN. Chloramphenicol inhibits the metabolism of phenytoin.

Monitor patients with concurrent therapy for signs of phenytoin toxicity: nystagmus, sedation, and lethargy. Serum levels may be ordered and the dosage of phenytoin reduced.

clindamycin (klin-dah-my′sin)
Cleocin (klee-o′sin), Dalacin C (dahl′ah-sin C)

Actions

Clindamycin is an antibiotic that acts by inhibiting protein synthesis.

Uses

Clindamycin is useful against infections caused by gram-negative aerobic organisms and a variety of gram-positive and gram-negative anaerobes.

Therapeutic Outcome

The primary therapeutic outcome expected from clindamycin therapy is elimination of bacterial infection.

Nursing Process

Premedication Assessment

1. Obtain baseline assessments of presenting symptoms.
2. Record temperature, pulse, respirations, blood pressure, and hydration status.
3. Record pattern of bowel elimination before initiation of drug therapy.
4. Assess for any allergies.
5. Obtain baseline laboratory studies ordered (for example, CBC with differential).

Planning

Availability. PO—75 and 150 mg capsules, 75 mg/5 ml suspension. IV—150 mg/ml in 2, 4, and 6 ml ampules.

Implementation

Dosage and administration. Adult: PO—150 to 450 mg every 6 hours. Do NOT refrigerate the suspension. It is stable at room temperature for 14 days. IM—600 to 2700 mg per 24 hours. Do NOT exceed 600 mg per injection. Pain, induration, and sterile abscesses have been reported. Deep IM injection is recommended to help minimize this reaction.

IV—600 to 2700 mg per 24 hours. Dilute to less than 6 mg/ml. Administer at a rate less than 30 mg per minute. Administration by IV push is not recommended.

Pediatric: PO—suspension: 8 to 25 mg/kg per 24 hours in 4 divided doses. Capsules: 8 to 20 mg/kg per 24 hours in 4 divided doses. Capsules should be taken with a full glass of water to prevent esophageal irritation. IM—15 to 40 mg/kg per 24 hours in 4 divided doses. IV—as for IM use. Dilute to less than 6 mg/ml and administer at a rate less than 30 mg per minute.

Evaluation

Side effects to report

DIARRHEA. These side effects are usually mild and tend to resolve with continued therapy. Encourage the patient not to discontinue therapy without first consulting the physician.

SEVERE DIARRHEA. Severe diarrhea may develop from the use of clindamycin. Report diarrhea of five or more stools per day to the physician. This may be an indication of drug-induced pseudomembranous colitis.

Blood or mucus in the stool should also be reported. *Warn patients not to treat diarrhea themselves when taking this drug.* The use of loperamide or paregoric may prolong or worsen the condition. Large doses of attapulgite (Kaopectate) may be effective in diminishing the diarrhea.

Drug interactions

IMPAIRED ABSORPTION. Kaopectate absorbs clindamycin. It is effective in stopping diarrhea that may occur with the administration of clindamycin.

NEUROMUSCULAR BLOCKADE. Label charts of patients scheduled for surgery who are taking clindamycin. When combined with surgical muscle relaxants or aminoglycosides, neuromuscular blockade may result.

These combinations may potentiate respiratory depression. Check the anesthesia record of surgical patients. Monitor postoperative patients for respiratory depression for a prolonged period. This may occur 48 hours or more after the drug administration.

THEOPHYLLINE TOXICITY. Clindamycin, when given with theophylline, may result in theophylline toxicity. Observe for vomiting, dizziness, restlessness, and cardiac arrhythmias. The dosage of theophylline may need to be reduced.

ERYTHROMYCIN. Therapeutic antagonism has been reported between clindamycin and erythromycin. Do not administer concurrently.

 imipenem/cilastatin (imee′pen-ehm si′la-stat′in)
Primaxin (pry-max-in)

Actions

Imipenem/cilastatin is a combination product containing a thienamycin antibiotic called imipenem and cilastatin, an inhibitor of the renal dipeptidase enzyme dehydropeptidase I. Cilastatin has no antimicrobial activity; it prevents the inactivation of imipenem by the renal enzyme.

Uses

Imipenem is an extremely potent, broad-spectrum antibiotic resistant to beta-lactamase enzymes secreted by bacteria. It acts by inhibition of bacterial cell wall synthesis. It is used in the treatment of lower respiratory tract and intraabdominal infections; infections of the urinary tract, bones, joints, and skin; gynecologic infections; endocarditis; and bacterial septicemia caused by gram-negative or gram-positive organisms. A primary therapeutic role of imipenem-cilastatin is in the treatment of severe infections caused by multiresistant organisms and in mixed anaerobic-aerobic infections, primarily those involving intraabdominal and pelvic sepsis in which *Bacteroides fragilis* is a common pathogen. It should be used in combination with antipseudomonal agents because of resistance of *Pseudomonas cepacia* and *P. aeruginosa* to imipenem.

Therapeutic Outcome

The primary therapeutic outcome expected from imipenen-cilastatin therapy is elimination of bacterial infection.

Nursing Process

Premedication Assessment

1. Obtain baseline assessments of presenting symptoms.
2. Record temperature, pulse, respirations, blood pressure, and hydration status.
3. Assess for and record any gastric symptoms present before initiation of therapy.
4. Assess for any allergies.
5. Obtain baseline laboratory studies ordered (for example, CBC with differential).
6. Perform a baseline assessment of the patient's degree of alertness and orientation to name, place, and time *before* initiating therapy.
7. Ask whether there is a history of any seizure disorders.

Planning

Availability. IV—250 mg/250 mg and 500 mg/500 mg imipenem-cilastatin powder in 13 ml vials or 120 ml infusion bottles for reconstitution. IM—500 mg/500 mg and 750 mg/750 mg imipenem-cilastatin powder in vials for reconstitution.

Implementation

Hypersensitivity. Although this antibiotic is a thienamycin, rather than a penicillin or cephalosporin, it also contains a beta-lactam nucleus. Cross-hypersensitivity may develop between these classes. Complete a history of hypersensitivity before starting therapy. If an allergic reaction to imipenem-cilastatin occurs, discontinue the infusion. Serious reactions may require epinephrine and other emergency measures.

Dosage and administration. Adult: IM, IV—250 mg (imipenem) every 6 hours for mild infections and up to 1 g every 6 hours for severe, life-threatening infections. Do not exceed 50 mg/kg per day or 4 g per day, whichever is lower. Dosage reduction is required in patients with creatinine clearance rates of less than 70 ml/min/1.73 m^2.

Preparation of Solution. Reconstitute the 120 mg infusion bottle with 100 ml of diluent and shake until dissolved. Reconstitute the 13 ml vial with 10 ml of diluent and shake until dissolved. Transfer the contents to a 100 ml infusion solution. DO NOT INFUSE THE SUSPENSION. IT MUST BE DILUTED TO AT LEAST 100 ML. A suggested procedure after reconstitution is to transfer the suspension and then rinse the 13 ml vial with another 10 ml of diluent and transfer again to the infusion solution. The resulting mixture should be agitated until clear.

Rate. Administer each 250 mg or 500 mg dose over 20 to 30 minutes and each 1 g dose over 60 minutes. If nausea develops, slow the infusion rate.

Evaluation

Side effects to expect

NAUSEA, VOMITING, DIARRHEA. These side effects are usually mild and tend to resolve with continued therapy.

Side effects to report

DIZZINESS. Provide for patient safety during episodes of dizziness; report for further evaluation.

CONFUSION, SEIZURES. Seizure activity, including myo-clonic activity, focal tremors, confusional states, and other seizures, has been reported with imipenem-cilastatin. These episodes occurred most frequently in patients with histories of seizure activity.

Perform a baseline assessment of the patient's degree of alertness and orientation to name, place, and time *before* initiating therapy. Make regularly scheduled subsequent mental status evaluations and compare findings. Report development of alterations.

Implement seizure precautions. Make sure the patient continues with anticonvulsant therapy. If seizures develop, provide for patient safety and then record the exact time of seizure onset and duration of each phase, a description of the specific body parts involved, and any progression of the affected parts. Describe the automatic responses seen during the clonic phase: altered, jerky respirations or frothy saliva-tion, dilated pupils and any eye movements, cyanosis, dia-phoresis, or incontinence.

PHLEBITIS. Carefully assess patients for the development of thrombophlebitis. Inspect the IV area frequently while providing care; inspect visually during dressing changes and at times the IV is changed to a new site. Report redness, warmth, tenderness to touch, and edema in the affected part; if in lower extremities, dorsiflexion of the foot may cause pain in the calf area (Homans' sign). Compare the affected limb with the unaffected limb.

Drug interactions

IMIPENEM/CILASTATIN should not be mixed with or added to other antibiotics, but it may be administered concomitantly with other antibiotics such as aminoglycosides.

metronidazole (met-row-nyd′a-zol)
Flagyl (fla′jil)

Actions

Metronidazole is a somewhat unusual medication in that it has antibacterial, trichomonacidal, and protozoacidal activity. Its mechanism of action is unknown.

Uses

Metronidazole is used to treat trichomoniasis, giardiasis, amebic dysentery, amebic liver abscess, and anaerobic bac-terial infections.

Therapeutic Outcome

The primary therapeutic outcome expected from metronida-zole therapy is elimination of infection.

Nursing Process

Premedication Assessment

1. Obtain baseline assessments of presenting symptoms.
2. Record temperature, pulse, respirations, blood pressure, and hydration status.
3. Assess for and record any gastric symptoms, peripheral neuropathy, or seizure disorders present before initiation of therapy.
4. Assess for any allergies.
5. Perform a baseline assessment of the patient's degree of alertness and orientation to name, place, and time *before* initiating therapy.
6. Obtain baseline laboratory studies ordered (for example, CBC with differential).

Planning

Availability. PO—250 and 500 mg tablets. IV—500 mg per vial.

Implementation

Dosage and administration. Adult: PO—trichomoniasis:
- Men and women—250 mg 3 times daily for 7 days. Sexual partners must be treated concurrently to prevent reinfection.
- Single doses of 2 g or 2 doses of 1 g each administered the same day appear to provide adequate treatment for tri-chomoniasis in both sexes.

Amebic dysentery: 750 mg 3 times daily for 5 to 10 days. Amebic liver abscess: 500 to 750 mg 3 times daily for 5 to 10 days. Giardiasis: 250 mg 2 to 3 times daily for 5 to 10 days. Anaerobic bacterial infections:
- Start with parenteral therapy initially.
- The usual *oral* dosage is 7.5 mg/kg every 6 hours. Do not exceed 4 g per 24 hours. The usual duration is 7 to 10 days. Infections of the bone and joint, lower respiratory tract, and endocardium may require longer treatment.

IV—anaerobic bacterial infections:
- Loading dose: 15 mg/kg infused over 1 hour.
- Maintenance dose: 7.5 mg/kg infused over 1 hour every 6 hours. Do not exceed 4 g per 24 hours. Convert to oral dosages when clinical condition is stable.
- Dosage reduction is necessary in patients with hepatic impairment but not renal impairment.

Pediatric: PO—trichomoniasis: 35 to 50 mg/kg per 24 hours in 3 divided doses for 7 days. Amebiasis: 35 to 50 mg/kg per 24 hours in 3 divided doses for 10 days. Giardiasis: 35 to 50 mg/kg per 24 hours in 3 divided doses for 7 days.

Evaluation

Side effects to expect

NAUSEA, VOMITING, DIARRHEA. These side effects are usually mild and tend to resolve with continued therapy.

Side effects to report

DIZZINESS. Provide for patient safety during episodes of dizziness; report for further evaluation.

CONFUSION, SEIZURES. Patients receiving high doses, those with histories of seizure activity, and those with significant hepatic impairment are at greater risk of confu-sion and seizures. Perform a baseline assessment of the patient's degree of alertness and orientation to name, place, and time *before* initiating therapy. Make regularly scheduled subsequent mental status evaluations and compare findings. Report development of alterations.

Implement seizure precautions. Make sure the patient continues with anticonvulsant therapy. If seizures develop, provide for patient safety and then record the exact time of seizure onset and duration of each phase, a description of the specific body parts involved, and any progression of the affected parts. Describe the automatic responses seen during the clonic phase: altered, jerky respirations, frothy salivation, dilated pupils and any eye movements, cyanosis, diaphoresis, or incontinence.

PHLEBITIS. Carefully assess patients for the development of thrombophlebitis. Inspect the IV area frequently while providing care; inspect visually during dressing changes and at times the IV is changed to a new site. Report redness, warmth, tenderness to touch, and edema in the affected part. If in lower extremities, dorsiflexion of the foot may cause pain in the calf area (Homans' sign). Compare the affected limb with the unaffected limb.

Drug interactions

IMIPENEM/CILASTATIN should not be mixed with or added to other antibiotics, but it may be administered concomitantly with other antibiotics such as aminoglycosides.

spectinomycin (spek-ti-no-my′sin)
Trobicin (tro′bi-sin)

Actions

Spectinomycin is a bacteriostatic agent thought to act by inhibiting protein synthesis.

Uses

Spectinomycin is used specifically for the treatment of gonorrhea in both men and women. It has the particular advantage that most bacterial strains of gonorrhea respond to one administration of the recommended dosage. It is not effective in the treatment of syphilis. Serology testing for syphilis should be done before initiation of therapy and should be repeated 3 months after spectinomycin therapy. This drug masks the symptoms of syphilis.

Therapeutic Outcome

The primary therapeutic outcome expected from spectinomycin therapy is elimination of gonorrhea.

Nursing Process

Premedication Assessment

1. Obtain baseline assessments of presenting symptoms.
2. Record temperature, pulse, respirations, blood pressure, and hydration status.
3. Assess for any allergies.

Planning

Availability. IM—400 mg/ml in 2 and 4 g vials.

Implementation

Dosage and administration. Adult: IM—a 20-gauge needle is recommended. Injections should be made deep into the upper outer quadrant of the gluteal muscle. The usual dose for both men and women is 2 g. In geographic areas in which penicillin-resistant gonorrhea is common, a dose of 4 g is recommended (2 g in each gluteal muscle).

Evaluation

Side effects to expect

PAIN AT THE INJECTION SITE. Pain at the injection site is common. Give deeply in a large muscle mass. Devise a plan for rotation of injection sites if more than one injection is administered.

Drug interactions

No significant drug interactions have been reported.

vancomycin (van-ko′my′sin)
Vancocin (van-ko′sin)

Actions

Vancomycin is an antibiotic that acts by preventing the synthesis of bacterial cell walls. This site of action is different from the sites sensitive to penicillin and other antibiotics interfering with cell wall synthesis.

Uses

Vancomycin is effective against only gram-positive bacteria such as streptococci, staphylococci, *Clostridium difficile*, *Listeria monocytogenes*, and *Corynebacterium* that may cause endocarditis, osteomyelitis, meningitis, pneumonia, or septicemia. It may be used orally against staphylococcal enterocolitis and antibiotic-associated pseudomembranous colitis produced by *C. difficile*. Because of potential adverse effects, vancomycin therapy is reserved for patients with potentially life-threatening infections who cannot be treated with less toxic agents such as the penicillins or cephalosporins.

The most prominent and severe adverse effects associated with the use of vancomycin are nephrotoxicity and ototoxicity. These occur with greater frequency and severity in patients with renal impairment or when large doses are administered. Hearing loss may be preceded by tinnitus and high-tone hearing loss and is often permanent. Elderly patients appear to be particularly susceptible to the ototoxic effects.

Therapeutic Outcome

The primary therapeutic outcome expected from vancomycin therapy is elimination of bacterial infection.

Nursing Process

Premedication Assessment

1. Obtain baseline assessments of presenting symptoms.
2. Record temperature, pulse, respirations, blood pressure, and hydration status.
3. Assess for normal renal function and hearing before initiation of therapy.
4. Assess for any allergies.
5. Obtain baseline laboratory studies ordered (for example, CBC with differential).

Planning

Availability. PO—125 and 250 mg capsules; 250 mg per 5ml powder for oral solution. IV—50 mg/ml in 10 ml vial.

Implementation

Red man syndrome. Rapid intravenous administration may result in a severe hypotensive episode. Patients develop a redneck syndrome, or red man syndrome, characteristic of vancomycin. It is manifested by a sudden and profound hypotension with or without a maculopapular rash over the face, neck, upper chest, and extremities. The rash generally resolves within a few hours after termination of the infusion. In rare cases the administration of fluids, antihistamines, or corticosteroids may be necessary. Administer the solution diluted to less than 5 mg/ml over at least 60 minutes. Monitor blood pressure during infusion.

PO reconstitution. Add 115 ml of distilled water to the contents of the 10 g container. Each 6 ml of solution provides approximately 500 mg of vancomycin.

Dosage and administration. Adult: PO—500 mg every 6 hours or 1 g every 12 hours. Pseudomembranous colitis produced by *C. difficile*—250 mg to 1 g per day in 3 or 4 divided doses for 7 to 10 days. IM—not recommended because of poor absorption and clinical response. IV—500 mg every 6 hours or 1 g every 12 hours. Dosage must be adjusted for patients with impaired renal function.

Pediatric: PO—neonates: 10 mg/kg per day in divided doses; children: 40 mg/kg per day in 4 divided doses not to exceed 2 g per day. IM—not recommended because of poor absorption and clinical response. IV—neonates: initial dose of 15 mg/kg followed by 10 mg/kg every 12 hours until 1 month of age, then every 8 hours thereafter; children: 40 mg/kg per day in divided doses.

Evaluation

Side effects to report

OTOTOXICITY. This may initially be manifested by dizziness, tinnitus, and progressive hearing loss. Assess patients for difficulty in walking unaided and assess the level of hearing daily. Intentionally speak to patients softly; note if they are aware that you said anything. Take particular notice of the patient who repeatedly says, "What did you say?" or who starts talking more loudly or progressively increases the volume on the television or radio.

NEPHROTOXICITY. Monitor urinalysis and kidney function tests for abnormal results. Report an increasing BUN and creatinine, decreasing urine output or decreasing urine specific gravity (despite amount of fluid intake), casts or protein in the urine, frank blood or smoky-colored urine, or RBCs in excess of 0 to 3 on the urinalysis report.

SERUM LEVELS. Serum levels of vancomycin should be routinely ordered to minimize these adverse effects. Notify the physician of any abnormal serum levels reported so that dosage adjustments may be made. Consult laboratory reports for normal range.

SECONDARY INFECTIONS. Oral thrush, genital and anal pruritus, vaginitis, and vaginal discharge may occur. Report promptly because these infections are resistant to the original antibiotic used.

Teach the importance of meticulous oral and perineal personal hygiene.

Drug interactions

NEPHROTOXICITY, OTOTOXICITY. Concurrent and sequential use of other ototoxic or nephrotoxic agents such as neomycin, streptomycin, kanamycin, gentamicin, viomycin, paromomycin, polymyxin B, colistin, tobramycin, amikacin, cisplatin, furosemide, and bumetanide requires careful monitoring.

Drug Class: Topical Antifungal Agents

Actions

The exact mechanisms by which antifungal agents act are unknown. However, it is known that cell membranes are altered, resulting in increased permeability, leakage of amino acids and electrolytes, and impaired uptake of essential nutrients needed for cell growth.

Uses

The common topical fungal infections caused by several different dermatophytes are tinea pedis (athlete's foot), tinea cruris (jock itch), tinea corporis (ringworm), and tinea versicolor. *Candida albicans* is the most common cause of oral candidiasis (thrush), cutaneous candidiasis (for example, diaper rash), and vaginal candidiasis (that is, moniliasis, or "yeast infection").

Therapeutic Outcome

The primary therapeutic outcome expected from topical antifungal therapy is elimination of fungal infection.

Nursing Process

Premedication Assessment

1. Obtain baseline assessments of presenting symptoms.
2. Assess for any allergies.

Planning

Availability. See Table 43-8.

Implementation

Dosage and administration. See Table 43-8.

Topical. Wash hands thoroughly before and immediately after application. Cleanse skin with soap and water and dry thoroughly.

For athlete's foot, the powder is most effective in intertriginous areas and in cases in which a dry environment may enhance the therapeutic response. Instruct patients to wear cotton socks (avoid nylon) if possible and change 2 to 3 times daily. Treatments may be required for 6 weeks or more with longstanding infections and in areas of thickened skin.

For jock itch or ringworm, wear well-fitting, nonconstrictive ventilated clothing.

For all fungal infections, instruct patients to avoid tight-fitting clothing or occlusive dressings unless otherwise instructed by the physician.

Eye contact. Instruct patient to avoid contact with the eye and wash eyes immediately if contact should occur.

Intravaginal. Give the patient the following instructions:
1. Wash the applicator in warm soapy water after each use so that it does not become a vehicle for reinfection.
2. A pad may be used to protect clothing.
3. Use the number of doses prescribed even if symptoms disappear or menstruation begins.
4. Refrain from sexual intercourse during therapy (or the male should wear a condom to avoid reinfection).

Table 43-8

Topical Antifungal Agents

GENERIC NAME	BRAND NAME	AVAILABILITY	ADULT DOSAGE RANGE
Butoconazole	Femstat-3	Vaginal cream: 2%	For vaginal candidiasis: Pregnant patients (second and third trimesters only): 1 applicatorful intravaginally at bedtime for 6 days Nonpregnant patients: 1 applicatorful intravaginally at bedtime for 3 days; may be extended to 6 days, if needed
Ciclopirox	Loprox	Cream: 1% Lotion: 1%	For ringworm, jock itch, athlete's foot, cutaneous candidiasis, and tinea versicolor: Massage cream or lotion into affected skin twice daily for at least 4 weeks
Clotrimazole	Gyne-Lotrimin	Vaginal tablets: 100, 500 mg	For vaginal candidiasis: Cream: 1 applicatorful at bedtime for 7-14 nights
	Mycelex-G	Vaginal Cream: 1%	Tablets: insert one 100 mg tablet intravaginally at bed time for 7 nights or two 100 mg tablets at bedtime for 3 nights; or one 500 mg tablet intravaginally, one time only, at bedtime
	Mycelex	Cream: 1% Solution: 1%	For ringworm, jock itch, athlete's foot: Apply topically to affected skin morning and evening; gently rub in
	Mycelex	Oral lozenges: 10 mg (troches)	For oral candidiasis: Allow 1 lozenge to dissolve slowly in mouth 5 times daily for 14 consecutive days.
Econazole	Spectazole	Cream: 1%	For ringworm, jock itch, athlete's foot, tinea versicolor: Apply over affected area once daily For cutaneous candidiasis: Apply twice daily, morning and evening
Haloprogin	Halotex	Cream: 1% Solution: 1%	For ringworm, jock itch, athlete's foot, cutaneous candidiasis, and tinea versicolor: Cover affected areas twice daily, morning and evening; treatment may require 2-4 weeks.
Ketoconazole	Nizoral	Cream: 2%	For ringworm, jock itch, athlete's foot, cutaneous candidiasis, and tinea versicolor: Massage in cream to affected and surrounding tissue once daily; may require 2-4 weeks of treatment For seborrheic dermatitis: Massage in cream to affected area twice daily for 4 weeks
		Shampoo: 2%	For dandruff: Moisten hair and scalp with water; apply shampoo and lather gently for 1 min; rinse and reapply, leaving lather on scalp for 3 min; rinse thoroughly and dry hair; apply shampoo twice weekly for 4 weeks with at least 3 days between shampooing
Miconazole	Monistat 3	Vaginal suppositories: 200 mg	For vaginal candidiasis: Monistat 3: insert 1 suppository intravaginally at bedtime for 3 days
	Monistat 7	Vaginal suppositories: 100 mg Vaginal cream: 2%	Monistat 7: insert 1 applicatorful or 1 suppository at bedtime for 7 days.
	Micatin	Cream: 2% Powder: 2% Spray: 2%	For ringworm, jock itch, athlete's foot, cutaneous candidiasis, and tinea versicolor: Cover affected areas twice daily, morning and evening; treatment may require 2-4 weeks

continued

Table 43-8

Topical Antifungal Agents—cont'd

GENERIC NAME	BRAND NAME	AVAILABILITY	ADULT DOSAGE RANGE
Naftifine	Naftin	Cream: 1% Gel: 1%	For ringworm, jock itch, athlete's foot: 　Cream: massage into affected area once daily 　Gel: massage into affected area twice daily
Nystatin	Mycostatin	Vaginal tablets: 100,000 U	For vaginal candidiasis: 　1 tablet intravaginally daily for 2 weeks
	Mycostatin, Nilstat, Nystex	Oral suspension: 100,000 U/ml	For oral candidiasis: 　4-6 ml 4 times daily; retain in mouth as long as possible before swallowing
	Mycostatin, Pastilles	Oral lozenges: 200,000 U (troches)	1-2 tablets 4 or 5 times daily; do not chew or swallow
	Mycostatin, Nilstat, Nystex	Cream, ointment, powder	For cutaneous candidiasis: 　Apply to affected area 2 to 3 times daily
Oxiconzole nitrate	Oxistat	Cream: 1% Lotion: 1%	For ringworm, jock itch, athlete's foot: 　Massage into affected areas once daily at bedtime
Sulconazole	Exelderm	Cream: 1% Solution: 1%	For ringworm, jock itch, athlete's foot: 　Massage into affected area twice daily
Terbinafine	Lamisil	Cream: 1%	Massage into affected area twice daily; treatment may require 2-4 weeks
Terconazole	Terazol 7 Terazol 3	Vaginal cream: 0.4% Vaginal cream: 0.8%	For vaginal candidiasis: 　Insert 1 applicatorful intravaginally daily at bedtime for 3 (Terazol 3) or 7 (Terazol 7) consecutive days
		Vaginal suppository: 80mg	Insert 1 suppository intravaginally once daily at bedtime for 3 consecutive days
Tioconazole	Vagistat-1	Vaginal ointment: 6.5%	For vaginal candidiasis: 　Insert 1 applicatorful intravaginally daily at bedtime
Tolnaftate	Tinactin	Cream: 1% Solution: 1% Gel: 1% Spray: 1% Powder: 1%	For ringworm, jock itch, athlete's foot, cutaneous candidiasis, and tinea versicolor: 　Cover affected areas twice daily, morning and evening; treatment may require 2-4 weeks

5. Contraception other than a diaphragm or condom should be used when the patient is being treated with the vaginal ointment (for example, Vagistat). Prolonged contact with petrolatum-based products may cause the diaphragm and condom to deteriorate.

Evaluation

Side effects to expect and report

IRRITATION. Some patients experience vulvar or vaginal burning, vulvar itching, or discharge, soreness, or swelling from the intravaginal products. These side effects are usually mild and tend to resolve with continued therapy. Encourage the patient not to discontinue therapy without first consulting the physician.

REDNESS, SWELLING, BLISTERING, OOZING. These signs may be an indication of hypersensitivity. Inform the physician.

Drug interactions

No clinically significant drug interactions have been reported.

Drug Class: Systemic Antifungal Agents

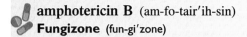

amphotericin B (am-fo-tair'ih-sin)
Fungizone (fun-gi'zone)

Actions

Amphotericin B is a fungistatic agent that disrupts the cell membrane of fungal cells, resulting in a loss of cellular contents.

Uses

Amphotericin B is used primarily for the treatment of systemic fungal infections and meningitis. It can also be used topically for candidal infections.

Therapeutic Outcome

The primary therapeutic outcome expected from amphotericin B therapy is elimination of fungal infection.

Nursing Process

Premedication Assessment
1. Obtain baseline assessments of presenting symptoms.
2. Record temperature, pulse, respirations, blood pressure, and hydration status.
3. Assess for normal renal function and normal electrolytes before initiation of therapy.
4. Assess for any allergies.
5. Gather baseline data about the patient's mental status (alertness, orientation, and confusion); muscle strength; presence of muscle cramps, tremors, and nausea; and general appearance (drowsy, anxious, or lethargic).

Planning
Availability. Topical—3% cream, lotion. IV—50 mg per vial.

Implementation
Dosage and administration. Adult: Topical—apply liberally to candidal lesions 2 to 4 times daily. Any clothing staining from cream or lotion preparations may be removed by soap and warm water, and any clothing staining from amphotericin ointment may be removed by standard cleaning fluids. IV—initially 250 µg/kg over 6 hours. The daily dose is gradually increased as the patient develops tolerance. Dosage may range between 1 and 1.5 mg/kg on alternate days.

Venous irritation may be diminished by the addition of 1200 to 1600 U of heparin or 10 to 15 mg of hydrocortisone or methylprednisolone to the infusion solution.

Amphotericin B must be reconstituted with sterile water for injection without bacteriostatic agent.

Filters. Do NOT use an in-line filter during infusion.

Light protection. The infusion must be protected from light during administration.

Concentration. The recommended infusion concentration is 1 mg per 10 ml of dextrose 5% in water.

Additives. Check for specific orders regarding the addition of heparin, hydrocortisone, or methylprednisone to diminish venous irritation.

Rate. Administer over 6 hours unless specifically ordered otherwise. Maintain close observation for thrombophlebitis.

Evaluation
Side effects to expect
TOPICAL CREAM OR LOTION. Side effects from topical preparations are usually minor. The cream may dry the skin. The lotion may cause slight irritation, manifested by erythema, pruritus, or a burning sensation. Allergic dermatitis is rare. If symptoms become severe, report for further evaluation by the physician.

Side effects to report
NEPHROTOXICITY. Nephrotoxicity may be manifested by increases in excretion of uric acid, potassium, and magnesium; oliguria; granular casts in the urine; proteinuria; and increased BUN and serum creatinine levels. Monitor urinalysis and kidney function tests for abnormal results. Report an increasing BUN and creatinine, decreasing urine output or decreasing urine specific gravity (despite amount of fluid intake), casts or protein in the urine, frank blood or smoky-colored urine, or RBCs in excess of 0 to 3 on the urinalysis report. Report intake and output, as well as a progressive decrease in daily urine volume or changes in visual characteristics.

ELECTROLYTE IMBALANCE. The electrolytes most commonly altered are potassium (K^+) and magnesium (Mg^{++}). Hypokalemia is most likely to occur.

Many symptoms associated with altered fluid and electrolyte balance are subtle and resemble general symptoms of drug toxicity or the disease process itself.

Gather data about changes in the patient's mental status (alertness, orientation, and confusion), muscle strength, muscle cramps, tremors, nausea, and general appearance (drowsy, anxious, and lethargic).

Always check the electrolyte reports for early indications of electrolyte imbalance.

Keep accurate records of intake and output, daily weights, and vital signs.

MALAISE, FEVER, CHILLS, HEADACHE, NAUSEA, VOMITING. These adverse effects tend to be dose related and may be minimized by slow infusion, reduction of dosage, and alternate-day administration. Check prn and standing orders for drugs (antihistamines, aspirin, and antiemetics) that may alleviate these symptoms.

THROMBOPHLEBITIS. Carefully assess patients receiving IV amphotericin B for the development of thrombophlebitis.

Inspect the IV area frequently while providing care; inspect during dressing changes and when the IV is changed to a new site. Always investigate pain at the IV site. Report redness, warmth, tenderness to touch, and edema in the affected part. If in lower extremities, dorsiflexion of the foot may cause pain in the calf (Homans' sign). Compare the affected limb with the unaffected one.

Drug interactions
CORTICOSTEROIDS (PREDNISONE, OTHERS). Corticosteroids may enhance the loss of potassium. Check potassium levels and monitor more closely for hypokalemia when these two agents are used concurrently.

NEPHROTOXIC POTENTIAL. Combining amphotericin B with other nephrotoxic agents such as aminoglycosides or diuretics should be done with extreme caution. Monitor closely for signs of nephrotoxicity.

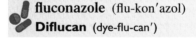

fluconazole (flu-kon′azol)
Diflucan (dye-flu-can′)

Actions
Fluconazole is an antifungal agent chemically related to ketoconazole and miconazole. It acts by inhibiting certain metabolic pathways in fungi that interfere with cell wall synthesis.

Uses
Fluconazole is used for oral and IV treatment of cryptococcal meningitis and oropharyngeal, esophageal, vulvovaginal, or systemic candidiasis. Fluconazole therapy is usually reserved for patients in whom other antifungal therapy was not tolerated or was ineffective. Fluconazole is also used prophylactically to prevent candidiasis in bone marrow transplant patients who are receiving radiation or chemotherapy treatment and in patients with human immunodeficiency virus

(HIV) infection. Fluconazole is also approved as a single-dose treatment of vaginal candidiasis in immunocompetent patients.

Therapeutic Outcomes

The primary therapeutic outcomes expected from fluconazole therapy are as follows:
* Prevention of systemic fungal infections
* Elimination of fungal infection

Nursing Process

Premedication Assessment

1. Obtain baseline assessments of presenting symptoms.
2. Record temperature, pulse, respirations, blood pressure, and hydration status.
3. Assess for and record any gastric symptoms and abnormal liver and renal function present before initiation of therapy.
4. Assess for any allergies.
5. Obtain baseline laboratory studies ordered (for example, CBC with differential).

Planning

Availability. PO—50, 100, 150, and 200 mg tablets; 50 and 200 mg per 5 ml suspension. IV—200 and 400 mg vials.

Implementation

Dosage and administration. PO—100 to 400 mg daily. Dosage must be individualized to type of infection being treated. IV—as for PO.

Evaluation

Side effects to expect

NAUSEA, VOMITING, DIARRHEA. These side effects are usually mild and tend to resolve with continued therapy. Encourage the patient not to discontinue therapy without first consulting the physician.

Side effects to report

RASH. Report symptoms for further evaluation by the physician. Do not administer any further doses until so ordered by the physician.

HEPATOTOXICITY. The symptoms of hepatotoxicity are anorexia, nausea, vomiting, jaundice, hepatomegaly, splenomegaly, and abnormal liver function tests (elevated bilirubin, AST, ALT, GGT, alkaline phosphatase, and prothrombin time).

Drug interactions

CIMETIDINE. Cimetidine inhibits the absorption of fluconazole. Concurrent use is not recommended.

DIURETICS. Diuretics inhibit the excretion of fluconazole. Monitor patients for an increase in frequency of side effects. The dosage of fluconazole may need to be decreased if concurrent therapy with diuretics is required.

TOXICITY INDUCED BY FLUCONAZOLE. Fluconazole can increase serum concentrations of cyclosporine, astemizole, terfenadine, phenytoin, zidovudine, and oral sulfonylurea hypoglycemic agents (tolbutamide, glipizide, and glyburide). Fluconazole can also potentiate the anticoagulant effects of warfarin. Read individual monographs for monitoring parameters of toxicity from these agents.

 flucytosine (flu-sy'toe-seen)
Ancobon (on-ko-bon'), **Ancotil** (ahn-co'til)

Actions

Flucytosine is an antifungal agent. Its mechanism of action is thought to be inhibition of RNA and protein synthesis.

Uses

Flucytosine is effective against susceptible candidal septicemia, endocarditis, urinary tract infections, cryptococcal meningitis, and pulmonary infections.

Therapeutic Outcome

The primary therapeutic outcome expected from flucytosine therapy is elimination of fungal infection.

Nursing Process

Premedication Assessment

1. Obtain baseline assessments of presenting symptoms.
2. Record temperature, pulse, respirations, blood pressure, and hydration status.
3. Assess for and record any gastric symptoms or abnormal liver or renal function present before initiation of therapy.
4. Assess for any allergies.
5. Record baseline mental status assessment data.

Planning

Availability. PO—250 and 500 mg capsules.

Implementation

Dosage and administration. Adult: PO—50 to 150 mg/kg per day divided into doses every 6 hours. Doses up to 250 mg/kg per day may be required in cryptococcal meningitis. Nausea may be reduced if the capsules are given a few at a time over 20 to 30 minutes.

Evaluation

Side effects to expect

NAUSEA, VOMITING, DIARRHEA. These side effects are usually mild and tend to resolve with continued therapy. Encourage the patient not to discontinue therapy without first consulting the physician.

Side effects may be reduced by administering a few capsules at a time over 30 minutes.

Side effects to report

HEMATOLOGIC, RASH. Monitor for the development of sore throat, fever, purpura, jaundice, or excessive and progressive weakness.

NEPHROTOXICITY. Monitor urinalysis and kidney function tests for abnormal results. Report an increasing BUN and creatinine, decreasing urine output or decreasing urine specific gravity (despite amount of fluid intake), casts or protein in the urine, frank blood or smoky-colored urine, or RBCs in excess of 0 to 3 on the urinalysis report.

HEPATOTOXICITY. The symptoms of hepatotoxicity are anorexia, nausea, vomiting, jaundice, hepatomegaly, splenomegaly, and abnormal liver function tests (elevated bilirubin, AST, ALT, GGT, alkaline phosphatase, and prothrombin time).

Drug interactions

AMPHOTERICIN B. Flucytosine and amphotericin B display enhanced activity when used concurrently.

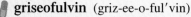

griseofulvin (griz-ee-o-ful′vin)
Fulvicin (ful′vi-sin), Grifulvin (gri-ful′vin)

Actions

Griseofulvin is a fungistatic agent that acts by stopping cell division and new cell growth.

Uses

Griseofulvin is used to treat ringworm of the scalp, body, nails, and feet. After griseofulvin is absorbed, it is incorporated into the keratin of the nails, skin, and hair in therapeutic amounts. The infecting fungus is not killed, but its growth into new cells is prevented. Once the cells are shed or removed, they are replaced by new cells that are free from the infection. Because of the slow growth of nails, treatment is often required for several months.

Therapeutic Outcome

The primary therapeutic outcome expected from griseofulvin therapy is elimination of fungal infection.

Nursing Process

Premedication Assessment

1. Obtain baseline assessments of presenting symptoms.
2. Record temperature, pulse, respirations, blood pressure, and hydration status.
3. Assess for and record any gastric symptoms or abnormal hematologic, liver, or renal function tests present before to initiation of therapy.
4. Assess for any allergies.
5. Obtain baseline laboratory studies ordered (for example, CBC with differential and liver and renal function tests).
6. Record results of baseline mental status examination.

Planning

Availability. PO—125, 165, 250, 330, and 500 mg tablets and capsules; 125 mg per 5 ml oral suspension.

Implementation

Dosage and administration. Adult: PO—depending on the specific organism and the location of the infection, 500 mg to 4 g in single or divided doses daily. Absorption from the gastrointestinal tract may be increased by administering with a meal high in fat content.

Evaluation

Side effects to expect

NAUSEA, VOMITING, ANOREXIA, ABDOMINAL CRAMPS. These side effects are usually mild and tend to resolve with continued therapy. Encourage the patient not to discontinue therapy without first consulting the physician.

Side effects to report

URTICARIA, RASH, PRURITUS. Hypersensitivity reactions, manifested by itching, urticaria, and rash, are relatively common. Report symptoms for further evaluation by the physician.

Pruritus may be relieved by adding baking soda to the bath water.

CONFUSION. Perform a baseline assessment of the patient's degree of alertness and orientation to name, place, and time *before* initiating therapy. Make regularly scheduled subsequent mental status evaluations and compare findings. Report development of alterations.

DIZZINESS. Provide for patient safety during episodes of dizziness; report for further evaluation.

SECONDARY INFECTIONS. With griseofulvin, oral thrush, genital and anal pruritus, vaginitis, and vaginal discharge may occur. Report promptly because these infections are resistant to the original antibiotic used.

Teach the importance of meticulous oral and perineal personal hygiene.

PHOTOSENSITIVITY. The patient should be cautioned to avoid exposure to sunlight and ultraviolet light. Suggest wearing long-sleeved clothing, hat, and sunglasses when exposed to sunlight. Discourage the use of artificial tanning lamps. Notify the physician for the advisability of continuing therapy.

HEMATOLOGIC. Routine laboratory studies (RBC, WBC, and differential counts) are scheduled for patients taking griseofulvin 30 days or longer. Stress the importance of returning for this laboratory work. Monitor for the development of sore throat, fever, purpura, jaundice, or excessive and progressive weakness.

NEPHROTOXICITY. Monitor urinalysis and kidney function tests for abnormal results. Report an increasing BUN and creatinine, decreasing urine output or decreasing urine specific gravity (despite amount of fluid intake), casts or protein in the urine, frank blood or smoky-colored urine, or RBCs in excess of 0 to 3 on the urinalysis report.

HEPATOTOXICITY. The symptoms of hepatotoxicity are anorexia, nausea, vomiting, jaundice, hepatomegaly, splenomegaly, and abnormal liver function tests (elevated bilirubin, AST, ALT, GTT, alkaline phosphatase, and prothrombin time).

Drug interactions

WARFARIN. Griseofulvin may diminish the anticoagulant effects of warfarin. Monitor the prothrombin time, and increase the dosage of warfarin if necessary.

BARBITURATES. The absorption of griseofulvin is impaired when combined with barbiturates. If concurrent therapy cannot be avoided, administer the griseofulvin in divided doses 3 times daily.

ORAL CONTRACEPTIVES. Griseofulvin may cause amenorrhea, increased breakthrough bleeding, and possibly decreased contraceptive efficacy when used concomitantly with oral contraceptives. Other methods of contraception such as condoms and foam should be considered during griseofulvin therapy.

itraconazole (it-rah-kon′a-zol)
Sporanox (spor-ahn-ox′)

Actions

Itraconazole is an antifungal agent chemically related to fluconazole, miconazole, and ketoconazole. It acts by interfering with cell wall synthesis, causing leakage of cellular contents.

Uses

Itraconazole is used orally to treat candidiasis, chronic mucocutaneous candidiasis, oral thrush, candiduria, coccidioidomycosis, histoplasmosis, chromomycosis, and paracoccidioidomycosis. It is also effective against *Aspergillus*.

Therapeutic Outcome

The primary therapeutic outcome expected from itraconazole therapy is elimination of fungal infection.

Nursing Process

Premedication Assessment

1. Obtain baseline assessments of presenting symptoms.
2. Record temperature, pulse, respirations, blood pressure, and hydration status.
3. Assess for and record any gastric symptoms or abnormal liver function tests present before initiation of therapy.
4. Assess for any allergies.
5. Obtain baseline laboratory studies ordered (for example, liver function tests).

Planning

Availability. PO—100 mg tablets.

Implementation

Dosage and administration. Adult: PO—200 to 400 mg daily. Dosages over 200 mg should be given in 2 divided doses. Instruct the patient to take with a full meal to ensure maximal absorption.

Evaluation

Side effects to expect

NAUSEA, VOMITING. These side effects are usually mild and tend to resolve with continued therapy. Encourage the patient not to discontinue therapy without first consulting the physician. Administer after a full meal for maximal absorption.

Side effects to report

HEPATOTOXICITY. Liver function tests are recommended before initiating therapy, with follow-up tests biweekly to monthly.

The symptoms of hepatotoxicity are anorexia, nausea, vomiting, jaundice, hepatomegaly, splenomegaly, and abnormal liver function tests (elevated bilirubin, AST, ALT, GGT, alkaline phosphatase, and prothrombin time).

PRURITUS, RASH. Report symptoms to the physician for further evaluation. Pruritus may be relieved by adding baking soda to the bath water.

Drug interactions

H_2 ANTAGONISTS. H_2 antagonists (cimetidine, famotidine, ranitidine, and nizatidine) inhibit the absorption of itraconazole. Concurrent use is not recommended.

CARBAMAZEPINE, PHENYTOIN, RIFAMPIN. Concurrent administration of itraconazole and these agents has resulted in a significant decrease in itraconazole activity and clinical failure. The mechanism is unknown, but it is suspected that these agents stimulate the metabolism of itraconazole. If these agents are to be used concurrently, itraconazole levels must be monitored to ensure therapeutic effect.

TOXICITY INDUCED BY ITRACONAZOLE. Itraconazole can increase serum concentrations of cisapride, cyclosporine, astemizole, terfenadine, isoniazid, digoxin, tacrolimus, quinidine, midazolam, triazolam, amlodipine, nifedipine, and oral sulfonylurea hypoglycemic agents (tolbutamide, glipizide, and glyburide). Itraconazole can also potentiate the anticoagulant effects of warfarin. Read individual monographs for monitoring parameters of toxicity from these agents.

ketoconazole (key-toe-kon′a-zol)
Nizoral (nis-o-ral′)

Actions

Ketoconazole is an antifungal agent chemically related to fluconazole, miconazole, and itraconazole. It acts by interfering with cell wall synthesis, causing leakage of cellular contents.

Uses

Ketoconazole is used orally to treat candidiasis, chronic mucocutaneous candidiasis, oral thrush, candiduria, coccidioidomycosis, histoplasmosis, chromomycosis, and paracoccidioidomycosis.

Therapeutic Outcome

The primary therapeutic outcome expected from ketoconazole therapy is elimination of fungal infection.

Nursing Process

Premedication Assessment

1. Obtain baseline assessments of presenting symptoms.
2. Record temperature, pulse, respirations, blood pressure, and hydration status.
3. Assess for and record any gastric symptoms or abnormal liver function tests present before initiation of therapy.
4. Assess for any allergies.
5. Obtain baseline laboratory studies ordered (for example, liver function tests).

Planning

Availability. PO—200 mg tablets; suspension: 100 mg per 5 ml.

Implementation

Note: Administer at least 2 hours before giving drugs that reduce stomach acidity.

Dosage and administration. Adults: PO—200 to 400 mg once daily. Absorption is improved when administered with food.

Pediatrics: PO—44 pounds or less: 50 mg once daily; 44 to 88 pounds: 100 mg once daily; more than 88 pounds: 200 mg once daily.

Evaluation

Side effects to expect

NAUSEA, VOMITING. These side effects are usually mild and tend to resolve with continued therapy. Encourage the patient not to discontinue therapy without first consulting the physician.

Administer with food or milk to reduce irritation.

Side effects to report

HEPATOTOXICITY. Liver function tests are recommended before initiating therapy with follow-up tests biweekly to monthly.

The symptoms of hepatotoxicity are anorexia, nausea, vomiting, jaundice, hepatomegaly, splenomegaly, and abnormal liver function tests (elevated bilirubin, AST, ALT, GGT, alkaline phosphatase, and prothrombin time).

PRURITUS, RASH. Report symptoms to the physician for further evaluation. Pruritus may be relieved by adding baking soda to the bath water.

Drug interactions

H_2 ANTAGONISTS, DICYCLOMINE, ANTACIDS. Anticholinergic agents (dicyclomine, Donnatal, and propantheline), antacids, and H_2 antagonists (cimetidine, ranitidine, nizatidine, and famotidine) diminish stomach acidity and decrease absorption of ketoconazole. Administer ketoconazole at least 2 hours before these medications.

RIFAMPIN. Administration of rifampin and ketoconazole decreases serum levels of both drugs. Avoid concurrent use if possible.

ALCOHOL. Instruct patients to avoid alcohol consumption during ketoconazole therapy. Patients ingesting alcohol during and for 24 to 72 hours after administration of ketoconazole will become flushed, tremulous, dyspneic, tachycardic, and hypotensive. Tell patients to avoid use of over-the-counter preparations containing alcohol, such as mouthwash (Cepacol) or cough preparations, because of their alcohol content.

TOXICITY INDUCED BY KETOCONAZOLE. Ketoconazole can increase serum concentrations of cisapride, cyclosporine, astemizole, terfenadine, loratadine, phenytoin, triazolam, and oral sulfonylurea hypoglycemic agents (tolbutamide, glipizide, and glyburide). Ketoconazole can also potentiate the anticoagulant effects of warfarin. Read individual monographs for monitoring parameters of toxicity from these agents.

miconazole (my-kon'a-zol)
Monistat (mon'i-stat), Micatin (my'ka-tin)

Actions

Miconazole is an antifungal agent chemically related to itraconazole, ketoconazole and fluconazole. It acts by interfering with cell wall synthesis, causing cellular contents to leak.

Uses

Parenteral miconazole is used to treat candidiasis, chronic mucocutaneous candidiasis, oral thrush, candiduria, coccidioidomycosis, histoplasmosis, chromomycosis, and paracoccidioidomycosis. Bladder irrigations may be used for fungal cystitis, and intrathecal injections may be used to treat fungal meningitis.

Therapeutic Outcome

The primary therapeutic outcome expected from miconazole therapy is elimination of fungal infection.

Nursing Process

Premedication Assessment

1. Obtain baseline assessments of presenting symptoms.
2. Record temperature, pulse, respirations, blood pressure, and hydration status.
3. Assess for and record any gastric symptoms present before initiation of therapy.
4. Assess for any allergies.
5. Obtain baseline laboratory studies ordered (for example, CBC with differential, hemoglobin, hematocrit, and electrolytes).
6. Check for premedication orders for an antiemetic or antihistamine to be administered before IV infusion.

Planning

Availability. IV—10 mg/ml in 20 ml ampules.

Implementation

Dosage and administration. Adult: IV—coccidioidomycosis, 1800 to 3600 mg divided into 3 doses daily; cryptococcosis, 1200 to 2400 mg divided into 3 doses daily; candidiasis, 600 to 1800 mg divided into 3 doses daily; paracoccidioidomycosis, 200 to 1200 mg divided into 3 doses daily.

Dilute all infusion solutions with at least 200 ml of 0.9% sodium chloride or dextrose 5% and administer over a period of 30 to 60 minutes.

Give antihistamines or antiemetics before infusion; slow the rate of miconazole administration if nausea and vomiting develop.

Intrathecal—20 mg every 3 to 7 days as an adjunct to intravenous treatment of fungal meningitis. Administer undiluted by alternating lumbar, cervical, and cisternal punctures.

Bladder instillation—using aseptic technique, catheterize and infuse via an indwelling catheter. Instill 200 mg of miconazole in a diluted solution into the bladder. Clamp catheter for a specified period; open and drain as ordered. Frequency of administration is determined by the infecting microorganism.

Evaluation

Side effects to report

PHLEBITIS. Avoid IV infusion in the lower extremities and areas with varicosities. Use proper technique in starting the IV solution.

Always assess complaints of pain at the infusion site. If signs of inflammation accompany complaints, discontinue and restart elsewhere.

PRURITUS, RASH, FEVER, CHILLS. Report symptoms to the physician for further evaluation. Pruritus may be relieved by adding baking soda to the bath water.

NAUSEA, VOMITING, EMESIS. Nausea and vomiting can be reduced by using antihistamines or antiemetic agents before infusion, reducing the dose, slowing the infusion rate, and avoiding administration after meals.

THROMBOCYTOPENIA. Assess for signs of bleeding: petechiae, ecchymoses, nosebleeds, bleeding gums, dark tarry stools, and bright red or coffee ground emesis.

Drug interactions

TOXICITY INDUCED BY MICONAZOLE. Miconazole can increase serum concentrations of cisapride, cyclosporine, carbamazepine, astemizole, terfenadine, phenytoin, and oral sulfonylurea hypoglycemic agents (tolbutamide, glipizide, and glyburide). Read individual monographs for monitoring parameters of toxicity from these agents.

WARFARIN. Parenteral miconazole may enhance the anticoagulant effects of warfarin. Observe for the development of petechiae, ecchymoses, nosebleeds, bleeding gums, dark tarry stools, and bright red or coffee ground emesis. Monitor the prothrombin time, and reduce the dosage of warfarin if necessary.

Drug Class: Antiviral Agents

acyclovir (a-sy′klo-veer)
Zovirax (zoh-veye′rahx)

Actions

Acyclovir is an antiviral agent that acts by inhibiting viral cell replication.

Uses

Acyclovir is used topically to treat initial infections of herpes genitalis and non–life-threatening cases of mucocutaneous herpes simplex virus infections in patients with suppressed immune systems. The intravenous form is used to treat initial and recurrent mucosal and cutaneous herpes simplex types 1 and 2 infections in immunosuppressed adults and children and to treat severe initial clinical episodes of herpes genitalis in patients who are not immunosuppressed.

Therapeutic Outcome

The primary therapeutic outcome expected from acyclovir therapy is elimination of symptoms of viral infection.

Nursing Process

Premedication Assessment

1. Obtain baseline assessments of presenting symptoms.
2. Record temperature, pulse, respirations, blood pressure, and hydration status.
3. Assess for and record any abnormal renal function present before initiation of therapy.
4. Assess for any allergies.
5. Obtain baseline laboratory studies ordered (for example, renal function tests).
6. Perform baseline mental status examination (for example, orientation).

Planning

Availability. Topical—5% ointment. PO—200 mg capsules; 400 and 800 mg tablets; 200 mg per 5 ml suspension. IV—500, 1000 mg per vial.

Implementation

Dosage and administration. Adult: Topical—apply to each lesion every 3 hours 6 times daily for 7 days. A finger cot or rubber gloves should be used to avoid the spread of virus to other tissues and persons. Use meticulous hand-washing technique before and after applying the ointment. Do NOT apply to the eyes—it is not an ophthalmic ointment. IV—*Note:* bolus or rapid intravenous infusions may result in renal tubular damage. Acyclovir is reconstituted with 10 ml of preservative-free sterile water for injection to provide a solution concentration of 50 mg/ml. The solution is stable for 12 hours. This solution should be further diluted by a glucose and electrolyte intravenous fluid to a concentration of 1 to 7 mg/ml before administration (stable for 24 hours). Infuse over at least 1 hour to well-hydrated patients to prevent renal damage. Observe for phlebitis at the infusion site.

Dose for patients with normal function: 5 mg/kg every 8 hours for 5 to 7 days.

PO—initial treatment of genital herpes: 200 mg every 4 hours while the patient is awake, for a total of 1000 mg daily for 10 days. Chronic suppressive therapy for recurrent disease: 400 mg 2 times daily for up to 12 months. Some patients require 200 mg 5 times daily. Intermittent therapy: 200 mg every 4 hours while awake the patient is awake, for a total of 1000 mg for 5 days. Therapy should be initiated at the earliest sign or symptom (prodrome) of recurrence.

Pediatric: topical—as for adult patients. IV—patients over 12 years of age: 250 mg/m^2 every 8 hours for 7 days at a constant infusion rate over 1 hour.

Evaluation

Side effects to report

PRURITUS, RASH, BURNING. Report symptoms to the physician for further evaluation. Pruritus may be relieved by adding baking soda to the bath water.

INTRAVENOUS THERAPY. Avoid IV infusion in the lower extremities and areas with varicosities. Use proper technique in starting the IV solution.

Carefully assess at regularly scheduled intervals for signs of developing phlebitis. Inspect for redness, warmth, tenderness to touch, edema, or pain.

RASH, HIVES. Assess, describe, and chart the location and extent of these presenting symptoms. Report for further evaluation.

DIAPHORESIS. Diaphoresis can be serious if the patient is not well hydrated. Assess hydration state, monitor electrolytes, and provide for nursing interventions (for example, clean, dry linens and adequate fluid intake).

NEPHROTOXICITY. Monitor urinalysis and kidney function tests for abnormal results. Report an increasing BUN and creatinine, decreasing urine output or decreasing urine specific gravity (despite amount of fluid intake), casts or protein in the urine, frank blood or smoky-colored urine, or RBCs in excess of 0 to 3 on the urinalysis report.

HYPOTENSION. Record the blood pressure in both supine and sitting positions before and during the administration of this drug. Caution the patient to rise slowly from a supine or sitting position.

CONFUSION. Perform a baseline assessment of the patient's degree of alertness and orientation to name, place, and time *before* initiating therapy. Make regularly scheduled subsequent mental status evaluations and compare findings. Report development of alterations.

Drug interactions

PROBENECID. Probenecid may reduce urinary excretion of acyclovir. Monitor closely for signs of toxicity from acyclovir.

ZIDOVUDINE. Patients may complain of severe drowsiness and lethargy when acyclovir and zidovudine are used concurrently. Observe for patient safety.

 amantadine hydrochloride (ah-man'tah-deen)
Symmetrel (sim'eh-trel)

Uses

Amantadine is an antiviral agent that has specific activity against the influenza A virus. Its current primary use, however, is as an anti–Parkinson's disease agent. It does not treat the underlying disease but reduces its clinical manifestations. It is described in greater detail in Chapter 13 (see p. 174).

didanosine (die-dahn-oh'seen)
Videx (veye'dex)

Actions

Didanosine (ddI) is an antiviral agent that acts by inhibiting viral cell replication.

Uses

Didanosine is used to treat pediatric and adult patients with advanced HIV infection who have received prolonged courses of zidovudine and have deteriorated clinically or who cannot tolerate zidovudine therapy. Zidovudine is still considered the drug of choice in HIV disease because it has been shown to prolong survival and decrease the incidence of secondary infections in patients with acquired immunodeficiency syndrome (AIDS).

Therapeutic Outcomes

The primary therapeutic outcomes expected from didanosine therapy are as follows:
• Slowed clinical progression of HIV infection
• Reduced frequency of opportunistic secondary infections

Nursing Process

Premedication Assessment

1. Obtain baseline assessments of presenting symptoms.
2. Record temperature, pulse, respirations, blood pressure, and hydration status.
3. Assess for and record any peripheral neuropathies or gastrointestinal symptoms present before initiation of therapy.
4. Assess for any allergies.
5. Obtain baseline laboratory studies ordered (for example, CBC with differential and serum amylase).

Planning

Availability. PO—25, 50, 100, and 150 mg chewable or dispersible buffered tablets; 100, 167, 250, and 375 mg buffered powder for oral solution; and 2 and 4 g powder for pediatric oral solution.

Implementation

Dosage and administration. Adult: PO—for patients over 60 kg, start with 200 mg tablets or 250 mg of buffered powder every 12 hours. For patients under 60 kg, start with 125 mg tablets or 167 mg of buffered powder every 12 hours. Administer on an empty stomach. Food significantly reduces absorption. *Note:* Tablets should be thoroughly chewed or crushed and well dispersed in at least 1 ounce of water. The buffered powder should be mixed with at least 4 ounces of water and thoroughly dispersed. Instruct the patient to drink the entire solution immediately. Do not mix with fruit juice or other acid-containing liquid.
Transmission of HIV. Didanosine therapy has not been shown to reduce the risk of transmission of HIV to others through sexual contact or blood contamination.

Evaluation

Side effects to expect

DIARRHEA. There appears to be a higher incidence of diarrhea associated with the buffered powder. If diarrhea develops, try switching to the oral tablet form.

Side effects to report

ABDOMINAL PAIN, NAUSEA, AND VOMITING. Patients receiving didanosine are susceptible to developing pancreatitis. If these symptoms develop, withhold further administration of didanosine and report to the physician.

NUMBNESS, TINGLING. Patients receiving didanosine are susceptible to developing peripheral neuropathies characterized by numbness, tingling, or pain in the feet or hands. Report to the physician for further evaluation.

Drug interactions

QUINOLONE AND TETRACYCLINE ANTIBIOTICS, DAPSONE. Do not administer quinolone or tetracycline antibiotics within 2 hours of administering didanosine tablets or pediatric powder for oral solution. The antacid present in these formulations inhibits the absorption of the quinolones, tetracyclines, and dapsone.

famciclovir (pham-sik'lo-veer)
Famvir (pham'veer)

Actions

Famciclovir is a prodrug of penciclovir, an antiviral agent that acts by inhibiting viral cell replication.

Uses

Famciclovir is used orally to treat recurrent infections of genital herpes and in the management of acute herpes zoster (shingles). In patients with genital herpes, famiciclovir reduces the time of viral shedding, the duration of symptoms, and the time of healing if started within 6 hours of the onset of symptoms and continued for 5 days. In patients with shingles, if therapy is begun within 72 hours and continued for 7 days, famciclovir reduces the times to full crusting, loss of vesicles, loss of ulcers, and loss of crusts more effectively than placebo treatment. Early treatment with famciclovir can also reduce the duration of postherpetic neuralgia.

Therapeutic Outcome

The primary therapeutic outcome expected from famciclovir therapy is elimination of symptoms of viral infection.

Nursing Process

Premedication Assessment

1. Obtain baseline assessments of presenting symptoms.
2. Record temperature, pulse, respirations, blood pressure, and hydration status.
3. Assess for and record any abnormal renal function present before initiation of therapy.
4. Assess for any allergies.
5. Perform baseline mental status examination (for example, orientation).

Planning

Availability. PO—125 and 250 mg tablets.

Implementation

Dosage and administration. Adult: PO—treatment of genital herpes: 125 mg 2 times daily for 5 days. Therapy should be started at the first sign or symptom of herpes breakout. Treatment of herpes zoster (shingles): 500 mg every 8 hours for 7 days. To be effective, therapy must be started within 72 hours of the onset of symptoms.

Evaluation

Side effects to expect

NAUSEA, VOMITING, HEADACHE. These side effects are usually mild and tend to resolve with continued therapy. Encourage the patient not to discontinue therapy without first consulting the physician.

Administer with food or milk to reduce irritation.

Side effects to report

CONFUSION. Perform a baseline assessment of the patient's degree of alertness and orientation to name, place, and time *before* initiating therapy. Make regularly scheduled subsequent mental status evaluations and compare findings. Report development of alterations.

Drug interactions

PROBENECID. Probenecid may reduce urinary excretion of penciclovir. Monitor closely for signs of toxicity from penciclovir.

lamivudine (lahm-ihv-u′deen)
Epivir (epi′vihr)

Actions

Lamivudine is an antiviral agent that acts by inhibiting replication of HIV.

Uses

Lamivudine (3TC) is used in combination with zidovudine for the treatment of HIV infection. Laboratory studies indicate that the two medicines should work together synergistically to prolong life expectancy in HIV-positive patients and reduce the frequency of secondary infections associated with AIDS. At present, there are no results from controlled clinical trials evaluating the effects of combined therapy on the clinical progression of HIV infection, such as longer-term survival or the incidence of secondary infections.

Therapeutic Outcomes

The primary therapeutic outcomes expected from lamivudine therapy are as follows:
- Slowed clinical progression of HIV infection
- Reduced frequency of opportunistic secondary infections

Nursing Process

Premedication Assessment

1. Obtain baseline assessments of presenting symptoms.
2. Record temperature, pulse, respirations, blood pressure, and hydration status.
3. Assess for and record any gastric symptoms present before initiation of therapy.
4. Assess for any allergies.
5. Obtain baseline laboratory studies ordered (for example, CBC with differential, platelets, hemoglobin, hematocrit, amylase, and liver function tests).

Planning

Availability. PO—150 mg tablets and 10 mg/ml oral solution in 240 ml bottles.

Implementation

Dosage and administration. Adult: PO—150 mg twice daily with zidovudine.

Transmission of HIV. Lamivudine therapy has not been shown to reduce the risk of transmission of HIV to others through sexual contact or blood contamination.

Evaluation

Side effects to report

ANEMIA, GRANULOCYTOPENIA. Monitor hematologic indices every 2 weeks to detect serious anemia or granulocytopenia. In patients developing bone marrow suppression, reduction in hemoglobin may occur as early as 2 to 4 weeks; granulocytopenia usually occurs after 6 to 8 weeks.

It is crucial that patients understand the importance of returning periodically for blood counts while receiving therapy.

ABDOMINAL PAIN, NAUSEA, AND VOMITING. Patients receiving lamivudine are susceptible to developing pancreatitis. If these symptoms develop, withhold further administration of lamivudine and report to the physician.

NUMBNESS, TINGLING. Patients receiving lamivudine are susceptible to developing peripheral neuropathies characterized by numbness, tingling, or pain in the feet or hands. Report to the physician for further evaluation.

Drug interactions

CO-TRIMOXAZOLE. Concurrent administration of lamivudine and co-trimoxazole results in a significant increase in lamivudine levels and potential for toxicity. Dosage levels of lamivudine may need to be reduced.

ZIDOVUDINE. Concurrent administration of lamivudine and zidovudine results in a significant increase in zidovudine levels and potential for toxicity. Dosage levels of zidovudine may need to be reduced.

ribavirin (ribe-ah-vi′rihn)
Virazole (vi-rah′zohl)

Actions

Ribavirin is the first antiviral agent available to be used effectively against respiratory viruses. The mechanisms of action are unknown.

Uses

Ribavirin has been shown to have inhibitory activity against members of the DNA-type viral families of *Adenoviridae*, *Herpesviridae*, and *Poxviridae*. The RNA viruses for which ribavirin exerts inhibitory activity are the influenza, parainfluenza, and respiratory syncytial viruses. Ribavirin has initially been given FDA approval to be used by aerosol administration to treat severe lower respiratory tract infections caused by respiratory syncytial virus.

Therapeutic Outcome

The primary therapeutic outcome expected from ribavirin therapy is elimination of viral infection.

Nursing Process

Premedication Assessment

1. Obtain baseline assessments of presenting symptoms.
2. Record temperature, pulse, respirations, blood pressure, and hydration status.
3. Assess for and record any gastric symptoms present before initiation of therapy.
4. Assess for any allergies.
5. Obtain baseline laboratory studies ordered (for example, pulmonary function tests).
6. Determine if the patient is pregnant; if pregnancy is suspected, check with physician before administering drug.

Planning

Availability. Aerosol powder—6 g vials of powder for reconstitution.

Implementation

Dosage and administration. Ribavirin must be administered through a specific, small-particle aerosol generator.

1. Using aseptic technique, reconstitute the 6 g of drug by adding 50 ml of sterile water for injection to the 100 ml vial.
2. When dissolved, transfer the contents to a clean, sterilized 500 ml widemouthed Erlenmeyer flask and further dilute with sterile water for injection to a final volume of 300 ml. The final concentration is 20 mg/ml.
3. Administer ribavirin at an initial concentration of 20 mg/ml through the reservoir of the small-particle aerosol generator. Treatment is carried out for 12 to 18 hours per day for at least 3 and no more than 7 days. The aerosol is delivered from the generator to the patient via an oxygen hood or face mask. It should not be administered concurrently with any other aerosolized medication.

Pregnancy. Ribavirin is contraindicated in women who are or may become pregnant during exposure to the drug. Ribavirin has been reported to cause birth defects in several animal species. It is not completely eliminated from human blood for at least 4 weeks after administration.

Patients on respirators. Ribavirin is not recommended for patients requiring assisted ventilation because precipitation of the drug in the respiratory equipment may interfere with safe and effective use of the ventilator by these patients. If it is deemed necessary to treat a patient with ribavirin who is also receiving ventilatory support, prefilters must be placed in the equipment to prevent precipitation in the endotracheal tube or on the valves and tubing.

Evaluation

Side effects to expect

RASH, CONJUNCTIVITIS. These adverse effects tend to occur because of local irritation from poorly placed inhalation equipment. Work with the patient for optimal fit. Methylcellulose eye drops may be applied to reduce conjunctival irritation.

Side effects to report

DIMINISHING PULMONARY FUNCTION. Perform baseline pulmonary function tests to assess whether the patient shows deterioration after therapy is initiated. If initiation of treatment appears to produce sudden deterioration of respiratory function, treatment should be discontinued immediately and reinstituted only with extreme caution and continuous monitoring. Immediately report complaints of chest soreness, shortness of breath, or other adverse effects.

ANEMIA. Reticulocytosis and anemia have been reported during therapy. The severity and significance are not known at this time.

Drug interactions

No significant drug interactions have been reported.

 valacyclovir (vahl-ah-syk'lo-veer)
Valtrex (vahl'trex)

Actions

Valacyclovir is a prodrug of acyclovir, an antiviral agent that acts by inhibiting viral cell replication.

Uses

Valacyclovir is used orally to treat acute herpes zoster (shingles) in immunocompetent patients.

Therapeutic Outcome

The primary therapeutic outcome expected from valacyclovir therapy is elimination of symptoms of viral infection.

Nursing Process

Premedication Assessment

1. Obtain baseline assessments of presenting symptoms.
2. Record temperature, pulse, respirations, blood pressure, and hydration status.
3. Assess for and record any abnormal renal function present before initiation of therapy.
4. Assess for any allergies.
5. Perform baseline mental status examination (for example, orientation).

Planning

Availability. PO—500 mg caplets.

Implementation

Dosage and administration. Adult: PO—treatment of herpes zoster (shingles), 1 g (two 500 mg caplets) 3 times daily for 7 days. To be effective, therapy must be started within 48 hours of the onset of the herpes rash.

Evaluation

See Acyclovir.

zidovudine (zid-ohv′u-deen)
Retrovir (ret′roh-veer)

Actions

Zidovudine (AZT) is the first of a new series of antiviral agents that has been shown to be effective for certain patients with HIV infections. It acts by inhibiting replication of the virus. In controlled clinical trials, zidovudine was shown to prolong the lives of patients with AIDS and AIDS-related complex (ARC), to reduce the risk and severity of opportunistic infections, and to improve immune status.

Uses

Zidovudine is indicated for patients who have confirmed histories of *Pneumocystis carinii* pneumonia or absolute CD4 lymphocyte counts of less than 200/mm3 in the peripheral blood before therapy. Unfortunately, zidovudine is not a cure for HIV infections, and patients may continue to acquire illnesses associated with AIDS.

Therapeutic Outcomes

The primary therapeutic outcomes expected from zidovudine therapy are as follows:
• Slowed clinical progression of HIV infection
• Reduced frequency of opportunistic secondary infections

Nursing Process

Premedication Assessment

1. Obtain baseline assessments of presenting symptoms.
2. Record temperature, pulse, respirations, blood pressure, and hydration status.
3. Assess for any allergies.
4. Obtain baseline laboratory studies ordered (for example, CBC with differential, platelets, hemoglobin, hematocrit, amylase, and liver function tests).

Planning

Availability. PO—100 mg capsules; 50 mg per 5 ml syrup. IV—10 mg/ml in 20 ml vial.

Implementation

Dosage and administration. Adult: PO—asymptomatic HIV infection: 100 mg every 4 hours while the patient is awake (500 mg per day). *Patients must understand the importance of taking the medication every 4 hours around the clock, even though it may interrupt normal sleep.* Patients must also understand that the drug is taken orally and must not be shared with other persons and that they must not exceed the recommended dose. Potentially fatal adverse effects may result. Symptomatic HIV infection: 200 mg every 4 hours in

a 24-hour period. After 1 month, reduce to 100 mg every 4 hours. IV—1 to 2 mg/kg infused over 1 hour; administer every 4 hours 6 times daily.

Transmission of HIV. Zidovudine therapy *has not been* shown to reduce the risk of transmission of HIV to others through sexual contact or blood contamination.

Evaluation

Side effects to report

ANEMIA, GRANULOCYTOPENIA. Monitor hematologic indices every 2 weeks to detect serious anemia or granulocytopenia. In patients developing bone marrow suppression, reduction in hemoglobin may occur as early as 2 to 4 weeks; granulocytopenia usually occurs after 6 to 8 weeks.

It is crucial that patients understand the importance of returning periodically for blood counts while receiving therapy.

NUMBNESS, TINGLING. Patients receiving zidovudine are susceptible to developing peripheral neuropathies characterized by numbness, tingling, or pain in the feet or hands. Report to the physician for further evaluation.

Drug interactions

NEPHROTOXIC, CYTOTOXIC, HEPATOTOXIC AGENTS. Use of drugs such as dapsone, pentamidine, amphotericin B, flucytosine, vincristine, vinblastine, adriamycin, or interferon may increase the risk of toxicity.

PROBENECID, ASPIRIN, ACETAMINOPHEN, INDOMETHACIN. These agents may inhibit the metabolism and excretion of zidovudine, enhancing the potential for toxicity.

Patients must be warned not to use these agents while receiving zidovudine therapy.

DRUG THERAPY FOR URINARY TRACT INFECTIONS

The urinary antiinfective agents, including cinoxacin, methenamine mandelate, nalidixic acid, nitrofurantoin, and norfloxacin, are mainstays in urinary antimicrobial therapy. They are discussed in greater detail in Chapter 39.

CHAPTER REVIEW

Antimicrobial agents are chemicals that eliminate living microorganisms that are pathogenic to the patient. If at all possible, the infecting organisms should first be isolated and identified. The antimicrobial therapy is then started based on the sensitivity results and the clinical judgment of the physician.

Nurses must consider the entire patient when administering and monitoring antimicrobial therapy. It is essential that the nurse be knowledgeable about the drugs themselves, including physiologic parameters for monitoring expected therapeutic activity and potential adverse effects. It is important to teach the individual with an infection basic principles of self-care that will enhance the recovery process and measures to prevent the spread of the infection. In the case of communicable diseases, exposed individuals must be contacted for follow-up testing and appropriate treatment.

MATH REVIEW

1. The physician ordered chloramphenicol 50 mg/kg per 24 hours intravenously in 4 equally divided doses for an infant 12 weeks old weighing 13 pounds.
The infant's weight in kg is: _____ kg.
The amount of chloramphenicol to be administered in a 24-hour period would be: _____ mg.
Each of the four divided doses is: _____ mg.
On hand: chloramphenicol sodium succinate 100 mg/ml.
Give: _____ mg for each single dose.

2. The doctor orders amoxicillin 150 mg q8h, PO. After establishing that this dose is safe for the weight of the infant, you proceed to prepare it:
On hand: amoxicillin oral suspension 125 mg per 5 ml.
Give: _____ ml.

3. Ordered: cefazolin (Kefzol) 400 mg, IM q6h.
On hand: cefazolin 330 mg/ml.
Give: _____ ml.

4. Ordered: an IV antibiotic for administration in 30 minutes. Volume to be given is 50 ml.
The administration set delivers 15 gtts/ml.
Set the drip rate at: _____ gtts/min.

5. Ordered: vancomycin 1 g in 150 ml D$_5$W over 1.5 hours. Using an infusion pump to deliver this IVPB, set the pump at: _____ ml/hr.

CRITICAL THINKING QUESTIONS

Situation:

1. In Math Review question 1, the infant is 12 weeks old. After calculating the drug dose, what type of syringe and what size needle would you use to administer the prescribed chloramphenicol? What site of administration would be best in an infant of this age? Give rationale. Explain correct technique for administration, including landmark identification.

2. While providing care to a patient diagnosed 3 months ago with tuberculosis, you suspect noncompliance with the prescribed regimen. How would you proceed to verify this, and what interventions would you attempt?

44

Miscellaneous Agents

MISCELLANEOUS AGENTS

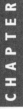

allopurinol (al-oh-pur′in-ol)

Zyloprim (zy′lo-prim)

Actions

Allopurinol blocks the terminal steps in uric acid formation by inhibiting the enzyme xanthine oxidase.

Uses

This agent can be used for the treatment of primary gout or gout secondary to antineoplastic therapy. It is not effective in the treatment of acute attacks of gouty arthritis.

Allopurinol has an advantage over uricosuric agents in that gouty nephropathy and the formation of urate stones are less likely with allopurinol because the drug inhibits the production of uric acid. It may also be used in patients with renal failure. Uricosuric agents should not be used in this case.

Therapeutic Outcome

The primary therapeutic outcome associated with allopurinol therapy is reduced serum uric acid levels with a lower frequency of acute gouty attacks.

Nursing Process

Premedication Assessment

1. Inquire about the time of onset of gouty attack; do not start the medication during an acute attack.
2. Assess for and record any gastrointestinal complaints present before initiation of drug therapy.
3. Obtain baseline blood studies, blood counts, and liver-function studies as requested.

Planning

Availability. PO—100 and 300 mg tablets.

Implementation

Dosage and administration. Adult: PO—initially 100 mg daily. Increase the daily dosage by 100 mg per week until the serum urate level falls to 6 mg/100 ml or a maximum dosage of 800 mg daily is achieved. The average maintenance dose is 300 mg daily.

Gastric Irritation. If gastric irritation occurs, administer with food or milk. If symptoms persist or increase in severity, report for physician evaluation.

Fluid Intake. Maintain fluid intake at 8 to 12 8-ounce glasses daily.

Evaluation

Side effects to expect

ACUTE GOUT ATTACKS. Patients should be told that the frequency of gout attacks may increase for the first few months of therapy. The patient should continue therapy without changing the doses during the attacks.

NAUSEA, VOMITING, DIARRHEA, DIZZINESS, HEADACHE. These side effects are usually mild and tend to resolve with continued therapy. Encourage the patient not to discontinue therapy without first consulting the physician.

Side effects to report

HEPATOTOXICITY. The symptoms of hepatotoxicity are anorexia, nausea, vomiting, jaundice, hepatomegaly, splenomegaly, and abnormal liver function tests (elevated bilirubin, aspartate aminotransferase [AST], alanine aminotransferase [ALT], gamma glutamyltransferase [GGT], alkaline phosphatase, and prothrombin time).

BLOOD DYSCRASIAS. Routine laboratory studies (red blood cell [RBC], white blood cell [WBC], and differential counts) should be scheduled. Stress the importance of returning for this laboratory work. Monitor for the development of sore throat, fever, purpura, jaundice, or excessive and progressive weakness.

FEVER, PRURITUS, RASH. Report symptoms for further evaluation by the physician. Pruritus may be relieved by adding baking soda to the bath water.

Drug interactions

THEOPHYLLINE DERIVATIVES. Allopurinol, when given with theophylline derivatives, may cause theophylline toxicity. Observe for vomiting, dizziness, restlessness, and cardiac arrhythmias. The dosage of theophylline may need to be reduced.

CHLORPROPAMIDE. Allopurinol may reduce the metabolism of chlorpropamide. Monitor for hypoglycemia (headache, weakness, decreased coordination, general apprehension, diaphoresis, hunger, and blurred or double vision). The dosage of the hypoglycemic agent may need to be reduced.

Notify the physician if any of the above-mentioned symptoms appears.

AZATHIOPRINE, MERCAPTOPURINE. When initiating therapy with azathioprine or mercaptopurine, start at one fourth to one third of the normal dosage and adjust subsequent dosages according to the patient's response.

AMPICILLIN, AMOXICILLIN. There is a high incidence of rash when patients are taking both allopurinol and ampicillin. Do not consider the patient allergic to either drug until sensitivity tests identify a hypersensitivity reaction.

CYCLOPHOSPHAMIDE. There is a greater frequency of bone marrow depression in patients receiving these agents concurrently. Monitor for the development of sore throat, fever, purpura, jaundice, or excessive and progressive weakness.

colchicine (kol'chi-sin)

Actions

The exact mechanism of action is not known, but colchicine does interrupt the cycle of urate crystal deposition in the tissues that results in an acute attack of gout. It does not affect the amount of uric acid in the blood or urine, therefore it is not a uricosuric agent.

Uses

Colchicine is an alkaloid that has been used for hundreds of years to prevent or relieve acute attacks of gout. Joint pain and swelling begin to subside within 12 hours and are usually gone within 48 to 72 hours after initiation of therapy.

Therapeutic Outcome

The primary therapeutic outcome expected from colchicine therapy is elimination of joint pain secondary to acute gout attack.

Nursing Process

Premedication Assessment
1. Assess for and record any gastrointestinal complaints present before initiation of drug therapy.
2. Obtain baseline complete blood count (CBC) and differential, uric acid level, and so on as requested by physician for future comparison and to monitor for development of blood dyscrasias and track progress in control of uric acid level.

Planning
Availability. PO—0.6 mg tablets, 0.5 mg granules. IV—1 mg/2 ml ampules.

Implementation
Note: Use with extreme caution in elderly or debilitated patients and in those patients with impaired renal, cardiac, or gastrointestinal function.

Dosage and administration. Adult: PO—acute gout: initially 0.5 to 1.3 mg, followed by 0.6 mg every 1 to 2 hours until pain subsides or nausea, vomiting, and diarrhea develop. A total dosage of 4 to 10 mg may be required. After the acute attack, 0.5 to 0.6 mg should be administered every 6 hours for a few days to prevent relapse. Do not repeat high-dose

therapy for at least 3 days. Prophylaxis for recurrent gout: 0.5 to 0.6 mg every 1 to 3 days depending on the frequency of gouty attacks. IV—acute gout: initially 2 mg diluted in 20 ml of saline solution administered slowly over 5 minutes. Follow with 0.5 mg every 6 to 12 hours to a maximum of 4 mg in 24 hours. If pain recurs, daily doses of 1 to 2 mg may be administered for several days. Do not repeat high-dosage therapy for at least 3 days. Avoid extravasation! Observe IV site for any change in the color, size, or skin integrity. Pain, swelling, or erythema signify infiltration.

DO NOT ADMINISTER SC OR IM!

Extravasation. Clamp, report, and follow hospital protocol for extravasation. Elevate the infiltrated area. Prepare to assist with administration of drugs to counteract the necrotizing effects.

Fluid intake. Monitor intake and output during therapy. Maintain fluid intake at 8 to 12 8-ounce glasses daily.

Evaluation
Side effects to expect
NAUSEA, VOMITING, DIARRHEA. These are common adverse effects of colchicine therapy. Discontinue therapy when gastrointestinal symptoms develop. Always report bright red blood in vomitus, coffee-ground vomitus, or dark tarry stools.

Side effects to report
BLOOD DYSCRASIAS. Serious, potentially fatal blood dyscrasias, including anemia, agranulocytosis, and thrombocytopenia, have been associated with colchicine therapy. Although the development of blood dyscrasias is rare, periodic differential blood counts are recommended if the patient requires prolonged treatment. Routine laboratory studies (RBC, WBC, and differential counts) should be scheduled. Stress to the patient the need to return for this laboratory work. Monitor for the development of sore throat, fever, purpura, jaundice, or excessive and progressive weakness. Report immediately.

Drug interactions
No clinically significant drug interactions have been reported.

lactulose (lak'tu-los)
Cephulac (sef'u-lak), Duphalac (du'fah-lak)

Actions

Lactulose is a sugar that acidifies the colon, thus preventing the absorption of ammonia. It also acts as a stool softener by increasing osmotic pressure and pulling water into the colon.

Uses

Elevated ammonia levels are thought to be a cause of portal-systemic (hepatic) encephalopathy and coma. Lactulose is used to reduce formation of ammonia in the gut. Lactulose may also be used as a laxative. Use with caution in patients with diabetes mellitus. Lactulose syrup contains small amounts of free lactose, galactose, and other sugars.

Therapeutic Outcomes

The primary therapeutic outcomes expected from lactulose therapy are as follows:
- Improved orientation to surroundings
- A gentle laxative effect with formed stool

Nursing Process

Premedication Assessment
1. Obtain baseline assessments of presenting symptoms.
2. Assess for and record any gastric symtoms present before the initiation of therapy.
3. Perform a baseline mental status examination (for example, orientation to time, place, and date).
4. Obtain baseline laboratory studies ordered (for example, electrolytes and serum ammonia levels).
5. Record temperature, pulse, respirations, blood pressure, and hydration status.

Planning
Availability. PO—10 g of lactulose per 15 ml of syrup.

Implementation
Dosage and administration. Adult: laxative, PO—initially 15 to 30 ml daily. Increase to 60 ml daily if necessary. Administer with fruit juice, water, or milk to make the syrup more palatable. It may take 24 to 48 hours to produce a normal bowel movement.

Portal-systemic encephalopathy, PO—initially 30 to 45 ml every hour for rapid laxation. Once the laxative effect is achieved, the dosage is reduced to 30 to 45 ml 3 to 4 times daily. Adjust the dose to produce two or three soft, formed stools daily. Rectal—mix 300 ml of syrup with 700 ml of water or normal saline. Instill rectally every 4 to 6 hours with a rectal balloon catheter. Instruct the patient to attempt to retain for 30 to 60 minutes. Do not use soap suds or cleansing enemas.

Evaluation
Side effects to expect
BELCHING, ABDOMINAL DISTENTION, FLATULENCE. These are common adverse effects frequently observed in the early stages of therapy. These side effects resolve with continued therapy, but dosage reduction may also be necessary. Diarrhea is a sign of overdosage and is corrected by dosage reduction.

Side effects to report
ELECTROLYTE IMBALANCE, DEHYDRATION. These effects may result from diarrhea. The electrolytes most commonly altered are potassium (K^+) and chloride (Cl^-). Hypokalemia is most likely to occur.

Many symptoms associated with altered fluid and electrolyte balance are subtle and resemble general symptoms of drug toxicity or the disease process itself.

Gather data relative to changes in the patient's mental status (that is, alertness, orientation, and confusion), muscle strength, muscle cramps, tremors, nausea, and general appearance (drowsy, anxious, and lethargic).

Always check the electrolyte reports for early indications of electrolyte imbalance.

Keep accurate records of intake and output, daily weights, and vital signs.

Patients on long-term lactulose therapy (6 months or longer) should have serum potassium and chloride levels measured periodically.

Drug interactions
LAXATIVES. Do not administer with other laxatives. Diarrhea makes it difficult to adjust to a proper dosage of lactulose.

ANTIBIOTICS. Antibiotic therapy may destroy too much of the bacteria in the colon necessary for lactulose to work. Monitor patients closely for reduced lactulose activity when concurrent antibiotic therapy is prescribed.

 probenecid (pro-ben'eh-sid)
Benemid (ben'eh-mid)

Actions
Uricosuric agents act on the tubules of the kidneys to enhance the excretion of uric acid. Probenecid promotes renal excretion of a number of substances, including uric acid. It inhibits the reabsorption of urate in the kidney, which results in reduction of uric acid in the blood.

Uses
Probenecid is used to treat hyperuricemia and chronic gouty arthritis. It is not effective in acute attacks of gout and is not an analgesic.

Therapeutic Outcome
The primary therapeutic outcome expected with probenecid therapy is prevention of acute attacks of gouty arthritis.

Nursing Process

Premedication Assessment
1. Inquire about time of onset of the last gout attack; do not administer medication during or within 2 to 3 weeks of an acute attack.
2. Assess for and record any gastrointestinal complaints present before initiation of drug therapy.
3. Ask about any history of blood dyscrasias or kidney stones; if present, withhold drug and contact physician.
4. Obtain baseline blood studies as requested (for example, uric acid level and serum creatinine) to assess appropriateness and to monitor response to therapy.

Planning
Availability. PO—500 mg tablets.

Implementation
Note: Do not start probenecid therapy during an acute attack of gout; wait 2 to 3 weeks.
Contraindication. Do NOT administer to patients with histories of blood dyscrasias or uric acid kidney stones.
Dosage and administration. Adult: PO—initially 250 mg twice daily for 1 week, then 500 mg twice daily. The dosage may be increased by 500 mg every few weeks to a maximum of 2 to 3 g daily. Administer with food or milk to diminish gastric irritation.

Maintain fluid intake at 2 to 3 L daily.

Do not administer to patients with a creatinine clearance of less than 40 ml per minute or a blood urea nitrogen (BUN) greater than 40 mg/100 ml.

Evaluation
Side effects to expect
ACUTE GOUT ATTACKS. Patients should be told that the frequency of gout attacks may increase for the first few

months of therapy. The patient should continue therapy without changing the doses during the attacks.

Side effects to report

NAUSEA, ANOREXIA, VOMITING. Use with caution in patients with histories of peptic ulcer disease. Individuals who experience symptoms of ulcers and are yet undiagnosed should be encouraged to report gastrointestinal symptoms if they increase in intensity or frequency. Always report bright red blood in vomitus, coffee-ground vomitus, or dark tarry stools.

HIVES, PRURITUS, RASH. These are signs of hypersensitivity. Notify the physician. Therapy may need to be discontinued.

Drug interactions

ORAL HYPOGLYCEMIC AGENTS. Monitor for hypoglycemia (headache, weakness, decreased coordination, general apprehension, diaphoresis, hunger, and blurred or double vision).

The dosage of the hypoglycemic agent may need to be reduced. Notify the physician if any of the above-mentioned symptoms appear.

ACYCLOVIR, FAMCICLOVIR, VALACYCLOVIR, ZIDOVUDINE, DAPSONE, INDOMETHACIN, SULFINPYRAZONE, RIFAMPIN, SULFONAMIDES, NAPROXEN, PENICILLINS, CEPHALOSPORINS, METHOTREXATE, AND CLOFIBRATE. Probenecid blocks the renal excretion of these agents. See individual drugs listed for side effects to report that may indicate development of toxicity.

SALICYLATES. Although occasional use of aspirin will not interfere with the effectiveness of probenecid, regular use of aspirin or aspirin-containing products should be discouraged. If analgesia is required, suggest acetaminophen.

ANTINEOPLASTIC AGENTS. Probenecid is not recommended for increased uric acid levels caused by antineoplastic therapy because of the potential development of renal uric acid stones.

CLINITEST. This drug may produce false-positive Clinitest results. Use Clinistix or Tes-Tape to measure urine glucose.

tacrine (tack′ rhin)
Cognex (cohg-nehx′)

Action

Tacrine is an acetylcholinesterase inhibitor that allows acetylcholine to accumulate at cholinergic synapses causing a prolonged and exaggerated cholinergic effect.

Uses

Although the causes are unknown, Alzheimer's disease is characterized by a loss of cholinergic neurons in the central nervous system resulting in memory loss and cognitive deficits (dementia). Tacrine is used in mild to moderate dementia to enhance cholinergic function.

Therapeutic Outcome

The primary therapeutic outcome expected from tacrine therapy is improved cognitive skills (for example, word recall, naming objects, language, word finding, and improved ability to do tasks).

Nursing Process

Premedication Assessment

1. Obtain baseline assessments of presenting symptoms.
2. Record baseline pulse, respirations, and blood pressure.

3. Assess for and record any gastric symptoms or abnormal liver function present before initiation of therapy.
4. Obtain baseline laboratory studies ordered (for example, liver function tests).

Planning

Availability. PO—10, 20, 30, and 40 mg tablets.

Implementation

Dosage and administration. Adult: PO—10 mg 4 times daily between meals and at bedtime. After at least 6 weeks, increase the dose to 20 mg 4 times daily. At 6-week intervals the dose can be increased up to a maximum of 40 mg 4 times daily.

Serum ALT levels should be measured to assess for the development of hepatotoxicity. The risk of hepatotoxicity is greatest in the first 12 weeks of tacrine treatment. Serum ALT levels should be monitored every other week during the first 16 weeks of therapy; thereafter, ALT serum concentrations can be monitored monthly. The manufacturer recommends specific guidelines on adjustment of treatment based on ALT levels.

Evaluation

Side effects to expect

NAUSEA, VOMITING, DYSPEPSIA, DIARRHEA. These are natural extensions of the pharmacologic effects of cholinergic agents. Dosage may need to be reduced if the patient has difficulty with these adverse effects.

Side effects to report

HEPATOTOXICITY. The symptoms of hepatotoxicity are anorexia, nausea, vomiting, jaundice, hepatomegaly, splenomegaly, and abnormal liver function tests (elevated bilirubin, AST, ALT, GGT, alkaline phosphatase, and prothrombin time). Stress the importance of returning for routine laboratory studies.

RASH, FEVER, JAUNDICE. The physician should be notified immediately if the patient develops a rash, fever, or jaundice. These signs are an indication of hypersensitivity or hepatotoxicity. The manufacturer recommends that tacrine be permanently discontinued.

BRADYCARDIA. Cholinergic agents cause a slowing of the heart. Notify the physician if the heart rate is regularly below 60 beats per minute.

Drug interactions

THEOPHYLLINE. Tacrine inhibits the metabolism of theophylline, substantially elevating theophylline serum levels and creating the potential for toxicity. Theophylline dosage adjustment is usually necessary.

CIMETIDINE. Cimetidine inhibits the metabolism of tacrine, substantially elevating tacrine serum levels and creating the potential for toxicity. Tacrine dosage adjustment is usually necessary.

ANTICHOLINERGIC AGENTS. As a cholinergic agent, tacrine has the potential to reduce the activity of anticholinergic agents (for example, benztropine, diphenhydramine, orphenadrine, procyclidine, and trihexyphenidyl).

SUCCINYLCHOLINE-TYPE MUSCLE RELAXANTS. As a cholinesterase inhibitor, tacrine is likely to exaggerate the actions of depolarizing muscle relaxants (for example, succinylcholine) during anesthesia.

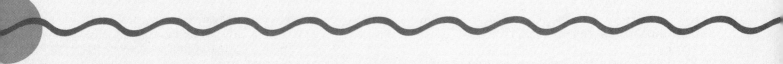

APPENDIX A

Prescription Abbreviations

aa, āā	of each (equal parts)	fl	fluid	qid	four times daily
ac	before meals	gtt	a drop	qod	every other day
ad	to; up to	hs	at bedtime	s̄	without
ad lib	as much as desired	od	right eye	sig.	label
bid	twice daily	os	left eye	ss	one half
c̄, c	with	ou	both eyes	stat	at once
caps	capsules	pc	after meals	tid	three times daily
d	day	prn	as needed	ung	ointment
et	and	q	every	ut dict.	as directed
ext	an extract	qd	once daily		

APPENDIX B

Medical Abbreviations

A	Assessment (POMR)
A_2	Aortic second sound
$A_2 > P_2$	Aortic sound larger than second pulmonary sound
AAL	Anterior axillary line
Ab	Abortion
Abd	Abdomen, abdominal
ABE	Acute bacterial endocarditis
ABG	Arterial blood gases
ACD	Anterior chest diameter
ADH	Antidiuretic hormone
ADT	Alternate-day therapy
AF	Atrial fibrillation; acid fast
AFB	Acid-fast bacteria; acid-fast bacilli
A/G	Albumin to globulin ratio
AGN	Acute glomerular nephritis
AHF	Antihemophilic factor
AHFS	American Hospital Formulary Service
AHG	Antihemophilic globulin
AI	Aortic insufficiency
AJ	Ankle jerk
AK	Above knee (amputation)
ALD	Alcoholic liver disease
ALL	Acute lymphocytic leukemia
ALS	Amyotrophic lateral sclerosis
AMA	Against medical advice
AMI	Acute myocardial infarction
ANA	Antinuclear antibodies
AODM	Adult-onset diabetes mellitus
A & P	Anterior and posterior; auscultation and percussion
ASAP	As soon as possible
AP	Apical pulse, anteroposterior
APB	Atrial premature beats
AS	Anal sphincter; arteriosclerosis
ASCVD	Arteriosclerotic cardiovascular disease
ASHD	Arteriosclerotic heart disease
ASO	Antistreptolysin titer; arteriosclerosis obliterans
ATN	Acute tubular necrosis
AV	Arteriovenous; atrioventricular
A & W	Alive and well
BAL	British anti-lewisite (dimercaprol)
bands	Banded neutrophils
BBB	Bundle branch block; blood-brain barrier
BBT	Basal body temperature
BE	Barium enema; base excess
BEI	Butanol-extractable iodine
bili	Bilirubin
BJ	Biceps jerk; bone and joint
BK	Below knee (amputation)
BLB	A type of oxygen mask
BLOBS	Bladder observation
BM	Bowel movement; basal metabolism
BMR	Basal metabolic rate

B & O	Belladonna and opium
BP	Blood pressure; British Pharmacopoeia
BPH	Benign prostatic hypertrophy
BRP	Bathroom privileges
BS	Bowel sounds; breath sounds
BSO	Bilateral salpingo-oophorectomy
BSP	Bromsulphalein
BT	Breast tumor; brain tumor
BTL	Bilateral tubal ligation
BTFS	Breast tumor frozen section
BU	Bodansky unit
BUN	Blood urea nitrogen
BVL	Bilateral vas ligation
BW	Body weight
Bx	Biopsy
C	Centigrade, Celsius
C_2	Second cervical vertebra
CA	Carbonic anhydrase
Ca	Cancer, calcium
C & A	Clinitest and Acetest
CAD	Coronary artery disease
CBC	Complete blood count
CC	Chief complaint
CCR	Creatinine clearance
CCU	Coronary care unit
Ceph floc	Cephalin flocculation
CF	Complement fixation
CHF	Congestive heart failure
CHO	Carbohydrate
Chol	Cholesterol
CI	Color index; contraindication
CK	Check
CLL	Chronic lymphocytic leukemia
CNS	Central nervous system
COAP	Cyclophosphamide, Oncovin, ARA-C, Prednisone
C/O	Complains of
Cong	Congenital
COP	Cyclophosphamide, Oncovin, Prednisone
COPD	Chronic obstructive pulmonary disease
CPK	Creatine phosphokinase
C & P	Cystoscopy and pyelography
CP	Cerebral palsy; cleft palate
CPR	Cardiopulmonary resuscitation
CR	Cardiorespiratory
CRF	Chronic renal failure
CRP	C-reactive protein
CS	Coronary sclerosis
C & S	Culture and sensitivity
CSF	Cerebrospinal fluid
C sect	Cesarean section
CT	Circulation time
CV	Cardiovascular; costovertebral angle
CVA	Cerebrovascular accident

CVP	Central venous pressure
CX	Cervix, cervical
CXR	Chest x-ray
DC(D/C)	Discontinue
D & C	Dilatation and curretage
DD	Differential diagnosis
DDD	Degenerative disc disease
DIC	Disseminated intravascular coagulation
Diff	Differential blood count
DJD	Degenerative joint disease
DM	Diabetes mellitus
DOA	Dead on arrival
DOE	Dyspnea on exertion
DPT	Diphtheria, pertussis, and tetanus
DSD	Dry sterile dressing
DT	Delirium tremens
DTR	Deep tendon reflex
Dx	Diagnosis
$D_5 W$	Dextrose 5% in water
E	Enema
EBL	Estimated blood loss
ECF	Extracellular fluid
ECG	Electrocardiogram
ECT	Electroconvulsive therapy
ECW	Extracellular water
EDC	Expected date of confinement (obstetrics)
EEG	Electroencephalogram
EENT	Eyes, ears, nose, throat
EFA	Essential fatty acids
EH	Enlarged heart
EKG	Electrocardiogram
EM	Electron microscope
EMG	Electromyography
ENT	Ears, nose, and throat
ER	Emergency room
ESR	Erythroctye sedimentation rate (sed rate)
EST	Electroshock therapy
EUA	Examine under anesthesia
F	Fahrenheit
FB	Finger breadths; foreign bodies
FBS	Fasting blood sugar
FEV_1	Forced expiratory volume in one second
FF	Filtration fraction
FFA	Free fatty acids
FH	Family history
FP	Family practice; family planning
FSH	Follicle-stimulating hormone
FTA	Fluorescent treponemal antibody
FUO	Fever of undetermined origin
Fx	Fracture; fraction

G	Gravida	LDH	Lactic dehydrogenase	PCN	Penicillin
GA	General appearance	LDL	Low density lipoproteins	PCV	Packed cell volume (hematocrit)
GB	Gallbladder	LE	Lupus erythematosus	PE	Physical examination
GC	Gonococcus; gonorrhea	LFTs	Liver function tests	PEEP	Positive end expiratory pressure
GFR	Glomerular filtration rate	LHF	Left heart failure	PEG	Pneumoencephalogram
GI	Gastrointestinal	LKS	Liver, kidneys, and spleen	PERRLA	Pupils equal, round, react to light and
G6PD	Glucose-6-phosphate dehydrogenase	LLE	Left lower extremity		accommodation
G-P-	Gravida-; para-	LLL	Left lower lobe	PH	Past history
GU	Genitourinary	LLQ	Left lower quadrant (abdomen)	PI	Present illness
GYN	Gynecology	LMD	Local medical doctor	PID	Pelvic inflammatory disease
		LML	Left middle lobe (lung)	PIE	Pulmonary infiltration with
H	Hypodermic; heroin	LMP	Last menstrual period		eosinophilia
HA	Headache	LOA	Left occipital anterior	PKU	Phenylketonuria
HAA	Hepatitis-associated antigen	LOM	Limitation of motion	PMH	Past medical history
HBP	High blood pressure	LOP	Left occipital posterior	PMI	Point of maximal impulse or
Hct	Hematocrit	LP	Lumbar puncture		maximum intensity
HCVD	Hypertensive cardiovascular disease	lpf	Low power field	PMN	Polymorphonuclear neutrophil
HEENT	Head, eyes, ears, nose, throat	LUQ	Left upper quadrant	PMT	Premenstrual tension
Hgb	Hemoglobin	LVH	Left ventricular hypertrophy	PND	Paroxysmal nocturnal dyspnea
HHD	Hypertensive heart disease	L & W	Living and well	PNX	Pneumothorax
HO	House officer	LWCT	Lee-White clotting time	POMR	Problem-oriented medical record
HOB	Head of bed	lytes	Electrolytes	Postop	After surgery
HPF	High power field			PO	By mouth
HPI	History of present illness			PP	Postpartum; postprandial
HSA	Human serum albumin	M	Murmur	PPD	Purified protein derivative
HTN	Hypertension	m^2	Square meters of body surface	PPL	Penicilloyl-polylysine conjugate
HTVD	Hypertensive vascular disease	M_1	First mitral sound	P & R	Pulse and respiration
Hx	History	MCH	Mean corpuscular hemoglobin	Preop	Before surgery
		MCHC	Mean corpuscular hemoglobin	PT	Physical therapy; prothrombin time
			concentration	PTA	Prior to admission
IASD	Intraatrial septal defect	MCL	Midclavicular line	PUD	Peptic ulcer disease
IBC	Iron-binding capacity	MCV	Mean corpuscular volume	PVC	Premature ventricular contraction
IBI	Intermittent bladder irrigation	MF	Myocardial fibrosis	PZI	Protamine zinc insulin
ICF	Intracellular fluid volume	MH	Marital history; menstrual history		
ICM	Intracostal margin	MI	Myocardial infarction; mitral		
ICS	Intercostal space		insufficiency	R	Respiration
ICU	Intensive care unit	MIC	Minimim inhibitory concentration	RA	Rheumatoid arthritis; right atrium
ICW	Intracellular water	MJT	Mead Johnson tube	RBC	Red blood cell
ID	Initial dose; intradermal	ML	Midline	RBF	Renal blood flow
I & D	Incision and drainage	MOM	Milk of Magnesia	RCM	Right costal margin
IDU	Idoxuridine	MS	Morphine sulfate; multiple sclerosis;	RF	Rheumatoid factor
I & O	Intake and output		mitral stenosis	RHD	Rheumatic heart disease; renal
IHSS	Idiopathic hypertrophic subaortic	MSL	Midsternal line		hypertensive disease
	stenosis			RISA	Radioactive iodine serum albumin
IM	Intramuscular			RLL	Right lower lobe
Imp	Impression	N	Normal	RLQ	Right lower quadrant
Int	Internal	NAD	No acute distress; no apparent distress	RO	Rule out
IP	Intraperitoneal	NG	Nasogastric	ROM	Range of motion
IPPB	Intermittent positive pressure breathing	NM	Neuromuscular	ROS	Review of systems; review of
ISW	Interstitial water	NPN	Nonprotein nitrogen		symptoms
ITh	Intrathecal	NPO	Nothing by mouth	RPF	Renal plasma flow; relaxed pelvic
IU	International unit	NR	No refill		floor
IUD	Intraterine device (contraceptive)	NS	Normal saline	RQ	Respiratory quotient
IVP	Intravenous pyelogram	NSFTD	Normal spontaneous full-term delivery	RR	Recovery room; respiratory rate
IVPB	Intravenous piggyback	NSR	Normal sinus rhythm	RSR	Regular sinus rhythm
IVSD	Intraventricular septal defect	NTG	Nitroglycerin	RTA	Renal tubular acidosis
		NVD	Nausea, vomiting, diarrhea; neck vein	RTN	Renal tubular necrosis
			distension	RUL	Right upper lobe
JRA	Juvenile rheumatoid arthritis	NYD	Not yet diagnosed	RUQ	Right upper quadrant
JVD	Jugular venous distension			RV	Right ventricle
				RVH	Right ventricular hypertrophy
K^+	Potassium	O_2	Oxygen		
KO	Keep open	O	Objective data (POMR)		
17-KS	17-Ketosteroids	OB	Obstetrics; occult blood	S	Subjective data (POMR)
KUB	Kidney, ureter, and bladder	OOB	Out of bed	S_1	First heart sound
K.W.	Keith Wagner (ophthalmoscopic	OOBBRP	Out of bed with bathroom privileges	S_2	Second heart sound
	findings)	OD	Overdose	SA	Sinoatrial
		OR	Operating room	SBE	Subacute bacterial endocarditis
		OT	Occupational therapy	SC	Subclavian, subcutaneous
L_2	Second lumbar vertebra			Sed rate	Erythrocyte sedimentation rate
LA	Left atrium			Segs	Segmented neutrophils
Lap	Laparotomy	P	Plan (POMR), pulse	SGOT	Serum glutamic oxaloacetic
LATS	Long-acting thyroid stimulator	P & A	Palpation and auscultation		transaminase
LBBB	Left bundle branch block	PA	Posteroanterior	SGPT	Serum glutamic pyruvic transaminase
LCM	Left costal margin	PAT	Paroxysmal atrial tachycardia	SH	Social history; serum hepatitis
LD	Longitudinal diameter (of heart)	PBI	Protein-bound iodine	SID	Sudden infant death
		PC	After meals		

SL	Sublingual	TEDS	Elastic stockings	VAH	Veterans' Administration Hospital
SLE	Systemic lupus erythematosus	TIA	Transient ischemic attack	VC	Vena cava
SLDH	Serum lactic dehydrogenase	TIBC	Total iron-binding capacity	VCU	Voiding cystourethrogram
SMA	Serial multiple analysis	TKO	To keep open	VDRL	Venereal Disease Research
SOAP	Subjective, objective, assessment plan	TLC	Tender loving care		Laboratories (for syphilis)
	(POMR)	TM	Tympanic membrane	VF	Ventricular fibrillation
SOB	Shortness of breath	TP	Total protein; thrombophlebitis	VMA	Vanillylmandelic acid
S/P	Status post	TPI	*Treponema pallidum* immobilization	VP	Venous pressure
SR	Sedimentation rate (ESR)	TPN	Total parenteral nutrition	VPC	Ventricular premature contraction
SSE	Saline solution enema; soapsuds	TPR	Temperature, pulse, and respiration	VS	Vital signs
	enema	TRA	To run at	VSD	Ventricular septal defect
SSPE	Subacute sclerosing panencephalitis	T-set	Tracheotomy set	VT	Ventricular tachycardia
STD	Skin test dose	TSH	Thyroid-stimulating hormone		
STS	Serologic test for syphilis	TUR	Transurethral resection	W	White; widow
SVC	Superior vena cava	TV	*Trichomonas vaginalis*	WBC	White blood cell; white blood count
				WDWN-	
t	Temperature	UA(U/A)	Urinalysis	WF	Well-developed, well-nourished, white
T_3	Triiodothyronine	U & C	Urethral and cervical		female
T_4	Thyroxin	UCHD	Unusual childhood diseases	WDWN-	
T & A	Tonsillectomy and adenoidectomy	UGI	Upper gastrointestinal	WM	Well-developed, well-nourished, white
TAH	Total abdominal hysterectomy	URI	Upper respiratory infection		male
TAO	Thromboangiitis obliterans	UTI	Urinary tract infection	WNL	Within normal limits
TB	Tuberculosis			Wt	Weight
TBW	Total body water	V	Vein		
TD	Transverse diameter (of heart)	Vag hyst	Vaginal hysterectomy		

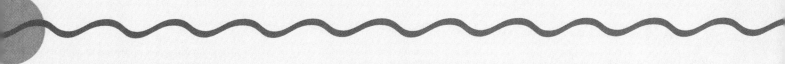

APPENDIX C

Nomogram for Calculating the Body Surface Area of Adults and Children

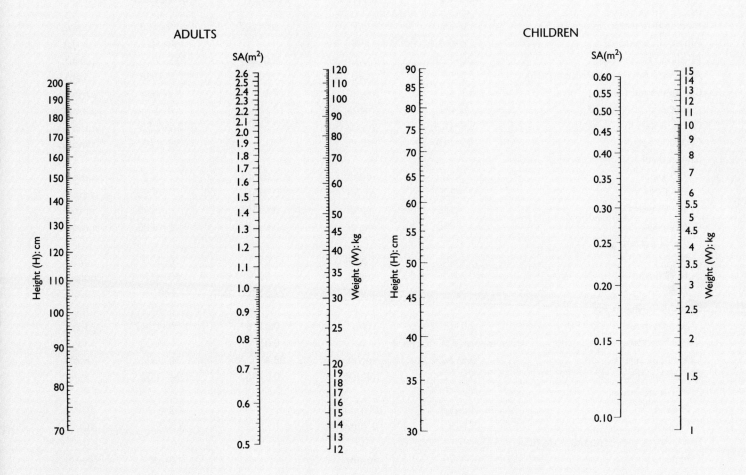

Align a ruler with the height and weight. The point at which the center line is intersected gives the corresponding value for surface area (SA). From Haycock GB: *J Pediatr* 93:62-66 1978.

APPENDIX D

Commonly Used Laboratory Test and Drug Values

TEST	RANGE	UNITS	CONVERSION FACTOR	SI RANGE	UNITS
Alanine Aminotransferase [ALT]	0–35	U/L	0.01667	0–0.58	μkat/L
Albumin, serum	4–6	g/dl	10	40–60	g/L
Alkaline Phosphatase	30–120	U/L	0.01667	0.5–2	μkat/L
Aspartate Aminotransferase [AST]	0–35	U/L	0.01667	0–0.58	μkat/L
Bilirubin, total (serum)	0.1–1	mg/dl	17.1	2–18	μmol/L
Bilirubin, conjugated	0–0.2	mg/dl	17.1	0–4	μmol/L
Calcium, serum	8.8–10.4	mg/dl	0.2495	2.2–2.58	mmol/L
Chloride, serum	95–110	mEq/L	1	95–110	mmol/L
Cholesterol					
<29 years	<200	mg/dl	0.02586	<5.2	mmol/L
30–39 years	<225	mg/dl	0.02586	<5.85	mmol/L
40–49 years	<245	mg/dl	0.02586	<6.35	mmol/L
>50 years	<265	mg/dl	0.02586	<6.85	mmol/L
Cortisol, serum					
0800 hours	4–19	μg/dl	27.59	110–520	nmol/L
1600 hours	2–15	μg/dl	27.59	50–410	nmol/L
2400 hours	5	μg/dl	27.59	140	nmol/L
Creatine kinase (CK)					
Isoenzymes	0–130	U/L	0.01667	0–2.167	μkat/L
MB fraction	>5 in myocardial infarction	%	0.01	>0.05	1
Creatinine, serum	0.6–1.2	mg/dl	88.4	50–110	μmol/L
Creatinine clearance	75–125	ml/min	0.01667	1.24–2.08	ml/s
Erythrocyte count					
Male	4.3–5.9	$10^6/mm^3$	1	4.3–5.9	$10^{12}/L$
Female	3.5–5	$10^3/mm^3$	1	3.5–5	$10^{12}/L$
Erythrocyte sedimentation rate (ESR)					
Male	0–20	mm/hr	1	0–20	mm/h
Female	0–30	mm/hr	1	0–30	mm/h
Gases, arterial blood					
PO_2	75–105	mm Hg	0.1333	10–14	kPa
PCO_2	33–44	mm Hg	0.1333	4.4–5.9	kPa
Gamma-glutamyltransferase (GGT)	0–30	U/L	0.01667	0–0.5	μkat/L
Glucose, plasma (fasting)	70–110	mg/dl	0.05551	3.9–6.1	mmol/L

From Young DS: Implementation of SI units for clinical laboratory data, *Ann In Med* 106:114–129, 1987.
"SI units" is the abbreviation of *système international d'unites*. It is a uniform system of reporting numerical values permitting interchangeability of information among nations and between disciplines.

continued

TEST	RANGE	UNITS	CONVERSION FACTOR	SI RANGE	UNITS
Hematocrit					
Male	39–49	%	0.01	0.39–0.49	l
Female	33–43	%	0.01	0.33–0.43	l
Hemoglobin					
Male	14–18	g/dl	10	140–180	g/L
Female	11.5–15.5	g/dl	10	115–155	g/L
Iron, serum					
Male	80–180	μg/dl	0.1791	14–32	μmol/L
Female	60–160	μg/dl	0.1791	11–29	μmol/L
Iron binding capacity	250–460	μg/dl	0.1791	45–82	mmol/L
Lactic dehydrogenase	50–150	U/L	0.01667	0.82–2.66	μkat/L
Leukocyte count differential	3200–9800	mm3	0.001	3.2–9.8	10^9/L
Number fraction (differential)		%	0.01		l
Lipoproteins					
Low density (LDL)	50–190	mg/dl	0.02586	1.3–1.9	mmol/L
High density (HDL)—male	30–70	mg/dl	0.02586	0.8–1.8	mmol/L
High density (HDL)—female	30–90	mg/dl	0.02586	0.8–2.35	mmol/L
Magnesium, serum	1.8–3	mg/dl	0.4114	0.8–1.2	mmol/L
	1.6–2.4	mEq/l	0.5	0.8–1.2	mmol/L
Mean corpuscular hemoglobin (MCH)	27–33	pg	1	27–33	l pg
Mean corpuscular hemoglobin concentration (MCHC)	33–37	g/dl	10	330–370	g/L
Mean corpuscular volume (MCV)	76–100	μm^3	1	76–100	fL
Osmolality, plasma	280–300	mOsm/kg	1	280–300	mmol/kg
Osmolality, urine	50–1200	mOsm/kg	1	50–1200	mmol/kg
Phosphate, serum	2.5–5	mg/dl	0.3229	0.8–1.6	mmol/L
Platelet count	130–400	10^3/mm^3	1	130–400	10^9/L
Potassium, serum	3.5–5	mEq/L	1	3.5–5	mmol/L
Reticulocyte count	1–24	#/1000 RBCs	0.001	0.001–0.024	l
Sodium, serum	135–147	mEq/L	1	135–147	mmol/L
Thyroid-stimulating hormone (TSH)	2–11	μU/ml	1	2–11	mU/L
Thyroxine (T$_4$)	4–11	μg/dl	12.87	51–142	nmol/L
Thyroid-binding globulin (TBG)	12–28	μg/dl	12.87	150–360	nmol/L
Thyroxine, free (serum)	0.8–2.8	ng/dl	12.87	10–36	pmol/L
Triiodothyronine (T$_3$)	75–220	ng/dl	0.01536	1.2–3.4	nmol/L
T$_3$ Uptake	25–35	%	0.01	0.25–0.35	l
Transferrin	170–370	mg/dl	0.01	1.7–3.7	g/L
Triglycerides	<160	mg/dl	0.01129	<1.8	mmol/L
Urea nitrogen [Blood urea nitrogen (BUN)]	8–18	mg/dl	0.357	3–6.5	mmol/L
Zinc, serum	75–120	μg/dl	0.153	11.5–18.5	μmol/L

continued

DRUG	RANGE	UNITS	CONVERSION FACTOR	SI RANGE	UNITS
Acetaminophen, toxic	>5	mg/dl	66.16	>330	μmol/L
Amitriptyline	50–200	ng/ml	3.605	180–720	nmol/L
Carbamazepine	4–10	mg/L	4.233	17–42	μmol/L
Chlordiazepoxide					
Therapeutic	0.5–5	mg/L	3.336	2–17	μmol/L
Toxic	>10	mg/L	3.336	>33	μmol/L
Desipramine	50–200	ng/ml	3.754	170–700	nmol/L
Diazepam					
Therapeutic	0.1–0.25	mg/L	3512	350–900	nmol/L
Toxic	>1	mg/L	3512	>3510	nmol/L
Digoxin					
Therapeutic	0.5–2	ng/ml	1.281	0.6–2.8	nmol/L
Toxic	>2.5	mg/ml	1.281	>3.2	nmol/L
Disopyramide	2–6	mg/L	2.946	6–18	μmol/L
Doxepin	50–200	ng/ml	3.579	180–720	nmol/L
Imipramine	50–200	ng/ml	3.566	180–710	nmol/L
Isoniazid					
Therapeutic	<2	mg/L	7.291	<15	μmol/L
Toxic	>3	mg/L	7.291	>22	μmol/L
Lidocaine	1–5	mg/L	4.267	4.5–21.5	μmol/L
Maprotiline	50–200	ng/ml	3.605	180–720	nmol/L
Phenobarbital	2–5	mg/dL	43.06	85–215	μmol/L
Phenytoin, therapeutic	10–20	mg/L	3.964	40–80	μmol/L
	>30	mg/L	3.964	>120	μmol/L
Procainamide					
Therapeutic	4–8	mg/L	4.249	17–34	μmol/L
Toxic	>12	mg/L	4.249	>50	μmol/L
N-acetylprocainamide	4–8	mg/L	3.606	14–29	μmol/L
Quinidine, therapeutic	1.5–3	mg/L	3.082	4.6–9.2	μmol/L
Toxic	>6	mg/L	3.082	>18.5	μmol/L
Theophylline	10–20	mg/L	5.55	55–110	μmol/L
Valproic acid	50–100	mg/L	6.934	350–700	μmol/L

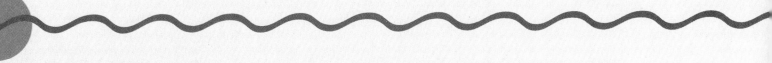

APPENDIX E

Recommended childhood vaccination schedule*—United States, January-June 1996

Vaccine		Age										
	Birth	1 Mo	2 Mo	4 Mo	6 Mo	12 Mo	15 Mo	18 Mo	4-6 Yr	11-12 Yr	14-16 Yr
Hepatitis B†	Hep B-1										
		Hep B-2			Hep B-3					Hep B§	
Diphtheria and tetanus toxoids and pertussis vaccine¶			DTP	DTP	DTP	DTP (DTaP at ≥15 mo.)			DTP or DTaP	Td	
Haemophilus influenzae type b**			Hib	Hib	Hib	Hib					
Poliovirus††			OPV	OPV	OPV				OPV		
Measels-mumps-rubella§§						MMR			MMR or MMR		
Varicella zoster virus¶¶						Var				Var***	

■ Range of Acceptable Ages for Vaccination

□ "Catch-Up" Vaccination §***

Source: Advisory Committee on Immunization Practices, American Academy of Pediatrics, and American Academy of Family Physicians.

Use of trade names and commercial sources is for identification only and does not imply endorsement by the Public Health Service or the U.S. Department of Health and Human Services.

*Vaccines are listed under the routinely recommended ages.

† **Infants born to hepatitis B surface antigen (HBsAg)–negative mothers** should receive 2.5 μg of Recombivax HB (Merck & Co.) or 10 μg of Engerix-B (SmithKline Beecham). The second dose should be administered ≥1 month after the first dose. **Infants born to HBsAg-positive mothers** should receive 0.5 ml hepatitis B immune globulin (HBIG) within 12 hours of birth, and either 5 μg of Recombivax HB or 10 μg of Engerix-B at a separate site. The second dose is recommended at age 1-2 months and the third dose at age 6 months. **Infants born to mothers whose HBsAg status is unknown** should receive either 5 μg of Recombivax HB or 10 μg of Engerix-B within 12 hours of birth. The second dose of vaccine is recommended at age 1 month and the third dose at age 6 months.

§ Adolescents who have not received three doses of hepatitis B vaccine should initiate or complete the series at age 11-12 years. The second dose should be administered at least 1 month after the first dose, and the third dose should be administered at least 4 months after the first dose and at least 2 months after the second dose.

¶ The fourth dose of diphtheria and tetanus toxoids and pertussis vaccine (DTP) may be administered at age 12 months, if at least 6 months have elapsed since the third dose of DTP. Diphtheria and tetanus toxoids and acellular pertussis vaccine (DTaP) is licensed for the fourth or fifth vaccine dose(s) for children aged ≥15 months and may be preferred for these doses in this age group. Tetanus and diphtheria toxoids, absorbed, for adult use (Td) is recommended at age 11-12 years if at least 5 years have elapsed since the last dose of DTP, DTaP, or diphtheria and tetanus toxoids, absorbed, for pediatric use (DT).

**Three Haemophilus influenzae type b (Hib) conjugate vaccines are licensed for infant use. If PedvaxHIB (Merck & Co.) Haemophilus b conjugate vaccine (Meningococcal Protein Conjugate) (PRP-OMP) is administered at ages 2 and 4 months, a dose at 6 months is not required. After completing the primary series, any Hib conjugate vaccine may be used as a booster.

†† Oral poliovirus vaccine (OPV) is recommended for routine infant vaccination. Inactivated poliovirus vaccine (IPV) is recommended for persons—or household contacts of persons—with a congenital or acquired immune deficiency disease or an altered immune status resulting from disease or immunosuppressive therapy, and is an acceptable alternative for other persons. The primary three-dose series for IPV should be given with a minimum interval of 4 weeks between the first and second doses and 6 months between the second and third doses.

§§ The second dose of measles-mumps-rubella vaccine (MMR) is routinely recommended at age 4-6 years or at age 11-12 years but may be administered at any visit provided at least 1 month has elapsed since receipt of the first dose.

¶¶ Varicella zoster virus vaccine (Var) can be administered to susceptible children any time after age 12 months.

***Unvaccinated children who lack a reliable history of chickenpox should be vaccinated at age 11-12 years.

MED**W**ATCH
THE FDA MEDICAL PRODUCTS REPORTING PROGRAM

For **VOLUNTARY** reporting
by health professionals of adverse
events and product problems

Page ____ of ____

Form Approved: OMB No. 0910-0291 Expires
See OMB statement on reverse

FDA Use Only (Pharm Let)

Triage unit
sequence #

A. Patient information

1. Patient Identifier	2. Age at time of event: or ____ Date of birth:	3. Sex ☐ female ☐ male	4. Weight ____ lbs or ____ kgs
In confidence			

B. Adverse event or product problem

1. ☐ Adverse event   and/or   ☐ Product problem (e.g., defects/malfunctions)

2. Outcomes attributed to adverse event
(check all that apply)

☐ death ____ (mo/day/yr)
☐ life-threatening
☐ hospitalization-initial or prolonged

☐ disability
☐ congenital anomaly
☐ required intervention to prevent permanent impairment/damage
☐ other: ____

3. Date of event (mo/day/yr)	4. Date of this report (mo/day/yr)

5. Describe event or problem

6. Relevant tests/laboratory data, including dates

7. Other relevant history, including preexisting medical conditions (e.g., allergies, race, pregnancy, smoking and alcohol use, hepatic/renal dysfunction, etc.)

C. Suspect medication(s)

1. Name (give labeled strength & mfr/labeler, if known)

#1 _____

#2 _____

2. Dose, frequency & route used	3. Therapy dates (if unknown, give duration) from/to (or best estimate)
#1	#1
#2	#2

4. Diagnosis for use (indication)	5. Event abated after use stopped or dose reduced
#1	#1 ☐ yes ☐ no ☐ doesn't apply
#2	#2 ☐ yes ☐ no ☐ doesn't apply

6. Lot # (if known)	7. Exp. date (if known)	8. Event reappeared after reintroduction
#1	#1	#1 ☐ yes ☐ no ☐ doesn't apply
#2	#2	#2 ☐ yes ☐ no ☐ doesn't apply

9. NDC # (for product problems only)
____ – ____ – ____

10. Concomitant medical products and therapy dates (exclude treatment of event)

D. Suspect medical device

1. Brand name

2. Type of device

3. Manufacturer name & address	4. Operator of device ☐ health professional ☐ lay user/patient ☐ other: ____
6. model # _____ catalog # _____ serial # _____ lot # _____ other # _____	5. Expiration date (mo/day/yr)
	7. If implanted, give date (mo/day/yr)
	8. If explanted, give date (mo/day/yr)

9. Device available for evaluation?   (Do not send to FDA)
☐ yes   ☐ no   ☐ returned to manufacturer on ____ (mo/day/yr)

10. Concomitant medical products and therapy dates (exclude treatment of event)

E. Reporter (see confidentiality section on back)

1. Name, address, & phone #

2. Health professional? ☐ yes ☐ no	3. Occupation	4. Also reported to ☐ manufacturer ☐ user facility ☐ distributor
5. If you do NOT want your identity disclosed to the manufacturer, place an "X" in this box. ☐		

FDA   Mail to: MED**W**ATCH   *or* FAX to
5600 Fishers Lane   1-800-FDA-0178
Rockville, MD 20852-9787

FDA Form 3500 (6/93)   Submission of a report does not constitute an admission that medical personnel or the product caused or contributed to the event.

ADVICE ABOUT VOLUNTARY REPORTING

Report experiences with:
- medications (drugs or biologics)
- medical devices (including in-vitro diagnostics)
- special nutritional products (dietary supplements, medical foods, infant formulas)
- other products regulated by FDA

Report SERIOUS adverse events. An event is serious when the patient outcome is:
- death
- life-threatening (real risk of dying)
- hospitalization (initial or prolonged)
- disability (significant, persistent, or permanent)
- congenital anomaly
- required intervention to prevent permanent impairment or damage

Report even if:
- you're not certain the product caused the event
- you don't have all the details

Report product problems — quality, performance, or safety concerns such as:
- suspected contamination
- questionable stability
- defective components
- poor packaging or labeling

How to report:
- just fill in the sections that apply to your report
- use section C for all products except medical devices
- attach additional blank pages if needed
- use a separate form for each patient
- report either to FDA or the manufacturer (or both)

Important numbers:
- 1-800-FDA-0178   to FAX report
- 1-800-FDA-7737   to report by modem
- 1-800-FDA-1088   for more information or to report quality problems
- 1-800-822-7967   for a VAERS form for vaccines

If your report involves a serious adverse event with a device and it occurred in a facility outside a doctor's office, that facility may be legally required to report to FDA and/or the manufacturer. Please notify the person in that facility who would handle such reporting.

Confidentiality: The patient's identity is held in strict confidence by FDA and protected to the fullest extent of the law. The reporter's identity may be shared with the manufacturer unless requested otherwise. However, FDA will not disclose the reporter's identity in response to a request from the public, pursuant to the Freedom of Information Act.

The public reporting burden for this collection of information has been estimated to average 30 minutes per response, including the time for reviewing instructions, searching existing data sources, gathering and maintaining the data needed, and completing and reviewing the collection of information. Send your comments regarding this burden estimate or any other aspect of this collection of information, including suggestions for reducing this burden to:

Reports Clearance Officer, PHS
Hubert H. Humphrey Building,
Room 721–B
200 Independence Avenue, S.W.
Washington, DC 20201
ATTN: PRA

and to:
Office of Management and Budget
Paperwork Reduction Project (0910–0291)
Washington, DC 20503

Please do NOT return this form to either of these addresses.

U.S. DEPARTMENT OF HEALTH AND HUMAN SERVICES
Public Health Service • Food and Drug Administration

FDA Form 3500-back   **Please Use Address Provided Below – Just Fold in Thirds, Tape, and Mail**

**Department of
Health and Human Services**
Public Health Service
Food and Drug Administration
Rockville, MD 20857

Official Business
Penalty for Private Use $300

NO POSTAGE
NECESSARY
IF MAILED
IN THE
UNITED STATES
OR APO/FPO

BUSINESS REPLY MAIL
FIRST CLASS MAIL   PERMIT NO. 946   ROCKVILLE, MD
POSTAGE WILL BE PAID BY FOOD AND DRUG ADMINISTRATION

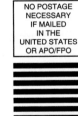

MEDWATCH
The FDA Medical Products Reporting Program
Food and Drug Administration
5600 Fishers Lane
Rockville, MD 20852-9787

APPENDIX G

Dyskinesia Identification System: Condensed User Scale (DISCUS)

NAME   **I.D.**

_____
(facility)

Dyskinesia Identification System: Condensed User Scale (DISCUS)

CURRENT PSYCHOTROPICS/ANTI-CHOLINERGIC AND TOTAL MG/DAY

_____ _____mg

_____ _____mg

_____ _____mg

_____ _____mg

See Instructions On Other Side

EXAM TYPE (check one)
- ❑ 1. Baseline
- ❑ 2. Annual
- ❑ 3. Semiannual
- ❑ 4. D/C — 1 Month
- ❑ 5. D/C — 2 Month
- ❑ 6. D/C — 3 Month
- ❑ 7. Admission
- ❑ 8. Other

COOPERATION (check one)
- ❑ 1. None
- ❑ 2. Partial
- ❑ 3. Full

SCORING

0 — **Not Present** (movements not observed or some movements observed but not considered abnormal)

1 — **Minimal** (abnormal movements are difficult to detect **or** movements are easy to detect but occur only once or twice in a short non-repetitive manner)

2 — **Mild** (abnormal movements occur infrequently **and** are easy to detect)

3 — **Moderate** (abnormal movements occur frequently **and** are easy to detect)

4 — **Severe** (abnormal movements occur almost continuously **and** are easy to detect)

NA — **Not Assessed** (an assessment for an item is not able to be made)

ASSESSMENT

DISCUS Item and Score (circle one score for each item)

		Item	0	1	2	3	4	NA
FACE	1.	Tics	0	1	2	3	4	NA
	2.	Grimaces	0	1	2	3	4	NA
EYES	3.	Blinking	0	1	2	3	4	NA
ORAL	4.	Chewing/Lip Smacking	0	1	2	3	4	NA
	5.	Puckering/Sucking/ Thrusting Lower Lip	0	1	2	3	4	NA
LINGUAL	6.	Tongue Thrusting/ Tongue in Cheek	0	1	2	3	4	NA
	7.	Tonic Tongue	0	1	2	3	4	NA
	8.	Tongue Tremor	0	1	2	3	4	NA
	9.	Athetoid/Myokymic/ Lateral Tongue	0	1	2	3	4	NA
HEAD/NECK/TRUNK	10.	Retrocollis/Torticollis	0	1	2	3	4	NA
	11.	Shoulder/Hip Torsion	0	1	2	3	4	NA
UPPER LIMB	12.	Athetoid/Myokymic Finger-Wrist-Arm	0	1	2	3	4	NA
	13.	Pill Rolling	0	1	2	3	4	NA
LOWER LIMB	14.	Ankle Flexion/ Foot Tapping	0	1	2	3	4	NA
	15.	Toe Movement	0	1	2	3	4	NA

COMMENTS/OTHER

_____

_____

_____

_____

_____

TOTAL SCORE _____

(items 1-15 only)

EXAM DATE _____

RATER SIGNATURE AND TITLE _____

NEXT EXAM DATE _____

EVALUATION (see other side)

1. Greater than 90 days neuroleptic exposure?   :   YES   NO

2. Scoring/intensity level met?   :   YES   NO

3. Other diagnostic conditions?   :   YES   NO
(if yes, specify)

_____

_____

_____

4. Last exam date: _____

    Last total score: _____

    Last conclusion: _____

Preparer signature and title for items 1-4 (if different from physician):

5. Conclusion (circle one):

A. No TD (if scoring pre-requisite met, list other diagnostic con-dition or explain in comments)   C. Masked TD
D. Withdrawal TD
E. Persistent TD
F. Remitted TD
G. Other (specify in comments)

B. Probable TD

6. Comments:

_____

_____

_____

_____

_____

_____

PHYSICIAN SIGNATURE _____   **DATE** _____

Sprague PL, Kalachnik JE: Reliability, validity, and a total score cutoff for the Dyskinesia Identification System: Condensed User Scale (DISCUS) with mentally ill and mentally retarded populations, *Psychopharmacol Bull* 27(1):51-58, 1991.

Simplified Diagnoses for Tardive Dyskinesia (SD-TD)

PREREQUISITES. — The 3 prerequisites are as follows. Exceptions may occur.

1. A history of at least three months' total cumulative neuroleptic exposure. Include amoxapine and metoclopramide in all categories below as well.

2. **SCORING/INTENSITY LEVEL.** The presence of a **TOTAL SCORE OF FIVE (5) OR ABOVE**. Also be alert for any change from baseline or scores below five that have at least a "moderate" (3) or "severe" (4) movement on any item or at least two "mild" (2) movements on two items located in different body areas.

3. Other conditions are not responsible for the abnormal involuntary movements.

DIAGNOSES. — The diagnosis is based upon the current exam and its relation to the last exam. The diagnosis can shift depending upon: (a) whether movements are present or not, (b) whether movements are present for 3 months or more (6 months if on a semi-annual assessment schedule), and (c) whether neuroleptic dosage changes occur and affect movements.

- **NO TD.**— Movements **are not** present on this exam **or** movements are present, but some other condition is responsible for them. The last diagnosis must be NO TD, PROBABLE TD, or WITHDRAWAL TD.

- **PROBABLE TD.** — Movements **are** present on this exam. This is the first time they are present **or** they have never been present for 3 months or more. The last diagnosis must be NO TD or PROBABLE TD.

- **PERSISTENT TD.** — Movements **are** present on this exam **and** they have been present for 3 months or more with this exam or at some point in the past. The last diagnosis can be any except NO TD.

- **MASKED TD.** — Movements **are not** present on this exam **but** this is due to a neuroleptic dosage increase or reinstitution after a prior exam when movements were present. Also use this conclusion if movements are not present due to the addition of a non-neuroleptic medication to treat TD. The last diagnosis must be PROBABLE TD, PERSISTENT TD, WITHDRAWAL TD, or MASKED TD.

- **REMITTED TD.** — Movements **are not** present on this exam **but** PERSISTENT TD has been diagnosed **and** no neuroleptic dosage increase or reinstitution has occurred. The last diagnosis must be PERSISTENT TD or REMITTED TD. If movements re-emerge, the diagnosis shifts back to PERSISTENT TD.

- **WITHDRAWAL TD.** — Movements **are not seen while** receiving neuroleptics or at the last dosage level **but are seen within** 8 weeks following a neuroleptic reduction or discontinuation. The last diagnosis must be NO TD or WITHDRAWAL TD. If movements continue for 3 months or more after the neuroleptic dosage reduction or discontinuation, the diagnosis shifts to PERSISTENT TD. If movements do not continue for 3 months or more after the reduction or discontinuation, the diagnosis shifts to NO TD.

INSTRUCTIONS

1. The rater completes the Assessment according to the standardized exam procedure. If the rater also completes Evaluation items 1-4, he/she must also sign the preparer box. The form is given to the physician. Alternatively, the physician may perform the assessment.

2. The physician completes the Evaluation section. The physician is responsible for the entire Evaluation section and its accuracy.

3. IT IS RECOMMENDED THAT THE PHYSICIAN EXAMINE ANY INDIVIDUAL WHO MEETS THE 3 PREREQUISITES OR WHO HAS MOVEMENTS NOT EXPLAINED BY OTHER FACTORS. NEUROLOGICAL ASSESSMENTS OR DIFFERENTIAL DIAGNOSTIC TESTS THAT MAY BE NECESSARY SHOULD BE OBTAINED.

4. File form according to policy or procedure.

OTHER CONDITIONS (partial list)

1. Age
2. Blind
3. Cerebral Palsy
4. Contact Lenses
5. Dentures/No Teeth
6. Down's Syndrome
7. Drug Intoxication (specify)
8. Encephalitis
9. Extrapyramidal Side-Effects (specify)
10. Fahr's Syndrome
11. Heavy Metal Intoxication (specify)
12. Huntington's Chorea
13. Hyperthyroidism
14. Hypoglycemia
15. Hypoparathyroidism
16. Idiopathic Torsion Dystonia
17. Meige Syndrome
18. Parkinson's Disease
19. Stereotypies
20. Syndenham's Chorea
21. Tourette's Syndrome
22. Wilson's Disease
23. Other (specify)

APPENDIX H

A Simple Method to Determine Tardive Dyskinesia Symptoms: AIMS* Examination Procedure

PATIENT IDENTIFICATION   DATE

RATED BY

Either before or after completing the examination procedure, observe the patient unobtrusively at rest (e.g., in waiting room).

The chair to be used in this examination should be a hard, firm one without arms.

After observing the patient, he may be rated on a scale of 0 (none), 1 (minimal), 2 (mild), 3 (moderate), and 4 (severe) according to the severity of symptoms.

Ask the patient whether there is anything in his/her mouth (i.e., gum, candy, etc.) and if there is to remove it.

Ask patient about the *current* condition of his/her teeth. Ask patient if he/she wears dentures. Do teeth or dentures bother patient *now?*

Ask patient whether he/she notices any movement in mouth, face, hands or feet. If yes, ask to describe and to what extent they *currently* bother patient or interfere with his/her activities.

*Abnormal Involuntary Movement Scale
From Sandoz Pharmaceuticals, East Hanover, NJ 07936.

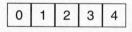

Ask patient to tap thumb, with each finder, as rapidly as possible for 10-15 seconds; separately with right hand, then with left hand. (Observe facial and leg movements.)

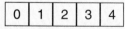

Flex and extend patient's left and right arms. (One at a time.)

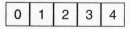

Ask patient to stand up. (Observe in profile. Observe all body areas again, hips included.)

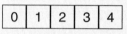

Have patient sit in chair with hands on knees, legs slightly apart, and feet flat on floor. (Look at entire body for movements while in this position.)

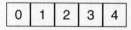

Ask patient to sit with hands hanging unsupported. If male, between legs, if female and wearing a dress, hanging over knees. (Observe hands and other body areas.)

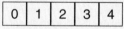

Ask patient to open mouth. (Observe tongue at rest within mouth.) Do this twice.

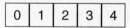

Ask patient to protrude tongue. (Observe abnormalities of tongue movement.) Do this twice.

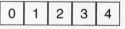

†Ask patient to extend both arms outstretched in front with palms down. (Observe trunk, legs, and mouth.)

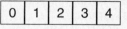

†Have patient walk a few paces, turn, and walk back to chair. (Observe hands and gait.) Do this twice.

*Activated movements.

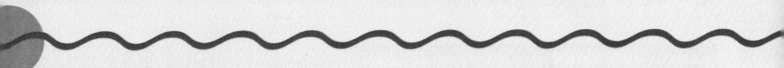

APPENDIX I

Self-Monitoring Drug Therapy Record

PATIENT EDUCATION AND MONITORING FORM   Self-Monitoring Drug Therapy Record

MEDICATIONS	COLOR	TO BE TAKEN

Name _____

Physician _____

Physician's phone _____

Next appt.* _____

PARAMETERS	DAY OF DISCHARGE						COMMENTS

From Clayton B, Stock Y: *Basic pharmacology for nurses,* 11 ed, St Louis, 1997, Mosby.
Permission given to make a limited number of copies for direct patient distribution.
*Please bring this record with you to your next appointment.
Use the back of this sheet for additional information.

BIBLIOGRAPHY

Abramowicz M, editor: *Medical letter,* New Rochelle, NY, 1996, The Medical Letter.

American Diabetes Association Day-By-Day Series: *Nutrition guide for people with diabetes,* 1994, American Diabetes Association.

Babcock DE, Miller MA: *Client education, theory and practice,* St Louis, 1993, Mosby.

Bates B: *A guide to physical examination and history taking,* ed 5, Philadelphia, 1991, Lippincott.

Beare PG, Myers JL: *Principles and practice of adult nursing,* ed 2, St Louis, 1994, Mosby.

Billups NF: *American drug index,* ed 40, St Louis, 1996, Facts and Comparisons.

Bobak I et al: *Maternity nursing,* ed 4, St Louis, 1995, Mosby.

Canobbio MM: *Cardiovascular disorders,* St Louis, 1991, Mosby.

Carlson JH et al: *Nursing diagnosis: a case study approach,* Philadelphia, 1991, Saunders.

Carpenito LJ: *Nursing diagnosis, application to clinical practice,* ed 6, Philadelphia, 1995, Lippincott.

Centers for Disease Control: Recommendations of the Immunization Practices Advisory Committee, *MMWR* 40:RR-1, 1991.

Centers for Disease Control: Recommended Childhood Immunization Schedule—United States, *MMWR* Jan-June, 44:940-943, 1996.

Covington TR: Birth of a drug: the US drug development and approval process, *Facts and Comparisons Drug Newsletter* 11:73-75, 1992.

Covington TR, editor: *Handbook of nonprescription drugs,* ed 10, Washington, DC, 1993, American Pharmaceutical Association.

Davis CM: Affective education for the health profession, *Phys Ther* 6(11):1587-1593, 1981.

DiPiro JT et al: *Pharmacotherapy, a pathophysiologic approach,* ed 2, Norwalk, Conn, 1993, Appleton & Lange.

Dracup K, Dunbar SB, Baker DW: Rethinking heart failure, *Am J Nurs* 23-27, 1995.

DSM-IV, diagnostic and statistical manual of mental disorders, ed 4, Washington, DC, 1994, American Psychiatric Association.

Engelking C: *Managing stomatitis: a nursing process approach, supportive care for the patient with cancer,* Richmond, Va, 1988, Robbins.

Ganong WF: *Review of medical physiology,* ed 16, Norwalk, Conn, 1993, Appleton & Lange.

Guyton AC: *Textbook of medical physiology,* ed 8, Philadelphia, 1991, Saunders.

Hardman JG, Limbird LL, editors: *Goodman and Gilman's the pharmacological basic of therapeutics,* ed 9, New York, 1996, Pergamon Press.

Hatcher RA et al: *Contraceptive technology,* ed 16, New York, 1994, Irvington.

Healy TEG, Cohen PJ: *Wylie and Churchill-Davidson's a practice of anesthesia,* ed 6, London, 1995, Edward Arnold.

Hegner BR, Caldwell E: *Geriatrics: a study of maturity,* ed 5, Albany, NY, 1991, Delmar.

Herberg P: Theoretical foundations of transcultural nursing. In Boyle JS, Andrews MM, editors: *Transcultural concepts in nursing care,* Boston, 1989, Scott, Foresman.

Herfindal ET, Gourley DR, Hart LL: *Clinical pharmacy and therapeutics,* ed 5, Baltimore, 1992, Williams & Wilkins.

Ignataviccius D, Bayne MV: *Medial surgical nursing: a nursing process approach,* Philadelphia, 1991, Saunders.

Illustrated manual of nursing practice, Springhouse, Pa, 1991, Springhouse.

James VE: Niacin, the need for monitoring, *US Pharmacist* 201:51-60, 1995.

Joint National Committee on Detection, Evaluation and Treatment of High Blood Pressure: The Fifth Report of the National Committee on Detection, Evaluation and Treatment of High Blood Pressure (JNC V), *Arch Intern Med* 153:154, 1993.

Kaluger G, Kaluger MF: *Human development: the span of life,* ed 3, St Louis, 1984, Mosby.

Keltner NL et al: *Psychiatric nursing,* ed 2, St Louis, 1995, Mosby.

Kirby RR, Granestein N: *Clinical anesthesia practice,* Philadelphia, 1994, Saunders.

Krogh CME, editor: *Compendium of pharmaceutical and specialties,* ed 30, Ottawa, Ontario, 1995, Canadian Pharmaceutical Association.

Leininger M: *Transcultural nursing: concepts, theories, and practices,* New York, 1978, Wiley.

LeMone P, Burke KM: *Medical surgical nursing, critical thinking in client care,* Menlo Park, Calif, 1996, Addison-Wesley.

Levine RR: *Pharmacology, drug actions, and reactions,* Boston, 1973, Little, Brown.

Lewis SM: *Medical-surgical nursing: assessment and management of clinical problems,* ed 4, St Louis, 1996, Mosby.

Luechkenotte AG: *Gerontologic nursing,* St Louis, 1996, Mosby.

MacDermott BL, Deglin JH: *Understanding basic pharmacology: practical approaches for effective application,* Philadelphia, 1994, Davis.

McEvoy G, editor: *AHFS drug information,* Bethesda, Md, 1996, American Society of Health System Pharmacists.

Medication administration and IV therapy manual process and procedures, Springhouse, Pa, 1988, Springhouse.

Melzack R: The McGill pain questionaire: major properties and scoring methods, *Pain* 1:277-299, 1975.

National Institutes of Health: Guidelines for the diagnosis and management of asthma. National Asthma Education Program Expert Panel Report, 1991, DHHS publication no. 91-3042.

National Institutes of Health: International consensus report on diagnosis and treatment of asthma, 1992, DHHS publication no. 92-3091.

Olin BR, Hebel SK, editors: *Facts and comparisons,* St Louis, 1996, Facts and Comparisons.

Physician's desk reference, ed 50, Montvale, NJ, 1996, Medical Economics.

Rhoades RA, Tanner GA: *Medical physiology,* Boston, 1995, Little, Brown.

Roffman DS: Heart failure, *US Pharmacist* 63-76, 1995.

Rumore MM: The decline in new drug development, *Am Pharm* NS32:353-358, 1992.

Seeley RR et al: *Essentials of anatomy and physiology,* St Louis, 1991, Mosby.

Sprague RL, Kalachnik JE: Reliability, validity and a total score cutoff for the Dyskinesia Identification System: Condensed User Scale (DISCUS) with mentally ill and mentally retarded populations, *Psychopharmacol Bull* 27(1):51-58, 1991.

Summary of the Second Report of the National Cholesterol Education Program (NCEP) Expert Panel on Detection, Evaluation, and Treatment of High Blood Cholesterol in Adults (Adult Treatment Panel II), *JAMA* 269(23):3015-3023, 1993.

Swearingen PL: *Photo atlas of nursing procedures,* ed 2, Redwood City, Calif, 1991, Addison-Wesley Nursing.

Trissel LA: *Handbook on injectable drugs,* ed 8, Bethesda, Md, 1990, American Society of Hospital Pharmacists.

USAN and USP dictionary of drug names, Rockville, Md, 1995, U.S. Pharmocopeial Convention.

U.S. Pharmacopeia, ed 23, Rockville, Md, 1995, U.S. Pharmacopeial Convention.

USP-DI-1996, ed 16, Rockville, Md, 1996, U.S. Pharmacopeial Convention.

Vallerand AH, Deglin JH: *Nurse's guide for IV medications,* Philadelphia, 1990, Davis.

Van De Graaff KM, Fox SI: *Concepts of human anatomy and physiology,* ed 3, Dubuque, Ia, 1992, William C Brown.

Wells PS et al: Interactions of warfarin with drugs and food, *Ann Intern Med* 121:676-683, 1994.

Williams AS: Adaptive diabetes education for visually impaired persons: teaching nonvisual diabetes self-care, *J Home Health Care Pract* 4:62-71, 1992.

Williams SR: *Nutrition and diet therapy,* ed 7, St Louis, 1993, Mosby.

Wyngaarden JB, Smith LH, editors: *Cecil's textbook of medicine,* ed 17, Philadelphia, 1985, Saunders.

Young, LY, Koda-Kimble MA, editors: *Applied therapeutics,* ed 6, Vancouver, Wash, 1995, Applied Therapeutics.

INDEX

"T" indicates table.